KV-338-389

Viral Hepatitis

For Churchill Livingstone

Publisher: Lucy Gardner
Copy Editor: Helen MacDonald
Design: Design Resources Unit
Production Controller: Mark Sanderson
Sales Promotion Executive: Douglas McNaughton

Viral Hepatitis
Scientific Basis and Clinical Management

Edited by

Arie J. Zuckerman MD DSc FRCP FRCPath
Professor of Microbiology and Dean,
Royal Free Hospital School of Medicine,
London, UK

Howard C. Thomas BSc PhD FRCP FRCPath
Chairman and Professor of Medicine,
St Mary's Hospital Medical School,
Imperial College of Science, Technology and Medicine,
London, UK

DR. M. CONTRERAS
DIRECTOR

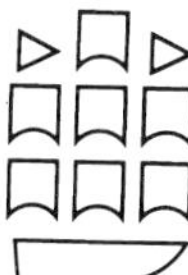

CHURCHILL LIVINGSTONE
EDINBURGH LONDON MADRID MELBOURNE NEW YORK AND TOKYO 1993

CHURCHILL LIVINGSTONE
Medical Division of Longman Group UK Limited

Distributed in the United States of America by Churchill Livingstone Inc., 650 Avenue of the Americas, New York, N.Y. 10011, and by associated companies, branches and representatives throughout the world.

© Longman Group UK Limited 1993

All rights reserved. No part of this publication may be reproduced, stored in a retrieval system, or transmitted in any form or by any means, electronic, mechanical, photocopying, recording or otherwise, without either the prior permission of the publishers (Churchill Livingstone, Robert Stevenson House, 1–3 Baxter's Place, Leith Walk, Edinburgh, EH1 3AF), or a licence permitting restricted copying in the United Kingdom issued by the Copyright Licensing Agency Ltd, 90 Tottenham Court Road, London, W1P 9HE.

First published 1993

ISBN 0-443-04708-1

British Library Cataloguing in Publication Data
A catalogue record for this book is available from the British Library.

Library of Congress Cataloging in Publication Data
A catalog record for this book is available from the Library of Congress.

The publisher's policy is to use **paper manufactured from sustainable forests**

Printed in Great Britain by The Bath Press, Avon

Contents

Contributors

Harvey J. Alter MD
Chief, Immunology Section; Associate Director for Research, Department of Transfusion Medicine, National Institutes of Health, Bethesda, Maryland, USA

John A. J. Barbara MSc PhD FIBiol MRCPath
Head of Microbiology, North London Blood Transfusion Centre, London, UK

Jean-Pierre Benhamou MD
Professeur à l'Université de Paris 7; Chef du Service D'Hepatologie à L'Hôpital Beaujon, Clichy, France

J. Bismuth MD
Hôpital Paul Brousse, Villejuif, France

Walter W. Bond MS
Supervisory Research Microbiologist, Hospital Infections Program, Centers for Disease Control and Prevention, Atlanta, Georgia, USA

Daniel W. Bradley PhD
Chief, Virology Laboratory Section, Hepatitis Branch, Division of Viral and Rickettsial Disease, National Center for Infectious Diseases, Centers for Disease Control and Prevention, Atlanta, Georgia, USA

Christian Brechot MD PhD
Professor of Cell Biology and Hepatology, CHU Necker, Inserm U370; Liver Unit, Necker Hospital; Hybridotest, Pasteur Institute, Paris, France

David Brown BSc MPhil
Clinical Scientist, University Department of Medicine, Royal Free Hospital, London, UK

Marie Annick Buendia PhD
Directeur de Recherche, Centre National de la Recherche Scientifique, Institut Pasteur, Paris, France

William F. Carman MB BCh MMed (Virology) MRCPath
Senior Lecturer, Institute of Virology, University of Glasgow; Honorary Consultant Virologist, Greater Glasgow Health Board, Glasgow, UK

Qui Lim Choo PhD
Senior Scientist, Chiron Corporation, California, USA

Anne Cockcroft MD FRCP DIH FFOM
Consultant/Senior Lecturer in Occupational Medicine, Royal Free Hampstead NHS Trust and Royal Free Hospital School of Medicine, University of London, UK

Hari S. Conjeevaram MD
National Institute of Health, Bethesda, Maryland, USA

Richard H. Decker PhD
Director, Diagnostic Biology Research, Abbott Laboratories, North Chicago, Illinois, USA

F. Deinhardt MD (deceased)
Formerly Director, Max V. Pettenkofer-Institut, Munich, Germany

Adrian M. Di Bisceglie MD FCP(SA) FACP
Chief, Liver Diseases Section, National Institute of Health, Bethesda, Maryland, USA

Jules L. Dienstag MD
Associate Physician, Massachusetts General Hospital; Associate Professor, Harvard Medical School, Boston, Massachusetts, USA

Geoffrey Dusheiko MB BCh FCP(SA) FRCP
Reader in Medicine, Royal Free Hospital School of Medicine, University of London, UK

Patrizia Farci MD
Visiting Scientist, Hepatitis Viruses Section, Laboratory of Infectious Diseases, National Institute of Allergy and Infectious Diseases, National Institute of Health, Besthesda, Maryland, USA; Associate Professor, Department of Internal Medicine, University of Cagliari, Cagliari, Italy

Martin S. Favero PhD
Associate Director for Laboratory Science, Hospital Infections, Program, Centers for Disease Control, Atlanta, USA

Lawrence S. Friedman MD
Gastrointestinal Unit, Massachusetts General Hospital and Harvard Medical School, Boston, Massachusetts, USA

Wolfram H Gerlich PhD
Professor and Head of Institute of Medical Virology, Justus Liebig University, Giessen, Germany

Germana V. Gregorio MD
Honorary Registrar in Paediatric Hepatology, Department of Child Health, King's College Hospital, London, UK

Ian A. O. Gust MD BS BSc Dip Bact(Lond) FRCP(A) FRACP FTS
Director, Research and Development Division, CSL Ltd, Parkville, Melbourne, Victoria, Australia

Jang H. Han PhD
Associate Director of Molecular Biology/Biochemistry, Chiron Corporation, Emeryville, California, USA

Phillip M. Harrison BSc MRCP
MRC Training Fellow, Molecular Medicine Unit and Institute of Liver Studies, King's College School of Medicine and Dentistry, London, UK

Tim J. Harrison PhD MRCPath
Reader in Molecular Virology, Royal Free Hospital School of Medicine, University of London, UK

Jay H. Hoofnagle MD
Director, Division of Digestive Diseases and Nutrition and Senior Investigator, Liver Diseases Section, National Institute of Diabetes and Digestive and Kidney Diseases, National Institute of Health, Bethesda, USA

Michael Houghton PhD
Director, Non-A, Non-B Hepatitis Research, Chiron Corporation, Emeryville, California, USA

Meron R. Jacyna MD MRCP
Honorary Senior Lecturer, St Mary's Hospital Medical School, London, UK, Consultant Gastroentrologist, Northwick Park Hospital, London, UK

Alan D. Kitchen PhD
Head of Microbiology, NE Thames Regional Blood Transfusion Centre, Brentwood, UK

K. Krawczynski MD PhD
Chief, Experimental Pathology Section, Hepatitis Branch, DVRD/NCID Centers for Disease Control and Prevention, Atlanta, Georgia, USA

G. Kuo PhD
Chiron Corporation, Emeryville, California, USA

Michael M. C. Lai MD PhD
Investigator, Howard Hughes Medical Institute; Professor, Department of Microbiology, University of Southern California, School of Medicine, Los Angeles, California, USA

Johnson Y. N. Lau MD MRCP
Assistant Professor, Section of Hepatobiliary Diseases, Division of Gastroenterology, Hepatology and Nutrition, Department of Medicine, University of Florida, Gainesville, Florida, USA

Christine A. Lee MA MD MRCPath FRCP
Consultant Haematologist and Director, Haemophilia Centre, Royal Free Hospital School of Medicine, London, UK

Stanley M Lemon MD
Professor of Medicine and Microbiology and Immunology, Associate Chairman for Research, Department of Medicine, The University of North Carolina at Chapel Hill, Chapel Hill, North Carolina, USA

Patrick Marcellin MD
Practicien Hospitalier, Service d'Hépatologie et Inserm U24 Hôpital Beaujon, Clichy, France

Paul Martin MD
Director of Clinical Hepatology and Assistant Professor of Medicine, UCLA School of Medicine, Los Angeles, California, USA

Giorgina Mieli-Vergani MD PhD
Senior Lecturer in Paediatric Hepatology, Department of Child Health, King's College School of Medicine and Dentistry, London, UK

J. Monjardino MB BS MSc PhD
Reader in Cell Studies, Department of Medicine, St Mary's Hospital Medical School, London, UK

Alex P. Mowat MB ChB FRCP DCH
Consultant Paediatric Hepatologist; Professor Paediatric Hapatology, Department of Child Health, King's College Hospital, London, UK

Kunio Okuda MD PhD
Eritus Professor of Medicine, Chiba University School of Medicine, Chiba, Japan

Patrizia Paterlini MD PhD
Assistant Associé, Université Necker, Paris, France

Robert H. Purcell MD
Head, Hepatitis Viruses Section, Laboratory of Infectious Diseases, National Institute of Allergy and Infectious Diseases, National Institute of Health, Bethesda, Maryland, USA

Michael A. Purdy PhD
Research Microbiologist, Hepatitis Branch, Division of Viral and Rickettsial Disease, National Center for Infectious Diseases, Centers for Disease Control and Prevention, Atlanta, Georgia, USA

Mario Rizzetto MD
Professor of Gastroenterology, Institute of Internal Medicine, University of Torino, Torino, Italy

Floriano Rosina MD
Assistant, Department of Gastroenterology, Molinette Hospital, Torino, Italy

Didier Samuel MD
Hepatologist, Practicien Hospitalier, Hepatobiliary Surgery and Liver Transplant Research Center, Hôpital Paul Brousse, Villejuif, France

Leonard B. Seeff MD
Chief, Gastroenterology and Hepatology, Veterans' Affairs Medical Center; Professor of Medicine, Georgetown University School of Medicine, Washington DC, USA

Sheila Sherlock *DBE* MD FRCP
Emeritus Professor of Medicine, Royal Free Hospital School of Medicine (University of London), London, UK

Gunter Siegl PhD
Professor and Head, Institute for Clinical Microbiology and Immunology, St Gallen, Switzerland

Jack T. Stapleton MD
Associate Professor, Departments of Internal Medicine, University of Iowa and Iowa City, Veterans Administration Medical Center, Iowa City, Iowa, USA

Howard C. Thomas BSc PhD FRCP FRCPath FRCPS
Chairman and Professor of Medicine, St Mary's Hospital Medical School, Imperial College of Science, Technology and Medicine, London, UK

Pierre Tiollais MD
Professor of Biochemistry, Institut Pasteur, Paris, France

Amy J. Weiner PhD
Chiron Corporation, Emeryville, California, USA

Manfred Weitz PhD
Head, Division of Experimental Microbiology, Institute of Clinical Microbiology and Immunology, St Gallen, Switzerland

Roger Williams MD FRCP FRCS FRCP(Edin) FRACP FACP(Hons)
Consultant Physician and Director, Institute of Liver Studies, King's College Hospital and King's College School of Medicine and Dentistry, London, UK

Reinhart Zachoval MD
Department of Internal Medicine 2, Klinikum Grosshadern, Ludwig-Maximilians University, Munich, Germany

Arie J. Zuckerman MD DSc FRCP FRCPath
Professor of Microbiology and Dean, Royal Free Hospital School of Medicine, University of London, UK

Jane N. Zuckerman MB BS
Occupational Health Unit, Royal Free Hospital School of Medicine, University of London, UK

Preface

Although the first reference to hepatitis was ascribed to Hippocrates, the observations leading to our current knowledge – identification and characterisation of five hepatotropic agents (hepatitis viruses A, B, C, D and E) – began with studies of hepatitis outbreaks during the First World War and the demonstration later by transmission studies with bacteria-free filtrates that the disease was caused by a virus.

The initial contributions by clinicians and epidemiologists distinguished between faecal-orally transmitted, short incubation, epidemic hepatitis – now known to be due to hepatitis A and E viruses – and the parenterally transmitted longer incubation hepatitis – now known to be due to hepatitis B, C and D viruses. The serologists, virologists and molecular biologists then isolated, and eventually characterised at a molecular level, the viruses concerned, starting with hepatitis B in 1963 and ending with hepatitis E in 1990.

This book deals with the virology, epidemiology, diagnostic serology, pathobiology, treatment and prevention of these diseases and also, to spread its appeal from virologists, epidemiologists and clinicians, to paediatricians, blood-bankers and public and occupational health specialists, we have added chapters on specific clinical areas.

The rapid progress of this field over the last three decades is an attraction and a challenge to any group of writers. We have tried to be comprehensive so that the book appeals to research workers, as well as practising virologists and clinicians, and have added 'update' sections to each chapter to allow addition of the most recent publications in each field. We hope that hepatitis F is not discovered in the three month 'last trimester' when the book is 'locked' in the hands of the publishers!

London, 1993

A. J. Z
H.C.T.

1. Clinical features of hepatitis

Sheila Sherlock

There are many varieties of viral hepatitis (Sherlock & Dooley 1993). Hepatitis A is a self-limiting faecal-spread infection caused by hepatitis A virus (HAV). Hepatitis B is a parenterally transmitted disease that often becomes chronic. Hepatitis D is spread parenterally, and affects only those with hepatitis B infection. Hepatitis C is a parenterally spread disease with a high chronicity rate. Hepatitis E resembles hepatitis A. It is spread enterically, usually via water, and causes a self-limiting hepatitis in those in underdeveloped countries. There will undoubtedly be other members of the hepatitis alphabet. General clinical features are common to all the virus infections. In general, type A, type B and type C run the same clinical course. Types B and C tend to be more severe and may be associated with a serum sickness-like syndrome.

The mildest attack is without symptoms, and is marked only by a rise in serum transaminase levels. Alternatively, the patient may be anicteric but suffer gastrointestinal and influenza-like symptoms. Such patients are likely to remain undiagnosed unless there is a clear history of exposure, or the patient is being followed up after a blood transfusion. Increasing grades of severity are then encountered, ranging from the icteric, from which recovery is usual, through to fulminant, fatal viral hepatitis.

The usual icteric attack in adults is marked by a prodromal period, usually about 3 or 4 days, but even up to 2–3 weeks, during which time the patient feels generally unwell, suffers digestive symptoms, particularly anorexia and nausea, and may, in the later stages, have a mild pyrexia. Rigors are unusual. An ache develops in the right upper abdomen. This is increased by jolting movements. There is loss of desire to smoke or to drink alcohol. Malaise is profound and increases towards evening; the patient feels wretched. Occasionally, headache may be severe, and in children its association with neck rigidity may suggest meningitis. Protein and lymphocytes in the cerebrospinal fluid (CSF) may be raised.

The prodromal period is followed by darkening of the urine and lightening of the faeces. Symptoms ameliorate and jaundice develops. The temperature returns to normal and there may be bradycardia. Appetite returns and abdominal discomfort and vomiting cease. Pruritus may appear transiently for a few days.

The liver is palpable with a smooth tender edge in 70% of patients. Heavy percussion over the right lower ribs posteriorly causes sickening discomfort. The spleen is palpable in about 20% of patients.

The adult loses about 4 kg in weight. A few vascular spiders may appear transiently. After an icteric period of about 1–4 weeks, the adult patient usually makes an uninterrupted recovery. In children, improvement is particularly rapid, and jaundice mild or absent. The stools regain their colour. The appetite returns to normal. After apparent recovery, lassitude and fatigue persist for some weeks. Clinical and biochemical recovery is usual within 6 months of the onset. However, chronic hepatitis may follow types B and C.

Neurological complications, including the Guillain–Barré syndrome, can complicate all forms of viral hepatitis.

Occasionally, prolonged jaundice is of cholestatic type. Onset is acute; jaundice appears and deepens, but within 3 weeks the patient starts to itch. After the first few weeks the patient feels well, gains weight and there are no physical signs apart from icterus and slight hepatomegaly. Jaundice persists for 8–29 weeks, and recovery is then complete. This type must be differentiated from surgical obstructive jaundice (Gordon et al 1984). The acute onset and only moderately enlarged liver are the most helpful points. Cholestatic drug jaundice is excluded by the history. Relapses occur in 1.8–15% of cases. In some, the original attack is duplicated, usually in a milder form. More often, relapse is simply shown by an increase in serum transaminases and sometimes bilirubin. Multiple episodes may occur. Recovery after relapse is usually complete. In some, relapses may indicate progression to chronic hepatitis.

Fulminant viral hepatitis usually overwhelms the patient within 10 days. It may develop so rapidly that jaundice is inconspicuous and the diagnosis is confused with an acute psychosis or meningoencephalitis. Alternatively, the patient, after a typical acute onset, becomes deeply jaundiced. Ominous signs are repeated vomiting, fetor hepaticus, confusion and drowsiness. The flapping tremor may be only transient, but rigidity is usual. Coma supervenes rapidly, and the picture becomes that of acute liver failure. Temperature rises, jaundice deepens and the liver shrinks. Widespread haemorrhages may develop.

HEPATITIS A

The disease occurs sporadically or in epidemic form and has an incubation time of 15–50 days (Fig. 1.1). It is usually spread by the faecal–oral route. Parenteral transmission is extremely rare, but can follow transfusion of blood from a donor who is in the incubation stage of the disease (Hollinger et al 1983).

Age 5–14 is the group most affected, and adults are often infected by spread from children. This is related to overcrowding, poor hygiene and poor sanitation. With improved standards of living the prevalence is decreasing worldwide. In urban areas, only about 30% of adults show IgG anti-HAV, whereas in underdeveloped countries 90% of children have the antibody by the age of 10. Young people, not previously exposed, and

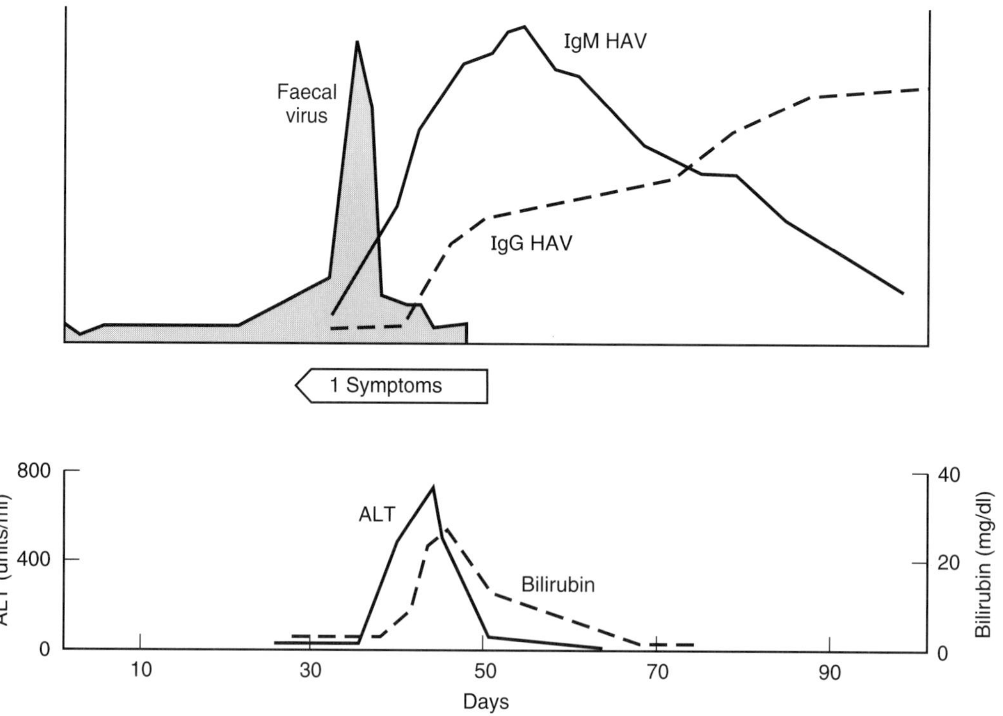

Fig. 1.1 The course of acute hepatitis A. ALT, alanine transferase; HAV, hepatitis A virus.

visiting endemic areas, are increasingly becoming affected. Medical staff in developed countries are at risk. A large outbreak among nurses and mothers in a nursery spread from an acute hepatitis A in a neonate with an ileostomy (Azimi et al 1986). In another outbreak, two infants in a neonatal intensive care unit received blood from a hepatitis A virus-infected donor (Rosenblum et al 1991). This resulted in infection of 13 infants, 22 nurses, eight other staff caring for the infants and four household contacts. The infants excreted virus for 4–5 months after they were infected.

Clinically, the hepatitis is usually mild, particularly in children, in whom it is frequently subclinical or passed off as gastroenteritis. The disease is more serious and prolonged in adults.

The rare fulminant course may be related to the dose of virus or impaired antibody responsiveness.

Cholestatic hepatitis A

This affects adults (Gordon et al 1984). The jaundice lasts 1–4 months and itching is severe. Serum IgM anti-HAV is positive. The prognosis is excellent.

Relapsing hepatitis A

Occasionally after 30–90 days the patient relapses. The serum transaminase levels have never returned to normal. The disease resembles the original attack clinically and biochemically, and virus A is found in the stools (Sjogren et al 1987). The relapse may last several months but recovery eventually ensues. Recently, 14 well-documented cases of relapsing HAV infection were described from Israel (Glikson et al 1992) (Fig. 1.2). They were confirmed by positive serum IgM anti-HAV tests. One or more relapses followed initial resolution of the clinical manifestations. This relapsing form may affect 3.8–20% of patients with an initial episode of acute HAV infection. Relapsing HAV is associated with continuing viraemia as well as shedding virus in stools during the relapse phase (Sjögren et al 1987). The pathogenesis probably involves an interaction between persistent viral infection and immune

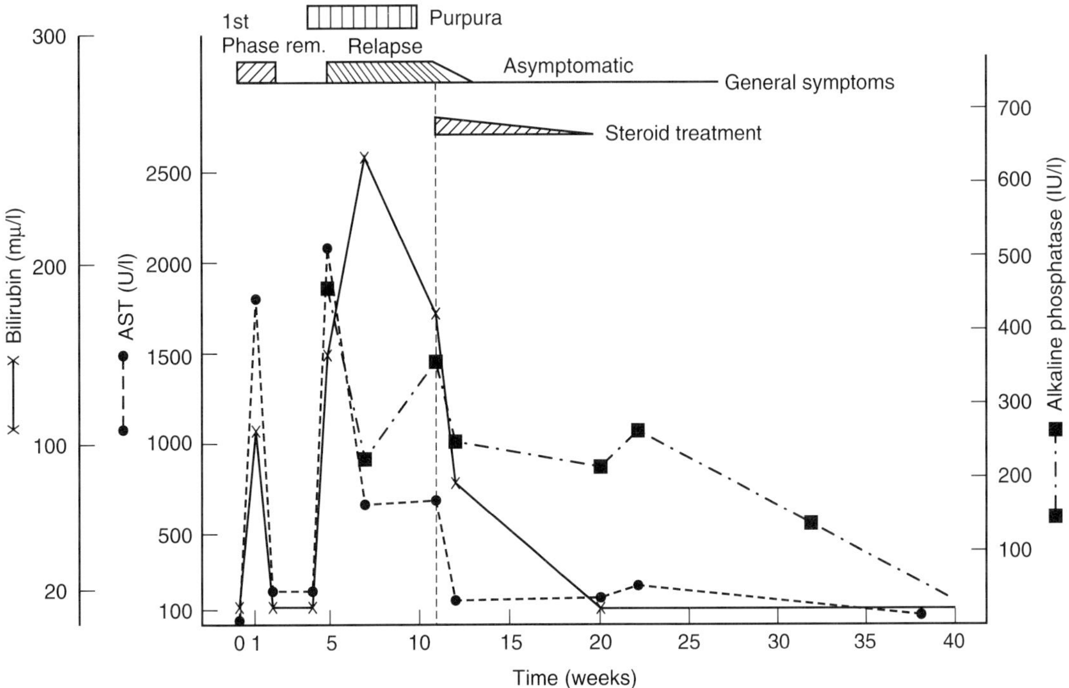

Fig. 1.2 Clinical and biochemical course of a patient with relapsing hepatitis A. (Rem, remission; AST, aspartate transaminase. (From Glikson et al 1992.)

mechanisms responding to the continuing antigenic stimulation. Rarely, the relapse can be associated with arthritis, vasculitis and cryoglobulinaemia (Dan & Yaniv 1990).

HEPATITIS B

The disease is transmitted parenterally or by intimate, often sexual, contact. The incubation period is about 6 weeks (Fig. 1.3). The carrier rate of hepatitis B surface antigen (HBsAg) varies worldwide from 0.1–0.2% in Britain, the USA and Scandinavia to more than 3% in Greece and southern Italy, and even up to 10–15% in Africa and the Far East. Carriage of HBsAg is even higher in some isolated communities such as Alaskan Eskimos or Australian Aborigines.

In high-carriage rate areas, infection is acquired by passage from the mother to the baby. The infection is usually not via the umbilical vein, but from the mother at the time of birth and during close contact afterwards. The risk of transmission increases as term approaches and is greater with acute than chronic carriers. The mother is HBsAg positive, and also, but not always, HBeAg positive. Antigenaemia develops in the baby within 2 months of birth and tends to persist (Bortolotti et al 1990). Several studies clearly document an inverse relationship between the risk of chronicity and the age of infection, the risks being 80–90% for infections before the age of 1, and 20–50% for infections in early childhood (Coursaget et al 1987). In contrast, recent surveys show that hepatitis B infection in adults gives rise to a carrier rate of only 1–2% (Seeff et al 1987, Tassopoulos et al 1987).

In high-endemic areas such as Africa, Greece and Hong Kong, the transmission is in childhood and is probably horizontal (Craven et al 1986), through kissing and shared utensils such as toothbrushes and razors. Contact in preschool day-care centres is possible. Sexual contacts in the family are at risk (M J Alter et al 1989). Infection is frequent in homosexuals, related to duration of homosexual activity, number of sexual contacts and anal contact.

Blood transfusion continues to cause hepatitis B in countries where donor blood is not screened

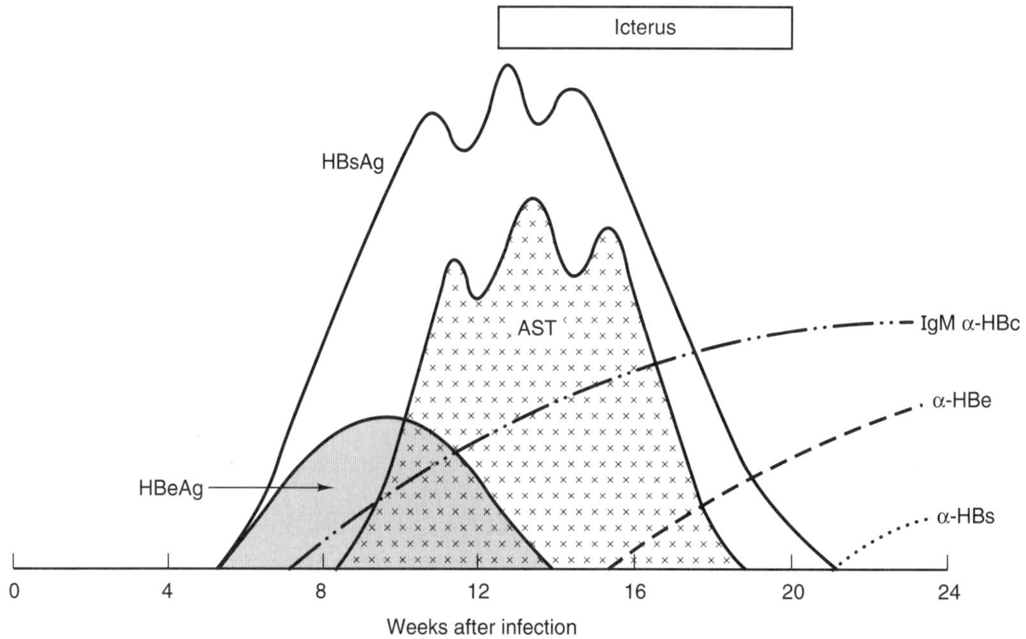

Fig. 1.3 The course of acute type B hepatitis. HBsAg, hepatitis B surface antigen. HBeAg, hepatitis B e antigen; α-HBs, antibody against hepatitis B surface antigen.

for HBsAg. Transmission is more likely with blood from paid donors than from volunteer blood.

Opportunities for parenteral infection include the use of non-sterile instruments for dental treatment, ear piercing and manicures, neurological examination, prophylactic inoculations, subcutaneous injections, acupuncture and tattooing. Parenteral drug abusers develop hepatitis from using shared, non-sterile equipment. The mortality may be very high in this group.

Hospital staff in contact with patients, and especially patients' blood, usually have a higher carrier rate than the general community. This applies particularly to staff on renal dialysis or oncology units. The patient's attendant is infected through contact with blood parenterally such as from pricking or through skin abrasions. Surgeons and dentists are particularly at risk in operating on HBsAg-positive patients with a positive HBeAg. Spread from a surgeon to a patient is rare, and usually involves major operations (Welch et al 1989).

Using standard cleansing procedures, there is no evidence that HBV infection is spread by endoscopes (Villa et al 1984).

Institutionalized mentally retarded children (especially with Down's syndrome) and their attendants have a high carrier rate.

Acute HBV infection

The clinical course may be anicteric. The high carriage rate of serum markers in those who give no history of acute hepatitis B suggests that subclinical episodes must be extremely frequent (Fig. 1.4). The non-icteric patient is more likely to become chronic than the icteric one.

The usual clinical attack diagnosed in the adult tends to be more severe than for hepatitis A or C. However, the overall picture is similar. The self-limited, benign icteric disease usually lasts less than 4 months; jaundice rarely exceeds 4 weeks. Occasionally, a prolonged benign course is marked by increased serum transaminase values for more than 100 days. Relapses are rare. Cholestatic hepatitis, with prolonged deep jaundice, is unusual.

There may be features suggesting immune

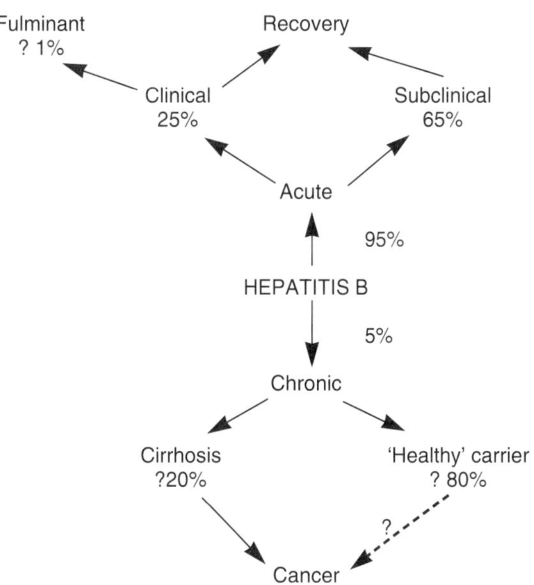

Fig. 1.4 The effect of exposure to hepatitis B virus (HBV).

complex disease. This is shown in the prodromal period by a serum sickness-like syndrome. This develops about 1 week before jaundice. It can be associated with an icteric or an anicteric attack. The syndrome has also been described with chronic hepatitis B. Fever is usual. The skin lesion is urticarial and, rarely, children show a papular acrodermatitis. The arthropathy is symmetrical, non-migratory and affects small joints. Serum rheumatoid factor is negative. It is usually transitory, but can persist.

A fulminant course of hepatitis B in the first 4 weeks is related to an enhanced immune response with more rapid clearing of virus. Antibodies to surface and 'e' antigen increase and multiplication of virus ceases (Brechot et al 1984). In fulminant hepatitis B, the surface antigen may be in low titre or undetectable. The diagnosis may be made only by finding serum IgM anti-HBC.

Another viral hepatitis, superimposed on a symptomless hepatitis B carrier, may precipitate a fulminant course. The new agent may be virus A or virus delta; hepatitis C is also a candidate.

Reactivation of hepatitis B viral replication is well recognized after cytotoxic therapy for malignant lymphoma and after organ transplantation requiring immunosuppression. The result is icteric hepatitis, non-fatal hepatic failure or death (Lok et al 1991). Spontaneous exacerbations may also occur as a result of reactivation of HBV replication (Lok et al 1987, Liaw et al 1991).

Chronic hepatitis B virus infection

The very young and the very old are at particular risk. Chronic HBV hepatitis is found predominantly in males.

The condition may follow an unresolved acute hepatitis B. The acute attack is usually mild and of 'grumbling' type. The patient having an explosive onset and deep jaundice usually recovers completely. Similarly, survivors of fulminant virus hepatitis seldom, if ever, develop progressive disease. Following the attack, serum transaminase levels fluctuate with intermittent jaundice. The patient may be virtually symptom-free with only biochemical evidence of continued activity, and may simply complain of fatigue and being generally unwell, the diagnosis being made after a routine medical check. Diagnosis may be made in a symptom-free patient at the time of a blood donation or routine blood screen, when the HBsAg is found to be positive and serum transaminases modestly increased.

Chronic hepatitis is often a silent disease. Symptoms do not correlate with the severity of liver damage. In about half of patients, presentation is as established chronic liver disease with jaundice, ascites or portal hypertension. Encephalopathy is unusual at presentation. The patient usually gives no history of a previous acute attack of hepatitis.

There are geographical and age-related differences in the natural history of HBV infection. In Taiwan, only 2% of healthy Chinese carriers or chronic hepatitis patients cleared HBsAg in a mean of 4 ± 2.3 years (Liaw et al 1991). Patients over 40 who were HBeAg negative and with established cirrhosis were more likely to clear HBsAg. In an Italian study in adults, 20% of patients presenting with chronic hepatitis developed cirrhosis in 1–13 years (Fattovich et al 1991). Older age, the presence of bridging hepatic necrosis on liver biopsy and persistence of serum HBV DNA implied a poor prognosis. In Spain, 26% of asymptomatic cases clear HBeAg every year (Morena-Otero et al 1991). A second liver biopsy shows negative hepatitis B core antigen and usually improved appearances, although in 6 of 15 patients studied chronic active hepatitis had progressed to cirrhosis.

Many patients, usually with established stable cirrhosis evolving slowly over many years, will present with hepatocellular carcinoma.

An apparently stable patient with chronic HBV disease may have a clinical relapse. This is marked by increasing fatigue, and usually increases in serum transaminase values. Relapse may be related to seroconversion from an HBeAg-positive state to an HBeAg- and HBV DNA-negative one. Liver biopsy shows an acute lobular-type hepatitis that ultimately subsides and the serum transaminase values fall. Seroconversion may be spontaneous in 10–15% of patients per annum (Viola et al 1981). HBV DNA can remain positive even when anti-HBe has developed (Fattovich et al 1986a, b). In some HBeAg-positive patients, flare-ups of viral replication and transaminase elevation are found without eventual clearing of HBeAg (Levy et al 1990).

Spontaneous reactivation from HBeAg negative to HBeAg and HBV DNA positive has also been described. The clinical picture ranges from absence of manifestations to fulminant liver failure (Levy et al 1990). Reactivation is particularly severe in those who are human immunodeficiency virus (HIV) positive.

Reactivation may be marked serologically simply by finding a positive IgM anti-HBc. In any severe exacerbation, superinfection with HDV, HAV or HCV must be considered.

Relation of HBV mutants to the clinical course

Variants of the hepatitis B genome are described owing to mutations in the various reading frames (Ch. 7) (Brunetto et al 1989; Carman et al 1989). An important one is in the pre-core region and is due to a mutation resulting in disturbed secretion of HBeAg (Bonino et al 1991). Patients have progressive liver disease, high serum HBV DNA levels and yet negative serum HBeAg. This variant is particularly frequent in the Mediterranean area and in the Far East. The disease may run a severe and a relapsing course (Brunetto et al 1989). Defects in pre-core may appear after seroconversion of HBeAg to anti-HBe, either spontaneously or after interferon treatment (Takeda et al 1990).

Fulminant hepatitis has been related to pre-core mutants (Carman et al 1991, Kosaka et al 1991, Omata et al 1991). In one report from Israel, a mutant pre-core HBV strain was transmitted from a common source to five patients who developed fatal fulminant hepatitis (Liang et al 1991). In another series, eight out of nine HBeAg-negative patients with fulminant hepatitis B harboured the pre-core variant, but none of six HBeAg-positive patients (Carman et al 1991). Encephalopathy was more common, but survival was better in those with the variant. The mutation may emerge spontaneously during fulminant hepatitis or, perhaps, less commonly, the patient may be infected with the variant *ab initio*.

Some HBV carrier mothers with pre-core region mutations and 'e' antibody, may transmit fulminant hepatitis to their babies (Terazawa et al 1991). There may be a high incidence of pre-core mutant viruses in anti-'e' carriers with chronic liver disease (Naoumov et al 1992). Anti-HBe-positive patients with predominant pre-core variant infection and high viraemia have more severe disease than patients with low viraemia and mixed infection with wild-type and pre-core mutant viruses. In two patients, a concomitant decrease in serum HBV DNA and transaminase levels occurred with the transition from pre-core mutant to mixed infection (Naoumov et al 1992). In patients with pre-core mutations, interferon treatment appears to be less effective and hepatocellular cancer development and mortality appear to be significantly higher than in patients infected with wild-type HBV (Hadziyannis et al 1991).

Extra hepatic associations

Some of these conditions are associated with circulating immune complexes containing HBsAg. The accompanying liver disease is usually mild, and, at the most, a chronic persistent hepatitis.

Polyarteritis

This involves largely medium and small arteries and appears early in the course of the disease. Immune complexes containing HBsAg are found in the vascular lesions and their blood levels correlate with disease activity. Polyarteritis is a rare complication of hepatitis B (Lisker-Melman et al 1989).

Membranous glomerulonephritis

This has been associated with hepatitis B infection, largely in children (Lin 1990). Liver disease is minimal. The patient are usually HBeAg positive. Immune complexes of HBsAg and HBsAb, HBcAg and anti-HBC or HBeAg and anti-HBe are found in glomerular and capillary basement membranes (Venkataseshan et al 1990). The ultrastructural changes correlate with HBeAg in the serum and glomeruli (Ito et al 1981). In children, interferon treatment may lead to a remission (Lisker-Melman et al 1989). The response to corticosteroids is poor (Lin 1990). Remission may precede HBe antigen seroconversion to anti-HBe.

In children, the glomerulonephritis usually resolves spontaneously in 6 months to 2 years. In adults, the disease is much worse, being slowly but relentlessly progressive in one-third. It presents as a nephrotic syndrome (Lai et al 1991). Treatment with prednisolone increases viral replication. In Chinese patients, treatment with interferon is disappointing. Spontaneous remission is uncommon, and the disease usually progresses relentlessly to renal failure.

Polymyalgia rheumatica

This has been connected with hepatitis B infection (Bacon et al 1975).

Essential mixed cryoglobulinaemia

A patient with peripheral neuropathy and cryoglobulinaemia showed cryoprecipitates with a high concentration of HBsAg. However, anti-HBsAg and complement were not found (Levo et al 1977). The relationship of hepatitis B to this condition has not been proved (Dienstag et al 1977).

Neuropathies

Neuropathies, including the Guillan–Barré syndrome, have been associated with HBV infection (Inoue et al 1987, Tabor 1987). Immune complexes containing HBsAg have been found in the serum and cerebrospinal fluid in Guillain-Barré syndrome (Penner et al 1982).

Myocarditis

This may have an immune complex basis (Ursell et al 1984).

Aplastic anaemia

Aplastic anaemia is usually fatal and has been associated with hepatitis B viral infection (McSweeney et al 1988). Suppression of haematopoietic stem cells has been shown in vitro in hepatitis B virus infection (Zeldis et al 1986).

Pancreatitis

Pancreatitis has been recorded in HBV infection, particularly following liver transplantation (Alexander et al 1988).

Semen abnormalities

Semen abnormalities have been found in patients with viral hepatitis B, presumably as a result of the virus (Huret et al 1986).

HEPATITIS D

The delta agent is a very small RNA particle coated with HBsAg. It is capable of infection only when activated by the presence of hepatitis B virus. It resembles satellite viruses of plants (viroids) that cannot replicate without another specific virus. The interaction between the two viruses is very complex. Synthesis of delta virus may depress the appearance of hepatitis B viral markers in infected cells and even lead to elimination of active viral replication.

Hepatitis B and delta infection may be simultaneous (*co-infection*) or delta may infect a chronic HBsAg carrier (*superinfection*).

Delta infection is strongly associated with intravenous drug abuse, but can affect all risk groups for hepatitis B infection. It can spread heterosexually. Intrafamilial spread has been noted from southern Italy (Bonino et al 1985) Delta infection is worldwide, but particularly in southern Europe, the Balkans, Middle East, South India and parts of Africa. In general, it is rare in the Far East (including Japan and South America). However, epidemics of delta infection have been reported from the Amazon Basin, Brazil (Labrea fever), Colombia (Santa Marta hepatitis), Venezuela and equatorial Africa. In these areas, children of the indigent population are affected and mortality is high.

With co-infection the acute delta hepatitis is usually self-limiting as the delta cannot outlive the transient HBV antigenaemia. The clinical picture is usually indistinguishable from hepatitis due to HBV alone. However, a biphasic rise in aspartate transaminase may be noted, the second rise being the result of the acute effects of delta (Rizzetto 1983).

With superinfection the acute attack may be severe and even fulminant, or may be marked only by a rise in serum transaminase levels. Delta infection should always be considered in any HBV carrier, usually clinically stable, who has a relapse.

Co-infection is more likely to be followed by recovery and the patient becoming immune to delta. Superinfection is followed by a complete recovery in only 10% and there is a high chronicity rate. Both modes of infection can have a fulminant course. Over the past 10 years, there have been reports that delta is associated with less severe underlying chronic liver disease than previously recorded. About equal numbers of patients show chronic active hepatitis/active cirrhosis, chronic persistent hepatitis–lobular hepatitis or inactive disease. The severity observed may depend on the case referral patterns, thus those coming to a specialized medical unit are likely to have more severe disease than if identified by population screening. A large study from the Greek island of Rhodes showed that only a minority of delta-infected patients had liver disease and the majority were healthy carriers (Hadziyannis et al 1991). In other areas, such as Los Angeles, the disease largely affects parenteral drug abusers and homosexuals. Biochemical reactivations (alanine transaminase greater than 10 times upper limit normal) affected 41%; in 58% this was due to HDV and in 16% to HBV (Ackerman et al 1992). In a hyperendemic region, such as Sicily, the natural history of delta infection may be indistinguishable from that of infections with wild-type HBV alone (Craxi et al 1992).

The HBV-infected patient who acquires delta virus has more active necroinflammation and develops cirrhosis more rapidly than those with chronic hepatitis of other viral aetiologies. However, the cirrhosis remains stable for long periods and there is prolonged survival.

In certain circumstances, delta virus can be present without HBsAg positivity. This is seen in HIV-infected patients and also after hepatic transplantation for HBV and HDV end-stage disease. Hepatocellular carcinoma is a complication of HDV infection.

HEPATITIS C

HCV infection is acquired in various ways. It could be the result of an infected blood transfusion, the indication for which may be trauma or obstetric complications, or all varieties of surgical operations. The amount of blood transfused can be as little as 1 unit. The condition is commoner in females, perhaps because they have more operations. Parenteral drug abusers and recipients of blood products such as haemophiliacs are at risk. In many instances the mode of infection is unknown. Of patients with community-acquired non-A, non-B hepatitis, 50% are anti-HCV-positive (M J Alter et al 1990, Bortolotti et al 1991a, b). These patients have no risk factor such as transfusion or drug abuse and their mode of infection is uncertain. Sexual and intrafamilial transmission is debated. Disease is rare in European homosexuals (Melbye et al 1990). Perinatal spread is also unusual unless the mother is also HIV infected (Thaler et al 1991).

Secretions from HCV RNA carriers, including semen, urine, stool, saliva and breast milk, are non-infectious (Hsu et al 1991, Fried et al 1992).

Acute HCV hepatitis

Time relationships have been assessed using post-transfusion hepatitis as the model, as the time of infection can be fixed. The incubation period is probably 5–12 weeks. Only 25% of sufferers are jaundiced and the patient may be completely asymptomatic. The disease in an anti-HIV-positive patient may have a rapidly progressive course (Martin et al 1989). However, a fulminant course is rare, and if it occurs co-infection with another virus must be considered. Post-transfusion hepatitis C is liable to be overlooked unless serum transaminases are monitored frequently. This is especially so in the post-operative setting, as malaise and fatigue are to be expected in the first few weeks after surgery.

Serum transaminase levels are only moderately elevated – about 15 times the upper limit of normal. This occurs 7–8 weeks after infection. Multiple peaks are usual for 3 months after the onset and occur in 70%; 21% have two peaks and only 0.5% a single peak. Serum hepatitis C RNA can be detected 1–2 weeks after infection (Garson et al 1990). In those that recover completely, serum HCV RNA is lost, but HCV antibody persists for months.

Chronic HCV hepatitis

Acute post-transfusion hepatitis, due to hepatitis C, is followed by chronic hepatitis in about 50%, and 20% will develop cirrhosis (Fig. 1.5). The blood transfusion may be as long as 25 years previously. Drug abusers and recipients of blood products are also at risk. The frequency of chronicity is the same in the community-acquired sporadic disease as in the parenterally transmitted one.

At the National Institutes of Health in the USA, patients contracting chronic non-A, non-B hepatitis as the result of transfusions administered during heart surgery were evaluated (Di Bisceglie et al 1991). Acute post-transfusion hepatitis developed in 65 of 1070 patients (6.1%), and became chronic in 45 (69%). Antibody to

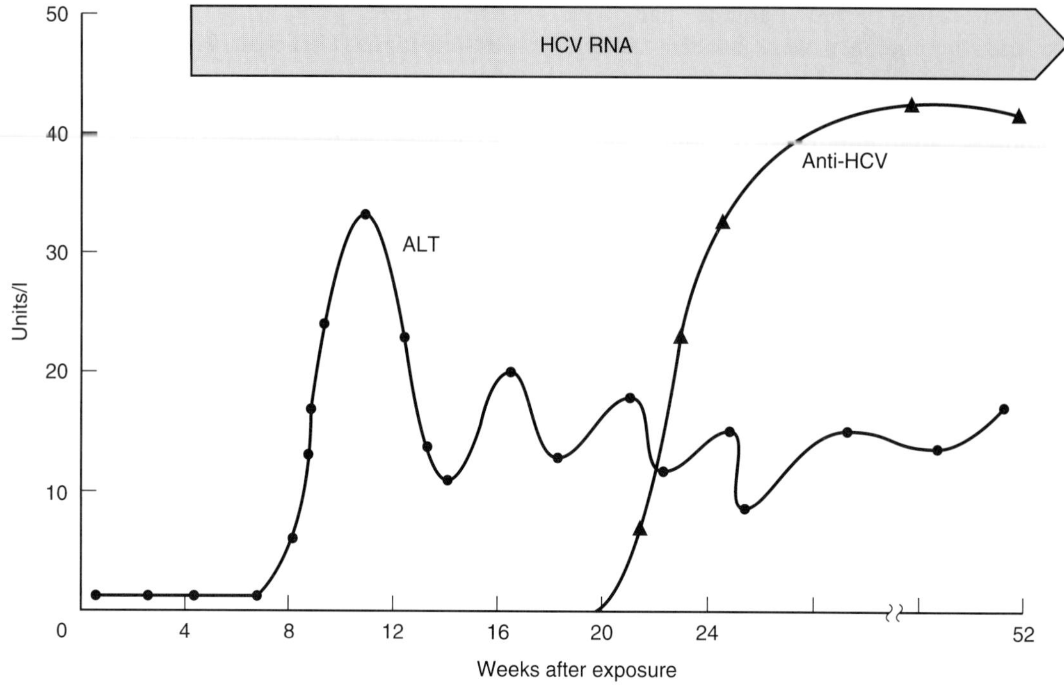

Fig. 1.5 The serological course of post-transfusion chronic HCV infection. Serum HCV RNA appears very early. Anti-HCV positivity is delayed. Serum alanine transferase (ALT) shows characteristic fluctuations.

HCV was detectable in 54 patients (82%) with post-transfusion non-A, non-B hepatitis. 39 patients were followed for between 1 and 24 years (mean 9.7 years) Cirrhosis developed in eight patients (20%) between 1.5 and 16 years after transfusion. The average time to develop cirrhosis is believed to be about 20 years (H J Alter 1990). In Italy, follow-up of 63 patients who developed post-transfusion hepatitis after open heart surgery showed that 17 recovered, whereas 46 developed chronic disease (Tremolada et al 1988). In Japan, 30 (81.1%) of 37 patients with HCV antibody-positive acute non-A, non-B hepatitis developed chronic liver disease by 12 months (Nishioka et al 1991). In southern California, HCV antibodies were found in 89% of cases of non-A, non-B chronic hepatitis in drug abusers, in 71% of those with transfusion-related non-A, non-B hepatitis and in 27% of patients with chronic, sporadic non-A, non-B hepatitis (McHutchison et al 1991).

In Japan, it has been estimated that only 2% of patients with HCV infection undergo spontaneous remissions, after 8 years 30% have chronic HCV infection, 20% will have progressed to cirrhosis and another 15% will develop hepatocellular carcinoma. In Japan, HCV infection is believed to be a more important antecedent of hepatocellular cancer than HBV.

Patients may present insidiously with fatigue as the major symptom. They complain of always feeling below par, and this varies from time to time. Diagnosis may be made only when increased serum transaminases are discovered during the course of a routine blood screen. Chronic hepatitis C is often asymptomatic.

The course is a slow one marked by fluctuating 'yo-yo' transaminases over many years (Fig. 1.5). Each elevation probably represents an episode of hepatitis C viraemia. At presentation, the serum transaminase levels rarely exceed six times the upper limit of normal and the mean is about three times (Fig. 1.6) (Patel et al 1991). In 24 post-transfusion patients, the mean was only 112 IU/l, and only rarely exceeded 200 IU/l (Patel et al 1991). Fluctuating transaminases in the absence

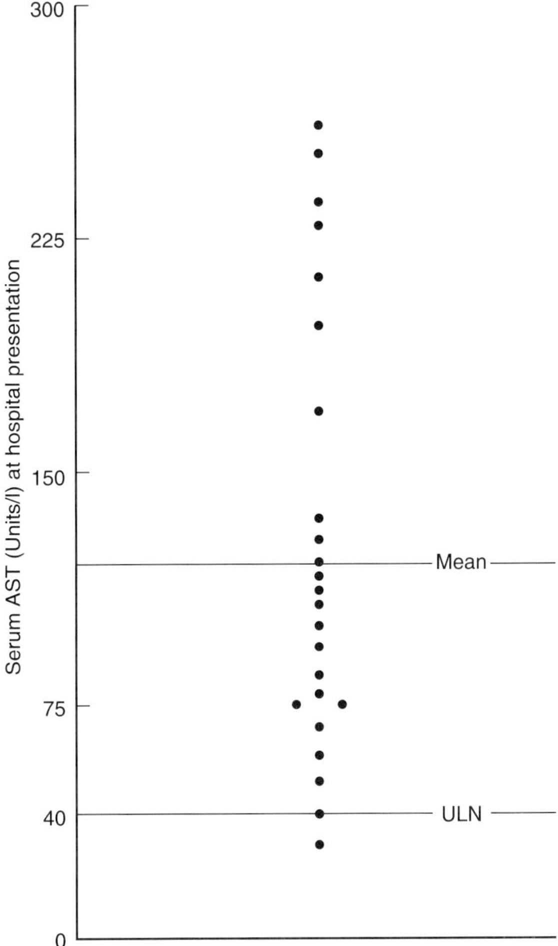

Fig. 1.6 Chronic HCV hepatitis. Serum aspartate transaminase (AST) values at time of referral.

of alcoholism are virtually diagnostic of HCV infection. During the peaks, symptoms, particularly fatigue, increase. Normal transaminase levels can be reported for weeks or months even though the HCV RNA remains positive.

Serum bilirubin and albumin concentrations are usually normal until the late stages of liver failure. Serum gamma glutamyltransferase and alkaline phosphatase levels show slight increases. Serum gammaglobulin levels are modestly increased but rarely exceed 2 g/l. Routine haematology is usually normal until splenomegaly leads to hypersplenism accompanied by thrombocytopenia, leucopenia and normocytic anaemia. Prothrombin time is maintained until late.

The spleen is only palpable in 50%. The sequelae of portal hypertension, particularly bleeding oesophageal varices, are rare (Patel et al 1991).

There is considerable heterogeneity in the hepatitis C virus, particularly in the viral envelope region. These HCV genotypes are highly related, but nevertheless distinct. Little has been published on the effect of different genomes on the clinical course. However, in Japan, 91 HCV RNA-positive patients were divided into two genotypes, HCV-K1-PT (80%) and HCV-K2 (20%) (Takada et al 1992). Detection of HCV antibody did not differ between the two. Patients with HCV-K2 were younger, and were less likely to have history of previous blood transfusion. This genotype may be more involved in sporadic cases.

Extrahepatic clinical features

These are rarer in association with hepatitis C than with hepatitis B infection. Urticaria and purpura were noted in one patient in a plasmapheresis-associated outbreak of non-A, non-B hepatitis (Martini et al 1979). Rashes were reported in 3% in one early report of acute non-A, non-B hepatitis (Perrillo et al 1981). First-generation anti-HCV tests gave false results in patients with the rheumatoid factor (Theilmann et al 1990), but HCV infection has not been reported in association with clinical rheumatoid arthritis. Erythema nodosa is believed to be rare with HCV infections. However, two cases of post-transfusion chronic HCV infection with recurrent purpuric eruptions have been described (Pappas et al 1991). Skin biopsies revealed leucocytoclastic vasculitis with IgM and complement deposition. Serum from one patient demonstrated mixed cryoglobulins, negative for HBV markers. This patient also had proteinuria and haematuria, and renal biopsy showed membranoproliferative glomerulonephritis with complement deposit. In both patients, prednisolone therapy proved ineffective, but alpha-interferon was beneficial.

Others have found HCV infection in patients with type II mixed cryoglobulinaemia (Pascual et al 1990). In a series of 29 patients with essential mixed cryoglobulinaemia, 14 reacted with two of more of the four antigens used for the second-generation anti-HCV test (Casato et al 1991). Some, but not all, of these patients had evidence of HBV infection. An association between HCV, HBV and mixed cryoglobulinaemia is suggested.

Aplastic anaemia is a well-recognized and common complication of acute non-A, non-B hepatitis (Zeldis et al 1983). However, there is some doubt whether the cause is actually HCV. In a survey of 118 patients with severe aplastic anaemia, in 19 of whom the disease was hepatitis-associated, anti-HCV levels did not differ significantly depending on whether the cause of the aplastic anaemia was hepatitis related or unknown (Pol et al 1990). There was no relation between HCV and HBV serologies regardless of cause. HCV RNA is not detected in serum (Hibbs et al 1992). This suggests that uncharacterized hepatotrophic viruses (namely non-A, non-B, non-C) are involved in most cases of post-hepatitis aplastic anaemia (Pol et al 1990).

HCV is known to be excreted in saliva, and it is of particular interest that HCV has been associated with Sjögren's syndrome of lymphocytic sialadenitis (Haddad et al 1992). The histological appearances of labial salivary glands in patients with proven HCV hepatitis or cirrhosis were compared with those from dead controls. Histological changes characteristic of Sjögren's syndrome were significantly more common in HCV infected patients (16 of 28; 57%) than in controls. Only 10 of 16 patients had a dry mouth and none complained of dry eyes. Of course, a direct link between HCV and sialadenitis is not proven, but an autoimmune reaction initiated by HCV is possible.

Relation of HCV infection to other viruses

Patients who have been infected with HCV are more likely to have past infection with HBV and to be HIV positive. This is especially so for drug abusers. Selection of the factors most likely to be the cause of the chronic liver disease is very difficult, and interaction between them must be taken into account (Sherlock 1989). In a selected group of patients with chronic HBV referred to the National Institutes of Health, Bethesda, for therapeutic trials, anti-HCV was detected in 11%, higher than the 0.9–1.4% prevalence in volunteer blood donors (Fong et al 1991), and similar to that reported in HBsAg-positive Italian patients (Fattovich et al 1991).

In HBsAg-positive patients, anti-HCV is more likely to be positive if the patient is anti-HBe positive, but HBV DNA negative (35% versus 8%) (Fattovich et al 1991). In this subgroup, HCV may play a leading role in causing the liver disease, and this diagnosis should be considered in HBV carriers who, in the integrated stage of their disease, unexpectedly deteriorate. Serum HBV DNA levels are lower in those that are anti-HCV positive, suggesting that HCV suppresses HBV infection.

Co-infection of patients with non-A, non-B hepatitis with HIV leads to a more severe course. In one series, three patients developed cirrhosis within 3 years of onset of hepatitis, an extremely rapid and unusual course for non-A, non-B hepatitis alone (Martin et al 1989). The HIV infection may have worsened the hepatitis C by its effects on host immune function, permitting greater viral replication and thus more liver injury.

Relation of HCV infection to alcohol

The problem is in deciding to what extent any liver damage is related to HCV and to what extent to alcohol, and how these factors can be related to the various socioeconomic risks to which the alcoholic is subjected. Depending on the population, 5–25% of alcoholics will have been exposed to HBV or HCV or both (Wands & Blum 1991).

Clearly, HCV antibody tests, first or second generation, do not truly represent the contribution of HCV to liver disease in alcoholics. There is need for HCV RNA studies. In one such a study from Japan of 80 patients with alcoholic liver disease, the prevalence of positive HCV antibody tests fell when more specific methods were used (Nishiguchi et al 1991). In alcoholic liver disease, antibody to HCV correlates with severity. Patients with a positive HCV RNA have more severe necroinflammatory changes in a liver biopsy (Nishiguchi et al 1991). HCV seems to be an important, although not essential, factor in the development of chronic hepatitis and cirrhosis in Japanese alcoholic individuals.

In a person consuming excess alcohol and also having markers for HCV, a positive HCV RNA suggests that this is the major culprit. The diagnosis of predominant HCV disease is also suggested if serum transaminase levels are persistently greater than 100 IU and mean aspartate to alanine transferase ratio is less than 1 (0.6), a finding that is characteristic of viral rather than alcoholic liver disease (Brillanti et al 1991). The effect of abstinence on serum transaminase levels may also be helpful (Nishiguchi et al 1991). 25 alcoholic patients with liver disease stopped drinking. In 11, with a positive HCV RNA, transaminases tended to decrease while in hospital, but increased on discharge. Of the 14 patients without HCV RNA, the transaminases decreased significantly during hospitalization, but increased only in 3 of the 14 after discharge. The increase in prevalence of HCV in alcoholics compared with the normal population is probably related to their lifestyles. Those alcoholics who have HCV markers have more severe liver disease (Caldwell et al 1991, Nishiguchi et al 1991, Nalpas et al 1991). The relationship between the two factors is unclear. It is impossible to predict which chronic alcoholic subject with liver disease will also have HCV infection, or to determine which factor is the more important.

Autoimmune chronic active hepatitis and chronic HCV infection

The diagnosis of chronic HCV disease can be confused with that of autoimmune chronic liver disease. First-generation anti-HCV tests gave false-positives in autoimmune chronic active hepatitis (McFarlane et al 1990), not confirmed by second-generation tests or by the presence of HCV RNA (Nishiguchi et al 1992). However, HCV infection results in a quite different clinical picture from genuine autoimmune chronic active hepatitis (Table 1.1). In chronic HCV, older people, largely male, are infected. Autoantibodies are usually negative, or present in low titre. However, a subgroup of HCV-positive patients with circulating autoantibodies has been described (Magrin et al 1991). Of 15 such patients, nine were serum antinuclear, three anti-LKM1 and three anti-smooth muscle antibody positive. None had associated autoimmune disease. Anti-HCV radioimmunoassay enzyme-linked immunosorbent assay (ELISA) results in all patients. HCV RNA was found in the serum from 10 patients. This subgroup is HCV-related, and clinically and aetiologically distinct from genuine autoimmune chronic active hepatitis. Nevertheless, it does seem that HCV can be associated with autoantibody positivity.

Hepatic histology in HCV chronic liver disease shows a mild chronic active hepatitis, and cirr-

Table 1.1 Chronic hepatitis C and autoimmune hepatitis contrasted

	Hepatitis C	Autoimmune hepatitis
Age	All ages	Young and middle age
Sex	Equal	Predominantly female
Contact blood	Frequent	Rare
Autoimmune diseases	Unusual	May be present
HLA-B8 Dr3 linkage	No	Yes
Serum transaminase		
>10 ×	Rare	Usual
Fluctuant	Usual	Very rare
Serum gammaglobulin >2.5 g/l	Unusual	Usual
Autoantibodies		
Antinuclear antibody (diffuse)	Absent or low titre	Usually positive
Smooth muscle	Absent or low titre	Usually positive
Response to corticosteroids	None or modest	Excellent
Response to interferon	50% respond	None (may exacerbate)

hosis develops late (Scheuer et al 1992). The picture is very different from the florid one of autoimmune chronic active hepatitis (Bach et al 1992). In chronic HCV disease, associated autoimmune diseases are exceedingly rare and serum gammaglobulin and transaminases are only moderately increased. In chronic HCV, the response to prednisolone is poor, and indeed can be hazardous, leading to deterioration in liver function. The subgroup of patients who are anti-HCV positive and also have circulating autoantibodies will still respond poorly to prednisolone, but may benefit from interferon therapy (Magrin et al 1991). It is possible that some patients with apparent type 1 autoimmune hepatitis who do not respond to corticosteroids may actually have chronic hepatitis C (or another non-A, non-B) virus infection (Nishiguchi et al 1992).

HEPATITIS E (HEV) INFECTION

This accounts for sporadic and major epidemics of viral hepatitis in underdeveloped countries. The disease is enterically transmitted, usually by sewage-contaminated water. The viral genome has been found in the stools of sufferers (Ray et al 1991). An ELISA for IgG and IgM anti-HEV has been developed and used to diagnose hepatitis E infection in rural Egyptian children (Goldsmith et al 1992).

In general, hepatitis E resembles hepatitis A. It affects young adults and has a self-limiting course. The mortality is very high (about 25%) in women in the last trimester of pregnancy. The course can be cholestatic and chronicity does not develop.

REFERENCES

Ackerman Z, Govindarajan S, Valinluck B et al 1992 Spontaneous exacerbation of disease activity in patients with chronic hepatitis delta infection: the role of hepatitis B, C, or D. Proceedings of the Fourth International Symposium on Hepatitis Delta Virus

Alexander J A, Demetrius A J, Gavaler J S Makowka L, Starzl T E, Van Thiel D H. 1988 Pancreatitis following liver transplantation. Transplantation 45: 1062–1065

Alter H J 1990 The hepatitis C virus and its relationship to the clinical spectrum of NANB hepatitis. Journal of Gastroenterology/Hepatology 5 (suppl. 1): 78–94

Alter M J, Hadler S C, Judson F N et al 1990 Risk factors for acute non-A, non-B hepatitis in the United States and association with hepatitis C virus infection. Journal of the American Medical Association 264: 2231–2235

Alter M J, Coleman P J, Alexander W J et al 1989 Importance of heterosexual activity in the transmission of hepatitis B and non-A, non-B hepatitis. Journal of the American Medical Association 162: 1201–1205

Azimi P H, Roberto R R, Guralnik J, Livermore T, Hoag S, Hagens S, Lugo N 1986 Transfusion-acquired hepatitis A in a premature infant with secondary nosocomial spread in an intensive care nursery. American Journal of Diseases of Children 140: 23–27

Bach N, Thung S N, Schaffner F 1992 The histological features of chronic hepatitis C and autoimmune chronic active hepatitis: a comparative analysis. Hepatology 15: 572–577

Bacon P A, Doherty S M, Zuckerman A J 1975 Hepatitis B antibody in polymyalgia rheumatica. Lancet ii: 476–478

Bonino F, Caporaso N, Dentico P et al 1985 Familial clustering and spreading of hepatitis delta virus infection. Journal of Hepatology 1: 221–226

Bonino F, Brunetto M R, Rizzetto M, Will H 1991 Hepatitis B virus unable to secrete 'e' antigen. Gastroenterology 100: 1138–1141

Bortolotti F, Cadrobbi P, Crivellaro C, Guido M, Rugge M, Noventa F, Calzia R, Realdi G 1990 Long-term outcome of chronic type B hepatitis in patients who acquire hepatitis B virus infection in childhood. Gastroenterology 99: 805–810

Bortolotti F, Tagger A, Cardrobbi P et al 1991a Failure to detect hepatitis C virus genome in human secretions with the polymerase chain reaction. Hepatology 14: 176–180

Bortolotti F, Tagger A, Cadrobbi C, Crivellaro C, Pregliasco F, Ribero M L, Alberti A. 1991b Antibodies to hepatitis C virus in community-acquired acute non-A, non-B hepatitis. Journal of Hepatology 12: 176–180

Brechot C 1992 Impact of genetic amplification in hepatitis diagnosis. Proceedings of the Vth International Symposium on Viral Hepatitis, Madrid. Journal of Hepatology (in press)

Brechot C, Bernuau J, Thiers V et al 1984 Multiplication of hepatitis B virus in fulminant hepatitis B. British Medical Journal 288: 270–271

Brillanti S, Masci C, Siringo S, Di Febo G, Miglioli M, Barbara L 1991 Serological and histological aspects of hepatitis C virus infection in alcoholic patients. Journal of Hepatology 13: 347–350

Brunetto M R, Stemler M, Schodel F et al 1989 Identification of HBV variants which cannot produce precore derived HBeAg and may be responsible for severe hepatitis. Italian Journal of Gastroenterology 21: 151–154

Caldwell S H, Jeffers L J, Ditomaso A et al 1991 Antibody to hepatitis C is common among patients with alcoholic liver disease with and without risk factors. American Journal of Gastroenterology 86: 1219–1223

Carman W F, Jacyna M R, Hadziyannis S et al 1989 Mutation preventing formation of Hbe antigen in patients with chronic hepatitis B infection. Lancet ii: 588–590

Carman W F, Fagan E A, Hadziyannis S, Karayiannis P, Tassopoulos N C, Williams R, Thomas H C 1991

Association of a precore genomic variant of hepatitis B virus with fulminant hepatitis. Hepatology 14: 219–222
Casato M, Taliani G, Pucillo L P, Goffredo F, Lagana B, Bonomo L 1991 Cryoglobulinaemia and hepatitis C virus. Lancet 337: 1047–1048
Coursaget P, Yvonnet B, Bourdil C et al 1987 HBsAg positive reactivity in man not due to the hepatitis B virus. Lancet ii: 1354–1358
Craven D E, Awdeh Z L, Kunches L M et al 1986 Nonresponsiveness to hepatitis B vaccine in health care workers. Annals of Internal Medicine 105: 356–360
Craxi A, Di Marco V, Lolacono O et al 1992 The natural history of chronic HDV infection. Proceedings of the Fourth International Symposium on Hepatitis Delta Virus and Liver Disease. Rhodes Island, Greece
Dan M, Yaniv R 1990 Cholestatic hepatitis, cutaneous vasculitis, and vascular deposits of immunoglobulin M and complement associated with hepatitis A virus infection. American Journal of Medicine 89: 103–104
Di Bisceglie A M, Goodman Z D, Ishak K G, Hoofnagle J H, Melpolder J J, Alter H J 1991 Long-term clinical and histopathological follow-up of chronic posttransfusion hepatitis. Hepatology 14: 969–974
Dienstag J L 1990 Hepatitis non-A, non-B: C at last. Gastroenterology 99: 1177–1180
Dienstag J L, Wands J R, Isselbacher K J 1977 Hepatitis B and essential mixed cryoglobulinemia. New England Journal of Medicine 197: 946–947
Farci P, Alter H J, Wong D, Miller R H, Shih J W, Jett B, Purcell R H 1991 A long-term study of hepatitis C virus replication in non-A, non-B hepatitis. New England Journal of Medicine 325: 98–104
Fattovich G, Rugge M, Brollo L et al 1986 Clinical virologic and histologic outcome following seroconversion from HBeAg to anti-HBe in chronic hepatitis type B. Hepatology 6: 167–172
Fattovich G, Tagger A, Brollo L et al 1991a Hepatitis C virus infection in chronic hepatitis B virus carriers. Journal of Infectious Diseases 163: 400–402
Fattovich G, Brollo L, Giustina G et al 1991b Natural history and prognostic factors for chronic hepatitis type B. Gut 32: 294–298
Fong T-L, Di Bisceglie A M, Waggoner J G, Banks S M, Hoofnagle J H 1991 The significance of antibody to hepatitis C virus in patients with chronic hepatitis B. Hepatology 14: 64–67
Fried M W, Shindo M, Fong T-L, Fox P C, Hoofnagle J H, Di Bisceglie A M 1992 Absence of hepatitis C viral RNA from saliva and semen of patients with chronic hepatitis C. Gastroenterology 102: 1306–1308
Garson J A, Tuke P W, Makris M, Briggs M, Machin S J, Preston F E, Tedder R S 1990 Demonstration of viraemia patterns in haemophiliacs treated with hepatitis C virus contaminated factor VIII concentrates. Lancet 336: 1022–1025
Glikson M, Galun E, Oren R, Tur-Kaspa R, Shouval D 1992 Relapsing hepatitis A. Review of 14 cases and literature survey. Medicine (Baltimore) 71: 14–23
Goldsmith R, Yarbough P O, Reyes G R et al 1992 Enzyme-linked immunosorbent assay for diagnosis of acute sporadic hepatitis E in Egyptian children. Lancet 339: 328–331
Gordon S C, Reddy R, Schiff L, Schiff E R 1984 Prolonged intrahepatic cholestasis secondary to acute hepatitis A. Annals of Internal Medicine 101: 635–637
Haddah J, Deny P, Munz-Gotheil C et al 1992 Lymphocytic sialadenitis of Sjogren's syndrome associated with chronic hepatitis C virus liver disease. Lancet 339: 321–323
Hadziyannis S, Bramou T, Alexopoulou A et al 1991 Immunopathogenesis and natural course of anti-HBc positive chronic hepatitis with replicating B virus in viral hepatitis and liver disease. In: Hollinger F B, Lemon S M, Margolis H S (eds) Viral hepatitis and liver disease. Williams & Wilkins, Baltimore, pp 673–676
Hibbs J R, Frickhofen N, Rosenfeld S J et al 1992 Aplastic anemia and viral hepatitis non-A, non-B, non-C? Journal of the American Medical Association 267: 2051–2054
Hollinger F B, Khan N C, Oefinger P E, Yawn D H, Schmulen A C, Dreesman G R, Melnick J L 1983 Post-transfusion hepatitis type A. Journal of the American Medical Association 250: 2313–2317
Huet J L, Jeulin C, Hadchou L M et al. 1986 Semen abnormalities in patients with viral hepatitis B. Archives of Andrology 17: 99–100
Hsu H H, Wright T L, Luba D, Martin M, Feinstone S M, Garcia G, Greenberg H B 1991 Failure to detect hepatitis C virus genome in human secretions with the polymerase chain reaction. Hepatology 14: 763–767
Inoue A, Tsukada N, Koh C-S, Yanagisawa N 1987 Chronic relapsing demyelinating polyneuropathy associated with hepatitis B infection. Neurology 37: 1663–1666
Ito H, Hattori S, Matsuda I et al 1981 Hepatitis B e antigen-mediated membranous glomerulonephritis. Correlation of ultrastructural changes with HBeAg in the serum and glomeruli. Laboratory Investigation 44: 214–220
Johnson R J, Gretch D R, Yamabe H 1993 Membranoproliferative glomerulonephritis associated with hepatitis C virus infection. New England Journal of Medicine 328, 7: 465–470
Kosaka Y, Takase K, Kojima M et al 1991 Fulminant hepatitis B: induction by hepatitis B virus mutants defective in the precore region and incapable of encoding e antigen. Gastroenterology 100: 1087–1094
Lai K N, Lai F M-M, Chan K W, Chow C B, Tong K L, Vallance-Owen J 1987 The clinico-pathologic features of hepatitis B virus-associated glomerulonephritis. Quarterly Journal of Medicine 240: 323–333
Lai K N, Li P K T, Lui S F, Au T C, Tam J S L, Tong K L, Lai FM-M 1991 Membranous nephropathy related to hepatitis B virus in adults. New England Journal of Medicine 324: 1457–1463
Levo Y, Gorevic P D, Kassab H J, Zucker-Franklin D, Franklin E C 1977 Association between hepatitis B virus and essential mixed cryoglobulinemia. New England Journal of Medicine 296: 1501–1504
Levy P, Marcellin P, Martinot-Peignoux M, Degott C, Nataf J, Benhamou J-P 1990 Clinical course of spontaneous reactivation of hepatitis B virus infection in patients with chronic hepatitis B. Hepatology 12: 570–574
Liang T J, Hasegawa K, Rimon N, Wands J R, Ben-Porath E 1991 A hepatitis B virus mutant associated with an epidemic of fulminant hepatitis. New England Journal of Medicine 324: 1705–1709
Liaw Y-F, Sheen I-S, Chen T-J, Chu C-M, Pao C-C 1991 Incidence, determinants and significance of delayed clearance of serum HBsAg in chronic hepatitis B virus infection: a prospective study. Hepatology 13: 627–631
Lin C-Y. 1990 Hepatitis B virus-associated membranous nephropathy: clinical features, immunological profiles and outcome. Nephron 55: 37–44
Lisker-Melman M, Webb D, Di Bisceglie A M et al 1989

Glomerulonephritis caused by chronic hepatitis B virus infection: treatment with recombinant human alpha-interferon. Annals of Internal Medicine 111: 479–483
Lok A S F, Lai C-L, Wu P-C, Leung E K Y, Lam T-S. 1987 Spontaneous hepatitis B e antigen to antibody seroconversion and reversion in Chinese patients with chronic hepatitis B virus infection. Gastroenterology 92: 1839–1843
Lok A S F, Liang R H S, Chiu E K W, Wong K-L, Chan T-K, Todd D 1991 Reactivation of hepatitis B virus replication in patients receiving cytotoxic therapy: report of a prospective study. Gastroenterology 100: 182–188
McFarlane I G, Smith H M, Johnson P J, Bray G P, Vergani D, Williams R 1990 Hepatitis C virus antibodies in chronic active hepatitis: pathogenetic factor or false-positive result? Lancet 335: 754–757
McHutchison J G, Kuo G, Houghton M, Choo Q-L, Redeker A G 1991 Hepatitis C virus antibodies in acute icteric and chronic non-A, non-B hepatitis. Gastroenterology 101: 1117–1119
McSweeney P A, Carter J M, Green G J, Romeril K R 1988 Fatal aplastic anemia associated with hepatitis B viral infection. American Journal of Medicine 85: 255–256
Magrin S, Craxi A, Fabiano C et al 1991 Hepatitis C virus replication in 'autoimmune' chronic hepatitis. Journal of Hepatology 13: 364–367
Martin P, Di Bisceglie A M, Kassianidies C, Lisker-Melman M, Hoofnagle J H et al 1989 Rapidly progressive non-A, non-B hepatitis in patients with human immunodeficiency virus infection. Gastroenterology 97: 1559–1561
Martini G A, Reiter H J, Kalbfleisch H 1979 Acute and chronic non-A, non-B hepatitis. Presented at the International Symposium on Viral Hepatitis, Munich, April 5–7
Melbye M, Biggar R J, Wantzin P, Krogsgaard K, Ebbesen P, Becker N G 1990 Sexual transmission of hepatitis C virus: cohort study (1981–9) among European homosexual men. British Medical Journal 301: 210–212
Moreno-Otero R, Garcia-Monzon C, Garcia-Sanchez A, Garcia-Buey L, Pajares J M, Di Bisceglie A M 1991 Development of cirrhosis after chronic type B hepatitis: a clinicopathologic and follow-up study of 46 HBeAg-positive asymptomatic patients. American Journal of Gastroenterology 86: 560–564
Nalpas B, Driss F, Pol S, Hamelin B, Housset C, Brechot C, Berthelot P 1991 Association between HCV and HBV infection in hepatocellular carcinoma and alcoholic liver disease. Journal of Hepatology 12: 70–74
Naoumov N V, Schneider R, Grotzinger T, Jung M C, Miska S, Pape G R, Will H 1992 Precore mutant hepatitis B virus infection and liver disease. Gastroenterology 102: 538–543
Nishiguchi S, Kuroki T, Yabusako T et al 1991 Detection of hepatitis C virus antibodies and hepatitis C virus RNA in patients with alcoholic liver disease. Hepatology 14: 985–989
Nishiguchi S, Kuroki T, Ueda T et al 1992 Detection of hepatitis C virus antibody in the absence of viral RNA in patients with autoimmune hepatitis. Annals of Internal Medicine 116: 21–25
Nishioka K, Watanabe J, Furuta S et al 1991 Antibody to the hepatitis C virus in acute hepatitis and chronic liver diseases in Japan. Liver 11: 65–70
Omata M, Ehata T, Yokosuka O, Hosoda K, Ohto M 1991 Mutations in the precore region of hepatitis B virus DNA in patients with fulminant and severe hepatitis. New England Journal of Medicine 324: 1699–1704
Pascual M, Perrin L, Giostra E, Schifferli J A 1990 Hepatitis C virus in patients with cryoglobulinaemia type II. Journal of Infectious Diseases 162: 569–570
Pappas S C, Lewtas J, Terrault N, Morgan-Bell C, Sauder D, Fam A 1991 Chronic hepatitis C associated with vasculitis, cryoglobulins and glomerulonephritis: clinical features and response to interferon therapy. Hepatology 14: 78A
Patel A, Sherlock S, Dusheiko G, Scheuer P J, Ellis L A, Ashrafzadeh P 1991 Clinical course and histological correlations in post-transfusion hepatitis C: the Royal Free Hospital experience. European Journal of Gastroenterology and Hepatology 3: 491–495
Penner E, Maida E, Mamoli B, Gangl A 1982 Serum and cerebrospinal fluid immune complexes containing hepatitis B surface antigen in Guillain–Barré syndrome. Gastroenterology 82: 576–580
Perrillo R P, Phol D A, Roodman S T, Tsai C C 1981 Acute non-A, non-B hepatitis with serum sickness-like syndrome and aplastic anemia. Journal of the American Medical Association 245: 494–496
Pol S, Driss F, Devergie A, Brechot C, Berthelot P, Gluckman E 1990 Is hepatitis C virus involved in hepatitis-associated aplastic anemia? Annals of Internal Medicine 113: 435–437
Ray R, Aggarwal R, Salunke P N, Mehrotra N N, Talwar G P, Naik S R 1991 Hepatitis E virus genome in stools of hepatitis patients during large epidemic in North India. Lancet 338: 783–784
Rizzetto M 1983 The delta agent. Hepatology 3: 729–737
Rosenblum L S, Villarino M E, Nainan O V et al 1991 Hepatitis A outbreak in a neonatal intensive care unit: risk factors for transmission and evidence of prolonged viral excretion among preterm infants. Journal of Infectious Diseases 164: 476–482
Scheuer P J, Ashrafzadeh P, Sherlock S, Brown D, Dusheiko G M 1992 The pathology of hepatitis C. Hepatology 15: 567–571
Seeff L B, Beebe G W, Hoofnagle J H et al 1987 A serologic follow-up of the 1942 epidemic of post-vaccination hepatitis in the United States Army. New England Journal of Medicine 316: 965–970
Sherlock S 1989 Classifying chronic hepatitis. Lancet ii: 1168–1170
Sherlock S, Dooley J S 1993 Acute and chronic hepatitis. In: Diseases of the liver and biliary system, 9th edn. Blackwell Scientific Publications, Oxford, pp 260–321
Sjögren M H, Tanno H, Fay O, Sileoni S, Cohen B D, Burke D S, Feighny R J 1987 Hepatitis A virus in stool during clinical relapse. Annals of Internal Medicine 106: 221–226
Tabor E 1987 Guillain–Barré syndrome and other neurologic syndromes in hepatitis A, B and non-A, non-B. Journal of Medical Virology 21: 207–216
Takada N, Takase S, Enomoto N, Takada A, Date T 1992 Clinical backgrounds of the patients having different types of hepatitis C virus genomes. Journal of Hepatology 14: 35–40
Takeda K, Akahane Y, Suzuki H, Okamoto H, Tsuda F, Miyakawa Y, Mayumi M 1990 Defects in the precore region of the HBV genome in patients with chronic hepatitis B after sustained seroconversion from HBeAg to anti-HBc induced spontaneously or with interferon therapy. Hepatology 12: 1284–1289
Tassopoulos N C, Papaevangelou G J, Sjogren M H,

Roumeliotou-Karayannis A, Gerin J L, Purcell R H 1987 Natural history of acute hepatitis B surface antigen-positive hepatitis in Greek adults. Gastroenterology 92: 1844–1850
Terazawa S, Kojima M, Yamanaka T et al 1991 Hepatitis B virus mutants with precore-region defects in two babies with fulminant hepatitis and their mothers positive for antibody to hepatitis B e antigen. Pediatric Research 29: 5–9
Thaler M M, Park C-K, Landers D V et al 1991 Vertical transmission of hepatitis C virus. Lancet 338: 17–18
Theilmann L, Blazek M, Gmelin K, Goeser T, Kommerell B, Fiehn W 1990 False-positive anti-HCV tests in rheumatoid arthritis. Lancet 335: 1346
Tremolada F, Loreggian M, Antona C et al 1988 Blood-transmitted and clotting-factor-transmitted non-A, non-B hepatitis. Journal of Clinical Gastroenterology 10: 413–418
Ursell P C, Habib A, Sharma P, Mesa-Tejada R, Lefkowitch J H, Fenoglio J J 1984 Hepatitis B virus and myocarditis. Human Pathology 15: 481–484
Venkataseshan V S, Liberman K, Kim D U et al 1990 Hepatitis-B-associated glomerulonephritis: pathology, pathogenesis, and clinical course. Medicine (Baltimore) 69: 200–216
Villa E, Pasquinelli C, Rigo G et al 1984 Gastrointestinal endoscopy and HBV infection: no evidence for a casual relationship. Gastrointestinal Endoscopy 30: 15–17
Viola L A, Barrison I G, Coleman J C, Paradinas F J, Fluker J L, Evans B A, Murray-Lyon I M 1981 Natural history of liver disease in chronic hepatitis B surface antigen carriers. Lancet ii: 1156–1159
Wands J R, Blum H E 1991 Hepatitis B and C virus and alcohol-induced liver injury. Hepatology 14: 730–733
Welch J, Webster M, Tilzey A J, Noah N D, Banatfala J E 1989 Hepatitis B infections after gynaecological surgery. Lancet i: 205–207
Zeldis J B, Mugishiuma H, Steinbert H N, Nir E, Gale R P 1986 In vitro hepatitis B virus infection of human bone marrow cells. Journal of Clinical Investigation 78: 411–417

UPDATE

- HCV infection causes both acute and chronic liver disease and is also associated with mixed cryoglobulinemia. A recent study suggests that, like HBV, it is also associated with renal disease. Eight patients with proteinuria, of which 7 had decreased renal function, revealed membranoproliferative glomerulonephritis on renal biopsy. Electron microscopy of the biopsy specimens showed cryoglobulin-like structures in 3 of 4 patients. All 8 patients had HCV RNA detected in their serum, elevated serum aminotransferase concentrations, and hypocomplementaemia, and the majority had cryoglobulins and circulating immune complexes in their serum. Cryoprecipitates from the 3 patients who were tested contained HCV RNA and IgG anti-HCV antibodies to the nucleocapsid core antigen (HCVc or c22–3). IgM rheumatoid factors, present in all patients, bound anti-HCV IgG in all 6 patients tested. Four patients received interferon alpha for 2–12 months; all had evidence of decreased HCV replication and improvement of their renal and liver disease.

  The pathogenesis of renal disease in HCV patients is unknown, but may relate to deposition within glomeruli of immune complexes containing HCV, anti-HCV IgG, and IgM rheumatoid factors.

- REFERENCE

Johnson RJ, Gretch DR, Yamabe H 1993 Membranoproliferative glomerulonephritis associated with hepatitis C virus infection. New England Journal of Medicine 328: 465–470

SECTION 1

Hepatitis A virus

2. Structure and molecular virology

Manfred Weitz   Günter Siegl

Hepatitis A virus (HAV) could not be cultivated in vitro for a long time, and even after successful adaptation to growth in cell cultures failed to replicate to large quantities. This situation has hampered characterization of the virus. In spite of these difficulties a considerable body of knowledge is now available proving that HAV is a picornavirus. Originally the virus was considered a member of the genus *Enterovirus* within this virus family (Melnick 1982). However, owing to specific features of its structure and molecular biology, HAV has recently been classified as a prototype virus of the new genus 'hepatovirus' (Minor 1991). The properties of HAV have already been extensively reviewed (Lemon 1985, Ticehurst 1986, Cohen 1989, Siegl & Lemon 1990, Ross et al 1991). This chapter presents an account of today's knowledge of the structure and molecular biology of the virus in the light of their biological functions.

STRUCTURE AND COMPOSITION OF HAV

The virion

The hepatitis A virion is a naked, spherical particle (Provost et al 1975, Siegl & Frosner 1978a) with a diameter of about 27 nm (Fig. 2.1) (Feinstone et al 1973). Although analysis of the virus by X-ray diffraction techniques has not yet been successfully performed, there is good evidence that the particle has icosahedral symmetry (Siegl 1984). The virion consists of a genome of linear, single-stranded RNA of messenger sense polarity and of a protein shell made up of three major proteins, VP1–VP3 (Siegl & Frosner 1978b, Gauss-Muller et al 1984).

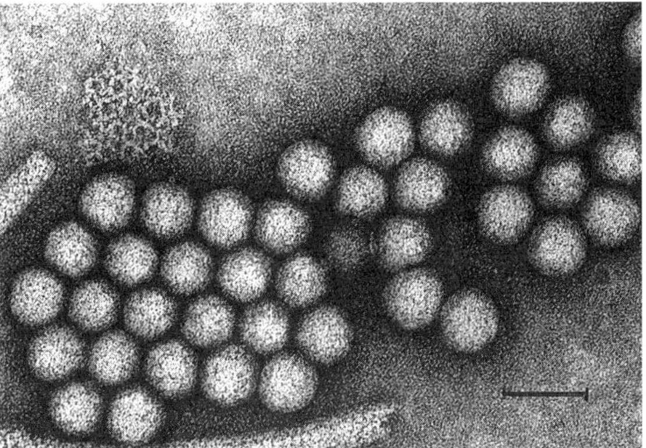

Fig. 2.1 Electron micrograph of hepatitis A virus particles. Virus was isolated from a human faecal specimen. The bar represents 50 nm.

The presence of a fourth protein VP4 has been repeatedly described, but the reported apparent molecular weights (7–14 kD) contrast sharply with those predicted from nucleic acid sequence data (1.5 kD or 2.3 kD). Conclusive physical identification of VP4 is still missing.

HAV has a buoyant density of 1.32–1.34 g/ml in caesium chloride and sediments with 156S during sucrose gradient centrifugation (Coulepis et al 1982). Additional infectious particles with higher (1.44 g/ml) as well as with lower (1.27 g/ml) buoyant density have also been described (Lemon et al 1985). The former appear to be more penetrable to caesium chloride; the latter have repeatedly been discussed as representing virions associated with residual membrane structures or lipids. The biological significance of both types of particles is unknown.

A major distinguishing feature of HAV among the picornaviruses is its exceptional stability (Parry

NHSBT
LIBRARY

& Mortimer 1984, Siegl et al 1984a). This physical feature is directly related to the structure of the virion and, obviously, has important implications for the biology and epidemiology of the virus. HAV has been found to resist heating to 60°C for 60 min. At higher temperatures infectivity is lost rapidly in a physiological, isotonic environment. However, in the presence of 1 M magnesium chloride, HAV retains its structural integrity and biological functions even at temperatures of up to 80°C. Variation in pH between 3 and 10 has no demonstrable effect on the stability of the virus. Survival of HAV in the environment is favoured at low relative humidity (Mbithi et al 1991), and inactivation of the virus in water requires higher concentrations of residual free chlorine (15–25 p.p.m.) than does inactivation of other picornaviruses (Peterson et al 1983, Siegl 1984).

Specific information on the physicochemical basis of HAV stability is not available. It may well be that the strength of interaction between capsid subunits is higher in HAV than in other picornaviruses. However, empty capsids of HAV have been found to be about as thermolabile as those of poliovirus (Ruchti et al 1991) and, hence, the presence of virus RNA seems to be an important stabilizing factor for the virion. Stabilization therefore may be related to regions of highly ordered RNA that specifically bind or interweave with capsid proteins. Such regionally highly structured RNA has recently been observed by X-ray crystallographic analysis of two positive-stranded RNA viruses (black beetle and flock house viruses) in which parts of the viral genomes protruded into the capsid protein shell (J Johnson, personal communication). Similarly structured RNA/protein elements have not yet been observed in picornaviruses of known atomic structure.

All attempts to resolve the structure of HAV by X-ray crystallography have failed. Therefore, the available structural information is mainly based on electron microscopical observations and on immunochemical data. Early in the study of HAV, Feinstone et al (1973) observed that both virions and empty capsids of HAV are agglutinated by human convalescent antisera. This implied immunogenicity of virions and empty particles but could not be taken as indication of a close antigenic relationship or even of the existence of identical antigenic structures on the surface of the virion and the empty protein shell. Very recently, however, both types of particles were shown to react to the same extent with anti-HAV monoclonal antibodies (Weitz et al 1991). Detailed analysis of the antigenic structure of the virion revealed a single immunodominant neutralizing site that is discontinuous and involves VP3 as well as VP1 (Ping et al 1988, Ping & Lemon 1992). This site is also present on empty capsids (Weitz et al 1991).

The topology of the HAV particle was assessed in addition by searching for proteinase-sensitive sites on the capsid surface and by analysing the effects of cleavage on particle antigenicity, infectivity and stability (Lemon et al 1991a). The results indicate that VP2 exposes a site sensitive to trypsin as well as to chymotrypsin on the virion surface. However, cleavage affected neither infectivity nor thermostability of HAV to a significant extent. Hence, the proteinase-sensitive site of VP2 is apparently not involved in virus attachment to susceptible cells and, consequently, seems to be distantly located to the putative receptor binding site. Cleavage of VP2 in the otherwise intact particle also failed to alter HAV antigenicity, as proteinase-treated virus continued to react fully with both human convalescent antibody and with murine neutralizing monoclonal antibodies specific for the immunodominant antigenic site of HAV.

Additional particles

The mature virion described previously is only one of several particle species present in faecal samples collected from naturally infected humans or experimentally infected non-human primates as well as in harvests from HAV-infected cell cultures (Bradley et al 1977, Siegl & Frosner 1978a, Siegl et al 1981). ‘Heavy’ and ‘light’ infectious particles with buoyant densities of about 1.42 g/ml and 1.27 g/ml, respectively, are usually only minor components of the particle spectrum. However, empty capsids banding in caesium chloride at buoyant densities of 1.29–1.31 g/ml, may account for as much as 60% of all viral structures present. The ‘heavy’ component is clearly less stable than the virion and, upon centrifugation through sucrose, dissociates into particles sedimenting with 230S, 156–160S, 90S and 50S (Bradley et al 1977, Siegl & Frosner 1978a, Siegl et al 1981). The last two particle species resemble the empty capsid structures that were shown to sediment with 79S and 59S respectively (Ruchti et al 1991). Empty capsids are made up of structural proteins VP1 and VP3 and, as would be predicted for a typical picornavirus, also of VP0. This protein is the precursor of VP2 and VP4 (see below) and can be expected to be processed to these end products during a final step of HAV maturation. Whether HAV empty capsids are precursors or dissociation products of the virion or whether they only represent an aberrant, terminal form of viral antigen produced in surplus during HAV replication is still unknown. In contrast, RNA-containing particles with a buoyant density of 1.32 g/ml and a sedimentation coefficient of 130S most likely represent an intermediate in the maturation of HAV. In analogy with the situation with poliovirus, they were putatively termed provirions (Ruchit et al 1991).

The last type of particles detectable in HAV-infected cell cultures as well as in faeces, blood and liver specimens from humans and monkeys suffering from hepatitis A are defective-interfering (Dl) particles (Nüesch et al 1988, 1989). These particles contain viral RNA and band close to the position of the mature virion in caesium chloride density gradients. Their genomes, however, are characterized by large internal deletions spanning the genetic information for viral structural proteins and extending even into the region coding for non-structural proteins. Genomes with 3' proximal truncations of variable length have also been described. HAV Dl particles are biologically active. They are able to interfere with replication of standard virus and, if present in high concentration during infection of cell cultures, may drastically reduce the yield of progeny infectious HAV (Siegl et al 1990).

THE HAV GENOME

General characteristics and variability

HAV contains a genome of linear single-stranded RNA composed of 7480 nucleotides. The RNA sediments with 33S and has a buoyant density of 1.64 g/ml in caesium chloride. The overall G+C composition is 38% (Cohen et al 1987a, Paul et al 1987). Among the picornaviruses this composition is the lowest and is only approximated by that of the rhinoviruses with a G+C content of 40%. Furthermore, the HAV genome shares a preference for A or U in the third position of codons with the genomes of the rhinoviruses. Information concerning type of nucleic acid and principle of its organization has initially been derived from molecules extracted from particles in clinical specimens or harvests from infected cell cultures (Provost et al 1975, Siegl & Frosner 1978b, Coulepis et al 1981, Siegl et al 1981). Virus RNA recovered under these conditions proved to be infectious and, hence, could be assumed to have messenger-sense polarity. However, detailed information on nucleotide composition, structure and functional organization only became available after molecular cloning of HAV RNA by Ticehurst et al (1983). The HAV strain (HM175) used by these authors was recovered during an outbreak of hepatitis A in Australia and had been passaged three times in marmosets prior to molecular cloning. It is assumed to represent wild-type (wt) human hepatitis A virus. In the meantime, a considerable number of cell culture-adapted derivatives of strain HM175 as well as wt and cell culture-adapted variants of other human hepatitis A virus isolates have been similarly cloned and sequenced (Baroudy et al 1985, Linemeyer et al 1985, Najarian et al 1985, Cohen et al 1987a, b, Paul et al 1987, Jansen et al 1988, Ross et al 1989). Two of the cloned variants represent cytolytic strains of HAV (Venuti et al 1985, Cromeans et al 1987). Furthermore, three independent simian isolates were recently molecularly characterized (Brown et al 1989, Nainan et al 1991, Tsarev et al 1991).

Cloning of the HAV genome was a necessary prerequisite for determination of the complete nucleotide sequence and also for assessment of the degree of genetic stability/variability of the virus, because authentic virus RNA was never recovered in amounts sufficient for direct sequence analysis. Early attempts to analyse by RNAase T1-mapping the genetic relatedness of HAV isolates from distant geographic locations met with extraordinary technical difficulties (Weitz & Siegl 1985). Nevertheless, the then investigated viruses were genetically closely related and differed in nucleotide sequence by no more than 10%. Results obtained by comparison of the complete nucleotide sequences of the HAV genomes cloned to date are in full agreement with this observation. Finally, introduction of antigen-capture–polymerase chain reaction (AC–PCR) by Jansen et al (1990) allowed genetic comparison of more than 150 HAV isolates via amplification and sequencing of a short, yet representative nucleotide stretch in the region VP1/2A of the viral genome (Robertson et al 1992). The results indicate that all human and simian HAV isolates can be grouped into seven unique genotypes distinguished by 15–25% sequence diversity. Within each of these genotypes subtypes that differ in approximately 7.5% of base positions can be defined. Viruses within these subtypes or those occurring in an epidemic or geographic cluster show <3% diversity over periods of up to 15 years. No sequence differences could be recorded in isolates for which serial specimens were available over a period of 41 days, and a single nucleotide substitution was identified in a HAV strain following 72 consecutive passages in cell culture. This is in striking contrast to the known genetic variability of other picornaviruses such as poliovirus, in which a variability of 1–2 base substitutions per week has been recorded (Rico-Hesse et al 1987).

Genome regions and biological function

The transfection of cultured cells with purified virus RNA and translation of authentic viral RNA in vitro demonstrated the messenger-sense polarity of the HAV genome (Locarnini et al 1981, Gauss-Muller et al 1984, Cohen et al 1987c). Nucleotide sequence analysis of cloned HAV cDNA also revealed that the genome is monocistronic and probably follows the translational strategy of other picornaviruses (Fig. 2.2) (Najarian

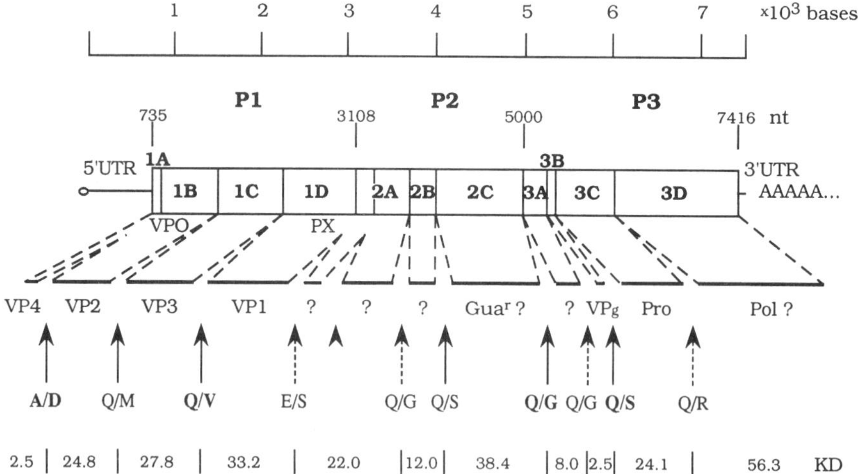

Fig. 2.2 Hepatitis A virus genome structure, products of proteolytic processing and functions of virus proteins. The hepatitis A virus genome is divided into a 5' untranslated region (5'-UTR), a giant open reading frame and a 3' untranslated region (3'-UTR). According to Rueckert & Wimmer (1984) the coding region can be subdivided into regions P1, P2 and P3, which specify proteins 1A–D, 2A–C and 3A–D. Figures above the genome structure represent nucleotide positions at the junctions of individual regions. 1A–D represents the structural proteins VP1–VP4. VPg represents the genome-linked virus protein, Pro the major virus protease and Pol may be an RNA-dependent RNA polymerase. The 2C gene carries a guanidine resistance maker (Guaʳ). The functions of all other proteins are so far unknown. Dipeptide cleavage sites within the polyprotein are indicated: full arrows with bold letters = confirmed sites, full arrows with normal letters = sites with strong evidence, broken arrows and normal letters = predicted sites, arrowhead = observed but unidentified cleavage site, kD = kilodalton.

et al 1985, Cohen et al 1987a). In consequence, the HAV genome may be divided into a 5' proximal untranslated region (5'-UTR) of 735 nucleotides, a coding region of 6681 nucleotides specifying one giant open reading frame for a polyprotein of 2227 amino acids, and a 3'-terminal untranslated region (3'-UTR) 63 nucleotides in length. Like the genomes of other picornaviruses, but in contrast to most eukaryotic messenger RNAs, the 5' end of the HAV genome is covalently linked to a small peptide, VPg (for genome-linked virus protein), instead of to the classical m^7G cap structure (Weitz et al 1986). At the 3' end HAV RNA contains a poly(adenylic acid) tail of 40–80 nucleotides (Siegl et al 1981).

5' untranslated region (5'-UTR)

For all picornavirus genera, the 5' untranslated region has been shown to contain essential regulatory functions for translation and, hence, for infectivity of the viral genome. The main structure of this region is compatible with a *cis*-acting element termed the internal ribosomal entry site (IRES) or ribosomal landing pad (Pelletier & Sonenberg 1988, Alsaadi et al 1989, Jang et al 1989, Belsham & Brangwyn 1990). This element directs initiation of cap-independent translation directly to a defined AUG triplet several hundreds of nucleotides downstream of the 5' terminus (Jackson 1988). The 5'-UTR of HAV is not homologous to those of other picornaviruses. Therefore, comparison of the primary structure of this region with that of other picornaviruses failed to identify an HAV-specific IRES. However, the combined results of phylogenetic analysis involving human and simian HAV strains, of digestion experiments applying specific nucleases and of thermodynamic modelling identified secondary and putative tertiary structures within the HAV 5'-UTR that are similar to those in the aphto- and cardiovirus 5'-UTRs (Brown et al 1991). The data can be interpreted in such a way that the equivalent of IRES in HAV RNA would direct initiation of translation to the 11th or the 12th AUG codon at nucleotide positions 735–737 and 741–743 respectively, of the genome. In vitro and in vivo translation studies with HAV RNA mutated at the position of AUG condons 11 or 12 have clearly indicated that each codon alone is sufficient to render RNA infectious (Tesar et al 1992). Furthermore, in BSC-1 cells, initiation of translation on synthetic transcripts of HAV cDNA seems to occur preferentially at the 12th AUG triplet.

Only little information is available concerning the significance of the 5'-UTR for the infectivity, replication and virulence of HAV. Thus, targeted mutational analysis of the three nucleotides UUC at its very 5' end seem to indicate that their presence in viral RNA is essential for productive infection (Harmon et al 1991). Furthermore, a specific point mutation at base position 687 (U → G) during adaptation of HAV to growth in BSC-1 cells has been found to have a positive effect on production of progeny virus (Day & Lemon 1990). Finally, mutations within the 5'-UTR most likely reduce hepatovirulence of HAV for susceptible non-human primates (Cohen et al 1989).

The 3' untranslated region (3'-UTR)

Whereas the 5'-UTR with 95% nucleotide identity among all HAV strains sequenced to date appears to be the most highly conserved region in the HAV genome, the 3'-UTR shows the highest (up to 20%) degree of variability. The function of the 3'-UTR within the picornavirus genome is widely unknown. However, on the basis of the actual concept of picornavirus replication, sequence elements within the 3'-UTR can be expected to play an important role in initiation and regulation of synthesis of progeny picornavirus RNA. A comparative analysis of 3'-UTR sequences of several HAV variants and of other picornaviruses was recently carried out under these aspects (Nüesch et al 1993). The results pointed to the presence of a short (only 23 nucleotides long), probably *cis*-acting element within the HAV genome that specifically interacted with proteins present during establishment and throughout persistent infection of HAV in vitro. A similar element (79% identity in nucleotides) is present in the 3'-UTR of poliovirus type 1; yet proteins binding to this region of the viral genome could not be detected in poliovirus-infected cells. Most interestingly, cell cultures infected with a cytolytic variant of HAV (strain HM175/18F; Lemon et al 1991b) also failed to yield these proteins. Therefore, protein–RNA interactions at the 23-nucleotide target site may indeed be involved in establishment and maintenance of the persistent type of infection characteristic for in vitro replication of most HAV isolates.

Coding region

The coding region of the HAV genome extends from nucleotide 735 to nucleotide 7415. It consists of a single open reading frame that specifies a giant polyprotein of 2227 amino acids as a primary translation product. There is only very distant overall similarity between the polyproteins of HAV and those of other picornaviruses. However, regional amino acid sequence similarities point to a very similar organization of the genetic information and to corresponding functions of the mature proteins that are derived from the polyprotein through processing by viral (or cellular?) proteinases. Therefore, in analogy with the situation with other picornaviruses, the coding region of the HAV genome can be subdivided into regions P1, specifying the four structural proteins VP1–4, P2, coding for three non-structural proteins 2A–C, and P3, coding for four additional non-structural proteins 3A–D (see Fig. 2.2).

HAV PROTEINS

Structural proteins

Capsid proteins VP1, VP2, VP3 and VP0, the putative peptide precursor protein of VP2 and VP4, were experimentally identified and mapped to the P1 region. To this end, VP1 and VP3 were isolated from virions, their N-termini were directly sequenced, and the corresponding codons were aligned with the nucleic acid sequence of the P1 region (Linemeyer et al 1985, Gauss-Muller et al 1986). In accordance with data obtained by electrophoretic separation of capsid proteins, VP1 (1D) is the largest structural protein (Wheeler et al 1986). It is 33 kD in size and maps to the 3' end of P1 (see Fig. 2.2). The information for VP3 (1C, 28 kD) and VP2 (1B, 25 kD) lies adjacent to VP1 towards the 5' end. Both location and size of VP2 were confirmed by use of antibodies that had been raised against synthetic peptides deduced from the presumed coding sequence of this protein. VP0 (1AB, 27 kD) was detected predominantly in empty capsids (Ruchti et al 1991).

Although there is evidence from computation of sequence data that the HAV genome codes for a fourth capsid protein, VP4, this peptide has not yet been physically identified. Following disruption and electrophoresis of highly purified virions, the presence of an additional small peptide in the range between 7 and 14 kD has been repeatedly reported (Coulepis et al 1980, Tratschin et al 1981). In contrast, molecular information suggests that the putative VP4 has a molecular weight of 1500–2500. Direct transformation of sequence data argues for a peptide consisting of 23 amino acids. However, identification of a myristoylation site (GXXXT/S) similar to the one defined by Chow et al (1987) for poliovirus at the N-terminus of the polyprotein is in favour of a molecule made up of 17 amino acids only. Under these conditions the remaining upstream information would specify a leader peptide of six amino acids for HAV.

Non-structural proteins

Size and location of the seven non-structural proteins within regions P2 and P3 of the HAV genome have originally been tentatively identified on the basis of sequence data and known cleavage sites within the polyproteins of other picornaviruses. However, because the genome of HAV lacks homology with the genomes of well-studied picornaviruses, the predictions are uncertain.

To the best of our knowledge, protein 2A of HAV consists of 189 amino acids. By analogy with other picornaviruses, it may be expected to function as a proteinase that co-translationally cleaves the polyprotein. However, region 2A of HAV shows extraordinarily low similarity to $2A^{pro}$ of other picornaviruses. Specifically, it neither contains the amino acid residues (catalytic triad) of the putative active site of rhino- and enteroviruses (Palmenberg 1990), nor shares any significant degree of similarity in its C-terminal region with cardio- and aphtoviruses. The latter viruses also have no catalytic triad but employ a stretch of C-terminal amino acid residues in the primary cleavage of the polyprotein (Ryan & King 1991). Protein 2B (107 amino acids) is also distinct from similar picornavirus proteins. Its function is unknown. The product of region 2C (335 amino acids) is assumed to play a role in RNA replication and, by comparison with the corresponding gene of other picornaviruses, carries a guanidine-resistant allele (Pincus et al 1986, Cohen et al 1987a). None of the proteins in region P2 of the HAV genome has to date been physically identified.

The proteins specified by P3 comprise VPg (3B, 23 amino acids), the peptide linked covalently to the 5' end of the viral genome, protease $3C^{pro}$ (219 amino acids) and an RNA-dependent RNA polymerase (3D, 489 amino acids). Protein 3A of HAV (74 amino acids) has been identified in context with the processing of the peptide precursor 3AB, and the generation of VPg (M Weitz, unpublished observation). Both 3A and 3B proteins are thought to be essential for picornavirus RNA replication. They are most likely anchored to the smooth endoplasmic reticulum via a hydrophobic domain of 3A. In agreement with this prediction, 3A of HAV, although overall not hydrophobic, contains 20 out of 30 C-terminal residues that are strongly hydrophobic.

By analogy with other picornaviruses, the proteinase $3C^{pro}$ represents a serine-like cysteine proteinase (Bazan & Fletterick 1988, Gorbalenya et al 1989). The protein has been identified experimentally as a proteinase that releases itself autocatalytically from the polyprotein. Very recently it was also shown to act in trans on sites within the P1 and P2 regions of the polyprotein (Gauss-Muller et al 1991, Jia et al 1991a, Harmon et al 1992, Malcolm et al 1992). Approaches to characterize HAV $3C^{pro}$ relied on in vitro translation of synthetic HAV RNAs encoding, besides $3C^{pro}$, a variable number of complete and truncated genes adjacent to 3C, and on heterologous expression of similar constructs. In agreement with predictions made on the basis of global alignments with encephalomyocarditis and foot-and-mouth disease viral proteins, these approaches identified a catalytically active cysteine residue at position 172. Further careful regional alignments including also $3C^{pro}$ amino acid sequences of polio- and rhinovirus $3C^{pro}$ point to histidine 44 and/or histidine 191, aspartic acid 98 and cysteine 172 as functionally most important residues in the HAV-specific protease (M Weitz, unpublished observation).

Replication of picornavirus RNA is performed by a highly specific, widely conserved, RNA-dependent RNA polymerase, $3D^{pol}$. Among all other regions of the HAV open reading frame, the region assumed to code for $3D^{pol}$ shows the highest degree (29%) of similarity to the corresponding sequence in the poliovirus type 1 polyprotein (Cohen et al 1987a). In addition, a region of 18 amino acids thought to be essential for an active polymerase is present in the HAV 3D region. This particular sequence contains a conserved motif of two aspartate residues flanked by hydrophobic amino acids (LKILCYG**DD**VLIVF) that might function as a GTP binding domain (Kamer & Argos 1984). However, a functional $3D^{pol}$ of HAV remains to be identified.

POLYPROTEIN PROCESSING

Proteolytic processing of the primary translation product of the viral genome plays a central role in the replication of picornaviruses (Palmenberg 1990). Knowledge of individual cleavage sites and of the cascade of proteolytic events is also essential to understand the translational strategy of the picornaviral genome. In this respect, three major steps can so far be distinguished. Firstly, a primary cleavage event mediated by $2A^{pro}$ occurs co-translationally at the P1/P2 junction in entero- and rhinoviruses or, alternatively, at the 2A/2B junction in cardio- and aphtoviruses. Secondly, the polyprotein is processed at most other sites in cis- and/or in trans by protease $3C^{pro}$ or the similarly proteolytic precursor 3CD. Thirdly, cleavage of VP0 to VP2 and VP4 appears to be a necessary, late event during maturation of the virion ('maturation cleavage').

As far as primary processing of the HAV polyprotein is concerned, neither the exact site nor the mechanism by which it is achieved is presently known. However, studies on HAV morphogenesis (Anderson & Ross 1990, Winokur et al 1991, Kusov et al 1992) revealed precursor structures of the hepatitis A virion and even small amounts of the mature virus particle which, instead of VP1 (1D, 33 kD), contained a larger protein, PX (38–42 kD). This protein is assumed to comprise 1D and at least part of the predicted protein 2A. Yet, because the exact size of 2A is unknown, it may well be that primary cleavage of the HAV polyprotein occurs not within 2A, but rather at the 2A/2B junction.

HAV proteinase $3C^{pro}$ is the only viral enzyme identified so far and characterized in some detail. Its role in processing of the polyprotein has recently been well established (Gauss-Muller et al 1991, Jia et al 1991a, Harmon et al 1992). The enzyme cleaves at most of the assumed sites and the following cleavages were directly proven on authentic HAV peptides: 2C/3A, 3A/3B, 3B/3C and 3C/3D. Less convincing evidence was reported for $3C^{pro}$-mediated processing at junctions VP0/VP3, VP3/VP1 and VP1/2A. Only indirect evidence is available for cleavage at junction 2B/2C (Malcolm et al 1992). Four of the 10 putative dipeptide cleavage sites within the polyprotein have been confirmed by amino acid sequence analysis (see Fig. 2.2); VP4/VP2 (Ala/Asp) (Gauss-Muller et al 1986, Wheeler et al 1986), VP3/VP1 (Gln/Val) (Linemeyer et al 1985, Gauss-Muller et al 1986, Wheeler et al 1986), 2C/3A (Gln/Gly) (Harmon et al 1992), and 3B/3C (Gln/Ser) (Gauss-Muller et al 1991, Harmon et al 1992). Strong evidence exists also for the nature of sequences at junctions VP2/VP3 (Gln/Met) (Wheeler et al 1986). The apparent variability in dipeptides that serve as substrates for $3C^{pro}$ within the HAV polyprotein implies an important role of peptide secondary structure as determining cleavage specificity.

The dynamics of $3C^{pro}$-mediated processing of the HAV polyprotein have been investigated by translation in vitro of RNA transcribed from recombinant constructs containing the information for the enzyme (Jia et al 1991a) as well as by expression of HAV proteins from similar constructs in prokaryotic (Gauss-Muller et al 1991, Petithory et al 1991) and recombinant vaccinia virus systems (M Weitz, unpublished observation). According to these studies, the speed at which individual cleavages occur is determined by the experimental system used. Thus, only inefficient processing of HAV peptide precursors has so far been observed in the course of translation in vitro or in recombinant prokaryotic expression. However expression of the same region from a recombinant vaccinia virus vector resulted in rapid and efficient accumulation of mature proteins.

Maturation cleavage, i.e. release of VP2 and VP4 from the peptide precursor VP0, has been proposed to be carried out as a last step in the generation of the mature picornavirus particle. The activity is provided by the virus itself in an autocatalytic, quasi-enzymatic reaction that involves viral RNA and amino acid residues located in the VP2- as well as in the VP4-specific regions of VP0 (Arnold et al 1987). A similar step is also likely to occur in the maturation of the hepatitis A virion. Empty capsids have been found to contain predominantly the peptide precursor VP0, and mature, infectious particles obviously include mainly structural protein VP2 instead (Ruchti et al 1991). In addition, sequence alignments of HAV VP0 with those of other picornaviruses revealed the quasi-active site of a proteinase that contains Ser-29 of VP2 as a putative catalytic residue (Palmenberg 1987). However, direct proof for the autocatalytic activity is still missing.

Information concerning the sequence of polyprotein cleavages is fragmentary. As outlined above, there is evidence that a primary cleavage occurs within 2A or at the 2A/2B junction. In addition, processing of P3 peptide precursor has been studied in some detail by in vitro translation (Jia et al 1991a) or recombinant eukaryotic expression (Gauss-Muller et al 1991). The results, however, are still controversial. It is thus not clear whether initial cleavage occurs at the 3B/3C junction to generate a fairly stable 3CD product (Jia et al 1991a) or at 3C/3D to yield 3ABC as the most prominent intermediate product of P3 polyprotein processing. Observations in HAV-infected cells and with recombinant vaccinia viruses are in favour of the latter situation (M Weitz, unpublished).

VIRUS REPLICATION

Kinetics and efficiency

One of the most distinguishing features between classical picornaviruses and HAV concerns viral replication. Viruses such as poliovirus or human rhinovirus replicate readily to high titres in susceptible cells and complete a full replication cycle within 8–10 h. In contrast, isolation of HAV from clinical samples and adaptation to growth in cell cultures is a lengthy, inefficient process that usually takes weeks or even months. Even after successful adaptation, replication of HAV is protracted over several days, and yields of progeny virus rarely exceed titres of 10^7 $TCID_{50}$/ml (Locarnini et al 1981, Siegl et al 1984b). Contrary to the situation in, for example, poliovirus-infected cells, HAV also fails to shut down host cell metabolism. Consequently, replication of practically all primary HAV isolates terminates in a state of persistent infection (Vallbracht et al 1984, de Chastonay & Siegl 1987, Siegl et al 1991). Cytopathic HAV strains have so far been only recovered from persistently infected cultures. They also fail to shut off host cell metabolism. The molecular basis of their cytolytic activity is unknown.

One-step replication of HAV strains establishing persistent infection typically occurs in three phases (de Chastonay & Siegl 1987). First evidence for virus replication is usually obtained after a lag period of 1–2 days. In a second phase, synthesis of both negative- and positive-strand viral RNA, synthesis of viral proteins and production of progeny virus proceed exponentially and reach highest rates over a period of 3–6 days. The end of this phase is signalled by down-regulation of viral RNA synthesis in the presence of a quantitatively unchanged, continuing synthesis of viral structural proteins. Finally, a state of persistent infection is stably established within 10–14 days of infection. It is characterized by minimal viral metabolic activity in virtually 100% of a culture's cells and can be maintained over weeks or even months without requirement for special culturing conditions.

The replicative events of cytolytic HAV variants are characterized by a shortened lag phase of 6–12 h (Anderson 1987, Anderson et al 1987, Nasser & Metcalf 1987, Cromeans et al 1989). Maximal levels of viral RNA synthesis can be observed as early as 24 h post infection (p.i.), and exponential production of progeny virus frequently continues up to day 4 p.i. Depending on the virus strain, lysis of infected cells may become apparent within 3–9 days after infection.

Factors controlling HAV replication

Attempts to identify and to characterize the conditions and factors responsible for the protracted, inefficient course of HAV replication have been made virtually since the first successful propagation of the virus in cell culture by Provost & Hilleman in 1979. The results available to date point to a close interaction of several viral and cellular functions as a prerequisite for efficient viral replication. Thus, comparative sequencing of the genomes of wt HAV strains that barely replicate in cell culture and those of efficiently replicating HAV strains derived thereof during multiple successive passages revealed that adaptation is consistent with the selection of variant viruses carrying up to 42 mutations (Cohen et al 1987a, b, Jansen et al 1988, Cohen et al 1989, Ross et al 1989). Of these, a point mutation within the 5'-UTR and three point mutations in regions 2B and 2C of the HAV genome were recently identified as being specifically important for enhanced growth of HAV in cell culture (Day & Lemon 1990, Emerson et al 1992a, b). None of these mutations alone proved able to determine differences in growth efficiency among HAV strains. Rather, each was found to interact with distantly located mutations and could also be functionally replaced by mutations elsewhere in the HAV genome.

Significant differences in sequence between cytolytic HAV strains and their non-cytolytic parent viruses were likewise localized in the 5'-UTR and in the regions of the genome coding for non-structural proteins. Most interestingly, however, such differences could also be identified in the 3'-UTR (Lemon et al 1991b).

The cellular functions contributing to efficient HAV replication are determined at the level of both the genotype and phenotype of the cell. In full support of this statement Emerson et al

(1992b) were able to select cell cultures with drastically enhanced competence for HAV replication by subcloning those cells that produced progeny virus most effectively. Moreover, susceptible cells, although infected simultaneously, were found to start HAV replication asynchronously (Harmon et al 1989). Synchrony in virus replication could not be accomplished by synchronization of cell growth (Gauss-Muller & Deinhardt 1984, Siegl et al 1984b, Cho & Ehrenfeld 1991). Consequently, the cellular factors obviously necessary for initiation of HAV replication are expressed independently of the cellular division cycle. However, for one distinct HAV strain replication could be synchronized and accelerated upon reversible treatment of infected cells with guanidine.

Regulation of HAV replication, specifically its attenuation to the low level of synthetic activity characteristic of persistently infected cells, may involve synthesis of viral RNA, translation and processing of viral proteins, as well as maturation of progeny virus. Of these major aspects, translation, processing and overall synthesis of viral proteins are assumed to be relatively inefficient. Detailed information on HAV protein synthesis in infected cells is not yet available as, owing to the inability of HAV to shut off host cell metabolism, newly produced viral proteins cannot be identified directly against the background of ongoing synthesis of cellular proteins. Results from in vitro translation of the HAV genome in rabbit reticulocyte lysates (Jia et al 1991b) or from recombinant prokaryotic expression of specific, truncated genomic constructs (Gauss-Muller et al 1991, Harmon et al 1992) have helped to understand some individual facets of protein processing. However, they failed to yield suggestive information concerning regulation of HAV protein synthesis.

The most likely critical step in HAV replication is synthesis of viral RNA. Down-regulation of synthesis of the negative-strand template of the HAV genome was found to be the first significant event prior to the slowdown of overall viral synthetic activity (de Chastonay & Siegl 1987). It was followed by a decrease in synthesis of the viral genome, which, in turn, was paralleled by cessation of the production of progeny virions. Anderson et al (1988) interpreted this sequence of events as the result of depletion of the pool of replicating viral genomes by rapid irreversible encapsidation of progeny positive-stranded RNA molecules. However, Nüesch et al (1993), provided suggestive evidence that down-regulation of viral RNA synthesis may be linked to the appearance of a so far undefined class of proteins binding specifically to a distinct sequence of 23 nucleotides in the 3'-UTR of the HAV genome as well as to the corresponding complementary sequence at the 5' terminus of the HAV antigenome. In accordance with accepted knowledge on picornavirus RNA replication, these regions in both types of RNA molecules can be assumed to play a significant role in initiation of synthesis and/or elongation of HAV RNA.

Finally, negative regulation of HAV replication may also be the effect of DI particles. As described above, three distinct types of DI particles with well-defined internal deletions in their genomes have been found in various HAV/cell culture systems and could also be recovered from clinical samples collected from HAV-infected humans and monkeys (Nuesch et al 1988, 1989). The presence of large concentrations of such DI particles in the inoculum of cell cultures led to reduction of synthesis of progeny virions by a factor of 10–100 (Siegl et al 1990). The most prominent type of defective viral genome could also be shown to reappear, even after infection of cells at a multiplicity of infection as low as 10^{-4}. It then accumulated to significant quantities in cell cultures concomitantly with establishment of persistent HAV infection (JPF Nuesch, M Weitz & G Siegl, unpublished observation).

Effects of antiviral substances on HAV replication

The unique position of HAV among the picornaviruses is well supported by the virus's distinct resistance to the inhibitory effects of chemical reagents known to interfere with the replication of poliovirus and other intensively studied members of this virus family. Among these reagents are arildone, disoxaril, 3'-methylquercitine, 2,4-dichloropyrimidine, guanidine and 2-(α-hydroxybenzyl)benzimidazol (Siegl & Eggers

1982, de Chastonay & Siegl 1988, Widell et al 1986, Lemon 1985). In contrast, HAV replication in cell culture can be inhibited by addition of ribavirin, amantadin and 2-deoxy-D-glucose (Biziagos et al 1987, 1990, Crance et al 1990). Enhanced production of HAV progeny and of antigen in vitro has been observed in the presence of prostaglandin E_1 and dexamethasone (Gauss-Muller & Deinhardt 1984a). Such effects were, however, restricted to particular virus/cell pairs. Widell et al (1988) also reported on improved yields of HAV in cell cultures when treated with 5,6-dichloro-1-β-D-ribofuranosylbenzimidazol (DRB).

REFERENCES

Alsaadi S, Hassard S, Stanway G 1989 Sequences in the 5' non-coding region of human rhinovirus 14 RNA that affect in vitro translation. Journal of General Virology 70: 2799–2804

Anderson D A 1987 Cytopathology, plaque assay, and heat inactivation of hepatitis A virus strain HM175. Journal of Medical Virology 22: 35–44

Anderson D A, Ross B C 1990 Morphogenesis of hepatitis A virus: isolation and characterization of subviral particles. Journal of Virology 64: 5284–5289

Anderson D A, Locarnini S A, Ross B C, Coulepis A G, Anderson B N, Gust I D 1987 Single growth kinetics of hepatitis A virus in BSC-1 cells. In: Brinton M A, Rueckert R R (eds) Positive strand RNA viruses. Alan R. Liss, New York, pp 497–507

Anderson D A, Ross B C, Locarnini S A 1988 Restricted replication of hepatitis A virus in cell culture: encapsidation of viral RNA depletes the pool of RNA available for replication. Journal of Virology 62: 4201–4206

Arnold E, Luo M, Vriend G, Rossmann M G, Palmenberg A C, Parks G D, Nicklin M J, Wimmer E 1987 Implications of the picornavirus capsid structure for polyprotein processing. Proceedings of the National Academy of Science USA 84: 21–25

Baroudy B M, Ticehurst J R, Miele T A, Maizel J V Jr, Purcell R H, Feinstone S M 1985 Sequence analysis of hepatitis A virus cDNA coding for capsid proteins and RNA polymerase. Proceedings of the National Academy of Science USA 82: 2143–2147

Bazan J K, Fletterick R J 1988 Viral cysteine proteases are homologous to the trypsin-like family of serine proteases: structural and functional implications. Proceedings of the National Academy of Science USA 85: 7872–7876

Belsham G J, Brangwyn J K 1990 A region of the 5' noncoding region of foot-and-mouth disease virus RNA directs efficient internal initiation of protein synthesis within cells: involvement with the role of L protease in translational control. Journal of Virology 64: 5389–5395

Biziagos E, Crance J M, Passagot J, Deloince R 1987 Effect of antiviral substances on hepatitis A virus replication in vitro. Journal of Medical Virology 22: 57–66

Biziagos E, Crance J M, Passagot J, Deloince R 1990 Inhibitory effects of atropine, protamine, and their combination on hepatitis A virus replication in PLC/PRF/5 cells. Antimicrobial Agents and Chemotherapy 34: 1112–1117

Bradley D W, McCaustland K A, Schreeder M T, Cook E H, Gravelle C R, Maynard J E 1977 Multiple buoyant densities of hepatitis A virus in cesium chloride gradients. Journal of Medical Virology 1: 219–226

Brown E A, Jansen R W, Lemon S M 1989 Characterization of a simian hepatitis A virus (HAV): antigenic and genetic comparison with human HAV. Journal of Virology 63: 4932–4937

Brown E A, Day S P, Jansen R W, Lemon S M 1991 The 5' nontranslated region of hepatitis A virus RNA: secondary structure and elements required for translation in vitro. Journal of Virology 65: 5828–5838

de Chastonay J, Siegl G 1987 Replicative events in hepatitis A virus-infected MRC-5 cells. Virology 157: 268–275

de Chastonay J, Siegl G 1988 Effect of three known antiviral substances on hepatitis A virus replication. In: Zuckerman A J (ed) Viral hepatitis and liver disease. Allan R. Liss, New York, pp 956–960

Cho M W, Ehrenfeld E 1991 Rapid completion of the replication cycle of hepatitis-A virus subsequent to reversal of guanidine inhibition. Virology 180: 770–780

Chow M, Newman J F, Filman D, Hogle J M, Rowlands D J, Brown F 1987 Myristylation of picornavirus capsid protein VP4 and its structural significance. Nature 327: 482–486

Cohen J I 1989 Hepatitis A virus: insights from molecular biology. Hepatology 9: 889–895

Cohen J I, Ticehurst J R, Purcell R H, Buckler-White A, Baroudy B M 1987a Complete nucleotide sequence of wild-type hepatitis A virus: comparison with different strains of hepatitis A virus and other picornaviruses. Journal of Virology 61: 50–59

Cohen J I, Rosenblum B, Ticehurst J R, Daemer R J, Feinstone S M, Purcell R H 1987b Complete nucleotide sequence of an attenuated hepatitis A virus: comparison with wild-type virus. Proceedings of the National Academy of Science USA 84: 2497–2501

Cohen J I, Ticehurst J R, Feinstone S M, Rosenblum B, Purchell R H 1987c Hepatitis A virus cDNA and its RNA transcripts are infectious in cell culture. Journal of Virology 61: 3035–3039

Cohen J I, Rosenblum B, Feinstone S M, Ticehurst J, Purcell R H 1989 Attenuation and cell culture adaptation of hepatitis A virus (HAV): a genetic analysis with HAV cDNA. Journal of Virology 63: 5364–5370

Coulepis A G, Locarnini S A, Gust I D 1980 Iodination of hepatitis A virus reveals a fourth structural polypeptide. Journal of Virology 35: 572–574

Coulepis A G, Tannock G A, Locarnini S A, Gust I D 1981 Evidence that the genome of hepatitis A virus consists of single-stranded RNA. Journal of Virology 37: 473–477

Coulepis A G, Locarnini S A, Westaway E G, Tannock G A, Gust I D 1982 Biophysical and biochemical

characterization of hepatitis V virus. Intervirology 18: 107–127
Crance J M, Biziagos E, Passagot J, van Cuyck-Gandre H, Deloince R 1990 Inhibition of hepatitis A virus replication in vitro by antiviral compounds. Journal of Medical Virology 31: 155–160
Cromeans T, Sobsey M D, Fields H A 1987 Development of a plaque assay for a cytopathic, rapidly replicating isolate of hepatitis A virus. Journal of Medical Virology 22: 45–56
Cromeans T, Fields H A, Sobsey M D 1989 Replication kinetics and cytopathic effect of hepatitis A virus. Journal of General Virology 70: 2051–2062
Day S P, Lemon S M 1990 A single base mutation in the 5' noncoding region of HAV enhances replication of virus in vitro. In: Brown F, Chanock R M, Ginsberg H S, Lerner R A (eds) Vaccines 90: modern approaches to new vaccines including prevention of AIDS. Cold Spring Harbor Laboratory Press, Cold Spring Harbor, pp 175–178
Emerson S U, Huang Y K, Mcrill C, Lewis M, Purcell R H 1992a Mutations in both the 2B-gene and 2C-gene of hepatitis-A virus are involved in adaptation to growth in cell culture. Journal of Virology 66: 650–654
Emerson S U, Huang Y K, Mcrill C, Lewis M, Shapiro M, London W T, Purcell R H 1992b Molecular basis of virulence and growth of hepatitis A virus in cell culture. Vaccine 10, S1: 36–39
Feinstone S M, Kapikian A Z, Purcell R H 1973 Hepatitis A: detection by immune electron microscopy of a viruslike antigen associated with acute illness. Science 182: 1026–1028
Gauss-Muller V, Deinhardt F 1984 Effect of hepatitis A virus infection on cell metabolism in vitro. Proceedings of the Society for Experimental Biology and Medicine 175: 10–15
Gauss-Muller V, von der Helm K, Deinhardt F 1984 Translation in vitro of hepatitis A virus RNA. Virology 137: 182–184
Gauss-Muller V, Lottspeich F, Deinhardt F 1986 Characterization of hepatitis A virus structural proteins. Virology 155: 732–736
Gauss-Muller V, Jurgensen D, Deutzmann R 1991 Autoproteolytic cleavage of recombinant 3C proteinase of hepatitis-A virus. Virology 182: 861–864
Gorbalenya A E, Donchenko A P, Blinov V M, Koonin E V 1989 Cysteine proteases of positive strand RNA viruses and chymotrypsin-like serine proteases. A distinct protein superfamily with a common structural fold. FEBS Letters 243: 103–114
Harmon S A, Summers D F, Ehrenfeld E 1989 Detection of hepatitis A virus RNA and capsid antigen in individual cells. Virus Research 12: 361–369
Harmon S A, Richards O C, Summers D F, Ehrenfeld E 1991 The 5'-terminal nucleotides of hepatitis-A virus RNA, but not poliovirus RNA, are required for infectivity. Journal of Virology 65: 2757–2760
Harmon S A, Updike W, Jia X Y, Summers D F, Ehrenfeld E 1992 Polyprotein processing in cis and in trans by hepatitis A virus 3C protease cloned and expressed in *Escherichia coli*. Journal of Virology 66: 5242–5247
Jackson R J 1988 RNA translation. Picornaviruses break the rules news. Nature 334: 292–293
Jang S K, Davies M V, Kaufman R J, Wimmer E 1989 Initiation of protein synthesis by internal entry of ribosomes into the 5' nontranslated region of encephalomyocarditis virus RNA in vivo. Journal of Virology 63: 1651–1660
Jansen R W, Newbold J E, Lemon S M 1988 Complete nucleotide sequence of a cell culture-adapted variant of hepatitis A virus: comparison with wild-type virus with restricted capacity for in vitro replication. Virology 163: 299–307
Jansen R W, Siegl G, Lemon S M 1990 Molecular epidemiology of human hepatitis A virus defined by an antigen-capture polymerase chain reaction method. Proceedings of the National Academy of Science USA 87: 2867–2871
Jia X Y, Ehrenfeld E, Summers D F 1991a Proteolytic activity of hepatitis-A virus 3C protein. Journal of Virology 65: 2595–2600
Jia X Y, Scheper G, Brown D et al 1991b Translation of hepatitis-A virus RNA in vitro – aberrant internal initiations influenced by 5' noncoding region. Virology 182: 712–722
Kamer G, Argos P 1984 Primary structural comparison of RNA-dependent polymerases from plant, animal and bacterial viruses. Nucleic Acids Research 12: 7269–7282
Kusov Y Y, Kazachkov Y A, Dzagurov G K, Khozinskaya G A, Balayan M S, Gauss-Muller V 1992 Identification of precursors of structural protein-VP1 and protein-VP2 of hepatitis-A virus. Journal of Medical Virology 37: 220–227
Lemon S M 1985 Type A viral hepatitis. New developments in an old disease. New England Journal of Medicine 313: 1059–1067
Lemon S M, Jansen R W, Newbold J E 1985 Infectious hepatitis A virus particles produced in cell culture consist of three distinct types with different buoyant densities in CsCl. Journal of Virology 54: 78–85
Lemon S M, Amphlett E, Sangar D 1991a Protease digestion of hepatitis-A virus – disparate effects on capsid proteins, antigenicity, and infectivity. Journal of Virology 65: 5636–5640
Lemon S M, Murphy P C, Shields P A, Ping L H, Feinstone S M, Cromeans T, Jansen R W 1991b Antigenic and genetic variation in cytopathic hepatitis-A virus variants arising during persistent infection – evidence for genetic recombination. Journal of Virology 65: 2056–2065
Linemeyer D L, Menke J G, Martin-Gallardo A, Hughes J V, Young A, Mitra S W 1985 Molecular cloning and partial sequencing of hepatitis A viral cDNA. Journal of Virology 54: 247–255
Locarnini S A, Coulepis A G, Westaway E G, Gust I D 1981 Restricted replication of human hepatitis A virus in cell culture: intracellular biochemical studies. Journal of Virology 37: 216–225
Malcolm B A, Chin S M, Jewell D A, Strattonthomas J R, Thudium K B, Ralston R, Rosenberg S 1992 Expression and characterization of recombinant hepatitis-A virus 3C-proteinase. Biochemistry 31: 3358–3363
Mbithi J N, Springthorpe V S, Sattar S A 1991 Effect of relative humidity and air temperature on survival of hepatitis-A virus on environmental surfaces. Applied and Environmental Microbiology 57: 1394–1399
Melnick J L 1982 Classification of hepatitis A virus as enterovirus type 72 and of hepatitis B virus as hepadnavirus type 1. Intervirology 18: 105–106
Minor P D 1991 Picornaviridae. In: Classification and nomenclature of viruses: Fifth Report of the International Committee on Taxonomy of Viruses. Archives of Virology, (suppl 2). Springer Verlag, Vienna, pp 320–326
Nainan O V, Margolis H S, Robertson B H, Balayan M, Brinton M A 1991 Sequence analysis of a new hepatitis a virus naturally infecting cynomolgus macaques

(*Macaca fascicularis*). Journal of General Virology 72: 1685–1689
Najarian R, Caput D, Gee W, Potter S J, Renard A, Merryweather J, Van Nest G, Dina D 1985 Primary structure and gene organization of human hepatitis A virus. Proceedings of the National Academy of Science USA 82: 2627–2631
Nasser A M, Metcalf T G 1987 Production of cytopathology in FRhK-4 cells by BS-C-1-passaged hepatitis A virus. Applied and Environmental Microbiology 53: 2967–2971
Nüesch J, Krech S, Siegl G 1988 Detection and characterization of subgenomic RNAs in hepatitis A virus particles. Virology 165: 419–427
Nüesch J, de Chastonay J, Siegl G 1989 Detection of defective genomes in hepatitis A virus particles present in clinical specimens. Journal of General Virology 70: 3475–3480
Nüesch J, Weitz M, Siegl G 1993 Proteins specifically binding to the 3' untranslated region of hepatitis A virus RNA in persistently infected cells. Archives of Virology 128: 65–79
Palmenberg A C 1987 Picornaviral processing: some new ideas. Journal of Cellular Biochemistry 33: 191–198
Palmenberg A C 1990 Proteolytic processing of picornaviral polyprotein. Annual Reviews of Microbiology 44: 603–623
Parry J V, Mortimer P P 1984 The heat sensitivity of hepatitis A virus determined by a simple tissue culture method. Journal of Medical Virology 14: 277–283
Paul A V, Tada H, von der Helm K, Wissel T, Kiehn R, Wimmer E, Deinhardt F 1987 The entire nucleotide sequence of the genome of human hepatitis A virus (isolate MBB). Virus Research 8: 153–171
Pelletier J, Sonenberg N 1988 Internal initiation of translation of eukaryotic mRNA directed by a sequence derived from poliovirus RNA. Nature 334: 320–325
Peterson D A, Hurley T R, Hoff J C, Wolfe L G 1983 Effect of chlorine treatment on infectivity of hepatitis A virus. Applied and Environmental Microbiology 45: 223–227
Petithory J R, Masiarz F R, Kirsch J F, Santi D V, Malcolm B A 1991 A rapid method for determination of endoproteinase substrate specificity – specificity of the 3C proteinase from hepatitis-A virus. Proceedings of the National Academy of Science USA 88: 11510–11514
Pincus S E, Diamond D C, Emini E A, Wimmer E 1986 Guanidine-selected mutants of poliovirus: mapping of point mutations of polypeptide 2C. Journal of Virology 57: 638–646
Ping L H, Lemon S M 1992 Antigenic structure of human hepatitis-A virus defined by analysis of escape mutants selected against murine monoclonal antibodies. Journal of Virology 66: 2208–2216
Ping L H, Jansen R W, Stapleton J T, Cohen J I, Lemon S M 1988 Identification of an immunodominant antigenic site involving the capsid protein VP3 of hepatitis A virus. Proceedings of the National Academy of Science USA 85: 8281–8285
Provost P J, Hilleman M R 1979 Propagation of human hepatitis A virus in cell culture in vitro. Proceedings of the Society for Experimental Biology and Medicine 160: 213–221
Provost P J, Wolanski B S, Miller W J, Ittensohn O L, McAleer W J, Hilleman M R 1975 Physical, chemical and morphologic dimensions of human hepatitis A virus strain CR326 (38578). Proceedings of the Society for Experimental Biology and Medicine 148: 532–539
Rico-Hesse R, Pallansch M, Nottay B K, Kew O M 1987 Geographic distribution of wild poliovirus type 1 genotypes. Virology 160: 311–322
Robertson B H, Jansen R W, Khanna B et al 1992 Genetic relatedness of hepatitis-A virus strains recovered from different geographical regions. Journal of General Virology 73: 1365–1377
Ross B C, Anderson B N, Edwards P C, Gust I D 1989 Nucleotide sequence of high-passage hepatitis A virus strain HM175: comparison with wild-type and cell culture-adapted strains. Journal of General Virology 70: 2805–2810
Ross B C, Anderson D A, Gust I D 1991 Hepatitis A virus and hepatitis A infection. Advances in Virus Research 39: 209–253
Ruchti F, Siegl G, Weitz M 1991 Identification and characterization of incomplete Hepatitis-A virus particles. Journal of General Virology 72: 2159–2166
Rueckert R R, Wimmer E 1984 Systematic nomenclature of picornavirus proteins. Journal of Virology 50: 957–959
Ryan M D, King A M Q, Thomas G P 1991 Cleavage of foot-and-mouth disease virus polyprotein is mediated by residues located within a 19 amino acid sequence. Journal of General Virology 72: 2727–2732
Siegl G 1984 Structure and biology of hepatitis A virus. In: Gerety R J (ed), Hepatitis A. Academic Press, New York, pp 9–32
Siegl G, Eggers H J 1982 Failure of guanidine and 2-(alpha-hydroxybenzyl)benzimidazole to inhibit replication of hepatitis A virus in vitro. Journal of General Virology 61: 111–114
Siegl G, Frosner G G 1978a Characterization and classification of virus particles associated with hepatitis A. I. Size, density, and sedimentation. Journal of Virology 26: 40–47
Siegl G, Frosner G G 1978b Characterization and classification of virus particles associated with hepatitis A. II. Type and configuration of nucleic acid. Journal of Virology 26: 48–53
Siegl G, Frosner G G, Gauss-Muller V, Tratschin J D, Deinhardt F 1981 The physicochemical properties of infectious hepatitis A virions. Journal of General Virology 57: 331–341
Siegl G, Lemon S M 1990 Recent advances in hepatitis A vaccine development. Virus Research 17: 75–92
Siegl G, Weitz M, Kronauer G 1984a Stability of hepatitis A virus. Intervirology 22: 218–226
Siegl G, de Chastonay J, Kronauer G 1984b Propagation and assay of hepatitis A virus in vitro. Journal of Virological Methods 9: 53–67
Siegl G, Nuesch J P F, de Chastonay J 1990 Dl-particles of hepatitis A virus in cell cultures and clinical specimens. In: Brinton M A, Heinz F X (eds) New aspects of positive-strand RNA viruses. American Society for Microbiology, Washington, pp 102–107
Siegl G, Nuesch J P F, Weitz M 1991 Replication and protein processing of hepatitis A virus. In: Hollinger F B, Lemon S M, Margolis H S (eds) Viral hepatitis and liver disease. Williams & Wilkins, Baltimore, pp 25–30
Tesar M, Harmon S A, Summers D F, Ehrenfeld E 1992 Hepatitis A virus polyprotein synthesis initiates from two alternative AUG codons. Virology 186: 609–618
Ticehurst J R 1986 Hepatitis A virus: clones, cultures, and vaccines. Seminars in Liver Disease 6: 46–55
Ticehurst J R, Racaniello V R, Baroudy B M, Baltimore D,

Purcell R H, Feinstone S M 1983 Molecular cloning and characterization of hepatitis A virus cDNA. Proceedings of the National Academy of Science USA 80: 5885–5889
Tratschin J D, Siegl G, Frosner G G, Deinhardt F 1981 Characterization and classification of virus particles associated with hepatitis A. III. Structural proteins. Journal of Virology 38: 151–156
Tsarev S A, Emerson S U, Balayan M S, Ticehurst J, Purcell R H 1991 Simian hepatitis A virus (HAV) strain AGM-27 – comparison of genome structure and growth in cell culture with other HAV strains. Journal of General Virology 72: 1677–1683
Vallbracht A, Hofmann L, Wurster K G, Flehmig B 1984 Persistent infection of human fibroblasts by hepatitis A virus. Journal of General Virology 65: 609–615
Venuti A, Di Russo C, del Grosso N et al 1985 Isolation and molecular cloning of a fast-growing strain of human hepatitis A virus from its double-stranded replicative form. Journal of Virology 56: 579–588
Weitz M, Siegl G 1985 Variation among hepatitis A virus strains. I. Genomic variation detected by T1 oligonucleotide mapping. Virus Research 4: 53–67
Weitz M, Baroudy B M, Maloy W L, Ticehurst J R, Purcell R H 1986 Detection of a genome-linked protein (VPg) of hepatitis A virus and its comparison with other picornaviral VPgs. Journal of Virology 60: 124–130
Weitz M, Finkel-Jimenez B, Siegl G 1991 Empty hepatitis A virus particles in vaccines. In: Hollinger F B, Lemon S M, Margolis H S (eds) Viral Hepatitis and Liver Disease. Williams & Wilkins, Baltimore, pp 104–108
Wheeler C M, Robertson B H, Van Nest G, Dina D, Bradley D W, Fields HA 1986 Structure of the hepatitis A virion: peptide mapping of the capsid region. Journal of Virology 58: 307–313
Widell A, Hansson B G, Oberg B, Nordenfelt E 1986 Influence of twenty potentially antiviral subtances on in vitro multiplication of hepatitis A virus. AntivirRes 6: 103–112
Widell A, Hansson B G, Nordenfelt E, Oberg B 1988 Enhancement of hepatitis A propagation in tissue culture with 5, 6-dichloro-1-beta-D-ribofuranosylbenzimidazole. Journal of Medical Virology 24: 369–376
Winokur P L, Mclinden J H, Stapleton J T 1991 The hepatitis-A virus polyprotein expressed by a recombinant vaccinia virus undergoes proteolytic processing and assembly into viruslike particles. Journal of Virology 65: 5029–5036

UPDATE

- Evidence for the myristoylation of the putative structural protein VP4 has been sought by mutational analysis. It was observed that neither myristoylation occurred nor that cleavage of a proposed leader peptide (amino acids 1–5 of VP4), which is required to functionally expose the acceptor site **GXXXT**, was essential for production of progeny virus (Tesar et al 1993). Borovec & Anderson (1993) have extended their work on HAV morphogenesis and polyprotein processing. The authors observed a lag period between synthesis of polyprotein and virus assembly, despite the presence of increased amounts of virus RNA. It was concluded that polyprotein processing is protracted but not rate limiting in early infection. Furthermore, the proposed HAV IRES in the 5'-UTR of virus RNA has been experimentally characterized as the site of ribosome entry (Glass et al 1993).
- REFERENCES

Borovec S V, Anderson D A 1993 Synthesis and assembly of hepatitis A virus specific proteins in BS-C1 cells. Journal of Virology 76: 3095–3102
Glass M J, Jia X Y, Summers D F 1993 Identification of the hepatitis A virus internal ribosome entry site: in vivo and in vitro analysis of bicistronic RNAs containing the HAV 5' noncoding region. Virology 193: 842–852
Tesar M, Jia X Y, Summers D F, Ehrenfeld E 1993 Analysis of a potential myristoylation site in hepatitis A virus capsid protein VP4. Virology 194: 616–626

3. Natural history and experimental models

R. Zachoval F. Deinhardt

Although hepatitis was known very early as an infectious disease (Zuckerman 1979), the observations leading to our current knowledge of human hepatitis began with studies of hepatitis outbreaks during the First World War, and the demonstration later by transmission studies with bacteria-free filtrates that the disease was caused by a virus. Human volunteer studies distinguished between a faecal–orally transmitted, short-incubation, epidemic (but also sporadic) hepatitis (hepatitis A) and a parenterally transmitted, long-incubation hepatitis (hepatitis B), and indicated the existence of further forms of hepatitis (non-A, non-B). Disease led to homologous immunity, with no cross-immunity between hepatitis A and B (Krugman et al 1962, 1967, 1979). Transmission of hepatitis A virus (HAV) to some non-human primate species led to the morphological, immunological and physicochemical characterization of the agent and its propagation in cell culture.

The molecular biology of HAV, viral diagnosis and prevention through immunization are discussed elsewhere in this book; this chapter discusses the epidemiology, clinical disease, including pathogenesis and pathology, and animal models of hepatitis A.

EPIDEMIOLOGY OF HEPATITIS A

The precise characterization of the epidemiology of hepatitis A began once specific laboratory assays for detecting antibodies (anti-HAV) and antigen (HAAg) of HAV were developed, thus allowing the human viral hepatitides to be distinguished from one another, at least in part, on the basis of viral markers. Before this time, even though cases were often grouped into infectious or serum hepatitis, epidemiological data could include not only the forms of hepatitis known today as hepatitis E (mostly grouped together with infectious hepatitis) and hepatitis C (in the group of serum hepatitis), but also hepatitides associated with agents other than hepatitis viruses.

The detection of HAV by electron microscopy in the faeces of hepatitis patients (Feinstone et al 1973) led to development of complement fixation, immune adherence agglutination tests (Hilleman et al 1975) and ultimately to radioimmunoassays (Hollinger et al 1975, Purcell et al 1976); today, hepatitis A is diagnosed by testing sera or plasma for specific IgM anti-HAV and total specific anti-HAV (IgG and IgM). Hepatitis A patients are usually anti-HAV IgM-positive by the onset of symptoms, and remain positive for 3–6 months (Roggendorf et al 1980); IgG anti-HAV antibody persists for many years, and indicates previous infection with HAV. It follows that epidemiological data gathered on the basis of assays for anti-HAV IgM and/or IgG are more reliable estimates of the prevalence of HAV infection, both at present and in the past, than data accumulated previously and not assayed retrospectively. For this reason, most of the epidemiological data discussed in this chapter is recent in origin, and is drawn from specific antibody surveys.

The natural history or biological characteristics of HAV determines the nature of its epidemiology: briefly, the significant characteristics are:

1. HAV is present in the faeces of acutely infected patients, and is transmitted by the faecal–oral route,
2. A reservoir of natural infection is unknown (but see below, Animal models),

3. Viraemia with persistent infection does not occur, and
4. HAV is a stable virus, maintaining its infectivity even under unfavourable environmental conditions.

Consequently, infection spreads from person to person, by serial transmission from acute cases to susceptible contacts, or through faecally contaminated food or water, leading to endemicity with widespread infection at an early age or outbreaks (to epidemic proportions) when susceptible adults are exposed to the virus.

By and large, surveys of hepatitis A infections cannot be regarded as precise, because in addition to the failure to evaluate all cases by specific HAV assays, under-reporting of overt clinical cases (i.e. acute disease) is common, and many infections are subclinical and would be detected only by specific laboratory tests. It may be that under-reporting is less important for an accurate estimate of the incidence of hepatitis A than for other forms of viral hepatitis (Alter et al 1987) but the non-A, non-B hepatitis category certainly contains non-diagnosed cases of hepatitis A. Data must, therefore, be interpreted with caution, and the influence of such factors as the introduction of new diagnostic assays or government regulations requiring notification of particular infectious diseases must be considered. In addition, extrapolation from data originating from surveys of small numbers of individuals belonging to groups such as prisoners or medical students in order to estimate national prevalence rates would be widely inaccurate. Nevertheless, the requirement by public health authorities, particularly in industrialized countries, to register hepatitis has provided data accumulating over decades (Sweden, for example, introduced notification requirements in 1928), and these data allow some identification and characterization of disease trends.

Global distribution and prevalence

HAV has a worldwide distribution. The first survey of 1297 subjects in countries from Europe, Africa, Asia, USA and the Middle East (Szmuness et al 1977) reported age-standardized anti-HAV prevalences ranging from 28.7% (Switzerland) to 96.9% (Yugoslavia), calculated mostly from data obtained in randomly selected, volunteer blood donors; the study indicated that, although HAV infections were widespread, distribution was uneven, and on a population-wide basis probably reflected determinants such as socioeconomic conditions and geographic factors. Many seroprevalence surveys of adults conducted in subsequent years complemented this pilot survey (Papaevangelou 1984), and wide differences in anti-HAV prevalence were reported in different areas of the world (Dienstag et al 1978).

Although, in general, prevalence and incidence are not significantly different between males and females, the age-specific prevalence varies widely in different countries. Here, too, comparison of different studies is difficult, and many studies are not representative, but prevalences in different age groups show marked differences. In countries with very low endemicity, the disease occurs almost exclusively in adults, and most cases occur in two groups, drug users and those returning from travel abroad to countries with high endemicities. At least five different patterns of age-specific seroprevalence have been described, although these patterns are neither absolute nor constant, and intermediate patterns and change with time occur (Hadler 1991): the patterns are very high anti-HAV seroprevalence, seen in countries such as Ethiopia, with over 90% of children infected by 5 years of age; the high pattern typified by the Amazonian region of Brazil with lower prevalence in 5-year-old children but 90% infected by the age of 10 years; an intermediate pattern in which 90% prevalence is reached in early adulthood; a low prevalence pattern, such as is seen in the USA, with prevalence at about 15% by 15 years of age and a gradual rise to over 75% by 50 years of age; and a very low pattern, seen for example in highly developed countries like Sweden, where seroprevalence increases only in later adulthood (Fig. 3.1). Such patterns can show great variation within countries; for example, in China a high seroprevalence pattern is seen north of the Yan-tse River, whereas in the south (Shanghai) seroprevalence in children and young adults is much lower and 50% prevalence is reached only after 30 years of age (Xu et al 1991).

Heterogeneity of prevalence rates and risk of infection is seen not only in different age groups

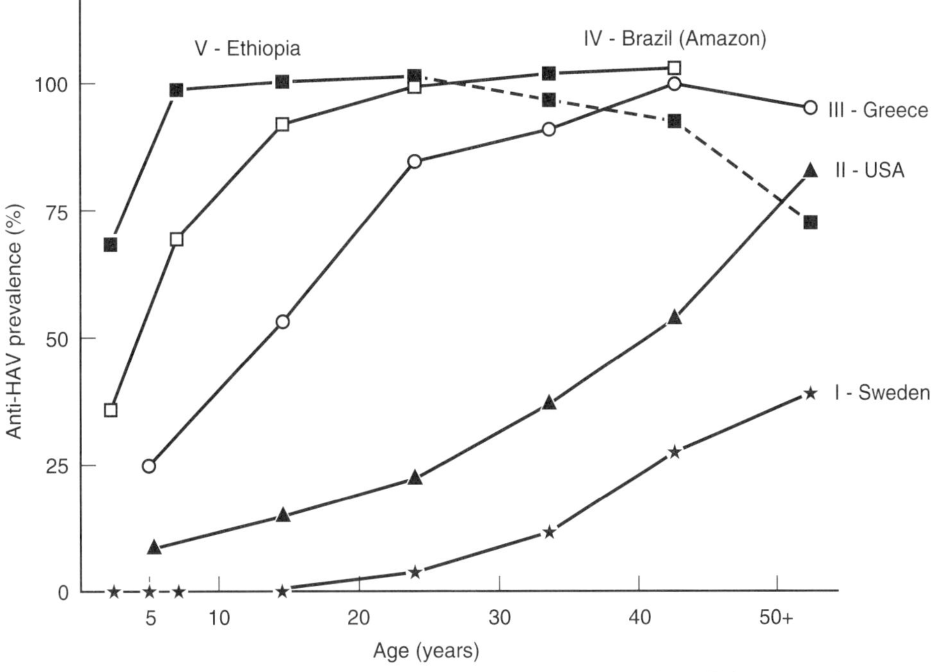

Fig. 3.1 Patterns of seroprevalence. V, very high; IV, high; III, intermediate; II, low; I, very low. (Reproduced with permission from Hadler 1991.)

but also within different population subgroups. This heterogeneity has been linked to ethnic origins, for example in Israeli military recruits prevalence is considerably higher in those of Eastern (mainly Middle East and North Africa) origin than in those of Western (European) origin (Kark & Bar-Shani 1980).

Magnitude of worldwide HAV infections

Estimating the global burden of HAV infections is difficult. Although many countries require the notification of hepatitis, frequently today subclassified into hepatitis A, B, non-A, non-B and unspecified, the numbers reported cannot be regarded as accurate. Subclinical cases, disinterest or inadequacies of local and national authorities, resistance by some population groups and administrative difficulties in developing countries all contribute to distortion of the true incidence of disease. Even so, the morbidity associated with HAV infection and disease is immense, causing a large loss of economic output in developed countries. Some idea may be obtained from nationwide data compiled by the Centers for Disease Control, US Public Health Service. With the exception of gonorrhoeal and syphilitic diseases, in 1990 viral hepatitis was the second most frequently reported infectious disease in the USA: in 1981, a total of 57 929 cases (25.3/100 000 population) was reported, of which 45% was categorized as hepatitis A (Gerety 1984), and in 1990 a total of 56 767 cases was reported (22.8/100 000 population), of which 31 441 (55%) (12.64/100 000 population) were cases of hepatitis A (Morbidity and Mortality Weekly Report 1991). With some fluctuation, figures for the whole decade were similar. These figures are likely to be representative of developed countries, but morbidity reflects the very different patterns of disease (see above) in countries at different levels of socioeconomic development, and loss of man–hours is considerably less in populations with almost universal infection in the childhood years.

Changes in seroprevalence and incidence

It is generally assumed that the level of seroprevalence is linked to socioeconomic conditions, since countries with crowded living conditions and the poorest sanitation and hygiene standards have the highest rates of HAV infection. With improvement of hygienic conditions (particularly by preventing faecal–oral transmission through better sanitation and control of food handling and water supplies), marked and rapid changes in HAV prevalence have been observed, and in countries with low or intermediate endemicity the risk of HAV infection has dropped considerably. An idea can be gathered of the pattern of hepatitis A infection in a large population (in 1990, 248 710 thousands) by examining data from the US Centers for Disease Control. The incidence of hepatitis A in the USA declined steadily after 1971 until 1984, when cases increased (Fig. 3.2), and this increase continued until 1989–90 (Morbidity and Mortality Weekly Report 1991). Increases in incidence were seen in all age groups, with the highest rates being observed in the 20–29 year age groups. Comparison of age-related anti-HAV prevalences in Europe and Australia first showed a decrease in disease prevalence in the younger age groups over a 10-year period (Frösner et al 1978, Gust et al 1978), and such shifts in seroprevalence have been seen in other parts of the world. In Japan, in random sera from healthy blood donors sampled in 1973 and 1984, the 25- to 34-year-old group had a statistically lower prevalence in 1984 (Taylor-Wiedeman et al 1987). A study in Finland, where epidemics of hepatitis A occurred in 1948 and 1954–57, showed a rapid decline from 24% to 0.3% positive over a 25-year period, and in 1980–82 only 3.2% of sera submitted for hepatitis A diagnosis were positive for IgM anti-HAV, and of these 68% were linked to travel abroad (Pohjanpelto & Lahdensivu 1984). Such shifts in the age-specific seroprevalence have important implications for controlling hepatitis A; a decrease in incidence in young children means that older children and young adults are susceptible, and vaccination strategies must be designed to protect this group by vaccination at an early age.

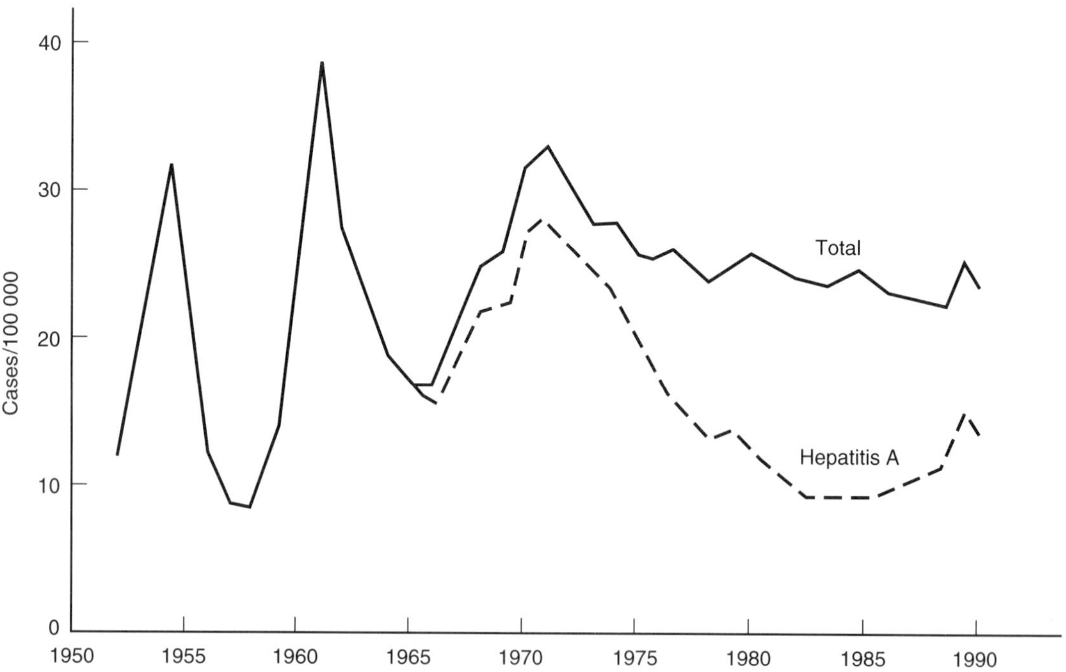

Fig. 3.2 Incidence of cases of viral hepatitis and hepatitis A in the USA from 1950 to 1990. (Data taken from Morbidity and Mortality Report 1991.)

Modes of transmission

Hepatitis A spreads primarily by faecal contamination. Virus is excreted in the faeces, mainly during the late incubation period and the first week of clinical illness, but viral shedding in faeces can recur during occasional relapses of acute hepatitis A (Sjögren et al 1987), and faeces may contain more than 10^8 infectious particles per ml (Purcell et al 1984). HAV in faeces remains viable for 30 days after drying and survives thermal, chlorine and formaldehyde treatment (Siegl 1984). Secondary in importance epidemiologically, the period of viraemia is short (7–10 days) (Krugman et al 1959), and viral particles are present in blood in relatively low concentrations (Hollinger et al 1975). Infective virus may be present in saliva: Cohen et al (1989) demonstrated virus in saliva and throat swabs 18 days after oral inoculation of a chimpanzee.

Person-to-person contact

Experimental oral transmission of HAV has shown that humans can be infected by this route (Krugman et al 1962), and the outbreaks of hepatitis A among people in close contact result from faecal (i.e. viral) contamination, directly through such routes as faeces–hand–mouth or indirectly through food or water contamination, and such spread of infection accounts for most cases of hepatitis A.

Intrafamilial and household spread of hepatitis A is well documented. Among household-associated susceptible contacts in a prospective study in Costa Rica, the infection rate was 70–83% with a final anti-HAV prevalence of 90–95% (Villarejos et al 1982). In recent years, anti-HAV prevalence has been falling in some population groups, and attack rates in parents (28%) and siblings (22%) of child index cases have been reported (Roumeliotou et al 1992).

Outbreaks of disease have been reported frequently in day care centres (Hadler & McFarland 1986), in institutions for the mentally handicapped (Mutton & Gust 1984), and occasionally in hospitals (Skidmore et al 1985), all of which share the same risk factors, i.e. the opportunity for faecal contamination and the difficulty of maintaining adequate standards of hygiene.

Food-borne and water-borne transmission

Most frequently associated with food-borne outbreaks and epidemics of hepatitis A are infection in a food handler with subsequent contamination during food preparation, and contamination of food (frequently shellfish) before its preparation. A wide variety of foods and drinks have been implicated in spread by food handlers, and in most cases uncooked or cooked and cooled food is involved (Mutton & Gust 1984). Outbreaks of disease are usually small, and easily contained.

Many outbreaks have been linked to contaminated bivalve molluscs, all of which are filter feeders, and process large volumes of seawater to obtain food and oxygen, during which HAV present in sewage-polluted water is concentrated. Bivalves tend to be harvested from shallow waters adjacent to highly populated areas where sewage contamination is more likely, and they are frequently eaten raw or undercooked, so that HAV is not inactivated. A recent, striking example of the potential dimensions of hepatitis A outbreaks linked to contaminated shellfish is that seen in Shanghai (Hu et al 1990). An outbreak of 20 000 cases of diarrhoea from December 1987 to early January 1988 indicated that hairy clams were likely to be contaminated, and their sale was banned. By the middle of January, cases of hepatitis A increased to a total of 292 301 (Fig. 3.3). The outbreak was shown not to be water-borne, epidemiological studies implicated hairy clam consumption as the cause, and HAV and HAV RNA were recovered from hairy clams.

The extent of water-borne transmission of HAV varies in different parts of the world. In developed countries, where contamination of drinking and recreational water with human faeces is infrequent, the risk is low, and even though the number of susceptibles in the population can lead to high attack rates (Bowen & McCarthy 1983) attack rates can be low and not statistically significant (Rosenberg et al 1980). In developing countries, water-borne transmission probably leads to the widespread infection at an early age and endemicity.

Extremely sensitive methods for monitoring HAV in shellfish and the waters in which they grow, in drinking and in recreational waters are in development (Metcalf & Jiang 1988, Papaevangelou et al 1991, Shieh et al 1991), and these will enable

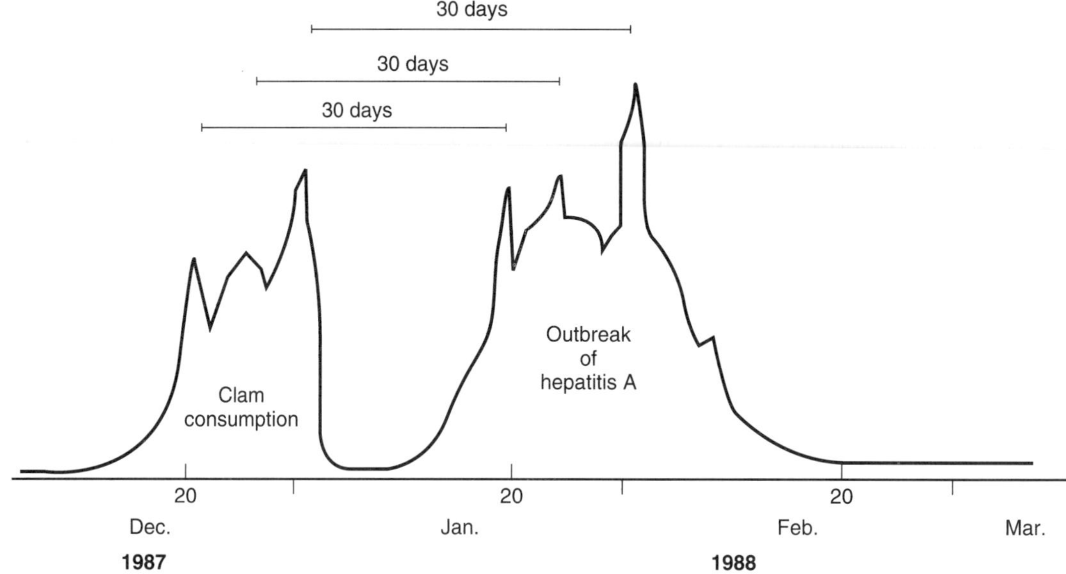

Fig. 3.3 Consumption of clams and outbreak of hepatitis A (HA) in Shanghai. (Reproduced with permission from Hu et al 1990.)

detection of contaminating HAV and the institution of public health measures to bring the danger of hepatitis A outbreaks under control.

CLINICAL FEATURES OF HEPATITIS A

The aetiological diagnosis of viral hepatitis is based on specific serological tests, and cannot be made on epidemiological or clinical grounds. Although different hepatitis viruses tend to induce discernible clinical features, when large patient groups are analysed there is considerable overlap in signs and symptoms.

Prodromal phase

The most useful definition of the incubation period in viral hepatitis is the time between infection and the appearance of dark urine, which is usually the first sign of hepatitis noticed by the patient. Based on experimental infections (Krugman et al 1959) and epidemiological observations in common source outbreaks (Routenberg et al 1979), the average incubation period in hepatitis A is about 4 weeks (2–7 weeks), independent of the route of infection (Krugman & Giles 1970). Variations in the incubation period may be related to the infectious dose (Purcell et al 1984), to differences in strain virulence or to host factors. Based on a large body of epidemiological data, there is convincing evidence that type A hepatitis is frequently a subclinical or unrecognized illness (Szmuness et al 1976), especially in children and young adults (Krugman et al 1959, Skinhoj & McNair 1972, Hadler 1991, Yao 1991). Patients developing symptomatic disease usually experience a prodromal period lasting several days, characterized in most cases by malaise, anorexia and fever. Nausea, vomiting, 'flu-like' complaints (headache, arthralgia, myalgia, upper respiratory tract symptoms), abdominal pain or discomfort and tenderness in the right upper quadrant, and diarrhoea or obstipation are common symptoms. Transient exanthematous skin eruptions have also been noted.

Acute disease

Clinical spectrum

Infection with HAV may result in a wide spectrum of clinical outcomes, ranging from silent anicteric infection only detectable by serological testing, through subclinical disease with biochemical abnormalities of liver function tests and classical icteric hepatitis, to fulminant hepatic failure with coma. The factors responsible for the different disease patterns are not fully understood, but the most important one seems to be age. Clinically, overt hepatitis A is more frequent with increasing age in almost all published reports (Skinhoj & McNair 1972, Benenson et al 1980, Hadler et al 1980, Villarejos 1982, Gingrich et al 1983, Friedman et al 1985, Lednar et al 1985, Hadler & McFarland 1986). Less than 5% of children below 3 years of age and 10% of children from 4 to 6 years old, but more than 80% of adults, develop icteric clinical illness. In contrast to these and numerous other reports, one recent Chinese study reported many serologically confirmed, acute HAV infections without symptoms or biochemical abnormalities in adults (Yang et al 1988); the reason for this difference is unclear.

Major symptoms

The first objective sign of hepatitis is the appearance of dark urine; this heralds an icteric phase, followed by acholic faeces and icterus of the sclera, skin and mucous membranes. In addition, 'flu-like' symptoms (fever, malaise, vomiting, headache) or right upper quadrant pain may outlast the prodromal phase and still prevail early in the course of illness. The incidence of major symptoms observed in an outbreak of hepatitis A by the Centers for Disease Control is given in Table 3.1.

Diarrhoea and vomiting seem to be more typical in children (Stewart et al 1978, Lemon 1985). Coloured faeces usually reappear after 2 or 3 weeks and are a reliable marker of clinical improvement. Many patients complain of itching, which sometimes requires symptomatic treatment but usually is tolerable and self-limiting. On physical examination, the liver may be enlarged and tender and the spleen palpable in a minority of patients (5–15%). Transient skin stigmata of liver disease such as spider naevi and signs of portal hypertension such as ascites develop rarely and are not bad prognostic markers.

The duration of illness is generally brief; clinical and biochemical indices of hepatitis A resolve fairly rapidly over several weeks (Krugman et al 1962). Malaise may sometimes persist for several months ('post-hepatitis syndrome').

Extrahepatic manifestations

Extrahepatic features of acute hepatitis A are rare. Transient arthralgias and skin rashes (erythematous, maculopapular, measles-like, petechial or urticarial) (Routenberg et al 1979, Bamber et al 1983), and single patients with arthritis and vasculitis (Inman et al 1986) have been reported. Neurological complications such as polyradiculopathy (Johnston et al 1981) and meningoencephalitis (Bromberg et al 1982, Hammond et al 1982) have also been described. Cardiac involvement indicated by ECG alterations (bradycardia, prolongation of the P–R interval, T-wave depression) usually resolves rapidly during convalescence (Hoaglund & Shank 1946). A severe haematological complication of acute hepatitis A is the development of aplastic anaemia in some patients (Le Moine Parker 1971, Hagler et al 1975).

Interestingly, in addition to the known echographic signs of all forms of viral hepatitis (liver

Table 3.1 Percentage of patients (n = 415) with hepatitis A presenting with symptoms (Gust & Feinstone 1988)

Symptom	Per cent	Symptom	Per cent
Dark urine	94	Drowsiness	49
Fatigue, anorexia	90	Irritability	43
Nausea	87	Itching	42
Weakness	77	Constipation	29
Fever	75	Diarrhoea	25
Vomiting	71	Arthralgia	21
Headache	70	Sore throat	20
Abdominal discomfort	65	Running nose	14
Paler faeces	52	Cough	7
Myalgia	52		

enlargement, thickening of the gall bladder wall, periportal hyperechogenicity), lymph node enlargement located near the hepatic hilum, pancreas and small omentum has been described as a unique ultrasonographic feature of acute hepatitis A in children (Toppet et al 1990).

Laboratory tests

Laboratory findings in acute hepatitis A are indistinguishable from those observed in other forms of viral hepatitis. Serum aminotransferases (also known as transaminases, e.g. alanine aminotransferase, ALT, and aspartate aminotransferase, AST), sensitive indicators of liver cell damage, rise rapidly during the incubation period, reaching peak levels (500–2000 U/l) within 1 week after the beginning of symptoms, and drop after the onset of jaundice. Owing to the altered permeability of the plasma membrane, ALT located in the cytosol is usually higher than AST, which resides in the mitochondria. High levels of AST indicate severe tissue necrosis. As acute illness subsides, transaminase levels return to normal (but occasionally may remain elevated for several weeks or months; see below). Generally, bilirubin reaches peak levels of 170–200 μmol/l after the maxima of transaminases, whereas the excretion enzymes alkaline phosphatase and γ-glutamyltranspeptidase are only slightly elevated during the course of acute hepatitis A. Non-specific elevation of IgM, IgG and smooth muscle antibodies may be noted, with IgM being mainly polyclonal; only a small fraction of IgM is directed against HAAg.

Minor coagulation defects and depressed fibrinogen levels without bleeding complications may occur. Severe depression of clotting factors is one of the hallmarks of fulminant hepatitis, and is not observed during uncomplicated acute hepatitis A. Mild lymphocytosis with atypical mononuclear cells, which is present early during the illness, subsides with disease evolution, and during recovery mild pancytopenia is not uncommon.

Outcome of disease

Uncomplicated course

Reports on the duration of acute hepatitis A are biased by the fact that most published studies deal with hospitalized patients, and this probably leads to overestimation of the duration and severity of acute, uncomplicated hepatitis A. By week 3 or 4, in most patients the transaminases are normal or close to normal, and symptoms have disappeared. Fatigability and depression, however, can persist longer.

Cholestatic form

Acute hepatitis A with prolonged cholestasis is a syndrome characterized by pruritus, fever, diarrhoea and weight loss, with bilirubin levels greater than 170 μmol/l and a clinical course of at least 12 weeks (Gordon et al 1984). In the few patients who have been biopsied, liver histology shows marked centrilobular cholestasis and portal inflammation (Gordon et al 1984, Sciot et al 1986a). Cholestatic hepatitis A is an unusual form of HAV infection with good prognosis and complete recovery. Cholestatic features have also been described during relapsing acute hepatitis A (Jacobson et al 1985, Tanno et al 1988).

Prolonged acute hepatitis A, relapse and chronicity

Although type A hepatitis is usually a benign disease of short duration (Krugman et al 1962, Norkrans 1978), prolonged elevation of liver function tests has been documented. Of 32 college students involved in a water-borne outbreak at Holy Cross College, six still had slightly elevated transaminases 5 months after acute illness and two even 9 months later (Wacker et al 1972, Dienstag 1979). In addition, of 130 recruits affected by a food-borne outbreak of hepatitis A, half showed complete biochemical recovery within 3.5 weeks, whereas 10 recruits had persistently elevated liver function tests after 14 weeks. Percutaneous liver biopsies showed slowly resolving hepatitis or chronic hepatitis, but resolution was complete 5–12 months after the outbreak (Dienstag 1979). Similar observations in six patients with elevated transaminases up to 15 months were made by Meier et al (1982). Lesnicar (1988) observed prolonged biochemical abnormalities up to 12 months in 73 of 451 patients with acute hepatitis A. Concomitantly with the protracted clinical and biochemical course of disease, the acute serological response to HAV (anti-HAV IgM) seems to last longer in these cases in man (Cornu et al 1984, Kao et al 1984, McDonald et al 1989) and in experimentally infected tamarins (Karayiannis et al 1990).

Hepatitis A may recur within a few weeks of apparent recovery, even after complete normalization of liver function tests; this second bout of disease may be icteric or anicteric, symptomatic or asymptomatic (Weir et al 1981, Gruer et al 1982, Bamber et al 1983, Jacobson et al 1985, Cobden & James 1986, Lesnicar 1988, Tanno et al 1988). In three cases, even a second relapse of acute hepatitis A has been described (Raimondo et al 1986). Sjögren and colleagues (1987) showed that during relapse of acute hepatitis A reactivation of viral shedding in the faeces could occur. Although tests for antibodies to hepatitis C virus (anti-HCV) were not available then, there is no doubt that true relapse in hepatitis A can occur; however, all data indicate that, although hepatitis A can be prolonged and may even show transient histological signs resembling chronic hepatitis A, there is no documented case of unresolved chronic hepatitis A or cirrhosis attributable to HAV.

Fulminant hepatitis

Fulminant hepatitis is a rare complication of HAV infection (Rakela et al 1978, Mathiesen et al 1980a, Yao 1991). The case fatality rate in a large study of more than 2000 hospitalized patients was < 0.2% (McNeill et al 1984). Mortality seems to correlate with age (Saunders et al 1979). Clinically and biochemically, fulminant hepatitis A is characterized by increasingly severe jaundice, deterioration in liver function (especially severely impaired synthesis of clotting factors) and eventual encephalopathy and coma. The treatment of choice when prognostic scores indicate a fatal outcome is liver transplantation. Viral persistence in two patients with fulminant hepatitis A treated by orthoptic liver transplantation as a peculiar course of HAV infection under immunosuppressive treatment has recently been described (Fagan et al 1990). In those patients who survive hepatic coma caused by acute hepatitis A without liver transplantation, there is no evidence of fibrosis or cirrhosis.

Clinical management and therapy

Isolation of patients with acute hepatitis A is unnecessary unless there is faecal incontinence or hygienic measures cannot be adequately implemented. For practical purposes, patients' faeces are unlikely to be infectious beyond 2 or 3 weeks after onset of icterus. Treatment is mainly symptomatic and supportive, with value claimed for bed rest during the acute phase but not proven by controlled trials; the same is true for nutritional intravenous supplementation and fluid replacement which may, however, be recommendable in older patients when nausea and vomiting are severe. Antiemetics, like other drugs, should be given cautiously at low dose. Cholestyramine may be tried in patients with protracted cholestatic hepatitis A in order to relieve pruritus; steroids given to reduce cholestasis were detrimental in a small controlled trial (Gregory et al 1976). In those rare cases where HAV infection runs a fulminant course, preference should be given to evaluation for liver transplantation (O'Grady et al 1989). Interferon in fulminant hepatitis A has been tried in an uncontrolled study but with only limited success (Levin & Hahn 1982).

Special issues

Hepatitis A in pregnancy

Unlike infection with hepatitis E virus (HEV), acute hepatitis A is not associated with increased mortality in pregnant women. In a large food-borne outbreak of hepatitis A in Shanghai involving more than 300 000 cases including more than 5000 pregnant women, no increase in morbidity or mortality was observed during pregnancy (Hu et al 1990). Moreover, there is no evidence that HAV infection gives rise to chromosomal abnormalities or deformities. Although there are no reports of HAV transmission to the newborn, there is general agreement that newborns of mothers with acute hepatitis A in the early acute phase should not be breast fed.

Hepatitis A in pre-existing liver disease and in chronic carriers of hepatitis B virus

It is possible that the benign course of acute

hepatitis A is altered in patients with pre-existing severe chronic, parenchymal liver disease of viral or non-viral origin. Akriviadis & Redeker (1989) reported four cases of fulminant hepatic failure associated with hepatitis A in intravenous drug users with evidence of superimposed acute hepatitis in a cirrhotic or fibrotic liver at autopsy. 15 of 47 patients who died with acute hepatitis A during the 1988 Shanghai epidemic had underlying chronic active hepatitis B or hepatitis B virus (HBV)-related cirrhosis: all 15 were positive for HBV surface antigen (HBsAg) and 11/15 were HBV e antigen-positive (Yao 1991). In contrast, several reports from areas of low to intermediate HBV endemicity did not find increased disease severity when HBV chronic carriers contracted acute hepatitis A (Hindman et al 1977, Viola et al 1982, Zachoval et al 1983, Tassopoulos et al 1985). A decrease of the HBsAg titre or HBV DNA, probably due to interferon induction during acute hepatitis A, was noted in some cases.

Histopathology

Most of our knowledge of liver morphology in hepatitis A is derived from experimental infection of chimpanzees in which the early histological lesions are periportal liver cell necrosis sparing the perivenular area of the lobule (Dienstag et al 1976, Popper et al 1980a, b). In those rare instances where a liver biopsy was performed, these histological findings have been confirmed in man (Tanikawa 1979, Tanaka et al 1981, Abe et al 1982). In a larger study by Schmid & Regli (1985), in 34 patients who were biopsied during different stages of acute hepatitis A, portal infiltration by lymphocytes, plasma cells and PAS-positive macrophages was a prominent feature in early biopsies (within 10 days), but it was also present and even more marked in later biopsies when a prolonged course or relapse was observed.

The infiltration of the portal triads may spill over into the lobular parenchyma, thus mimicking piecemeal necrosis and chronic hepatitis (Teixeira et al 1982). Very severe periportal necrosis may lead to portoportal bridging. Another characteristic, light microscopic finding in hepatitis A is iron storage in Kupffer cells and clusters of macrophages, findings atypical in acute hepatitis B or hepatitis non-A, non-B (Schmid & Regli 1985). In addition, a variety of bile duct lesions (regressive changes and focal destruction) have been described. The changes in liver morphology usually resolve within 8–12 weeks, leaving the lobular architecture intact. There are no chronic changes. Although certain morphological trends are typical for acute hepatitis A, there is a large overlap of the histological changes with those of other forms of viral hepatitis so that, for diagnostic purposes, liver biopsy is neither indicated nor helpful.

Pathogenesis

The pathogenetic mechanism underlying hepatocellular injury in acute hepatitis A is poorly understood. The successful propagation in vitro of HAV in different cell lines (Frösner et al 1979, Provost & Hilleman 1979) was a prerequisite for designing experiments to evaluate the interactions of HAV and the host cell. With very rare exceptions, replicating HAV does not induce a cytopathic effect but leads to a persistent inapparent infection in vitro. As there is general agreement that HAV infection does not evolve to chronic liver disease in man, immune mechanisms have been suspected of playing a major role in eliminating virus-infected liver cells.

In an attempt to clarify the role of cell-mediated immunity in acute hepatitis A, Vallbracht and co-workers (1986) used peripheral blood lymphocytes (PBLs) of patients as effectors and autologous ^{51}Cr-labelled HAV-infected and uninfected skin fibroblasts as targets in a microcytotoxicity assay. Cytotoxic PBLs capable of lysing autologous HAV-infected fibroblasts were detected in all patients with hepatitis A but not in controls. During the course of the illness, cytolytic activity peaked 2–3 weeks after onset of icterus. The effector cells mediating this cytolytic activity were found to reside in the $CD8^+$, HLA class I-dependent T-cell subset and were able to produce interferon-γ (IFN-γ) (Maier et al 1988). Both functions (cytotoxicity and IFN-γ release) were virus specific. Even more important, after cloning human T lymphocytes from liver biopsies of hepatitis A patients, most T-cell clones obtained again belonged to the $CD8^+$ subset, and were HAV-specific, IFN-γ-producing, HLA class I-dependent, self-restricted cytotoxic T-cell clones (Vallbracht et al 1989, Fleischer et al 1990). It was concluded that IFN-γ, in addition to its antiviral effect, stimulates HLA class I expression on hepatocytes, thus enabling a more efficient cytotoxic T-cell response against virus-infected liver cells.

In one patient, from whom a biopsy was obtained later in the course of illness, in addition to $CD8^+$ clones $CD4^+$ T-cell clones were also generated in a substantial number. This observation is supported by the demonstration of $CD4^+$ cells in the portal tracts during acute hepatitis A by immunohistological staining (Govindarajan et al 1983, Sciot et al 1986b). The specificity and functional capacity of these $CD4^+$ cells remain to be determined. Taken together, the experimental data support the hypothesis that liver cell injury in acute HAV infection is mediated by HAV-specific cytotoxic T cells accumulating at the site of tissue injury in the liver and is not a viral cytopathic effect. However, humoral immune effector mechanisms, such as the induction of neutralizing anti-HAV antibodies as well as antiviral cytokines like IFN-α (Davis et al 1984, Zachoval et al 1986, 1990) or tumour necrosis factor (R Zachoval, unpublished observations), may also play an important role in the network of immunological interactions bringing HAV infection under control.

ANIMAL MODELS OF HEPATITIS A

Despite alternatives to the use of experimental animals that have become available in biomedical research recently, animal models remain essential for the study of hepatitis A. Experimentally infected animals are needed for studying the pathogenesis of hepatitis A; obtaining biopsy materials for such studies from patients suffering from natural infections would be unethical in most circumstances.

Animal models of disease are also needed for vaccine development. Although hepatitis A has a very low mortality and a generally benign outcome, the infection is responsible for considerable morbidity and subsequent economic loss. Inactivated whole-virus vaccines have undergone extensive safety and antigenicity studies in man, and are in clinical trials (Andre et al 1992, Werzberger et al 1992), and several candidate live, attenuated hepatitis A vaccines have been developed, at least two of which are in clinical evaluation (Mao et al 1989, Midthun et al 1991). Such vaccines must be assessed continually for safety, stability and efficacy, and this assessment can only be achieved in vivo in experimental animal model systems, at least until other measures of attenuation, perhaps on a molecular basis, become available.

Early searches for animal models

The search for animal models of hepatitis in general has a long history. Early attempts to transmit human hepatitis to laboratory animals and other species were largely unsuccessful (MacCallum 1951), and only the use of human volunteers led to the confirmation of the transmissible, infectious nature of hepatitis A (Voegt 1942) and the differentiation between hepatitis A and B and their causative viruses (Krugman et al 1967). The Willowbrook studies of Krugman, Ward and Giles in the 1950s were a watershed in the process of identifying and characterizing animal models for hepatitis A because the MS-1 materials containing HAV provided defined inocula for testing the susceptibility of experimental animals to human hepatitis A. Even so, it was only after laboratory tests for HAV antigen and antibodies made it possible to determine whether animals were preimmune that the search for animal models was placed on a scientific basis. The result is that only non-human primates, and of these only a few genera, are valuable as animal models for hepatitis A. Early transmission studies had already indicated this, and as these studies have been reviewed (Deinhardt & Deinhardt 1984), only the principal findings and recent studies will be discussed here.

Non-human primate experimental models of hepatitis A

Several lines of evidence indicated that non-human primates might be animal models for human hepatitis A: for example, association of non-human primates with outbreaks of hepatitis A, and identification of antibodies to HAV in surveys of non-human primate species.

In the early 1960s, infectious hepatitis was reported among personnel caring for newly imported chimpanzees, and the animals exhibited biochemical and histological abnormalities characteristic of human hepatitis (Hillis 1963). During subsequent years, many outbreaks of viral hepatitis were associated with close contact with non-human primates, mostly with recently imported chimpanzees (Deinhardt 1976). In general, outbreaks were clinically and epidemiologically typical of hepatitis A, with short incubation periods; later chimpanzee and human outbreaks were shown to be negative for hepatitis B antigens and antibodies.

These associations of non-human primates with cases of human hepatitis led to renewed efforts to transmit the disease to non-human primates. Several South American marmoset and tamarin species (Deinhardt et al 1975), chimpanzees (Dienstag et al 1975), lesser bushbabies (*Galago senegalensis*) (Grabow & Prozesky 1975), stump-tailed monkeys (*Macaca speciosa*) (Mao et al 1981) and owl monkeys (*Aotus trivirgatus*) (LeDuc et al 1983) were shown to be susceptible to HAV, and to a large extent studies in these primate species have replaced human volunteers.

Other non-human primate species are very likely to be susceptible to human hepatitis A; anti-HAV has been detected in several species, inside and outside captivity, although numbers examined in early studies were small (Deinhardt & Deinhardt 1984). More recently, larger surveys have been conducted: 24 of 106 cynomolgus monkeys were positive for anti-HAV (Burke & Heisey 1984); among 700 Old World monkeys of five different species, clinical disease, excretion of HAV in faeces, anti-HAV, HAV in the liver and abnormal liver enzymes were observed (Lapin & Shevtsova 1989); and abnormal aminotransferase levels were correlated with IgM anti-HAV and typical liver histology in immature rhesus monkeys (Lankas & Jensen 1987). The group of 106 wild cynomolgus monkeys studied by Burke & Heisey (1984) was particularly interesting because most animals weighing more than 2 kg (i.e. adults) were positive for anti-HAV, indicating that age-specific prevalence had reached 50% by that age. This age-specific prevalence of adult animals negative for IgM anti-HAV seen in animals trapped in virgin forest suggests that animals became infected months before capture and raises the possibility that a sylvatic cycle of HAV infection occurs in these animals, of either a virus identical to HAV or very closely related to it. Strains antigenically indistinguishable from human HAV have been isolated from several species believed to be naturally infected, and the question of whether these isolates are human or simian strains has been approached by comparing the genomes (see below).

Experimental infections in marmosets and tamarins

Several species of marmosets or tamarins (*Saquinus* spp.) are regularly susceptible to parenteral or oral infection with HAV, with *S. mystax*, *S. labiatus* (*rufiventer*) and *S. fuscicollis* the most susceptible. The disease is generally mild, with a course similar to hepatitis A in man. Incubation times range from about 14 to up to 50 days with a median between 17 and 28, HAV is excreted in the stool during the early acute phase of disease, and a chronic carrier state does not develop. HAV antigen has been detected in liver and faeces, and identified by immunofluorescence not only in hepatocytes but also in monocytes and Kupffer cells of the hepatic sinusoids and in the bile canaliculi (see Deinhardt & Deinhardt 1984).

Attempts to identify experimentally in marmosets the primary sites of HAV infection and replication, to determine secondary sites, and to establish the mode of hepatocyte destruction have been extensive but largely unsuccessful. However, hepatitis A antigen was detected in the liver of a marmoset (*Callithrix jacchus*) experimentally infected 2 weeks earlier, at a time when histology was still normal (Shibayama et al 1985). In another study with *S. labiatus* marmosets, HAV antigen appeared in stool at 6–7 days after intravenous inoculation and persisted to 20 days, with highest levels between days 11 and 17; HAV antigen was detected by immunofluorescence in liver at about the time of maximum ALT levels (by 4 weeks post inoculation), and in kidney, spleen and (most interestingly) duodenum (Karayiannis et al 1986). Attempts previously to demonstrate HAV antigen in the gastrointestinal tract of marmosets were negative (Mathiesen et al 1980b, Krawczynski et al 1981) but these animals were inoculated orally, and as the oral route must be supposed to be the natural means of infection the significance of detecting viral antigen in the gastrointestinal tract of intravenously inoculated animals must be questioned. A further interesting observation in these studies was that peak antibody titres and liver damage coincided, as also seen in man (Dienstag 1981), supporting the idea that liver damage is immune-mediated rather than caused by direct viral cytopathic interaction. Marmosets monitored for longer than 6 months exhibited a form of relapsing hepatitis with abnormal ALT levels and persistent IgM anti-HAV (Karayiannis et al 1990), a pattern observed in up to 25% of human patients. Although activation of a second, marmoset hepatitis virus could be responsible for these relapsing episodes, it seems more likely that an autoimmune response causes the liver pathology.

In summary, marmosets are useful experimental models of human hepatitis A; they provide model systems for studying hepatitis A pathogenesis, and their use allowed the first development of an experimental vaccine against hepatitis A (Provost & Hilleman 1978). Evaluation and monitoring of the efficacy of future hepatitis A vaccines in marmosets is certain to continue (Karayiannis et al 1991), as these animals are available in sufficient numbers from captive breeding colonies and their maintenance presents no great difficulties.

Experimental hepatitis A in chimpanzees

Despite the restrictions caused by the need for conservation, and the constraints imposed by maintenance of chimpanzees, this non-human primate model remains essential for hepatitis A research.

The course of experimental HAV infection in chimpanzees is similar to marmosets, and to natural infection in man (Deinhardt & Deinhardt 1984). Neither experimental infection nor natural infection with HAV (seen earlier quite frequently in chimpanzees) is usually associated with reliable clinical signs or symptoms, but seroconversion, excretion of HAV in faeces, elevation of serum enzyme levels and histological parameters (Dienstag et al 1975) and histopathological changes are typical although less pronounced than those in man (Popper et al 1980a). Chronic hepatitis does not develop.

Fulminant hepatitis associated with spontaneous HAV has been reported in a chimpanzee (Abe & Shikata 1982), and it was speculated that localization of immune complexes in hepatocytes led to necrosis. HAV antigen was shown to localize primarily in the liver cell cytoplasm obtained from an acutely infected chimpanzee (Khan et al 1984), and IgM immune complexes were detected in experimentally infected chimpanzees (Margolis et al 1988); use of such experimental models could resolve the role of immunopathogenetic mechanisms in hepatic damage.

A further example of the usefulness of chimpanzees as models for human hepatitis A is illustrated by studies to identify extrahepatic replication sites of HAV. Although man is relatively easily infected by the oral route, viral replication has not been shown to occur in the gastrointestinal tract, but HAV has been detected in saliva of patients (Purcell et al 1984), suggesting an oropharyngeal replication site. A chimpanzee orally inoculated with HAV was monitored every 2–4 days; HAV was present in blood from 14–28 days after infection, in pharyngeal swabs from 18–21 days, and antigen was detected in the tonsils on days 16 and 18 and liver on day 21 (Cohen et al 1989). Such a study in man would be difficult, but it was comparatively easy to obtain sequential samples and biopsies from a chimpanzee. Similarly, attenuated HAV was shown to protect chimpanzees from challenge with virulent HAV, indicating that attenuated vaccines against human hepatitis A were feasible (Provost et al 1983).

Chimpanzees are susceptible not only to HAV but also to HBV (progressing sometimes to chronic infection), HCV and HDV (Shimizu et al 1991) and HEV (Krawczynski 1991). This allows experimental analysis of the course of disease and interference in acute HAV infection in HBV carrier chimpanzees (a not infrequent combination in man), and simultaneous infection with two or more human hepatotrophic viruses. (Bradley et al 1983, 1987, Tsiquaye et al 1984).

Susceptibility of bushbabies to HAV

Lesser bushbabies (*Galago senegalensis moholi*) inoculated with HAV-positive materials responded with elevated serum transaminase levels, seroconversion and excretion of HAV antigen in faeces; these responses were not observed in all experimentally infected animals and, although the pattern of disease resembled that in man, marmosets and chimpanzees, in general lesser bushbabies seem to be less susceptible to HAV (Grabow et al 1981), and this coupled with their limited availability has impeded wider use of bushbabies as experimental models.

Experimental transmission of HAV to stump-tailed monkeys

A stump-tailed monkey (*Macaca speciosa*) was infected with human HAV: clinical hepatitis was not observed but liver pathology, seroconversion, excretion of HAV antigen in the faeces and serum enzyme elevations were typical of human hepatitis A (Mao et al 1981). The infection was passaged with virus isolated from the stool of the primary animal to two more monkeys, and similar patterns of disease resulted.

These findings, together with the observations of naturally occurring antibodies to HAV in several other Old World non-human primates (see above), indicate that macaque monkeys could be useful experimental models for human hepatitis A. This is supported by the susceptibility of cynomolgus macaques to HEV, another enterically transmitted human hepatitis virus (Bradley et al 1988, Krawczynski 1991). As with the experimental models of different types of hepatitis in chimpanzees, this susceptibility to more than one human agent may offer the possibility of examining double infection in a single model.

Hepatitis A infection in owl monkeys

Owl monkeys (*Aotus trivirgatus*) are susceptible to experimental infection with HAV isolated from a naturally infected owl monkey, to HAV isolated from man (LeDuc et al 1983) and to an antigenic variant, neutralization-escape mutant of HAV (Lemon et al 1990). The course of experimental infection and histological changes (Keenan et al 1984) was similar to but milder than in man, and their size and availability make these non-human primates an attractive alternative to marmosets and chimpanzees.

Simian hepatitis A virus

Molecular studies of HAV shed new light on primate-associated cases of hepatitis and the nature of the hepatitis-like viruses isolated from non-human primates. Initially, it was assumed that primate-associated cases of human viral hepatitis had originated with an initial transmission from man to primate and subsequent transmission back to man. This assumption came about because primates after capture often had close contact to man in high endemic areas of hepatitis A, and animals were frequently inoculated with pooled human blood obtained locally to protect them from human disease. In addition, clusters of hepatitis in primate handlers were usually observed after introduction of new animals to existing groups. Without doubt, such a chain of HAV transmission from man to primate to man remains valid for some outbreaks, but from detailed genomic analyses of various human and non-human primate hepatitis A-like viruses it has become clear recently that some non-human primates are infected with simian hepatitis A-like viruses. Viruses with clear genomic heterogeneity from human strains have been isolated from owl monkeys, cynomolgus macaques and from African green monkeys.

Two viruses (PA 21 and PA 33) have been isolated from naturally infected, recently captured Panamanian owl monkeys (LeDuc et al 1983): although antigenically similar to human HAV (HM 175) by analysis with monoclonal antibodies, cross-protection and neutralization, PA 21 is substantially different at the genomic level, suggesting that this strain is native to owl monkeys (Lemon et al 1987, Brown et al 1989). However, this genotype has now been identified in human patients (Robertson et al 1991), and the precise nature of this agent is still unclear.

Isolates were also obtained from cynomolgus macaques, one directly from a case of spontaneous hepatitis A (CY-145) and the other (CY-55) from an animal inoculated with materials from an Indonesian macaque with hepatitis A (Andjaparidze et al 1985). Sequence analysis of both of these strains identified diversities between the macaque viruses but distinct antigenic and genetic divergence from human isolates (Nainan et al 1991).

A spontaneously infected African green monkey

was the source of yet another simian isolate (AGM-27); sequencing identified substantial differences from human and other simian strains, and differences in growth in cell culture (Tsarev et al 1991). The data suggest that AGM-27 is a genuine simian HAV strain, and certain similarities between CY-55 and AGM-27 may indicate that the African green and cynomolgus monkeys had been infected by the same simian virus.

Although considerable differences between the various isolates and human HAV have been found at the nucleotide level, there is little antigenic change and cross-neutralization between these isolates and human HAV can be expected, making the simian strains possible candidates for attenuated live vaccine strains in man. Cross-neutralization between the owl monkey strain PA 33 has been shown to induce partial protection to later challenge with human HAV (Lemon et al 1987), and two simian strains failed to induce hepatitis in chimpanzees (Purcell 1991), suggesting the possibility that the agents could be naturally attenuated for man.

REFERENCES

Abe H, Benninger P R, Ikejiri N, Setoyama H, Sata M, Tanikawa K 1982 Light microscopic findings of liver biopsy specimens from patients with hepatitis type A and comparison with type B. Gastroenterology 82: 938–947

Abe K, Shikata T 1982 Fulminant type A viral hepatitis in a chimpanzee. Acta Pathologica Japonica 32: 143–148

Akriviadis E A, Redeker A G 1989 Fulminant hepatitis A in intravenous drug users with chronic liver disease. Annals of Internal Medicine 110: 838–839

Alter M J, Mares A, Hadler S C, Maynard J E 1987 The effect of underreporting on the apparent incidence and epidemiology of acute viral hepatitis. American Journal of Epidemiology 125: 133–139

Andjaparidze A G, Poleshchuk V F, Zamyatina N A, Savinov A P, Gavriloskaya I N, Balayan M S 1985 Spontaneous hepatitis in *Macacus fascicularis* treated with immunosuppressing drugs. Voprosy Virusologii 4: 468–474

Andre F E, Hepburn A, Safary A, D'Hondt E 1992 Development of an inactivated vaccine against hepatitis A. In: Rhodes J, Arroyo V (eds) Therapy in liver diseases. Ediciones Doyma, Barcelona, pp 33–37

Bamber M, Thomas H C, Bannister B, Sherlock S 1983 Acute type A, B and non-A, non-B hepatitis in a hospital population in London: clinical and epidemiological features. Gut 24: 561–564

Benenson M W, Takafuji E T, Bancroft W H, Lemon S M, Callahan M C, Leach D A 1980 A military community outbreak of hepatitis type A related to transmission in a child care facility. American Journal of Epidemiology 112: 471–481

Bowen G S, McCarthy M A 1983 Hepatitis A associated with a hardware store water fountain and a contaminated well in Lancaster County, Pennsylvania, 1983. American Journal of Epidemiology 117: 695–705

Bradley D W, Maynard J E, McCaustland K A, Murphy B L, Cook E H, Ebert J W 1983 Non-A, non-B hepatitis in chimpanzees: interference with acute hepatitis A virus and chronic hepatitis B virus infections. Journal of Medical Virology 11: 207–213

Bradley D W, Krawczynski K, Humphrey C D, McCaustland K A 1987 Biochemically silent posttransfusion non-A, non-B hepatitis interferes with superinfection by hepatitis A virus. Intervirology 27: 86–90

Bradley D, Andjaparidze A, Cook E H Jr et al 1988 Aetiological agent of enterically transmitted non-A, non-B hepatitis. Journal of General Virology 69: 731–738

Bromberg K, Newhall D N, Peter G 1982 Hepatitis A and meningoencephalitis. Journal of the American Medical Association 247: 815

Brown E A, Jansen R W, Lemon S M 1989 Characterization of a simian hepatitis A virus (HAV): antigenic and genetic comparison with human HAV. Journal of Virology 63: 4932–4937

Burke D S, Heisey G B 1984 Wild Malaysian cynomolgus monkeys are exposed to hepatitis A virus. American Journal of Tropical Medicine and Hygiene 33: 940–944

Cobden I, James O F W 1986 A biphasic illness associated with acute hepatitis A virus infection. Journal of Hepatology 2: 19–23

Cohen J I, Feinstone S, Purcell R H 1989 Hepatitis A virus infection in a chimpanzee: duration of viremia and detection of virus in saliva and throat swabs. Journal of Infectious Diseases 160: 887–890

Cornu C, Lamy M E, Geubel A, Galanti L 1984 Persistence of immunoglobulin M antibody to hepatitis A virus and relapse of hepatitis A infection. European Journal of Clinical Microbiology 3: 45–46

Davis G L, Hoofnagle J H, Waggoner J G 1984 Acute hepatitis A during chronic HBV infection: association of depressed HBV replication with appearance of endogenous alpha interferon. Journal of Medical Virology 14: 141–147

Deinhardt F 1976 Hepatitis in primates. Advances in Virus Research 20: 113–157

Deinhardt F, Deinhardt J B 1984 Animal Models. In: Gerety R J (ed) Hepatitis A. Academic Press, London, pp 185–204

Deinhardt F, Peterson D, Cross G, Wolfe L, Holmes A W 1975 Hepatitis in marmosets. American Journal of Medical Sciences 270: 73–80

Dienstag J L 1979 The Pathobiology of hepatitis A virus. In: International Review of Experimental Pathology 20: 1–48

Dienstag J L 1981 Hepatitis A virus: virologic, clinical and epidemiologic studies. Human Pathology 12: 1097–1106

Dienstag J L, Feinstone S M, Purcell R H et al 1975 Experimental infection of chimpanzees with hepatitis A virus. Journal of Infectious Diseases 132: 532–545

Dienstag J L, Popper H, Purcell R H 1976 The pathology of

viral hepatitis type A and B in chimpanzees. American Journal of Pathology 85: 131–148

Dienstag J L, Szmuness W, Stevens C E, Purcell R H 1978 Hepatitis A virus infection: new insights from seroepidemiologic studies. Journal of Infectious Diseases 137: 328–340

Fagan E, Yousef G, Brahm J et al 1990 Persistence of hepatitis A virus in fulminant hepatitis and after liver transplantation. Journal of Medical Virology 30: 131–136

Feinstone S M, Kapikian A Z, Purcell R H 1973 Hepatitis A: detection by immune electron microscopy of a viruslike antigen associated with acute illness. Science 182: 1026–1028

Fleischer B, Fleischer S, Maier K, Wiedmann K H, Sacher M, Thaler H, Vallbracht A 1990 Clonal analysis of infiltrating T lymphocytes in liver tissue in viral hepatitis A. Immunology 69: 14–19

Friedman L S, O'Brien T F, Morse L J, Chang L W, Wacker W E C, Ryan D M, Dienstag J L 1985 Revisiting the Holy Cross Football team hepatitis outbreak (1969) by serological analysis. Journal of the American Medical Association 254: 774–776

Froesner G G, Willers H, Müller R et al 1978 Decrease in incidence of hepatitis A infections in Germany. Infection 6: 259–260

Froesner G G, Deinhardt F, Scheid R et al 1979 Propagation of human hepatitis A virus in a hepatoma cell line. Infection 7: 303–305

Gerety R J 1984 Introduction. In: Gerety R J (ed) Hepatitis A. Academic Press, London, pp 1–8

Gingrich G A, Hadler S C, Elder H A, Ash K O 1983 Serologic investigation of an outbreak of hepatitis A in a rural day-care center. American Journal of Public Health 73: 1190–1193

Gordon S C, Reddy K R, Schiff L, Schiff E R 1984 Prolonged intrahepatic cholestasis secondary to acute hepatitis A. Annals of Internal Medicine 101: 635–637

Govindarajan S, Uchida T, Peters R L 1983 Identification of T lymphocytes and subsets in liver biopsy cores of acute viral hepatitis. Liver 3: 13–18

Grabow W O K, Prozesky O W 1975 Lesser bushbabies (*Galago senegalensis*) may be susceptible to the CR 326 hepatitis A virus. South African Journal of Science 71: 310–311

Grabow W O K, Prozesky O W, Bradley D W, Maynard J E 1981 Response of *Galago* bushbabies to the hepatitis A virus. South African Journal of Science 77: 314–318

Gregory P B, Knauer C M, Kempson R L, Miller R 1976 Steroid therapy in severe viral hepatitis A: a double-blind, randomized trial of methyl-prednisolone versus placebo. New England Journal of Medicine 294: 681–687

Gruer L D, McKendrick M W, Beeching N J, Geddes A M 1982 Relapsing hepatitis associated with hepatitis A virus. Lancet 2: 163

Gust I D, Feinstone S M 1988 Clinical features. In: Gust I D, Feinstone S M (eds) Hepatitis A. CRC Press, Boca Raton, pp 145–162

Gust I D, Lehmann N I, Lucas C R 1978 Relationship between prevalence of antibody to hepatitis A antigen and age: a cohort effect? Journal of Infectious Diseases 138: 425–426

Hadler S C, McFarland L 1986 Hepatitis in day care centers: epidemiology and prevention. Reviews of Infectious Diseases 8: 548–557

Hadler S C, Webster H M, Erben J J, Swanson J E, Maynard J E 1980 Hepatitis A in day-care centers: a community-wide assessment. The New England Journal of Medicine 302: 1222–1227

Hadler S C 1991 Global impact of hepatitis A virus infection changing patterns. In: Hollinger F B, Lemon S M, Margolis H (eds) Viral hepatitis and liver disease. Williams & Wilkins, Baltimore, pp 14–20

Hagler L, Pastore R A, Bergin J J 1975 Aplastic anemia following viral hepatitis. Report of two fatal cases and literature review. Medicine 54: 139–164

Hammond G W, McDougall B K, Plummer F, Sekla L H 1982 Encephalitis during the prodromal stage of acute hepatitis A. Journal of the Canadian Medical Association 126: 269–270

Hilleman M R, Provost P J, Miller W J, Villarejos V M, Ittensohn O L, McAleer W J 1975 Immune adherence and complement-fixation tests for human hepatitis A. Diagnostic and epidemiologic investigations. Developments in Biological Standardization 30: 383–389

Hillis W D 1963 Viral hepatitis associated with subhuman primates. Transfusion 3: 445–454

Hindman S, Maynard J, Bradley D, Berquist K, Denes A 1977 Simultaneous infection with type A and B hepatitis viruses. American Journal of Epidemiology 105: 135–139

Hoaglund C L, Shank R E 1946 Infectious hepatitis: a review of 200 cases. Journal of the American Medical Association 130: 615–621

Hollinger F B, Bradley D W, Maynard J E, Dreesman G R, Melnick J L 1975 Detection of hepatitis A viral antigen by radioimmunoassay. Journal of Immunology 115: 1464–1466

Hu M, Kang L, Yao G 1990 An outbreak of viral hepatitis A in Shanghai. In: Bianchi L, Gerok W, Maier K-P, Deinhardt F (eds) Infectious Diseases of the Liver. Kluwer Academic Publishers, Dordrecht, pp 361–372

Inman R D, Hodge M, Johnston M E A, Wright J, Heathcote J 1986 Arthritis, vasculitis and cryoglobulinaemia associated with relapsing hepatitis A virus infection. Annals of Internal Medicine 105: 700–703

Jacobson I M, Nath B J, Dienstag J L 1985 Relapsing viral hepatitis type A. Journal of Medical Virology 16: 163–169

Johnston C L W, Schwartz M, Wansborough-Jones M H 1981 Acute inflammatory polyradiculoneuropathy following type A viral hepatitis. Postgraduate Medical Journal 57: 647–648

Kao H W, Ashcavai M, Redeker A G 1984 The persistence of hepatitis A IgM antibody after acute clinical hepatitis A. Hepatology 5: 933–936

Karayiannis P, Jowett T, Enticott M et al 1986 Hepatitis A virus replication in tamarins and host immune response in relation to pathogenesis of liver cell damage. Journal of Medical Virology 18: 261–276

Karayiannis P, Chitranukroh R, Fry M et al 1990 Protracted alanine aminotransferase levels in tamarins infected with hepatitis A virus. Journal of Medical Virology 30: 151–158

Karayiannis P, O'Rourke S, McGarvey M J et al 1991 Vaccination of tamarins with a recombinant vaccinia-hepatitis A virus protects against HAV infection. In: Hollinger F B, Lemon S M, Margolis H (eds) Viral hepatitis and liver disease. Williams & Wilkins, Baltimore, pp 101–104

Kark J D, Bar-Shani S 1980 Hepatitis A antibody in Israel defence forces recruits. Journal of Medical Virology 6: 341–345

Keenan C M, Lemon S M, LeDuc J W, McNamee G A, Binn L N 1984 Pathology of hepatitis A infection in the owl monkey (*Aotus trivirgatus*). American Journal of Pathology 115: 1–8
Khan N C, Hollinger F B, Melnick J L 1984 Localization of hepatitis A virus antigen to specific subcellular fractions of hepatitis-A-infected chimpanzee liver cells. Intervirology 21: 187–194
Krawczynski K 1991 Antigens and antibodies of hepatitis E virus infection in experimental primate models and man. In: Hollinger F B, Lemon S M, Margolis H (eds) Viral hepatitis and liver disease. Williams & Wilkins, Baltimore, pp 517–521
Krawczynski K K, Bradley D W, Murphy B Y et al 1981 Pathogenetic aspects of hepatitis A virus infection in enterically inoculated marmosets. American Journal of Clinical Pathology 76: 698–706
Krugman S, Giles J P 1970 Viral hepatitis: new light on an old disease. Journal of the American Medical Association 212: 1019–1029
Krugman S, Ward R, Giles J P, Bodansky O, Jacobs A M 1959 Infectious hepatitis: detection of virus during the incubation period and in clinically inapparent infections. New England Journal of Medicine 261: 729–734
Krugman S, Ward R, Giles J P 1962 The natural history of infectious hepatitis. American Journal of Medicine 32: 717–728
Krugman S, Giles J P, Hammond J 1967 Infectious hepatitis: evidence for two distinctive clinical, epidemiological and immunological types of infection. Journal of the American Medical Association 200: 365–373
Krugman S, Overby L R, Mushahwar I K, Ling C M, Frösner G G, Deinhardt F 1979 Viral hepatitis, type B. Studies on natural history and prevention re-examined. New England Journal of Medicine 300: 101–106
Lankas G R, Jensen R D 1987 Evidence of hepatitis A infection in immature rhesus monkeys. Veterinary Pathology 24: 340–344
Lapin B A, Shevtsova Z V 1989 Sensitivity of the Old World monkeys to hepatitis A virus (spontaneous and experimental infection). Experimental Pathology 36: 63–64
Lednar W M, Lemon S M, Kirkpatrick J W, Redfield R R, Fields M L, Kelley P W 1985 Frequency of illness associated with epidemic hepatitis A virus infections in adults. American Journal of Epidemiology 122: 226–233
LeDuc J W, Lemon S M, Keenan C M, Graham R R, Marchwicki R H, Binn L N 1983 Experimental infection of the New World owl monkey (*Aotus trivirgatus*) with hepatitis A virus. Infection and Immunity 40: 766–772
Le Moine Parker M, 1971 Aplastic anemia and infectious hepatitis. Lancet ii: 261–262
Lemon S M 1985 Type A viral hepatitis. New developments in an old disease. New England Journal of Medicine 313: 1059–1067
Lemon S M, Chao S F, Jansen R W, Binn L N, LeDuc J W 1987 Genomic heterogeneity among human and nonhuman strains of hepatitis A virus. Journal of Virology 61: 735–742
Lemon S M, Binn L N, Marchwicki R et al 1990 In vivo replication and reversion to wild type of a neutralization-resistant antigenic variant of hepatitis A virus. Journal of Infectious Diseases 161: 7–13
Lesnicar G 1988 A prospective study of viral hepatitis A and the question of chronicity. Hepato-Gastroenterology 35: 69–72
Levin S, Hahn T, 1982 Interferon system in acute viral hepatitis. Lancet i: 592–594
MacCallum F O 1951 Transmission experiments. In: MacCallum F O, McFarlan A M, Miles J A R, Pollock M R, Wilson C (eds) Infective hepatitis. MRC, Special Report No 273, HMSO, London
McDonald G S A, Courtney M G, Shattock A G, Weir D G 1989 Prolonged IgM antibodies and histopathological evidence of chronicity in hepatitis A. Liver 9: 223–228
McNeill M, Hoy J F, Richards M J, Lehmann N J, Dimitrikakis M, Gust I D 1984 Etiology of fatal hepatitis in Melbourne. Medical Journal of Australia 141: 637–640
Maier K, Gabriel P, Koscielniak E et al 1988 Human gamma interferon production by cytotoxic T lymphocytes sensitized during hepatitis A virus infection. Journal of Virology 62: 3756–3763
Mao J S, Go Y Y, Huang H Y et al 1981 Susceptibility of monkeys to human hepatitis A virus. Journal of Infectious Diseases 144: 55–60
Mao J S, Dong D X, Zhang H Y et al 1989 Primary study of attenuated live hepatitis A vaccine (H2 strain) in humans. Journal of Infectious Diseases 159: 621–624
Margolis H S, Nainan O V, Krawczynski K et al 1988 Appearance of immune complexes during experimental hepatitis A infection in chimpanzees. Journal of Medical Virology 26: 315–326
Mathiesen L R, Skinhoj P, Nielsen J O, Purcell R H, Wong D, Ranek L 1980a Hepatitis type A, B and non-A, non-B in fulminant hepatitis. Gut 21: 72–77
Mathiesen L R, Moller A M, Purcell R H, London W T, Feinstone S M 1980b Hepatitis A virus in the liver and intestine of marmosets after oral inoculation. Infection and Immunity 28: 45–48
Meier E, Richter K, Frühmorgen P 1982 Vorübergehend-chronische Hepatitis nach akuter Virushepatitis A. Deutsche Medizinische Wochenschrift 107: 46–50
Metcalf T G, Jiang X 1988 Detection of hepatitis A virus in estuarine samples by gene probe assay. Microbiological Sciences 5: 296–300
Midthun K, Ellerbeck E, Gershman K et al 1991 Safety and immunogenicity of a live attenuated hepatitis A virus vaccine in seronegative volunteers. Journal of Infectious Diseases 163: 735–739
Morbidity and Mortality Weekly Report 1991 Summary of notifiable diseases, United States 1990. US Department of Health and Human Services, PHS, CDC, 39: 3–61
Mutton K J, Gust I D 1984 Public health aspects of hepatitis A. In: Gerety R J (ed) Hepatitis A. Academic Press, London, pp 133–161
Nainan O V, Margolis H S, Robertson B H, Balayan M, Brinton M A 1991 Sequence analysis of a new hepatitis A virus naturally infecting cynomolgus macaques (*Macaca fascicularis*). Journal of General Virology 72: 1685–1689
Norkrans G 1978 Clinical epidemiological and prognostic aspects of hepatitis A, B and non-A, non-B. Scandinavian Journal of Infectious Diseases (suppl. 17): 1–44
O'Grady J G, Alexander G J M, Hayllar K M, Williams R 1989 Early indicators of prognosis in fulminant hepatic failure. Gastroenterology 97: 439–445
Papaevangelou G J 1984 Global epidemiology of hepatitis A. In: Gerety R J (ed) Hepatitis A. Academic Press, London, pp 101–132
Papaevangelou G J, Biziagos E, Stathopoulos G, Crance J M, Vayona T, Deloince R 1991 Detection of hepatitis A virus from shellfish and seawater: one-year study in Thermaicos

Gulf (Thessaloniki, Greece). In: Hollinger F B, Lemon S M, Margolis H (eds) Viral hepatitis and liver disease. Williams & Wilkins, Baltimore, pp 78–81

Pohjanpelto P, Lahdensivu R 1984 Rapid decline of hepatitis A in Finland. Scandinavian Journal of Infectious Diseases 16: 229–233

Popper H, Dienstag J L, Feinstone S M, Alter H J, Purcell R H 1980a Lessons from the pathology of viral hepatitis in chimpanzees. In: Bianchi L, Gerok W, Sickinger K, Stalder G A (eds) Virus and the Liver. MTP Press, Lancaster, pp 137–150

Popper H, Dienstag J L, Feinstone S M, Alter H J, Purcell R H 1980b The pathology of viral hepatitis in chimpanzees. Virchows Archiv A, Pathological Anatomy and Histology 387: 91–106

Provost P J, Hilleman M R 1978 An inactivated hepatitis A virus vaccine prepared from infected marmoset liver. Proceedings of the Society for Experimental Biology and Medicine 159: 201–203

Provost P J, Hilleman M R 1979 Propagation of human hepatitis A virus in cell culture in vitro. Proceedings of the Society for Experimental Biology and Medicine 160: 213–221

Provost P J, Conti P A, Giesa P A et al 1983 Studies in chimpanzees of live, attenuated hepatitis A vaccine candidates. Proceedings of the Society for Experimental Biology and Medicine 172: 357–363

Purcell R H, Wong D C, Moritsugu Y, Dienstag J L, Routenberg J A, Boggs J D 1976 A microtiter solid-phase radioimmunoassay for hepatitis A antigen and antibody. Journal of Immunology 116: 349–356

Purcell R H, Feinstone S M, Ticehurst J R, Daemer R J, Baroudy B M 1984 Hepatitis A virus. In: Vyas G N, Dienstag J L, Hoofnagle J H (eds) Viral hepatitis and liver disease. Grune & Stratton, Orlando, pp 9–22

Purcell R H, 1991 Approaches to immunization against hepatitis A virus. In: Hollinger F B, Lemon S M, Margolis H (eds) Viral hepatitis and liver disease. Williams & Wilkins, Baltimore, pp 41–46

Raimondo G, Longo G, Caredda F, Saracco G, Rizzetto M 1986 Prolonged, polyphasic infection with hepatitis A. Journal of Infectious Diseases 153: 172–173

Rakela J, Redeker A G, Edwards V M, Decker R, Overby L R, Mosley J W 1978 Hepatitis A virus infection in fulminant hepatitis and chronic active hepatitis. Gastroenterology 74: 879–882

Robertson B H, Khanna B, Nainan O V, Margolis H S 1991 Epidemiologic patterns of wild-type hepatitis A virus determined by genetic variation. Journal of Infectious Diseases 163: 286–292

Roggendorf M, Frösner G G, Deinhardt F, Scheid R 1980 Comparison of solid phase test systems for demonstrating antibodies against hepatitis A virus (anti-HAV) of the IgM-class. Journal of Medical Virology 5: 47–62

Rosenberg M L, Koplan J P, Pollard R A 1980 The risk of acquiring hepatitis from sewage-contaminated water. American Journal of Epidemiology 112: 17–22

Roumeliotou A, Papachristopoulos A, Alexiou D, Papaevangelou G 1992 Intrafamilial spread of hepatitis A. Lancet 339: 125

Routenberg J A, Dienstag J L, Harrison W O et al 1979 Foodborne epidemic of hepatitis A: clincial and laboratory features of acute and protracted illness. American Journal of Medical Sciences 278: 123–137

Saunders S J, Seggie J, Kirsch R E, Terblanche J 1979 Acute liver failure. In: Wright R, Alberti K G M M, Karran S, Millward-Sadler G H (eds) Liver and biliary disease. W B Saunders, Philadelphia, pp 569–584

Schmid M, Regli J 1985 The morphology of hepatitis A in man. In: Bianchi L, Gerok W, Popper H (eds) Trends in hepatology, MTP Press, Lancaster, pp 201–207

Sciot R, van Damme B, Desmet V J 1986a Cholestatic features in hepatitis A. Journal of Hepatology 3: 172–181

Sciot R, van den Oord J J, De Wolf-Peeters C, Desmet V J 1986b In situ characterization of the (peri)portal inflammatory infiltrate in acute hepatitis A. Liver 6: 331–336

Shibayama T, Kojima H, Ashida M et al 1985 Localization of hepatitis A virus in marmoset liver tissue during the acute phase of experimental infection. Gastroenterologia Japonica 20: 564–572

Shieh Y-S C, Baric R S, Sobsey M D et al 1991 Detection of hepatitis A virus and other enteroviruses in water by ssRNA probes. Journal of Virological Methods 31: 119–136

Shimizu Y K, Weiner A J, Rosenblatt J et al 1991 Early events in hepatitis C virus infection of chimpanzees. In: Hollinger F B, Lemon S M, Margolis H (eds) Viral hepatitis and liver disease. Williams & Wilkins, Baltimore, pp 393–396

Siegl G 1984 The biochemistry of hepatitis A virus. In: Gerety R J (ed) Hepatitis A. Academic Press, Orlando, pp 9–32

Sjögren M H, Tanno H, Fay O et al 1987 Hepatitis A virus in stool during clinical relapse. Annals of Internal Medicine 106: 221–226

Skidmore S J, Gully P R, Middleton J D, Hassam Z A, Singal G M 1985 An outbreak of hepatitis A on a hospital ward. Journal of Medical Virology 17: 175–177

Skinhoj P, McNair A 1972 An outbreak of infectious hepatitis in Southwest Greenland. Scandinavian Journal of Infectious Diseases 4: 73–77

Stewart J S, Farrow L J, Clifford R E et al 1978 A three year survey of viral hepatitis in West London. Quarterly Journal of Medicine 47: 365–384

Szmuness W, Dienstag J L, Purcell R H, Harley E J, Stevens C E, Wong D C 1976 Distribution of antibody to hepatitis A antigen in urban adult populations. New England Journal of Medicine 295: 755–759

Szmuness W, Dienstag J L, Purcell R H et al 1977 The prevalence of antibody to hepatitis A antigen in various parts of the world: a pilot study. American Journal of Epidemiology 106: 392–398

Tanaka T, Tanaka I, Koga M et al 1981 Morphologic findings of acute hepatitis A. Acta Hepatologica Japonica 22: 494–507

Tanikawa K 1979 Acute viral hepatitis. Type A hepatitis. Its epidemiology, clinical pictures and pathologic changes of the liver. Gastroenterologia Japonica 14: 168

Tanno H, Fay O H, Rojman J A, Palazzi J 1988 Biphasic form of hepatitis A virus infection: a frequent variant in Argentina. Liver 8: 53–57

Tassopoulos N, Papaevangelou G, Roumeliotou-Karayannis A, Kalafatas P, Engle R, Gerin J, Purcell R H 1985 Double infections with hepatitis A and B viruses. Liver 5: 348–353

Taylor-Wiedeman J, Moritsugu Y, Miyamura K, Yamazaki S 1987 Seroepidemiology of hepatitis A virus in Japan. Japanese Journal of Medical Science and Biology 40: 119–130

Teixeira M R, Weller I V D, Murray A, Bamber M, Thomas H C, Sherlock S, Scheuer P J 1982 The pathology of hepatitis A in man. Liver 2: 53–60

Toppet V, Souayah H, Delplace O, Alard S, Moreau J, Levy J, Spehl M 1990 Lymph node enlargement as a sign of acute hepatitis A in children. Pediatric Radiology 20: 249–252

Tsarev S A, Emerson S U, Balayan M S, Ticehurst J, Purcell R H 1991 Simian hepatitis A virus (HAV) strain AGM-27: comparison of genome structure and growth in cell culture with other HAV strains. Journal of General Virology 72: 1677–1683

Tsiquaye K N, Harrison T J, Portmann B, Hu S, Zuckerman A J 1984 Acute hepatitis A infection in hepatitis B chimpanzee carriers. Hepatology 4: 504–509

Vallbracht A, Gabriel P, Maier K et al 1986 Cell-mediated cytotoxicity in hepatitis A virus infection. Hepatology 6: 1308–1314

Vallbracht A, Maier K, Stierhof Y-D, Wiedmann K H, Flehmig B, Fleischer B 1989 Liver-derived cytotoxic T cells in hepatitis A virus infection. Journal of Infectious Diseases 160: 209–217

Vento S, Garofano T, Di Perri G, Dolci L, Concia E, Bassetti D 1991 Identification of hepatitis A virus as a trigger for autoimmune chronic hepatitis type 1 in susceptible individuals. Lancet i: 1183–1187

Villarejos V M, Serra J, Anderson-Visona K, Mosley J W 1982 Hepatitis A virus infection in households. American Journal of Epidemiology 115: 577–586

Viola L, Barrison I, Coleman J, Murray-Lyon I 1982 The clinical course of acute type A hepatitis in chronic HBsAg carriers. A report of three cases. Postgraduate Medical Journal 58: 80–81

Voegt H 1942 Zur aetiologie der hepatitis epidemica. Münchener Medizinische Wochenschrift 89: 76–79

Wacker W E C, Riordan J F, Snodgrass P J et al J 1972 The Holy Cross hepatitis outbreak. Archives of Internal Medicine 130: 357–360

Weir W R C, Mellor J A, Smith H, Tyrell D A J 1981 Significance of hepatic enzyme levels at discharge in acute viral hepatitis. Journal of Infection 3: 309-315

Werzberger A, Mensch B, Kuter B, et al 1992 A controlled trial of a formalin-inactivated, hepatitis A vaccine in healthy children. New England Journal of Medicine 327: 453–457

Xu Z Y, Fu T Y, Margolis H S et al 1991 Impact and control of viral hepatitis in China. In: Hollinger F B, Lemon S M, Margolis H (eds) Viral hepatitis and liver disease. Williams & Wilkins, Baltimore, pp 700–706

Yang N-Y, Yu P-H, Mao Z-X, Chen N-L, Chai S-A, Mao J-S 1988 Inapparent infection of hepatitis A virus. American Journal of Epidemiology 127: 599–604

Yao G 1991 Clinical spectrum and natural history of viral hepatitis A in a 1988 Shanghai epidemic. In: Hollinger F B, Lemon S M, Margolis H S (eds) Viral hepatitis and liver disease. Williams & Wilkins, Baltimore, pp 76–78

Zachoval R, Roggendorf M, Deinhardt F 1983 Hepatitis A infection in chronic carriers of hepatitis B virus. Hepatology 3: 528–531

Zachoval R, Abb J, Zachoval V, Deinhardt F 1986 Circulating interferon in patients with acute hepatitis A. Journal of Infectious Diseases 153: 1174-1175

Zachoval R, Kroener M, Brommer M, Deinhardt F 1990 Serology and interferon production during the early phase of acute hepatitis A. Journal of Infectious Diseases 161: 353–354

Zuckerman A J 1979 Chronicle of viral hepatitis. Abstracts on Hygiene 54: 1113–1135

UPDATE

- An interesting new aspect of HAV infection has been raised by Vento et al (1991). When healthy relatives of patients with type I autoimmune (classical 'lupoid') hepatitis were followed prospectively, clinically overt auto-immune hepatitis following acute HAV infection in two individuals who had a pre-existing specific suppressor/inducer T-cell defect against the asialoglycoprotein-receptor was observed. From these data, it could be speculated that HAV is one of the factors triggering autoimmune liver disease in predisposed individuals.

  A formalin-inactivated hepatitis A vaccine prepared from tissue culture virus according to WHO requirements is now available for clinical use. This vaccine is highly immunogenic, safe and protective (Vento et al 1991).

- REFERENCE

Vento S, Garofano T, Di Perri G, Dolci L, Concia E, Bassetti D 1991 Identification of hepatitis A virus as a trigger for autoimmune chronic hepatitis type 1 in susceptible individuals. Lancet i: 1183–1187

4. Diagnosis

I. Gust

DIFFERENTIATION OF THE DISEASE ON THE BASIS OF CLINICAL AND EPIDEMIOLOGICAL FEATURES

Hepatitis A is an acute infection with generalized symptoms accompanied by jaundice. The course of the disease is affected by the patient's age, so that infections in childhood are frequently anicteric.

Patients who develop a typical illness often describe several days of vague symptoms, such as fatigue, malaise, loss of appetite, nausea and vomiting. The prodrome is often flu-like and may be accompanied by chills, a slight fever and headache. Loss of appetite is common and the patient may be nauseated by the sight or smell of certain foods. Smokers often lose interest in cigarettes.

In most patients, the first objective sign of illness is the onset of dark urine, accompanied by clay-coloured faeces and gradual yellowing of the sclera and skin. The disease is usually self-limiting, with jaundice subsiding and colour returning to the faeces within 4 weeks of the onset of symptoms.

While most of these symptoms are shared by patients with other forms of viral hepatitis, some features may be helpful to an astute clinician. A small proportion of patients with prolonged acute hepatitis A develop complications, of which the most common are cholestasis, relapse and extra-hepatic manifestations (cutaneous vasculitis and arthritis), while the disease has sometimes been found to trigger autoimmune hepatitis. Hepatitis A may occasionally present with a cholestatic picture and prolonged jaundice, although serum AST levels are usually ≥ 500 IU/ml, peak bilirubin levels may exceed 10 mg/ml (Gordon et al 1984). While liver biopsies show centrilobular cholestasis, the condition usually resolves completely. Steroids may speed this process.

In some studies, up to 6–10% of patients with hepatitis A have been found to develop biochemical evidence of relapse within 4–15 weeks of their initial illness (Weir et al 1981, Bamber et al 1983). ALT levels may reach 1000 IU/ml and remain elevated for weeks or months. Hepatitis A-specific IgM remains detectable during this period, and HAV particles have been reported in the faeces of some patients.

LABORATORY DIAGNOSIS OF HEPATITIS A

Confirmation of a clinical diagnosis of hepatitis A usually requires two groups of tests – an initial set of tests to confirm that the symptoms are due to acute inflammation of the liver and a second set aimed at defining the aetiological agent. Most of these can be performed on a simple blood sample (5–10 cm^3) collected when the patients first seek treatment, which is usually about the time their urine becomes dark and they or their family or friends notice they are becoming jaundiced.

Biochemical tests of liver function (subsidiary)

Diagnosis of hepatitis is usually made by liver function tests, in particular by testing the patient's serum for the presence of total and direct bilirubin, alanine aminotransferase (ALT), aspartate amino-transferase (AST) and alkaline phosphatase (Clermont & Chalmers 1967). Aminotransferase levels are sensitive markers of liver damage and usually reach peak levels about the time the patient seeks medical attention. Levels generally range from 50 to 2000 IU/ml, although the degree of elevation does not appear to correlate with outcome.

Alkaline phosphatase levels are mildly elevated in patients with acute hepatitis A and in other forms of viral hepatitis. High levels are indicative of cholestasis and suggest other causes of jaundice.

Elevated levels of IgM have been noted in more than three-quarters of patients with acute hepatitis A and may be useful in distinguishing the disease from other forms of viral hepatitis when specific serological tests are unavailable (Giles & Krugman 1968, Zhuang et al 1982).

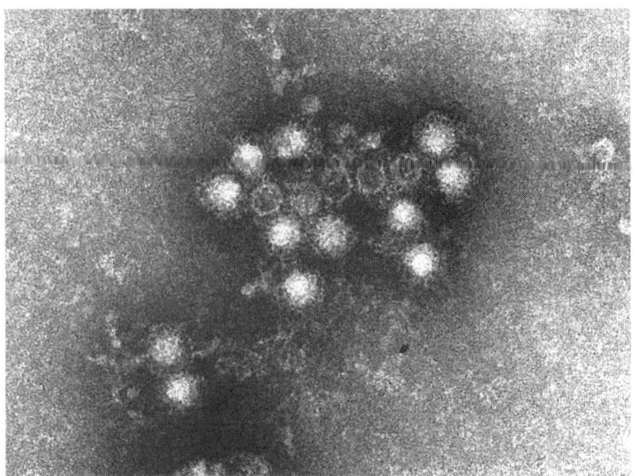

Fig. 4.1 Electron micrograph showing an immune electron microscope preparation of HAV. Note the heavy coating of antibody around the virus particles. (Courtesy of Dr J Marshall, Fairfield Hospital, Melbourne, Australia.)

Specific diagnostic tests (subsidiary)

Tests for confirmation of the diagnosis of hepatitis A fall into two broad categories: detection of the virus or viral components (such as specific antigens or HAV RNA) and detection of a specific antibody response (either a rising titre of antibodies at the time of the disease or the presence of specific IgM or IgA antibodies).

Detection of HAV particles or components of the virus

Immune electron microscopy

HAV was originally recognized by immune electron microscopy (IEM) (Feinstone et al 1973, Locarnini et al 1974) – a process in which clarified suspensions of faeces, collected from patients in the late incubation period or acute phase of the illness, were mixed with sera known to contain high titres of anti-HAV and the resultant virus–antibody complexes detected by examination with a transmission EM (see Fig. 4.1). Although various techniques have been used, most involve mixing preparations of HAV with dilutions of human serum, incubating the mixture at 37°C for 1 h and overnight at 4°C, then staining the sample with, for example, 3% phosphotungstic acid (PTA) at Ph 7 on a Formvar carbon-coated grid (Kiernan et al 1987).

Immune electron microscopy is a tedious and time-consuming process which, while useful as an experimental tool, makes it extremely difficult to screen large numbers of samples. The technique requires an experienced operator and considerable patience (as many grid squares need to be examined before declaring a sample negative). Because of the subjectivity of the process, even when confirmatory photographs are made, it is wise to review samples under code.

Studies in several laboratories have demonstrated that the limit of sensitivity of IEM is approximately 10^5–10^6 particles per ml. As a consequence, virus particles are more likely to be detectable in the late incubation period before the patient needs medical attention.

Recently, Humphrey et al (1990) have developed a solid-phase form of IEM for detection of virus particles in faecal extracts (or cell culture supernatants), which appears to increase the number of particles in immune aggregates so that they are more readily detectable. The technique, which appears to be both simple and sensitive, uses monoclonal antibodies to aggregate the particles, which are then bound to a carbon–plastic grid by protein A or anti-immunoglobulin. This technique has been found to be useful for detecting other enteric viruses, including hepatitis E virus.

Thus, while detection of virus particles is a useful experimental tool and may assist in confirming a diagnosis, our inability to detect particles in every patient with serologically confirmed disease means that the absence of particles cannot be used to preclude a diagnosis.

In an attempt to overcome the limited sensitivity of IEM, assays have been developed for the detection of specific viral antigens and HAV RNA.

Hepatitis A antigen

Although strains of HAV collected from individual patients may differ slightly in nucleotide sequences and in the amino acid sequences of some of their structural proteins, these differences are not important at the level of immunogenicity. To date, only one serotype of HAV has been recognized, so that specific antibodies collected from patients in one country appear to be capable of neutralizing strains of virus collected from other parts of the world.

Several groups have developed sensitive immunoassays, either radioimmunoassays (RIAs) or enzyme-linked immunosorbent assays (ELISA) for detection of HAAg in faecal samples and for quantitation of virus during vaccine production (Hollinger et al 1975, Purcell et al 1976, Locarnini et al 1978). A number of workers have used ELISAs or RIAs to define the pattern of virus shedding in experimentally infected animals and patients with naturally acquired hepatitis A. In one large study in which serial faecal samples from patients with acute hepatitis A were examined by RIA, HAAg was detected in 45% of samples collected within a week of the onset of dark urine, and in 11% of samples collected in the following week (Coulepis et al 1980).

Detection of HAV RNA

Molecular hybridization has been used to detect HAV RNA in faecal samples from patients with hepatitis A (Jansen et al 1985, Ticehurst et al 1987) and, occasionally, in the blood of patients seen early in the disease (Oren et al 1989). This technique has been found to be more sensitive than ELISA or RIA for detection of HAAg and to demonstrate evidence of viral shedding for longer periods of time. Tassopoulos et al (1986) have demonstrated that this technique is 4–10 times more sensitive than RIA for detection of HAV in faecal samples, although it is still less sensitive than assays for viral infectivity in primates or cell culture (Ticehurst et al 1987).

Improved methods of detection of HAV by dot-blot hybridization have been described (Jiang et al 1987, 1989) involving ^{32}P-labelled single-stranded (ss) RNA probes, and have been used to detect virus in oysters and clams grown in contaminated water (Zhou et al 1991). After separation of shellfish polysaccharide and concentration of virus particles by precipitation with polyethylene glycol, viral RNA was detected by dot-blot hybridization. This assay, which is capable of detecting as few as 10^3 infectious particles in a 20 g sample of shellfish meat, is likely to become extremely valuable for detecting evidence of environmental contamination and has been adapted as a semiquantitative technique (Jiang et al 1989).

Recently, Shieh et al (1991) have used ssRNA probes to detect HAV and other enteroviruses in contaminated water collected during an outbreak of water-borne hepatitis. These samples were negative for HAAg by solid-phase RIA. The development of gene probes for detection of HAV particles in environmental samples is very important because these particles are very stable and less readily removed than faecal indicator bacteria.

Detection of a specific antibody response

Antibodies to HAV can be detected by a variety of serological tests, including immune electron microscopy, complement fixation, immune adherence haemagglutination, immunofluorescence, radioimmunoassay and enzyme-linked immunosorbent assay. In recent years, ELISAs for total (and class-specific) antibodies have become available from a number of manufacturers, at least one of which presents the assay as part of a fully automated system (Eble et al 1991, Robbins et al 1991).

Because antibodies to HAV develop early in the course of the illness, it is only possible to demonstrate a conventional fourfold rise in titre, if the first blood sample is collected early. A large proportion of patients with hepatitis A do not seek attention until their urine becomes dark, by which time anti-HAV titre may be reaching peak levels (Gust & Feinstone 1988). Thus, while rising titres of antibody may be detected in patients who seek attention early in their illness, failure to detect a fourfold or greater rise in titre between acute and convalescent samples does not preclude the diagnosis. The corollary to this is that, if patients do not have detectable levels of anti-HAV in their serum at the time they seek medical attention, they are unlikely to have hepatitis A.

The most reliable single assay for diagnosis of infection with HAV is detection of hepatitis A-specific IgM. The first indication that specific IgM was produced early in infection was the observation by Locarnini et al (1974) that complexes of HAV and acute-phase sera examined by IEM contain IgM-like bridges between adjoining particles. A variety of assays have been developed for detection of HA-specific IgM, of which the most widely used are ELISA and RIA. The most popular assays involve attachment of anti-human IgM (μ chain specific) to a solid phase. After addition of the test serum, any IgM present is bound to the solid phase and anti-HAV-specific IgM can be detected by the addition of purified HAAg and labelled anti-HAV (Locarnini et al 1979).

The sensitivity of commercial assays for HA IgM has been adjusted so that, in uncomplicated infections, these antibodies are only detectable for 3 to 4 months after the onset of illness. Thus, under most circumstances, the presence of hepatitis A-specific IgM in a patient with acute hepatitis is sufficient to confirm the diagnosis. Recently, Parry et al (1989) have investigated the use of saliva specimens as an alternative to serum samples for the detection of total and class-specific antibodies to HAV. Preliminary studies indicate that, in experienced hands, saliva collected with an appropriate device can serve as a suitable sample for defining current or past infection with the virus. This technique may be of particular value in the investigation of epidemics among children.

Bull et al (1989) recently described a small outbreak of hepatitis A in a private boarding school, in which salivary antibody testing was used to detect current or past infection with HAV and to determine which children should be given immunoglobulin to limit the spread of the disease.

Other tests

While strains of HAV have been adapted to growth in cell culture, the isolation rate is relatively low, so that this technique is not a practical method of establishing the diagnosis.

REFERENCES

Bamber M, Thomas H C, Bannister B, Sherlock S 1983 Acute type A, B and non-A, non-B hepatitis in a hospital population in London: clinical and epidemiological features. Gut 24: 561–564

Bull A R, Kimmance K J, Parry J V, Perry K R 1989 Investigation of an outbreak of hepatitis A simplified by salivary antibody testing. Epidemiological Infections 103: 371–376

Clermont R J, Chalmers T C 1967 The transaminase tests in liver disease. Medicine, Baltimore 46: 197–207

Coulepis A G, Locarnini S A, Lehmann N I, Gust I D 1980 Detection of hepatitis A virus in the faeces of patients with naturally-acquired infections. Journal of Infectious Diseases 141: 151–156

Eble K, Clemens J, Krenc C et al 1991 Differential diagnosis of acute viral hepatitis using rapid, fully automated immunoassays. Journal of Medical Virology 33: 139–150

Feinstone S M, Kapikian A Z, Purcell R H 1973 Hepatitis A: detection by immune electron miroscopy of a virus-like antigen associated with acute illness. Science 182: 1026–1028

Giles J P, Krugman S 1968 Viral hepatitis: immunoglobulin response during the course of the disease. Journal of the American Medical Association 208: 497–503

Gordon S C, Reddy K R, Schiff L, Schiff E R 1984 Prolonged intrahepatic cholestasis secondary to acute hepatitis A. Annals of Internal Medicine 101: 635–637

Gust I D, Feinstone S M 1988 Detection of rising titres of anti-HAV. Hepatitis A. CRC Press, Boca Raton, pp 153–154

Hollinger F B, Bradley D W, Maynard J E, Dreessman G R, Melnick J L 1975 Detection of hepatitis A viral antigen by radioimmunoassay. Journal of Immunology 115: 1464–1468

Humphrey C D, Cook E H Jr, Bradley D W 1990 Identification of enterically transmitted hepatitis virus particles by solid phase immune electron microscopy. Journal of Virological Methods 29: 177–188

Jansen R W, Newbold J E, Lemon S M 1985 Combined immunoaffinity CDNA–RNA hybridization assay for detection of hepatitis A virus in clinical specimens. Journal of Clinical Microscopy 221: 984–989

Jiang X I, Estes M K, Metcalf T G 1987 Detection of hepatitis A virus by hybridization with single-stranded RNA probes. Applied and Environmental Microbiology 53: 2487–2495

Jiang X I, Estes M K, Metcalf T G 1989 In situ hybridization for quantitative assay of infectious hepatitis A virus. Journal of Clinical Microbiology 27: 874–879

Kiernan R E, Marshall J A, Coulepis A G, Anderson D A, Gust I D 1987 Cellular changes associated with persistent hepatitis A infection in vitro. Archives of Virology 94: 81–95

Locarnini S A, Ferris A A, Stott A C, Gust I D 1974 The relationship between a 27 nm virus-like particle and hepatitis A as demonstrated by immune electron microscopy. Intervirology 4: 110–118

Locarnini S A, Garland S M, Lehmann N I, Pringle R C, Gust I D 1978 Solid-phase enzyme-linked immunoabsorbent assay for detection of hepatitis A virus. Journal of Clinical Microscopy 8: 277–282

Locarnini S A, Coulepis A G, Stratton A M, Kaldor J, Gust I D 1979 Solid-phase enzyme immunoassay for detection of hepatitis A specific immunoglobulin M. Journal of Clinical Microscopy 9: 459–465

Oren R, Shouval D, Tur-Kaspa T 1989 Detection of hepatitis A virus RNA in serum from patients with acute hepatitis. Journal of Medical Virology 28: 261–263

Parry J V, Perry K R, Panday S, Mortimer P P 1989 Diagnosis of hepatitis A and B by testing saliva. Journal of Medical Virology 28: 255–260

Purcell R H, Wong D C, Moritsugu Y, Dienstag J L, Routenberg J A, Boggs J D 1976 A microtitre solid-phase radioimmunoassay for hepatitis A antigen and antibody. Journal of Immunology 116: 349–356

Robbins D J, Krater J, Kiang W, Alcalde X, Helgesen S, Carlos J, Mimms L 1991 Detection of total antibody against hepatitis A virus by an automated microparticle enzyme immunoassay. Journal of Virological Methods 32: 255–263

Shieh Y S C, Baric R S, Sobsey M D, Ticehurst J, Miele T A, DeLeon R, Walter R 1991 Detection of hepatitis A virus and other enteroviruses in water by ssRNA probes. Journal of Virological Methods 31: 119–136

Tassopoulos N C, Papavangelou G J, Ticehurst J C, Purcell R H 1986 Faecal excretion of Greek strains of hepatitis A virus in patients with hepatitis A and in experimentally-infected chimpanzees. Journal of Infectious Diseases 154: 231–237

Ticehurst J, Feinstone S M, Chestnut T, Tassopoulos N C, Popper H, Purcell R H 1987 Detection of hepatitis A virus by extraction of viral RNA molecular hybridization. Journal of Clinical Microbiology 25: 1822–1829

Weir W R C, Mellor J A, Smith H, Tyrell D A J 1981 Significance of hepatic enzyme levels at discharge in acute viral hepatitis. Journal of Infection 3: 309–315

Zhou Y J, Estes M K, Jiang X I, Metcalf T G 1991 Concentration and detection of hepatitis A virus and rotavirus from shellfish by hybridization tests. Applied and Environmental Microbiology 57: 2963–2968

Zhuang H, Kaldor J, Locarnini S A, Gust I D 1982 Serum immunoglobulin levels in acute A, B and non-A, non-B hepatitis. Gastroenterology 82: 549–553

5. Prevention

Stanley M. Lemon Jack T. Stapleton

There are three general strategies by which hepatitis A may be prevented. First, because hepatitis A virus (HAV) is generally transmitted by the faecal–oral route, hygienic measures such as the sanitary disposal of human waste and the maintenance of adequate standards for purity of drinking water reduce the risk of HAV infection. These simple lessons have often been learned the hard way by camp directors and military surgeons charged with maintaining the health of fighting forces. On a larger scale, because of the high levels of sanitation achieved in many northern European countries, hepatitis A has become an uncommon disease, occurring mostly in travellers to less developed countries or in certain high-risk groups such as illicit drug users.

As a second general approach, hepatitis A may be prevented by timely administration of normal human immune globulin (NHIG) to those known to be exposed to the virus (*passive immunization*). This has been the mainstay of medical prevention since 1945 (reviewed by Winokur & Stapleton 1991). In certain settings, NHIG may prevent infection with HAV as well as the occurrence of clinical hepatitis A. However, protection is short-lived and requires early recognition of exposure. A third strategy for prevention of hepatitis A is offered by the development of HAV vaccines (*active immunization*). An inactivated HAV vaccine is already available in several European countries, and other inactivated, attenuated or recombinant HAV vaccines are under development (reviewed by Siegl & Lemon 1990).

In contrast to previously available measures, active immunization against HAV should offer many new opportunities for prevention of hepatitis A. Because most cases of hepatitis A occur in individuals who do not have a specific exposure history (Francis et al 1984), passive immunization offers no hope for control of endemic hepatitis A. In contrast, it is likely that endemic hepatitis A could be effectively eliminated with universal active immunization. Because there is no human chronic carrier state and no well-documented animal reservoirs for HAV, the virus may even be eradicated from human populations by such a strategy.

PASSIVE IMMUNIZATION FOR PREVENTION OF HEPATITIS A

History

In 1944, Stokes & Neefe (1945) administered NHIG to residents of a summer camp that was in the midst of an extensive hepatitis outbreak. Three of 53 NHIG recipients (5.7%) compared with 125 of 278 non-immunized controls (45%) developed hepatitis, representing an 87% reduction in the attack rate among NHIG recipients. Shortly thereafter, additional studies of passive immunoprophylaxis demonstrated protection against hepatitis in adults in the Armed Forces, and in children in an institutional setting (Havens & Paul 1945, Gellis et al 1945). These and other early studies of NHIG suffer from the fact that virus-specific serological tests were not available. The viral aetiology of hepatitis cases could not be established, and asymptomatic infections could not be documented. Also, plasma donor screening practices have changed significantly since the time these studies were carried out, and these changes may have implications for the anti-HAV content of NHIG preparations.

Efficacy of NHIG: pre-exposure *vs.* post-exposure prophylaxis

Evidence supports the use of NHIG in either pre-exposure or post-exposure settings, although a higher dose of NHIG may be warranted in pre-exposure situations when a longer period of protection is desired. Because of the limited supply and high cost of NHIG during the 1950s, several attempts were made to define the lowest dose that was effective under post-exposure conditions. Two studies demonstrated that a dose of 0.02 ml/kg was effective in preventing hepatitis when administered during epidemics or to household contacts of patients with hepatitis (Stokes et al 1951, Hsia et al 1954). This has since become accepted practice for post-exposure prophylaxis (Immunization Practices Advisory Committee 1990). Most studies suggest that post-exposure administration of NHIG is only effective if given within the first 2 weeks following exposure. Efficacy is considerably reduced if NHIG is given later in the incubation period, presumably because extensive secondary infection of the liver has already occurred (Lemon 1985).

In 1967, a programme was initiated to assess pre-exposure passive immunoprophylaxis of viral hepatitis among American military personnel assigned to duty in Korea (Cooperative Study 1971). At that time, viral hepatitis was a substantial problem among US soldiers stationed in Korea, although the viruses responsible for this hepatitis were not known. Upon arrival in Korea for a 1-year tour of duty, more than 107 000 soldiers received an intramuscular injection that contained either NHIG (2-, 5- or 10-ml dose) or placebo solution. Administration of as little as 2 ml of NHIG provided protection against clinical hepatitis, although the extent of protection was less than that afforded by 5- or 10-ml doses. A subsequent retrospective serological analysis revealed that the incidence of acute hepatitis A was significantly greater in the placebo group than in the groups that had received any dose of NHIG (Conrad & Lemon 1987). This study thus provided clear evidence for the prevention of hepatitis A by pre-exposure administration of NHIG. While the NHIG used in this study was prepared from a donor pool that was not screened for HBV surface antigen (HBsAg), similar results would be expected with currently available commercial lots of NHIG prepared in the United States. Several additional studies have confirmed the efficacy of NHIG in preexposure prophylaxis of hepatitis A (reviewed by Winokur & Stapleton 1991).

The duration of pre-exposure protection resulting from administration of NHIG appears to be dose related, with a 0.05–0.06 ml/kg dose providing good protection for 4–6 months (Woodson & Clinton 1969, Weiland et al 1981, Conrad & Lemon 1987, Pierce et al 1990). The duration of protection obtained with smaller doses of NHIG is not well defined, but one study found that an NHIG dose of 0.014 ml/kg prevented clinical hepatitis for 3 months (Kluge 1990). It is probably safe to assume that a 0.02 ml/kg dose provides protection for approximately 3 months. Thus, for pre-exposure prophylaxis, the choice between 0.02 or 0.06 ml/kg doses should be based on the length of protection required. For travellers who will be resident in high-risk areas for extended periods of time, repetitive administration of the higher dose of NHIG (0.06 ml/kg) should be considered at intervals of 4–6 months (Immunization Practices Advisory Committee 1990).

Modification of disease *vs.* prevention of infection with NHIG

An important question is whether NHIG prevents HAV infection or merely ameliorates its clinical manifestations, as it does in the case of measles (Janeway 1945). Several studies suggest that when hepatitis occurs despite previous NHIG administration, the illness tends to have its onset within 10 days of the administration of NHIG and may be less severe than in people who have not received NHIG (Stokes & Neefe 1945, Woodson & Clinton 1969, Weiland et al 1981). Two early studies found that the frequency of abnormal liver function tests was virtually identical among NHIG recipients and controls, suggesting that NHIG may not have prevented virus infection at all (Drake & Ming 1954, Schneider & Mosley 1959). The length of protection observed following administration of NHIG led Krugman and co-workers to question whether administration of NHIG may ameliorate the clinical manifestations of hepatitis A, but not prevent infection with the responsible virus (Ward et al 1958). Infection that was clinically inapparent or otherwise modified by administration of NHIG could nonetheless lead to long-standing immunity, a process these authors termed *passive–active immunity*. More recent studies are consistent with this hypothesis, as they suggest that the proportion of HAV infections that are anicteric is increased following administration of NHIG (Lednar et al 1985, Pierce et al 1990). Nevertheless, several studies have demonstrated a very low rate of HAV infection among people receiving NHIG, suggesting that infection is actually prevented. For example, symptomatic seroconversion was rare in Scandinavian soldiers assigned United Nations peace-keeping duties in the Sinai (Weiland et al 1981). Only one of 540 (0.1%) susceptible soldiers acquired serological evidence of HAV infection during the first 5 months of service. In addition, as the protection conferred by NHIG declines over time following its administration, the probability of both overt, clinical hepatitis and subclinical disease increases (Rakela et al 1977, Weiland et al 1981).

While many clinical studies of NHIG have perforce not been well controlled, most evidence suggests that NHIG largely prevents HAV infection when given prior to exposure. However, there are undoubtedly a small number of HAV infections that still occur despite administration of NHIG. In such cases, the critical variables are probably the magnitude of the HAV inoculum, the level of circulating anti-HAV antibody provided by NHIG, and the timing of NHIG administration in relation to virus exposure.

Safety of NHIG

NHIG is prepared by ethanol fractionation of pooled human serum (Cohn et al 1944), and contains IgG at a concentration of approximately 15 g/dl along with trace quantities of IgM, IgA and other serum proteins (Stiehm 1979). Passive immunization with NHIG has proven to be very safe. However, individuals who are IgA deficient or who have received multiple transfusions may rarely experience anaphylactic reasons (Vyas et al. 1968, Ellis & Henney 1969). Although there has been concern about the potential of NHIG to transmit blood-borne viruses, this has happened only on rare occasions. The Cohn ethanol fractionation method effectively excludes HBsAg as well as human immunodeficiency virus (HIV) (Schroeder & Mozen 1970, Mitra et al 1986, Trepo et al 1986, Wells et al 1986). Before the screening of plasma donors for HBsAg, transmission of HBV may have resulted occasionally from administration of NHIG (Tabor & Gerety 1979), perhaps from HBV immune complexes partitioning with the IgG fraction during purification. However, since the institution of HBsAg screening in the early 1970s, there have been no further reports of HBV transmission due to administration of NHIG. In part, this may reflect the presence of significant quantities of HBV-neutralizing antibodies that are now present in current lots of NHIG. There is no evidence that HIV transmission has ever been related to NHIG, and two studies demonstrated that conditions occurring during the preparation of NHIG inactivate this virus (Piszkiewics et al 1985, Wells et al 1986). Transmission of hepatitis C virus (HCV) by NHIG also does not appear to be a problem, although there may be rare exceptions (Ochs et al 1985, Welch et al 1988). In fact, some evidence suggests that NHIG may protect against HCV infection in the setting of multiple transfusions, although this has yet to be confirmed (Knodell et al 1977).

Anti-HAV content of NHIG

Although the immune response to HAV infection is complex and involves both cellular and humoral limbs of the immune system (Lemon et al 1991), it is clear that the efficacy of NHIG is related solely to circulating antibodies of HAV (anti-HAV). At least three primary mechanisms have been proposed for antibody-mediated neutralization of picornaviruses such as HAV (Mosser et al 1989). Neutralizing antibodies can interfere with attachment of virus to a specific cellular receptor, reduce infectivity as a result of aggregation of viral particles, or inhibit uncoating of the virus following attachment of antibody to the capsid. One or more of these mechanisms may contribute to the efficacy of NHIG in the pre-exposure setting. It is less clear how anti-HAV antibodies modify disease in individuals who become infected despite the administration of NHIG. Circulating antibodies probably act by limiting the secondary viraemia that follows initial replication of virus in the liver, and may thereby reduce the extent of secondary hepatic infection (Lemon 1985). There is as yet no evidence for an antibody-dependent mechanism for clearance of virus from infected cells, although such mechanisms certainly exist for other viruses.

Commercial lots of NHIG contain variable concentrations of antibody to HAV (summarized by Winokur & Stapleton 1991). Owing to decreases in the proportion of blood donors who are immune to HAV in many developed countries, concern has been raised that NHIG effectiveness may eventually decline (Stapleton 1992). Thus, some European countries that have a low seroprevalence of antibodies to HAV presently import special lots of NHIG which are designated for use in hepatitis A prophylaxis.

To assist in standardizing the anti-HAV content of NHIG, an international reference reagent for HAV immunoglobulin was developed under the auspices of the World Health Organization (Gerety et al 1983). This reference NHIG preparation has a geometric mean HAV antibody titre of about 1:600 by HAVAB radioimmunoassay (Abbott Laboratories, N. Chicago IL, USA), and a virus-neutralizing antibody titre of approximately 1:800 000 by radioimmunofocus reduction assay (Stapleton et al 1985). One millilitre of this preparation has been assigned the value of 100 international units (IU). This reference reagent has been very useful in comparing NHIG lots, as well as in monitoring the immune response following passive and active immunization.

Minimal protective antibody levels

As described above, antibody to HAV is readily detected in NHIG preparations. However, in people who have received standard doses of NHIG, antibody cannot be detected by standard, commercially available, competitive inhibition immunoassays for anti-HAV, such as HAVAB, which has an anti-HAV detection threshold of approximately 100 mIU/ml (Rakela et al 1977, Stapleton et al 1985). Using the more sensitive radioimmunofocus reduction assay, HAV-neutralizing antibody was evaluated in 18 individuals passively immunized with NHIG in the midst of an HAV outbreak (Stapleton et al 1985) (Fig. 5.1). All sera were negative for HAV antibodies by radioimmunoassay prior to, and 3 and 55 days following, NHIG administration. However, each of the post-immunization samples contained low levels of neutralizing antibodies against HAV (detectable at serum dilutions of 1:10 to 1:40). Subsequent studies suggest that a standard dose of NHIG (0.02 ml per kg body weight) results in a peak serum antibody response of approximately 20 mIU/ml (Ambrosch et al 1991). This level of antibody is within the range of detection by specially modified immunoassays, such as the 'modified HAVAB' test, which measures antibody present in a 10-fold greater volume of serum than usually tested in the standard HAVAB assay (Provost et al 1986).

The minimum levels of neutralizing antibody that are protective against HAV infection and disease are unknown. A very conservative estimate of a minimal protective antibody level would be 10–20 mIU/ml. Such levels are very low, however, and may be difficult to measure reproducibly with solid-phase immunoassays.

Limitations to passive immunization against hepatitis A

Although NHIG has proven to be safe and effective for preventing hepatitis A when given either before or after exposure to virus, timely recognition of exposure is critical to its success. This fact severely limits the value of NHIG for control of hepatitis A, as the majority of endemically acquired cases of hepatitis A have no definitive history of exposure (Francis et al 1984). The usefulness of NHIG is also limited in common source outbreaks of hepatitis A, because

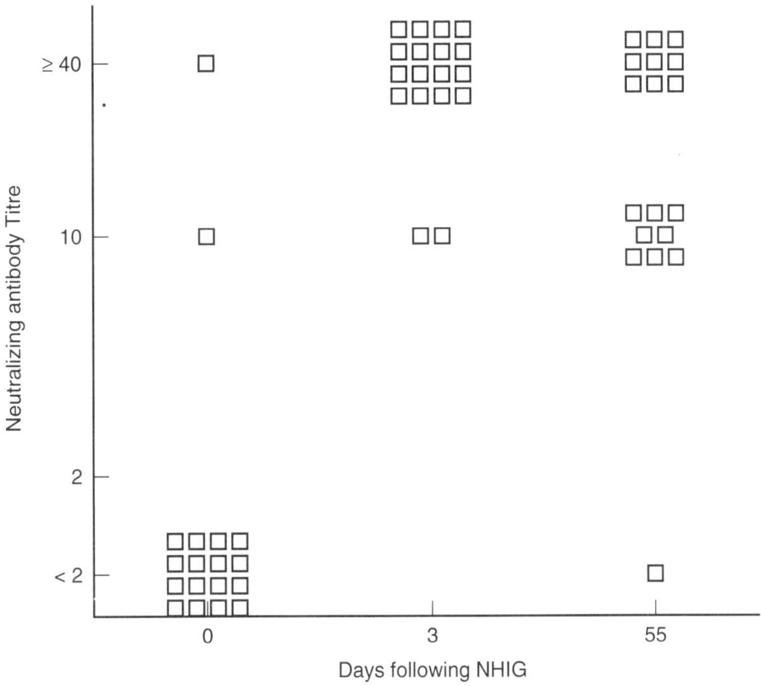

Fig. 5.1 Titres of neutralizing antibody to HAV present in sera collected from 18 individuals prior to (day 0) and 3 and 55 days after administration of NHIG (0.02 ml/kg). (Data from Stapleton et al 1985.)

exposure is usually recognized only late in the incubation period when NHIG is thought to have little protective efficacy (Immunization Practices Advisory Committee 1990). In addition, NHIG has a relatively short duration of action, and the HAV antibody content of future lots of NHIG may decrease as the proportion of HAV-immune individuals continues to decline due to changes in the prevalence of hepatitis A. However, NHIG is inexpensive, safe and highly effective when used properly, and it is likely to remain an important preventive measure for years to come.

Indications for prophylaxis with NHIG

Reasonable indications for administration of NHIG for prevention of hepatitis A have evolved over time and are generally well accepted. Table 5.1 lists those individuals who should be considered candidates for NHIG immunoprophylaxis, under current recommendations of the US Public Health Service (Immunization Practices Advisory Committee 1990).

ACTIVE IMMUNIZATION AGAINST HEPATITIS A VIRUS

History

Unlike passive immunization for hepatitis A, which was developed empirically in the absence of any understanding of the nature of HAV, vaccines capable of inducing active immunity have emerged from several decades of research concerning the pathogenesis of hepatitis A and the physical and biological characteristics of HAV (reviewed by Siegl & Lemon 1990). Several past research advances stand out as having made HAV vaccines possible. These advances include the development of primate models for HAV infection by Dienhardt et al (1975), the identification of the HAV particle by Feinstone et al (1973) and the development of methods for the propagation of HAV in cell cultures by Provost & Hilleman (1979). Provost & Hilleman (1978) were also the first to demonstrate the feasibility of an inactivated HAV vaccine, by purifying and inactivating virus present in the liver of infected

Table 5.1 People who should be considered candidates for NHIG prophylaxis

*Pre-exposure prophylaxis** (0.02 ml/kg for $<$ 3 months, 0.06 ml/kg for $>$ 3 months)
- Travellers to developing countries
- Animal handlers working with newly captured primates

Post-exposure prophylaxis (0.02 ml/kg, much better if $<$ 2 weeks from exposure)
- Close personal (household) contact of hepatitis A case
- Sexual contact with hepatitis A patient
- Children and staff in day-care facilities where HAV infection is documented
- Household contacts of children in nappies in day care if HAV transmission in day-care centre
- Schoolchildren if HAV transmission documented in classroom
- Institutionalized subjects if HAV transmission documented in institution

*Active immunization with inactivated HAV vaccine preferable if available.

marmosets. Although poorly immunogenic, this early HAV vaccine induced anti-HAV antibodies in immunized animals and protected these animals from hepatitis following live virus challenge.

Inactivated HAV vaccines

Active immunization against hepatitis A is now available. A number of inactivated HAV vaccines have been developed by academic research groups, institutes and commercial vaccine manufacturers (Binn et al 1986, Provost et al 1986, Flehmig et al 1989, Andre et al 1990). These vaccines consist of HAV that has been propagated in cell culture, purified to a greater or lesser extent by one of several possible methods and inactivated, usually by exposure to formaldehyde. These inactivated HAV vaccines have often been adsorbed to alum to enhance immunogenicity. The discussion in this chapter will focus on the vaccines produced by two commercial manufacturers, SmithKline Beecham (SKB vaccine, containing the HM175 strain of HAV) (Andre et al 1990) and Merck Sharp & Dohme (MSD vaccine, containing the CR326 virus strain) (Lewis et al 1991), as the greatest amount of information is available concerning these vaccines. These are also the vaccines that are likely to be used most widely within Europe and North America although other inactivated HAV vaccines are likely to be manufactured in Europe. The SKB vaccine has already been licensed in five European countries at the time this manuscript was prepared, while the MSD vaccine was well along in the development process. In addition, a third inactivated vaccine has been developed by the Chemo-Sero-Therapeutic Research Institute of Japan (KRM003 strain), and has undergone preliminary clinical evaluation (Iino et al 1992).

Seed viruses

Because both the HM175 and CR326 virus strains contained within the SKB and MSD vaccines have been adapted to growth in cell culture, they are substantially attenuated in terms of their ability to cause disease in otherwise susceptible primates (see below) (Karron et al 1988, Lewis et al 1991). This provides an additional level of safety with respect to the inactivation process, although there is no evidence that inactivation failures occur if formalin inactivation procedures are carefully followed. Generally, the capsid protein-encoding region of the HAV genome has a low frequency of mutation during cell culture adaptation (Jansen et al 1988), and available data suggest these cell culture-adapted strains remain antigenically indistinguishable from wild-type virus.

Purity

Inactivated vaccines that have undergone clinical trials vary widely in their degree of purity. The prototype Walter Reed Army Institute of Research vaccine, one of the first inactivated HAV vaccines to be administered to humans, was simply a clarified lysate of infected cells (Sjögren et al 1991). In contrast, virus present in the MSD vaccine is greater than 90% purified, as only viral protein bands are identified by silver staining following separation in sodium dodecyl sulphate–polyacrylamide gel electrophoresis (SDS-PAGE) (Lewis et al 1991). Most other vaccines being tested on a worldwide scale probably fall somewhere between these two extremes. Although it makes good sense to use as purified a product as possible, there is no direct evidence that the inclusion of cellular impurities impairs immunogenicity, enhances reactogenicity or reduces safety.

Inactivated HAV vaccines contain both 155S viral particles (complete virions) as well as 70S empty capsids. These 70S particles have been shown to be natural 'empties' containing unprocessed VP0 rather than VP2 (Anderson & Ross 1990), and have antigenicity that is indistinguishable from that of native virus (Ruchti et al 1991). The empty capsids present in inactivated vaccines may represent the majority of the particles, and are an important component of the total antigenic mass.

Inactivation

The inactivation procedures used for manufacture of killed HAV vaccines are largely derived from methods established for manufacture of formalin-inactivated poliovirus vaccines (Lewis et al 1991, Peetermans 1992). HAV shows a typical inactivation profile in the presence of 1:4000 formalin (Fig. 5.2) (Binn et al 1986, Lewis et al 1991). There is an approximate 5 $\log_{10}$ drop in infectivity over a 24-h period at 37°C. Inactivation is carried out for 12–20 days, a length of time extending well beyond the theoretical limit of survival of infectious virus. Under these conditions, viral inactivation has been proven by serial negative blind passages of relatively large quantities of inactivated vaccine in permissive cells (Binn et al 1986). Formalin inactivation of HAV does not significantly alter the antigenicity of the virus.

Viral antigen content

The antigen content of inactivated vaccines is not standardized, nor is it readily determined in terms of absolute protein mass. Comparison of vaccines prepared by different manufacturers is difficult as there is as yet no international antigen reference reagent. The prototype inactivated vaccine developed at the Walter Reed Army Institute of Research probably contained less than 10–20 ng of viral protein per dose, based on

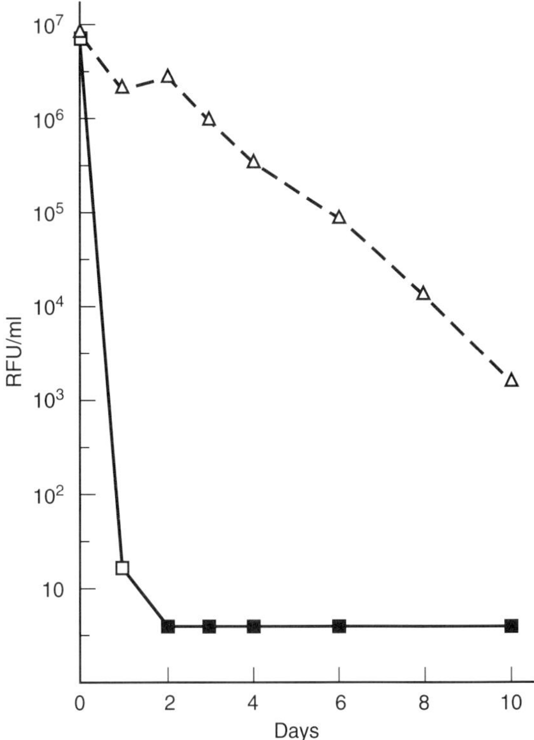

Fig. 5.2 Inactivation of the infectivity of cell culture-propagated HAV in the presence of 1:4000 formalin at 35°C (solid line), compared with non-specific loss of infectivity at the same temperature (dashed line). Solid symbols indicate samples that were negative for infectious virus following three blind cell culture passages. (Data from Binn et al 1986.)

quantitative cDNA–RNA hybridization and an estimate of the proportion of 155S and 70S particles. Even at this low dose, this vaccine was immunogenic following administration of several doses to volunteers (Sjögren et al 1991). The highest dose formulation of the MSD vaccine evaluated in clinical trials was estimated initially to have a viral protein content of 400 ng based on ultraviolet spectroscopy (J Lewis, personal communication). This estimate was subsequently reduced to 25 ng of viral protein following quantitative amino acid analysis of a new, highly purified standard (Ellerbeck et al 1992). Vaccine lots containing equivalent antigenic activity are now considered by the manufacturer to contain 25 'antigen units'. The viral protein content of the SKB vaccine has been quantified similarly in terms of 'ELISA units' established by the manufacturer according to an in-house reference preparation (Peetermans 1992). The highest dose formulation contains 1440 ELISA units. To date, there are no direct comparative data that allow an accurate assessment of the relative antigen content of the SKB and MSD, or any other, inactivated vaccines. An effort is now being taken to develop an international HAV antigen reference reagent, which may help to alleviate this problem.

Adjuvants

The SKB and MSD vaccines are adsorbed to aluminium hydroxide in an effort to enhance antigenicity (Lewis et al 1991, Peetermans 1992). The effect of the adjuvant on the immunogenicity of the inactivated virus is not dramatic, however, and the Japanese KRM003 vaccine is not adsorbed to alum.

Immunogenicity

The immune response to inactivated HAV vaccines has been measured in terms of antibody to HAV. There is no evidence that a human leucocyte antigen class I-restricted, virus-specific T-cell response is stimulated by administration of inactivated HAV vaccine, nor would such a cellular immune response be expected following administration of a non-replicating antigen. Antibodies elicited by inactivated vaccines have been assayed by solid-phase immunoassays or virus neutralization tests (Fig. 5.3). It is possible that neutralization assays provide a more meaningful measure of protective immunity, but available data suggest that antibody detected by any type of assay is predictive of immunity.

The magnitude of the antibody response to inactivated vaccines is proportional to the dose of

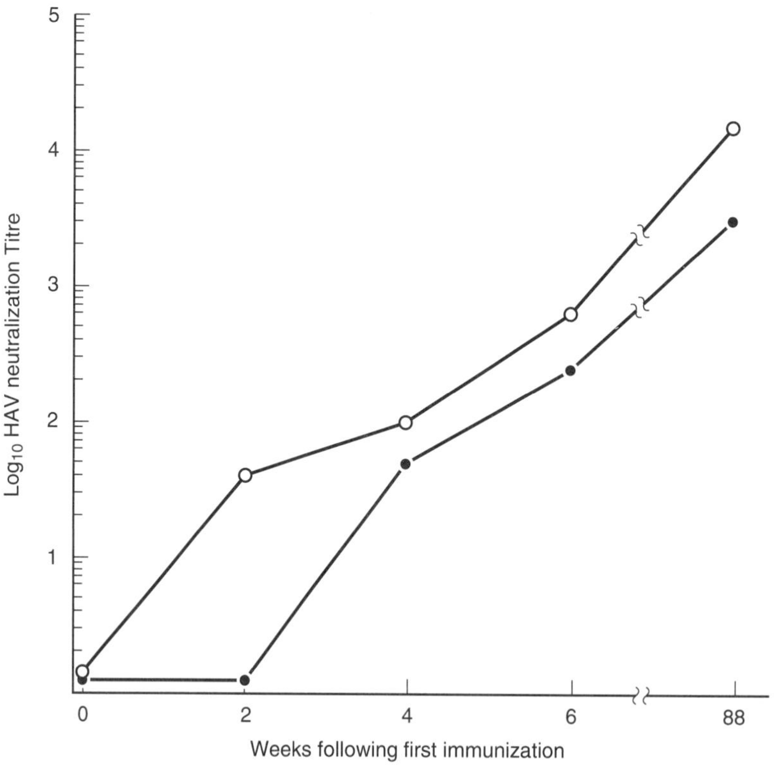

Fig. 5.3 HAV-neutralizing antibody responses in two chimpanzees that were immunized with three doses of the MSD inactivated HAV vaccine given at 0, 4 and 24 weeks (each dose contained approximately six antigen units). Neutralizing antibody was determined by a radioimmunofocus inhibition assay. Compare with data in Figure 5.1. Sera were provided by J. Lewis (see Lewis et al 1991).

antigen administered (Andre et al 1990, Ellerbeck et al 1991, Lewis et al 1991, Kallinowski et al 1992). A single dose of either the MSD or SKB vaccines usually results in seroconversion that is detectable in either modified solid-phase immunoassays or virus neutralization tests. Direct comparisons of the immunogenicity of these two vaccines are not yet available, but there is little to suggest any practical difference in immunogenicity. The levels of antibody obtained with one dose of either vaccine, generally in the range of 40 to 350 mIU/ml, are significantly in excess of the level conferred by passive administration of immune serum globulin, and thus likely to be protective. The same may be said for the Japanese KRM003 vaccine (Iino et al 1992). Indeed, the protective effect of these low levels of antibody have been demonstrated in a recent efficacy trial of the MSD vaccine (see below).

Primary immunization has been achieved with two doses given at 0 and 2 weeks, 0 and 4 weeks, and 0 and 8 weeks, as well as with a single dose of inactivated HAV vaccine (Werzberger et al 1992). Booster responses occur with subsequent doses of inactivated vaccine (Ellerbeck et al 1992, Iino et al 1992, Kallinowski et al 1992). Late booster doses given at 6–12 months following primary immunization result in substantial titres of anti-HAV, ranging from 1000 to 10 000 mIU/ml and even higher. These antibody levels are readily detectable in conventional commercial immunoassays such as the standard HAVAB and are likely to persist for 5–10 years, or longer (Ambrosch et al 1991). Further studies are required to optimally define the dosage and schedule for inactivated HAV vaccine. It may be that two doses of vaccine will be sufficient for protection in most individuals.

Preliminary data suggest that the immunogenicity of the MSD vaccine may be lower in males who weigh more than 86 kg (D Nalin, personal communication). Such data suggest that the deposition of vaccine into adipose tissue may be detrimental to immunogenicity, as observed previously with hepatitis B vaccine.

It is important to note that even the most substantial antibody response to inactivated HAV vaccine is well below the response which follows infection with wild-type virus (Fig. 5.4). Although this difference in the concentration of serum antibody to HAV is unlikely to be of significance in terms of protection against hepatitis A in the first few years after immunization, additional experience with these vaccines will be required before we know whether the lower level immunization responses reflect a similarly lower level of immunological memory and shorter terms of immunity.

Reactogenicity

The reactogenicity of inactivated HAV vaccines is generally very low, and similar to that of recombinant or plasma-derived hepatitis B vaccines. The most common adverse effects of vaccine administration are local tenderness and pain at the injection site (Andre et al 1990, Ellerbeck et al 1991, 1992, Kallinowski et al 1992). These complaints are generally minimal, of short duration and occur at a frequency similar to that seen with other alum-adsorbed vaccines (25–60% with the first dose, and generally decreasing with subsequent doses). Significant systemic complaints are very rare. Low-grade fever has been noted in less than 1–4% of recipients of inactivated HAV vaccine.

Efficacy of inactivated vaccines

The more immunogenic of the inactivated HAV vaccines were predicted to be capable of eliciting a protective antibody response following administration of a single dose, as the levels of antibodies induced by these vaccines exceeded those observed following administration of protective doses of NHIG (see above). This conjecture has since been proven in a double-blind, randomized field trial documenting the clinical efficacy of the MSD vaccine (Werzberger et al 1992). The first efficacy trial of an inactivated vaccine to be completed, this study involved the administration of the MSD vaccine to a cohort of children living within a Hassidic Jewish community in Monroe County in lower New York state, where hepatitis A had been a common and persistent problem among children of school age. The 1037 children enrolled in this randomized, placebo-controlled

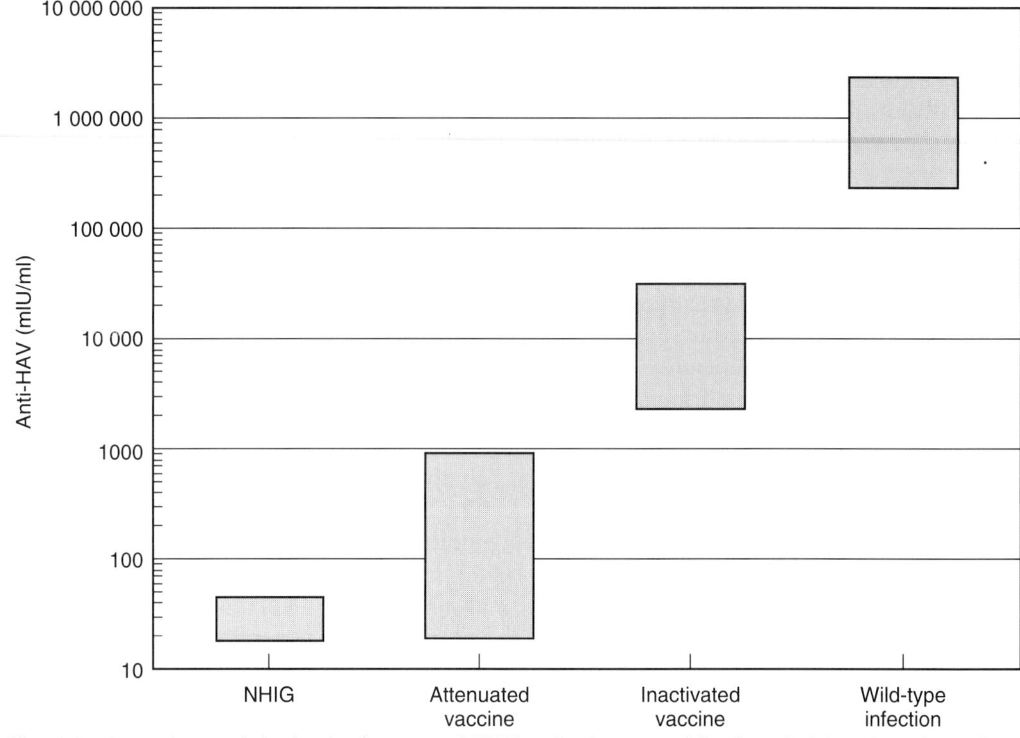

Fig. 5.4 Approximate relative levels of serum anti-HAV antibody present following administration of NHIG inactivated and attenuated HAV vaccines, or natural HAV infection. (From Lemon 1992.)

study were between the ages of 2 and 16. The vaccine used in the trial contained 25 units of viral antigen per dose (see above); each child received a single dose. A substantial epidemic of hepatitis A occurred among the children of this community shortly after the study commenced.

A very high level of protection was noted among immunized children in the Monroe trial (Fig. 5.5). In fact, protection against clinical disease was complete within 3 weeks of administration of a single dose of the vaccine (the lower 95% confidence limit for clinical efficacy 50 days after vaccine administration was 88%) (Werzberger et al 1992). Among those children who did in fact become ill within 18 days of administration of the vaccine, there was no evidence that either the risk or severity of hepatitis A was enhanced. Serological evaluation of a subset of the immunized children who did not become ill demonstrated the presence of antibody in 99%, with a geometric mean titre of 42 mIU/ml (Werzberger et al 1992). Continued observation of this cohort of children will document the antibody response to booster doses of vaccine given at several different intervals after the primary injection and, hopefully, the long-term persistence of antibody and protective immunity.

A field trial evaluating the efficacy of the SKB vaccine in children of school age has also been under way in Thailand (B Innis, personal communication). This study is larger than the Monroe trial, involving approximately 20 000 children in each of the vaccine and placebo control arms. The immunization schedule was three doses of the SKB vaccine, 360 ELISA units of antigen each, given at months 0, 1 and 12. Primary immunization was with two vaccine doses, so that the efficacy of a single dose of vaccine could not be evaluated in this trial. Nevertheless, a determination of the rates of hepatitis between the second and third vaccine doses has shown that administration of the SKB vaccine also results in virtually complete protection against symptomatic hepatitis A. When efficacy was

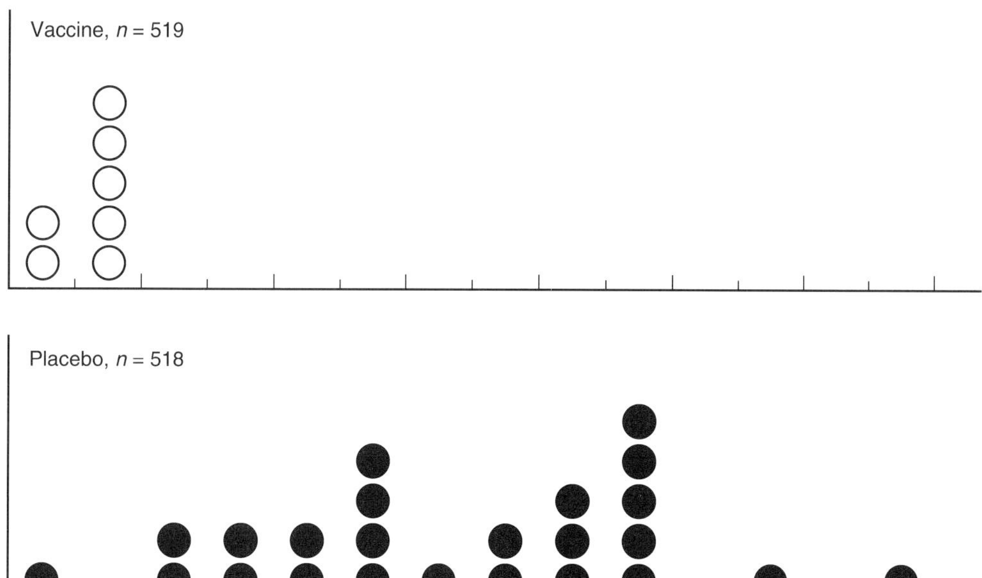

Fig. 5.5 The Monroe, NY, trial of the MSD inactivated HAV vaccine. Each symbol represents a case of clinically evident hepatitis A, grouped according to the interval between administration of the vaccine (single dose at day ○) or placebo and onset of symptoms. (Data from Werzberger et al 1992.)

assessed beginning approximately 5 months following the first vaccine dose, the 95% confidence limits for protective efficacy were 75–99%. In addition, the Thai study provided convincing evidence that vaccine administration prevents subclinical infections as well as symptomatic hepatitis A (B Innis, personal communication).

These two clinical studies demonstrated similar efficacy of the MSD and SKB inactivated vaccines in children who were immunized under somewhat different circumstances. Although two late cases of hepatitis A were observed in children immunized with the SKB vaccine, these cases were mild, symptoms lasted only a few days and ALT elevations were minimal (B Innis, personal communication). A small number of clinical breakthroughs is not unexpected given the very large size of the Thai study population and the inherent power of the study. Thus, the occurrence of these cases in children immunized with the SKB vaccine does not necessarily indicate a difference in the efficacy of the two vaccines.

It is very likely that similar levels of clinical protection would be found in adults immunized with either vaccine, provided that levels of antibodies induced in adults are similar to those found in children following immunization. In fact, these two clinical trials are so convincing that further field trials to document the efficacy of other inactivated HAV vaccines are probably not necessary. Efficacy could be established by analysis of the levels of anti-HAV antibodies induced, and a comparison of these levels with those obtained following administration of either the MSD or SKB vaccine. Modified immunoassays and quantitative measures of HAV-neutralizing activity are well suited to this task.

No significant antigenic variation has yet been found among strains of HAV recovered from humans (Lemon et al 1991). Thus, the available data suggest that inactivated HAV vaccines derived from either the CR326 or HM175 virus strain, or for that matter any other human HAV strain, will provide protection against human

HAV strains circulating anywhere in the world.

Unlike inactivated poliovirus vaccines, which have a limited impact on transmission of poliovirus due to poor induction of secretory IgA antibodies to the virus, inactivated HAV vaccines are likely to have a major effect on transmission. It is worth noting that infection with wild-type HAV does not regularly induce detectable levels of secretory neutralizing antibodies to the virus (Stapleton et al 1991). Secretory immunity thus does not appear to be important in prevention of disease. As faecal shedding of virus is due largely or exclusively to virus replicated within the liver, levels of circulating antibodies that are capable of preventing infection of the liver will sharply reduce or eliminate virus shedding. Older studies with NHIG as well as preliminary observations with the SKB vaccine (B Innis, personal communication) suggest that inactivated vaccines will not only protect against disease but also prevent inapparent infection. If so, faecal shedding of virus and virus transmission should be similarly reduced.

Remaining problems

Despite the dramatic success of inactivated HAV vaccines, important questions remain. The first of these is the cost of production and safety testing of inactivated vaccines. While this is likely to be reduced by large-scale purchases from manufacturers, widespread use of the vaccine in other than very high-risk individuals cannot be anticipated at the present cost (approximately US$27.00 for one dose of the SKB vaccine). Additionally, the length of protection conferred by these vaccines remains unknown. While this can be predicted from the observed rate of decay of anti-HAV antibodies in immunized individuals (Ambrosch et al 1991), it will be difficult to determine the protective benefits conferred by immunological memory following administration of a full course of inactivated vaccine. Such protection may extend well beyond the period when antibody is measurably present. However, studies determining the extent of immunological memory are likely to take years to complete, if in fact they are ever accomplished. Until such time, there will be doubts about the wisdom of using these vaccines in regions where hepatitis A infection is currently occurring in very young individuals, and is not at present associated with a great deal of disease (Kane 1990).

The findings of the Monroe study suggest that a single dose of the MSD vaccine might be capable of providing protection to overseas travellers within several weeks of administration (Werzberger et al 1992). This raises questions concerning whether a single dose of vaccine could be used in lieu of NHIG for pre-exposure prophylaxis of travellers, or whether vaccine might actually provide effective post-exposure prophylaxis. The latter seems very unlikely unless vaccine is given almost immediately after exposure, but there is a need to carefully examine the administration of a combination of NHIG and vaccine where both immediate and lasting protection is desired. Preliminary data suggest that very large doses of NHIG may reduce the immunogenicity of simultaneously administered vaccine, but this requires confirmation.

Attenuated HAV vaccines

An attenuated HAV vaccine may have several advantages over inactivated vaccines, including cost, the need for only a single dose and perhaps the induction of longer lasting immunity. Several candidate attenuated vaccines have been developed. Attenuated variants of both the CR326 and HM175 strains of HAV have undergone testing in primates as well as limited clinical trials (Karron et al 1988, Midthun et al 1991), while an attenuated H2 strain vaccine has been administered to a large number of children and adults in China (Mao et al 1989). However, only very limited data have been published concerning the attenuation properties of the H2 strain.

Mechanism of attenuation

Each of these candidate attenuated HAV vaccine strains has been derived by passage in cell culture, at either 37°C or at lower temperatures. The molecular basis for their attenuation phenotype remains inadequately explained, but it is associated with a reduced capacity for replication in otherwise susceptible primates. Molecular studies of the attenuation phenotype are limited to the HM175 strain. Comparisons of the genomic sequences of wild-type and attenuated, cell culture-adapted variants of the HM175 strain indicate that mutations are particularly likely to accumulate in the 5' untranslated (5'-UTR) and P2 (proteins 2B and 2C) regions of the genome during adaptation of the virus to growth in cell culture (Cohen et al 1987, Jansen et al 1988). These mutations have been shown to be responsible for the growth properties of cell culture-adapted viruses (Day et al 1992, Emerson et al 1992). The mutations responsible for attenuation of the HM175 variant appear to be confined to the P2 and P3 regions of the genome (Cohen et al 1989). However, the data do not completely exclude a role for the 5'-UTR mutations in determining the attenuation phenotype. Notably, mutations within the 5'-UTR play an important role in the attenuation of multiple other picornaviruses, in some cases through induced alterations in the virus-specific translation mechanism.

Virological events during infection with attenuated variants

One of the first wild-type traits to be lost by HAV during its adaptation to growth in cell culture is the ability to infect primates by oral challenge. No credible explanation has yet been offered for this observation, but cell culture-adapted vaccine candidates must thus be administered by parenteral injection.

The replication of attenuated viruses in chimpanzees or humans is severely limited and may be difficult to demonstrate at all. With more highly passaged CR326 variants, there is no evidence for replication of the virus in primates even after parenteral inoculation of substantial titres of virus (Provost et al 1982). In contrast, with less highly passaged candidate viruses, varying degrees of replication competence have been noted in primates, at times with elevations of liver enzymes (Provost et al 1982). Primate studies with attenuated variants of the CR326 (CR326/F') and HM175 strains indicate that limited faecal shedding of virus follows inoculation (Provost et al 1986, Karron et al 1988). Similarly, faecal shedding of the attenuated H2 vaccine virus has been documented in immunized humans (Mao et al 1989).

Immunogenicity

Antibody responses to attenuated viruses are typically delayed in comparison to those that follow infection with wild-type virus, and are usually relatively meagre. Infection of human volunteers with a 10^7 $TCID_{50}$ dose of the attenuated CR326/F' vaccine candidate results in a low-level antibody response (less than 1000 mIU/ml 6 months after infection) (Midthun et al 1991). This level is higher than that induced by a single dose of inactivated vaccine, but much lower than that found in most recipients of a full course of inactivated HAV vaccine (see above) (Fig. 5.4). However, it is likely that administration of an attenuated HAV vaccine that replicates in human hosts would lead to induction of class I-restricted cytotoxic T-cell responses (Maier et al 1988, Vallbracht et al 1989) as well as circulating antibodies. Such T-cell responses may be equally or perhaps even more important than the antibody response in determining the extent of protective immunity, but data that address this issue are not available.

Although other attenuated HAV vaccines have undergone extensive testing in China, only limited information is available concerning the degree of attenuation of these vaccine candidates and the levels of antibodies these viruses induce. However, the available data suggest that the Chinese H2 vaccine candidate might be somewhat less attenuated than the CR326/F' vaccine virus (greater faecal shedding), and capable of inducing higher antibody levels (Mao et al 1989).

Reactogenicity of attenuated vaccines

With respect to reactogenicity, the major concern with attenuated HAV vaccines is the development of mild hepatitis following administration. In early studies carried out in primates, this occurred more often with candidate vaccine viruses that had undergone a lower number of passages in cell culture (Provost et al 1982). However, it is likely that low-level enzyme elevations in the absence of symptoms are of no clinical significance. Moreover, significant hepatotoxicity was not described in clinical trials of either the attenuated CR326/F' vaccine carried out in adults or of the H2 vaccine conducted in children in China (Mao et al 1989, Midthun et al 1991). Other manifestations of reactogenicity were minimal. A second major safety concern with any attenuated vaccine virus is the potential for reversion of the virus to virulence. HAV is an RNA virus, and thus prone to a high frequency of mutation during replication of its genome. However, available evidence suggests that cell culture-adapted viruses have a stable attenuation phenotype when passaged up to three times in primates (Provost et al 1986, 1991). The inability of cell culture-passaged virus to establish infection via oral challenge would represent an important safety feature, if it is shown that this phenotypic trait is also preserved following passage in humans.

Efficacy

Both the CR326/F' and H2 attenuated vaccines are capable of eliciting levels of antibody that should be protective in immunized subjects (Mao et al 1989, Midthun et al 1991) (see above). A brief report from China indicates that the H2 vaccine, administered to school-age children in the face of epidemic disease, is capable of conferring clinical protection (Mao et al 1991). The CR326/F' and HM175 vaccine candidates have not been evaluated for efficacy in humans, but both are able to protect immunized primates against challenge with virulent virus (Provost et al 1986, Karron et al 1988).

Remaining problems

While the development of attenuated HAV vaccines appears to be continuing in China, commercial efforts in this direction have been largely halted in the developed countries of the West because of the imminent availability of inactivated vaccines. As mentioned above, attenuated vaccines have a number of potential advantages over inactivated vaccines, and may be the only type of vaccine that would make widespread use feasible in underdeveloped countries where hepatitis A is endemic. However, concerns over relatively poor immunogenicity or potential for induction of mild hepatitis with the candidate vaccines now under evaluation suggest a need to develop alternative approaches to attenuation of HAV.

Alternative approaches to vaccine development

Recombinant protein and synthetic peptide vaccines

A considerable body of experimental data attests to the fact that the major neutralization epitopes present on the surface of the HAV particle are conformationally defined (reviewed by Lemon et al 1991). Isolated, purified capsid proteins have a very limited ability to induce neutralizing antibodies in small animals. Furthermore, monoclonal neutralizing antibodies to HAV do not recognize HAV capsid proteins in immunoblot assays. Careful analysis of mutant HAVs that have been selected for their ability to escape neutralization by monoclonal antibodies has resulted in the identification of a number of amino acid residues within the capsid proteins which are involved in forming neutralization epitopes (Ping & Lemon 1992). The results of these studies suggest that both VP3 and VP1 contribute to a major antigenic site that is composed of several distinct neutralization epitopes. It is likely that the native antigenicity of the virus is thus dependent upon higher ordered structures, including quaternary interactions between individual capsid proteins. For this reason, with a notable exception described in the next section, attempts to produce a recombinant HAV vaccine have been generally unsuccessful. Although a recent report suggests that unprocessed protein expressed from cDNA representing part of the capsid proteins of HAV is capable of inducing significant titres of HAV antibodies in marmosets (Karayiannis et al 1991), this report stands in contrast to results obtained in several other laboratories and has yet to be confirmed (Grace et al 1991, Winokur et al 1991). Recombinant proteins have generally failed to induce neutralizing antibodies, although VP1, VP2 and VP3 may prime the rabbit immune system to respond to subsequent sub-immunogenic doses of intact HAV (Ostermayr et al 1987, Gauss-Muller et al 1990, Powdrill & Johnston 1991).

Experimental recombinant HAV particle-based vaccines

Since the neutralization epitopes of HAV are assembled, conformationally defined structures, attempts have been made to express the capsid proteins of HAV in either baculovirus or vaccinia virus eukaryotic expression systems under conditions favouring the processing and assembly of these proteins into antigenic capsids (Gao et al 1989, Stapleton et al 1991, Winokur et al 1991). The vaccinia-expressed HAV polyprotein has been shown to undergo processing into individual capsid proteins, and to assemble into empty capsids and pentameric structures (a subunit in virus assembly containing five copies of each of the capsid proteins), which are specifically recognized by HAV monoclonal or polyclonal antibodies (Gao et al 1989, Winokur et al 1991). When the structural precursor protein (P1) was expressed by vaccinia virus in the absence of the viral protease ($3C^{pro}$), it did not undergo processing or assembly, and was not antigenic when evaluated by polyclonal- or monoclonal-based solid-phase radioimmunoassays (Winokur et al 1991). Purified HAV particles expressed by baculovirus elicited neutralizing antibodies in mice, as did infection of mice with recombinant vaccinia viruses expressing the entire polyprotein. Thus, the assembly of antigenic empty particles in cells infected with recombinant vaccinia virus represents an alternative approach to cell culture production of a non-infectious HAV vaccine, although substantial questions remain concerning the cost and stability of such an immunogen. Alternatively, recombinant vaccinia strains might be capable of inducing immunity when administered directly to humans as live vector vaccines.

The 'Jennerian' approach

Several unique HAV strains have been recovered recently from naturally infected Old World monkeys (Nainan et al 1991, Tsarev et al 1991). These simian strains of HAV differ significantly from human HAV strains both in nucleotide sequence and in antigenicity. While reactive with polyclonal antibody, these strains do not bind some monoclonal antibodies raised against human HAV strains and moreover have amino acid substitutions at critical capsid protein amino acid residues that contribute to putative antibody binding sites on the virus surface. Recent evidence suggests that these simian strains do not cause liver disease in inoculated chimpanzees, but may induce protective immunity against subsequent challenge with human HAV. These observations have suggested the possibility that such simian HAVs might serve as 'Jennerian' vaccines (Purcell 1991).

WHO SHOULD RECEIVE HAV VACCINES?

Given the likelihood that safe and effective, inactivated HAV vaccines will soon be widely available, there is a need to carefully formulate strategies for the optimal utilization of these products. The simple answer to this question is to consider immunization of individuals shown to be at increased risk of acquiring HAV infection. Such people include travellers (both civilian and military) from well-developed countries to lesser developed regions, young children attending day-care centres and the staff supervising these centres, homosexually active men, users of illicit drugs and individuals held in penal or other institutions where the risk of HAV transmission may be increased. In addition, immunization of food handlers would seem well worthwhile, as it should prevent the possibility of food-borne, common-source outbreaks of hepatitis A. It is likely, however, that such a targeted immunization strategy would have a minimal impact on the overall incidence of hepatitis A, as the majority of infected subjects do not fall into any of these high-risk groups (Francis et al 1984). We do not know whether the vaccine will be able to replace the use of NHIG in household or other close personal contacts of people with hepatitis A, but this seems an unlikely possibility at present. Such subjects actually constitute the largest identified risk group for hepatitis A.

Recent experience with the hepatitis B vaccine

in the United States has demonstrated the ineffectiveness of immunization strategies that are targeted at high-risk groups (AAP Committee on Infectious Diseases 1992). The failure of targeted hepatitis B immunization to reduce the incidence of this disease stems from the inability to both recognize and deliver vaccine to those at risk. It is very likely that the situation would be much the same with hepatitis A, and that general childhood immunization will be required for effective control of this disease. Whether or not such a strategy is adopted in any particular country will be dependent upon increasing confidence in the safety and efficacy of these vaccines (which is likely to follow their initial use in high-risk groups), the incidence of hepatitis A and the magnitude of its perceived threat to the general health and well-being of society, the cost of the vaccine and the resources available to national immunization authorities. At present, in view of the cost of the vaccine, it is unlikely that general childhood immunization will be recommended by any national authority.

As suggested above, the finding of anti-HAV in a person considered at risk for hepatitis A would indicate previous infection, solid immunity and the absence of a need for immunization. However, whether or not preimmunization antibody screening will represent a useful and cost-effective strategy will depend upon the cost of the antibody test, the cost of vaccine, and the expected prevalence of antibody in the specific population under consideration. Formal cost–benefit analyses, of the type done previously for antibody screening in hepatitis B immunization programmes (Mulley et al 1982), have yet to be reported for hepatitis A. However, it is likely that preimmunization antibody testing might be cost-effective in some high-risk groups.

ACKNOWLEDGEMENTS

The authors are indebted to Bruce Innis, David Nalin, John Lewis and Francis Andre for helpful discussions and/or for providing information in advance of publication. The authors are supported in part by grants from the US Army Medical Research and Development Command (DAMD 17-89-Z-9022) (SML), Merck & Co. (SML) and SmithKline Beecham (JTS).

REFERENCES

AAP Committee on Infectious Diseases 1992 Universal hepatitis B immunization. Pediatrics 89: 795

Ambrosch F, Widermann G, Andre F E, D'Hondt E, Delem A, Safary A 1991 Comparison of HAV antibodies induced by vaccination, passive immunization, and natural infection. In Hollinger F B, Lemon S M, Margolis H S (eds) Viral hepatitis and liver disease. Williams & Wilkins, Baltimore, p 98

Anderson D A, Ross B C 1990 Morphogenesis of hepatitis A virus: isolation and characterization of subviral particles. Journal of Virology 64: 5284

Andre F E, Hepburn A, D'Hondt E 1990 Inactivated candidate vaccines for hepatitis A. Progress in Medical Virology 37: 72

Binn L N, Bancroft W H, Lemon S M et al 1986 Preparation of a prototype inactivated hepatitis A virus vaccine from infected cell cultures. The Journal of Infectious Diseases 153: 749

Cohen J I, Rosenblum B, Ticehurst J R, Daemer R J, Feinstone S M, Purcell R H 1987 Complete nucleotide sequence of an attenuated hepatitis A virus: comparison with wild-type virus. Proceedings of the National Academy of Sciences of the USA 84: 2497

Cohen J I, Rosenblum B, Feinstone S M, Ticehurst J, Purcell R H 1989 Attenuation and cell culture adaptation of hepatitis A virus (HAV): a genetic analysis with HAV cDNA. Journal of Virology 63: 5364

Cohen E J, Oncley J L, Strong L E, Hughes W L, Armstrong S H 1944 Chemical, clinical, and immunological studies on the products of human plasma fractionation. Journal of Clinical Investigation 23: 417

Conrad M E, Lemon S M 1987 Prevention of endemic icteric viral hepatitis by administration of immune serum gamma globulin. The Journal of Infectious Disease 156: 56

Cooperative Study 1971 Prophylactic gamma globulin for prevention of endemic hepatitis. Archives of Internal Medicine 128: 723

Day S P, Murphy P, Brown E A, Lemon S M 1992 Mutations within the 5' nontranslated region of hepatitis A virus RNA which enhance replication in BS-C-1 cells. Journal of Virology 66: 6533–6540

Deinhardt F, Peterson D, Cross G, Wolfe L, Holmes A W 1975 Hepatitis in marmosets. American Journal of the Medical Sciences 270: 73

Drake M E, Ming C 1954 Gamma globulin in epidemic hepatitis comparative value of two dosage levels, apparently

near the minimal effective level. Journal of the American Medical Association 155: 1302
Edgar W M, Campbell A D 1985 Nosocomial infection with hepatitis A. The Journal of Infectious Diseases 10: 43
Ellerbeck E, Lewis J, Midthun K et al 1991 Safety and immunogenicity of an inactivated hepatitis A virus vaccine. In Hollinger F B, Lemon S M, Margolis H S (eds) Viral hepatitis and liver disease. Williams & Wilkins, Baltimore, p 91
Ellerbeck E F, Lewis J A, Nalin D et al 1992 Safety profile and immunogenicity of an inactivated vaccine derived from an attenuated strain of hepatitis A virus. Vaccine 10 (10): 668–672
Ellis E F, Henney C S 1969 Adverse reactions following administration of human gamma globulin. Journal of Allergy 43: 45
Emerson S U, Huang Y K, McRill C, Lewis M, Purcell R H 1992 Mutations in both the 2B and 2C genes of hepatitis A virus are involved in adaptation to growth in cell culture. Journal of Virology 66: 650
Feinstone S M, Kapikian A Z, Purcell R H 1973 Hepatitis A: detection by immune electron microscopy of a viruslike antigen associated with acute illness. Science 182: 1026
Flehmig B, Heinricy U, Pfisterer M 1989 Immunogenicity of a killed hepatitis A vaccine in seronegative volunteers. Lancet i: 1039
Francis D P, Hadler S C, Prendergast T J et al 1984 Occurrence of hepatitis A, B, and non-A/non-B in the United States: CDC Sentinel County hepatitis study I. American Journal of Medicine 76: 69
Gao F, Liu C, Yi Y, Ruan L, Zhu J 1989 Expression of hepatitis A virus proteins by recombinant vaccinia virus. Chinese Journal of Virology 5: 303
Gauss-Muller V, Zhou M Q, von der Helm K, Deinhardt F 1990 Recombinant proteins VP1 and VP3 of hepatitis A virus prime for neutralizing response. Journal of Medical Virology 31: 277
Gellis S S, Stokes Jr, J., Brother G M et al 1945 The use of human immune serum globulin (gamma globulin). Journal of the American Medical Association 128: 1062
Gerety R J, Smallwood L A, Finlayson J S, Tabor E 1983 Standardization of the antibody to hepatitis A virus (anti-HAV) content of immunoglobulin. Developments in Biological Standardization 54: 411
Grace K, Amphlett E, Day S et al 1991 In vitro translation of hepatitis A virus subgenomic RNA transcripts. Journal of General Virology 72: 1081
Havens W P, Paul J R 1945 Prevention of infectious hepatitis with gamma globulin. Journal of the American Medical Association 129: 270
Hsia D Y, Lonsway M, Gellis S S 1954 Gamma globulin in the prevention of infectious hepatitis. Studies on the use of small doses in family outbreaks. New England Journal of Medicine 250: 417
Iino S, Fujiyama S, Horiuchi K et al 1992 Clinical trial of a lyophilized inactivated hepatitis A candidate vaccine in healthy adult volunteers. Vaccine 10: 323
Immunization Practices Advisory Committee 1990 Protection against viral hepatitis. Morbidity and Mortality Weekly Report 39 (No. RR-2)
Janeway C A 1945 Use of concentrated human serum gamma globulin in the prevention and attenuation of measles. Bulletin of the New York Academy of Sciences 21: 202
Jansen R W, Newbold J E, Lemon S M 1988 Complete nucleotide sequence of a cell culture-adapted variant of hepatitis A virus: comparison with wild-type virus with restricted capacity for in vitro replication. Virology 163: 299
Kallinowski B, Gmelin K, Kommerell B et al 1992 Immunogenicity, reactogenicity and consistency of a new, inactivated hepatitis A vaccine – a randomized multicentre trial with three consecutive vaccine lots. Vaccine 10: 500
Kane M A 1990 Prospects for the introduction of hepatitis A vaccine into public health use. Progress in Medical Virology 37: 96
Karayiannis P, O'Rourke S, McGarvey M J et al 1991 A recombinant vaccinia virus expressing hepatitis A virus structural polypeptides: characterization and demonstration of protective immunogenicity. Journal of General Virology 72: 2167
Karron R A, Daemer R J, Ticehurst J R et al 1988 Studies of prototype live hepatitis A virus vaccine in primate models. Journal of Infectious Diseases 157: 338
Kluge T. Gamma-globulin in the prevention of viral hepatitis. A study on the effect of medium-size doses. Acta Medica Scandinavica, 1990: 174: 469–477
Knodell R G, Conrad M E, Ishak K G 1977 Development of chronic liver disease after acute non-A, non-B post-transfusion hepatitis: role of [γ]-globulin prophylaxis in its prevention. Gastroenterology 72: 902
Lednar W M, Lemon S M, Kirkpatrick J W et al 1985 Frequency of illness associated with epidemc hepatitis A virus infections in adults. American Journal of Epidemiology 122: 226
Lemon S M 1985 Type A viral hepatitis: new developments in an old disease. New England Journal of Medicine 313: 1059
Lemon S M 1992 Immunological approaches to assessing the response to inactivated hepatitis A vaccine. European Journal of Hepatology (suppl.)
Lemon S M, Ping L-H, Day S et al 1991 Immunobiology of hepatitis A virus. In Hollinger F B, Lemon S M, Margolis H S (eds) Viral hepatitis and liver disease. Williams & Wilkins, Baltimore, p 20
Lewis J A, Armstrong M E, Larson V M et al 1991 Use of a live attenuated hepatitis A vaccine to prepare a highly purified, formalin-inactivated hepatitis A vaccine. In Hollinger F B, Lemon S M, Margolis H S (eds) Viral hepatitis and liver disease. Williams & Wilkins, Baltimore, p 94
Maier K, Gabriel P, Koscielniak E et al 1988 Human gamma interferon production by cytotoxic T lymphocytes sensitized during hepatitis A virus infection. Journal of Virology 62: 3756
Mao J S, Dong D X, Zhang H Y et al 1989 Primary study of attenuated live hepatitis A vaccine (H2 strain) in humans. The Journal of Infectious Diseases 159: 621
Mao J S, Dong D X, Zhang S Y et al 1991 Further studies of attenuated live hepatitis A vaccine (H2 strain) in humans. In: Hollinger F B, Lemon S M, Margolis H S (eds) Viral hepatitis and liver disease. Williams & Wilkins, Baltimore, p 110
Midthun K, Ellerbeck E, Gershman K et al 1991 Safety and immunogenicity of a live attenuated hepatitis A virus vaccine in seronegative volunteers. The Journal of Infectious Diseases 163: 735
Mitra G, Wong M F, Mozen M M, McDougal J S, Levy J A 1986 Elimination of infectious retroviruses during preparation of immunoglobulins. Transfusion 26: 394
Mosser A G, Leippe D M Rueckert R R 1989 Neutralization

of Picornaviruses: Support for the Pentamer Bridging Hypothesis. In Semler B L Ehrenfeld E (eds) Molecular aspects of picornavirus infection and detection. American Society of Microbiology, Washington, p 155

Mulley A G, Silverstein M D, Dienstag J L 1982 Indications for use of hepatitis B vaccine, based on cost effectiveness analysis. New England Journal of Medicine 307: 644

Nainan O V, Margolis H S, Robertson B H, Balayan M, Brinton M A 1991 Sequence analysis of a new hepatitis A virus naturally infecting cynomolgus macaques (*Macaca fascicularis*). Journal of General Virology 72: 1685

Ochs H D, Fischer s H, Virant F S, Lee M L, Kingdom H S, Wedgwood R J 1985 Non-A, non-B hepatitis and intravenous immunoglobulin. Lancet i: 404

Ostermayr R, von der Helm K, Gauss-Muller V, Winnacker E L, Deinhardt F 1987 Expression of hepatitis A virus cDNA in *Escherichia coli*: antigenic VP1 recombinant protein. Journal of Virology 61: 3645

Peetermans J 1992 Production, quality control and characterization of an inactivated hepatitis A vaccine. Vaccine (suppl.) 1: S99–101

Pierce P F, Cappello M, Bernard K W 1990 Subclinical infection with hepatitis A in Peace Corps volunteers following immune globulin prophylaxis. American Journal of Tropical Medicine and Hygeine 42: 465

Ping L-H, Lemon S M 1992 Antigenic structure of human hepatitis A virus defined by analysis of escape mutants selected against murine monoclonal antibodies. Journal of Virology 66: 2208

Piszkiewicz D, Kingdom H, Apfelzweig R et al 1985 Inactivation of HTLV-III/LAV during plasma fractionation. Lancet ii: 1188

Powdrill T F, Johnston J M 1991 Immunologic priming with recombinant hepatitis A virus proteins produced in *E. coli*. Journal of Virology 65: 2686

Provost P J, Hilleman M R 1978 An inactivated hepatitis A virus vaccine prepared from infected marmoset liver. Proceedings of the Society for Experimental Biology and Medicine 159: 201

Provost P J, Hilleman M R 1979 Propagation of human hepatitis A virus in cell culture in vitro. Proceedings of the Society for Experimental Biology and Medicine 160: 213

Provost P J, Banker F S, Giesa P A, McAleer W J, Buynak E B, Hilleman M R 1982 Progress toward a live, attenuated human hepatitis A vaccine. Proceedings of the Society for Experimental Biology and Medicine 170: 8

Provost P J, Bishop R P, Gerety R J et al 1986 New findings in live, attenuated hepatitis A vaccine development. Journal of Medical Virology 20: 165

Provost P J, Hughes J V, Miller W J, Giesa P A, Banker F S, Emini E A 1986 An inactivated hepatitis A viral vaccine of cell culture origin. Journal of Medical Virology 19: 23

Provost P J, Banker F S, Wadsworth C W, Krah D L 1991 Further evaluation of a live hepatitis A vaccine in marmosets. Journal of Medical Virology 34: 227

Purcell R H 1991 Approaches to immunization against hepatitis A virus. In Hollinger F B, Lemon S M, Margolis H S (eds) Viral hepatitis and liver disease. Williams & Wilkins, Baltimore, p 41

Rakela J, Nugent E, Mosley J W 1977 Viral hepatitis: Enzyme assays and serologic procedures in the study of an epidemic. American Journal of Epidemiology 106: 493

Ruchti F, Siegl G, Weitz M 1991 Identification and characterization of incomplete hepatitis A virus particles. Journal of General Virology 72: 2159

Schneider A J, Mosley J W 1959 Studies of variations of glutamic-oxaloacetic transminase in the serum in infectious hepatitis. Pediatrics 24: 367

Schroeder D D, Mozen M M 1970 Australia antigen: distribution during Cohn ethanol fractionation of human plasma. Science 168: 1162

Siegl G, Lemon S M 1990 Recent advances in hepatitis A vaccine development. Virus Research 17: 75

Sjögren M H, Hoke C H, Binn L N et al 1991 Immunogenicity of an inactivated hepatitis A vaccine. Annals of Internal Medicine 114: 470

Stapleton J T 1992 Passive immunization against hepatitis A. Vaccine (suppl.) 1: S45–47

Stapleton J T, Jansen R, Lemon S M 1985 Neutralizing antibody to hepatitis A virus in immune serum globulin and in the sera of human recipients of immune serum globulin. Gastroenterology, 89: 637

Stapleton J T, Lange D K, LeDuc J W, Binn L N, Jansen R W, Lemon S M 1991 The role of secretory immunity in hepatitis A virus infection. The Journal of Infectious Diseases 163: 7

Stapleton J T, Rosen E McLinden J 1991 Detection of hepatitis A virus capsid proteins in insect cells infected with recombinant baculoviruses encoding the entire hepatitis A virus open reading frame. In Hollinger F B, Lemon S M Margolis H S (eds) Viral hepatitis and liver disease. Williams & Wilkins, Baltimore p 50

Stiehm E R 1979 Pediatrics for the clinician. Standard and special human immune serum globulins as therapeutic agents. Pediatrics 63: 301

Stokes J Jr, Neefe J R 1945 The prevention and attenuation of infectious hepatitis by gamma globulin. Journal of the American Medical Association 127: 144

Stokes Jr J, Farquhar J A, Drake M E, Capps R B, Ward C S Jr, Kitts A W 1951 Length of protection by immune serum globulin (gamma globulin) during epidemics. Journal of the American Medical Association 147: 714

Tabor E, Gerety R J 1979 Transmission of hepatitis B by immune serum globulin. Lancet ii: 1293

Trepo C, Hantz O, Vitvitski L 1986 Non-A, non-B hepatitis after intravenous gammaglobulin. Lancet i: 322

Tsarev S A, Emerson S U, Balayan M S, Ticehurst J, Purcell R H 1991 Simian hepatitis A virus (HAV) strain AGM-27: Comparison of genome structure and growth in cell culture with other HAV strains. Journal of General Virology 72: 1677

Vallbracht A, Maier K, Stierhof Y-D, Wiedmann K H, Flehmig B, Fleischer B 1989 Liver-derived cytotoxic T cells in hepatitis A virus infection. The Journal of Infectious Diseases 160: 209

Vyas G N, Perkins H A, Fudenberg H H 1968 Anaphylactoid transfusion reactions associated with anti-IgA. Lancet ii: 312

Ward R, Krugman S, Giles J P, Jacobs A M, Bodansky O 1958 Infectious hepatitis: studies of its natural history and prevention. New England Journal of Medicine 258: 407

Weiland O, Niklasson B, Berg R, Lundbergh P, Tidestrom L 1981 Clinical and subclinical hepatitis A occurring after immunoglobulin prophylaxis among Swedish UN soldiers in Sinai. Scandinavian Journal of Gastroenterology 16: 967

Welch A G, Cuthbertson B, McIntosh R V, Foster P R 1988 Non-A, non-B hepatitis from intravenous immunoglobulin. Lancet ii: 1488

Wells M A, Wittek A E, Epstein J S et al 1986 Inactivation

and partition of human T-cell lymphotrophic virus, type III, during ethanol fractionation of plasma. Transfusion 26: 210

Werzberger A, Mensch B, Kuter B et al 1992 A controlled trial of a formalin-inactivated hepatitis A vaccine in healthy children. New England Journal of Medicine 327: 453–457

Winokur P L, Stapleton J T 1992 Immunoglobulin prophylaxis for hepatitis A. Clinical Infectious Diseases 14: 580

Winokur P L, McLinden J H, Stapleton J T 1991 The hepatitis A virus polyprotein expressed by a recombinant vaccinia virus undergoes proteolytic processing and assembly into virus-like particles. Journal of Virology 65: 5029

Woodson R D, Clinton J J 1969 Hepatitis prophylaxis abroad. Effectiveness of immune serum globulin in protecting Peace Corps volunteers. Journal of the American Medical Association 209: 1053

UPDATE

- Hepatitis A virus (HAV) has an immunodominant neutralization antigenic site. By using a panel of monoclonal antibodies targetted against the HAV neutralization antigenic site, it was shown that three epitopes within this site are present on 14S subunits (pentamers of the structural unit). In contrast, two other epitopes within this site are formed upon assembly of 14S subunits into capsids. Thus, the epitopes recognized by these two monoclonal antibodies are formed either by a conformational change in the antigenic site or by the juxtaposition of epitope fragments present on different 14S subunits during assembly of 14S into 70S particles. Both 14S and 70S particles elicited HAV-neutralizing antibodies in mice; thus, these particles may be useful for HAV vaccine development (Stapleton et al 1993).
- REFERENCE

Stapleton J T, Raina V, Winokur P L, Walters K, Klinzman D, Rosen E, McLinden J H 1993 Antigenic and immunogenic properties of recombinant hepatitis A virus 14S and 70S subviral particles. Journal of Virology 67, 2: 1080–1085

SECTION 2

Hepatitis B virus

6. Structure and molecular virology

Wolfram Gerlich

HISTORICAL BACKGROUND

Discovery of hepatitis B virus

Hepatitis B virus (HBV) was the first human hepatitis virus from which the proteins and genome could be identified and characterized. Before discovery of the viruses, two types of hepatitis transmission were differentiated on the basis of epidemiological observations: type A was considered to be predominantly transmitted by the faecal–oral route, while type B was transmitted parenterally. In 1963, B S Blumberg, in a search for polymorphic serum proteins, discovered a previously unknown antigen in the blood of an Australian aborigine (Australia antigen). Soon thereafter, it was recognized that the appearance of this antigen was related to type B hepatitis (Blumberg et al 1967). Using immune electron microscopic methods, D S Dane eventually discovered virus-like particles that carried this antigen on their surface, in the serum of hepatitis B patients (Dane et al 1970). These particles were consequently considered to be 'the' hepatitis B virus (HBV). Further non-related viruses that caused parenterally transmissible hepatitis in humans were discovered subsequently, but HBV retained its name. In 1973 the viral nature of the particles discovered by Dane was confirmed by the detection of an endogenous, DNA-dependent DNA polymerase within their core (Kaplan et al 1973). This enzyme allowed Robinson et al (1974a,b) to detect and characterize the HBV genome as a small, circular DNA that was partially double-stranded and partially single-stranded.

Hepadnaviridae

HBV infection was known to result in acute and chronic liver disease and, based on epidemiological data, it was postulated as early as the 1970s that this virus might represent a cause of liver cancer. This led to a search for an HBV-like agent in woodchucks (marmot-like animals from North America), which have been observed to develop liver cancer. Woodchuck hepatitis virus (WHV) was subsequently discovered (Summers et al 1978), and a similar virus was found in seemingly healthy ground squirrels (GSHV) (Marion et al 1980), a species that is distantly related to marmots. In addition, an HBV-like virus was also found in Pekin ducks, which also occasionally develop liver cancer (Zhou et al 1980), and in grey herons living in their natural wild habitat (Sprengel et al 1988). HBV and its relatives throughout the animal kingdom now comprise an officially recognized virus family termed hepadnaviridae, the name derived from their hepatotropism and DNA genome (Howard 1991). The hepadnaviruses of animals are currently not of particular interest to veterinary medicine, but they serve as important models for human HBV. A highlight was the discovery of reverse transcription of viral RNA into DNA within core particles of duck HBV (DHBV) as an essential step of the viral genome replication (Summers & Mason 1982). This replication strategy is used by all hepadnaviruses. Thus, hepadnaviruses are also termed pararetroviruses, in contrast to orthoretroviruses, which have an RNA genome.

BIOLOGY OF HEPADNAVIRIDAE

Immune pathogenesis

Human hepatitis virus was recognized as a pathogen that causes acute hepatitis. However, in order to understand the biology of hepadnaviruses, it is necessary to keep in mind that the members of this virus family are not highly cytotoxic per se, certainly not to the extent of causing massive cell death. Acute and chronic hepatitis B are the result of the host defence mechanisms against HBV, which result in the death of HBV protein-expressing cells and the neutralization of circulating virus (see Ch. 10). Immunologically immature or deficient individuals do not develop a typical hepatitis, but they become chronic carriers of the virus. In this case, the virus continues to replicate in hepatocytes and, to a lesser extent, in other organs or cell types, without destroying tissues or severely impeding organ function.

Viraemia

The infected hepatocytes continue secreting complete virus particles (virions) until titres typically as high as 10^8–10^{10} particles per ml of serum are reached. The great majority of the virions are not cell bound, but a minor number may exist in certain subpopulations of leucocytes. The significance of the persistent viraemia for the virus appears obvious; if these viruses are unable to replicate in cells of the mucosa, but only replicate further within the organism, they require the bloodstream of the host to leave their site of replication as well as to reach it in a newly infected individual. Blood-to-blood contact is not very frequent between individuals and may lead to exchange of only minute amounts of serum. Thus, long-lasting, high-level viraemia seems to be useful for the spread and survival of hepadnaviruses in the population of its host species.

Host range

Typical for hepadnaviruses is their narrow host range. Human HBV infects only higher primates such as chimpanzees. The hepadnaviruses of marmot-like animals do not infect other rodents, and even the duck virus DHBV does not infect all species of ducks. Important transmission-effective contacts such as sexual activity, squabbles and similar activities would usually occur between individuals of the same species. Thus, a wide host range would not be useful for a virus that is transmitted by blood, unless an insect vector was involved. It must be noted, however, that replication of mammalian hepadnaviruses in insects has never been reported nor have hepadnaviruses been found in insects. Hepadnaviruses are relatively stable against heat and can, therefore, maintain infectivity while circulating in the blood. They do, however, appear to be sensitive to detergents and proteases. Thus, passage through the bile to the faeces, if it occurs at all, would not lead to spread of infections as it does so efficiently for hepatitis A virus.

Antigenaemia

The unusually high level of viraemia is accompanied by antigenaemia. In typical individuals with severe viraemia of all host species, the hepadnaviral surface (HBs) proteins are present at concentrations of 10–1000 μg per ml of serum. The HBs proteins are secreted by the infected cells as particles of variable morphology and size (see below). Moreover, it appears that all hepadnaviruses are able to induce secretion of their core protein (HBc protein) in a non-assembled soluble form that is referred to as HBe protein. This molecule reaches also such high concentrations that it can be detected by a technique as insensitive as agar-gel immunodiffusion, indicating levels of 10 μg/ml and more (Magnius & Espmark 1972). The origin and meaning of the 'e' in the name of this protein is a mystery.

Immune tolerance

It appears that, even in immunologically competent individuals who are able to resolve the infection, the onset of the immune response is delayed by several weeks. Among HBV-infected humans with normal immune systems several per cent never develop an effective cytotoxic immune response and proceed directly to persistent infection with high-level viraemia and antigenaemia. The mechanisms by which hepadnaviruses suppress or escape immune elimination are not known, but it appears that variability of the surface proteins, as occurs in hepatitis C virus (see Chs 13 and 14) does not play a major role during the high-level viraemic phase. Several serological subtypes and genotypes of HBV are recognized, but variability within these types is very low, even at those genomic sites that are known to vary most between genotypes. Infection of immune cells has been described (Korba et al 1988), but a general decrease in immune functions has not been observed in HBV carriers. Induction of a specific tolerance toward HBs and HBe proteins, however, appears to be a possibility.

Immune complex disease

High-dose tolerance induction may be one possible function of the viral proteins that are excessively produced and secreted. However, this immune tolerance is not complete since circulating immune complexes of HBsAg or HBeAg and their antibodies are often detectable in viraemic carriers (Madalinski et al 1991). Glomerulonephritis, periarteritis nodosa and acrodermatitis are immune complex diseases that are occasionally found in viraemic carriers.

HBe seroconversion

In HBV carriers a state of low-level viraemia may often develop after elimination of HBeAg from the blood while HBsAg persists to circulate in the blood. Disappearance of HBeAg seems to indicate that HBc protein-expressing cells are no longer tolerated by the immune system. Once most of the HBV-producing cells are eliminated, the state of 'healthy' HBsAg carrier is reached. However, some latent HBV genomes seem to remain and are able to become reactivated when the immune system is weakened. Certain variants that cannot synthesize HBeAg may be selected out during immune pathogenesis and lead to considerable viraemia. Such variants are often found in fulminant hepatitis or chronic hepatitis B without HBeAg (see Ch. 7).

Integration of HBV DNA and oncogenesis

As will be pointed out later, integration of its DNA is, in contrast to orthoretroviruses, not an essential step in the replication of HBV. However, integration of HBV DNA in fragments occurs often. In some cases cells may gain an illegitimate growth advantage by this event, if genetic elements of growth control are disturbed by the insertion of viral DNA. Furthermore, viral proteins themselves, if expressed by integrated HBV DNA fragments in a dysregulated manner, may favour uncontrolled growth. There can be no doubt that hepadnaviruses have oncongenic potential, but it varies from species to species: WHV has the highest oncogenicity, DHBV and GSHV the lowest (see Ch. 15).

STRUCTURE OF HEPADNAVIRIDAE

Electron microscopy (EM)

Figure 6.1 shows the three types of virus-associated particles that are present in the blood of HBV-infected subjects. Similar particles are also found in the serum of hepadnavirus-infected woodchucks or ground squirrels.

Virion morphology

The virus is spherical with a diameter of 42 nm. Using negative staining of virions adsorbed to the EM grids the double-shelled structure of the virions becomes apparent. The outer protein shell (or envelope) is formed by the HBs proteins (Dane et al 1970). Apparent surface structure details such as knobs or spikes, as observed on many other enveloped viruses, are not found on HBV. The inner protein shell is referred to as the core particle or capsid (Almeida et al 1971). It is composed of HBc protein. The capsid encloses the viral DNA, which is often positively stained as in Figure 6.1.

HBs particles

The sera of highly viraemic carriers contain very large numbers of non-infectious particles, composed of excessive HBs protein. Most abundant are spherical particles of 17–25 nm that typically

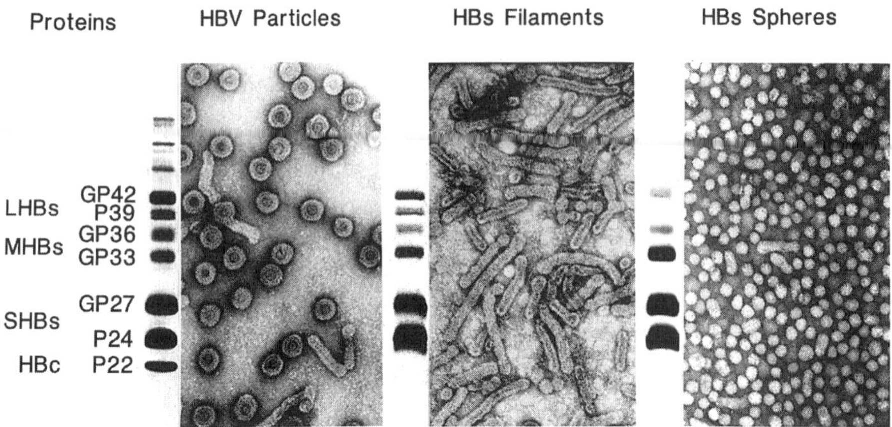

Fig. 6.1 *Morphology and protein composition of purified HBV and HBs particles.* The particles were isolated from high-titred HBV carrier plasma and separated from each other using ultracentrifugation and gel chromatography. The HBV particles were enriched approximately 1000-fold and the filaments approximately 10-fold, while the HBs spheres were slightly diluted for preparation of these three negatively stained electron micrographs. The same purified particle preparations were denatured by SDS/DTT and run through a 13% polyacrylamide gel and stained with colloidal silver. The apparent size and the nomenclature of the viral proteins are shown at the left. The viral surface antigen contains small, middle-sized and large proteins (SHBs, M, L), which appear in variably glycosylated forms. The core protein (HBc) forms a single P22 band in gel electrophoresis.

reach numbers of 10^{13}/ml. The spheres seem to be small vesicles with walls approximately 4 nm thick and an interior diameter of 10–15 nm. Less numerous (up to 10^{11}/ml or 1 μg/ml) are the filamentous (or tubular) particles of 20 nm diameter and variable length. Sera from low-viraemic HBsAg carriers contain up to 10^{12}/ml HBs spheres and few or no HBs filaments.

Avian hepadnaviridae

DHBV has a similar virion morphology as the mammalian hepadnaviruses (Mason et al 1980). The serum from DHBV-infected ducks also contains excessive HBs particles but their morphology is different in that the vesicles have a variable diameter of 40–60 nm. No filaments are detectable.

HBs particles in the liver

The virion envelope and the HBs particles are synthesized and assembled at the membrane of the endoplasmic reticulum (ER). From the ER, the particles are transported and excreted by vesicles. However, when the largest of the three HBs proteins (LHBs) is overproduced in comparison with the smaller HBs proteins, filamentous particles are formed that are retained within the ER (Ganem 1991). This may lead to the accumulation of HBs protein to the point that the ER becomes dilated (Chisari et al 1987). In light microscopy such LHB-storing hepatocytes appear opaque like ground glass.

Core particles in liver

The core particles are synthesized and assembled independently from the HBs proteins in the cytosol. Thereafter they probably attach to patches of HBs protein in the ER membrane. By enclosing the whole core particle, the HBs proteins would mediate budding of the virions to the ER lumen, but these processes have not yet been studied. Non-enveloped core particles of human HBV are often found in the nucleus where they are obviously stored (Gudat et al 1975). In highly viraemic individuals without high disease activity virtually all hepatocytes may contain considerable numbers of core particles, which can be extracted, purified and visualized by EM as 27-nm spherical particles. Both empty core particles without nucleic acid and full particles with DNA are found. Non-enveloped core particles are not detectable in the serum. However, a certain HBV-producing cell line, HepG2.2.15, secretes not only virions and HBs particles but also naked core particles (Sells et al 1987).

PROTEIN COMPOSITION OF HBV PARTICLES

Purification of HBs particles

The typical density of HBs particles and virions is between 1.16 and 1.19 g/ml in sucrose gradients or 1.19–1.24 in caesium chloride gradients. This density is only shared by high-density lipoproteins, which are, however, much smaller than the HBs particles. Thus, a combination of isopycnic and rate-zonal centrifugation is suitable to purify virions and HBs particles. Size chromatography using wide-pore gels is also useful for separation of HBs spheres from HBs filaments and virions. Virions can be partially separated from filaments because of their higher density (Heermann et al 1984). The particles shown in Figure 6.1 were separated by this method.

SDS gel electrophoresis of proteins

Virions and large structures like the HBs or HBc particles are built from protein subunits that are held together by non-covalent interactions and, in the case of HBV proteins, by disulphide bonds between cysteines of different protein molecules. These interactions can be disrupted by the anionic detergent sodium dodecyl sulphate (SDS) and disulphide cleaving reagents such as ß-mercaptoethanol or dithiothreitol (DTT). Moreover, the protein subunit is denatured to form a random coil. For analysis of HBs proteins gel electrophoresis after treatment with SDS/DTT was applied to separate them by size. Thereafter, the gel slabs were stained with colloidal silver, as shown in Figure 6.1.

In the HBs filaments, six protein bands are visible ranging from 24 000 to 42 000 daltons apparent molecular weight. All of these proteins can also be stained specifically by the immunoblotting technique with an antibody against the smallest component, P24 (data not shown), which demonstrates that at least one epitope of the smallest protein is present in the larger proteins. Four of the proteins contain an oligosaccharide linked to one or two of their asparagine residues (*N*-linked glycan). These glycoproteins migrate as somewhat larger molecules in electrophoresis than the non-glycosylated forms. Enzymatic removal of the glycan shows that HBs filaments contain only three different HBs polypeptides:

1. The largest (LHBs) is converted by partial glycosylation in vivo from P39 to GP42.
2. A middle-sized protein (MHBs) that is either single or double glycosylated as GP33 or GP36.
3. A small protein (SHBs) that may be glycosylated as GP27 or non-glycosylated as P24.

SHBs is the most abundant polypeptide in all three HBV-associated particles, whereas MHBs is a minor component in all three. LHBs is more prevalent than MHBs in virions and filaments, but less prevalent in HBs spheres. It appears that the proportion of LHBs determines the morphology of the HBs particles (Marquardt et al 1987), while the ratio of SHBs to MHBs does not significantly alter morphology. A model of the HBs particles is shown in Figure 6.2.

Core particles

In addition to the HBs proteins, purified virions possess a non-glycosylated protein, P22, which builds up the core particle. Naked core particles from liver show the same P22 HBc protein in SDS gel electrophoresis (Gerlich et al 1982).

Virion cores are known to contain the viral DNA polymerase, a protein covalently bound to the minus DNA strand (Gerlich & Robinson 1980), and a protein kinase (Albin & Robinson 1980), but the identity of these proteins has not

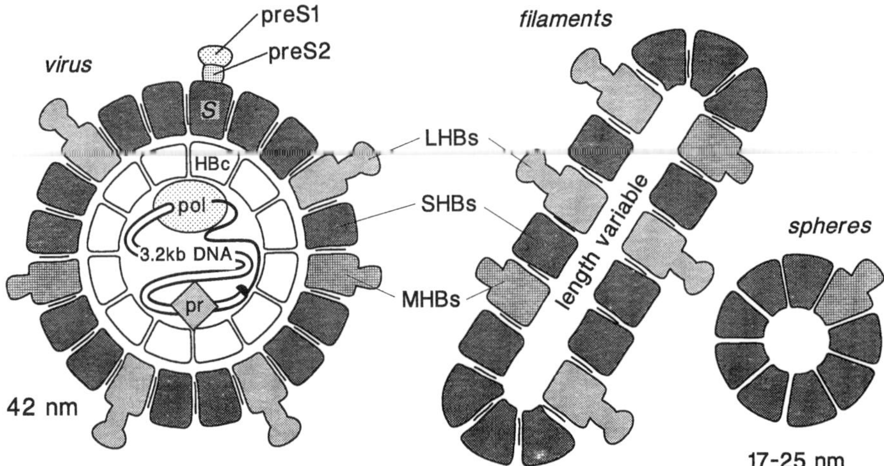

Fig. 6.2 *Schematic model of the HBV and HBs particles.* The SHBs protein of the viral envelope is identical to the S domain of MHBs and LHBs. MHBs contains a small pre-S2 domain facing toward the outside of the particle. LHBs contains, above pre-S2, a pre-S1 domain. The viral envelope encloses a symmetrical capsid consisting of 180 HBc protein subunits. These encapsidate the 3.2- kb-long DNA genome of HBV to which a primase protein (pr) and a DNA polymerase (pol) are associated. It is not completely clear whether the pol and pr are part of one polyprotein or of two separate proteins. The filaments consist of the same proteins as the virion envelope. The spheres contain less LHBs. The virion envelope and the HBs particles contain small amounts of lipid between the protein subunits.

yet been verified by gel electrophoresis. A model of the virions is shown in Figure 6.2.

Host proteins

Numerous human proteins can be found in purified preparations of HBs particles or virions. Well documented is the binding of modified serum albumin to human HBV and HBsAg (Machida et al 1983). Moreover, a small amount of antibodies to HBs antigen may simultaneously be produced with HBsAg, even in high-viraemic carriers. Thus, virions and HBs particles isolated from virus carrier serum often contain immunoglobulin. The significance of the three protein bands in the virion preparation shown in Figure 6.1 is not known.

GENOME OF HBV

Endogenous DNA polymerase of HBV

The first hint regarding the nature of the HBV genome came from the discovery of an endogenous DNA polymerase activity in ultracentrifugation pellets from HBV-containing sera (Kaplan et al 1973). The reaction was dependent on all four desoxynucleotide triphosphates and divalent cations, but no primer or template was necessary. It could be inhibited by actinomycin D, which intercalates into DNA templates. The enzyme was precipitable with antibodies against HBc protein if the HBs envelope was removed from virions by treatment with a non-ionic detergent. The DNA template was not accessible to DNAase unless the core protein was lysed by SDS or digested by proteinase. The existence and the properties of the endogenous DNA polymerase provided evidence that the virus contained a DNA genome.

Structure of the virion DNA

Using electron microscopy, the DNA of HBV was shown to be circular, partially double stranded and 3200 nucleotides in length (Robinson et al 1974). The endogenous DNA polymerase reaction is possible because one of the DNA strands is incomplete (Landers et al 1977). The remaining gap is filled by the viral DNA polymerase if the dNTPs are added in vitro. In vivo, HBV particles are obviously secreted from the infected cell before the double strand is completed. Thus the incomplete plus strand has a defined 5' end but a variable 3' end, as shown in Figure 6.3 a.

The complete minus stand has defined 5' and 3' ends, with a terminal redundancy of nine bases, in the region in which the genome is triple stranded (Will et al 1987). A protein is covalently bound, probably via a tyrosine-linked phosphodiester bridge to the 5' end of the minus strand. This linkage causes extraction of virion-derived DNA to the phenol phase during classical DNA extraction, unless the sample is thoroughly digested with proteinase (Gerlich & Robinson 1980).

The 5' end of the plus DNA strand is formed by 18 ribonucleotides that are capped in the same manner as an mRNA (Seeger et al 1986). The genome is held in an open circular structure because there is an overlap between the two DNA strands (Sattler & Robinson 1979). The genome contains two directly repeated sequences of bases, DR1 and DR2 (Dejean et al 1984). This genome structure is typical for all hepadnaviridae, but in the case of the avian hepadnaviruses the overlap and the distance between the DRs is shorter.

The structure of the hepadnaviral genome does not abide by the usual classification criteria for viruses (Francki et al 1991) in two respects: it contains both DNA *and* RNA and its genome contains partially single-stranded, double-stranded and even triple-stranded DNA. These unusual features are a direct consequence of its replication mechanism, which will be explained below.

Cloning of HBV DNA

In the late 1970s only minute amounts of virion DNA were available. These samples were used for cleavage with a restriction enzyme (often *Eco*RI) and the DNA was ligated to plasmid DNA. The recombinant DNA was introduced into *Escherichia coli*, and bacterial clones carrying the inserted HBV DNA molecules were identified and multiplied (Galibert et al 1979, Pasek et al 1979, Valenzuela et al 1979). By this technique unlimited amounts of HBV DNA became available. During replication of the recombinant DNA within the bacteria all the unusual features of the HBV DNA were removed by the bacterial enzymes for DNA repair. Thus, covalently closed DNA circles of recombinant plasmids were obtained from the bacteria. From these plasmids the HBV DNA or defined fragments thereof could be recovered by cleavage with suitable restriction enzymes. Such fragments were used to determine the complete DNA sequence and virtually all studies on the HBV genome have subsequently been performed using cloned DNA.

Definition of open reading frames (ORFs)

From the nucleotide sequence of a double-stranded version of the DNA genome it is possible to derive six different sequences of amino acid-encoding triplets of nucleotides (codons). If a sequence of potential codons does not encode a protein, it is randomly interrupted by one of the three possible stop codons, whereas protein-encoding sequences are free of stop codons for a distance of at least 50 codons. These stretches of codons are called open reading frames (ORFs). Protein biosynthesis additionally requires a start codon (AUG) in messenger RNA (mRNA). By applying these rules, all genomes of mammalian hepadnaviruses must contain four ORFs, which are encoded by the same DNA strand (Fig. 6.3b). Virologists define the polarity of viral nucleic acid strands in such a way that the mRNA has plus polarity. Thus, the protein-encoding DNA strand of the HBV genome, which is transcribed into mRNA, has minus polarity. Additional ORFs can be identified both on the minus and plus strands, but they are not conserved and are probably generated by statistical sequence variations.

Compact genome structure of HBV

Most functional ORFs of cellular organisms as well as those from larger viruses are arrayed in a linear fashion on the genomes and encode one protein. Moreover, they are interspersed by large

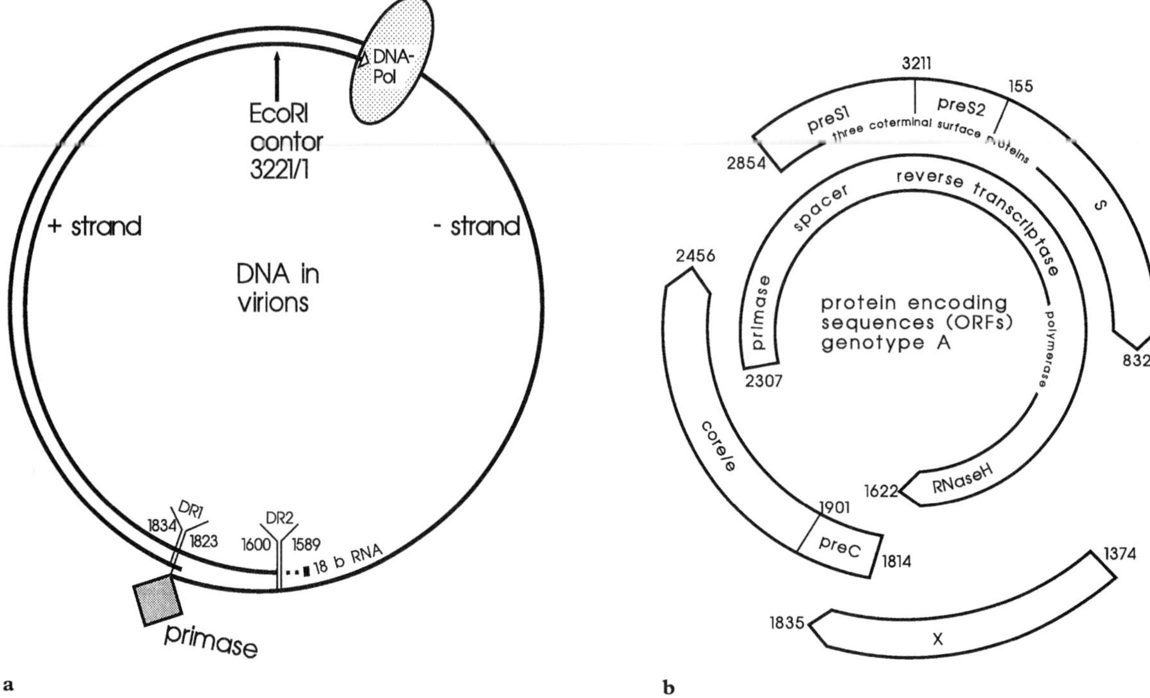

a

b

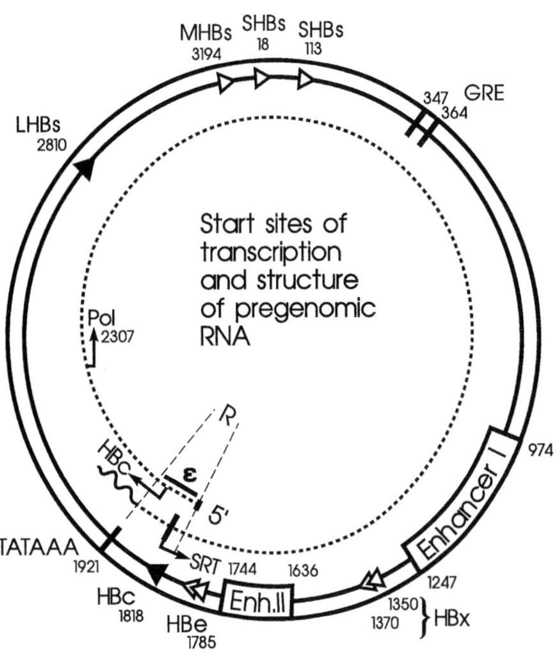

c

Fig. 6.3 *Physical structure (a), open reading frames (b), transcription signals and pregenomic RNA (c) of HBV.* (a) All known complete HBV genomes are circular and between 3182 and 3221 bases long. The figure shows one of the longer examples. Numbering begins at a cleavage site of *Eco*RI. Within the virion, the DNA strand that encodes the viral proteins (i.e. the minus strand) is of full length but is not covalently closed. It has a small redundancy of 9–10 bases at the ends. At its 5' terminus it contains a covalently bound protein known as primase because it is necessary for priming of the minus strand synthesis. The plus strand starts with an 18-base-long RNA piece containing a methylated base (cap) at its 5' end. The plus strand keeps the minus strand in a circular conformation because it bridges the discontinuity of the minus strand. The 3' end of the plus strand is not at a fixed position, and is still connected with the HBV DNA polymerase. Most virion-bound genomes contain a single-stranded gap of 300–2000 bases in length. (b) The ORFs shown here are defined by the first start codon of protein synthesis and the first stop codon. Some internal start codons are also shown. The longest ORF with its four continguous domains encodes the polymerase polyprotein of HBV. (c) The initiation sites of mRNA synthesis for the various HBV proteins in hepatocytes are shown as triangles within the covalently closed genome. Initiation sites that are also used in non-hepatic cells are shown as open triangles. The common termination signal for all mRNAs is the TATAAA box at base 1921. Only the pregenomic HBV RNA is shown as a dashed line. It has a terminal redundancy R, and within the 5' terminal R the encapsidation signal sequence ε. A short sequence within the 3' terminal R is the signal for reverse transcription (SRT). The pregenome is polyadenylated (wavy line) and encodes the HBc and pol protein. Shown are the start sites of these proteins (→).

non-coding regions (introns) that are removed after transcription by splicing. Regulatory and protein-coding regions are well separated. However, the genomes of hepadnaviruses seem to have evolved towards minimal length. Thus, the genome is not much longer than its longest ORF, P, which encodes the viral DNA *p*olymerase and its accessory functions. ORF S is completely located within the ORF P. ORF C and ORF X overlap partially with ORF P. HBV encodes more than one protein from one ORF by using internal AUG codons in an ORF as starting sites for protein biosynthesis. Thus, nested sets of proteins with different amino ends and a common carboxy end are synthesized. ORF S encodes the three HBs proteins (Heermann et al 1984). ORF C encodes the HBe protein and the HBc protein (Ou et al 1986). ORF X also appears to encode more than one protein (Kwee et al 1992). Furthermore the numerous genetic elements that regulate transcription of the viral DNA into RNA are placed within coding regions.

Complete HBV genomes are between 3182 and 3221 bases long (Tiollais et al 1981). The numbering of the bases starts in most publications (as it does here) at the cleavage site for the restriction enzyme *Eco*RI or at homologous sites if a particular genome type does not have such an *Eco*RI site. Other numberings, e.g. beginning at the ATG of the HBc protein or the first base of the RNA pregenome (see below), are also in use.

STRUCTURE OF HBs PROTEINS

Protein sequence of small HBs

The amino acid sequence of small HBs (SHBs) at the amino and carboxy ends has been determined by Edman degradation (Peterson et al 1977, Peterson 1981). The internal sequences could only be partially analysed by this approach. However, together with the protein sequence predicted by the nucleotide sequence, it became clear that the sequence of SHBs begins at the third conserved AUG of ORF S, and that it ends at the stop codon of ORF S. The function of the 5' terminal part of ORF S was originally unknown and was named region pre-S, simply to indicate its location upstream of gene S (Tiollais et al 1981). It is important to note that proteins containing the pre-S sequence are *not* precursors of SHBs.

SHBs are very rich in hydrophobic amino acids. They have many tryptophans but few tyrosines, and, thus, unlike most proteins possess an ultraviolet absorption spectrum similar to tryptophan. Furthermore, they contain the unusually high number of 14 cysteines, which are all cross-linked with each other. At asparagine 146 there is a signal for addition of an *N*-linked glycan, which is present in approximately half of the molecules (Peterson 1981). This glycan has two complex antennas with terminal sialic acids (Heermann & Gerlich 1991). In SDS gel electrophoresis, SHBs have a microheterogeneity, the pattern of which is typical of a virus carrier (Stibbe & Gerlich 1982). The origin of this microheterogeneity is unknown.

Subtypes

SHBs occur in stable subtypes that were originally defined by antibodies. Antigen reactivities that were present on all known HBs isolates were considered as determinant *a*. The best-known subtype determinants are *d* or *y* (Le Bouvier et al 1972) and *w* or *r* (Bancroft et al 1972). Determinant *d* has a lysine at position 122, *y* an arginine (Peterson et al 1984). Likewise, determinant *w* has a lysine at position 160, *r* an arginine (Okamoto et al 1988). Recently, a further subtype allele that has either isoleucine or threonine in position 126 of SHBs has been identified (Ohnuma et al 1993). These type-specific amino acid exchanges may, however, occur in quite divergent HBV genomes. Recently, subtyping has been done by DNA sequencing of the SHBs gene. At least six genotypes, A–F, which differ by more than 8% in the protein sequence, have been identified (Okamoto et al 1988, Norder et al 1992). These possess group-specific amino acids that have not yet been clearly assigned to serological determinants. In contrast, the determinants *d* and *w* occur in four different genotypes. Since all SHBs subtypes are able to induce cross-protection after immunization, the significance of serological or other subtyping is mainly of epidemiological and phylogenetic interest. However, it cannot be excluded that some of the neutralizing antibodies are subtype specific, as is the case with most other viruses.

Topology of SHBs

Circular dichroism of HBs spheres suggests that 50–60% of the polypeptide chain are folded into α-helices. Computer programs used to model the secondary structure of proteins predict that these α-helices are formed by four hydrophobic stretches of SHBs, as shown in Figure 6.4 (Stirk et al 1992). Biosynthetic studies suggest that α-helix I is inserted co-translationally into the ER membranes and furthermore that it is able to trans-

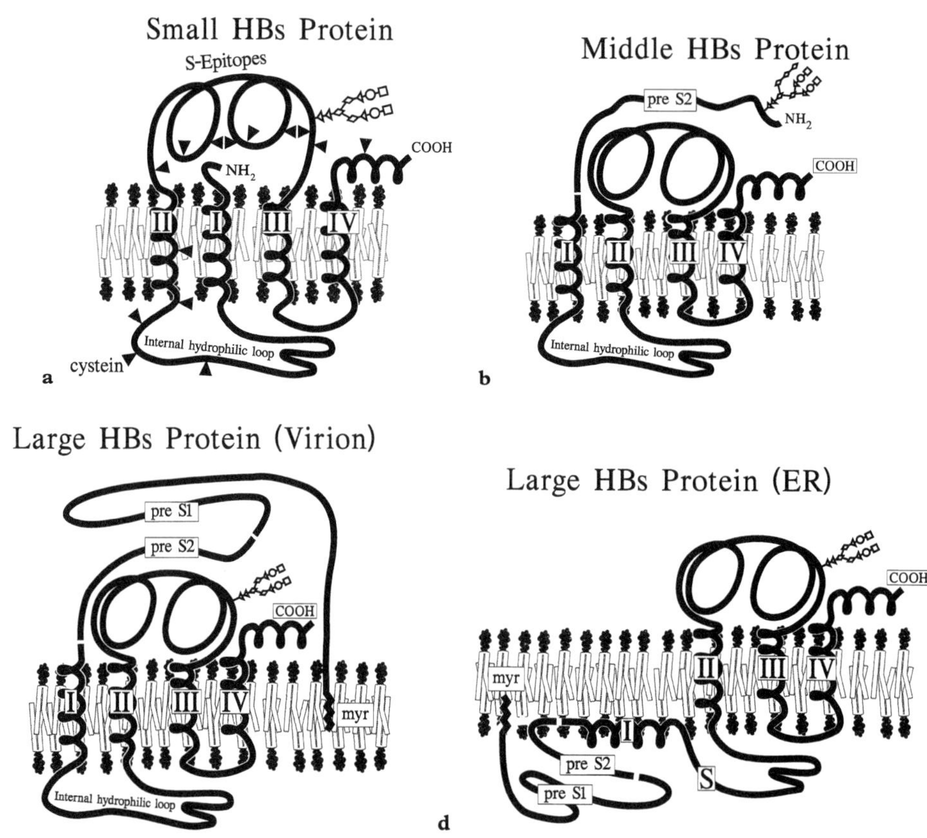

Fig. 6.4 *Topological models of the three HBs proteins.* The polypeptide thread is shown as thick black line. The lipid bilayer of the ER membrane is symbolized by the lipid molecules. The top of the figures corresponds to the lumen of the ER or – after multimerization and budding of the HBs protein – to the surface of the virus particles. The bottom of the figure corresponds to the cytosol or to the interior of the particles. It is assumed that the ER membrane is crossed at least four times by hydrophobic α-helical segments of the S domain. (a) Structure of SHBs. The branched structure at top right is a complex two-antenna glycoside present in GP27 but not in P24. The black triangles represent cysteines that are linked with each other, but the exact nature of the linkage is not known. The HBs epitopes are generated by the complex folding of the external hydrophilic loop between α-helices II and III and are stabilized by cysteine bonds. The amino end seems to be hidden within the molecule. (b) Structure of MHBs. The arrangement of the transmembraneous α-helices of the S domain seems to be slightly altered in that the amino end is more accessible and its hydrophilic loop is less often glycosylated. The pre-S2 domain carries a three-antenna glycoside. (c) Structure of LHBs in the virion. The structure seems to be similar to MHBs, but the pre-S2 domain is *not* glycosylated. The pre-S1 domain partially covers the pre-S2 domain and is linked at methionine 2 with myristic acid (myr). (d) Presumed structure of LHBs soon after its synthesis. At the early phase of LHBs folding it appears that the entire pre-S domain stays in the cytosol. Schematically, the proposed structure would result, but the true folding of the cytoplasmic pre-S domain is not known. At later phases of virion or HBs filament maturation the entire pre-S domain is translocated through the particle membrane to the surface as shown in (c).

locate amino-terminal sequences to the lumen of the ER if they are not too long (Eble et al 1986). Helix II is also inserted into the ER membrane, but it translocates the carboxy-terminal sequences (Eble et al 1987). This topology implies that the hydrophobic sequence between helix I and II remains cytoplasmic. After budding of HBs particles to the lumen of the ER, this sequence is in the interior of the particles. In agreement with this evidence, B-cell epitopes have not been found in this region. The sequence from amino acids 99 to 168 forms the HBs antigen region.

Most of the SHBs epitopes depend upon the presence of disulphide bonds. Mild treatment with DTT first destroys subtype-specific epitopes and at higher concentrations also the *a* epitopes. Completely reduced HBs particles are almost non-immunogenic. Thus, SHBs is virtually undetectable in immunoblots in which reduced and denatured proteins are reacted with antisera against HBs particles (Neurath et al 1984).

Computer modelling of the following hydrophobic regions suggests formation of two membrane-spanning helices III and IV, which may insert post-translationally into the ER membrane. Owing to their polarity with one hydrophobic and one hydrophilic side, these two helices are predicted to multimerize (Stirk et al 1992, A Berting & W H Gerlich, unpublished). Multimerization may possibly also occur between different HBs subunits, and this event would potentially mediate budding of the HBs particles. In agreement with that presumption, truncated HBs proteins without this region no longer form HBs particles, but remain at the ER (Bruss & Ganem 1991a). Genes for such truncated HBs proteins have been found in certain hepatoma cells (Lauer et al 1992). The carboxy-terminal part is dispensable for HBs particle formation (Bruss & Ganem 1991a, Prange et al 1992).

Middle HBs (MHBs)

This minor component of the virion or HBs particles is composed of the S domain, the sequence of which is identical to that of SHBs, and of the 55 amino acid long pre-S2 domain (Stibbe & Gerlich 1983). The pre-S2 domain is hydrophilic and does not contain cysteines. It is very sensitive to proteases, and can be removed selectively from HBs particles without destroying the S domain. Thus, pre-S2 is virtually absent in HBV vaccines that contain protease-treated HBs particles from carrier plasma. The asparagine at position 4 is linked with a glycan of the mixed type (Fig. 6.4). It contains a mannose chain in addition to two complex chains (X Lu & W H Gerlich, unpublished). The amino-terminal part of the pre-S domain is relatively conserved, but sequence 32–54 is highly variable.

The pre-S2 domain is located at the surface and partially covers the S domain of MHBs. It may be slightly more immunogenic than the HBs antigen. Furthermore, the epitopes are not conformation dependent and can (in contrast to HBsAg) easily be generated by synthetic peptides. Peptides with the sequence of the amino-terminal half of pre-S2 were found to induce protective immunity (Itoh et al 1986, Neurath et al 1986a, Neurath & Kent 1988). Pre-S2-containing HBs particles from transfected Chinese hamster ovary cells (CHO) have been introduced in some countries as a vaccine (Tron et al 1989).

The central part of the pre-S2 domain, which also forms the major epitopes, binds a modified form of serum albumin (Machida et al 1984, Krone et al 1990). In vivo, approximately 1 in 10 000 serum albumin molecules is able to bind to pre-S2. HBV carriers with more than 10 μg of HBsAg per ml usually have free albumin binding sites on their particles, while at lower HBsAg concentrations all binding sites are occupied. The nature of the modification is not known, but it can be mimicked by cross-linking of albumin with glutaraldehyde (Yu et al 1985). Serum albumin of non-primate origin does not bind (Machida et al 1984).

Large HBs (LHBs)

The largest HBs protein contains the three domains: pre-S1, pre-S2 and S. In the mature virions or HBs particles the pre-S domains are accessible for antibodies (Heermann et al 1984), receptors (Neurath et al 1992) and proteases (Heermann et al 1987). The S domain and parts of the pre-S2 domain are hidden by the pre-S1 domain of LHBs (Fig. 6.4). During biosynthesis, the entire pre-S domain of LHBs seems to stay initially at the cytoplasm (V Bruss, personal communication, 1992). Thus, the asparagine 4 of the pre-S2 domain is not glycosylated in LHBs (Heermann et al 1984), because this modification occurs co-translationally in the ER lumen. The pre-S1 domain, however, probably becomes membrane attached by another modification. The amino end of the pre-S1 domain carries the sequence methionine–glycine which, together with other less well-defined neighbouring amino acids, serves as a signal for the replacement of the methionine by the C_{14} fatty acid, myristic acid (Persing et al 1987). During virion or HBs particle maturation, the pre-S1 domain is obviously reconfigured and translocated to the surface of the particle.

Overexpression of LHBs relative to expression of SHBs prevents secretion of HBs particles (Persing et al 1986). Instead, filaments become enriched in the ER (Chisari et al 1987). Expression of MHBs and SHBs is independently regulated from expression of LHBs (see below). Hepatocytes that express and secrete SHBs predominantly appear to exist, whereas others express more LHBs and store it intracellularly. It is known that the degree of hepatic immune staining for HBsAg does not correlate with the level of HBsAg in the serum. Only hepatocytes that express LHBs, SHBs and the other viral components in a well-balanced manner are able to assemble and secrete virions (Bruss & Ganem 1991b).

The pre-S1 domain is one of the most variable regions of the HBV genome. One reason for this may be that the part of the polymerase protein that is encoded by the same DNA region as pre-S1 is not essential for replication. The other reason is that this may be *the* surface structure that is most intensively selected for by immune pressure. However, within a chronically infected person or within a defined chain of infection pre-S1 is not mutated (Uy et al 1992). Thus, it is not similar to the hypervariable domains of human immunodeficiency virus (HIV) or HCV envelope proteins.

STRUCTURE OF CORE PROTEINS

Products of ORF C

The essential product of ORF C is the HBc protein of either 183 or 185 amino acids, depending upon the genotype of the virus. In most isolates from highly viraemic carriers, ORF C has 212 or 214 codons, but translation of HBc protein starts only at the AUG, 29 codons downstream of the first AUG (Ou et al 1986). The region upstream is termed pre-C for historical reasons (Tiollais 1981). This name is misleading because the product of the entire ORF C is *not* a precursor of HBc protein but of the secretory form of the core protein, which is termed HBe protein.

HBc protein

This protein contains many hydrophilic and charged amino acids. It does not contain lipid or glycan, but if expressed in eukaryotic cells it becomes phosphorylated (Roosinck & Siddiqui 1987, Lanford & Notvall 1990). It is synthesized in the cytoplasm of the infected cells. As an essential step in the viral life cycle it packages its own mRNA and the viral polymerase and assembles into core particles. A protein kinase, most likely of cellular origin, is also packaged. These particles are then enveloped by patches of the ER membrane that contain the three HBs proteins.

HBc protein expressed in bacteria such as *E. coli* packages RNA in a non-specific manner. The ability to assemble to particles resides in the first 147 amino acids (Gallina et al 1989), while the four arginine clusters of the last 36 or 38 amino acids are involved in packaging of nucleic acids (Hatton et al 1992, Nassal 1992a). Phosphorylation of serine 170 or 172 between arginine clusters 3 and 4 may interfere with nucleic acid binding (Machida et al 1991).

It appears that a critical concentration of HBc protein is necessary for assembly. First, dimers of HBc protein are formed (Zhou & Standring 1992), which then assemble at 0.8 μM concentration (Seifer et al 1993) to isometric particles of T3 symmetry, i.e. 180 HBc subunits form one particle (Birnbaum & Nassal 1990). It has been postulated that HBc protein folds in a similar manner to the subunits of other viral capsids with T3 symmetry into two apposed β-sheets, each with four anti parallel strands, but experimental data for this have not yet been obtained (Argos & Fuller, 1988). Once the core particles are assembled, their structure is stabilized by disulphide bonds (Zhou & Standring 1992, Nassal 1992b).

HBe protein

All hepadnaviruses have evolved the ability to express a secretory form of their HBc protein. They achieve this by the 5' terminal part of the ORF C, called the pre-C sequence. The pre-C sequence encodes a hydrophobic α-helix that is a secretion signal and allows for translocation of the HBe protein into the lumen of the ER (Bruss & Gerlich 1988, Standring et al 1988). During that process, 19 of the 29 pre-C amino acids are cleaved off by the signal peptidase (Fig. 6.5). The 10 remaining amino acids of the pre-C sequence

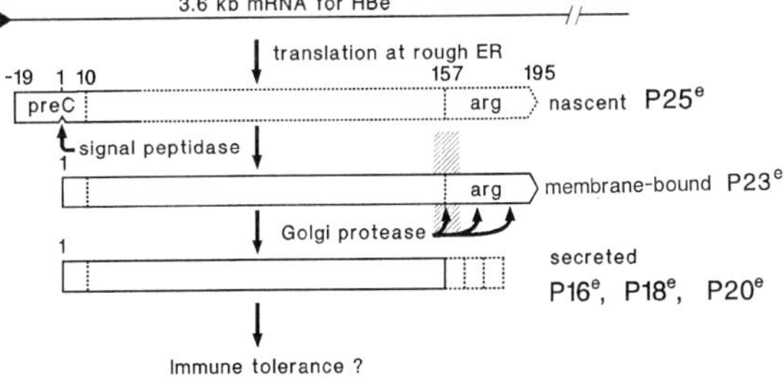

Fig. 6.5 *Biosynthesis of HBe proteins.* When the more-than-genome-length mRNA starts upstream of the HBe start codon, translation of the pre-C region prevents the necessary folding of ε. Thus, the HBe mRNA does not usually function as a pregenome. It is translated to the HBe precursor P25^e, which may be co-translationally cleaved to a membrane-associated P23^e. The 10 remaining amino acids of the pre-C sequence prevent folding of P23^e to core particles. Secretion requires partial or complete removal of the arginine-rich carboxy-terminal domain by a Golgi protease. Thus, secreted HBe protein may be of variable size between 16 and 20 kD. The HBe protein is *not* essential for virion replication or assembly, but may modulate the host's immune response to HBV.

prevent assembly of HBe to core particles by interaction with the HBc protein sequence (Wasenauer et al 1992). Thus, HBe protein differs in almost all aspects from HBc protein, although the primary sequence of these two molecules is almost identical. Part of the HBe protein is transported to the plasma membrane (Schlicht & Schaller 1989); another part is further cleaved within the arginine-rich domain by a Golgi protease and then secreted (Standring et al 1988). Another part of the HBe protein does not reach the ER lumen and is not cleaved at all. The P25^e protein exposes a nuclear transport signal (Ye et al 1990, Wang et al 1991). Thus, HBe proteins of variable length are found in practically all compartments of the cell and furthermore are secreted.

Function of HBe protein

HBe protein is not essential for the viral life cycle. Variants without functional pre-C sequence and HBe protein arise often during acute or chronic HBV infection (see Ch. 7). Nevertheless, all known hepadnaviruses from duck to man have an HBe protein. Using a different expression strategy, murine leukaemia viruses have also developed the ability to produce a secretory form of their nucleoprotein, the glycosylated gag protein.

High levels of secreted HBe protein are found in highly viraemic virus carriers with few symptoms. Elimination of HBeAg is usually accompanied by a flare-up of immune pathogenesis and a decrease of viraemia (see Ch. 10). An HBe-minus variant of woodchuck hepatitis B virus was infectious for newborn woodchucks but it could not induce persistent infection, whereas the HBe-expressing virus resulted in persistent infection (Chen et al 1992). These observations suggest that HBe protein may somehow suppress the immune elimination of HBV-producing hepatocytes. Because HBe protein is probably able to pass the placenta, it may make the T cells of the fetus tolerant of the HBc protein, thus preventing a cytotoxic T-cell response against HBc/e epitopes (Milich et al 1990). However, the tolerogenic effect of HBe protein is not dependent on maternal transmission to the newborn.

PRODUCTS OF ORF P

While the products of ORFs S and C have been identified and well characterized within virions, evidence regarding the products of ORF P is quite circumstantial. There is no doubt that such (a) product(s) (is) are expressed during infection in vivo, but the exact mode of transcription, translation and post-translational processing is not known.

Domains of ORF P

As will be discussed below, mutational analysis of the 834–845 codon-spanning ORF P, sequence homologies with well-studied reverse transcriptases (Toh et al 1983), together with studies on the mechanism of genome replication of HBV, show that most parts of the ORF are indispensable for the virus. These studies suggest that ORF P has four clearly distinguishable domains (Schlicht et al 1991):

1. The amino-terminal domain, which encodes the terminal protein, which is linked to the 5' end of the minus-strand of virion DNA. This part of ORF P is necessary for priming of minus-strand synthesis and is, thus, also termed primase.
2. The next domain has no specific function except as a spacer or tether.
3. The following domain encodes the RNA- or DNA-dependent polymerase, i.e. the reverse transcriptase.
4. The last carboxy-terminal domain is an RNAase H, which cleaves the RNA if it is present in hybrids of RNA and DNA.

The ORF P of hepadnaviruses differs from the ORF P of retroviridae in that it has most likely no protease and integrase domain, but it has a primase domain that is absent in retroviridae.

Products of ORF P in virions

Until now, extraction of ORF P products from virions has only yielded controversial results. Extraction of an active endogenous DNA polymerase from virion core particles has been difficult, because disruption of cores requires harsh treatment. Moreover, it has been noted that a template switch of the viral polymerase to exogenously added templates and primers is difficult or impossible (Radziwill et al 1990).

Bavand & Laub (1988) finally succeeded in extracting DNA polymerase from virions and demonstrated in situ its enzymatic activity together with 90-kD and 70-kD protein bands using so-called activity gels. A 70-kD band was also observed in immune blots using antisera against the conserved active centre of the reverse transcriptase (Mack et al 1988) or against the C-terminal peptide (Bavand et al 1989). These observations suggest either post-translational cleavage of the entire ORF-P product or a separate expression of the DNA polymerase domain without from the amino-terminal part. However, recent data from Bartenschlager & Schaller (1992) suggest that a 90-kD protein encoded by the entire ORF P is predominant in virions.

The polymerase protein is only packaged together with the pregenomic RNA within core particles (Bartenschlager & Schaller 1992). Since the pregenome contains only one packaging signal (Junker Niepmann et al 1990), and core particles seems to have only a packaging capacity for 3300 nucleotides (Melegari et al 1991) probably one polymerase molecule is packaged. It cannot be excluded, however, that the polymerase is packaged as dimer or even oligomer.

HBx PROTEIN

The 154 amino acid-spanning ORF X is conserved in similar form in the hepadnaviruses of woodchucks and ground squirrels. The absence of HBx in the avian hepadnaviruses suggests that it does not participate in the mechanism of genome replication or virion assembly. Furthermore, analysis of codon usage suggests that phylogenetically the HBx gene was introduced quite recently from the eukaryotic genome into the genome of the primordial hepadnaviral genome, which itself seems, in contrast, to be very old (Miller 1991).

Occurrence of HBx

Mutational studies suggest that the HBx protein is dispensable for virus production after transfection of permanent cell cultures in vitro (Blum et al 1992). However, transfection of WHV DNA without a functional X ORF into livers of susceptible woodchucks did not cause infection, which shows that HBx is essential for replication in vivo (Chen et al 1993). Detection of antibodies toward HBx protein in a large number of HBV-infected humans demonstrates that HBx is expressed in vivo, but detection of HBx protein in naturally infected liver specimens or serum presents certain problems because the antibodies used for its detection tend to react non-specifically with other proteins. There is no clear indication that HBx protein is a structural component of virions or core particles. The amino acid sequence suggests that HBx is a cytosolic protein without a specific intracellular transport signal. Thus, reports on the occurrence of HBx protein in the serum of virus carriers (Horiike et al 1991) are difficult to explain.

Function of HBx

In vitro-expressed HBx is highly unstable in animal cells, with a short half-life of 20 min, during which time it becomes phosphorylated (Schek et al 1992). Reports on various biochemical activities of HBx protein, such as protein kinase (Wu et al 1990), dinucleotide kinase (Shaul 1991), protease inhibitor (Arii et al 1992) or squelching factor (Shaul 1991) are preliminary and need confirmation. It is now clear that HBx protein activates transcription of many genes in a somewhat non-specific manner when it is introduced artificially into cells by co-transfection with reporter systems (Rossner 1992). The in vivo function of HBx protein remains, however, completely obscure. The size and number of HBx proteins expressed from ORF in vivo are also unknown, but the conservation of its three start codons and the results of mutational studies suggest that the smaller potential proteins are expressed and transcription activating.

One of the most significant side-effects of HBx protein may be its tumurigenic activity, which has been shown in immortalized mouse hepatocyte cultures (Seifer et al 1992) and transgenic mice (Kim et al 1991). In the immortalized hepatocyte cell line FMH 202, HBx protein is associated with cytoplasmic retention of the tumour-suppressor protein p53 (Höhne et al 1993).

REPLICATION OF HBV

The life cycle of the virus

As with all other viruses, the life cycle of HBV and its relatives in the animal kingdom can be divided into several steps: attachment of the virus to the host cell, virus penetration into the cell, release of the viral genome, expression of viral gene products, replication of the viral genome, formation of virions, release of the virus. A discussion of these various steps follows, and they are schematically shown in Figure 6.6.

Attachment of the virus to the host cell

Virus attachment is one of the crucial steps that determines among other factors the host range and organ tropism of viruses. Furthermore, blocking of attachment by neutralizing antibodies against surface epitopes is a major component of protective immunity and is the basis of many antiviral vaccines. Thus, it is interesting to identify the viral attachment site(s) and the corresponding cellular receptor(s).

Lack of infectivity systems. A great drawback of many of the studies on the attachment of HBs proteins to cell surface proteins is that the target cells were not *susceptible* for HBV infection even if they were *permissive* for HBV replication after transfection. A most striking example is the human hepatoma cell line HepG2, which could not be infected by most – but not all (Bchini et al 1990) – investigators but replicates and secretes HBV quite efficiently after transient or stable introduction of HBV DNA (Sureau et al 1986, Sells et al 1987). Even primary cultures of chimpanzee hepatocytes were found to be non-susceptible to HBV infection (Sureau et al 1992). Somewhat better results were reported with polyethylene glycol-treated primary cultures of human hepatocytes from adult liver (Gripon et al 1988,

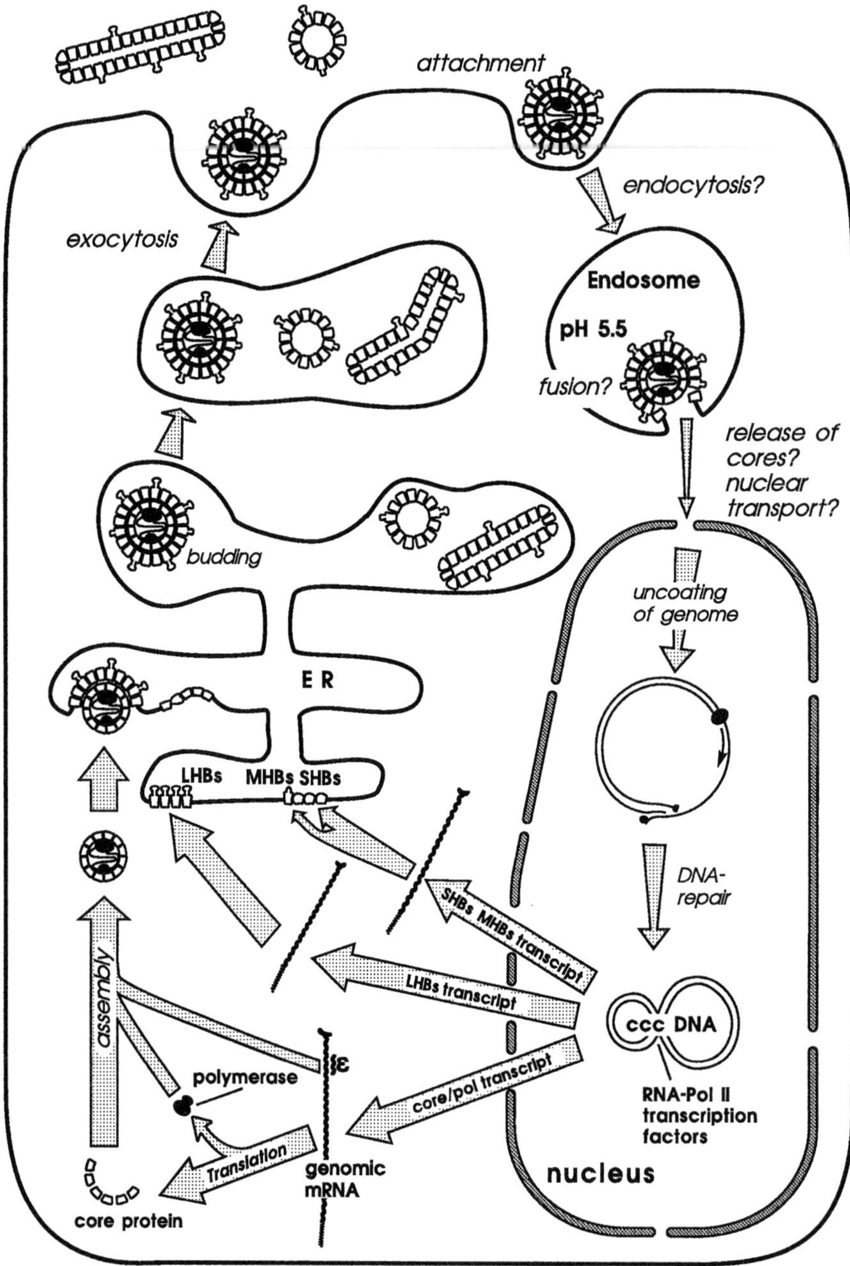

Fig. 6.6 *Schematic view of the life cycle of HBV.* In many details this model is still speculative. It is assumed that the virus is endocytosed after attachment, and the genome or nucleocapsid is released to the cytosol after acidification in the endosome. The genome is repaired in the nucleus and transcribed to three essential classes of mRNA. The non-essential HBe and HBx synthesis is omitted for the sake of simplicity. Translation of the core/pol transcript in the cytosol allows for assembly of core particles that contain the pregenome. The transcripts for LHBs and M/SHBs are translated at the rough ER and the HBs proteins are inserted in that membrane. The HBs particles bud to the lumen of the ER, and at least a part of LHBs-rich ER membrane areas envelopes core particles. The HBV and HBs particles are secreted thereafter by the constitutive pathway.

1993). This relatively high resistance of hepatocytes in culture contrasts sharply with the high infectivity of HBV in vivo.

An effective infectivity system exists for DHBV, for which primary hepatocytes from newly hatched ducklings are a highly susceptible target (Tuttleman et al 1986a). Primary woodchuck hepatocyte cultures are also susceptible for WHV (Aldrich et al 1989). However, these animal hepatocytes also rapidly lose their susceptibility within several days in culture. The reason for the non-susceptibility of long-term hepatocyte cultures to HBV infection is not fully known, but it appears that it is caused by a block in attachment and/or virus entry.

Pre-S1-mediated attachment. An organ- and species-specific attachment of serum-derived HBs particles was found by Neurath et al (1986b) with HepG2 cells, but not with animal liver cells or human carcinoma cells of non-hepatic origin. The binding could be *blocked* by antibodies to the pre-S1 sequence 21–47, and *competed* for by the peptide sequence itself. The relevance of this attachment site was confirmed by studies using natural, purified HBV–particles and plasma membrane preparations from surgically obtained human liver specimens (Pontisso et al 1989). Furthermore, antibodies to peptide pre-S1 (21–47) were able to neutralize in vitro HBV inocula that were no longer infectious (Neurath et al 1989). Monoclonal antibodies to this region could block attachment to HepG2 cells or infectivity for primary human hepatocyte cultures (Petit et al 1991, 1992). Many monoclonal neutralizing antibodies against duck HBV are also directed against the pre-S region of DHBV.

Recently, Neurath et al (1992) suggested that the pre-S1 (21–47) sequence binds to a novel form of membrane-bound interleukin 6, the occurrence of which can be induced on white blood cells. Pontisso et al (1992) observed that IgA competed with pre-S1 (21–47) for the receptor on liver plasma membranes, but they could not identify the receptor. While the pre-S1 sequence 21-47 seems to be essential for the infection process, its attachment to the cell surface is obviously not sufficient for infectivity, or HepG2 cells would be more susceptible to HBV.

Pre-S2-glycan mediated attachment. Three potential candidates for attachment sites have been found in the pre-S2 domain. The pre-S2-linked glycan of MHBs has a weak but distinct affinity for HepG2 cells, but not for permanent mouse hepatocyte cultures or the human carcinoma cell line HeLa. This binding depends on the hybrid structure of the glycan with one mannose antenna and two complex antennas (Y Lu & W H Gerlich, unpublished). With plasma membranes from human liver no such binding was detectable, but it cannot be excluded that in vivo hepatocytes may bind this glycan in certain states of growth or differentiation. Irrespective of this, such binding is probably not sufficient for infectivity because the HepG2 cell is not highly susceptible.

Pre-S2-pHSA-mediated attachment. It is possible that the attachment that can be mediated by modified human serum albumin is more important. Human liver specimens contain receptors for polymerized human serum albumin (pHSA), and pretreatment of liver plasma membranes with pHSA strongly enhances binding of HBV (Pontisso et al 1989). The absence of pHSA receptors on HepG2 cells (Y Lu & W H Gerlich, unpublished) may be one reason why these cells are refractory to infection. The fate of the attached pHSA is probably uptake and digestion within the hepatocyte. HBV may therefore use this altered serum protein as a vehicle for entry into the hepatocyte. Unfortunately, an in vitro system for this possible mode of entry has not yet been established. Recent observations suggest that MHBs may be dispensible for infectivity in vivo and in vitro (H Will, personal communication).

Transferrin-mediated uptake of pre-S2. Binding and uptake of HBs particles has recently been demonstrated with T lymphocytes. It was suggested that these processes are mediated by the transferrin receptor and are dependent upon the amino-terminal portion of the pre-S2 domain (Franco et al 1992). These observations do not explain the hepatotropism of HBV, but may be relevant for the interactions of HBV with the immune systems and for the latency of HBV in liver-transplanted hosts.

SHBs and attachment. Studies with HepG2 cells and liver plasma membranes suggested that

SHBs is not directly involved in attachment (Neurath et al 1986b, Pontisso et al 1989), but Leenders et al (1990, 1992) observed attachment of SHBs particles to primary hepatocytes. Furthermore, a specific attachment of SHBs to Vero cells, a permanent primate kidney cell line, has been reported (Komai & Peeples 1990). While it cannot be excluded that such a cell may accidentally express a relevant receptor for HBV, the significance of that binding remains unclear. The existence of neutralizing antibodies toward SHBs, and of escape mutants to those antibodies (see Ch. 7), suggests that SHBs structures participate in the attachment, entry or both. Alternatively, such antibodies may mediate aggregation and immune elimination of HBV, or sterically hinder the pre-S domains.

Regulation of attachment. One reason for the unsatisfactory understanding of the attachment process may be that it is indeed of low affinity and possibly more non-specific than specific. Since high-titred viraemia and HBs antigenaemia belong to the evolutionary strategy of hepadnaviruses, a highly abundant and avid receptor should theoretically not exist. Otherwise, viraemia and antigenaemia could be never established and the potential target cells would be completely overloaded by regurgitated virus and HBs antigen. Binding to inducible receptors of low abundance would be one possible mechanism, and the membrane-bound interleukin or the pre-S2-glycan binding receptor of HepG2 would be candidates for such receptors. Alternatively, the natural ligand of the receptor would compete with the HBs protein, as may be the case with transferrin or IgA. Binding may also be mediated by a partially degraded serum protein that is destined for recycling in the liver, for example serum albumin. Finally, it may be considered that entry of HBV into hepatocytes is completely non-specific and may be compared to the hepatic uptake and biliary excretion of Indian ink particles. The species specificity of hepadnaviruses would then be more a matter of gene expression and immunotolerance, and the attachment sites mentioned above may be only an auxiliary factor.

Virus penetration into the cell

Two principal mechanisms by which animal viruses can enter a cell are known. The first is only used by certain enveloped viruses that possess fusion proteins. The fusion protein inserts a hydrophobic sequence into the lipid bilayer of the target cell and causes fusion of the viral membrane with the cellular membrane, thereby releasing the viral nucleocapsid into the cytoplasm. However, most enveloped and non-enveloped viruses use the second method, which requires receptor-mediated endocytosis into endosomal vesicles. The physiological acidification and/or proteases in the endosome activate(s) processes that allow(s) transition of the viral nucleocapsid or the genome alone to the cytosol. The mechanism of HBV entry into hepatocytes is not known. As mentioned above, the transferrin receptor allows not only for attachment to T lymphocytes but also for endocytosis and proteolytic processing of HBs particles, but the behaviour of virions and potential genome release have not yet been studied.

In the duck it was originally reported that infection could be blocked by substances that inhibit acidification of endosomes (Offensperger et al 1991), but recent data suggest that this is not the case (Rigg & Schaller 1992). Circumstantial evidence suggests that uptake of human HBV into hepatocytes may require proteolysis and acid pH, because the low-susceptible hepatoma cell HepG2 became more susceptible after proteolytic removal of the pre-S domains and incubation at pH 5.5 (Y Lu & W H Gerlich, unpublished).

Release of the viral genome

Even more obscure than penetration are the further steps of capsid transport and genome release. It is known that 24 h after infection DHBV DNA occurs in the nucleus and is converted to covalently closed circular molecules (Tuttleman et al 1986b). However, it is not known whether the free DNA or core particles are transported to the nucleus. An involvement of the cytoskeleton during that process appears very likely.

Generation of episomal DNA

Currently, it is presumed that the replication of hepadnaviridae requires conversion of the virion DNA with its gap, terminal protein, RNA sequence and triple-stranded structure into a double-stranded covalently closed circle as shown in Figure 6.3c (Seeger et al 1991). It appears likely that the virion polymerase helps to close the single-stranded gap, but possibly further functions of virus proteins may contribute to this repair process. From the result of the cloning experiments in *E. coli* it is known that bacterial enzymes are able (1) to remove all unusual structural elements from the virion DNA, (2) to fill up the gap, (3) to close the nicks and (4) to supercoil the covalently closed HBV DNA. Analogous enzymes of the natural host cell, e.g. hepatocytes, probably also have this capability. Whether the HBV DNA in eukaryotic cells becomes associated with histones and forms nucleosomes has not yet been shown experimentally. A question of clinical relevance is the half-life of the episomal HBV DNA. In cell culture a half-life of 2–4 days has been found, but in vivo the extended latency period of HBV reactivation after liver transplantation suggests a longer survival time.

In contrast to the retroviridae, an integration of HBV DNA into host cell DNA is not only unneccessary for replication of HBV but even detrimental, because linearization of the circular HBV DNA would disrupt at least one gene and would prevent transcription of a functional RNA pregenome. Such a RNA pregenome can, however, be transcribed from linear DNA that is longer than the genome. Such artificial HBV DNA constructs have often been used to transfect cell lines in vitro, but such integrated replication-competent HBV DNA molecules are not found in HBV-infected liver or hepatocellular carcinomas (HCCs). What is occasionally found are fusions between HBV genes and host cell genes. The resulting neoproteins may acquire novel properties, and have been found in certain HCC as potentially oncogenic factors (see Ch. 15).

Transcription of HBV DNA into RNA

General aspects of transcription. Transcription of double-stranded DNA into RNA is a highly regulated process that controls the expression of all genes – whether from the host or the virus – in a timely and structurally ordered manner. Thus, all genomes including those of the smallest replication-competent DNA elements contain not only structural genes that encode protein sequences but also regulatory elements. These DNA sequences bind a number of cellular or viral proteins that act as positive or negative transcription factors. Positive factors bind the cellular RNA polymerase II at a more or less defined position of the DNA sequence, where it initiates RNA synthesis. The RNA polymerase transcribes one strand of the double-stranded DNA into RNA until a termination signal for this enzyme in the DNA sequence occurs.

There are two types of DNA sequence elements that contribute to the binding of transcription factors. *Promoters* are necessary for binding of essential transcription factors, and bring the RNA polymerase into a position where it begins to transcribe only one DNA strand at a defined site. Many promoters contain the so-called TATA box, which binds transcription factor (TF) IID. This factor binds RNA polymerase II in a way that transcription initiates approximately 30 bases downstream. *Enhancers* are DNA segments that enhance transcription initiation at a given promoter, but they do not need to be in an exactly defined position next to the promoter, and their sequence orientation may even be inverted without impairing their function. Thus, promoters are a clearly defined part of one gene, but enhancers, such as those of HBV, may act on expression of several genes.

The rate of RNA synthesis beginning at a promoter is controlled by the amount, type, and activity of positive transcription factors which are available in the host cells, and by the accessibility of enhancers and promoters. There are some essential ubiquitous transcription factors, others are organ specific and a third group is inducible by intra- or extra-cellular signals. Most regulatory gene sequences also contain negative elements that counteract the effect of promoters and enhancers by binding negative transcription factors. Such sequence elements are termed *silencers*.

Methods for the study of transcriptional control elements. When studying their function, transcription-regulating DNA elements are usually separated from the other parts of the genome and linked to the structural gene of a protein that is not naturally present in the cell used for the experiment. These 'reporter genes' encode proteins which can be easily detected by their enzymatic activity. Typical reporter genes are the ones for chloramphenicol acetyltransferase (CAT) or bacterial luciferase. The DNA constructs are made in vitro and are transfected into the target cell, which is then analysed for the expression of the reporter gene. For the study of enhancers, these molecules are linked to a basal promoter that has a low activity in the target cell. Enhancers and promoter are called *cis-acting* transactivating elements because they must be on the same DNA strand as the gene that is to be expressed. *Trans-acting* elements are those DNA segments that also activate transcription when they are present on a separate DNA strand. Usually their effect is exerted by expression of a transcription factor.

Enhancers and promoters are usually composed of modular elements consisting of 6–10 bases, sometimes palindromic or a direct repeat. These elements bind single or dimerized transcription factors that need to cooperate for activation or suppression of transcription. Binding of such proteins to their target DNA can be studied by the reduced accessibility of this DNA to modifying reagents such as DNAase or methylating chemicals. They leave a so-called *footprint* in a sequence ladder of a DNA.

Promoters of HBV. Using the above-mentioned techniques, four promoters and two enhancers have been identified in the HBV genome (Siddiqui 1991, Schaller & Fischer, 1991). These promoters direct initation of RNA synthesis upstream of the HBc/e gene, LHBs gene, M/SHBs gene and the HBx gene as shown in Figure 6.3c. Only the LHBs promoter (often referred to as S promoter I, SpI) has a typical TATA box, and only the mRNA encoding LHBs protein has a sharply defined 5' end. The TATA-less promoters usually have multiple initiation sites, and this is indeed the case for the HBc/e, M/SHBs and X mRNAs. As a result the corresponding sets of mRNAs are able to encode nested sets of co-terminal proteins. The two longer of the HBc/e mRNAs encode HBe protein; the shorter starts four bases after the start codon for the the HBe protein. In this case the ribosome can only use the next start codon for protein synthesis, which defines the amino end of HBc protein. A similar phenomenon occurs for the mRNAs encoding MHBs and SHBs. Only the largest of three mRNAs that are initiated at this promoter (known also as SPII promoter) contains the start codon for MHBs; the other two mRNAs contain only the proximal start codon of SHBs. Whether there are mRNAs that encode only smaller HBx proteins but not full-length HBx protein is not clear.

The relative activity of the four promoters and the fine specificity of the heterogenous 5' ends is dependent on the cell type in which the HBV genome or fragments thereof are expressed. It appears that the M/SHBs promoter and the HBx promoter can be active in all mammalian cell lines (Seifer et al 1990a). The M/SHBs promoter contains, for example, four binding sites for ubiquitous constitutive transcription factor SpI (Raney et al 1992). The LHBs promoter requires the hepatic nuclear factor I (HNF I) (Chang et al 1989). The HBc/e promoter (as well as enhancer II) binds other liver-specific transcription factors such as HNF III and C/EBP in order to be activated (Yuh et al 1992).

Because the proteins expressed by the corresponding mRNAs are absolutely necessary for genome replication and virion assembly, the specificity of the transcription signals in the HBV genome may already be sufficient to explain its organ tropism. Replacement of the liver-specific HBc/e promoter by a ubiquitously active promoter such as the immediate-early promoter of cytomegalovirus allows replication of the HBV genome and assembly of complete core particles in non-hepatic cell lines (Seeger et al 1989). Addition of the SV40 enhancer to the HBV genome also allows for generation of virus-like particles in mouse fibroblasts (Seifer et al 1990b).

Termination of transcription. Not only the start but also the stop of transcription is a well-defined and regulated process. The genomes of all mammalian hepadnaviruses contain one TATAAA stop signal shortly after the start of the HBc gene as shown in Fig. 6.3c. It needs an additional sequence element upstream of the HBc/e promoter and, furthermore, it only becomes active if the initiation site of the RNA is more than 400 bases distant (Cherrington et al 1992). Thus, the stop signal is ignored during the first pass of the RNA polymerase II after initiation at the HBc/e promoter. An RNA of supergenomic length is generated, starting upstream or within the pre-C sequence and ending within the core gene. It has redundant ends ('R'), which are essential for the genome replication of hepadnaviridae (see Fig. 6.3c). All other RNAs of HBV are shorter than genome length. Thus, RNAs of 3.5 kb for HBc/e, 2.4 kb for LHBs, 2.1 kb for M/SHBs and 0.8 kb for HBx are formed. They are all co-terminal. The existence of several promoters and one common stop signal is an elegant way to express several different translation products from one very compact genome with overlapping genes. This expression strategy is unique for hepadnaviridae.

Enhancers. Transcription of HBV RNAs would probably be very low without the enhancer I. This DNA sequence element enhances the initiation of transcription by a factor of 10–50 in liver cells. Its effect is much lower in non-hepatic cells but it is not strictly liver specific (Shaul 1991, Siddiqui 1991). The effect of enhancer II is more liver specific (Yuh et al 1992). Extracellular factors may influence transcription as well. Addition of dexamethasone activates the glucocorticoid receptor, which then binds to the glucocorticoid-responsive elements (GREs) of the HBV genome and enhances transcription further by a factor of 2–5. This effect may be also present in vivo, because glucocorticoid-treated patients express very high levels of HBV, HBeAg and HBsAg.

Viral transcription activator proteins. All double-stranded DNA viruses and retroviruses contain positive sequence signals for initiation of transcription, but – at least in mammalian viruses – these cis-acting elements are obviously insufficient to warrant highly efficient expression and replication of the viral genome. For most viruses the first gene products to be expressed are transcription factors, which activate promoters of other viral genes in a time-ordered manner. Such products are called *immediate early* (*IE*) genes. The time order of HBV gene expression has not yet been fully analysed, but it appears that HBx protein is the first protein to be expressed (Wu et al 1991) and it has been shown that HBx activates many enhancers (Rossner 1992). It links cellular transcription factors together and stabilizes their binding to enhancer I (Maguire et al 1991). Furthermore, HBx protein activates formation of diacylglycerol. This activates protein kinase C, which then phosphorylates the transcription factor AP1 (Kekulé et al 1993). AP1 acts on many promoter/enhancers, including the HBV enhancer and the promoters of cellular proto-oncogenes c-*myc* and c-*fos* (Balsano et al 1991). Furthermore, other transcription-activating pathways can be opened by HBx protein, e.g. one that uses reactive oxygen intermediates for activation of the transcription factor NFKB (Meyer et al 1992).

Oncogenic transcription factors of HBV. In this respect HBx is similar to the IE proteins of oncogenic DNA viruses, such as E6/E7 of papillomaviruses or E1A/B of adenoviruses. These viral transcription activators are also quite non-specific and act also on cellular growth-controlling genes. Furthermore they have the ability to inactivate the cellular tumour-suppressor protein p53 or Rb. HBx inactivates p53 in that p53 is hyperphosphorylated and retained in the cytoplasm (Höhne et al 1993). An HBV protein that inactivates Rb has not yet been observed. However, a further transcription activator of HBV has been discovered in HBV DNA-containing hepatocellular carcinomas. These are truncated LHBs (Caselmann et al 1990) or MHBs (Kekulé et al 1990) proteins that have lost the sequences necessary for budding and secretion of HBs particles. Whether this type of protein has a function in the normal viral life cycle is questionable, because the genes for these proteins are generated only by integration of HBV DNA fragments with a truncated S domain.

Expression of IE proteins is down-regulated by

negative feedback on their transcription by the gene products that are induced by them. It appears that this is also the case in HBV infection. This may explain why in vivo mRNA for HBx is not very abundant during acute infection or is even is undetectable (Will et al 1987). A dangerous situation for the host occurs when viral DNA fragments are integrated into a host genome that is able to express IE proteins but not the genes exerting the negative feedback. Such a situation is found in tumorigenesis by oncogenic adeno- or papillomaviruses and may also occur with HBV, because HBV-associated HCCs often contain HBx genes but no HBc gene, which may represent a candidate for a negative feedback factor on transcription of HBx (Twu & Schloemer, 1989).

Processing of HBV RNAs. After transcription, RNAs are modified by addition of methylated bases to the 5' end (known as a cap) and addition of a poly-(A) tail at the 3' end. Most eukaryotic RNAs are further modified by splicing, i.e. removal of internal non-coding RNA regions (introns) and ligation of the remaining fragments (exons), which finally constitute the mRNA. However, all known HBV genes are contiguous and, thus, the mRNA precursors mentioned above must not be spliced, although numerous potential splice signals are present in the RNA. Spliced HBV RNAs are, however, found in HCCs (Su et al 1989). It appears possible that as yet unrecognized spliced mRNAs lead to fused HBV gene products that may contain portions of different ORFs.

Transport of HBV mRNAs does not seem to be restricted. The half-life of the mRNAs in the plasma has not been well studied, but it has been reported that fusion of viral RNA with a 3' terminal portion derived from host cell DNA may enhance the stability of such a hybrid RNA (von Loringhoven et al 1985).

Translation

General aspects of translation. Protein synthesis in eukaryotic cells is predominantly regulated by the site and frequency of its initiation at the mRNA. The scanning model of this process applies to most mRNAs. The small ribosome subunit binds to the 'capped' 5'-end of the mRNA and thereafter scans the sequence until an AUG start codon for methionine occurs. Protein biosynthesis starts from this site after binding of initiation factors and the large subunit of the ribosomes. The efficiency of protein synthesis at a start codon is influenced by flanking bases. A purine at the +4 and/or -3 position is usually found in initiation codons, but not in internal codons for methionine (Kozak 1989). Synthesis stops at one of the three possible stop codons, UAA, UAG or UGA, that occur first in this particular ORF. Thus, the position of the 5'-ends of the mRNAs in the HBV genome determines which gene product is expressed.

Exceptions to this rule are: internal ribosome entry sites (IRES), leaky scanning for start codons, use of atypical start codons, readthrough of stop codons, frame shifting and reinitiation. Some of these exceptions may apply to the translation of certain HBV proteins.

An important early step in protein biosynthesis is the distribution of the protein synthetic complex between the cytosol and the endoplasmic reticulum (ER). Nascent protein chains that contain a hydrophobic α-helical stretch of 16–20 amino acids bind to a signal recognition particle, which attaches the ribosome to a pore-like structure at the ER. The growing peptide is transported through this pore to the lumen of the ER. The particular structure and number of such hydrophobic signal sequences determines the intracellular distribution or secretion of the protein. Proteins without signal sequence are synthesized by free ribosomes and released after completion to the cytotosol. Enveloped viruses with subgenomic mRNAs, such as HBV, normally use free ribosomes for synthesis of their nucleocapsid proteins, and ER-bound ribosomes for synthesis of the envelope proteins, as shown in Figure 6.6

HBe protein. As mentioned above, the pre-C sequence encodes a signal sequence that makes HBe protein into a secreted protein. As with many secreted proteins, the amino-terminal signal sequence of HBe is cleaved by the cellular signal peptidase at the ER lumen (Standring et al 1988). Further proteolytic processing of the HBe protein probably occurs in the trans-Golgi apparatus (Wang et al 1991). This cellular compartment contains proteases (e.g. furin) that cleave within the arginine-rich carboxy-terminal domain of the HBe protein. Since the signal peptide of HBe protein is not particularly strong, a significant part of the HBe protein remains cytoplasmic (Yang et al 1992). The amount of synthesized HBe protein relative to other HBV proteins is probably regulated by the level of mRNA containing the start codon of an uninterrupted HBe gene. It is likely that the HBe mRNA may be used for synthesis of the polymerase protein (Seifer et al 1990b).

HBc protein. The start codon of HBc protein has two guanosines at positions -3 and +4, which is a relatively good but not optimal context for initiation. A highly efficient translation of the HBc mRNA is necessary, because at a critical level of HBc protein and polymerase protein this mRNA is encapsidated into core particles and is no longer available for protein synthesis (Bartenschlager & Schaller 1992). Co-translational modifications probably do not occur.

Polymerase. An intensive search for an mRNA containing a 5'-end slightly upstream of the presumed amino end of the polymerase (pol) sequence was not successful. Most orthoretroviridae have developed the strategy of pol expression to induce a frame shift between the ORFs of gag (i.e. the analogue of HBc protein) and pol, thus generating a gag–pol fusion protein. Mutational analysis excluded this possibility for HBV. Instead, an unusual internal initiation of the pol protein synthesis at the HBc mRNA is assumed. This would generate a full-length non-fused HBV polymerase (Schlicht et al 1991). A leaky scanning mechanism appears possible, because an optimal start codon of ORF C reduces the efficiency of pol expression (Lin & Lo 1992). There are, however, several stronger initiation codons upstream in the HBc mRNA. The existence of a weak internal ribosome entry site in proximity to the pol start codon would be another obvious explanation (Jean-Jean et al 1989). Ideally, the relative frequency of initiation at the HBc or pol start should regulate the required proportion of HBc to pol protein, which is probably 180:1. Mutational analysis suggests that pol protein initiates encapsidation of the HBc mRNA and itself into core particles predominantly (but not exclusively) in cis (Hirsch et al 1990). This means that the pol protein binds to its own template directly after its completion.

LHBs. Initiation of LHBs protein synthesis follows the usual rules (Gallina et al 1992). It occurs initially in the cytosol because the pre-S domains do not contain an ER translocation signal peptide. The signal peptides I and II of the S domain insert the growing LHBs into the ER membrane, but possibly the entire pre-S domain is too long to be translocated to the ER lumen during protein synthesis (V Bruss, personal communication). In agreement with this conclusion is the absence of glycoside in the pre-S2 domain of LHBs. However, another co- or post-translational modification occurs with all LHBs molecules. The amino-terminal methionine is replaced by myristic acid, which links it to the cytosolic side of cellular membranes. The central hydrophilic part of the S domain is, however, in the lumen of the ER and more efficiently glycosylated than the S domain of MHBs or SHBs. The mRNA for LHBs is not translated well into MHBs or SHBs (Masuda et al 1990, Gallina et al 1992).

MHBs and SHBs. These two gene products are usually coexpressed because of the common promoter for their mRNAs. It is not clear which factors control the relative ratio of the mRNAs containing a start for MHBs or only for SHBs. Irrespective of this transcriptional regulation, the ratio of MHBs to SHBs is also regulated at the translational level. The start codon of MHBs does not have the optimal flanking bases, whereas that of SHBs is optimal for initiation of protein synthesis. Thus, mRNAs for MHBs also always express some SHBs unless the start codon of SHBs has been mutated away.

Signal I of the S domain is obviously able to translocate the pre-S2 domain of MHBs to the ER lumen rapidly, because MHBs is always glycosylated in secreted HBs particles (Eble et al 1990). However, the folding of the nascent S domains seems to be slightly different in MHBs and SHBs, because the S domain is only rarely glycosylated in MHBs (Heermann & Gerlich 1991).

HBx. Translation of HBx protein(s) may occur also from mRNAs that contain or do not contain the first start codon of ORF X (Seifer et al 1990a), but the size of naturally occurring HBx proteins has not yet been reliably elucidated. Sequence predictions suggest that it is a cytosolic protein. Overexpression of HBx protein using vaccinia vectors suggests that it is a very labile phosphoprotein within the cell, with a half-life of 20 min (Schek et al 1991). The insolubility of HBx protein suggests that it oligomerizes rapidly or binds to other cellular proteins.

Formation of virions

Encapsidation of pregenomic RNA. After translation of sufficient amounts of HBc proteins and at least one polymerase protein molecule, these proteins assemble together with their mRNA to form the core particle, as shown in Figure 6.6. Encapsidation occurs only when the polymerase interacts with a specific RNA sequence present at the 5' end (base 1846 to base 1907) of the HBc mRNA (Junker-Niepmann et al 1990). This signal is termed ε (for encapsidation). It is characterized by a secondary structure consisting of a stem, a bulge, a loop and a non-paired U. These elements and the sequence of the loop are required and sufficient for encapsidation. The signal sequence ε is also present in the mRNA for HBe, but there it is obviously not folded to the required secondary structure because of the movement of the ribosome during synthesis of HBe protein (Nassal et al 1990). Since the sequence of ε is also present in the 3' terminal part of all known subgenomic mRNAs of HBV, an unknown interaction of this ε* with 3' terminal sequences in HBV mRNAs may be postulated which prevents encapsidation.

Empty core particles. Empty or nearly empty core particles are found in the hepatocyte nuclei of patients with severe viraemia (Gerlich et al 1982). They probably do not contain HBV DNA, RNA or polymerase. It is not known whether these empty particles are primary assembly products of HBc protein, or whether they are remnant or reassembled from complete core particles that have migrated to the nucleus and released their nucleic acid. Both complete and empty particles contain phosphorylated HBc protein and an endogenous protein kinase activity. It is likely that the kinase is packaged while it is bound to HBc protein.

Envelopment of core particles. The assembly of core particles occurs in the cytosol, but after assembly HBc protein seems to exhibit an affinity for ER membranes that contain inserted LHBs molecules (Bruss & Ganem 1991b). It appears that only the last 16 carboxy-terminal amino acids of the pre-S1 domain in LHBs are necessary for envelopment (V Bruss, personal communication). This length of the pre-S sequence seems to be sufficient to keep LHBs in a conformation such that it can promote binding of core particles. For secretion of enveloped virions an excess of SHBs protein is necessary. It appears that the envelope is formed by mixed aggregates of LHBs, MHBs and SHBs. For secretion, virions and accompanying HBs particles move from the ER via the Golgi apparatus to the cell surface (Ganem 1991). During this migration within transport vesicles the HBs protein is further modified similar to normal cellular secreted proteins. The glycoside side chains of the HBs proteins are trimmed and modified, and covalent disulphide bridges are formed within and between HBc and HBs subunits. It appears that the release of virions and HBs particles from secretory vesicles does not require any specific signal and follows the constitutive pathway of secretion.

Human hepatoma cell lines such as HepG2 and Huh7 express a suitable ratio of all HBV proteins to allow for virion assembly and secretion. Immortalized mouse hepatocyte cultures (Höhne et al 1990) are also able to produce HBV. In vivo, not all hepatocytes may be able to express all HBV proteins in a suitable ratio. Thus, in histological specimens from persistently infected liver only few cells contain HBV DNA, HBcAg and HBsAg, while many cells contain HBsAg and HBcAg alone.

Replication of the viral genome

General strategy. The actual multiplication of the HBV genome occurs in the nucleus of the infected cell by the cellular RNA polymerase II, which transcribes the circular HBV DNA to more than genome-length mRNA with redundant ends (see Fig. 6.3 c). HBx protein may possibly support or enhance this process but is not essential in cell culture. All other essential gene products of HBV are used to encapsidate that RNA, transcribe it to a circular DNA and secrete it as an enveloped virion with attachment sites for new target cells. An overview is given in Figure 6.7.

Signal for reverse transcription. In the woodchuck hepatitis virus model it has been shown that the 3' terminal direct repeat 1 (DR*) in the pregenomic RNA is the natural site of initiation. Essential elements of this site are a short sequence UUUC, within the seven bases that extend from -1 to +6 of DRI*. However this signal for reverse transcription needs to be in the context of 1000 bases upstream of DR1* (Seeger & Maragos, 1990, 1991).

Priming of DNA minus strand. Previously, it was believed that reverse transcription would only occur after encapsidation (Schlicht et al 1991), but recently a DHBV polymerase protein translated in vitro was found to reversely transcribe its own mRNA, beginning at the cytosine within DR1* of the RNA. As with virion DNA, the newly synthesized product was linked to the polymerase protein itself. The first step was addition of guanosine monophosphate to the polymerase protein. Previous studies have shown that virion DNA was linked via an alkali-resistant bond to the amino-terminal domain of the polymerase, probably to a tyrosine. The priming of this reaction is resistant to the polymerase inhibitor

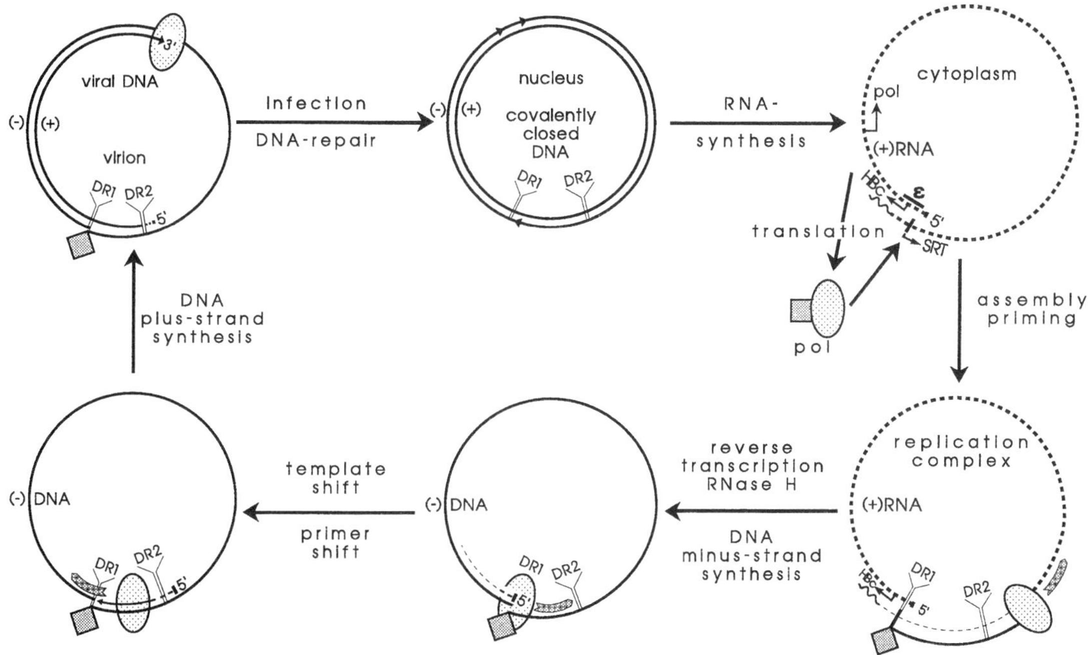

Fig. 6.7 *Replication of the HBV genome.* The virion DNA (top left, see also Fig. 6.3a) is brought by the mechanism shown in Figure 6.6 to the cell nucleus and is converted to covalently closed DNA. This episomal DNA is transcribed to various RNAs (see also Figures 6.3c and 6.6), one ofwhich serves as template for the polymerase protein (→) and HBc protein (→). These two proteins assemble together with their mRNA to the replication complex. The encapsidation signal e at its 5' end governs the packaging of the RNA. The redundant part of the 3' end serves as a signal for reverse transcription (SRT). The primase domain of the polymerase (♦) serves as a primer for the reverse transcriptase. Thus, the growing minus DNA strand (see bottom right) is linked at its 5' end to the primase. The reverse transcription proceeds until the 5' end of the RNA template is reached (bottom centre). Thus, a short redundancy is generated in the minus strand. The RNAase H activity associated with the reverse transcriptase degrades the RNA tempalte, and leaves at its 5' end an 18-base-long capped RNA fragment. This fragment has a six base homology to the direct repeat DR1 and DR2. This weak interaction allows shifting of the fragment and of the reverse transcriptase/DNA polymerase from DR1 to DR2. There, the RNA fragment functions as primer for the plus-strand DNA. The DNA polymerase is able to cross the discontinuity in the minus-strand template owing to its short terminal redundancy. Thereafter, the structure of the virion DNA is reproduced. The multiplication effect originates from the fact that one episomal HBV genome can be transcribed to many pregenome molecules by the cellular RNA polymerase II.

phosphonoformic acid, but elongation of the DNA is not (GH Wang & Seeger 1992).

Elongation of DNA minus strands. DNA minus strands of heterogeneous length with less than 3200 bases are often found as replicative intermediates in HBV-producing cells. Presumably most of these intermediates are within core particles, but in view of the above-mentioned results it cannot be excluded that there are also free intermediates. Normally, the pol-expressing RNA would contain ε and would be encapsidated. In a full cycle of DNA synthesis, reverse transcription will proceed until the pregenome is completely transcribed. This generates a nine-base-long redundancy (r) in the DNA minus strand (Seeger et al 1991).

RNAase H and priming of the DNA plus strand. All reverse transcriptases are associated with an RNAase H activity, which cleaves the RNA of RNA–DNA hybrids into oligoribonucleotides. Mutational inactivation of the RNAase H domain in the HBV polymerase results in a block of DNA plus-strand synthesis (Radziwill et al 1990). Most important for plus-strand synthesis is the generation of an 18-base-long capped RNA fragment from the 5' end of the pregenome. This fragment dissociates for unknown reasons from its DR1 site in the DNA counterstrand and is translocated to DR2 of the same strand. Here it functions as a primer for the DNA plus strand. The DNA begins with the last base of DR2 (Seeger et al 1991).

Circularization of the genome. In Figure 6.7 the pregenome has been drawn as a circle for the sake of simplicity, although the tertiary structure of the pregenome is not known. It is, however, reasonable to assume a structure in which the 5' and 3' short redundances (r) come into close proximity. Otherwise the plus-strand DNA synthesis would stop at the 5' end of the minus strand. However, the polymerase is able to switch at r to the 3' terminal part of the minus strand as template. The circular structure of the non-covalently linked minus strand is then stabilized by the plus strand, which bridges the discontinuity.

Normally, the plus strand is not completed within the core particle or the virion. It is not clear whether this is due to steric hindrance within the core particle, due to inverted repeats within the minus strand acting as pause sites, or due to secretion of the virion to the extracellular space where no deoxynucleotide triphosphates are available.

Conclusion

With minor variations all hepadnaviridae replicate in the same manner. One of the most surprising results in the study of their replication was the finding that all of the seemingly strange properties of these viruses are a logical consequence of their biological strategy as a small persistent virus in the bloodstream.

REFERENCES

Albin C, Robinson W S 1980 Protein kinase activity in hepatitis B virus. Journal of Virology 34: 297–302

Aldrich C E, Coates L, Wu T T, Newbold J, Tennant B C, Summers J, Seeger C, Mason W S 1989 In vitro infection of woodchuck hepatocytes with woodchuck hepatitis virus and ground squirrel hepatitis virus. Virology 172: 247–252

Almeida J D, Rubenstein D, Stott E J 1971 New antigen–antibody system in Australia-antigen-positive hepatitis. Lancet ii: 1225–1227

Argos P, Fuller S D 1988 A model for the hepatitis B virus core protein: prediction of antigenic sites and relationship to RNA virus capsid proteins. EMBO Journal 7: 819–824

Arii M, Takada S, Koike K 1992 Identification of three essential regions of hepatitis B virus X protein for trans-activation function. Oncogene 7: 397–403

Balsano C, Avantaggiati M L, Natoli G, De Marzio E, Will H, Perricaudet M, Levrero M 1991 Full-length and truncated versions of the hepatitis B virus (HBV) X protein (pX) transactivate the cmyc protooncogene at the transcriptional level. Biochemical and Biophysical Research Communications 176: 985–992

Bancroft W H, Mundon F K, Russell P K 1972 Detection of additional antigenic determinants of hepatitis B antigen. Journal of Immunology 109: 842–848

Bartenschlager R, Schaller H 1988 The amino-terminal domain of the hepadnaviral P-gene encodes the terminal protein (genome-linked protein) believed to prime reverse transcription. EMBO Journal 7: 4185–4192

Bartenschlager R, Schaller H 1992 Hepadnaviral assembly is initiated by polymerase binding to the encapsidation signal in the viral RNA genome. EMBO Journal 11: 3413–3420

Bavand M R, Laub O 1988 Two proteins with reverse transcriptase activities associated with hepatitis B virus-like particles. Journal of Virology 62: 626–628

Bavand M, Feitelson M, Laub O 1989 The hepatitis B virus-associated reverse transcriptase is encoded by the viral pol gene. Journal of Virology 63: 1019–1021

Bchini R, Capel F, Dauguet C, Dubanchet S, Petit M A 1990 In vitro infection of human hepatoma (HepG2) cells with hepatitis B virus. Journal of Virology 64: 3025–3032

Birnbaum F, Nassal M 1990 Hepatitis B virus nucleocapsid assembly: primary structure requirements in the core protein. Journal of Virology 64: 3319–3330

Blum H E, Zhang Z S, Galun E, von Weizsäcker F, Garner B, Liang T J, Wands J R 1992 Hepatitis B virus X protein is not central to the viral life cycle in vitro. Journal of Virology 66: 1223–1227

Blumberg B S, Gerstley B S J, Hungerford D A, London W T, Sutnick A J 1967 A serum antigen (Australia antigen) in Down's syndrome, leukemia, and hepatitis. Annals of Internal Medicine 66: 924–931

Bruss V, Ganem D 1991a Mutational analysis of hepatitis B surface antigen particle assembly and secretion. Journal of Virology 65: 3813–3820

Bruss V, Ganem D 1991b The role of envelope proteins in hepatitis B virus assembly. Proceedings of the National Academy of Sciences of the USA 88: 1059–1063

Bruss V, Gerlich W H 1988 Formation of transmembranous hepatitis B e-antigen by cotranslational in vitro processing of the viral precore protein. Virology 163: 268–275

Caselmann W H, Meyer M, Kekule A S, Lauer U, Hofschneider P H, Koshy R 1990 A trans-activator function is generated by integration of hepatitis B virus preS/S sequences in human hepatocellular carcinoma DNA. Proceedings of the National Academy of Sciences of the USA 87: 2970–2974

Chang H K, Wang B Y, Yuh C H, Wei C L, Ting L P 1989 A liver-specific nuclear factor interacts with the promoter region of the large surface protein gene of human hepatitis B virus. Molecular and Cellular Biology 9: 5189–5197

Chen H S, Kew M C, Hornbuckle W E et al 1992 The precore gene of the woodchuck hepatitis virus genome is not essential for vial replication in the natural host. Journal of Virology 66: 5682–5684

Cherrington J, Russnak R, Ganem D 1992 Upstream sequences and cap proximity in the regulation of polyadenylation in ground squirrel hepatitis virus. Journal of Virology 66: 7589–7596

Chen H S, Kaneko S, Girones R et al 1993 The woodchuck hepatitis virus X gene is important for establishment of virus infection in woodchucks. Journal of Virology 66: 1218–1226

Chisari F V, Filippi P, Buras J et al 1987 Structural and pathological effects of synthesis of hepatitis B virus large envelope polypeptide in transgenic mice. Proceedings of the National Academy of Sciences of the USA 84: 6909–6913

Dane D S, Cameron C H, Briggs M 1970 Virus-like particles in serum of patients with Australia-antigen-associated hepatitis. Lancet i: 695–698

Dejean A, Sonigo P, Wain Hobson S, Tiollais P 1984 Specific hepatitis B virus integration in hepatocellular carcinoma DNA through a viral 11-base-pair direct repeat. Proceedings of the National Academy of Sciences of the USA 81: 5350–5354

Eble B E, Lingappa V R, Ganem D 1986 Hepatitis B surface antigen: an unusual secreted protein initially synthesized as a transmembrane polypeptide. Molecular and Cellular Biology 6: 1454–1463

Eble B E, Macrae D R, Lingappa V R, Ganem D 1987 Multiple topogenic sequences determine the transmembrane orientation of the hepatitis B surface antigen. Molecular and Cellular Biology 7: 3591–3601

Eble B E, Lingappa V R, Ganem D 1990 The N-terminal (pre-S2) domain of a hepatitis B virus surface glycoprotein is translocated across membranes by downstream signal sequences. Journal of Virology 64: 1414–1419

Francki R I B, Fauquet C M, Knudson D L, Brown F 1991 Classification and nomenclature of viruses. Springer, Vienna

Franco A, Paroli M, Testa U, Benvenuto R, Peschle C, Balsano F, Barnaba V 1992 Transferrin receptor mediates uptake and presentation of hepatitis B envelope antigen by T lymphocytes. Journal of Experimental Medicine 175: 1195–1205

Galibert F, Mandart E, Fitoussi F, Tiollais P, Charnay P 1979 Nucleotide sequence of the hepatitis B virus genome (subtype ayw) cloned in *E. coli*. Nature 281: 646–650

Gallina A, Bonelli F, Zentilin L, Rindi G, Muttini M, Milanesi G 1989 A recombinant hepatitis B core antigen polypeptide with the protamine-like domain deleted self-assembles into capsid particles but fails to bind nucleic acids. Journal of Virology 63: 4645–4652

Gallina A, De Koning A, Rossi F, Calogero R, Manservigi R, Milanesi G 1992 Translational modulation in hepatitis B virus preS-S open reading frame expression. Journal of General Virology 73: 139–148

Ganem D 1991 Assembly of hepadnaviral virions and subviral particles. Current Topics in Microbiology and Immunology 168: 61–83

Gerlich W H, Robinson W S 1980 Hepatitis B virus contains protein attached to the 5' terminus of its complete DNA strand. Cell 21: 801–809

Gerlich W H, Goldmann U, Müller R, Stibbe W, Wolff W 1982 Specificity and localization of the hepatitis B virus-associated protein kinase. Journal of Virology 42: 761–766

Gripon P, Diot C, Theze N, Fourel I, Loreal O, Brechot C, Guguen Guillouzo C 1988 Hepatitis B virus infection of adult human hepatocytes cultured in the presence of dimethyl sulfoxide. Journal of Virology 62: 4136–4143

Gripon P, Diot C, Guguen-Guilhozo C 1993 Reproducible high level infection of cultured adult human hepatocytes by hepatitis B virus: effect of polyethylene glycol on adsorption and penetration. Virology 192: 534–540

Gudat F, Bianchi L, Sonnabend W, Thiel G, Aenishaenslin W, Stalder G A 1975 Pattern of core and surface expression in liver tissue reflects state of specific immune response in hepatitis B. Laboratory Investigations 32: 1–9

Hatton T, Zhou S, Standring D N 1992 RNA- and DNA-binding activities in hepatitis B virus capsid protein: a model for their roles in viral replication. Journal of Virology 66: 5232–5241

Heermann K H, Gerlich W S 1991 Surface proteins of hepatitis B viruses. In: McLachlan A (ed) Molecular Biology of the hepatitis B viruses. CRC Press, Boca Raton pp 109–144

Heermann K H, Goldmann U, Schwartz W, Seyffarth T, Baumgarten H, Gerlich W H 1984 Large surface proteins of hepatitis B virus containing the pre-S sequence. Journal of Virology 52: 396–402

Heermann K H, Kruse F, Seifer M, Gerlich W H 1987 Immunogenicity of the gene S and pre-S domains in hepatitis B virions and HBsAg filaments. Intervirology 28: 14–25

Hirsch R C, Lavine J E, Chang L J, Varmus H E, Ganem D 1990 Polymerase gene products of hepatitis B viruses are required for genomic RNA packaging as well as for reverse transcription. Nature 344: 552–555

Höhne M, Schaefer S, Seifer M, Feitelson M A, Paul D, Gerlich W H 1990 Malignant transformation of immortalized transgenic hepatocytes after transfection with hepatitis B virus DNA. EMBO Journal 9: 1137–1145

Horiike N, Blumberg B S, Feitelson M A 1991 Characteristics of hepatitis B X antigen, antibodies to X antigen, and antibodies to the viral polymerase during hepatitis B virus infection. Journal of Infectious Diseases 164: 1104–1112

Howard C R 1991 Hepadnaviridae. In: Francki RIB, Fauquet C M, Knudson, P L, Brown F (eds) Classification and nomenclature of viruses. Springer, Vienna, pp 111–116

Itoh Y, Takai E, Ohnuma H et al 1986 A synthetic peptide vaccine involving the product of the pre-S(2) region of hepatitis B virus DNA: protective efficacy in chimpanzees. Proceedings of the National Academy of Sciences of the USA 83: 9174–9178

Jean-Jean O, Levrero M, Will H, Perricaudet M, Rossignol J M 1989 Expression mechanism of the hepatitis B virus (HBV) C gene and biosynthesis of HBe antigen. Virology 170: 99–106

Junker Niepmann M, Bartenschlager R, Schaller H 1990 A short cis-acting sequence is required for hepatitis B virus pregenome encapsidation and sufficient for packaging of foreign RNA. EMBO Journal 9: 3389–3396

Kaplan P M, Greenman R L, Gerin J L, Purcell R H, Robinson W S 1973 DNA polymerase associated with human hepatitis B antigen. Journal of Virology 12: 995–1005

Kekulé A S, Lauer U, Meyer M, Caselmann W H, Hofschneider P H, Koshy R 1990 The preS2/S region of integrated hepatitis B virus DNA encodes a transcriptional transactivator. Nature 343: 457–461

Kekulé A S, Lauer U, Weiss L, Luber B, Hofschneider P H 1993 Hepatitis B virus transactivator HBx uses a tumour promoter signalling pathway. Nature 361: 742–745

Kim C M, Koike K, Saito I, Miyamura T, Jay G 1991 HBx gene of hepatitis B virus induces liver cancer in transgenic mice. Nature 351: 317–320

Komai K, Peeples M E 1990 Physiology and function of the vero cell receptor for the hepatitis B virus small S protein. Virology 177: 332–338

Korba B E, Cote P J, Gerin J L 1988 Mitogen-induced replication of wood-chuck hepatitis virus in cultured peripheral blood lymphocytes. Science 241: 1213–1216

Kozak M 1989 The scanning model for translation and uptake. Journal of Cellular Biology 108: 229–241

Krone B, Lenz A, Heermann K H, Seifer M, Lu X, Gerlich W H 1990 Interaction between hepatitis B surface proteins and monomeric human serum albumin. Hepatology 11: 1050–1056

Kwee L, Lucito R, Aufiero B, Schneider R J 1992 Alternate translation initiation on hepatitis B virus X mRNA produces multiple polypeptides that differentially transactivate class II and III promoters. Journal of Virology 66: 4382–4389

Landers T A, Greenberg H B, Robinson W S 1977 Structure of hepatitis B Dane particle DNA and nature of the endogenous DNA polymerase reaction. Journal of Virology 23: 368–376

Lanford R E, Notvall L 1990 Expression of hepatitis B virus core and precore antigens in insect cells and characterization of a core-associated kinase activity. Virology 176: 222–233

Lauer U, Weiss L, Hofschneider P H, Kekule A S 1992 The hepatitis B virus pre-S/S(t) transactivator is generated by 3' truncations within a defined region of the S gene. Journal of Virology 66: 5204–5209

Le Bouvier G L, McCollum R W, Hierholzer W J J, Irwin G R, Krugman S, Giles J P 1972 Subtypes of Australia antigen and hepatitis-B virus. Journal of the American Medical Association 222: 928–930

Leenders W P, Glansbeek H L, de Bruin W C, Yap S H 1990 Binding of the major and large HBsAg to human hepatocytes and liver plasma membranes: putative external and internal receptors for infection and secretion of hepatitis B virus. Hepatology 12: 141–147

Leenders W P, Hertogs K, Moshage H, Yap S H 1992 Host and tissue tropism of hepatitis B virus. Liver 12: 51–55

Lin C G, Lo S J 1992 Evidence for involvement of a ribosomal leaky scanning mechanism in the translation of the hepatitis B virus pol gene from the viral pregenome RNA. Virology 188: 342–352

Machida A, Kishimoto S, Ohnuma H et al 1983 A hepatitis B surface antigen polypeptide (P31) with the receptor for polymerized human as well as chimpanzee albumins. Gastroenterology 85: 268–274

Machida A, Kishimoto S, Ohnuma H et al 1984 A polypeptide containing 55 amino acid residues coded by the pre-S region of hepatitis B virus deoxyribonucleic acid bears the receptor for polymerized human as well as chimpanzee albumins. Gastroenterology 86: 910–918

Machida A, Ohnuma H, Tsuda F 1991 Phosphorylation in the carboxyterminal domain of the capsid protein of hepatitis B virus: evaluation with a monoclonal antibody. Journal of Virology 12: 1017–1021

Mack D H, Bloch W, Nath N, Sninsky J J 1988 Hepatitis B virus particles contain a polypeptide encoded by the largest open reading frame: a putative reverse transcriptase. Journal of Virology 62: 4786–4790

Madalinski K, Burczynska B, Heermann K H, Uy A, Gerlich W H 1991 Analysis of viral proteins in circulating immune complexes from chronic carriers of hepatitis B virus. Clinical and Experimental Immunology 84: 493–500

Magnius L O, Espmark A 1972 A new antigen complex co-occurring with Australia antigen. Acta Pathologica Microbiologica Scandinavia B 80: 335–337

Maguire H F, Hoeffler J P, Siddiqui A 1991 HBV X protein alters the DNA binding specificity of CREB and ATF-2 by protein–protein interactions. Science 252: 842–844

Marion P L, Oshiro L S, Regnery D C, Scullard G H, Robinson W S 1980 A virus in Beechey ground squirrels that is related to hepatitis B virus of humans. Proceedings of the National Academy of Sciences of the USA 77: 2941–2945

Marquardt O, Heermann K H, Seifer M, Gerlich W H 1987 Cell type specific expression of pre S 1 antigen and secretion of hepatitis B virus surface antigen. Archives of Virology 96: 249–256

Mason W S, Seal G, Summers J 1980 Virus of Pekin ducks with structural and biological relatedness to human hepatitis B virus. Journal of Virology 36: 829–836

Masuda M, Yuasa T, Yoshikura H 1990 Effect of the preS1 RNA sequence on the efficiency of the hepatitis B virus preS2 and S protein translation. Virology 174: 320–324

Melegari M, Bruss V, Gerlich W H 1991 The arginine-rich

carboxyterminal domain is necessary for RNA packaging by hepatitis B core protein. In: Hollinger F B, Lemon S M, Margolis H (eds) Viral hepatitis and liver disease. Williams & Wilkins, Baltimore, pp 164–168

Meyer M, Caselmann W H, Schlüter V, Schreck R, Hofschneider P H, Baeuerle P A 1992 Hepatitis B virus transactivator MHBs^{t}: activation of NF-kappa B, selective inhibition by antioxidants and integral membrane localization. EMBO Journal 11: 2991–3001

Milich D R, Jones J E, Hughes J L, Price J, Raney A K, McLachlan A 1990 Is a function of the secreted hepatitis B e antigen to induce immunologic tolerance in utero? Proceedings of the National Academy of Sciences of the USA 87: 6599–6603

Miller R H 1991 Evolutionary relationship between hepadnaviruses and retroviruses. In: McLachlan A (ed) Molecular biology of the hepatitis B virus. CRC Press, Boca Raton, pp 227–244

Nassal M 1992a The arginine-rich domain of the hepatitis B virus core protein is required for pregenome encapsidation and productive viral positive-strand DNA synthesis but not for virus assembly. Journal of Virology 66: 4107–4116

Nassal M 1992b Conserved cysteines of the hepatitis B virus core protein are not required for assembly of replication-competent core particles nor for their envelopment. Virology 190: 499–505

Nassal M, Junker Niepmann M, Schaller H 1990 Translational inactivation of RNA function: discrimination against a subset of genomic transcripts during HBV nucleocapsid assembly. Cell 63: 1357–1363

Neurath A R, Kent S B 1988 The pre-S region of hepadnavirus envelope proteins. Advances in Virus Research 34: 65–142

Neurath A R, Kent S B, Strick N 1984 Location and chemical synthesis of a pre-S gene coded immunodominant epitope of hepatitis B virus. Science 224: 392–395

Neurath A R, Kent S B, Parker K, Prince A M, Strick N, Brotman B, Sproul P 1986a Antibodies to a synthetic peptide from the preS 120–145 region of the hepatitis B virus envelope are virus neutralizing. Vaccine 4: 35–37

Neurath A R, Kent S B, Strick N, Parker K 1986b Identification and chemical synthesis of a host cell receptor binding site on hepatitis B virus. Cell 46: 429–436

Neurath A R, Seto B, Strick N 1989 Antibodies to synthetic peptides from the preS1 region of the hepatitis B virus (HBV) envelope (env) protein are virus-neutralizing and protective. Vaccine 7: 234–236

Neurath A R, Strick N, Sproul P 1992 Search for hepatitis B virus cell receptors reveals binding sites for interleukin 6 on the virus envelope protein. Journal of Experimental Medicine 175: 461–469

Norder H, Hammas B, Löfdahl S, Courouce A M, Magnius L O 1992 Comparison of the amino acid sequences of nine different serotypes of hepatitis B surface antigen and genomic classification of the corresponding hepatitis B virus strains. Journal of General Virology 73: 1201–1208

Offensperger W B, Offensperger S, Walter E, Blum H E, Gerok W 1991 Inhibition of duck hepatitis B virus infection by lysosomotropic agents. Virology 183: 415–418

Ohnuma H, Machida A, Okamoto et al 1993 Allelic subtypic determinants of hepatitis B surface antigen (i and t) that are distinct from d/y or w/r. Journal of Virology 67: 927–932

Okamoto H, Tsuda F, Sakugawa H, Sastrosoewignjo R I, Imai M, Miyakawa Y, Mayumi M 1988 Typing hepatitis B virus by homology in nucleotide sequence: comparison of surface antigen subtypes. Journal of General Virology 69: 2575–2583

Ou J H, Laub O, Rutter W J 1986 Hepatitis B virus gene function: the precore region targets the core antigen to cellular membranes and causes the secretion of the e antigen. Proceedings of the National Academy of Sciences of the USA 83: 1578–1582

Pasek M, Goto T, Gilbert W, Zink B, Schaller H, MacKay P, Leadbetter G, Murray K 1979 Hepatitis B virus genes and their expression in *E. coli*. Nature 282: 575–579

Persing D H, Varmus H E, Ganem D 1986 Inhibition of secretion of hepatitis B surface antigen by a related presurface polypeptide. Science 234: 1388–1391

Persing D H, Varmus H E, Ganem D 1987 The preS1 protein of hepatitis B virus is acylated at its amino terminus with myristic acid. Journal of Virology 61: 1672–1677

Peterson D L 1981 Isolation and characterization of the major protein and glycoprotein of hepatitis B surface antigen. Journal of Biological Chemistry 256: 6975–6983

Peterson D L, Roberts I M, Vyas G N 1977 Partial amino acid sequence of two major component polypeptides of hepatitis B surface antigen. Proceedings of the National Academy of Sciences of the USA 74: 1530–1534

Peterson D L, Paul D A, Lam J, Tribby II, Achord D T 1984 Antigenic structure of hepatitis B surface antigen: identification of the "d" subtype determinant by chemical modification and use of monoclonal antibodies. Journal of Immunology 132: 920–927

Petit M A, Dubanchet S, Capel F, Voet P, Dauguet C, Hauser P 1991 HepG2 cell binding activities of different hepatitis B virus isolates: inhibitory effect of anti-HBs and anti-preS1(21–47). Virology 180: 483–491

Petit M A, Capel F, Dubanchet S, Mabit H 1992 PreS1-specific binding proteins as potential receptors for hepatitis B virus in human hepatocytes. Virology 187: 211–222

Pontisso P, Ruvoletto M G, Gerlich W H, Heermann K H, Bardini R, Alberti A 1989 Identification of an attachment site for human liver plasma membranes on hepatitis B virus particles. Virology 173: 522–530

Pontisso P, Ruvoletto M G, Tiribelli C, Gerlich W H, Ruol A, Alberti A 1992 The preS1 domain of hepatitis B virus and IgA cross-react in their binding to the hepatocyte surface. Journal of General Virology 73: 2041–2045

Prange R, Nagel R, Streeck R E 1992 Deletions in the hepatitis B virus small envelope protein: effect on assembly and secretion of surface antigen particles. Journal of Virology 66: 5832–5841

Radziwill G, Tucker W, Schaller H 1990 Mutational analysis of the hepatitis B virus P gene product: domain structure and RNase H activity. Journal of Virology 64: 613–620

Raney A K, Le H B, McLachlan A 1992 Regulation of transcription from the hepatitis B virus major surface antigen promoter by the Sp1 transcription factor. Journal of Virology 66: 6912–6921

Rigg R J, Schaller H 1992 Duck hepatitis B virus infection of hepatocytes is not dependent on low pH. Journal of Virology 66: 2829–2836

Robinson W S, Greenman R L 1974a DNA polymerase in the core of the human hepatitis B virus candidate. Journal of Virology 13: 1231–1236

Robinson W S, Clayton D A, Greenman R L 1974b DNA of a human hepatitis B virus candidate. Journal of Virology 14: 384–391

Roossinck M J, Siddiqui A 1987 In vivo phosphorylation and

protein analysis of hepatitis B virus core antigen. Journal of Virology 61: 955–961
Rossner M T 1992 Review: hepatitis B virus X-gene product: a promiscuous transcriptional activator. Journal of Medical Virology 36: 101–117
Sattler F, Robinson W S 1979 Hepatitis B viral DNA molecules have cohesive ends. Journal of Virology 32: 226–233
Schaller H, Fischer M 1991 Transcriptional control of hepadnaviruses gene expression. In: Mason W S, Seeger C (eds) Hepadnaviruses molecular biology and pathogenesis. Current Topics in Microbiology and Immunology 168: 21–39
Schek, N, Bartenschlager R, Kuhn C, Schaller H 1991 Phosphorylation and rapid turnover of hepatitis B virus X-protein expressed in HepG2 cells from a recombinant vaccinia virus. Oncogene 6: 1735–1744
Schlicht H J, Schaller H 1989 The secretory core protein of human hepatitis B virus is expressed on the cell surface. Journal of Virology 63: 5399–5404
Schlicht H J, Bartenschlager R, Schaller H 1991 Biosynthesis and enzymatic functions of the hepadnaviral reverse transcriptase. In: McLachlan A (ed) Molecular biology of the hepatitis B virus, CRC Press, Boca Raton, pp 171–180
Seeger C, Maragos J 1990 Identification and characterization of the woodchuck hepatitis virus origin of DNA replication. Journal of Virology 64: 16–23
Seeger C, Maragos J 1991 Identification of a signal necessary for initiation of reverse transcription of the hepadnavirus genome. Journal of Virology 65: 5190–5195
Seeger C, Ganem D, Varmus H E 1986 Biochemical and genetic evidence for the hepatitis B virus replication strategy. Science 232: 477–484
Seeger C, Baldwin B, Tennant BC 1989 Expression of infectious woodchuck hepatitis virus in murine and avian fibroblasts. Journal of Virology 63: 4665–4669
Seeger C, Summers J, Mason W S 1991 Viral DNA synthesis. Current Topics in Microbiology and Immunology 168: 41–60
Seifer M, Gerlich W H 1992 Increased growth of permanent mouse fibroblasts in soft agar after transfection with hepatitis B virus DNA. Archives of Virology 126: 119–128
Seifer M, Heermann K H, Gerlich W H 1990a Expression pattern of the hepatitis B virus genome in transfected mouse fibroblasts. Virology 179: 287–299
Seifer M, Heermann K H, Gerlich W H 1990b Replication of hepatitis B virus in transfected nonhepatic cells. Virology 179: 300–311
Seifer M, Höhne M, Schaefer S, Gerlich W S 1992 In vitro tumorigenicity of hepatitis B virus DNA and HBx protein. Journal of Hepatology 13 (suppl. 4): S61–S65
Seifer M, Zhou S, Standring D N 1993 A micromolar pool of antigenically distinct precursors is required to initiate cooperative assembly of hepatitis B virus capsids in *Xenopus* oocytes. Journal of Virology 67: 249–257
Sells M A, Chen M L, Acs G 1987 Production of hepatitis B virus particles in Hep G2 cells transfected with cloned hepatitis B virus DNA. Proceedings of the National Academy of Sciences of the USA 84: 1005–1009
Shaul Y 1991 Regulation of hepadnaviruses transcription In: McLachlan A (ed) Molecular biology of the hepatitis B viruses. CRC Press, Boca Raton, pp 193–212
Siddiqui A 1991 Transcription of hepadnaviruses. In: McLachlan A (ed) Molecular biology of the hepatitis B viruses. CRC Press, Boca Raton, pp 95–104
Sprengel R, Kaleta E F, Will H 1988 Isolation and characterization of a hepatitis B virus endemic in herons. Journal of Virology 62: 3832–3839
Standring D N, Ou J H, Masiarz F R, Rutter W J 1988 A signal peptide encoded within the precore region of hepatitis B virus directs the secretion of a heterogeneous population of e antigens in *Xenopus* oocytes. Proceedings of the National Academy of Sciences of the USA 85: 8405–8409
Stibbe W, Gerlich W H 1982 Variable protein composition of hepatitis B surface antigen from different donors. Virology 123: 436–442
Stibbe W, Gerlich W H 1983 Structural relationships between minor and major proteins of hepatitis B surface antigen. Journal of Virology 46: 626–629
Stirk H J, Thornton J M, Howard C R 1992 A topological model for hepatitis B surface antigen. Intervirology 33: 148–158
Su T S, Lai C J, Huang J L, Lin L H, Yauk Y K, Chang C M, Lo S J, Han S H 1989 Hepatitis B virus transcript produced by RNA splicing. Journal of Virology 63: 4011–4018
Summers J, Mason W S 1982 Replication of the genome of a hepatitis B-like virus by reverse transcription of an RNA intermediate. Cell 29: 403–415
Summers J, Smolec J M, Snyder R 1978 A virus similar to human hepatitis B virus associated with hepatitis and hepatoma in woodchucks. Proceedings of the National Academy of Sciences of the USA 75: 4533–4537
Sureau C, Romet Lemonne J L, Mullins J I, Essex M 1986 Production of hepatitis B virus by a differentiated human hepatoma cell line after transfection with cloned circular HBV DNA. Cell 47: 37–47
Sureau C, Moriarty A M, Thornton G B, Lanford R E 1992 Production of infectious hepatitis delta virus in vitro and neutralization with antibodies directed against hepatitis B virus pre-S antigens. Journal of Virology 66: 1241–1245
Tiollais P, Charnay P, Vyas G N 1981 Biology of hepatitis B virus. Science 213: 406–411
Toh H, Hayashida H, Miyata T 1983 Sequence homology between retroviral reverse transcriptase and putative polymerases of hepatitis B virus and cauliflower mosaic virus. Nature 305: 827–829
Tron F, Degos F, Brechot C et al 1989 Randomized dose range study of a recombinant hepatitis B vaccine produced in mammalian cells and containing the S and preS2 sequences. Journal of Infectious Diseases 160: 199–204
Tuttleman J S, Pugh J C, Summers J W 1986a In vitro experimental infection of primary duck hepatocyte cultures with duck hepatitis B virus. Journal of Virology 58: 17–25
Tuttleman J S, Pourcel C, Summers J 1986b Formation of the pool of covalently closed circular viral DNA in hepadnavirus-infected cells. Cell 47: 451–460
Twu J S, Schloemer R H 1989 Transcription of the human beta interferon gene is inhibited by hepatitis B virus. Journal of Virology 63: 3065–3071
Uy A, Wunderlich G, Olsen D B, Heermann K H, Gerlich W H, Thomssen R 1992 Genomic variability in the preS1 region and determination of routes of transmission of hepatitis B virus. Journal of General Virology 73: 3005–3009
Valenzuela P, Gray P, Quiroga M, Zaldivar J, Goodman H M, Rutter W J 1979 Nucleotide sequence of the gene coding for the major protein of hepatitis B virus surface antigen. Nature 280: 815–819
von Loringhoven A F, Koch S, Hofschneider P H, Koshy R

1985 Co-transcribed 3' host sequences augment expression of integrated hepatitis B virus DNA. EMBO Journal 4: 249–255
Wang G H, Seeger C 1992 The reverse transcriptase of hepatitis B virus acts as a protein primer for viral DNA synthesis. Cell 71: 663–670
Wang J, Lee A S, Ou J H 1991 Proteolytic conversion of hepatitis B virus e antigen precursor to end product occurs in a postendoplasmic reticulum compartment. Journal of Virology 65: 5080–5083
Wasenauer G, Köck J, Schlicht H J 1992 A cysteine and a hydrophobic sequence in the noncleaved portion of the pre-C leader peptide determine the biophysical properties of the secretory core protein (HBe protein) of human hepatitis B virus. Journal of Virology 66: 5338–5346
Will H, Reiser W, Weimer T, Pfaff E, Büscher M, Sprengel R, Cattaneo R, Schaller H 1987 Replication strategy of human hepatitis B virus. Journal of Virology 61: 904–911
Wu J Y, Zhou Z Y, Judd A, Cartwright C A, Robinson W S 1990 The hepatitis B virus-encoded transcriptional trans-activator hbx appears to be a novel protein serine/threonine kinase. Cell 63: 687–695
Wu H L, Chen P J, Lin M H, Chen D S 1991 Temporal aspects of major viral transcript expression in HepG2 cells transfected with cloned hepatitis B virus DNA: with emphasis on the X transcript. Virology 185: 644–651
Yang S Q, Walter M, Standring D N 1992 Hepatitis B virus p25 precore protein accumulates in *Xenopus* oocytes as an untranslocated phosphoprotein with an uncleaved signal peptide. Journal of Virology 66: 37–45
Yeh C T, Liaw Y F, Ou J H 1990 The arginine-rich domain of hepatitis B virus precore and core proteins contains a signal for nuclear transport. Journal of Virology 64: 6141–6147
Yu M W, Finlayson J S, Shih J W 1985 Interaction between various polymerized human albumins and hepatitis B surface antigen. Journal of Virology 55: 736–743
Yuh C H, Chang Y L, Ting L P 1992 Transcriptional regulation of precore and pregenomic RNAs of hepatitis B virus. Journal of Virology 66: 4073–4084
Zhou Y Z 1980 A virus possibly associated with hepatitis and hepatoma in ducks. Shanghai Medical Journal 3: 641–649
Zhou S, Standring D N 1992 Hepatitis B virus capsid particles are assembled from core-protein dimer precursors. Proceedings of the National Academy of Sciences of the USA 89: 10046–10050

7. Molecular variants

William F. Carman Howard C. Thomas Arie J. Zuckerman Tim Harrison

All virus isolates consist of a mixture of viral genotypes; multiple variants are found in a single host. This is particularly evident in the case of RNA viruses and retroviruses (Holland et al 1982). Such population heterogeneity occurs because of the high rate of incorporation of incorrect nucleotides during RNA replication or reverse transcription, coupled with an inability to correct these mistakes – the enzymes lack proof-reading functions. The mutation rate averages 1 in 100 000 to 1 in 1000 point replacements, deletions or insertions per nucleotide and round of copying (Steinhauer & Holland 1987). It has been estimated that, considering substitutions, deletions and insertions together, about one-half of the progeny of a single cycle of retrovirus replication will have some mutation (Temin 1989).

The rate of replication is an important factor in the genetic evolution of a virus population. Viruses that cause acute infections in numerous members of a large host population or chronic infections, will undergo rapid change. Whether these variants are transmitted together and then replicate independently at different levels until one predominates, or whether new genotypes are new mutants that arise by random mutation followed by selection, is not clear. It seems likely that both situations occur; for HBV, it is not known whether the former takes place, but there is good evidence that selection occurs (Carman & Thomas 1992). It is possible, but probably unusual, that some of these 'mixed infections' are due to superinfection.

After the random mutation process, selection by the host for the 'fittest' genotypes occurs (Fig. 7.1). Fitness may be defined at the cellular level (viruses that replicate most efficiently in a cell type will predominate) or at the extra-cellular level (viruses that avoid immune elimination will become dominant). The immune selection process is probably determined by the host's immune response genes. Random mutations may be lethal or deleterious to the virus and therefore be selected against, termed negative selection. However,

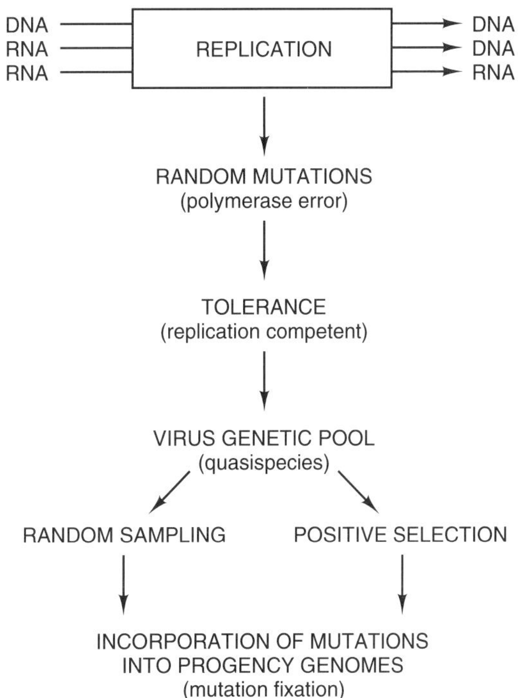

Fig. 7.1 Evolution of viral genotype within individuals. Random mutations occur during replication of DNA viruses, retroviruses and RNA viruses due to transcription error. For these mutant viruses to persist in the viral pool, the mutation must leave the virus replication competent. From this pool of quasispecies various selection pressures are applied altering the proportions of these quasispecies (mutation fixation).

individual point mutations frequently have no phenotypic effect, either because of the redundancy of the genetic code such that the nucleotide change may not result in an amino acid change or because the change does not affect the secondary structure of the RNA or protein. Some of these phenotypically silent mutations may become incorporated into the mixture of genotypes by 'random sampling' of genotypes with equal fitness (Domingo et al 1988). However, the major force for evolutionary change within a virus population is positive selection by the host. This subject is covered in more depth in recent reviews (Carman et al 1993a, Domingo 1985).

HBV replicates through an RNA intermediate, rendering it liable to a high mutation rate. The potential for variation is, however, constrained by the compact organization of the genome. All the nucleotides code for protein, and approximately half are in regions where two open reading frames overlap. For example, the surface open reading frame is entirely overlapped by that encoding the polymerase, and any nucleotide change that leads to loss of function of either protein will be lethal. Further constraints are imposed by the need to conserve the direct repeats which are involved in replication of the genome, promoters and other cis-acting elements. Despite these constraints, up to 12% of nucleotides may vary between isolates of HBV.

The issue of the nomenclature of genetic variation is unresolved. For some viruses, the sequence divergence is so great that the term 'strains' may be appropriate; at what level of divergence this term should be used needs further discussion. The terms 'variant' and 'mutant' are not strictly interchangeable; a virus should only be called mutant if a previous isolate from the patient has been shown to be different. What is a variant? And when does a variant become a strain? Should all genotypes that have the same replication strategy, protein expression and antigenic reactivities which have been defined for the virus be termed 'wild type'? A number of variants have only a single mutation, yet this is sufficient, for example, to prevent the synthesis of HBeAg; this virus is obviously not 'wild type', yet some evidence exists that it can be transmitted to a new host! In this chapter, we review recent data on genetic variation of HBV and use the term variant for any genotype that has an obviously changed biology.

IMMUNE RESPONSE AGAINST HBV

Response to a viral B-cell or T-cell epitope is dependent upon the ability of the antigen-presenting cell to process and present the epitope and of the immunocytes to recognize the epitopes: these functions are genetically determined. The presentation and recognition of viral epitopes are dependent on the presentation of peptides in the cleft of MHC class I or II molecules, which present to CD4 helper and CD8 cytotoxic T cells respectively. The inflammatory process associated with HBV infection is thought to be due to the immune response recognizing either whole proteins that contain B-cell epitopes or peptides which constitute T-cell epitopes. There is little evidence in vivo or in vitro that B-cell epitopes play a major role in clearance of the virus during episodes of hepatitis, but there is growing evidence that T-cell epitopes are recognized by cytotoxic T cells, at least during the acute phase. Both HBcAg (Mondelli et al 1982, Bertoletti et al 1991) and HBsAg (Penna et al 1992) have been shown to contain CTL epitopes, and undoubtedly other viral proteins will play a role in this process.

It is becoming apparent that there are a number of mechanisms involved in the maintenance of chronic infection by HBV. Immune modulation by secreted proteins (Thomas et al 1988), escape mutation (Carman 1992) and integration of viral DNA into the cellular genome (Shafritz et al 1981) probably all play an important role (Fig. 7.2). The core protein is able to suppress production of β-interferon in vitro (Twu & Schloemer 1989) and the polymerase gene product can inhibit the interferon response of hepatocytes (Foster et al 1991). The contribution of each of these phenomena to viral persistence remains to be clarified.

ESCAPE MUTATION

Escape mutation is the process by which a viral epitope that has attracted immune attention is altered so that it is antigenically different from the initial epitope and therefore the virus can persist in the presence of an adequate immune response to

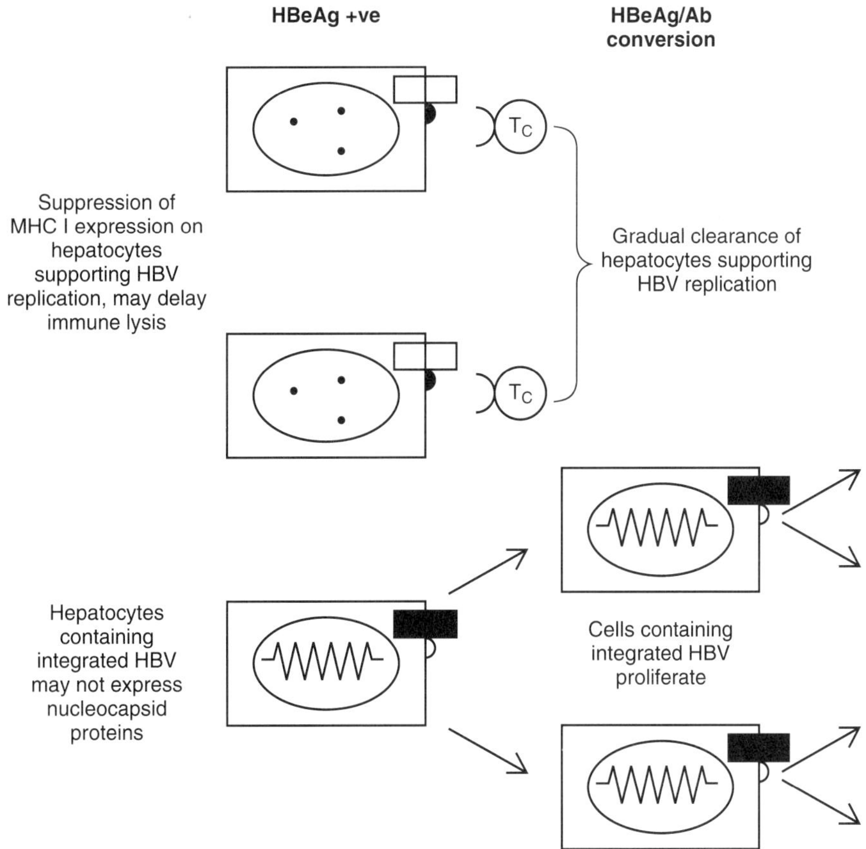

Fig. 7.2 HBV-infected hepatocytes may evade immune lysis by suppression of MHC class I expression and then failure to express HBcAg. □ = diminished MHC class 1 expression; ■ = normal or increased MHC class 1 expression; ◓ = HBc peptides; ◠ = HBs peptides.

the initial epitope. The first epitope is recognized by the immune response, leading to the destruction of infected cells or neutralization of free virus. Viruses that encode for the expression of a mutated epitope (or cells that present it on their surface) will survive and take over the infective process (Fig. 7.3). Escape mutation occurs in numerous viral infections, and can be induced in cell culture, when monoclonal antibodies of restricted specificity are added (Brocade Wu et al 1990, Lemon et al 1990). Subsequent growth of these viruses shows that the antigenic epitopes have changed and no longer react with the monoclonal antibodies. If the selecting antibody is withdrawn, the original genotype will reappear (back selection) (Lemon et al 1990).

T-cell epitopes, both helper and CTL, can also undergo mutation, allowing viral escape. The latter was first described in a transgenic mouse model of lymphochoriomeningitis virus infection (Pircher et al 1990) and confirmed in vivo in patients with human immunodeficiency virus (HIV) infection (Phillips et al 1991, Johnson et al 1992). Over time, HIV-infected patients with particular MHC types show changes both within and around the viral epitopes presented by the MHC I molecules present in that patient. The mutated peptide sequences were shown to be unreactive with the CTL that recognized the original peptides (Fig. 7.3).

In HBV infection, most adults suffer symptomatic or asymptomatic hepatitis following the clearance of the virus. Less than 5% develop persistent infection with chronic hepatitis, and most of these will eventually seroconvert to anti-HBe. During these years of chronic infection, changes occur in all the genes of HBV; some of

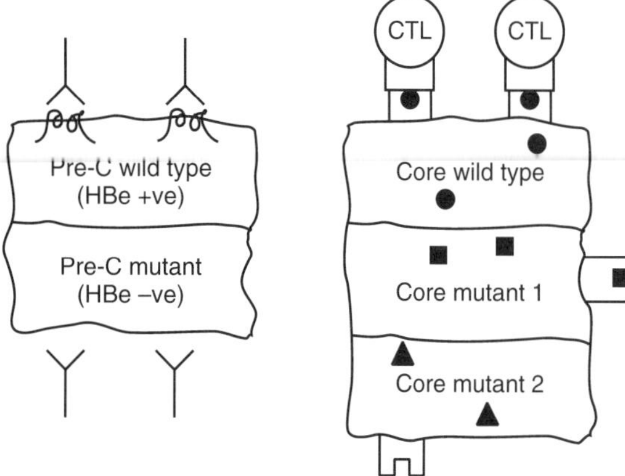

Fig. 7.3 Mechanisms of avoidance of immune lysis of infected cells. Avoidance of lysis by antibody is shown on the left (using HBeAg as a hypothetical example) and cytotoxic T-cell escape on the right (using core antigen as a hypothetical example). If HBeAg is no longer secreted, then antibodies will not bind to the hepatocyte surface. If peptides within core were to change, this may have two effects on immune surveillance. Either the mutant peptide will be picked up by the MHC molecule but will not be recognized by CTL or the peptide will no longer be able to bind to the MHC molecule. Both situations would constitute CTL escape.

these changes will result in evasion of the immune response. Such variation seems to be distinct from the substitutions which define the subtypes of HBV – these will be discussed later.

PRE-CORE MUTANTS

Pre-core/core proteins and the host

Hepatitis B e antigen (HBeAg) is derived from the translation product of the pre-core and core regions. It is secreted from the infected hepatocyte by virtue of the presence of a secretory signal sequence at the beginning of the pre-core region (Ou et al 1986) (Fig. 7.4). The core protein (HBcAg) is translated from the second ATG of this gene and thus shares a large number of amino acids with HBeAg (from the core methionine to the carboxy terminus of HBeAg). These proteins contain B- and T-cell epitopes, of which some are shared between the two proteins and others are peculiar to one polypeptide. The finding of antigenic epitopes that are different between the two proteins, even though they share so many amino acids, is based on conformational differences related to the 10 amino acid pre-core peptide at the amino terminus of HBeAg and the carboxy-terminal arginine-rich domain of core.

HBeAg is highly conserved both between HBV isolates and within the members of the hepadnavirus family. It is secreted from the infected cell but is not part of the virion. Why should it be advantageous for the virus to conserve such translated genetic material that is not part of the virion and plays no role in replication? It has been suggested that HBeAg, by crossing the placenta, is a tolerogen in the neonate born to an HBV-infected mother (Thomas et al 1988). It may also serve immunomodulatory functions after infection in adult life. Tolerogenic proteins induce a state of non-responsiveness. In the case of HBeAg-induced tolerance, if this non-responsiveness includes the cellular response to all the nucleocapsid (pre-core/core)-derived epitopes, elimination of HBV-infected cells would not occur. There is evidence from a transgenic mouse model that HBeAg can be tolerogenic in fetal mice (Milich et al 1990). Another way in which HBeAg influences the host response is by down-regulating interferon production, which has been shown to occur with ß-interferon in vitro (Twu & Schloemer 1989). After the tolerogenic effect has been lost, virus escape from the cellular or humoral response to HBeAg may occur by suppression of expression of the protein, giving rise to HBeAg-negative viraemia (pre-core mutant viraemia) (Fig. 7.5).

Pre-core mutants in chronic hepatitis

When patients with chronic hepatitis seroconvert to anti-HBe, a peak in liver transaminases usually occurs, probably due to immune-mediated killing of infected hepatocytes. It seems likely that the target of the immune response is HBeAg on the surface of hepatocytes (Schlicht & Schaller 1989, Yamada et al 1990). However, not all patients lose serum HBV DNA (by dot-blot hybridization) and some continue to have elevated transaminases after such seroconversion. A significant proportion of chronic hepatitis patients in Mediterranean countries (Hadziyannis et al 1983, Bonino et al 1986) and in the Far East (Chu et al 1985) retain high-level viraemia, have liver disease and may

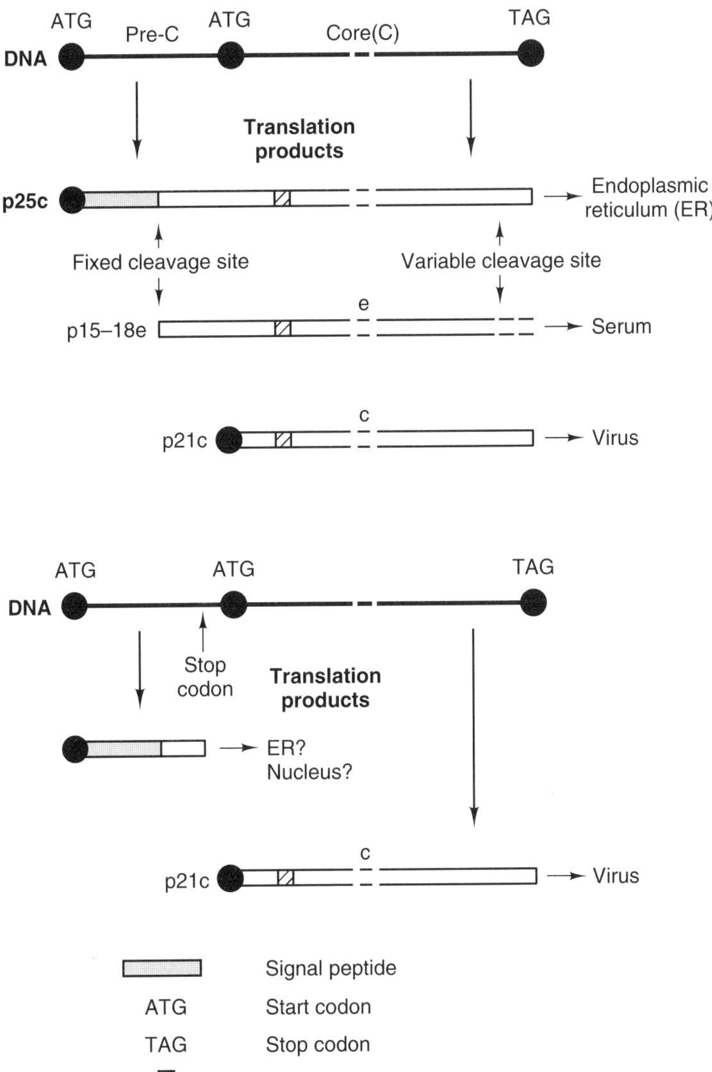

Fig. 7.4 Synthesis of core and HBe proteins. Two translational start codons (ATG) are found in the pre-core/core open reading frame. Should translation begin at the first, a long protein will be synthesized, of which the first 19 amino acids are a signal peptide, enabling secretion into the endoplasmic reticulum. After modification of the carboxy terminus, this constitutes HBeAg. If translation begins at the second, then core protein is generated. Thus for protein purposes, pre-core is dispensable for virion production, as HBeAg is not found in virus particles. The stop codon mutant (A1896) is at the end of pre-core, giving rise to the protein products suggested in the lower half of the figure.

rapidly progress to cirrhosis (Fig. 7.6). As HBeAg is usually associated with high-level viraemia, a molecular explanation has to be found for the continued viraemia in the absence of the HBe antigenaemia. The pre-core region is necessary for the production of HBeAg but is not necessary for the production of virions. HBcAg is translated from the second ATG of the pre-core/core gene

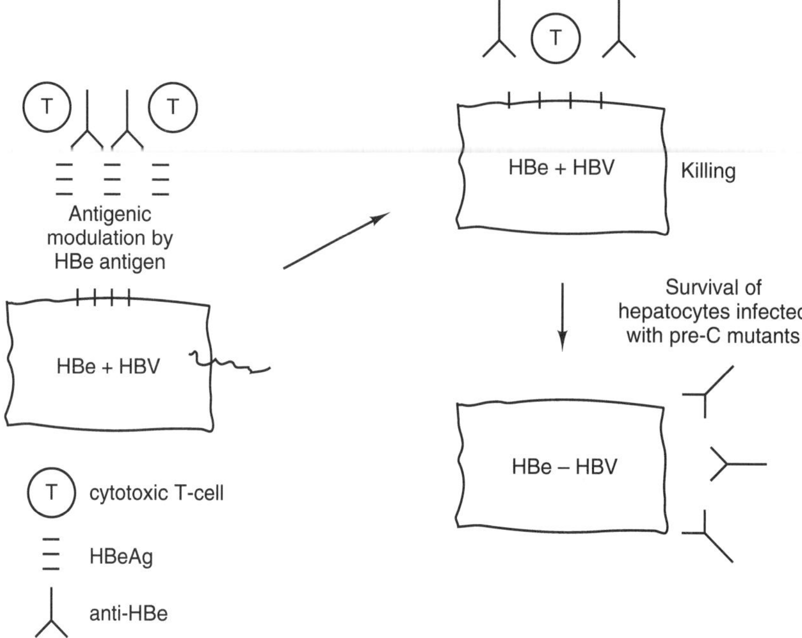

Fig. 7.5 Selection of pre-core mutants. Initially, the predominant HBV genotype is HBe-positive virus. The secreted HBeAg in some way 'modulates' the immune system such that killing of hepatocytes does not occur. With time, this modulation subsides and HBeAg is recognized as foreign: a humoral response occurs to HBe. HBV generates mutants randomly; some of these are HBeAg non-producing genotypes. These survive the immune killing of HBeAg-producing cells and the population seen in serum correspondingly changes.

and is assembled into nucleocapsids (Fig. 7.4). A variety of mutations have now been described in the pre-core region in most of these anti-HBe-positive, high-level viraemic patients. The most common of these is a G to A mutation at position 1896 from the unique *Eco*RI site (mutant A_{1896}) that changes codon 28 from TGG to TAG, the latter being a translational stop codon (Brunetto et al 1989a, Carman et al 1989, Fiordalisi et al 1990, Okamoto et al 1990, Tong et al 1990). A G to A mutation at 1897 (A_{1897}) results in TGA, also a stop codon. Another mutation of interest is found in the first codon, in which the ATG (the translational start codon) is mutated to ACG (Fiordalisi et al 1990, Okamoto et al 1990) so that the pre-core region is not translated. Failure to initiate translation or premature termination of translation results in loss of HBeAg production. There are a number of places within the pre-core where stop codons can be generated by single mutations, but studies to date have shown these to be rare. Additionally, a number of pre-core amino acid substitutions have been detected in HBeAg-minus genotypes (Fiordalisi et al 1990, Carman et al 1992a). Often they are associated with the stop codon at the end of pre-core. Nucleotides 1896–1899 are G residues, all of which have been documented to mutate to A. Only the first two give rise to stop codons, as mentioned above; the other two G to A mutations, A_{1898} (Carman et al 1992a) and A_{1899} (Carman et al 1989) are of unknown significance but are strongly linked with, respectively, T_{1856} and A_{1896}. It seems likely that this run of four Gs is a 'hotspot' for mutation, where the polymerase is particularly liable to misincorporate a nucleotide.

A_{1896} is selected from the wild-type, HBeAg-producing genotype, at or after seroconversion to anti-HBe (Carman et al 1989, Okamoto et al 1990, Carman et al 1993b). This process can take years, during which a mixture of strains is seen. Translation of a key antigenic protein thus ceases;

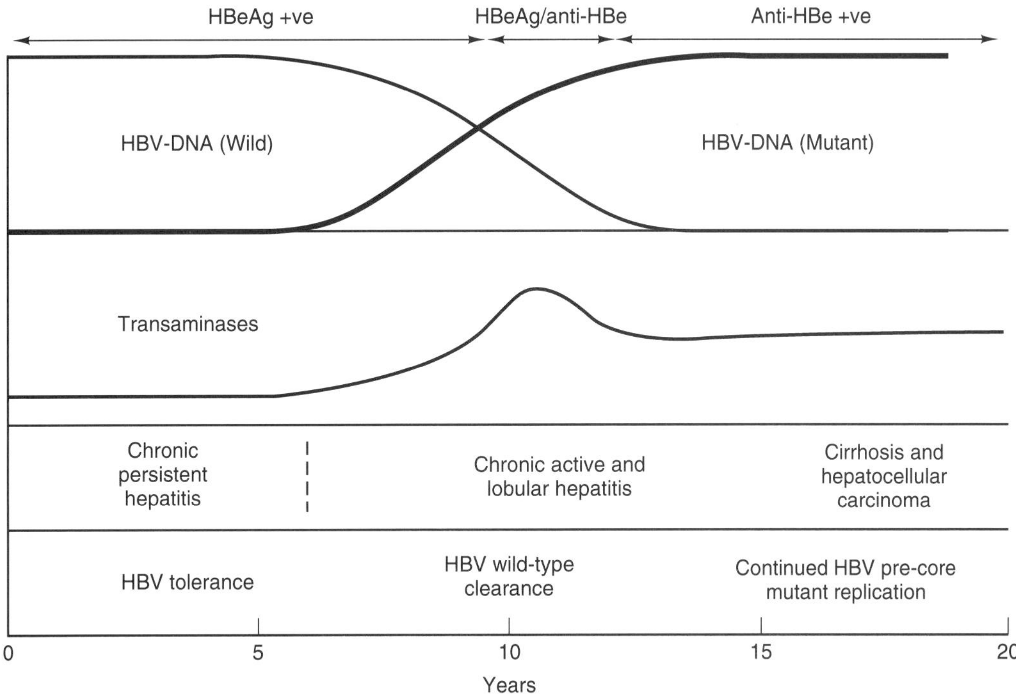

Fig. 7.6 Emergence of the HBe-negative mutant during HBe/anti-HBe seroconversion in chronic HBV infection.

this is an example of a random genetic event followed by survival of the fittest strain in the presence of immune pressure. It should be noted that patients in whom HBeAg and anti-HBe are intermittently detected tend to be infected with the HBeAg-producing genotype (Carman et al 1992a).

The link between severity of disease and such pre-core mutations is presently incompletely defined. The mutations occur both in patients with progressive disease as well as in those who have seroconverted to anti-HBe with normalization of liver transaminases (Okamoto et al 1990). The level of viraemia in the latter case is extremely low – detectable only by polymerase chain reaction (PCR). One group has shown that there is a temporal association with peaks in transaminases and selection of pre-core mutants (Brunetto et al 1991a). The explanation given for increased severity of disease in those who have selected such mutants is that the immune-modulating effect of HBeAg has been lost, exposing the hepatocytes to normal immune activity (Fig. 7.5).

Mixtures of the wild-type and A_{1896} mutant virus have been observed to be related to mild disease (Carman et al 1989, Naoumov et al 1992). This may represent an intermediate stage, with complete selection occurring later. Alternatively, it may be that these patients are not able to mount an effective response against HBeAg, resulting in mild disease and less selection pressure on HBeAg.

The importance of A_{1899} remains unclear. It is only seen (except for rare examples) in those with A_{1896}, implying that a second selection pressure is exerted on the carboxy terminal of pre-core after emergence of A_{1896}. It was linked with severe disease in early studies, but subsequent work has failed to confirm this association (Akahane et al 1990). A weak correlation exists between A_{1899} and poor interferon response (Carman et al 1993b), as discussed below.

Pre-core mutants in fulminant hepatitis

Fulminant hepatitis has a strong linkage with A_{1896}. Many patients with fulminant hepatitis, in particular those who are HBeAg negative, are infected with such a mutant (Carman et al 1991, Kosaka et al 1991, Liang et al 1991, Omata et al 1991). Furthermore, the source of infection for the fulminant cases has also been shown to be infected with the mutant; similar sequences in other regions of the genome from both source and fulminant patients indicate that they are infected with the same genotype. Most patients with fulminant hepatitis are HBeAg negative, and thus it can be said that most fulminant hepatitis is associated with infection by the pre-core mutants. However, one group (Carman et al 1991) and isolated cases from the work of other groups have shown that those who have fulminant hepatitis in the presence of HBeAg are infected with wild-type HBV. Thus, two possibilities exist to explain the linkage of this severe disease with pre-core mutant virus infection. Firstly, it may be that the pre-core mutant infects de novo, resulting in enhanced immune activity because of the absence of HBeAg as an immune modulator. Secondly, it may be that patients with a genetic predisposition to fulminant hepatitis are infected with wild-type HBV (which produces HBeAg) and an enhanced immune response is directed against HBeAg on the surface of hepatocytes. There follows a severe hepatitis with rapid clearance of HBeAg and, in some cases, selection of the mutant. The link between fulminant hepatitis and infection with the pre-core mutation is far from clear. In a limited study, mutation A_{1896} was not seen in patients from Britain, Hong Kong (Lo et al 1992) or the USA (Hasegawa et al 1991a). Thus, geographical differences in the incidence of specific mutations, as discussed later for core mutations and the proline to serine change at amino acid 15 of the pre-core (T_{1856}) (Carman et al 1992a), are seen. The issue of core mutations in fulminant hepatitis will also be discussed later. Experimentation in animal models will be required to define the linkage between severity of liver disease and such mutations.

The incidence of pre-core mutation during acute hepatitis is presently unclear. Two groups (Carman et al 1991, Hasegawa et al 1991b) have noted selection of these strains during non-fulminant acute disease. This is consistent with the appearance of anti-HBe exerting a selection pressure. After this stage, most patients would then go on to clear the virus by other immune mechanisms. Other groups were unable to find evidence for this process during acute hepatitis (Okamoto et al 1990, Kosaka et al 1991), and in fact found that years were sometimes needed for emergence of pre-core variants. In patients with non-fulminant acute disease and pre-core mutant viraemia, the initial inoculum may be mixed, containing wild-type and mutant virus, and in those without pre-core mutant viraemia, the initial inoculum may only have contained the wild-type virus and the duration of application of the selection pressure may be too short to select pre-core mutant viraemia occurring by random mutation during the acute infection.

The condition of fibrosing cholestatic hepatitis has been described recently in liver transplant patients (Davies et al 1991). These patients undergo a fulminant course and the hepatocytes contain large amounts of HBsAg and HBcAg. Preliminary evidence is that there are multiple mutations in the HBcAg of these patients (A Ackrill, personal communication). The issue is raised from time to time that HBV may be cytopathic, rather than immune lysis of infected cells being primarily responsible for the hepatitis. In particular, mutation may result in truncated proteins which have secretory signal sequences or nuclear binding activity (Fig. 7.4). These proteins are not generated by wild-type virus, and it may be that they have toxic effects on cells, explaining how HBV can escape the immune response and yet continue to cause hepatitis.

Pre-core mutants, relationship to interferon therapy

Mediterranean patients with chronic hepatitis who are anti-HBe positive and have circulating HBV DNA may respond poorly to interferon therapy (Brunetto et al 1989b), although a more recent study has shown that they may respond with equal efficacy to HBeAg-positive carriers (Fattovich et al 1992). Therapeutic interferon is believed to amplify immune activity against infected hepatocytes, perhaps by enhancing MHC expression and therefore presentation of peptides to CTL. HBeAg-positive patients who respond to interferon already have evidence of immune activity, as shown by raised transaminases and declining HBV DNA levels. Patients at this stage may have minor populations of pre-core mutants, indicating an active immune response and the beginning of the immune selection process. If this were shown to be the case, patients could be selected for therapy on the basis of sequencing studies. One small study has shown that those with pre-core mutants in the HBeAg-positive stage are more likely to respond to interferon (Takeda et al 1990), although this was not confirmed in two other studies (Xu et al 1992, Carman et al 1993b). These studies showed no pre-core mutations detectable in HBeAg-positive patients before seroconversion, whether or not they responded to interferon. One of these studies (Carman et al 1993b) also compared the frequency of selection of mutants after successful interferon therapy, with natural seroconversion in HBeAg-positive patients. There were no significant differences in the emergence of mutations, although there was a trend towards slower emergence of mutants in those who seroconverted during infection therapy.

The issue of the association of pre-core mutations and efficacy of therapy in anti-HBe-positive, viraemic patients is presently unclear. One group has shown a weak association between the presence of A_{1896} and A_{1899} and poor response (Brunetto et al 1991b) and another group has found that the presence of pre-core mutants before therapy in those who are anti-HBe positive is linked at a low level of significance with poor response (Carman et al 1993b). It cannot at this stage be recommended that all patients should be sequenced before therapy to determine who is likely to respond; many patients who would have responded would be missed by such a protocol.

A pre-core variant that produces HBeAg

The sole proline of the pre-core region has been found to be replaced by serine at amino acid 15 (a C to T mutation at 1856; T_{1856}) in at least three areas of the world. This is within the signal peptide, so is not part of HBeAg. This mutation was found by chance while sequencing the complete HBV genome of an HIV-positive patient with a strange serological profile (Liang et al 1990). These authors felt that it may have been related to the poor anti-HBc response seen in this patient, but there is no direct evidence for this.

A second group found this mutation both in Canadian patients (Carman, Heathcote, unpublished observations) and in Hong Kong Chinese patients with chronic hepatitis (Carman et al 1992a). T_{1856} or A_{1896} was found in about half each of the studied Chinese population, but these mutations were mutually exclusive. T_{1856} was found both in the HBeAg-and the anti-HBe-positive phases of the illness, quite unlike A_{1896}. On long follow-up during the anti-HBe-positive phase, no selection for A_{1896} was seen in those with T_{1856}. There was also a weak association with progressive disease after seroconversion to anti-HBe in those who had a serine at amino acid 15 of pre-core during the HBeAg positive phase. The unresolved question here is why there is no selection for a non-functional pre-core in anti-HBe-positive patients who are infected with T_{1856}. It may be that there is no pressure on infected hepatocytes to select a strain that cannot produce HBeAg; one possible explanation is that HBeAg in patients with this mutation is not displayed on the surface of the hepatocyte, yet is found in serum. Thus, there would be no immune elimination of HBeAg-expressing cells. How HBeAg could be secreted through the endoplasmic reticulum into serum and yet not be expressed on the hepatocyte membrane is speculative. A_{1898} was associated only with T_{1856}, but there was no correlation with disease severity.

Pre-core mutants: replication efficiency and detection methods

Anti-HBe-positive patients with A_{1896} often have high titres of HBV DNA in serum as determined by dot-blot hybridization. It would thus seem that replication efficiency is not lowered by selection of this mutation. In vitro studies using cloned HBV DNA containing A_{1896} have confirmed the replicative competence of A_{1896} (Ulrich et al 1990). Replication is not enhanced by A_{1899} (Will, personal communication).

As sequencing can be time-consuming, various approaches have been tried to screen PCR products for A_{1896}. Hybridization with oligoprobes has met with success (Li et al 1990) and has been applied to clinical material to assess the relative importance of mutants to clinical severity (Brunetto et al 1991a). The alternative is to employ a common primer at one end of the DNA of interest and a second that contains either a G or an A at the 3' end (Lo et al 1992). The latter binds to either the wild-type or the variant genotype. In this way, using the correct reaction conditions, PCR products will only be generated with one or the other of the primers. This technique has been applied to paraffin-fixed sections with some success.

CORE MUTANTS

The finding that pre-core mutants can be found in those with both mild and severe disease after seroconversion has led to the investigation of changes in other genes that may be linked with progression of disease. Attention has been focused on the core gene because an HLA-A2-restricted CTL epitope is located in this region (Bertoletti et al 1991). A number of groups have now described mutations that are selected in the core gene of patients with chronic hepatitis that are linked with progression. One group has found that the virus infecting Japanese HBeAg-positive chronic hepatitis patients has many more amino acid substitutions, clustered between amino acid positions 84 and 101, than that infecting those who have mild disease (Ehata et al 1992) (Fig. 7.7). A few amino acid substitutions were seen in the virus of patients with liver disease, while in those patients without disease the virus had identical sequences to the 'prototype'. A second group found that deletions in multiples of three bases occur in this area of core (Wakita et al 1991). Most of the Japanese patients were HBeAg positive, but both HBeAg-and anti-HBe-positive Mediterranean patients with chronic hepatitis have also been studied (Carman et al 1992c). In these Greek and Italian patients, those in the HBeAg group had one or two amino acid substitutions each compared to the consensus sequence of all 20 patients in the study. A similar number of changes were noted in the anti-HBe-positive patients with minimal hepatitis. In HBeAg-positive patients, these mutations were clustered in a similar area of HBcAg as for Japanese patients. By contrast, five or six substitutions were seen in the anti-HBe-positive

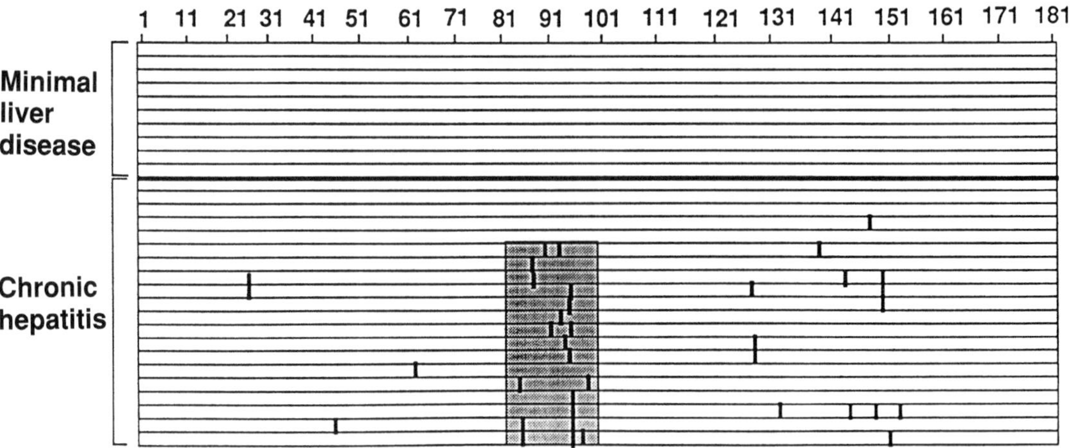

Fig. 7.7 Core mutations seen in Japanese HBeAg-positive chronic hepatitis patients. Ehata et al (1992) described amino acid substitutions seen only in those HBeAg-positive patients with chronic disease. Patients without disease (carriers with minimal liver disease) had no mutations away from the prototype. The substitutions were clustered between amino acids 84 and 101.

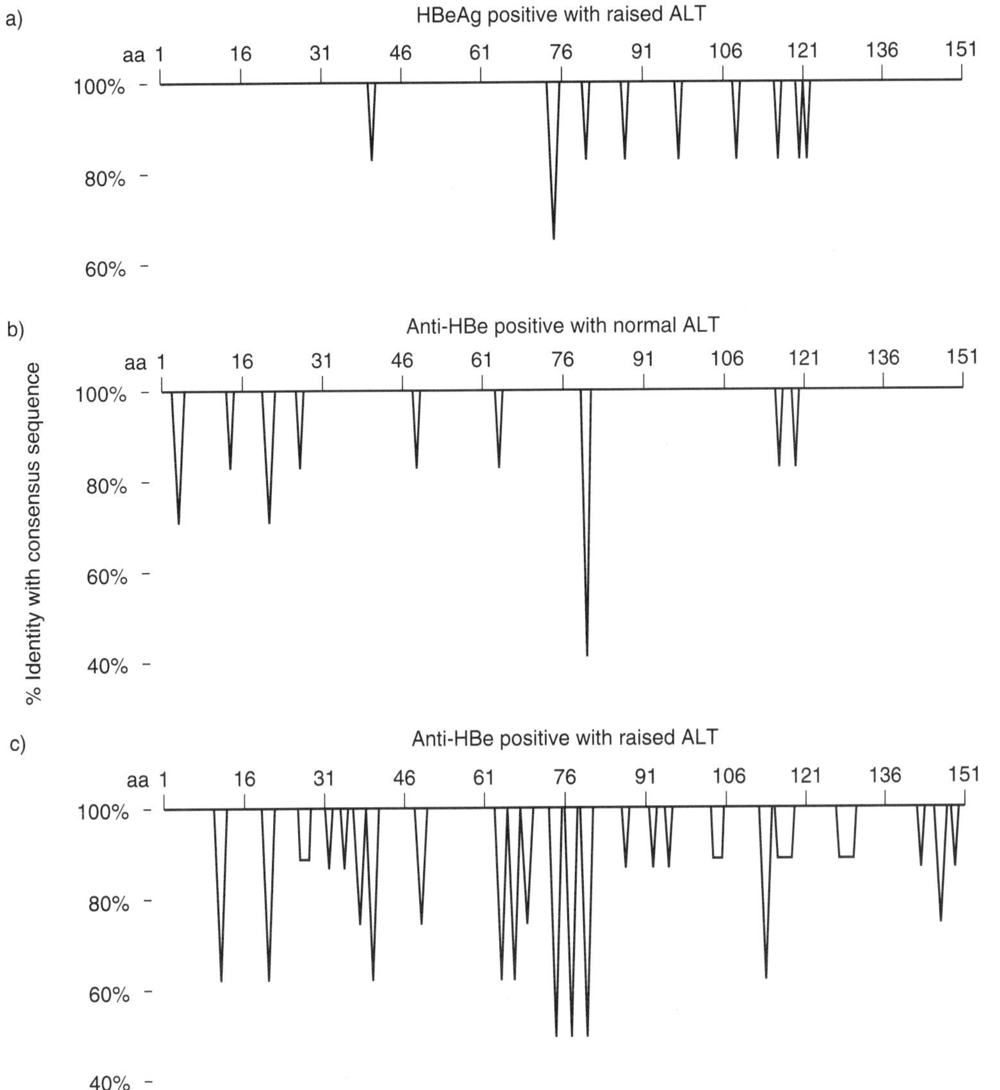

Fig. 7.8 The frequency of mutation of each amino acid in the amino-terminal part of the core protein (aa 1–151) in patients with HBe antigenaemia, and in patients after seroconversion to anti-HBe with and without hepatitis (raised ALT). Pattern c is seen mostly in the Mediterranean countries and in the Far East and is associated with severe disease: mutations are most common in this group of patients. It is with this group that the pre-core stop codon was first associated (Carman et al 1989).

group with progressive disease; these were not clustered (Fig. 7.8). Those in the fulminant hepatitis group had more than six changes each. Thus, severe disease is linked with multiple amino acid changes, only if associated with anti-HBe.

In Mediterranean patients, an amino acid change from threonine to serine at the 12th position of core, very close to the CTL epitope (although there is no association with HLA type), is significantly associated with progressive disease. These patients selected virus with a serine at this position only after they had seroconverted to anti-HBe *and* selected a pre-core stop codon mutant. Yet, in all the HBeAg-positive Japanese patients infected with a wild-type pre-core, serine was found at amino acid 12. The implication of these conflicting results from different geographical areas is that the host is also an important factor in viral evolution. Thus, in Mediterranean patients, there are two linked mutations in two protein products, one of which, it seems, must precede the other: HBeAg must be switched off before threonine will be replaced by serine in the core. A hypothesis to explain this begins by suggesting that HBeAg acts as a humoral target on the surface of hepatocytes, resulting in selection of A_{1896}. Because HBeAg shares common amino acids and T-cell epitopes with HBcAg, and HBeAg is believed to be an immune modulator, it may be that HBeAg 'protects' hepatocytes from immune activity directed against HBcAg. With the absence of HBeAg in a pre-core mutant-infected patient, this immune activity is restored, with attendant selective pressure on the epitope. As this change is near to an HLA-A2 CTL epitope, it is reasonable to suggest that this change results in an altered CTL response. The mutation itself is a few amino acids before the epitope, thus raising the possibility that it is the processing of the peptide with non-presentation that is involved rather than a change in the epitope itself (Fig. 7.3). This would imply that CTL escape, as described for HIV (Phillips et al 1991, Johnson et al 1992), has occurred. An alternative possibility is that anti-HBc antibodies are exerting this pressure; the role of anti-HBc has not been formally evaluated in this process.

Why should these patients go on to have more severe disease if they no longer exhibit the appropriate CTL epitope? This suggests the possibility that, like the clusters of core mutations noted in Japanese patients during the transition to severe disease, these mutations result in presentation of secondary epitopes which attract further immune attention.

One further type of genetic event that occurs in HBV core should be mentioned. Two groups (Bhat et al 1990, Tran et al 1991) have described a 36-bp insertion found around and including the core ATG. In association with this is mutation A_{1896}; it has been seen in both an HIV-infected patient and a carrier who was treated with interferon. The significance of an extra 12 amino acids at the beginning of core is unclear at present, as is the association with interferon treatment. Why two patients should have an almost identical insertion is also unexplained. It may be that these are previously undescribed variants of HBV which may be widespread. Alternatively, they may have arisen independently within each patient by some mechanism such as recombination with the host genome.

ENVELOPE MUTANTS

The envelope genes of HBV

A single open reading frame (ORF) that occupies more than one-third of the HBV genome encodes the three HBsAg-containing polypeptides. Comparison of the coding potential of a number of HBV sequences reveals that the pre-*S* and *S* proteins are highly conserved at the amino acid level, although regions of variability are apparent (Neurath & Kent 1985). The domain within pre-S1 (aa 21–47) which may be involved in binding to the receptor on the hepatocyte (Neurath et al 1986) is highly conserved.

HBV subtypes

Before the sequence of the HBV genome was determined, a number of antigenic subtypes of HBsAg had been defined. In addition to the highly conserved, major antigenic determinant, *a*, two pairs of mutually exclusive subdeterminants, *d* and *y* (Le Bouvier 1971) and *w* and *r* (Bancroft et al 1972), were detected using appropriate antisera. Thus, four subtypes of HBV, *adw*, *ayw*, *adr* and (rarely) *ayr*, are recognized. Rare examples of unusual specificity, such as *adwr* or *adyr*, may be the result of mixed infections. While there are clear differences in the geographical distributions of the subtypes (Courouce-Pauty et al 1983), there seems to be no correlation between virus subtype and virulence.

Recently, specific nucleotide changes have been associated with variation between the pairs of determinants. In each case, a single nucleotide change results in alternative specification of the corresponding codon of arginine or lysine. The epitope responsible for *d/y* specificity seems to lie near residue 122 of the major surface protein – *adw* and *adr* subtypes have lysine at this position, while *ayw* and *ayr* have arginine (Fig. 7.9). Similarly, residue 160 seems to be central to *w/r* specificity – *adw* and *ayw* have lysine at this

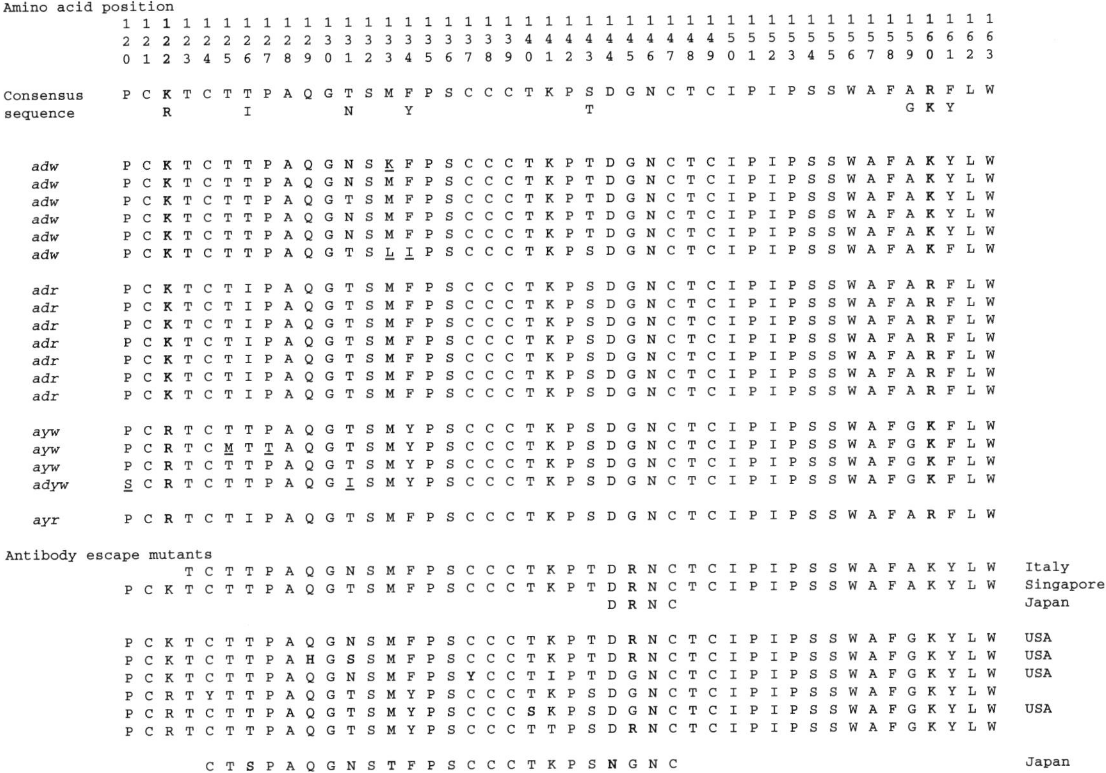

Fig. 7.9 Amino acid sequences of the antigenic domains of the major form of HBsAg. The upper portion shows amino acid positions and the consensus sequence, includes common alternatives. Amino acid sequences in the central portion of the figure are derived from nucleotide sequences deposited in the EMBL database. Positions 122 and 160, which seem to be involved in subtype specificity (see text for details), are emboldened. The sequence designated *adyw* apparently was derived from a mixed infection and has *ady* characteristics. Residues that differ from the consensus are underlined. Sequences of anti-HBs escape variants of HBsAg are given in the lower part of the figure: changed amino acids are emboldened. Sequences are from isolates derived from Italy (Carman et al 1990), Singapore (Harrison et al 1991), Japan (Moriyama et al 1991, Fujii et al 1992) and the USA (McMahon et al 1991, 1992). Sequences from Okamoto et al (1992) are not shown.

The EMBL accession numbers and references relating to Fig. 7.9 are as follows:

For the 6 adw sequences:

1. HBVADW standard; DNA; VRL; 3200 BP. AC V00866; X00715 (Ono et al 1983)
2. HBVADW2 standard; DNA; VRL; 3221 BP. AC X02763 (Valenzuela et al 1980)
3. HPBADWZ standard; DNA; VRL; 3215 BP. AC M54923 (Satrosoewignjo et al 1987)
4. HPBADWZCG standard; DNA; VRL; 3221 BP. AC M57663 (Estacio et al 1988)
5. HPBS standard; DNA; VRL; 681 BP. AC M21030 (Rivkina et al 1988)
6. HPBVCG standard; DNA; VRL; 318 BP. AC D00220 (Vaudin et al 1988)

For the 7 adr sequences:

1. HBVADR standard; DNA; VRL; 3188 BP. AC V00867 (Ono et al 1983)
2. HBVADR4 standard; DNA; VRL; 3214 BP. AC X01587 (Fujiyama et al 1983)
3. HBVADRM standard; DNA; VRL; 3213 BP. AC X14193 (Rho et al 1989)
4. HPBADRA standard; RNA; VRL; 3215 BP. AC M12906 (Kobayashi & Koike 1984)
5. HPBADRC standard; DNA; VR:L; 3215 BP. AC D00630 (Ono et al 1983)
6. HPBCGADR standard; DNA; VRL; 3213 BP. AC M38636 (Kim et al 1988)
7. HPBSADR standard; DNA; VRL; 1279 BP. AC M54892 (Renbao et al 1984)

For the 5 further wild type sequences:

1. HPBHBSAG standard; DNA; VRL; 829 BP. AC M12393; X00715 (Pumpen et al 1984)
2. XXHEPA standard; DNA; VRL; 3182 BP. AC V01460; J02203 (Galibert et al 1979)
3. XXHEPAV standard; DNA; VRL; 3182 BP. AC X02496 (Bichko et al 1985)
4. NCADYW standard; xxx; VRL; 2743 BP. AC J02202 (Pasek et al 1979)
5. HEHBVAYR standard; DNA; VRL; 3215 BP. AC X04615 (Okamoto et al 1986)

position, while *adr* and *ayr* have arginine (Fig. 7.9). These allocations have been confirmed by expression in cell culture of HBsAg from clones of various sequence (Okamoto et al 1987) and by site-directed mutagenesis (Okamoto et al 1989). In addition, variation at residues 113 and 134 (Ashton-Rickardt & Murray 1989a) and residues 144 and 145 (Okamoto et al 1989) may also be involved in *d/y* specificity. Specificity of codon 126 further correlates with *w/r* variation: *w* isolates have threonine and *r* isolates have isoleucine at this position (Fig. 7.9). Minor subtype specificities have also been defined and have been recently correlated with sequence (Norder et al 1992).

Anti-HBs escape mutants

The group-specific determinant, *a*, is located between residues 124 and 147 and seems to have a double loop structure (Brown et al 1984, Waters et al 1987, Howard et al 1988) (Fig. 7.10). The affinity of antibodies in anti-HBs-positive human sera for a linear synthetic peptide representing residues 139–147 was found to be significantly higher than for a peptide representing residues 124–137. Furthermore, if the former peptide was cyclized by formation of a disulphide bond between the terminal cysteine residues, antibody affinity was increased, implying a better fit between the combining site and the peptide (Brown et al 1984). As cysteines can be cross-linked by disulphide bridges, those in this region of HBsAg may be important for maintaining the double loop structure in vivo. The importance of the cysteines at positions 124 and 147, along with the proline at position 142, for antigenic reactivity has been demonstrated by expression of HBsAg following site-directed mutagenesis of the DNA (Ashton-Rickardt & Murray 1989b). The amino acid sequence of this region, particularly the second loop, is highly conserved (Fig. 7.9). The subdeterminants *d/y* and *w/r* seem to flank, and perhaps overlap, this region, forming a cluster of epitopes.

Antibodies which recognize the *a* determinant are a major component of the anti-HBs response following infection or immunization. Isolated cases of HBV mutants with variation in this region which escape neutralization by antibody have been described, and cases of HBsAg positivity have been missed because of failure of current serological assays to detect some variant forms of the antigen.

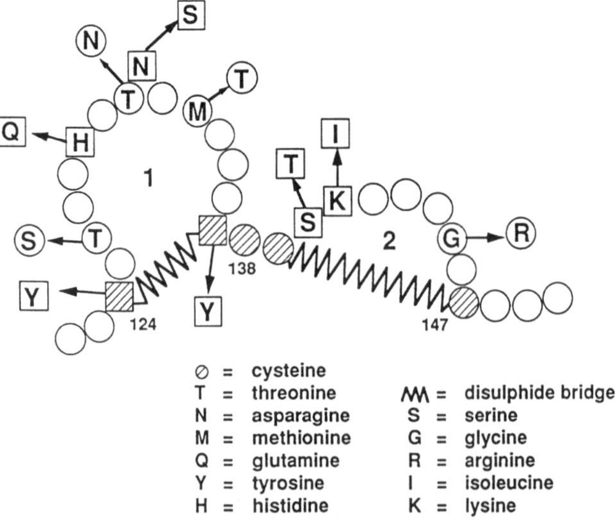

Fig. 7.10 The proposed double loop structure of the 'a' determinant of HBsAg. Cysteines 124–137 and 139–147 form the two loops. Mutations identified in circles are from Moriyama et al (1991). Those in squares are seen in transplant patients receiving monoclonal anti-HBs (McMahon et al 1991).

Variants which escape neutralization by monoclonal anti-HBs have been selected both during immunoprophylaxis of liver transplant recipients and in vaccinees.

Responses to the first-generation (plasma-derived) vaccine were studied in 1590 subjects, mostly infants from two regions of southern Italy, where the prevalence of HBsAg is greater than 5% (Zanetti et al 1988, Carman et al 1990). 44 of the vaccinees became HBsAg-positive, 32 with additional markers of HBV replication, in the presence of anti-HBs. Sera from several of these cases were investigated further, including PCR amplification and nucleotide sequencing of the region of the HBV genome encoding the major antigenic epitopes of HBsAg (Carman et al 1990). One case was of particular interest. The child of an HBeAg-positive mother was given HBIG at birth and at 1 month and a course of vaccine at 3, 4 and 9 months. Despite immunoprophylaxis, he became chronically infected with HBV. HBsAg present at 11 months and at 5 years (when anti-HBs was no longer detectable) showed reduced reactivity with a panel of monoclonal antibodies which were known to bind to the *a* determinant, although antigen from the mother exhibited normal levels of binding with two of the monoclonal antibodies and only slightly reduced binding with a third. Nucleotide sequence studies of HBV in the sample taken from the child at 5 years revealed a point mutation which predicted a change from glycine to arginine at residue 145 in the second loop of the *a* determinant (Carman et al 1990). The mother had glycine at this position.

An identical mutation has subsequently been described in HBV from similar cases from Singapore and Japan (Harrison et al 1991, Fujii et al 1992, Okamoto et al 1992). Again combined immunoprophylaxis (hepatitis B hyperimmune globulin and vaccine) was given in attempt to protect the offspring of HBeAg-positive mothers, but they became chronically infected with coexistent HBsAg and anti-HBs. In these cases, similarity of nucleotide sequence of viruses from mother and child at sites other than aa145, indicated maternal–infant transmission. It has been impossible to demonstrate the mutant in the virus population of the mother, although it may have constituted a minority component. If so, the wild-type virus in the inoculum from the mother may have been neutralized by the hepatitis B immune globulin, leaving the mutant to become established. In no case has horizontal transmission of the mutant HBV been proven, although this must be regarded as a potential problem since anti-HBs-positive vaccinees are likely to be susceptible to infection.

Another mutation has been noted at position 126 in vaccinated children (two siblings), in which an asparagine was selected in the infant (Okamoto et al 1992). However, unlike the Arg-145 cases, this was also seen in 12 of 17 clones taken from the mother.

Selection of mutation Arg-145 by antibody has been observed in the USA. A patient with end-stage liver disease attributable to HBV was transplanted and treated with human monoclonal anti-HBs in an attempt to prevent infection of the graft (McMahon et al 1991). After several months, HBsAg again became detectable in the serum and a number of variant sequences were determined after PCR sequencing of HBV DNA (Figs 7.9 & 7.10). These authors have described further examples of selection of anti-HBs escape mutants following liver transplantation and treatment with monoclonal antibody (McMahon et al 1992). Three of six patients so treated exhibited reactivation of HBV in the graft and the surface gene of the virus was sequenced. The mutation causing the change from glycine to arginine was present in a mixture of genotypes in a second patient; other genotypes present simultaneously in this patient exhibited changes of threonine to serine at residue 140 and cysteine to tyrosine at residue 124. In the case of the third patient, virus escaping neutralization by the monoclonal antibody had a mutation leading to a substitution of tyrosine for the cysteine at residue 137. These are the only natural genotypes of HBV that have lost the cysteines proposed to be involved in the loop structure of the *a* determinant. Whether these are independently viable genotypes was not addressed by this study.

A single case of Arg-145 mutation has been seen in a patient who developed fulminant hepatitis after withdrawal of cytotoxic therapy for lymphoma. No anti-HBs was administered nor was this patient known to have been vaccinated. This may therefore represent the first natural, circulating example of such a variant and indicates that such strains may be more widespread than previously believed (W F Carman, unpublished observations). Of interest is that HBsAg was not detectable using standard monoclonal assays (R Decker et al, unpublished observations).

Substitution of arginine for glycine at amino acid 145 in the yeast vaccine markedly reduced binding by monoclonal and polyclonal antibodies (Waters et al 1992), indicating that this change alone maybe important in the cases of vaccine escape described to date.

Another case of persistence of HBV replication in the presence of anti-HBs has been reported (Moriyama et al 1989, 1991). Here, sequence analysis revealed a mutation affecting amino acid residue 144 with a substitution of asparagine for aspartate. Changes at positions 126, 131 and 133 (Fig. 7.9) may also have affected the antigenicity of the protein. The patient also lacked pre-*S*2 antigen and antibodies and sequence analysis of the relevant region of the HBV genome revealed a large deletion and other mutations (Moriyama et al 1991).

That monoclonal antibody can select HBsAg mutants is not surprising. However, polyclonal antibody in the form of hepatitis B hyperimmune globulin (HBIG) can also lead to different gentoypes after therapy. In a limited study (Carman et al 1992b), HBsAg gene sequences were established in four patients who had infected the homograft during or after HBIG therapy. Comparing the sequences before and after, 1–6 nucleotide changes with 1–4 amino acid substitutions were seen. Overall, 80% of the nucleotide changes led to amino acid changes. Two were in the *a* determinant, including Arg-145, albeit as a mixture after therapy. The other change was at amino acid 130. In the other patients, substitutions were randomly distributed, with one patient having two adjacent alterations. Amino acid changes have been seen at positions 129 and 131 in other patient groups (as described above), perhaps indicating that this is an antigenic area. The significance of these results is in doubt however, because some of the changes seen after therapy were seen before therapy in other patients. This may merely mean that a mutant to one patient is a normal sequence to another.

The issue of diagnostic assays and variants is particularly pertinent. With most of the current HBsAg assays using monoclonal antibodies, it would not be surprising if some variants are not detectable. Mutations of the second loop are most likely to be important in this regard.

It is clear that a number of mutations that alter the amino acid sequence of the *a* domain of the major surface protein may lead to escape from neutralization by anti-HBs. The most common mutation seems to be that which changes residue 145 from glycine to arginine, and it should be possible to include this variant in future formulations of hepatitis B vaccine. However, it is clear that other changes may occur in patients with both HBsAg and anti-HBs; whether these lead to escape has not been formally shown as for the amino acid 145 substitution.

PRE-S

Mutations in the pre-*S* region of the surface ORF have been described in a patient with chronic hepatitis B and hepatocellular carcinoma who died of end-stage liver failure (Gerken et al 1991). Serum HBV DNA was not detected by nucleic acid hybridization but could be amplified by PCR using several primer pairs. Amplification of the DNA encoding the pre-S domains yielded a shorter product than expected, and sequence analysis of that product revealed a plethora of nucleotide substitutions and deletions. The most significant deletion of 183 bp was found in 9 of 12 clones and resulted in the predicted loss of 61 amino acid residues from the carboxy-terminal half of the pre-*S*1 domain and of the promoter for the mRNA for the middle and major forms of the hepatitis B virus envelope proteins. The authors also presented electron microscopical evidence of aberrant forms of virions. Interestingly, the region of the genome encoding the domain in the amino portion of pre-*S*1, which is believed to be responsible for attachment to the receptor on the hepatocyte (Neurath et al 1986), was conserved in all of the clones.

Analysis of HBV from an infected patient without HBeAg in Sardinia revealed a 21-nt deletion as well as mutations in the pre-core region (Lai et al 1991). The deletion resulted in the loss of seven amino acid residues from the pre-S2 region of HBsAg and the polymerase. Mutations in the pre-S2 region seem to be common in HBV genomes isolated in Italy (Fernholz et al 1991, Sanantonio et al 1992). In some of the sequences described, the pre-S2 initiation codon was lost, preventing pre-S2 synthesis, and the pre-*S*1 region was truncated.

SERONEGATIVE HBV

A number of reports have described the serological profiles of infections in patients which may be attributable to variants of HBV. However, this hypothesis has not always been confirmed by sequence analysis. Two such cases were studied by Wands et al (1986). One patient was seropositive for anti-HBs and anti-HBc and weakly positive for HBV DNA as determined by hybridization. HBsAg was detected using radioimmunoassay (RIA) based on monoclonal anti-HBs but not by assays using polyclonal antiserum. The other also had HBsAg detectable only by the monoclonal antibody-based test and was weakly positive for HBV DNA by hybridization but had no other markers of HBV infection. Virus from both patients was able to infect chimpanzees which were anti-HBs positive following immunization. Furthermore, a non-immune chimpanzee infected with virus from the first case was later challenged with wild-type HBV and succumbed to infection (Wands et al 1986). It seems likely that the structural proteins of these viruses lack at least some of the epitopes of wild-type HBV, but nucleotide sequence data have not been reported.

Three further cases of infection negative for conventional HBV markers have been investigated by Thiers et al (1988). All were positive for HBV DNA by PCR. One patient was positive for HBsAg using a monoclonal RIA, and transmission to a chimpanzee resulted in acute hepatitis with normal markers of infection. Transmission from another patient, in whom HBsAg was not detectable using the monoclonal assay, produced an acute hepatitis with raised ALT and HBV DNA detectable by PCR. However, HBsAg and anti-HBc were not detected in the chimpanzee, although seroconversion to anti-HBs accompanied clinical recovery. Limited nucleotide sequence analysis of the highly conserved 3' portion of the surface open reading frame revealed only a single point mutation in the latter case (Thiers et al 1988). Sequencing of the region encoding the major antigenic domains of HBsAg was not reported. The complete nucleotide sequence of a further isolate of HBV from a patient without serological markers and which was transmitted to a chimpanzee has been determined (Liang et al 1990). Numerous point mutations were detected throughout the genome and some of these may have accounted for the lack of serological reactivity.

Other cases characterized by unusual serological profiles were first described in Senegal (Coursaget et al 1987) and have since been recorded elsewhere. These are distinguished by the absence of anti-HBc or HBeAg, HBsAg positivity and without seroconversion to anti-HBs after recovery and, in some cases, infection despite vaccine-induced anti-HBs. The agent responsible for such infections has been designated HBV_2 (Coursaget et al 1987), but again sequencing studies have not been reported and it is not clear how different this virus is from wild-type HBV. Virus from an individual case in the Senegalese series was transmitted to two chimpanzees and produced apparently normal infections (Gallagher et al 1991). It has been suggested that 'HBV_2-like' infections may be explained, at least in part, by abnormal immune responses in the patient. However, others continue to postulate that a variant strain of HBV, perhaps with an altered mode of transmission, is responsible (Echevarria et al 1991).

HBx MUTANTS

HBx has transactivating properties, but its role in the biology of HBV is unclear. HBx protein and antibody can be detected in serum, and these assays have been used to study samples from renal dialysis patients in the USA (M Feitelson et al, unpublished observations). The patients were from a cohort that was dialysed during the period when HBV was endemic in dialysis units. It was noted that many had circulating HBx or anti-HBx; unexpectedly, patients without any markers of HBV but raised transaminases were also positive. The presence of these markers was intermittent. PCR studies showed that HBV DNA was positive, but that the HBx PCR product on electrophoresis was shorter than expected. In many cases, mixtures of deleted and normal-length HBx were present. An examination of known HBV-infected dialysis patients revealed HBx deletions in a wide range of individuals, but usually in those with low-level HBV DNA in serum or after seroconversion to anti-HBx. It was hypothesized that these deletions were allowing avoidance of immune surveillance: they were in some way linked to the low level of viraemia and the absence of the usual markers of HBV infection such as HBsAg and anti-HBc. Pre-core mutant A_{1896} was also seen in patients without HBsAg, either with or without anti-HBV antibodies, and very seldom simultaneously with HBx deletions (W F Carman et al, unpublished observations). Patients remained PCR positive for long periods after seroconversion, and pre-core mutants were not seen in any anti-HBe seroconverters. This may relate to the renal dialysis therapy. Further work is needed to define the importance of these mutations.

CONCLUSIONS

HBV seems to be highly evolved. It has a small genome, makes very efficient use of its nucleic acid and many regions are highly conserved, even between different hepadnaviruses. Yet the potential for significant change is also present. The changes described above may not be 'evolution'; it may be that viruses containing mutations with significant structural or functional effects are not the 'preferred' strains and either a minor wild type virus population infects the next host or the wild-type virus is back-selected upon infection of a new host. The most important selection pressure affecting HBV seems to be the immune response. The mutations seen in the pre-core/core gene and their effect on the antigenicity of the encoded proteins are giving important insights into the pathogenesis of chronic HBV infection, by delineating the epitopes under immune pressure. Variants of HBV with altered antigenicity of the envelope protein (large, middle and major) have shown that HBV is not as antigenically singular as previously believed and that humoral escape mutation can occur in vivo. They are a cause for concern on two accounts. Firstly, failure to detect HBsAg may lead to transmission through donated blood or organs. Secondly, HBV may infect individuals who are anti-HBs positive following immunization. Variation in the second loop of the *a* determinant seems to be of particular importance. Mutants, variants, altered genotypes and unusual strains are now being sought in many laboratories and we must be wary of the significance of findings that do not have a strong clinical association or proven in vitro effect.

REFERENCES

Akahane Y, Yamanaka T, Suzuki H et al 1990 Chronic active hepatitis with hepatitis B virus DNA and antibody against e antigen in the serum. Gastroenterology 90: 1113–1119

Ashton-Rickardt P G, Murray K 1989a Mutations that change the immunological subtype of hepatitis B virus surface antigen and distinguish between antigenic and immunogenic determination Journal of Medical Virology 29: 916–203

Ashton-Rickardt P G, Murray K 1989b Mutants of the Hepatitis B virus surface antigen that define some antigenically essential residues in the immunodominant *a* region. Journal of Medical Virology 29: 196–203

Bancroft W H, Mundon F K, Russell P K 1972 Detection of additional antigenic determinants of hepatitis B antigen. Journal of Immunology 109: 842–848

Bertoletti A, Ferrari C, Fiaccadori F et al 1991 HLA class I–restricted human cytotoxic T cells recognize endogenously synthesized HBV core antigens. Proceedings of the National Academy of Sciences of the USA 88: 10445–10449

Bhat R A, Ulrich P P, Vyas G N 1990 Molecular characterization of a new variant of hepatitis B virus in a persistently infected homosexual man. Hepatology 11: 271–276

Bichko V, Dreilina D, Pushko P M, Pumpen P P, Gren F 1985 Subtype ayw variant of hepatitis B virus. FEBS Letters 185: 208–212

Bonino F, Rosina F, Rizzetto M et al 1986 Chronic hepatitis in HBsAg carriers with serum HBV-DNA and anti-HBe. Gastroenterology 90: 1268–1273

Brocade Wu C-T, Levine M, Homa F, Highlander S L, Glorioso J C 1990 Characterisation of the antigenic structure of herpes simplex virus type 1 glycoprotein C through DNA sequence analysis of monoclonal antibody-resistant mutants. Journal of Virology 64: 856–863

Brown S E, Howard C R, Zuckerman A J, Steward M W

1984 Affinity of antibody responses in man to hepatitis B vaccine determined with synthetic peptides. Lancet ii: 184–187

Brunetto M R, Stemmler M, Schodel F et al 1989a Identification of HBV variants which cannot produce precore-derived HBeAg and may be responsible for severe hepatitis. Italian Journal of Gastroenterology 21: 151–154

Brunetto M R, Oliveri F, Rocca G et al 1989a Natural course and response to interferon of chronic hepatitis B accompanied by antibody to hepatitis e antigen. Hepatology 10: 198–202

Brunetto M R, Giarin M M, Oliver F et al 1991a Wild-type and e antigen-minus hepatitis B viruses and course of chronic hepatitis. Proceedings of the National Academy of Sciences of the USA 88: 4186–4190

Brunetto M R, Saracco G, Oliveri F et al 1991b HBV heterogeneity and response to interferon. Journal of Hepatology 13: S15

Carman W F 1992 Genetic variation in hepatitis B virus. Recent Advances in Gastroenterology 9: 217–230

Carman W F, Thomas H C 1992 Genetic variation in hepatitis B virus. Gastroenterology 102: 711–719

Carman W F, Jacyna M R, Hadziyannis S et al 1989 Mutation preventing formation of e antigen in patients with chronic HBV infection. Lancet ii: 588–591

Carman W F, Zanetti A R, Karayiannis P et al 1990 Vaccine-induced escape mutant of hepatitis B virus. Lancet 336: 325–329

Carman W F, Hadziyannis S, Karayiannis P et al 1991 Association of the precore variant of HBV with acute and fulminant hepatitis B infection. In: Hollinger F B, Lemon S M, Margolis H S (eds) Viral hepatitis and liver disease Williams & Wilkins, Baltimore pp 216–219

Carman W F, Ferrao M, Lok A S F, Ma O C K, Lai C L, Thomas H C 1992a Pre-core sequence variation in Chinese isolates of hepatitis B virus. Journal of Infectious Disease 165: 127–133

Carman W F, McIntyre G, Klein H 1992b Mutation of HBsAg in homograft recipients receiving hyperimmune globulin. Journal of Hepatology 16: S9.

Carman W F, McIntyre G, Hadzinyannis S, Alberti A, Fattovich G, Thomas H C 1992c Mutation of HBcAg after loss of HBeAg. Journal of Hepatology 16: S25

Carman W F, Thomas H C, Domingo E 1993a Genetic variation in viruses; clinical relevance to HBV. Lancet 341: 349–353

Carman W F, Fattovich G, McIntyre G et al 1993b Hepatitis B virus pre-core variation and interferon therapy. Hepatology (in press)

Chu C-M, Karayiannis P, Fowler M J F, Monjardino J, Liaw Y-F, Thomas H C 1985 Natural history of chronic hepatitis B virus infection in Taiwan: Studies of hepatitis B virus DNA in serum. Hepatology 5: 431–434

Courouce Pauty A M, Plancon A, Soulier J P 1983 Distribution of HBsAg subtypes in the world. Vox Sanguis 44: 197–211

Coursaget P, Yvonnet B, Bourdil C 1987 HBsAg positive reactivity in man not due to hepatitis B virus. Lancet ii: 1354–1358

Davies S E, Portmann B C, O'Grady J G et al 1991 Hepatic histological findings after transplantation for chronic hepatitis B virus infection, including a unique pattern of fibrosing cholestatic hepatitis. Hepatology 13: 150–157

Domingo E, Martinez-Salas E, Sobrino F et al 1985 The quasispecies (extremely heterogenous) nature of viral RNA genome populations: biological relevance – a review. Gene 40: 1–8

Domingo E, Holland J J, Ahlquist P (eds) 1988 RNA genetics. CRC Press, Boca Raton

Echevarria J M, Leon P, Domingo C J, Contreras G, Fuertes A, Lopez J A, Echeverria J E 1991 Characterization of HBV2-like infections in Spain. Journal of Medical Virology 33: 240–247

Ehata T, Omata M, Yokosuka O, Hosodo K, Ohto M 1992 Variations in codons 84–101 in the core nucleotide sequence correlate with hepatocellular injury in chronic hepatitis B virus infection. Journal of Clinical Investigation 89: 332–338

Estacio R C, Chavez C C, Okamoto H, Lingao A L, Reyes M T, Domingo E, Mayumi M 1988 Nucleotide sequence of a hepatitis B virus genome of subtype adw isolated from a Philippino: comparison with the reported three genomes of the same subtype. Journal of Gastroenterology and Hepatology 3: 215–222

Fattovich G, Farci P, Rugge M et al 1992 Chronic hepatitis B positive for anti-HBe and with hepatitis B viral DNA in serum can be successfully treated with alpha interferon. Hepatology 15: 584–589

Fernholz D, Stemler M, Brunetto M et al 1991 Replicating and virion secreting hepatitis B mutant virus unable to produce preS2 protein. Journal of Hepatology 13: S102–S104

Fiordalisi G, Cariani E, Mantero G et al 1990 High genomic variability in the pre-C region of hepatitis B virus in anti-HBe, HBV-DNA positive chronic hepatitis. Journal of Medical Virology 31: 297–300

Foster G R, Ackrill A M, Goldin R D, Kerr I M, Thomas H C, Stark G R 1991 Expression of the terminal protein region of hepatitis B virus and inhibits cellular responses to interferons α and ß and double-stranded RNA. Proceedings of the National Academy of Sciences of the USA 88: 2888–2892

Fujii H, Moriyama K, Sakamoto N et al 1992 Gly 145 to Arg substitution in HBs antigen of immune escape mutant of hepatitis B virus. Biochemical and Biophysics Research Communications 184: 1152–1157

Fujiyama A, Miyanohara A, Nozaki C, Yoneyama T, Ohtomo N, Matsubara K 1983 Cloning and structural analyses of hepatitis B virus DNAs, subtype adr. Nucleic Acids Research 11: 4601–4610

Galibert F, Mandart E, Fitoussi F, Tiollais P, Charnay P 1979 Nucleotide sequence of the hepatitis B virus genome (subtype ayw). cloned in *E. Coli.* Nature 281: 646–650

Gallagher M, Fields H A, De La Torre N et al 1991 Characterization of HBV2 by experimental infection of primates. In: Hollinger F B, Lemon S M, Margolis H S (eds) Viral hepatitis and liver disease. Williams & Wilkins Baltimore, pp 227–229

Gerken G, Kremsdorf D, Petit M A et al 1991 Hepatitis B defective virus with rearrangements in the preS gene during HBV chronic infection. Journal of Hepatology 13: S93–S96

Hadziyannis S J, Lieberman H M, Karvountzis M G, Shafritz D 1983 Analysis of liver disease, nuclear HBcAg, viral replication and hepatitis B virus in liver and serum of HBeAg vs anti-HBe positive chronic hepatitis B virus infection. Hepatology 3: 652–662

Harrison T J, Hopes E A, Oon C J, Zanetti A R, Zuckerman A J 1991 Independent emergence of a vaccine-induced escape mutant of hepatitis-B virus. Journal of Hepatology 13: S105–S107

Hasegawa K, Shapiro C N, Alter M S, Liang T S 1991 Lack of an association of hepatitis B virus precore mutation with fulminant hepatitis B in the USA. Hepatology 14: 78A

Hasegawa K, Huang J, Wands J R, Obata H, Liang T J 1991b Association of hepatitis B viral precore mutations with fulminant hepatitis B in Japan. Virology 185: 460–463

Holland J J, Spindler K, Horodyski F, Grabau E, Nichol S, VandePol S 1982 Rapid evolution of RNA genomes. Science 215: 1577–1585

Howard C R, Stirk H J, Brown S E et al 1988 Towards the development of synthetic Hepatitis B Vaccines. In: Zuckerman A J (ed) Viral hepatitis and liver disease. Alan R Liss, New York, pp 1094–1101

Johnson R P, Trocha A, Buchanan T M, Walker B D 1992 Identification of overlapping HLA class- I-restricted cytotoxic T cell epitopes in a conserved region of the human immunodeficiency virus type 1 envelope glycoprotein: definition of minimum epitopes and analysis of the effects of sequence variation. Journal of Experimental Medicine 175: 961–971

Kim K T, Hyun S W, Kim Y S, Rho H M 1988 Complete nucleotide sequence of hepatitis B virus (subtype adr). Korean Journal of Biochemistry 21: 319–331

Kobayashi M, Koike K 1984 Complete nucleotide sequence of hepatitis B virus DNA of subtype adr and its conserved gene organization. Gene 30: 227–232

Kosaka Y, Takase K, Kojima M et al 1991 Fulminant hepatitis B: Induction by hepatitis B virus mutants defective in the precore region and incapable of encoding e antigen. Gastroenterology 324: 1087–1094

Lai M E, Melis A, Mazzoleni A P, Farci P, Balestrieri A 1991 Sequence analysis of hepatitis B virus genome of a new mutant of ayw subtype isolated in Sardinia. Nucleic Acids Research 19: 5078

Le Bouvier G L 1971 The heterogeneity of Australia antigen. Journal of Infectious Diseases 123: 671–675

Lemon S M, Binn L N, Marchwicki R et al 1990 *In vivo* replication and reversion to wild type of a neutralization-resistant antigenic variant of hepatitis A virus. Journal of Infectious Diseases 161: 7–13

Li J, Tong S, Vitviski L et al 1991 Rapid detection and further characterization of infection with hepatitis B virus variants containing a stop codon in the distal pre-C region. Journal of General Virology 71: 1993–1998

Liang T J, Blum H E, Wands J R 1990 Characterization and biological properties of a hepatitis B virus isolated from a patient without hepatitis B virus serologic markers. Hepatology 12: 204–212

Liang T J, Hasegawa K, Rimon N, Wands J R, Ben-Porath E 1991 A hepatitis B virus mutant associated with an epidemic of fulminant hepatitis. New England Journal of Medicine 324: 1705–1709

Lo E S-F, Lo Y-M D, Tse C H, Fleming K A Detection of hepatitis B pre-core mutant by allele-specific polymerase chain reaction. Journal of Clinical Pathology 45: 689–692

McMahon G, Ehrlich P H, Moustafa Z A et al 1992 Genetic alterations in the gene encoding the major HBsAg: DNA and immunological analysis of recurrent HBsAg derived from monoclonal antibody-treated liver transplant patients. Hepatology 15: 757–766

McMahon G, McCarthy L A, Dottavio D, Ostberg L 1991 Surface antigen and polymerase gene variation in hepatitis B virus isolates from a monoclonal antibody treated liver transplant patient. In: Hollinger F B, Lemon S M, Margolis H S (eds) Viral hepatitis and liver disease. Williams & Wilkins, Baltimore, pp 219–221

Milich D R, Jones J E, Hughes J L, Price J, Raney A K, McLachlan A 1990 Is a function of the secreted hepatitis B e antigen to induce immunologic tolerance in utero? Proceedings of the National Academy of Sciences of the USA 87: 6599–6603

Mondelli M, Vergani G M, Alberti A, Eddleston A L W F, Williams R 1982 Specificity of T cell cytotoxicity to autologous hepatocytes in chronic hepatitis B virus infection: evidence that T cells are directed against HBV core antigen exposed on hepatocytes. Journal of Immunology 129: 2773–2779

Moriyama K, Ishibashi H, Kashiwagi S et al 1989 Presence of HBV DNA and HBeAg in serum of an anti-HBs-positive individual (letter). Gastroenterology 97: 1068–1069

Moriyama K, Nakajima E, Hohjoh H, Asayama R, Okochi K 1991 Immunoselected hepatitis B virus mutant. Lancet 337: 125

Naoumov N V, Schneider R, Grötzinger T et al 1992 Precore mutant hepatitis B virus infection and liver disease. Gastroenterology 102: 538–543

Neurath A R and Kent S B H 1985 Antigenic structure of human hepatitis viruses. In: vanRegenmortel M V H, Neurath A R (eds) Immunohistochemistry of viruses. Elsevier, Amsterdam, pp 325–366

Neurath A R, Kent S B, Strick N, Parker K 1986 Identification and chemical synthesis of a host cell receptor binding site on hepatitis B virus. Cell 46: 429–436

Okamoto H, Imai M, Shimozaki M, Hoshi Y, Iizuka H, Gotanda T, Tsuda F, Miyakawa Y, Mayumi M 1986 Nucleotide sequence of a cloned hepatitis B virus genome, subtype ayr: comparison with genomes of the other three subtypes. Journal of General Virology 67: 2305–2314

Okamoto H, Imai M, Miyakawa Y, Mayumi M, 1987 Site-directed mutagenesis of hepatitis B surface antigen sequence at codon 160 from arginine to lysine for conversion of subtypic determinant from r to w. Biochemical and Biophysics Research Communications 148: 500–504

Okamoto H, Omi S, Wang Y et al 1989 The loss of subtypic determinants in alleles, d/y or w/r on hepatitis B surface antigen. Molecular Immunology 26: 197–205

Okamoto H, Yotsumoto S, Akahane Y et al 1990 Hepatitis B viruses with pre-core region defects prevail in persistently infected hosts along with seroconversion to the antibody against e antigen. Journal of Virology 64: 1298–1303

Okamoto H, Yano K, Nozaki Y et al 1992 Mutations within the s gene of hepatitis-B virus transmitted from mothers to babies immunized with hepatitis-B immune globulin and vaccine. Pediatric Research 32: 264–268

Omata M, Ehata T, Yokosuka O, Hosoda K, Ohto M 1991 Mutations in the precore region of hepatitis B virus DNA in patients with fulminant and severe hepatitis. New England Journal of Medicine 324: 1699–704

Ono Y, Onda H, Sasada R, Igarashi K, Sugino Y, Nishioka K 1983 The complete nucleotide sequences of the cloned hepatitis B virus DNA: subtype adr and adw. Nucleic Acids Research 11: 1747–1757

Ou J-H, Laub O, Rutter W J 1986 Hepatitis B virus gene function: the precore region targets the core antigen to cellular membranes and causes the secretion of the e antigen. Proceedings of the National Academy of Sciences of the USA 83: 1578–1582

Pasek M, Goto T, Gilbert W et al 1979. Hepatitis B virus genes and their expression in *E. coli* Nature 282: 575–579

Penna A, Fowler P, Bertoletti A et al 1992 Hepatitis B virus (HBV)-specific cytotoxic T-cell (CTL) response in humans. Characterization of HLA class II-restricted CTLs that recognize endogenously synthesized HBV envelope antigens. Journal of Virology 66, 1193–1198

Phillips R E, Rowland-Jones S, Nixon D F et al 1991 Human immunodeficiency virus genetic variation that can escape cytotoxic T cell recognition. Nature 354: 453–459

Pircher H, Moskophidis D, Rohrer U, Bürki K, Hengartner H, Zinkernagel R M 1990 Viral escape by selection of cytotoxic T cell-resistant virus variants in vivo. Nature 346: 629–633

Pumpen P P, Kozlovskaya T M, Borisova G L et al 1984. Synthesis of the surface antigen of hepatitis B virus in *Escherichia coli* Dokl. Biochem. 271: 246–249

Renbao G, Leuping S, Meijin C, Zaiping L 1984 The nucleotide sequence of surface antigen gene of hepatitis B virus subtype adr. Sci. Sin., B, Chen Biol. Agric. Med. Earth Sci. 27: 926–935

Rho H M, Kim K, Hyun S W, Kim Y S 1989 The nucleotide sequence and reading frames of a mutant hepatitis B virus adr. Nucleic Acids Research 17: 2124–2124

Rivkina M B, Lunin V G, Mahov A M, Tikchonenko T I, Kukain R A 1988 Nucleotide sequence of integrated hepatitis B virus DNA and human flanking regions in the genome of the PLC/PRF/5 cell line. Gene 64: 285–296

Santantonio T, Jung M C, Schneider R et al 1992 Hepatitis-B virus genomes that cannot synthesize pre-S2 proteins occur frequently and as dominant virus populations in chronic carriers in Italy. Virology 188: 948–952

Satrosoewignjo R I, Omi S, Okamoto H, Mayumi M, Rustam M, Sujudi 1987 The complete nucleotide sequence of HBV DNA clone of subtype adw (pMND122) from Menado in Sulawesi Island, Indonesia. ICMR Ann. 7: 51–60

Schlicht H-J, Schaller H 1989 The secretory core protein of human hepatitis B virus is expressed on the cell surface. Journal of Virology 63: 5399–5404

Shafritz D A, Shouval D, Sherman H, et al 1981. Integration of hepatitis B virus DNA into the genome of liver cells in chronic liver disease and hepatocellular carcinoma New England Journal of Medicine 305: 1067–1073

Steinhauer D A, Holland J J 1987 Rapid evolution of RNA viruses. Annual Reviews of Microbiology 41: 409–433

Takeda K, Akahane Y, Suzuki H et al 1990 Defects in the precore region of the HBV genome in patients with chronic hepatitis B after sustained seroconversion from HBeAg to anti-HBe induced spontaneously or with interferon therapy. Hepatology 12: 1284–1289

Temin H 1989 Is HIV unique or merely different? Journal of AIDS 2: 1–9

Thiers V, Nakajima E, Kremsdorf D 1988 Transmission of hepatitis B from hepatitis-B-seronegative subjects. Lancet ii: 1273–1276

Thomas H C, Jacyna M, Waters J, Main J 1988 Virus–host interaction in chronic hepatitis B virus infection. Seminars in Liver Disease 8: 342–349

Tong S, Li J, Vitvitski L, Trepo C 1990 Active hepatitis B virus replication in the presence of anti-HBe is associated with viral variants containing an inactive pre-C region. Virology 176: 596–603

Tran A, Kremsdorf D, Capel F et al 1991 Emergence of and takeover by hepatitis B virus (HBV) with rearrangements in the pre-S/S and pre-C/C genes during chronic HBV infection. Journal of Virology 65: 3566–3574

Twu J S, Schloemer R H 1989 Transcription of the human beta interferon gene is inhibited by hepatitis B virus. Journal of Virology 63: 3065–3071

Ulrich P P, Bhat R A, Kelly I et al 1990 A precore-defective mutant of hepatitis B virus associated with e antigen-negative chronic liver disease. Journal of Medical Virology 32: 109–118

Valenzuela P, Quiroga M, Zalvidar J, Gray P, Rutter W J 1980 The nucleotide sequence of the hepatitis B viral genome and the identification of the major viral genes. In: Fields B N et al (eds) Animal virus genetics, Academic Press, pp 57–70

Vaudin M, Wolstenholme A J, Tsiquaye K N, Zuckerman A J, Harrison T J 1988 The complete nucleotide sequence of the genome of a hepatitis B virus isolated from a naturally infected chimpanzee. Journal of General Virology 69: 1383–1389

Wakita T, Kakumu S, Shibata M et al 1991 Detection of pre-C and core region mutants of hepatitis B virus in chronic hepatitis B virus carriers. Journal of Clinical Investigation 88: 1793–1801

Wands J R, Fujita Y K, Isselbacher K J 1986 Identification and transmission of hepatitis B virus-related variants. Proceedings of the National Academy of Sciences of the USA 83: 6608–6612

Waters J A, O'Rourke S M, Richardson S C et al 1987 Qualitative analysis of the humoral immune response to the 'a' determinant of HBs antigen after inoculation with plasma-derived or recombinant vaccine. Journal of Medical Virology 21: 155–160

Waters J, Kennedy M, Voet P et al 1992 Loss of the common 'a' determinant of hepatitis B surface antigen by a vaccine induced escape mutant. Journal of Clinical Investigation 90: 2543–2547

Xu J, Brown D, Harrison T, Lin Y, Dusheiko G 1992 Absence of hepatitis B virus precore mutants in patients with chronic hepatitis B responding to interferon-α. Hepatology 15: 1002–1006

Yamada G, Takaguchi K, Matsueda K et al 1990 Immunoelectron microscopic observation of intrahepatic HBeAg in patients with chronic hepatitis B. Hepatology 12: 133–140

Zanetti A R, Tanzi E, Manzillo G et al 1988 Hepatitis B variant in Europe (letter). Lancet ii: 1132–1133

UPDATE

- *Mutants and fulminant hepatitis.* Further cases have been reported that weaken the association between pre-core mutants and fulminant hepatitis. Two of 22 patients were positive for HBeAg. Four anti-HBe positive cases had pre-core changes that precluded translation of HBeAg; 2 only had A_{1896}. The core promoter region was altered in 10 of 37 cases (Laskus et al 1993). A strain of HBV isolated from a fulminant case was transmitted to chimpanzees; an identical strain was recovered that had multiple changes in the *cis*-acting regulatory elements (6 of 13 such changes were seen in the enhancer II-core promoter region). The pre-core stop codon was also present (Ogata et al 1993). Core genes were sequenced in acute hepatitis (no changes seen), severe acute and fulminant cases. The latter two groups had mutations clustered to codons 84–99 and 48–60 (Chuang et al 1993).

- *Pre-core mutant transmission.* Pre-core mutants containing woodchuck hepatitis viruses (WHV) replicte well in their natural hosts (Chen et al 1992). Newborn woodchucks infected with wild-type WHV developed chronic infections and those infected with pre-core mutant, self-limited infection (Bonino & Brunetto 1993). Similarly, newborn humans developed self-limited infections after transmission from their mothers with pre-core mutant virus (Raimondo et al 1993).

- *Core mutants.* Further work in Mediterranean patients shows that the core amino-acid to nucleotide substitution ratio is 2 in anti-HBe positive patients with severe liver disease, compared to 7 in those with normal transaminases. This implies selection at the protein level (by the immune response) in the former group. Core mutations appeared after selection of a pre-core stop codon, not only after the appearance of anti-HBe. This is further evidence of the immunomodulatory effect of HBeAg.

- *Vaccine associated mutants.* Further cases of arginine 145 in vaccinees have been seen in Japan (Hino et al 1993) and Singapore (Harrison et al 1993). In Singapore, some 7 cases have now been identified. One case was associated with recombinant vaccine. In the Gambia (Howard et al 1993), 2 cases with lysine 141 to glutamic acid have been seen in vaccinated individuals. This genotype was not present some years ago in unvaccinated people (when these sera were collected), but has been noted recently. Perhaps this is becoming the dominant genotype under pressure of mass vaccination.

- REFERENCES

Bonino F, Brunetto M R 1993 Hepatitis B virus heterogeneity, one of many factors influencing the severity of hepatitis B. Journal of Hepatology 18: 5–8

Chen H S et al 1993 The precore gene of woodchuck hepatitis virus genome is not essential for viral replications in the natural host. Journal of Virology 66: 5682–5684

Chuang W-L et al 1993 Precore mutations and core clustering mutations in chronic hepatitis B virus infection. Gastroenterology 104: 263–271

Harrison T J et al 1993 Mutations in hepatitis B virus (HBV) in carriers with co-existent surface antigen and antibody. International Symposium on Viral Hepatitis and Liver Disease, Abstract 93, p 124

Hino K et al 1993 A vaccine-induced escape mutant of hepatitis B virus (HBV) in a family clustered with HBV infection. International Symposium on Viral Hepatitis and Liver Disease, Abstract 96, p 124

Howard C R et al 1993 Hepatitis B virus variants with altered α determinants causing infections in immunised children. International Symposium on Viral Hepatitis and Liver Disease, Abstract 95, p 75

Laskus et al 1993 Prevalence and nucleotide sequence analysis of pre-core mutations among patients with fulminant hepatitis B in the USA. International Symposium on Viral Hepatitis and Liver Disease, Abstract 769, p 74

Ogata et al 1993 Complete nucleotide sequence of a pre-core mutant of hepatitis B virus, implicated in fulminant hepatitis, and its biological characteristics in chimpanzees. International Symposium on Viral Hepatitis and Liver Disease, Abstract 768, p 74

Raimondo et al 1993 Is the course of perinatal hepatitis B infection influenced by genetic heterogeneity of the virus? Journal of Medical Virology

8. Liver cancer

Marie Annick Buendia   Patrizia Paterlini   Pierre Tiollais
Christian Bréchot

Hepatocellular carcinoma (HCC) is among the most common cancers in the world, and one of the rare human cancers showing sero-epidemiological association with viral infection. The role of hepatitis B virus (HBV) as a major aetiological agent of HCC has been firmly established, and the increased risk of developing HCC has been estimated to be 100-fold for chronic HBV carriers as compared with non-infected populations, placing HBV in the first rank among known human carcinogens (Szmuness 1978, Beasley et al 1981). Apart from epidemiological evidence, another factor linking HBV and liver cancer comes from related animal viruses, which with HBV form the hepadnavirus group, and induce acute and chronic infections of the liver and eventually HCC (reviewed by Schödel et al 1989, Robinson 1990). Whether HBV acts through any recognized oncogenic mechanism, either directly or indirectly, represents an important unsolved question.

It is generally considered that HBV has no direct oncogenic or cytopathic effect on the infected hepatocyte. Malignant transformation occurs after a long period of chronic liver disease, frequently associated with cirrhosis, suggesting a non-specific mechanism triggered by the immune response against infected hepatocytes. Chronic inflammation of the liver, continuous cell death and consequent cell proliferation might increase the risk factors for cancer. In a more specific pathway, persistent production of viral proteins might interfere with endogenous metabolic processes and sensitize liver cells to endogenous or exogenous mutagens; recent data using transgenic mouse models support the hypothesis that unregulated expression of the viral X protein, a promiscuous transcriptional activator, or that of the large surface protein might be involved in hepatocarcinogenesis (Chisari et al 1989, Kim et al 1991). Alternatively, the virus might play a direct role as an insertional mutagen: integration of viral DNA into the host genome might cause direct activation of proto-oncogenes or secondary chromosomal alterations. Such a role has been suggested by the repeated finding of integrated viral sequences in the cellular DNA of HBV-associated HCC; insertional activation of potential oncogenes has been described only in rare cases (Dejean et al 1986, Wang et al 1990), and the consequences of genetic instability resulting from viral integration events have not been determined. Integrated HBV sequences might also alter the host cell growth control 'in trans', through unregulated expression of native or modified viral proteins. All these potential mechanisms might not be mutually exclusive. To date, although information on risk factors causally linked to HCC has accumulated, the role of viral agents and carcinogenic co-factors is only partially elucidated, and no unifying model accounting for the contribution of viral and cellular factors to liver oncogenesis has been established.

In contrast, recent studies of naturally occurring models for hepatitis B virus and liver cancer have outlined a predominant role of the *myc* oncogenes in hepatocarcinogenesis induced by rodent hepadnaviruses. Woodchuck hepatitis virus (WHV), a virus closely related to HBV, acts mainly as an insertional mutagen, activating *myc* family genes (c-*myc* and N-*myc*) in about 50% of the woodchuck tumours analysed (T Y Hsu et al 1988, Fourel et al 1990, Wei et al 1992a); this virus represents the first example of a DNA virus producing insertional events at such a frequency. Another related virus, the ground squirrel hepatitis virus (GSHV), shows weaker oncogenic properties; integration of GSHV DNA has not been implicated in the tumourigenic process in the natural host, but frequent amplifications of the c-*myc* oncogene have been described in squirrel tumours (Transy et al 1992). In human HCCs, there is no published evidence for a key role of activated *myc* genes, albeit amplification of c-*myc* has been occasionally described, suggesting a different transformation pathway. Whether these striking differences are related to viral determinants, or to species-specific factors, remains to be determined.

This chapter reviews the different mechanisms that may be implicated in the development of HBV-related hepatocellular carcinoma, with reference to naturally occurring animal models.

EPIDEMIOLOGICAL ASSOCIATION BETWEEN HBV AND HEPATOCELLULAR CARCINOMA

Epidemiological research has contributed largely to the understanding of the aetiology of HCC. By the end of the 1970s, it became evident that chronic HBV infection was by far the major risk factor of liver cancer (Szmuness 1978). These conclusions stimulated the search for the molecular mechanisms linking HBV and HCC, and pointed out the importance of vaccination against HBV infection as the appropriate strategy to prevent HCC. Other carcinogenic factors, such as exposure to dietary aflatoxins and excessive alcohol intake, have also been implicated in human hepatocarcinogenesis, and preliminary epidemiological data support a correlation between chronic infection with the human hepatitis C virus (HCV), cirrhosis and HCC (Tanaka et al 1991).

Primary liver cancer, predominantly HCC, ranks among the most frequent cancers of males in many countries. A recent estimate (Bosch & Munoz 1991), indicates that HCC represents the eighth most common cancer, with about 250 000 new cases each year, 70% of which occur in Asia.

Several lines of evidence associate chronic HBV infection with the development of HCC:

1. The incidence of HCC and the prevalence of HBV serological markers follow the same general geographic pattern of distribution. HCC is common in regions where HBV is endemic, but comes far behind other types of cancer in regions where HBV infection is uncommon (Szmuness 1978, Hollinger 1990, Tabor 1991).
2. Serological evidence of HBV infection is detected in about 70% of HCC patients in Africa, and more than 90% in mainland China, as compared with 10–20% of the total population residing in the same areas (Tabor 1991).
3. A marked increased risk of HCC has been shown among HBsAg carriers compared with non-carriers (risk factors up to 200 have been reported in different ethnic or social groups, using different methodologies of investigation; Obata et al 1980, Beasley et al 1981, Iijima et al 1984, Chen et al 1991).

A long period of chronic HBV infection generally precedes the onset of liver tumours, but HCC may also affect, less frequently, HBsAg-positive children under 12 years of age. In contrast, a large number of HBsAg carriers remain unaware of their carrier status before they die at an old age (Beasley 1988). In the Far East, early detection of HCC is now frequent in asymptomatic carriers (Chen et al 1991, Lok et al 1991). Epidemiological data have shown not only that HBV is causally related to HCC, but also that there is a great variation in HCC incidence among different carrier populations. This variation may be attributed both to differences in the intrinsic properties of HBV infection patterns observed among chronic carriers, and to additional, genetic and environmental determinants.

Chronic infections resulting from maternal–neonatal transmission present a greater risk of HCC than those acquired as adults, probably reflecting differences in the incubation time (Popper et al 1987a, Beasley 1988) (Fig. 8.1). Among HBsAg carriers infected at an early age, an additional HCC risk has been associated with HBeAg carriage, with significant liver damage and high level of anti-HBcAg antibodies in chronic active hepatitis and with the presence of

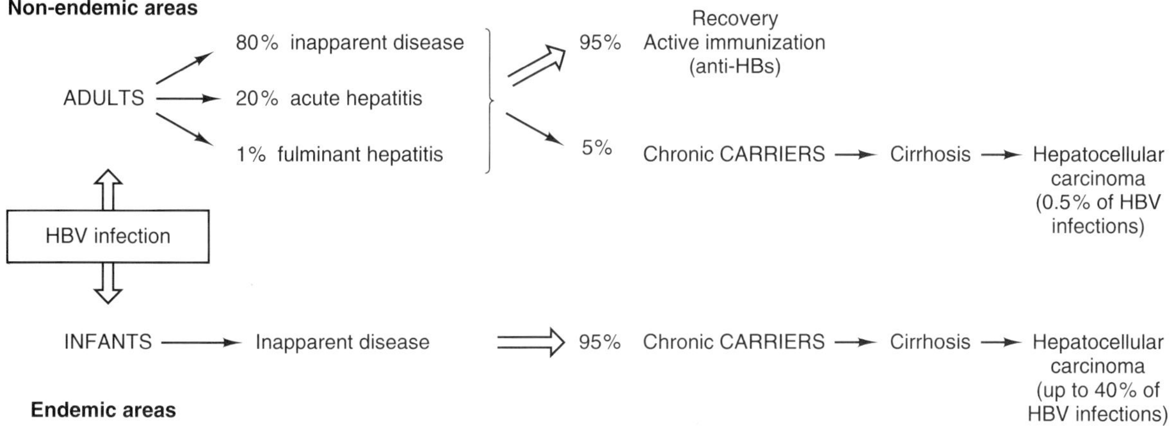

Fig. 8.1 Epidemiological association between HBV and HCC. Description of HBV transmission, progression to chronicity and HCC incidence in endemic and non-endemic countries.

cirrhosis. A gender discrepancy (males have a two- to eight-fold elevated risk of developing HCC compared with females) and familial tendency (familial clusters of HCC are common in Asia) have also been documented as factors involved in the frequency of tumour development (Chang et al 1984, Lok et al 1991, Shen et al 1991).

In addition, inconsistent geographical variations in HCC mortality and HBsAg prevalence have been observed in endemic regions, suggesting that other independent or cooperative factors might be implicated. In highly endemic regions, particularly in South Africa and in southern provinces of mainland China, an association of dietary aflatoxins and HCC has been recognized in several reports (Yeh et al 1989, Bosch & Munoz 1991). The carcinogenic potential of aflatoxin B1 in liver cells is well known in many species. Excessive alcohol intake also increases the risk of HCC in HBV carriers as well as in cirrhotic males at advanced ages in regions of low prevalence for HBV (Austin 1991, Chen et al 1991). However, the coexistence of HBV infection, often undetectable by conventional serological assays, and/or of HCV infection in more than 90% of patients from various countries has called in question the prevalence of chronic hepatitis induced by alcohol (Bréchot et al 1985, Takase et al 1991). The potential role of cigarette smoking and of long-term use of oral contraceptives is still debated. In addition, preliminary data indicate that infection with the human hepatitis delta virus (HDV), which causes extremely severe hepatic injury and cirrhosis, might be associated with a more rapid onset of liver tumours (Oliveri et al 1991).

It is important to point out that HBV infection, alone or associated with cooperative factors, can be implicated in only 20% of HCC cases in low endemic regions (North America and Europe) and in Japan. In that country, the incidence of liver cancer has been continuously increasing during the past decade, but the number of cases related to HBV remains constant. It now seems probable that infection with hepatitis C virus (HCV), a human RNA virus related to flaviviridae and pestiviridae, plays an increasing part in the development of HCC in these regions, as well as in countries highly endemic for HBV, e.g. China. With the development of HCV markers, evidence of an association between HCV infection, cirrhosis and HCC is now increasing (Okuda 1991). The relationship between cirrhosis and HCC appears to be complex, and the degree of correlation varies with aetiology of cirrhosis. Macronodular cirrhosis precedes or accompanies a majority of HBV (over 80% in Asia and 40–60% in Africa) and HCV-associated HCCs in children as well as at older ages. The risk of HCC has been considered to be lower in HBsAg-negative micronodular cirrhosis observed in alcoholics (Beasley 1988, Kew 1989, Craig et al 1991). Whether cirrhosis and carcinogenesis result from the action of common factors, or whether increased risk of HCC can be related to some mechanism like regenerative stimulation, which occurs in cirrhotic livers, remains an unsolved problem.

THE HEPATITIS B VIRUS GENOME

Since the earliest studies of the genetic organization of HBV and of the viral replication by reverse transcription of an RNA intermediate, there has been constant interest in the unique properties of hepatitis B viruses. Virological and molecular studies have outlined the structural organization of the HBV genome, its coding potential, the mode of transcription of individual viral genes and their functional capacities; the main aspects of viral DNA replication and virion assembly within infected hepatocytes have been unravelled (reviewed by Tiollais et al 1985, Ganem & Varmus 1987). Less is known about the viral–cellular interactions that control virus attachment, uncoating and entry into susceptible cells, and the cell-surface receptor for HBV has not been identified.

Nucleotide and deduced amino acid sequences of cloned HBV DNA from different virus subtypes (*adw*, *adr*, *ayw*, *ayr*) have revealed a genome size of 3.2 kb and the presence of four open reading frames, localized on one viral strand in the same transcriptional orientation (Galibert et al 1979, Pasek et al 1979, Valenzuela et al 1980, Fujiyama et al 1983, Ono et al 1983, Kobayashi & Koike 1984) (Fig. 8.2). The C and S regions specify structural proteins of the virion core and surface (or envelope); the longest one, P, encodes a polyprotein necessary for viral replication, which contains primase and replicase activities; the smallest, termed X, codes for a transcriptional transactivator. The entire viral genome is coding, and a large portion of the genome harbours two different reading frames. More striking than the overlapping of the P gene with the other viral genes, a feature common to all structures presenting reverse transcriptase activity (Toh et al 1983), is the constant and

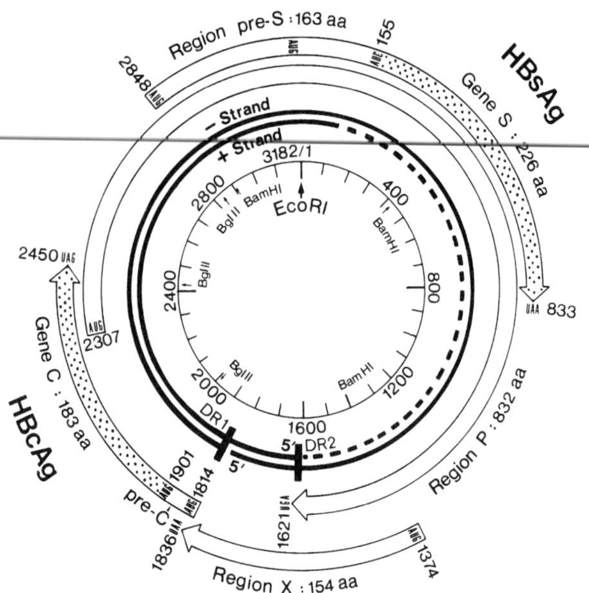

Fig. 8.2 Genetic organization of HBV. The inner cycle shows a restriction map of the *ayw* genome (Galibert et al 1979). The partially double-stranded genome is represented as a thick line. Four open reading frames encoding seven peptides are indicated by large arrows. DR1 and DR2 are two directly repeated sequences located at the extremities of the viral DNA strands.

unusual overlapping of coding and regulatory sequences (promoters, enhancers and termination signal). The genomes of different HBV subtypes differ mainly by single nucleotide substitutions or by addition of multiples of three nucleotide blocks, preserving the reading frames and leading primarily to conservative amino acid changes. Genomic variability among viruses of the same subtype has been characterized in different patients, and also in the same patient at different times during chronic infection. These genetic variations can be attributed to errors during synthesis of the minus-strand DNA by reverse transcriptase, an enzyme that lacks polymerase-associated proof-reading functions. A number of mutations, however, lead to the outcome of HBV variants with modified immunological and pathological properties: altered immunological response has been correlated with HBV-related variants (Wands et al 1986, Thiers et al 1988, Blum et al 1991, Tran et al 1991), and severe liver injury with e-minus mutant-associated hepatitis (Liang et al 1991a, Omata et al 1991). Defective viral particles carrying a deleted genome have been described (Okamoto et al 1987, Gerken et al 1991, Terré et al 1991), showing that HBV shares with other viruses, and notably with retroviruses, the property to develop defective variants in the natural host. Although deleted viral forms have been observed in a human HCC, creating core/polymerase fusion proteins (Will et al 1986), there is no experimental evidence that free defective HBV genomes might present oncogenic properties, or that particular HBV subtypes might be more oncogenic than others.

Comparison of the HBV genome with those of animal hepadnaviruses reveals extensive homologies among mammalian hepadnaviruses, which share a basically identical genomic organization. The best-conserved regions are located in the C and S genes and in the viral polymerase. The extent of homology is weaker in the pre-S1 region, which however retains the same general conformation and hydrophobicity profile. The rather strict host range of the different hepadnaviruses suggests that the cellular receptor for these viruses, which has not been characterized, might be poorly conserved during evolution. Accordingly, viral sequences implicated in the interaction of the virion with the cellular membrane are located in the amino-terminal part of the pre-S1 domain (Neurath et al 1986), a variable region among hepadnaviral genomes. Finally, the internal domain of the X protein is the less conserved region. Two strong homology blocks in the amino- and carboxy-terminal parts of X might correspond to a conservative pressure for functional activity of the X transactivator, and of the viral RNAase H encoded by C-terminal P sequences that overlap with the 5' end of X (Radziwill et al 1990, Takada & Koike 1990, Arii et al 1992).

The hepadnaviral genome, isolated from infectious extracellular virions, is made of two complementary DNA strands of different length, maintained in a circular configuration by base pairing at their 5' extremities (Summers et al 1975). The viral replication pathway, virtually identical for all hepadnaviruses, takes place in the nucleus and cytoplasm of infected cells, and although it can be instructively compared with the retroviral life cycle it is entirely extrachromosomal (Summers & Mason 1982, Seeger et al 1986, Will et al 1987). Hepadnaviruses, like retroviruses and caulimoviruses, use a reverse transcription step during replication. Significant homologies between reverse transcriptases encoded by these viruses have suggested that they display a common evolutionary origin (Toh et al 1983, Miller & Robinson 1986).

In productive hepadnavirus infections, a strict balance in the amount of individual viral gene products is necessary for active viral replication and release of infectious virions as well as for survival of infected host cells. Despite the small size of the HBV genome and a very compact organization of coding sequences, the expression of the different viral genes is subjected to a complex regulation at various levels, both transcriptionally and post-transcriptionally. Each individual HBV gene is controlled by an independent set of regulatory signals, probably acting in cooperation with HBV elements that coordinate the relative level of viral gene expression. In chronically infected livers and in cell lines supporting active viral replication, two major HBV transcripts of molecular size 3.5 and 2.1 kb are produced from ccc DNA template at roughly similar levels (Gough 1983, Cattaneo et al 1984) and minor 2.4- and 0.8-kb transcripts have been described (Ou & Rutter 1985, Siddiqui et al 1986, 1987, Treinin & Laub 1987). These polyadenylated RNAs direct the synthesis of seven viral proteins: the 3.5-kb species encode the core protein, the e antigen and the polymerase; the 2.1-kb RNA encodes the middle and major surface glycoproteins; and the large surface protein and the viral X transactivator activity are specified by the 2.4- and 0.8-kb transcripts respectively. The transcription patterns of WHV and GSHV in chronically infected livers are strikingly similar, whereas that of DHBV differs mainly by higher levels of 2.4-kb RNA (Büscher et al 1985, Enders et al 1985, Möröy et al 1985). Two enhancer elements stimulate transcription from the viral promoters: EN I, positioned about 450 bp upstream of the core promoter, and EN II, located in the X gene coding region (Shaul et al 1985, Yee 1989).

ONCOGENIC PROPERTIES OF VIRAL PROTEINS

It has been accepted for a long time that prolonged expression of viral genes may have no direct cytotoxic effects on the infected hepatocytes. Transfection of cultured cells with HBV DNA has not usually been associated with tumorigenic conversion, and most transgenic lines of mice bearing the full-length HBV genome or subgenomic constructs never show any sign of liver cell injury. However, recent studies in particular experimental systems have indicated that abnormal overexpression of different viral proteins, including the X gene product and the surface proteins in native or modified forms, might play a part in malignant transformation of infected hepatocytes.

The X transactivator

The smallest HBV open reading frame was initially designated 'X', because it was unclear at that time that it might encode a protein produced during HBV infection (Galibert et al 1979). Examination of the nucleotide and amino acid sequences of HBx has led to the prediction of a regulatory function for the deduced X polypeptide and has revealed a codon usage similar to that used in eukaryotic cell genes, suggesting that X might have been transduced by the HBV genome (Miller & Robinson 1986). The strong conservation of X sequences among HBV subtypes and the presence of homologous reading frames in the WHV and GSHV genomes suggest that their products may be of importance for viral replication.

Evidence for expression of the HBx gene has been obtained by Moriarty et al (1985) and by Kay et al (1985), who reported that the sera of HBV-related HCC patients recognize synthetic peptides based on X sequences. Expression of the X reading frame in prokaryotic and eukaryotic cells, using various vectors, has allowed the identification of a 16.5-kD polypeptide that reacts with serum samples from a number of HBV-infected individuals (Elfassi et al 1986, Meyers et al 1986, Pfaff et al 1987, Schek et al 1991a). Anti-HBx antibodies have been detected in acutely infected patients about 3–4 weeks after the onset of clinical signs (Vitvitski-Trepo et al 1990), and more frequently in chronic HBsAg carriers showing markers of active viral replication and chronic liver disease (Haruna et al 1991, Levrero et al 1991, Wang et al 1991). The X protein is localized mainly in the cytoplasm of in vivo–infected cells, at or near the plasma membrane and at the nuclear periphery (Vitvitski-Trepo et al 1990, Wang et al 1991). The X protein has been detected in the nuclear compartment only in transfected cell lines (Höhne et al 1990).

The recent finding that the X gene product can transactivate transcription from a number of HBV and heterologous promoters is of considerable importance in defining its role in viral replication and in pathogenesis (for a review, see Rossner 1992). The X protein behaves as a broad-range transactivator: it stimulates transcription from the viral promoters coupled to HBV enhancer, from heterologous viral promoters like the SV40 early promoter, the herpes simplex virus – thymidine kinase (HSV-Tk) promoter and the Rous sarcoma virus (RSV) and human immunodeficiency virus (HIV) long terminal repeats (LTRs), and from cellular promoters including the β-interferon, HLA-DR, c-*fos* and c-*myc* promoters (Twu & Schloemer 1987, Spandau & Lee 1988, Colgrove et al 1989, Balsano et al 1991). The X protein has been shown to interact, directly or indirectly, with transcriptional activators such as AP-1, AP-2, CREB, ATF-2, NF-kB and possibly Sp1 (Seto et al 1990, Maguire et al 1991, Lucito & Schneider 1992). It is unlikely that the X protein directly binds to its DNA target sequences; activation of cellular and viral genes, which occurs at the level of transcription, might be mediated by protein–protein interactions, either in the cytoplasm or in the nucleus of the cell. Regions of X protein essential for transactivation are included in the amino acid sequences conserved among hepadnavirus X proteins (Arii et al 1992). It has been shown that HBx can be phosphorylated in vivo and that it displays an intrinsic serine/threonine protein kinase activity (Schek et al 1991b, Wu et al 1990), two features also shared by a number of proteins implicated in intracellular signalling pathways. HBx might therefore directly activate cellular transcription factors.

Although present at very low levels in chronically infected livers, the X protein has been shown to stimulate the production of viral particles in transient transfection assays (Yaginuma et al 1987). However, it has not been established that the expression of cellular genes showing X-responsive promoters is stimulated in HBV-infected hepatocytes in vivo. More clues to the possible role of HBx in HBV-associated pathogenesis have been provided by three recent lines of studies, including both in vitro and in vivo studies and direct analysis of human liver and HCC biopsy samples.

It has been shown that high levels of X expression may induce malignant transformation of certain cultured cells, like the NIH3T3 cell line (Shirakata et al 1989), and immortalized hepatocytes expressing the SV40 large tumour antigen (Höhne et al 1990). Studies of transgenic mice carrying the X reading frame controlled by its natural HBV enhancer/promoter sequences or by heterologous liver-specific promoters have given rise to conflicting results. In two lines of mice derived from the inbred CD1 strain, carrying a 1.15-kb HBV fragment (spanning the enhancer, the complete X coding region and the polyadenylation signal), the development of preneoplastic lesions has been observed in the liver, followed by malignant carcinomas at 8–10 months of age (Kim et al 1991). In contrast, another transgene, in which the X coding domain was placed under the control of α_1-antitrypsin regulatory region, failed to induce serious liver damage in ICR × B6C3 F1 transgenic animals, although X mRNAs were detected in liver tissues (Lee et al 1990). Analysis of integrated viral sequences in tumour DNA has shed new light on one of the mechanisms leading to overexpression of HBx in chronically infected livers and in HCCs. It has been shown that HBV sequences are frequently interrupted between the viral direct repeats DR1 and DR2 upon integration into host cell DNA (see p. 145) and that overproduction of hybrid viral/host transcripts may result from HBV DNA integration in a hepatoma cell line (Ou & Rutter 1985). The presence of viral/host transcripts containing a 3' truncated version of the X coding region fused with flanking cellular sequences and retaining transactivating capacity was first described in a human HCC (Wollersheim et al 1988). Moreover, enhanced transactivating capacity of the integrated X gene product has been related to the substitution of viral carboxy-terminal residues by cellular amino acids (Koshy & Wells 1991). Transactiving ability of similarly truncated X products made from fusion of integrated HBV sequences with adjacent cell DNA has also been shown in many chronic hepatitis tissues (Takada & Koike 1990). This suggests that the integrated X gene might be essential for maintaining the tumour phenotype that develops at the early stages of carcinogenesis. Consistent with this model, viral/host junctions have been mapped in the carboxy-terminal region of X in a majority of human HCCs (Nagaya et al 1987, Shih et al 1987). Further studies are now necessary to better delineate the contribution of X gene product to malignant transformation in persistent HBV infections.

Surface glycoproteins

In natural HBV infections, the production of infectious virions and HBsAg particles depends on a tight regulation of the relative levels of the three envelope glycoproteins (Fig. 8.3). Neither liver lesions nor HCC have been observed in any of the published transgenic lineages that produce the middle and major surface proteins from HBV-derived regulatory sequences (Babinet et al 1985, Chisari et al 1985, Burk 1988, Farza et al 1988, Araki et al 1989). However, it has been shown that the number and rate of appearance of preneoplastic nodules and primary tumours following carcinogen administration are slightly increased in HBsAg-positive transgenic mouse livers as compared with negative littermates, suggesting that HBsAg expression might enhance the effects of the hepatocarcinogens (Dragani et al 1989). When the endogenous pre-S1 promoter is replaced by an exogenous promoter (the metallothionien or albumin promoter) the production of roughly equimolar ratios of large S protein with respect to middle and major

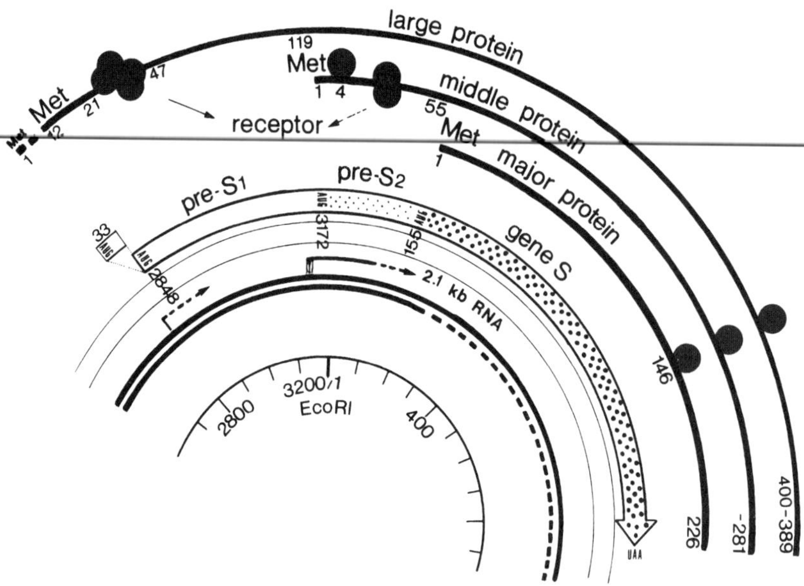

Fig. 8.3 Genetic map of the three HBs proteins (subtype *ayw*). The inner circles represent a part of the HBV genome shown in Figure 8.1. The transcription start sites are indicated. The outer circles denote the large (LHBs), middle (MHBs) and major or small (SHBs) proteins of the envelope. Numbers refer to the amino acids of the primary translation products. Met, methionine initiator codon. The large black round spots mark the positions of the glycosylated residues, and the black hemispheres correspond to regions probably involved in the binding to the cell membrane.

S leads to intracellular accumulation of non-secretable filamentous envelope particles within the endoplasmic reticulum of transgenic mouse hepatocytes (Chisari et al 1986, 1987). This results in histological and ultrastructural features of 'ground glass' hepatocytes, which have been described in some cases of chronic human liver diseases and are considered to be typical of chronic hepatitis B, ultimately killing the cells.

In the transgenic mouse lineages, mild persistent hepatitis was followed by the development of regenerative nodules and eventually HCCs by 12 months of age (Chisari et al 1989, Dunsford et al 1990). The preneoplastic nodules and tumours displayed a marked reduction in transgene expression, suggesting that hepatocytes that express low levels of the large S polypeptide would have a selective survival advantage. Exogenous, chemical co-factors are not required for tumorigenic induction in this model, but exposure of adult transgenic mice to hepatocarcinogens produced more rapid and extensive development of preneoplastic lesions and HCC under conditions that do not alter the liver morphology of non-transgenic controls (Teeter et al 1990). These data show that inappropriate expression of the large S protein has the potential to be directly cytotoxic to the hepatocyte and may initiate a cascade of events that ultimately progress to malignant transformation, although the molecular mechanism connecting viral and host factors in this process has not been elucidated.

Studies of integrated HBV sequences in human liver tumours have also suggested a possible role for abnormal expression of rearranged viral S genes in HCC development. It has been shown that deletion of the carboxy-terminal region of the S gene generates a novel transcriptional transactivation activity (Caselmann et al 1990, Kekulé et al 1990). Integrated HBV sequences from a human tumour and a hepatoma-derived cell line, as well as different constructs bearing similarly truncated pre-S2/S sequences (Lauer et al 1992), can stimulate the SV40 promoter in transient transfection assays. Although the mutated S polypeptide is retained in the endoplasmic reticulum and Golgi membranes, transactivation occurs at the transcriptional level and is dependent on the SV40 enhancer. The c-*myc* P2 promoter is also activated in trans (Koshy et al 1991). These findings support the hypothesis that accidental 3' truncation of integrated pre-S2/S genes could be a causative factor in HBV-associated oncogenesis.

VIRAL INTEGRATIONS IN HEPATOCELLULAR CARCINOMA

The hepadnavirus replication pathway in infected cells has been shown to take place within nuclear and cytoplasmic compartments and does not require a step of viral DNA integration in the host cell genome. However, hepadnaviruses share with other retroelements of common evolutionary origin (Xiong & Eickbush 1990) the ability to integrate their DNA into cellular chromosomes. The molecular events leading to the invasion of cell DNA by hepadnaviral DNA have not been fully elucidated.

The main question is whether viral integrations might play a part in the virally induced transformation process, either by conferring a selective growth advantage on targeted cells, leading to the onset of preneoplastic nodules, or by providing an additional step in tumour progression. Whereas insertional activation of proto-oncogenes now emerges as a common event in WHV-induced woodchuck HCC, a related mechanism has been observed only in rare examples of human HCCs, in which different activities for integrated HBV sequences have been proposed.

Integrated HBV sequences

Integrated HBV sequences have been observed in established hepatoma cell lines and in about 80% of human HCCs (Bréchot et al 1980, 1981, 1982, Chakraborty et al 1980, Edman et al 1980, Shafritz et al 1981). HBV DNA integrations occur at early stages in natural acute infections and in experimental infections of cultured cells (Lugassy et al 1987, Yaginuma et al 1987, Ochiya et al 1989). As a result of multiple integrations in chronic hepatitis tissues (Boender et al 1985, Tanaka et al 1988), integrated HBV sequences have been detected in most HBV-related HCCs that arise from clonal outgrowth of one or a few transformed liver cells (see Matsubara & Tokino 1990). Single HBV insertions are common in childhood HCCs but are rather uncommon later in life, suggesting that multiple integrations occurring during the course of long-standing HBV infections might accumulate within single cells (Chang et al 1991), as also indicated by sequence divergence among HBV inserts in the same tumour (Imai et al 1987). Studies of the organization of cloned HBV inserts in liver tissues and HCCs have shown that HBV sequences are fragmented and rearranged and that integration and recombination sites are dispersed over the viral genome, indicating that HBV integration does not occur through a unique mechanism, as in the case of other retro-elements and retroviruses (Dejean et al 1984, Koch et al 1984a, Shaul et al 1984, Ziemer et al 1985). The absence of complete genomes in virtually all HBV inserts, which consist either of linear subgenomic fragments or of rearranged fragments in different orientations, shows that these sequences cannot serve as a template for viral replication. Integrated forms made of a sub-genomic fragment, which are frequent in HCC and hepatitis tissues from children (Yaginuma et al 1987), are believed to represent primary products of integration. They are of particular interest in the study of the molecular mechanisms responsible for HBV DNA integration.

Highly preferred integration sites have been mapped in the HBV genome within the 'cohesive ends' region, which lies between two 11-bp direct repeats (DR1 and DR2) highly conserved among hepadnaviruses (Koshy et al 1983, Nagaya et al 1987). A narrow region encompassing DR1 has been shown to be particularly prone to recombination (Shih et al 1987, Yaginuma et al 1987, Nakamura et al 1988, Hino et al 1989). This region coincides with a short terminal redundancy of the minus-strand DNA, which confers a triple-stranded structure to the circular viral genome. Integration sites are tightly clustered at both the 5' and 3' ends of minus-strand DNA, suggesting that replication intermediates and specially relaxed circular DNA might be preferential preintegration substrates

(Nagaya et al 1987, Shih et al 1987). Invasion of cellular DNA by single-stranded HBV DNA, using mainly free 3' ends, might take place through a mechanism of illegitimate recombination, also suggested by frequent patch homology between HBV and cellular sequences at the recombination breakpoints. Although different minor changes in flanking cellular DNA have been associated with viral integration (both microdeletions and short duplications have been described) (Yaginuma et al 1985, Dejean et al 1986, Berger & Shaul 1987, Nakamura et al 1988, Hino et al 1989), more precise mechanisms have been proposed. The recombination-proficient region spanning DR1 is located close to a U5-like sequence highly conserved between hepadnaviruses, suggesting that sequences necessary for precise recombination with cellular DNA have been retained from a common ancestor with retroviruses, despite the absence of a gene coding for an integrase in the HBV genome (Miller & Robinson 1986). Mapping of a set of preferred topoisomerase I (topo I) sites near DR1 and DR2 and in vitro studies of WHV DNA integration into cloned cellular DNA have sustained the hypothesis that topo I might promote illegitimate recombination of hepadnavirus DNA in vivo (Wang & Rogler 1991).

As a consequence of the viral integration process, sequences of the S and X genes and of the enhancer I element are almost systematically present in HBV inserts, whereas those of the C gene are less frequently represented. It has been shown that the pre-S2/S promoter is transcriptionally active in its integrated form in HCCs (Ou & Rutter 1985, Caselmann et al 1990) and that HBsAg may be produced from viral inserts (Dejean et al 1984, Zhou et al 1987). Highly rearranged HBV inserts show virus junctions scattered throughout the viral genome, and in some of them recombination breakpoints have been mapped in the S coding region (Nagaya et al 1987). It has been recently shown that truncation of the S gene between residues 77 and 221 confers a transcriptional activation activity to the mutated pre-S2/S products (Lauer et al 1992). The shorter pre-S2/S protein lacks carboxy-terminal signals for translocation through the endoplasmic reticulum membrane and should be retained in the bilayer. Activation of the c-*myc* oncogene promoter, demonstrated in in vitro assays, might result from an indirect transacting action of the truncated viral proteins (Kekulé et al 1990). Whether this or some related mechanism participates in liver cell transformation remains to be determined. Other studies have shown that a significant percentage of viral junctions are localized in the carboxy-terminal part of the viral X gene, predicting a fusion of the X open reading frame to flanking cellular sequences in a way that might preserve the functional capacity of the X transactivator. Evidence for transcriptional activity at integrated X sequences has been provided in tumours and chronically infected livers (Wollersheim et al 1988, Takada & Koike 1990, Hilger et al 1991) and might be correlated with the detection of HBxAg in a number of human HCCs. It has also been shown that a number of viral X/cell fusion peptides harbour transcriptional activation activity. The contribution of downstream cellular sequences to activated expression and/or to enhanced transactivating capacities of the integrated HBV sequences has been suggested (Wollersheim et al 1988). These data indicate that abnormal expression of integrated and truncated X gene might play a part in HBV-associated oncogenesis, by deregulating the normal expression of cellular genes in trans (Fig. 8.4).

Cellular target sites

Studies of different viral insertions in many human HCCs have revealed that integration can take place at multiple sites on various chromosomes (reviewed by Matsubara & Tokino 1990). These studies failed to demonstrate the presence of a known dominant oncogene or tumour-suppressor gene in the immediate vicinity of any integration site. It has been reasoned that integration of HBV DNA occurs at random in the human genome and that it has no direct mutagenic effect on growth control genes in most cases. However, contrary to a widely held opinion, integration of retroelements and viruses might not be entirely random; it has been shown that the possible sites for retroviral integration in eukaryotic DNA are numerous but not limited

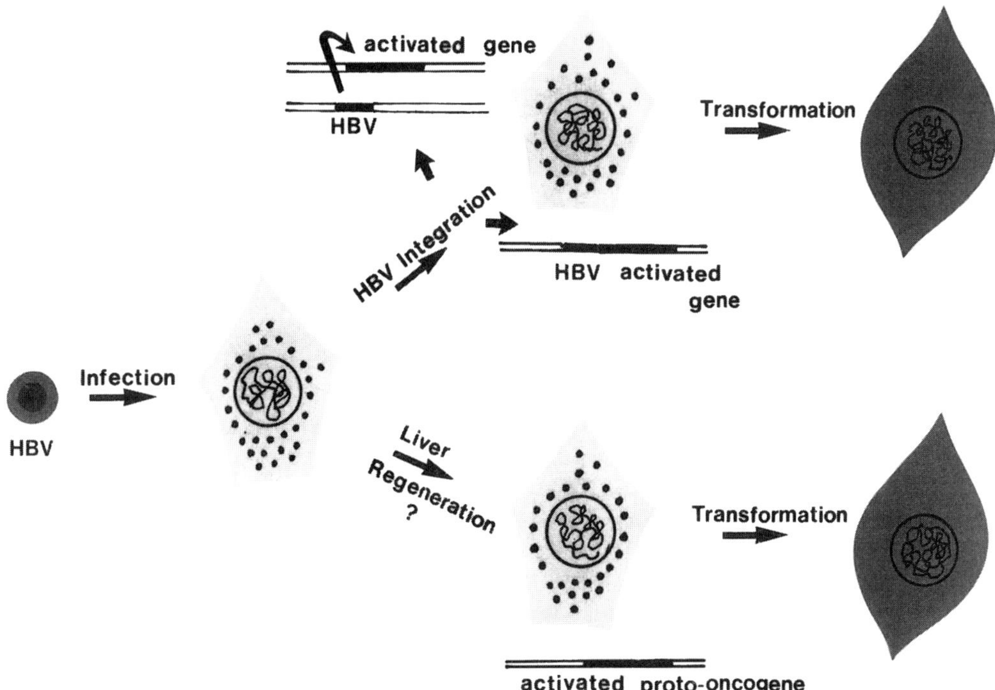

Fig. 8.4 Hypothetical transformation pathways associated with HBV infection in human hepatocytes. Viral DNA may turn on cellular growth genes either 'in trans', through modified protein products of integrated viral sequences (truncated X or pre-S2/S genes) (top pathway), or directly 'in cis' by integration adjacent to those genes (middle pathway). Alternatively, continuous cell death and regeneration due to persistent infection may trigger aberrant activation of cellular proto-oncogenes (bottom pathway).

(about 500–1000) (Shih et al 1988). It has been proposed that simple repetitive elements are hotspots for HBV insertion in the human genome. Indeed, Alu-type repeats, minisatellite-like, satellite III or variable number of tandem repeat (VNTR) sequences have frequently been identified near HBV insertion sites (Shaul et al 1986, Berger & Shaul 1987, Nagaya et al 1987), suggesting that chromosomal regions accessible to specific families of mobile repeated sequences are also preferential targets for HBV insertion. A small cellular DNA compartment (H3) characterized by a base composition close to that of HBV DNA and a high concentration of Alu repeats has been designated as a major target for stable HBV integration (Zerial et al 1986).

It has been shown that HBV DNA integration may enhance chromosomal instability: in many tumours, large inverted duplications, deletions, amplifications or chromosomal translocations have been associated with HBV insertions, suggesting that this process may function as a random mutagen, promoting chromosomal defects in hepatocytes (Koch et al 1984b, Mizusawa et al 1985, Rogler et al 1985, Yaginuma et al 1985, Hino et al 1986, Tokino et al 1987, Hatada et al 1988). In addition, HBV DNA may promote homologous recombination at a distance from the insertion site (Hino et al 1991). However, a role for most of these chromosomal abnormalities has not been assigned as yet, although in a few cases the p53 or *Hst* I loci have been altered as a sequel of HBV integration in the same chromosomal region (Hatada et al 1988, Zhou et al 1988, Slagle et al 1991).

Evidence for a direct cis-acting promoter insertion mechanism has been provided in two independent HCCs (Dejean et al 1986, de Thé et al 1987, Dejean & de Thé 1990, Wang et al

1990). These investigators analysed early tumours that developed in non-cirrhotic livers from clonal proliferation of a cell containing a single specific viral integration. In one case, the HBV insertion occurred in an exon of the retinoic acid receptor β gene (RAR-β) and fused 29 amino-terminal residues of the viral pre-S1 gene to the DNA-binding and hormone-binding domains of RAR-β (Dejean et al 1986). Retinoic acid and retinoids are vitamin A-derived substances that have striking effects on differentiation and proliferation in a large variety of systems (Brockes 1990). RARs are members of the steroid thyroid hormone receptors family, which includes the c-*erb*A proto-oncogene. Recently, the chromosomal translocation t(15; 17) fusing the RAR-α gene to a cellular gene termed PML has been implicated in acute promyelocytic leukaemias (de Thé et al 1990, 1991). In the human HCC, it seems most probable that inappropriate activation of RAR-β resulted in expression of a chimeric HBV/RAR-β protein at greater levels than that of the native protein, and participated in the tumorigenic process. In a second HCC, HBV DNA integration occurred in an intron of the human cyclin A gene, resulting in a strong expression of hybrid HBV/cyclin transcripts (Wang et al 1990, 1992). Cyclins are conserved though evolution from yeast to man, and their association with cyclin-dependent kinases (cdks) is central to the mechanism controlling the cell cycle (Nurse 1990). Furthermore, the cyclin A protein and cdk2 participate in a growth regulatory network that regulates the S phase (Girard et al 1991). Two different lines of evidence connecting cyclins and oncogenesis have recently been obtained: cyclin A can form a complex with the oncoprotein E1A in adenovirus-transformed cells and cyclin D is overexpressed in parathyroid adenomas (Giordano et al 1989, Motokura et al 1991). There are several hypotheses to explain the potential role of a chimeric HBV/cyclin A protein in the development of the human HCC. The replacement of the amino-terminal part of the cyclin A protein, which contains signals for its degradation, by HBV sequences may stabilize a chimeric protein retaining the ability to complex with specific kinases. Its constitutive expression driven by the strong viral pre-S2/S promoter may lead to uncontrolled DNA synthesis and cell proliferation.

In the two cases reported above, analysis of single HBV insertion sites has allowed the identification of new genes involved in the control of cell growth and differentiation. Both studies have opened the way to novel approaches of the cellular pathways regulating cell division and differentiation. In addition, they have provided evidence for a potential role of HBV as an insertional mutagen in primary liver cancer; in the two examples, a direct cis-acting promoter insertion mechanism has been described. However, such examples are still exceptional, and further analysis of other tumours selected on similar criteria is now necessary to better delineate the relative contribution of insertional mutagenesis over other mechanisms in the transformation process induced by chronic HBV infection (Fig. 8.4).

Insertional activation of *myc* genes in woodchuck HCC

The availability of naturally occurring animal models for HBV-induced liver disease and cancer has been largely exploited for a better understanding of the viral/host interactions. In the WHV/woodchuck model in particular, the natural history of viral infections, the presence and state of viral DNA and the patterns of viral gene expression have been extensively investigated. Experimental inoculation of newborn woodchucks with infectious virions has given conclusive information on the oncogenic activity of WHV: this virus now appears to be the most potent inducer of liver cancer among the hepadnavirus group (Popper et al 1987b, Seeger et al 1991). The ground squirrel hepatitis virus (GSHV) appears to be more weakly oncogenic (Marion et al 1986).

Search for transcriptional activation of known proto-oncogenes and for viral insertion sites in woodchuck HCCs has revealed that WHV acts as an insertional mutagen, activating *myc* family genes (c-*myc* or N-*myc*) in more than one-half of the tumours examined (Hsu et al 1988, Fourel et al 1990, Wei et al 1992a, b). Analysis of the mutated c-*myc* alleles in two individual tumours has shown integration of WHV sequences in the vicinity of the c-*myc* coding domain, either 5' of the first exon or in the 3' untranslated region (Hsu et al 1988). Deregulated expression of the oncogene driven by its normal promoters resulted from deletion or displacement of c-*myc* regulatory regions known to exert a negative effect on c-*myc* expression, and their replacement by viral sequences encompassing the enhancer I element. Such a mechanism is highly reminiscent of that previously reported for c-*myc* activation in murine T-cell lymphomas induced by murine leukaemia viruses (MuLV) (Corcoran et al 1984, Selten et al 1984). Evidence for a direct role of WHV DNA integration into c-*myc* in hepatocyte transformation has been provided by the development of hepatocellular carcinoma in transgenic lines of mice bearing WHV and *myc* sequences from the mutated allele of a woodchuck HCC (J Etiemble, C Babinet, P Tiollais & M A Buendia, unpublished results). Expression of the transgene in liver cells was correlated with the occurrence of primary liver tumours at 5–12 months of age in more than 80% of cases.

The insertional activation of N-*myc* genes was observed more frequently. In contrast to human and mouse, the woodchuck genome contains two distinct N-*myc* genes: N-*myc* 1, the homologue of known mammalian N-*myc* genes similarly organized into three exons, and N-*myc* 2, a functional processed pseudogene or 'retroposon', which has retained extensive coding and transforming homology with parental N-*myc* (Fourel et al 1990). In woodchuck HCCs, N-*myc* 2 represents by far the most frequent target for WHV DNA integrations. As shown in Figure 8.5, in about one-half of cases viral inserts were detected either upstream of the gene or in a short sequence of the 3' untranslated region, also identified as a unique hotspot for retroviral insertions into the murine N-*myc* gene in T-cell lymphomas (Dolcetti et al 1989, Setoguchi et al 1989, van Lohuizen et al 1989). Activated expression of the N-*myc* 2 retroposed oncogene, frequently correlated with overexpression of c-*fos* and c-*jun*, was observed in a large majority of woodchuck HCCs (Hsu et al 1990). Significantly enhanced expression of the human N-*myc*, c-*fos* or c-*jun* proto-oncogenes has been observed only occasionally in HBV-associated HCCs (our unpublished results), underlining the importance of host cell factors in the differences observed between the tumorigenic processes induced by hepadnaviruses in humans and woodchucks.

Further evidence that *myc* family genes are predominantly implicated in rodent liver tumours associated with hepadnavirus infection comes from other studies of woodchuck and ground squirrel HCCs. In two independent woodchuck tumours, a genetic rearrangement fusing the coding domain of c-*myc* with the promoter and 5' translated sequences of a cellular locus termed '*hcr*' has been observed (Möröy et al 1986, Etiemble et al 1989, Hino 1992). In a recent study of ground squirrel HCCs, frequent amplifications of c-*myc* were found in tumour cell DNA (11/24 cases examined) and associated with enhanced expression of the oncogene (Transy et al 1992). Integration of GSHV DNA into host cell genome, which occurs only rarely in squirrel tumours, has not been correlated with the observed genetic alterations of c-*myc*. It is noticeable that similar alterations have also been described in rodent liver tumours (Chandar et al 1989). Although amplification of c-*myc* has been observed on rare occasions in HBV-positive human liver tumours (Trowbridge et al 1988, and our unpublished results), there is no experimental demonstration, until now, that deregulated expression of *myc* genes might be generally associated with HBV-induced tumorigenesis in human livers, by any known cis- or trans-acting mechanism.

The strategy used by WHV in liver cell transformation now appears strikingly similar to that of some non-acute retroviruses, such as Moloney murine leukaemia virus (MoMuLV), which induce disease (usually leukaemias) slowly, emphasizing the described similarities between hepadnaviruses and retroviruses (Wain-Hobson 1984, Miller & Robinson 1986) (Fig. 8.5). These conclusions raise two different albeit related questions. What are the factors driving the oncogenic potential of WHV exclusively towards hepatocytes, as we know that this virus can infect a wide variety of woodchuck tissues? How can the apparent differences in the strategies of the closely related mammalian hepadnaviruses be

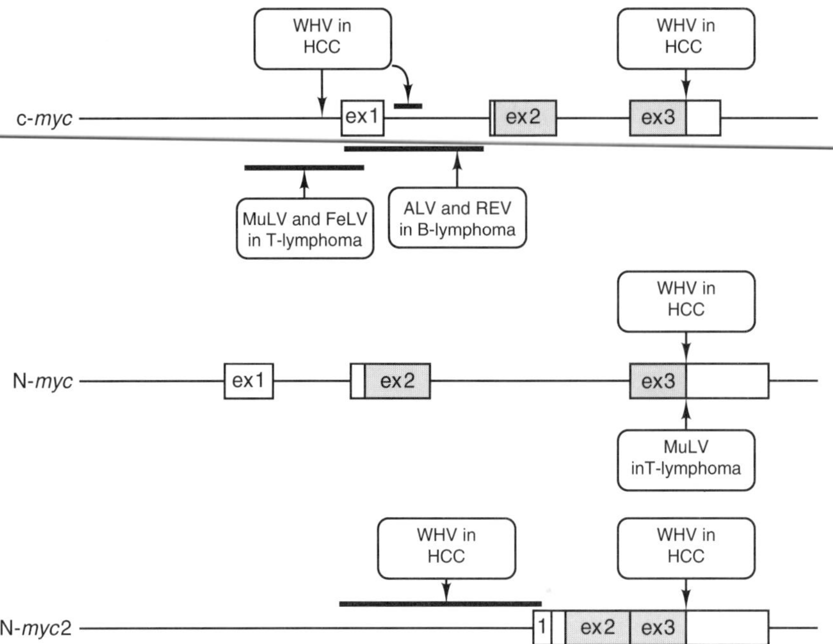

Fig. 8.5 Comparison of hepadnaviral and retroviral insertion sites in the c-*myc* and N-*myc* genes. Preferred target sites for WHV in the *myc* family genes are indicated above the corresponding genes and those of murine and avian retroviruses are shown under the genes. The processed N-*myc* 2 oncogene, generated by retrotransposition of the parental woodchuck N-*myc* gene (N-*myc* 1), is specific of the 'Sciuridae' family of rodents. Insertional activation of *myc* family genes by WHV DNA was observed in about 50% of the woodchuck HCCs analysed.

explained at the molecular level? To address these issues and identify the genomic variations responsible for such discrepancies, it would probably be instructive to re-examine the retroviral genetic elements influencing disease specificity and latency of different MuLVs (Li et al 1987, Thiesen et al 1988, Portis et al 1991) or the oncogenic properties of HPV strains in different tissues (Münger et al 1989, Romanczuk et al 1991).

HEPATOCELLULAR CARCINOMA IN HBsAg-NEGATIVE PATIENTS

As stated above (p. 138), there are striking geographical variations in the association between chronic infection by HBV and HCC. In Western countries (i.e. Northern Europe, USA, Japan), only 15–20% of the tumours occur in HBsAg-positive patients, and other environmental factors, such as alcohol and infection by hepatitis C virus (HCV), are clearly major risk factors. A number of epidemiological studies previously showed a high prevalence of anti-HBs and anti-HBc antibodies in the group of HBsAg-negative subjects (around 40–50% in France), indicating exposure to the virus (see Table 8.1 and Kew & Popper 1984, Bréchot 1987, Tabor 1989, Blum et al 1991, Colombo 1992). These antibodies generally reflect past and resolved HBV infection; however, in HBsAg-negative subjects with HCC, HBV DNA sequences can be detected in the tumours, demonstrating the persistence of the viral infection and suggesting its implication in liver carcinogenesis (see Table 8.2 and Bréchot 1987). With this view, it is indeed important to realize that the improvement in the sensitivity of assays for HBsAg detection, together with the introduction of sensitive tests for HBV DNA identification, have modified the

Table 8.1 Total prevalence of HBV markers in patients with HCC

	HCC (%)	HCC on alcoholic cirrhosis (%)
Zambie, Taiwan	100	NT
China	98	NT
Philippines	97	NT
Senegal	96	NT
Uganda	89	NT
Japan	81	NT
Greece	80	NT
USA	74	NT
Italy (North)	49	81.5
France (South)	43	58
Great Britain	32	27

Sources: Tabor (1989), Bréchot (1987), Colombo (1992), Nalpas et al (1992), Okuda (1992). NT, not tested.

criteria for the diagnosis of HBV infection; thus there is a spectrum of chronic HBV infections with a low replication rate, which might also be a risk factor for liver cancer (Bréchot et al 1985, 1991, Liang et al 1989, 1991b, Kremsdorf et al 1991).

HBV and HCV can interact with chronic alcohol consumption, and there is circumstantial evidence for a high prevalence of HBV and HCV infections in alcoholics. The increased prevalence of anti-HCV in alcoholics with cirrhosis (around 40–50%) as compared with those with minimal liver damage (around 20%) suggests that HCV infection might be implicated in the development of the cirrhosis in some of these patients; this observation may also account for the high prevalence of anti-HCV (50%) in alcoholics with HCC (Pares et al 1990, Mendenhall et al 1991, Nalpas et al 1991, 1992, Colombo 1992). In contrast, there is no evidence for a role of HBV in the development of alcoholic cirrhosis, since the prevalence of anti-HBs and anti-HBc, although higher than in the general population, does not significantly differ whether or not a cirrhosis is diagnosed (around 20%); however, there is evidence for the role of HBV in the liver cancers occurring in alcoholics, since the prevalence of HBV serological markers is significantly increased in these patients (around 50%) and the tumours frequently contain HBV DNA sequences (Attali et al 1981, Saunders et al 1983, Nalpas et al 1985, Poynard et al 1991).

The actual prevalence of these HBV DNA-positive HCCs in HBsAg-negative subjects has been a matter of debate, owing to the presence in the tumours of a low copy number per cell of the viral DNA sequences (estimated at around 0.1 to 0.001). Thus, studies performed in different geographical areas showed very different results (Table 8.2), these discrepancies probably being the result of different technical conditions (specificity and sensitivity) as well as distinct epidemiological situations. The sensitivity of the polymerase chain reaction (PCR) has now allowed confirmation of the previous observations, demonstration of the transmission of HBV particles present in the serum of these HBsAg-negative patients to chimpanzees, and determination of the nucleotide sequences of the HBV genomes. For example, in a study performed in patients from areas of high (South Africa) and low (France, Italy) HBV prevalence, HBV DNA was shown in 8 out of 10 serologically recovered subjects and in 6 of 13 patients without any detectable HBV serological marker (Paterlini et al 1990). Similar results were also recently obtained in Spain, Africa and the USA (see Table 8.3). It is striking from these studies that there is no real correlation between the serological HBV profiles and the presence or absence of HBV DNA detection in serum or tumour. Taken together, they show a persistent HBV infection in a large number of subjects with HBsAg-negative HCCs. It is interesting to note that related findings have been reported in the woodchuck and ground squirrel models of HCC. Liver cancer occurs in 17% of serologically recovered woodchucks, a figure to be compared with a 0% rate in uninfected animals (Korba et al 1989); WHV DNA was detected in the tumour tissues of seroconverted woodchucks, with a much lower number of copies per cell (about 0.1–0.3) than in HCCs from WHsAg-positive animals (100–1000 copies per cell).

In the ground squirrel model, about 25% of serologically recovered animals develop HCC (Marion 1986, 1991), and integrated GSHV sequences have been characterized in 2/5 tumours analysed (Transy et al 1992). In addition, HCC has also been observed in about 20% (6/30) of aged, seronegative squirrels. In these tumours,

Table 8.2 HBV DNA in HBsAg-negative patients with HCC: Southern and dot blot*

Geographical area	Tumour	Serum	Reference
France	17(6)/20	0/9	Bréchot et al 1985
	NT	3/54	Pol et al 1987
	4(4)/21†	NT	Marcellin et al 1989
Italy	0/6	NT	Pontisso et al 1987
	2/8‡	NT	Pontisso et al 1991
Germany	0/17	NT	Walter et al 1988
UK	1(1)/7	NT	Cobden et al 1986
	0/8	NT	Dunk et al 1988
	1/6	NT	White et al 1990
USA	0/5	NT	Fong et al 1988
Japan	2(2)/15	NT	Hino et al 1984
	4(3)/21	NT	Hino et al 1985
	5/13	NT	Koike et al 1985
	0/13	NT	Horiike et al 1989
China	1/2	NT	Chen et al 1986
	1/3	NT	Zhou et al 1987
	3/3	NT	Hsu et al 1991
Hong Kong	3/5	0/12	Lok et al 1990
Taiwan	4/21	NT	Lai et al 1990
South Africa	0/5	NT	Shafritz et al 1981
	3/8	NT	Shafritz et al 1981

*Positive cases/tested cases. Numbers in parenthesis indicate patients without any serological HBV marker.
†patients with HCC developing on histologically normal adjacent liver.
‡HCC developing in children.
NT, not tested.

Table 8.3 HBV DNA in HBsAg-negative patients with HCC: polymerase chain reaction*

Geographical area	Tumour	Serum	Reference
France	5(2)/10	NT	Paterlini et al 1990
	5(3)/8	11(6)/22	Paterlini et al 1993
Italy	5(4)/9	NT	Paterlini et al 1990
	2/3†	NT	Pontisso et al 1992
Spain	NT	12(5)/54	Ruiz et al 1992
Japan	8/22‡	NT	Ohkoshi et al 1991
South Africa	6/8	NT	Paterlini et al 1990
Senegal	18/31	NT	Coursaget et al 1991
Mozambique	4(1)/11	NT	Dazza et al 1991
USA	14/38	25/105	Liang et al 1992

*Positive cases/tested cases. Numbers in parenthesis indicate patients without any serological HBV marker.
†HCC developing in children.
‡Non-tumorous tissue analysed only.
NT, not tested.

GSHV DNA is undetectable by conventional methods; however, low levels of GSHV DNA have been found in two different cases by using PCR (Transy et al 1992), reinforcing the established association between HCC development in ground squirrels and infection with GSHV.

While all these observations point to an association between viral infection and tumour occurrence. It is not understood why only a small fraction of the tumour cells actually contain viral DNA. In view of a potential role of HBV in these tumours, it is noteworthy that, although most of the patients have cirrhosis associated with the tumour, HBV DNA was also subsequently identified in some subjects in tumours developed on histologically normal adjacent livers (Paterlini et al 1991). In addition, PCR, performed with a combination of different primers, has recently provided evidence for the presence in the tumour tissue of defective HBV genomes (Fig. 8.6), together with HBV RNA, in a clonally expanded population of cells and probably integrated in the host genome (Paterlini et al 1993). It is not

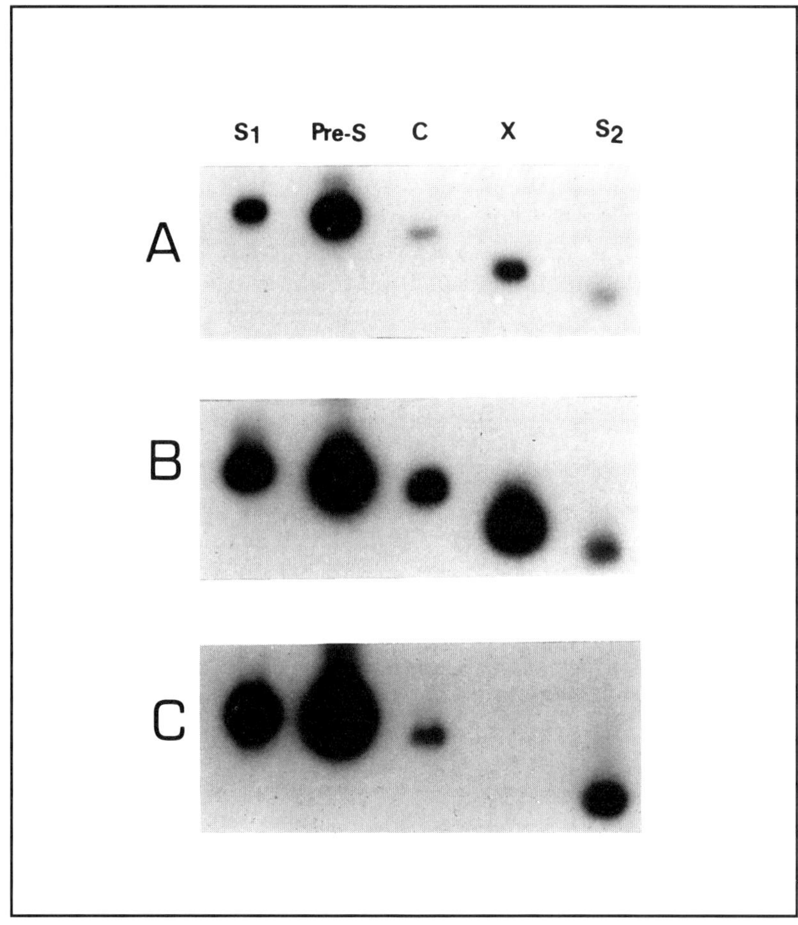

Fig. 8.6 Detection of HBV DNA in serum, non-tumorous and tumorous liver samples from an HBV-DNA positive patient (Paterlini et al 1993). The amplification products were obtained with various sets of HBV primers on the S (5' part, S1; 3' part, S2), pre-S, C and X viral genes, analysed electrophoretically, transferred to a nylon membrane and hybridized with a whole ^{32}P-labelled HBV probe (exposure time 12 h). A, B and C respectively show the results obtained in serum, non-tumour and tumour samples. The absence of amplification with primers in the X gene (C) suggests the presence of integrated HBV DNA molecules in the tumour tissue.

presently known if the low HBV DNA copy number in the tumours is the result of progressive rearrangements and deletions of integrated HBV DNA sequences, possibly in individuals infected with a low amount of viral particles. Further studies are also mandatory to determine whether HBV acts through a 'hit and run' mechanism (Galloway 1983, Smith et al 1988) in the liver carcinogenesis, initiating some of the early carcinogenic events but being unnecessary for the maintenance of the transformed phenotype.

In any case, it is clear that chronic infection by HCV is an important aetiological factor in HBsAg-negative HCCs, although the prevalence of anti-HCV antibodies varies considerably from one area to the other (80% in Japan, 60–70% in south Europe, 40–50% in France and 10–30% in Africa) (Bruix et al 1989, Dazza et al 1990, Hasan et al 1990, Kew et al 1990, Nalpas et al 1991, Nishioka et al 1991, Colombo 1992). The presence of HCV RNA sequences has been demonstrated in the tumour tissue, and there is evidence for an ongoing HCV multiplication at the time of tumour development; as for HBV, the number of HCV RNA copies per cell is apparently low but, in contrast to HBV, no HCV DNA sequences can be detected and thus the virus cannot be integrated into cellular DNA (Ohkoshi et al 1990, Yoneyama et al 1990, Paterlini et al 1993).

A recent study, conducted in France, has shown that most HBsAg-negative liver cancer tissues (from alcoholics as well as non-alcoholics) contain either HCV RNA (7/22), HBV DNA (7/22) or both (4/22) (Paterlini et al 1993). Similar results were found in the USA, where around half of these cancers are associated with either HCV, HBV or both (Liang et al 1992). Thus primary liver cancer in low endemic areas shows a strong association with both viral infections, a result that should have implications for prevention strategies.

GENETIC ALTERATIONS IN HBV-RELATED HCC

Different genetic alterations that cannot be clearly associated with a direct effect of viral infection have been described in human HCCs. These somatic changes include allele losses on several chromosomal regions, mutation and activation of cellular genes showing oncogenic potential and deletion or mutation of a tumour-suppressor gene. Search for activated oncogenes using the NIH3T3 cells in transformation assays has not been conclusive for most HCC DNAs analysed. In rare cases, a transforming DNA called '*lca*' has been obtained in the transformation assays (Ochiya et al 1986). This novel oncogene, located on the human chromosome 2, is expressed at a proliferative stage in fetal liver, and its activation in liver cancer has not been associated with gross rearrangements of the gene (Shiozawa et al 1988). A very low incidence of point mutations in the c-Ha-*ras*, c-Ki-*ras* and N-*ras* genes has been described in liver tumours (Tsuda et al 1989).

Loss of heterozygosity on chromosomes 1p, 4q, 11p, 13q and 16q occurs frequently in human liver tumours, suggesting that these parts of the human genome might contain some genes whose functional loss might be involved in hepatocellular carcinogenesis (Pasquinelli et al 1988, Buetow et al 1989, Tsuda et al 1990, Simon et al 1991). Because the large-scale chromosomal alterations that arise in cancer cells occur infrequently in normal cells, it is probable that control mechanisms that safeguard chromosomal integrity are abrogated in the development of malignancy (Wright et al 1990). Such changes might represent secondary events linked to tumour progression and reflect a general property of transformed cells; whether HBV DNA integration, known to promote genetic instability (Hino et al 1991), contributes to these events has not been elucidated.

Allele loss of the short arm of chromosome 17, which include the p53 gene, have been commonly observed in human HCCs and hepatoma-derived cell lines (Fujimori et al 1991, Slagle et al 1991). Studies of the p53 gene at the DNA, RNA and protein levels have revealed abnormal structure and expression in most established HCC cell lines; these alterations, including partial deletions or DNA rearrangements and abnormal expression patterns, may not occur as a late 'in vitro' event and are not correlated with integration of HBV DNA (Bressac et al 1990). Although viral insertions in chromosome 17p have been described in some liver tumours (Hino et al 1986, Tokino et al 1987, Zhou et al 1988), it seems most probable that the genetic alterations observed in a majority of human HCCs are not due to a direct action of the virus. The wild-type p53 gene seems to negatively regulate cellular growth and has therefore been designated a tumour-suppressor gene or 'antioncogene' (see Levine et al 1991). Mutant forms of p53 frequently gain a growth stimulatory function, and genetic alterations of the gene, a common feature in human neoplasms, generally consist in the deletion of one p53 allele and in the mutation of the second allele. Point mutations that would alter the functional properties of p53 have not been reported so far in HBV-related HCCs, with the exception of a mutation affecting codon 249 and leading to a G–T transversion in most liver cancers from patients residing in South Africa and in the Qidong province of China (Bressac et al 1991, Hsu et al 1991). In these countries, exposure to high levels of dietary aflatoxins is well documented and the G to T substitution appears to be specific for the mutagenic action of the hepatocarcinogen. Evidence indicating that HBV infection does not contribute to the p53 mutation at codon 249 has been provided in a recent report showing that this mutation is not observed in HBV-related HCCs from patients that have not accumulated high exposure to aflatoxin B1 (Hayward et al 1991). Other studies of early and advanced HCCs from Japan have suggested that changes in the p53 may be related to tumour progression (Murakami et al 1991). Structural aberrations of the p53 gene (mutations at different codons and loss of one allele) have been observed only in advanced, less differentiated HCCs, frequently associated with abnormalities of another tumour-suppressor gene, RB. More recently, the frequency of p53 mutations has been evaluated in a large collection of tumours from diverse geographical and ethnic sources (Buetow et al 1992) and found to be much lower than previously reported. In particular, codon 249 mutations were not specifically related to high aflatoxin B1 exposure. In none of these studies could a contribution of HBV infection to genetic changes in DNA encoding p53 be established.

CONCLUSIONS

Several lines of evidence contribute in linking chronic HBV infection and primary liver cancer. First, a strong epidemiological association has been provided by extensive prospective and retrospective studies in many parts of the world. Second, a network of indirect, but convincing, arguments has further supported the connection between HBV and HCC, including the existence of related animal viruses that induce HCC in their hosts, the weak oncogenicity of the viral X transcriptional transactivator, the long-term tumorigenic effect of surface glycoproteins and the mutagenic action of viral integration into the cell genome, which may, directly or indirectly, contribute in deregulating the normal cell growth control.

The exponential relationship between HCC incidence and age indicates that, as in other human cancers, multiple steps, probably involving independent genetic lesions, are required. In particular, the long latency of HCC development after the initial HBV infection may be interpreted as a sign of an indirect action of the virus: a long-term toxic effect of viral gene products and/or the immune response against infected hepatocytes would trigger continuous necrosis and cell regeneration, which would in turn favour the accumulation of genetic alterations. In this model, productive HBV infections might potentiate the action of exogenous carcinogenic factors, like aflatoxins and alcohol. It might also be speculated that the latency period depends on the occurrence of a decisive HBV integration event that would promote genetic instability or lead to cis- or transactivation of relevant genes. Recent investigations of the functional and pathological properties of HBV gene products and of the consequences of HBV integration in the liver DNA suggest that various and probably cooperative mechanisms may operate in the development of liver cancer, and that HBV may share with other human oncogenic viruses a number of basic strategies. The HBV genome encodes at least seven different polypeptides;

none of them seems to act as a strong, dominant oncogene, but several lines of evidence indicate that the surface glycoproteins and the viral X transactivator might participate in carcinogenesis, in a native or modified state. In this respect, it is noteworthy that in human oncogenic viruses such as HTLV-1, EBV and HPV-16 and -18, transforming capacity is associated with the transcriptional transactivation activity of viral gene products. Comparative analyses of the different viral transactivators may help to guide future work in this field. Studies of mammalian HBV-related viruses have revealed strikingly different mechanisms and pointed out the importance of the activation of *myc* family genes in rodent hepatocarcinogenesis. However, a role for HBV in activating the c-*myc* oncogene, suggested by in vitro assays, has not been established in vivo, and recent data support a predominant role of tumour-suppressor genes such as p53 in human HCCs. The identification of the cellular effectors connecting HBV infection and liver cell transformation remains the main unsolved question.

REFERENCES

Araki K, Miyazaki J I, Hino O, Tomita N, Chisaka O, Matsubara K, Yamamura K I 1989 Expression and replication of hepatitis B virus genome in transgenic mice. Proceedings of the National Academy of Sciences of the USA 86: 207–211

Arii M, Takada S, Koike K 1992 Identification of three essential regions of hepatitis B virus X protein for trans-activation function. Oncogene 7: 397–403

Attali P, Thibault N, Buffett C, Briantais M J, Papoz L, Chaput J C, Etienne J P 1981 Les marqueurs du virus B chez les alcooliques chroniques. Clinical Biology 5: 1095–1102

Austin H 1991 The role of tobacco use and alcohol consumption in the etiology of hepatocellular carcinoma. Advances in Applied Biotechnology Series 13: 57–76

Babinet C, Farza H, Morello D, Hadchouel M, Pourcel C 1985 Specific expression of hepatitis B surface antigen (HBsAg) in transgenic mice. Science 230: 1160–1163

Balsano C, Avantaggiati M L, Natoli G, De Marzio E, Elfassi E, Will H, Levrero M 1991 Transactivation of c-fos and c-myc protooncogenes by both full-length and truncated versions of the HBV-X protein. In: Hollinger F B, Lemon S M, Margolis H (eds) Viral hepatitis and liver disease. Williams & Wilkins, Baltimore, pp 572–576

Beasley R P 1988 Hepatitis B virus – the major etiology of hepatocellular carcinoma. Cancer 61: 1942–1956

Beasley R P, Lin C C, Hwang L Y, Chien C S 1981 Hepatocellular carcinoma and hepatitis B virus: a prospective study of 22,707 men in Taiwan. Lancet ii: 1129–1133

Berger I, Shaul Y 1987 Integration of hepatitis B virus: analysis of unoccupied sites. Journal of Virology 61: 1180–1186

Blum H E, Liang T J, Galun E, Wands J R 1991 Persistence of hepatitis B virus DNA after serological recovery from hepatitis B virus infection. Hepatology 14: 56–63

Boender P J, Schalm S W, Heijtink R A 1985 Detection of integration during active replication of hepatitis B virus in the liver. Journal of Medical Virology 16: 47–54

Bosch F X, Munòz N 1991 Hepatocellular carcinoma in the world: epidemiologic questions. Advances in Applied Biotechnology Series 13: 35–56

Bréchot C 1987 Hepatitis B virus (HBV) and hepatocellular carcinoma, HBV status and its implication. Journal of Hepatology 4: 269–279

Bréchot C, Pourcel C, Louise A, Rain B, Tiollais P 1980 Presence of integrated hepatitis B virus DNA sequences in cellular DNA of human hepatocellular carcinoma. Nature 286: 533–535

Bréchot C, Hadchouel M, Scotto J, Degos F, Charnay P, Trépo C, Tiollais P 1981 Detection of hepatitis B virus DNA in liver and serum: a direct appraisal of the chronic carrier state. Lancet ii: 765–768

Bréchot C, Pourcel C, Hadchouel M, Dejean A, Louise A, Scotto J, Tiollais P 1982 State of hepatitis B virus DNA in liver diseases. Hepatology 2: 27S-34S

Bréchot C, Degos F, Lugassy C et al 1985 Hepatitis B virus DNA in patients with chronic liver disease and negative test for hepatitis B surface antigen. New England Journal of Medicine 312: 270–276

Bréchot C, Kremsdorf D, Paterlini P, Thiers V 1991 Hepatitis B virus DNA in HBsAg-negative patients. Molecular characterization and clinical implications. Journal of Hepatology 13: S49-S55

Bressac B, Galvin K M, Liang T J, Isselbacher K J, Wands J R, Ozturk M 1990 Abnormal structure and expression of p53 gene in human hepatocellular carcinoma. Proceedings of the National Academy of Sciences of the USA 87: 1973–1977

Bressac B, Kew M, Wands J, Ozturk M 1991 Selective G to T mutations of p53 gene in hepatocellular carcinoma from Southern Africa. Nature 350: 429–431

Brockes J 1990 Reading the retinoid signals. Nature 345: 766–768

Bruix J, Calvet X, Costa J et al 1989 Prevalence of antibodies to hepatitis C virus in Spanish patients with hepatocellular carcinoma and hepatic cirrhosis. Lancet 28: 1004–1008

Buetow K H, Murray J, Israel J et al 1989 Loss of heterozygosity suggests tumor suppressor gene responsible for primary hepatocellular carcinoma. Proceedings of the National Academy of Sciences of the USA 86: 8852–8856

Buetow K H, Sheffield V C, Zhu M et al 1992 Low frequency of p53 mutations observed in a diverse collection of primary hepatocellular carcinomas. Proceedings of the National Academy of Sciences of the USA 89: 9622–9626

Burk R D, DeLoia J A, ElAwady M K, Gearhart J D 1988 Tissue preferential expression of the hepatitis B virus (HBV) surface antigen gene in two lines of HBV transgenic mice. Journal of Virology 62: 649–654

Büscher M, Reiser W, Will H, Schaller H 1985 Transcripts and the putative RNA pregenome of duck hepatitis B virus: implications for reverse transcription. Cell 40: 717–724

Caselmann W H, Meyer M, Kekulé A S, Lauer U, Hofschneider P H, Koshy R 1990 A trans-activator function is generated by integration of hepatitis B virus pre-S/S sequences in human hepatocellular carcinoma DNA. Proceedings of the National Academy of Sciences of the USA 87: 2970–2974

Cattaneo R, Will H, Schaller H 1984 Hepatitis B virus transcription in the infected liver. EMBO Journal 3: 2191–2196

Chakraborty P R, Ruiz Opazo H, Shouval D, Shafritz D A 1980 Identification of integrated hepatitis B virus DNA and expression of viral RNA in an HBsAg-producing human hepatocellular carcinoma cell line. Nature 286: 531–533

Chandar N, Lombardi B, Locker J 1989 C-myc gene amplification during hepatocarcinogenesis by a choline-devoid diet. Proceedings of the National Academy of Sciences of the USA 86: 2703–2707

Chang M H, Hsu C, Lee C Y, Chen D S, Lee C H, Lin K S 1984 Fraternal hepatocellular carcinoma in young children in two families. Cancer 53: 1807–1810

Chang M H, Chen P J, Chen J Y et al 1991 Hepatitis B virus integration in hepatitis B virus-related hepatocellular carcinoma in childhood. Hepatology 13: 316–320

Chen C, Diani A, Brown P, Kaluzny M, Epps D 1986 Detection of hepatitis B virus DNA in hepatocellular carcinoma. The British Journal of Experimental Pathology 67: 1868

Chen C J, Liang K Y, Chang A S et al 1991 Effects of hepatitis B virus, alcohol drinking, cigarette smoking and familial tendency on hepatocellular carcinoma. Hepatology 13: 398–406

Chisari F V, Pinkert C A, Milich D R, Filippi P, McLachlan A, Palmiter R and Brinster R 1985 A transgenic mouse model of the chronic hepatitis B surface antigen carrier state. Science 230: 1157–1159

Chisari F V, Filippi P, MaLachlan A et al 1986 Expression of hepatitis B virus large envelope polypeptide inhibits hepatitis B surface antigen secretion in transgenic mice. Journal of Virology 60: 880–887

Chisari F V, Filippi P, Buras F et al 1987 Structural and pathological effects of synthesis of hepatitis B virus large envelope polypeptide in transgenic mice. Proceedings of the National Academy of Sciences of the USA 84: 6909–6913

Chisari F V, Klopchin K, Moriyama T et al 1989 Molecular pathogenesis of hepatocellular carcinoma in hepatitis B virus transgenic mice. Cell 59: 1145–1156

Cobden I, Bassendine M, James O 1986 Hepatocellular carcinoma in North-East England: importance of hepatitis B infection and ex-tropical military service. Quarterly Journal of Medicine 855–863

Colgrove R, Simon G, Ganem D 1989 Transcriptional activation of homologous and heterologous genes by the hepatitis B virus X gene product in cells permissive for viral replication. Journal of Virology 63: 4019–4026

Colombo M 1992 Hepatocellular carcinoma. Journal of Hepatology 15: 225–236

Corcoran L M, Adams J M, Dunn A R, Cory S 1984 Murine T lymphomas in which the cellular myc oncogene has been activated by retrovirus insertion. Cell 37: 113–122

Coursaget P, Le Cann P, Leboulleux D, Diop M T, Bao O, Coll A M 1991 Detection of hepatitis B virus DNA by polymerase chain reaction in HBsAg negative Senegalese patients suffering from cirrhosis or primary liver cancer. FEMS Letters 35–38

Craig J R, Klatt E C, Yu M 1991 Role of cirrhosis and the development of HCC: evidence from histologic studies and large population studies. Advances in Applied Biotechnology Series 13: 177–190

Dazza M C, Meneses L V, Giarad P M, Villaroel C, Bréchot C, Larouzé M D 1990 Hepatitis C virus antibodies in Mozambican patients with hepatocellular carcinoma and cirrhosis. Lancet 335: 1216

Dazza M C, Meneses L V, Girard P M, Paterlini P, Villaroel C, Bréchot C, Larouzé B 1991 Polymerase chain reaction for detection of hepatitis B virus DNA in HBsAg seronegative patients with hepatocellular carcinoma from Mozambique. Annals of Tropical Medicine and Parasitology 85: 277–279

Dejean A, De Thé H 1990 Hepatitis B virus as an insertional mutagen in a human hepatocellular carcinoma. Molecular Biology and Medicine 7: 213–222

Dejean A, Sonigo P, Wain-Hobson S, Tiollais P 1984 Specific hepatitis B virus integration in hepatocellular carcinoma DNA through a viral 11 base pair direct repeat. Proceedings of the National Academy of Sciences of the USA 81: 5350–5354

Dejean A, Bougueleret L, Grzeschik K H, Tiollais P 1986 Hepatitis B virus DNA integration in a sequence homologous to v-erbA and steroid receptor genes in a hepatocellular carcinoma. Nature 322: 70–72

de Thé H, Marchio A, Tiollais P, Dejean A 1987 A novel steroid/thyroid hormone receptor-related gene inappropriately expressed in human hepatocellular carcinoma. Nature 330: 667–670

de Thé H, Chomienne C, Lanotte M, Degos L, Dejean A 1990 The t(15;17) translocation of acute promyelocytic leukaemia fuses the retinoic acid receptor alpha gene to a novel transcribed locus. Nature 347: 558–561

de Thé H, Lavau C, Marchio A, Chomienne C, Degos L, Dejean A 1991 The PML-RAR-alpha fusion mRNA generated by the t(15,17) translocation in acute promyelocytic leukaemia encodes a functionally altered retinoic acid receptor. Cell 66: 675–684

Dolcetti R, Rizzo S, Viel A, Maestro R, De Re V, Feriotto G, Boiocchi M 1989 N-*myc* activation by proviral insertion in MCF 247-induced murine T-cell lymphomas. Oncogene 4: 1009–1014

Dragani T, Manenti G, Della Porta G, Tiollais P, Farza H, Pourcel C 1989 Hepatitis B transgenic mice are more susceptible to carcinogen-induced hepatocarcinogenesis. Carcinogenesis 11: 953–956

Dunk A, Spiliadis H, Sherlock S, Fowler M, Monjardino J, Scheuer P, Thomas H 1988 Hepatocellular carcinoma: clinical, aetiological and pathological features in British patients. International Journal of Cancer 41: 17–23

Dunsford H A, Sell S, Chisari F V 1990 Hepatocarcinogenesis due to chronic liver cell injury in hepatitis B virus transgenic mice. Cancer Research 50: 3400–3407

Edman J C, Gray P, Valenzuela P, Rall L B, Rutter W J 1980 Integration of hepatitis B virus sequences and their expression in a human hepatoma cell. Nature 286: 535–537

Elfassi E, Haseltine W A, Dienstag J L 1986 Detection of hepatitis B virus X product using an open reading frame *Escherichia coli* expression vector. Proceedings of the National Academy of Sciences of the USA 83: 2219–222

Enders G H, Ganem D, Varmus H 1985 Mapping the major transcripts of ground squirrel hepatitis virus: the presumptive template for reverse transcriptase is terminally redundant. Cell 42: 297–308

Etiemble J, Möröy T, Jacquemin E, Tiollais P, Buendia M A 1989 Fused transcripts of c-*myc* and a new cellular locus, hcr, in a primary liver tumor. Oncogene 4: 51–57

Farza H, Hadchouel M, Scotto J, Tiollais P, Babinet C, Pourcel C 1988 Replication and gene expression of hepatitis B virus in a transgenic mouse that contains the complete viral genome. Journal of Virology 62: 4144–4152

Fong T, Govindarajan S, Valinluck B, Redeker A 1988 Status of hepatitis B virus DNA in alcoholic liver disease: a study of a large urban population in the United States. Hepatology 8: 1602–1604

Fourel G, Trépo C, Bougueleret L, Henglein B, Ponzetto A, Tiollais P, Buendia M A 1990 Frequent activation of N-*myc* genes by hepadnavirus insertion in woodchuck liver tumours. Nature 347: 294–298

Fujimori M, Tokino T, Hino O et al 1991 Allelotype study of primary hepatocellular carcinoma. Cancer Research 51: 89–93

Fujiyama A, Miyanohara A, Nozaki C, Yoneyama T, Ohtomo N, Matsubara K 1983 Cloning and structural analyses of hepatitis B virus DNAs, subtype adr. Nucleic Acids Research 11: 4601–4610

Galibert F, Mandart E, Fitoussi F, Tiollais P, Charnay P 1979 Nucleotide sequence of hepatitis B virus genome (subtype ayw) cloned in *E. coli*. Nature 281: 646–650

Galloway D J K 1983 The oncogenic potential of herpes simplex viruses: evidence for a hit and run mechanism. Nature 302: 21–24

Ganem D, Varmus H E 1987 The molecular biology of the hepatitis B viruses. Annual Review in Biochemistry 56: 651–693

Gerken G, Kremsdorf D, Capel F et al 1991 Hepatitis B defective virus with rearrangements in the preS gene during chronic HBV infection. Virology 183: 555–565

Giordano A, Whyte P, Harlow E, Franza B R, Beach D, Draetta G 1989 A 60 kd cdc2-associated polypeptide complexes with the E1A proteins in adenovirus-infected cells. Cell 58: 981–990

Girard F, Strausfeld U, Fernandez A, Lamb N J C 1991 Cyclin A is required for the onset of DNA replication in mammalian fibroblasts. Cell 67: 1169–1179

Gough N M 1983 Core and E antigen synthesis in rodent cells transformed with hepatitis B virus DNA is associated with greater than genome length viral messenger RNAs. Journal of Molecular Biology 165: 683–699

Haruna Y, Hayashi N, Katamaya K et al 1991 Expression of X protein and hepatitis B virus replication in chronic hepatitis. Hepatology 13: 417–421

Hasan F, Jeffers L J, Medina M et al 1990 Hepatitis C associated hepatocellular carcinoma. Hepatology 12: 589–591

Hatada I, Tokino T, Ochiya T, Matsubara K 1988 Co-amplification of integrated hepatitis B virus DNA and transforming gene *hst*-1 in a hepatocellular carcinoma. Oncogene 3: 537–540

Hayward N K, Walker G J, Graham W, Cooksley E 1991 Hepatocellular carcinoma mutation. Nature 352: 764

Hilger C, Velhagen I, Zentgraf H, Schröder C H 1991 Diversity of hepatitis B virus X gene-related transcripts in hepatocellular carcinoma: a novel polyadenylation site on viral DNA. Journal of Virology 65: 4284–4291

Hino O, Kitagawa T, Koike K, Kobayashi M, Hara M, Mori W, Nakashima T et al 1984 Detection of hepatitis B virus DNA in hepatocellular carcinomas in Japan. Hepatology 4: 90–95

Hino O, Kitagawa T, Sugano H 1985 Relationship between serum and histochemical markers for hepatitis B virus and rate of viral integration in hepatocellular carcinomas in Japan. International Journal of Cancer 35: 5–10

Hino O, Shows T B, Rogler C E 1986 Hepatitis B virus integration site in hepatocellular carcinoma at chromosome 17;18 translocation. Proceedings of the National Academy of Sciences of the USA 83: 8338–8342

Hino O, Ohtake K, Rogler C E 1989 Features of two hepatitis B virus (HBV) DNA integrations suggest mechanisms of HBV integration. Journal of Virology 63: 2638–2643

Hino O, Tabata S, Hotta Y 1991 Evidence for increased in vitro recombination with insertion of human hepatitis B virus DNA. Proceedings of the National Academy of Sciences of the USA 88: 9248–9252

Hino O, Kitagawa T, Nomura K, Ohtake K, Yasui H, Okamoto N, Hirayama Y 1992 Comparative molecular pathogenesis of hepatocellular carcinomas. In: Klein-Szanto A J P, Anderson M W, Barrett J C and Slaga T J (eds) Comparative molecular carcinogenesis. Wiley–Liss, New York, pp 173–185

Höhne M, Schaefer S, Seifer M, Feitelson M A, Paul D, Gerlich W H 1990 Malignant transformation of immortalized transgenic hepatocytes after transfection with hepatitis B virus DNA. EMBO Journal 9: 1137–1145

Hollinger F B 1990 Hepatitis B virus. In: Fields B N, Knipe D M et al (eds) Fields virology, Vol. 2. Raven Press, New York, pp 2171–2236

Horiike N, Michitaka K, Onji M, Murota T, Ohta Y 1989 HBV DNA hybridization in hepatocellular carcinoma associated with alcohol in Japan. Journal of Medical Virology 28: 189–192

Hsu H C, Chiou T J, Chen J Y, Lee C S, Lee P H, Peng S Y 1991 Clonality and clonal evolution of hepatocellular carcinoma with multiple nodules. Hepatology 13: 923–928

Hsu I C, Metcalf R A, Sun T, Welsh J A, Wang N J 1991 Mutational hotspot in the p53 gene in human hepatocellular carcinomas. Nature 350: 427–428

Hsu T Y, Möröy T, Etiemble J, Louise A, Trépo C, Tiollais P, Buendia M A 1988 Activation of c-myc by woodchuck hepatitis virus insertion in hepatocellular carcinoma. Cell 55: 627–635

Hsu T Y, Fourel G, Etiemble J, Tiollais P, Buendia M A 1990 Integration of hepatitis virus DNA near c-myc in woodchuck hepatocellular carcinoma. Gastroenterologia Japonica 25: 43–48

Iijima T, Saitoh N, Nobutomo K, Nambu M, Sakuma K 1984 A prospective cohort study of hepatitis B surface antigen carriers in a working population. Gann 75: 571–573

Imai M, Hoshi Y, Okamoto H et al 1987 Free and integrated forms of hepatitis B virus DNA in human hepatocellular carcinoma cells (PLC/342) propagated in nude mice. Journal of Virology 61: 3555–3560

Kay A, Mandart E, Trepo C, Galibert F 1985 The HBV HBx gene expressed in *E. coli* is recognized by sera from hepatitis patients. EMBO Journal 4: 1287–1292

Kekulé A S, Lauer U, Meyer M, Caselmann W H, Hofschneider P H, Koshy R 1990 The pre-S2/S region of

integrated hepatitis B virus DNA encodes a transcriptional transactivator. Nature 343: 457–461
Kew M C 1989 Role of cirrhosis in hepatocarcinogenesis. In: Bannasch P, Keppler D, Weber G (eds) Liver cell carcinoma. Kluwer Academic Publishers, Dordrecht, pp 37–45
Kew M, Popper H 1984 Relationship between hepatocellular carcinoma and cirrhosis. Seminars in Liver Disease 4: 136–145
Kew M, Houghton M, Choo Q L, Kuo G 1990 Hepatitis S virus antibodies in southern African blacks with hepatocellular carcinoma. Lancet 335: 873–874
Kim C M, Koike K, Saito I, Miyamura T, Jay G 1991 HBx gene of hepatitis B virus induces liver cancer in transgenic mice. Nature 351: 317–320
Kobayashi M, Koike K 1984 Complete nucleotide sequence of hepatitis B virus DNA of subtype adr and its conserved gene organization. Gene 30: 227–232
Koch S, Freytag von Loringhoven A, Kahmann R, Hofschneider P H, Koshy R 1984a The genetic organization of integrated hepatitis B virus DNA in the human hepatoma cell line PLC/PRF/5. Nucleic Acids Research 12: 6871–6876
Koch S, Freytag von Loringhoven A, Hofschneider P H, Koshy R 1984b Amplification and rearrangement in hepatoma cell DNA associated with integrated hepatitis B virus DNA. EMBO Journal 3: 2185–2189
Koike K, Yaginuma K, Mizusawa H, Kobayashi M 1985 Structure of integrated HBV DNA in human hepatomas. In: Nishioka K, Blumberg B S, Ishida N, Koike K (eds) Hepatitis viruses and hepatocellular carcinoma: approaches through molecular biology and ecology. Academic Press, Tokyo, pp 99–115
Korba B E, Wells F V, Baldwin B, Cote P J, Tennant B C, Popper H, Gerin J L 1989 Hepatocellular carcinoma in woodchuck hepatitis virus-infected woodchucks: presence of viral DNA in tumor tissue from chronic carriers and animals serologically recovered from acute infections. Hepatology 9: 461–470
Koshy R, Wells J 1991 Deregulation of cellular gene expression by HBV transactivators in hepatocarcinogenesis. Advances in Applied Biotechnology Series 13: 159–170
Koshy R, Koch S, Freytag von Loringhoven A, Kahmann R, Murray K, Hofschneider P H 1983 Integration of hepatitis B virus DNA: evidence for integration in the single-stranded gap. Cell 34: 215–223
Koshy R, Meyer M, Kékulé A, Lauer U, Caselmann W H, Hofschneider P H 1991 Altered functions of hepatitis B virus proteins as a consequence of viral DNA integration may lead to hepatocyte transformation. In: Hollinger F B, Lemon S M, Margolis H (eds) Viral hepatitis and liver disease. Williams & Wilkins, Baltimore, pp 566–572
Kremsdorf D, Thiers V, Garreau F 1991 Nucleotide sequence analysis of hepatitis B virus genomes isolated from serologically negative patients. In: Hollinger F B, Lemon S M, Margolis H (eds) Viral hepatitis and liver disease. Williams & Wilkins, Baltimore, pp 222–226
Lai M, Chen P, Yang P, Sheu J, Sung J, Chen D 1990 Identification and characterization of intrahepatic B virus DNA in HBsAg-seronegative patients with chronic liver disease and hepatocellular carcinoma in Taiwan. Hepatology 3: 575–581
Lauer U, Weiss L, Hofschneider P H, Kekulé A S 1992 The hepatitis B virus pre-S/St transactivator is generated by 3' truncations within a defined region of the S gene. Journal of Virology 66: 5284–5289
Lee T H, Finegold M J, Shen R F, DeMayo J L, Woo S L C, Butel J S 1990 Hepatitis B virus transactivator X protein is not tumorigenic in transgenic mice. Journal of Virology 64: 5939–5947
Levine A J, Momand J, Finlay C A 1991 The p53 tumour suppressor gene. Nature 351: 453–456
Levrero M, Stemler M, Pasquinelli C et al 1991 Significance of anti-HBx antibodies in hepatitis B virus infection. Hepatology 13: 143–149
Liang T J, Isselbacher K J, Wands J R 1989 Rapid identification of low level hepatitis B-related viral genome in serum. Journal of Clinical Investigation 84: 1367–1371
Liang T J, Hasegawa K, Rimon N, Wands J R, Ben-Porath E 1991a A hepatitis B virus mutant associated with an epidemic of fulminant hepatitis. New England Journal of Medicine 324: 1705–1709
Liang T J, Baruch Y, Ben-Porath E et al 1991b Hepatitis B virus infection in patients with idiopathic liver disease. Hepatology 13: 1044–1051
Liang T J, Jeffers L, Cheinquer H et al 1992 Viral etiology of hepatocellular carcinoma in the United States. Hepatology 16: 128A
Li Y, Golemis E, Hartley J W, Hopkins N 1987 Disease specificity of non defective Friend and Moloney murine leukemia viruses is controlled by a small number of nucleotides. Journal of Virology 61: 693–700
Lok A, Ma O 1990 Hepatitis B virus replication in Chinese patients with hepatocellular carcinoma. Hepatology 12: 582–588
Lok A S F, Lai C L, Chung H, Lau J Y N, Leung E K Y, Wong L S K 1991 Morbidity and mortality from chronic hepatitis B virus infection in family members of patients with malignant and non-malignant hepatitis B virus-related chronic liver diseases. Hepatology 13: 834–837
Lucito R, Schneider R J 1992 Hepatitis B virus X protein activates transcription factor NF-κB without a requirement for protein kinase C. Journal of Virology 66: 983–991
Lugassy C, Bernuau J, Thiers V et al 1987 Sequences of hepatitis B virus DNA in the serum and liver of patients with acute benign and fulminant hepatitis. Journal of Infectious Diseases 155: 64–71
Maguire H F, Hoeffler J P, Siddiqui A 1991 HBV X protein alters the DNA binding specificity of CREB and ATF-2 by protein–protein interactions. Science 252: 842–844
Marcellin P, Thiers V, Degott C, Franco D, Belghitti J, Castaing D, Fagniez P, Zafrani S, Benhamou J P, Bismuth H, Tiollais P, Bréchot C 1989 Hepatocellular carcinoma with normal adjacent liver hepatitis B virus DNA status. Journal of Hepatology 8: 249–253
Marion P L 1991 Ground squirrel hepatitis virus. In: McLachlan A (ed) Molecular biology of the hepatitis B virus. CRC Press, Boca Raton, pp 39–51
Marion P L, Van Davelaar M J, Knight S S, Salazar F H, Garcia G, Popper H, Robinson W S 1986 Hepatocellular carcinoma in ground squirrels persistently infected with ground squirrel hepatitis virus. Proceedings of the National Academy of Sciences of the USA 83: 4543–4546
Matsubara K, Tokino T 1990 Integration of hepatitis B virus DNA and its implications for hepatocarcinogenesis. Molecular Biology and Medicine 7: 243–260
Mendenhall C L, Seeff L, Diehl A M et al 1991 Antibodies to hepatitis B virus and hepatitis C virus in alcoholic hepatitis and cirrhosis: their prevalence and clinical relevance. Hepatology 14: 581–589
Meyers M L, Vitvitski Trépo L, Nath N, Sninsky J J 1986

Hepatitis B virus polypeptide X: expression in *Escherichia coli* and identification of specific antibodies in sera from hepatitis B virus-infected humans. Journal of Virology 57: 101–109

Miller R H, Robinson W S 1986 Common evolutionary origin of hepatitis B virus and retroviruses. Proceedings of the National Academy of Sciences of the USA 83: 2531–2535

Mizusawa H, Taira M, Yaginuma K, Kobayashi M, Yoshida E, Koike K 1985 Inversely repeating integrated hepatitis B virus DNA and cellular flanking sequences in the human hepatoma-derived cell line huSP. Proceedings of the National Academy of Sciences of the USA 82: 208–212

Moriarty A M, Alexander H, Lerner R A 1985 Antibodies to peptides detect new hepatitis B antigen: serological correlation with hepatocellular carcinoma. Science 227: 429–433

Möröy T, Etiemble J, Trépo C, Tiollais P, Buendia M A 1985 Transcription of woodchuck hepatitis virus in the chronically infected liver. EMBO Journal 4: 1507–1514

Möröy T, Marchio A, Etiemble J, Trépo C, Tiollais P, Buendia M A 1986 Rearrangement and enhanced expression of c-myc in hepatocellular carcinoma of hepatitis virus infected woodchucks. Nature 324: 276–279

Motokura T, Bloom T, Kim H G, Jüppner H, Ruderman J V, Kronenberg H M, Arnold A 1991 A novel cyclin encoded by a bcl-1-linked candidate oncogene. Nature 350: 512–515

Münger K, Phelps W C, Bubb V, Howley P M, Schlegel R 1989 The E6 and E7 genes of the human papillomavirus type 16 together are necessary and sufficient for transformation of primary human keratinocytes. Journal of Virology 63: 4417–4421

Murakami Y, Hayashi K, Hirohashi S, Sekiya T 1991 Aberrations of the tumor suppressor p53 and retinoblastoma genes in human hepatocellular carcinomas. Cancer Research 51: 5520–5525

Nagaya T, Nakamura T, Tokino T et al 1987 The mode of hepatitis B virus DNA integration in chromosomes of human hepatocellular carcinoma. Genes and Development 1: 773–782

Nakamura T, Tokino T, Nagaya T, Matsubara K 1988 Microdeletion associated with the integration process of hepatitis B virus DNA. Nucleic Acids Research 16: 4865–4873

Nalpas B, Berthelot P, Thiers V, Duhamel G, Courouce A M, Tiollais P, Bréchot C 1985 Hepatitis B virus multiplication in the absence of usual serological markers. A study of 146 alcoholics. Journal of Hepatology 1: 89–97

Nalpas B, Driss F, Pol S, Hamelin B, Housset C, Bréchot C, Berthelot P 1991 Association between HCV and HBV infection in hepatocellular carcinoma and alcoholic liver disease. Journal of Hepatology 12: 70–74

Nalpas B, Thiers V, Pos S, Driss F, Thepot V, Berthelot P, Bréchot C 1992 Hepatitis C viremia and anti-HCV antibodies in alcoholics. Journal of Hepatology 14: 381–384

Neurath A R, Kent S B H, Strick N, Parker K 1986 Identification and chemical synthesis of a host cell receptor binding site on hepatitis B virus. Cell 46: 429–436

Nishioka K, Watanabe J, Furuta S et al 1991 A high prevalence of antibody to the hepatitis C virus in patients with hepatocellular carcinoma in Japan. Cancer 67: 429–433

Nurse P 1990 Universal control mechanism regulating onset of M-phase. Nature 344: 503–508

Obata H, Hayashi N, Motoike Y, Hisamitsu T, Okuda H, Kobayashi S, Nishioka K 1980 A prospective study on the development of hepatocellular carcinoma from liver cirrhosis with persistent hepatitis B virus infection. International Journal of Cancer 25: 741–747

Ochiya T, Fujiyama A, Fukushige S, Hatada I, Matsubara K 1986 Molecular cloning of an oncogene from a human hepatocellular carcinoma. Proceedings of the National Academy of Sciences of the USA 83: 4993–4997

Ochiya T, Tsurimoto T, Ueda K, Okubo K, Shiozawa M, Matsubara K 1989 An in-vitro system for infection with hepatitis B virus that uses primary human fetal hepatocytes. Proceedings of the National Academy of Sciences of the USA 86: 1875–1879

Ogata N, Tokino T, Kamimura T, Asakura H 1990 A comparison of the molecular structure of integrated hepatitis B virus genomes in hepatocellular carcinoma cells and hepatocytes derived from the same patient. Hepatology 11: 1018–1023

Ohkoshi S 1991 Detection of HBV DNA in non-A, non-B hepatic tissues using the polymerase chain reaction assay. Gastroenterologia Japanica 26: 728–733

Ohkoshi S, Kato N, Kinoshita T et al 1990 Detection of hepatitis C virus RNA in sera and liver tissues of non-A, non-B hepatitis patients using the polymerase chain reaction. Japanese Journal of Experimental Medicine 81: 862–865

Okamoto H, Imai M, Kametani M, Nakamura T, Mayumi M 1987 Genomic heterogeneity of hepatitis B virus in a 54-year-old woman who contracted the infection through materno-fetal transmission. Japanese Journal of Experimental Medicine 57: 231–236

Okuda K 1991 Hepatitis C virus and hepatocellular carcinoma. Advances in Applied Biotechnology Series 13: 119–126

Okuda K 1992 Hepatocellular carcinoma: recent progress. Hepatology 15: 948–963

Oliveri F, Brunetto M R, Baldi M et al 1991 Hepatitis delta virus (HDV) infection and hepatocellular carcinoma. In: Gerin J L, Purcell R H, Rizetto M (eds) The hepatitis delta virus. Wiley–Liss, New York, pp 217–222

Omata M, Ehata T, Yokosuka O, Hosoda K, Ohto M 1991 Mutations in the precore region of hepatitis B virus DNA in patients with fulminant and severe hepatitis. New England Journal of Medicine 324: 1699–1704

Ono Y, Onda H, Sasada R, Igarashi K, Sugino Y, Nishioka K 1983 The complete nucleotide sequences of the cloned hepatitis B virus DNA; subtype adr and adw. Nucleic Acids Research 11: 1747–1756

Ou J H, Rutter W J 1985 Hybrid hepatitis B virus–host transcripts in a human hepatoma cell. Proceedings of the National Academy of Sciences of the USA 82: 83–87

Pares A, Barrera J M, Caballeria J et al 1990 Hepatitis C virus antibodies in chronic alcoholic patients association with severity of liver injury. Hepatology 12: 1295–1299

Pasek M, Goto T, Gilbert W et al 1979 Hepatitis B virus genes and their expression in *Escherichia coli*. Nature 282: 575–579

Pasquinelli C, Garreau F, Bougueleret L et al 1988 Rearrangement of a common cellular DNA domain on chromosome 4 in human primary liver tumors. Journal of Virology 62: 629–632

Paterlini P, Gerken G, Nakajima E et al 1990 Polymerase

chain reaction to detect hepatitis B virus DNA and RNA sequences in primary liver cancers from patients negative for hepatitis B surface antigen. New England Journal of Medicine 323: 80–85

Paterlini P, Gerken G, Khemeny F et al 1991 Primary liver cancer in HBsAg-negative patients: a study of HBV genome using the polymerase chain reaction. In: Hollinger F B, Lemon S M, Margolis H (eds) Viral hepatitis and liver disease. Williams & Wilkins, Baltimore pp 605–610

Paterlini P, Driss F, Nalpas B, Pisi E, Franco D, Berthelot P, Bréchot C 1993 Persistence of hepatitis B and hepatitis C viral genomes in primary liver cancers from HBsAg-negative patients: a study of a low-endemic area. Hepatology 17: 20–29

Pfaff E, Salfeld J, Gmelin K, Schaller H, Theilmann L 1987 Synthesis of the X protein of hepatitis B virus in vitro and detection of anti-X antibodies in human sera. Virology 158: 456–460

Pol S, Thiers V, Nalpas B, Degos F, Gazengel C, Carnot F, Tiollais P et al 1987 Monoclonal anti-HBs antibodies radioimmunoassay and serum HBV-DNA hybridization as diagnostic tools of HBV infection: relative prevalence among HBsAg-negative alcoholics, patients with chronic hepatitis or hepatocellular carcinomas and blood donors. European Journal of Clinical Investigation 17: 515–521

Pontisso P, Stanico D, Diodati G, Marin G, Caldironi M V, Giacchino R, Realdi G, Alberti A 1987 HBV DNA sequences are rarely detected in the liver of patients with HBsAg negative chronic active liver disease and with hepatocellular carcinoma in Italy. Liver 7: 211–215

Pontisso P, Basso G, Perilongo G, Morsica G, Ceccheto G, Ruvoletto M G, Alberti A 1991 Does hepatitis B virus play a role in primary liver cancer in children of western countries? Cancer Detection and Prevention 15: 363–368

Pontisso P, Morsica G, Ruvoletto M G, Barzon M, Perilongo G, Basso G, Cecchetto G et al 1992 Latent hepatitis B virus infection in childhood hepatocellular carcinoma. Cancer 69: 2731–2735

Popper H, Shafritz D A, Hoofnagle J H 1987a Relation of the hepatitis B virus carrier state to hepatocellular carcinoma. Hepatology 7: 764–772

Popper H, Roth L, Purcell R H, Tennant B C, Gerin J L 1987b Hepatocarcinogenicity of the woodchuck hepatitis virus. Proceedings of the National Academy of Sciences of the USA 84: 866–870

Portis J L, Perryman S, McAtee F J 1991 The R-U5-5' leader sequence of neurovirulent wild mouse retrovirus contains an element controlling the incubation period of neurodegenerative disease. Journal of Virology 65: 1877–1883

Poynard T, Aubert A, Lazizi Y et al 1991 Independent risk factors for hepatocellular carcinoma in French drinkers. Hepatology 13: 896–901

Radziwill G, Tucker W, Schaller H 1990 Mutational analysis of the hepatitis B virus P gene product: domain structure and RNase H activity. Journal of Virology 64: 613–620

Robinson W S 1990 Hepadnaviridae and their replication. In: Fields B N, Knipe D M, Chanock R M, Hirsch M S, Melnick J L, Monath T P, Roizman B (eds) Fields virology. Raven Press, New York, pp 2137–2169

Rogler C E, Sherman M, Su C Y et al 1985 Deletion in chromosome 11p associated with a hepatitis B integration site in hepatocellular carcinoma. Science 230: 319–322

Romanczuk H, Villa L L, Schlegel R, Howley P M 1991 The viral transcriptional regulatory region upstream of the E6 and E7 genes is a major determinant of the differential immortalization activities of human papillomavirus types 16 and 18. Journal of Virology 65: 2739–2744

Rossner M T 1992 Hepatitis B virus X-gene product: a promiscuous transcriptional activator. Journal of Medical Virology 36: 101–117

Ruiz J, Sangro B, Guende J I, Beloqui O, Riezu-Boj J I, Herrero J I, Prieto J 1992 Hepatitis B and C viral infections in patients with hepatocellular carcinoma. Hepatology 3: 637–640

Saunders J B, Wodak A D, Morgan-Capner P, Whyte Y S, Portmann B, Davis M, Williams R 1983 Importance of markers of hepatitis B virus in alcoholic liver disease. British Medical Journal 286: 1851–1854

Schek N, Fischer M, Schaller H 1991a The hepadnaviral X protein. In: McLachlan A (ed) The hepadnaviral X protein. CRC Press, Boca Raton, pp 181–192

Schek N, Bartenschlager R, Kuhn C, Schaller H 1991b Phosphorylation and rapid turnover of hepatitis B virus X-protein expressed in HepG2 cells from a recombinant vaccinia virus. Oncogene 6: 1735–1744

Schödel F, Sprengel R, Weimer T, Fernholz D, Schneider R, Will H 1989 Animal hepatitis B viruses. In: Klein G (ed) Advances in viral oncology. Raven Press, New York, pp 73–102

Seeger C, Ganem D, Varmus H E 1986 Biochemical and genetic evidence for the hepatitis B virus replication strategy. Science 232: 477–484

Seeger C, Baldwin B, Hornbuckle W E et al 1991 Woodchuck hepatitis virus is a more efficient oncogenic agent than ground squirrel hepatitis virus in a common host. Journal of Virology 65: 1673–1679

Selten G, Cuypers H T, Zijlstra M, Melief C, Berns A 1984 Involvement of c-myc in MuLV-induced T cell lymphomas in mice: frequency and mechanisms of activation. EMBO Journal 3: 3215–3222

Seto E, Mitchell P J, Yen T S B 1990 Transactivation by the hepatitis B virus X protein depends on AP-2 and other transcription factors. Nature 344: 72–74

Setoguchi M, Higuchi Y, Yoshida S, Nasu N, Miyazaki Y, Akizuki S I, Yamamoto S 1989 Insertional activation of N-myc by endogenous Moloney-like murine retrovirus sequences in macrophage cell lines derived from myeloma cell line–macrophage hybrids. Molecular and Cellular Biology 9: 4515–4522

Shafritz D A, Shouval D, Sherman H, Hadziyannis S, Kew M C 1981 Integration of hepatitis B virus DNA into the genome of liver cells in chronic liver disease and hepatocellular carcinoma. New England Journal of Medicine 305: 1067–1073

Shaul Y, Ziemer M, Garcia P D, Crawford R, Hsu H, Valenzuela P, Rutter W J 1984 Cloning and analysis of integrated hepatitis virus sequences from a human hepatoma cell line. Journal of Virology 51: 776–787

Shaul Y, Rutter W J, Laub O 1985 A human hepatitis B viral enhancer element. EMBO Journal 4: 427–430

Shaul Y, Garcia P D, Schonberg S, Rutter W J 1986 Integration of hepatitis B virus DNA in chromosome-specific satellite sequences. Journal of Virology 59: 731–734

Shen F-M, Lee M K, Gong H M, Cai X Q, King M C 1991 Complex segregation analysis of primary hepatocellular carcinoma in Chinese families: interaction of inherited susceptibility and hepatitis B viral infection. American Journal of Human Genetics 49: 88–93

Shih C, Burke K, Chou M J et al 1987 Tight clustering of human hepatitis B virus integration sites in hepatomas near a triple-stranded region. Journal of Virology 61: 3491–3498

Shih C C, Stoye J P, Coffin J M 1988 Highly preferred targets for retrovirus integration. Cell 53: 531–537

Shiozawa M, Ochiya T, Hatada I, Imamura T, Okudaira Y, Hiraoka H, Matsubara K 1988 The 1ca as an onco-fetal gene: its expression in human fetal liver. Oncogene 2: 523–526

Shirakata Y, Kawada M, Fujiki Y et al 1989 The X gene of hepatitis B virus induced growth stimulation and tumorigenic transformation of mouse NIH3T3 cells. Japanese Journal of Cancer Research 80: 617–621

Siddiqui A, Jameel S, Mapoles J E 1986 Transcriptional control elements of hepatitis B surface antigen gene. Proceedings of the National Academy of Sciences of the USA 83: 566–570

Siddiqui A, Jameel S, Mapoles J 1987 Expression of the hepatitis B virus X gene in mammalian cells. Proceedings of the National Academy of Sciences of the USA 84: 2513–2517

Simon D, Knowles B B, Weith A 1991 Abnormalities of chromosome 1 and loss of heterozygosity on 1p in primary hepatomas. Oncogene 6: 765–770

Simonetti R G, Camma C, Fiorello F et al 1992 Hepatitis C virus infection as a risk factor for hepatocellular carcinoma in patients with cirrhosis. A case control study. Annals of Internal Medicine 116: 97–102

Slagle B L, Zhou Y Z, Butel J S 1991 Hepatitis B virus integration event in human chromosome 17p near the p53 gene identifies the region of the chromosome commonly deleted in virus-positive hepatocellular carcinomas. Cancer Research 51: 49–54

Smith K T, Campo M S 1988 'Hit and run' transformation of mouse C127 cells by bovine papillomavirus type 4: the viral DNA is required for the initiation but not for maintenance of the transformed phenotype. Virology 64: 39–47

Spandau D F, Lee C H 1988 Trans-activation of viral enhancers by the hepatitis B virus X protein. Journal of Virology 62: 427–434

Summers J, Mason W S 1982 Replication of the genome of a hepatitis B-like virus by reverse transcription of an RNA intermediate. Cell 29: 403–415

Summers J A, O'Connell A, Millman I 1975 Genome of hepatitis B virus: restriction enzyme cleavage and structure of DNA extracted from Dane particles. Proceedings of the National Academy of Sciences of the USA 72: 4597–4601

Szmuness W 1978 Hepatocellular carcinoma and the hepatitis B virus: evidence for a causal association. Progress in Medical Virology 24: 40–69

Tabor E 1989 Hepatocellular carcinoma: Possible etiologies in patients without serologic evidence of hepatitis B virus infection. Journal of Medical Virology 27: 1–6

Tabor E 1991 Strongly supported features of the association between hepatitis B virus and hepatocellular carcinoma. Advances in Applied Biotechnology Series 13: 107–118

Takada S, Koike K 1990 Trans-activation function of a 3' truncated X gene–cell fusion product from integrated hepatitis B virus DNA in chronic hepatitis tissues. Proceedings of the National Academy of Sciences of the USA 87: 5628–5632

Takase S, Takada N, Enomoto N, Yasuhara M, Takada A 1991 Different types of chronic hepatitis in alcoholic patients: does chronic hepatitis induced by alcohol exist? Hepatology 13: 876–881

Tanaka K, Hirohata S, Koga S et al 1991 Hepatitis C and hepatitis B in the etiology of hepatocellular carcinoma in the Japanese population. Cancer research 51: 2842–2847

Tanaka Y, Esumi M, Shikata T 1988 Frequent integration of hepatitis B virus DNA in noncancerous liver tissue from hepatocellular carcinoma patients. Journal of Medical Virology 26: 7–14

Teeter L D, Becker F F, Chisari F V, Li D, Kuo M T 1990 Overexpression of the multidrug resistance gene mdr3 in spontaneous and chemically induced mouse hepatocellular carcinomas. Molecular and Cellular Biology 10: 5728–5735

Terré S, Petit M A, Bréchot C 1991 Defective hepatitis B virus particles are generated by packaging and reverse transcription of spliced viral RNAs in vivo. Journal of Virology 65: 5539–5543

Thiers V, Nakajima E, Kremsdorf D et al 1988 Transmission of hepatitis B from hepatitis B negative subjects. Lancet ii: 1273–1276

Thiesen H J, Bosze Z, Henry L, Charnay P 1988 A DNA element responsible for the different tissue specificities of Friend and Moloney retroviral enhancers. Journal of Virology 62: 614–618

Tiollais P, Pourcel C, Dejean A 1985 The hepatitis B virus. Nature 317: 489–495

Toh H, Hyashida H, Miyata T 1983 Sequence homology between retroviral reverse transcriptase and putative polymerases of hepatitis B virus and cauliflower mosaic virus. Nature 305: 827–829

Tokino T, Fukushige S, Nakamura T et al 1987 Chromosomal translocation and inverted duplication associated with integrated hepatitis B virus in hepatocellular carcinomas. Journal of Virology 61: 3848–3854

Tran A, Kremsdorf D, Capel F, Housset C, Dauguet C, Petit M A, Bréchot C 1991 Emergence of and takeover by hepatitis B virus (HBV) with rearrangements in the pre-S/S and pre-C/C genes during chronic HBV infection. Journal of Virology 65: 3566–3574

Transy C, Fourel G, Robinson W S, Tiollais P, Marion P L, Buendia M A 1992 Frequent amplification of c-myc in ground squirrel liver tumors associated with past or ongoing infection with a hepadnavirus. Proceedings of the National Academy of Sciences of the USA 89: 3874–3878

Treinin M, Laub O 1987 Identification of a promoter element located upstream from the hepatitis B virus X gene. Molecular and Cellular Biology 7: 545–548

Trowbridge R, Fagan E A, Davison F, Eddleston A, Williams R, Linskens M, Farzaneh F 1988 Amplification of the c-myc gene locus in a human hepatic tumor containing integrated hepatitis B virus DNA. In: Zuckerman, A J (ed) Viral hepatitis and liver disease. Alan R. Liss, New York, pp 764–768

Tsuda H, Hirohashi S, Shimosato Y, Ino Y, Yoshida T, Terada 1989 Low incidence of point mutation of c-Ki-ras and N-ras oncogen in human hepatocellular carcinoma. Japanese Journal of Cancer Research 196–199

Tsuda H, Zhang W, Shimosato Y et al 1990 Allele loss on chromosome 16 associated with progression of human hepatocellular carcinoma. Proceedings of the National Academy of Sciences of the USA 87: 6791–6794

Twu J S, Schloemer R H 1987 Transcriptional trans-

activating function of hepatitis B virus. Journal of Virology 61: 3448–3453
Valenzuela P, Quiroga M, Zaldivar J, Gray J, Rutter W J 1980 The nucleotide sequence of the hepatitis B virus genome and the identification of the major viral genes. In: Fields B, Jaenisch R, Fox C F (eds) Animal virus genetics. Academic Press, New York, pp 57–70
Van Lohuizen M, Breuer M, Berns A 1989 N-myc is frequently activated by proviral insertion in MuLV-induced T-cell lymphomas. EMBO Journal 8: 133–136
Vitvitski-Trepo L, Kay A, Pichoud C et al 1990 Early and frequent detection of HBxAg and/or anti-HBxAg in hepatitis B virus infection. Hepatology 12: 1278–1283
Wain-Hobson S 1984 Molecular Biology of the hepadna viruses. In: Chisari F V (ed) Advances in hepatitis research. Masson Publishing, New York, pp 49–53
Walter E, Blum H, Meier P, Huonker M, Schmid M, Maier K, Offensperger W, Offensperger S, Gerok W 1988 Hepatocellular carcinoma in alcoholic liver disease: no evidence for a pathogenetic role of hepatitis B virus infection. Hepatology 8: 745–748
Wands J R, Fujita Y K, Isselbacher K J et al 1986 Identification and transmission of hepatitis B virus-related variants. Proceedings of the National Academy of Sciences of the USA 83: 6608–6612
Wang H P, Rogler C E 1991 Topoisomerase I-mediated integration of hepadnavirus DNA in vitro. Journal of Virology 65: 2381–2392
Wang J, Chenivesse X, Henglein B, Bréchot C 1990 Hepatitis B virus integration in a cyclin A gene in a human hepatocellular carcinoma. Nature 343: 555–557
Wang J, Zindy F, Chenivesse X, Lamas E, Henglein B, Bréchot C 1992 Modification of cyclin A expression by hepatitis B virus DNA integration in a hepatocellular carcinoma. Oncogene 7: 1653–1656
Wang W, London W T, Lega L, Feitelson M A 191 HBxAg in the liver from carrier patients with chronic hepatitis and cirrhosis. Hepatology 14: 29–37
Wei Y, Fourel G, Ponzetto A, Silvestro M, Tiollais P, Buendia M A 1922a Hepadnavirus integration: mechanisms of activation of the N-myc2 retrotransposon in woodchuck liver tumors. Journal of Virology 66: 5265–5276
Wei Y, Ponzetto A, Tiollais P, Buendia M A 1992b Multiple rearrangements and activated expression of c-myc induced by woodchuck hepatitis virus integration in a primary liver tumor. Research in Virology 143: 89–96
White Y S, Johnson P J, Davison F, Williams R 1990 Frequency of hepatic HBV-DNA in patients with cirrhosis and hepatocellular carcinoma: relation to serum HBV markers. British Journal of Cancer 61: 909–912
Will H, Salfeld J, Pfaff E, Manso C, Theilmann L, Schaller H 1986 Putative reverse transcriptase intermediates of human hepatitis B virus in primary liver carcinoma. Science 231: 594–596
Will H, Reiser W, Weimer T et al 1987 Replication strategy of human hepatitis B virus. Journal of Virology 61: 904–911
Wollersheim M, Debelka U, Hofschneider P H 1988 A transactivating function encoded in the hepatitis B virus X gene is conserved in the integrated state. Oncogene 3: 545–552
Wright J A, Smith H S, Watt F M, Hancock C, Hudson D L, Stark G R 1990 DNA amplification is rare in normal human cells. Proceedings of the National Academy of Sciences of the USA 87: 1791–1795
Wu J Y, Zhou Z Y, Judd A, Cartwright C A, Robinson W S 1990 The hepatitis B virus-encoded transcriptional trans-activator hbx appears to be a novel protein serine/threonine kinase. Cell 63: 687–695
Xiong Y, Eickbush T H 1990 Origin and evolution of retroelements based upon their reverse transcriptase sequences. EMBO Journal 9: 3353–3362
Yaginuma K, Kobayashi M, Yoshida E, Koike K 1985 Hepatitis B virus integration in hepatocellular carcinoma DNA: duplication of cellular flanking sequences at the integration site. Proceedings of the National Academy of Sciences of the USA 82: 4458–4462
Yaginuma K, Kobayashi H, Kobayashi M, Morishima T, Matsuyama K, Koike K 1987 Multiple integration site of hepatitis B virus DNA in hepatocellular carcinoma and chronic active hepatitis tissues from children. Journal of Virology 61: 1808–1813
Yee J K 1989 A liver-specific enhancer in the core promoter region of human hepatitis B virus. Science 246: 658–661
Yeh F S, Yu M C, Mo C C, Luo S, Tong M J, Henderson B E 1989 Hepatitis B virus, aflatoxins and hepatocellular carcinoma in southern Guangxi, China. Cancer Research 49: 2506–2509
Yoneyama T, Takeuchi K, Watanabe Y et al 1990 Detection of hepatitis C virus cDNA sequence by the polymerase chain reaction in hepatocellular carcinoma tissues. Japanese Journal of Medicine Science and Biology 43: 89–94
Zerial M, Salinas J, Filipski J, Bernardi G 1986 Genomic localization of hepatitis B virus in a human hepatoma cell line. Nucleic Acids Research 14: 8373–8385
Zhou Y Z, Butel J S, Li P J, Finegold M J, Melnick J L 1987 Integrated state of subgenomic fragments of hepatitis B virus DNA in hepatocellular carcinoma from mainland China. Journal of the National Cancer Institute 79: 223–231
Zhou Y Z, Slagle B L, Donehower L A, VanTuinen P, Ledbetter D H, Butel J S 1988 Structural analysis of a hepatitis B virus genome integrated into chromosome 17p of a human hepatocellular carcinoma. Journal of Virology 62: 4224–4231
Ziemer M, Garcia P, Shaul Y, Rutter W J 1985 Sequence of hepatitis B virus DNA incorporated into the genome of a human hepatoma cell line. Journal of Virology 53: 885–892

UPDATE

- HBV transactivator protein HBx is enigmatic in that it stimulates a striking variety of promoters which do not share a common *cis*-regulatory element. As it does not bind to DNA, it has been speculated that HBx acts indirectly through cellular pathways. Under certain conditions HBx can have an oncogenic potential, which may be relevant for HBV-associated liver carcinogenesis, but until now the mechanism for transactivation and cell transformation by HBx was unclear. HBx uses a complex signal transduction pathway for transactivation. An increase in the endogenous protein kinase C (PKC) activator sn-1, 2-diacylglycerol and the subsequent activation of PKC give rise to activation of the transcription factor AP-1 (Jun-Fos). As a result, HBx transactivates through binding sites for AP-1 and other PKC-dependent transcription factors (AP-2, NF-kappa B), thereby explaining the as-yet incomprehensible variety of HBx-inducible genes. As the PKC signal cascade also mediates cell transformation by tumour-promoting agents, the mechanism presented here might account for the oncogenic potential of HBx (Kekule et al 1993).
- REFERENCE

Kekule A S, Lauer U, Weiss L, Luber B, Hofschneider P H 1993 Hepatitis B virus transactivator HBx uses a tumour promoter signalling pathway. Nature 361, 6414: 742–745

9. Diagnosis

Richard H. Decker

When a patient presents with clinical symptoms that are characteristic of an acute infection and liver involvement, the physician looks for a history of risk factors of viral hepatitis and sends the patient's blood for laboratory analysis. If the results reveal that the patient has elevated levels of alanine aminotransferase (ALT), bilirubin and the presence of HBsAg, there is a strong probability that the physician's initial diagnosis of acute hepatitis was correct and that it is viral hepatitis B. However, diagnosis of other patients with hepatitis B may not be so straightforward. While the presence of serum HBsAg in acute disease is common, a few patients may have undetectable levels at the time they are tested. Some cases of acute or subacute hepatitis B remain undiagnosed and the outcome is uneventful. Still other patients may develop an unrecognized chronic, asymptomatic carrier state. The chance finding of HBsAg in such patients at a later time may confound the diagnosis of another acute disease. While the presence of HBsAg in serum remains the primary diagnostic and screening marker for hepatitis B, it is now possible to use several other serological tests in a work-up of patients suspected of hepatitis B in order to avoid errors and to resolve the complexities of the diagnostic staging in chronic hepatitis B. This chapter will review the markers and tests used in the serodiagnosis of acute and chronic hepatitis B.

ACUTE HEPATITIS

The sera of patients with acute hepatitis B may display an entire spectrum of antigens, antibodies and DNA related to the virus at one time or another. These markers are in dynamic change (Fig. 9.1) and the changes are a reflection of virus replication and the patient's immune responses, as will be discussed in more detail later. The serological patterns that can be defined by diagnostic tests help to assess accurately the stages of the acute illness and its progression to recovery or chronicity. In newly infected subjects there is an incubation period of 6–8 weeks from exposure to clinical symptoms, and the length of time depends upon the size of inoculum and host factors. In 10% of acute cases, patients will have a prodromal phase with flu-like symptoms (Perrillo 1992). HBsAg appearance accompanies this phase, and the symptoms of arthralgias and skin rash that sometimes appear are thought to be related to formation of HBsAg-anti-HBs complexes. All of this occurs prior to elevation of ALT and other manifestations of liver involvement. HBsAg concentrations peak at or shortly after an increase in serum ALT. The duration of HBsAg positivity can be highly variable and usually has little relationship to clinical recovery, but ALT and HBsAg decline and disappear together. HBsAg is cleared early in 10% of patients by the time they present to physicians (Gerlich et al 1980). Such a serological event can cause diagnostic problems, but in such cases the detection of IgM anti-HBc can help to confirm the diagnosis. Both IgM and IgG anti-HBc appear prior to symptoms. The presence of a strong IgM anti-HBc is indicative of acute-phase infection. IgG anti-HBc is eventually present in high titres in acute infections or in chronic disease, but it often persists in recovered patients for their lifetime at lower levels.

HBeAg and HBV DNA appear in sera of patients prior to symptoms and about the same

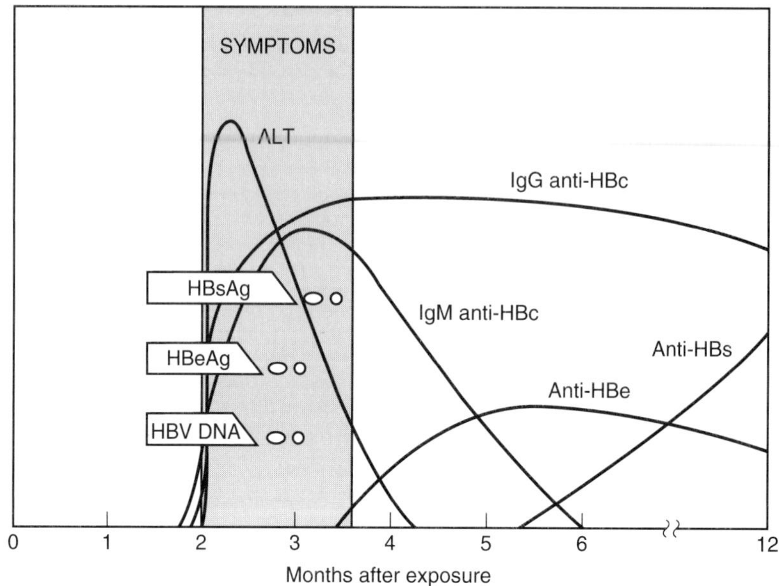

Fig. 9.1 Profile of serological markers of hepatitis B during the course of infection and convalescence.

time as HBsAg is detected. They are considered to be markers of viral replication. The disappearance of these markers and the seroconversion to anti-HBe precedes clearance of HBsAg, and such events predict recovery. The best indicator of recovery is the appearance of anti-HBs, but in many cases this is not detected before clinical recovery is already evident. Less than 1% of patients with acute hepatitis B develop fulminant hepatitis, but the majority of them will die. In such patients, the period of viraemia and antigenaemias is substantially shorter than usual, but IgM anti-HBc remains prominent. It has been observed that the few survivors of fulminant disease seldom if ever progress to chronic disease. This is consistent with the currently held belief that HBV is not cytopathic to the hepatocyte, but rather that it induces cellular and humoral immune reactions that cause the damage to liver (Eddleston 1988, Thomas 1991).

CHRONIC OUTCOMES OF HBV INFECTION

In most adult cases of acute hepatitis B, serum HBsAg disappears within 3–4 months after exposure, but in about 5% of patients antigenaemia will be detected for more than 6 months. A 6-month persistence of HBsAg by convention defines the carrier state because these patients have a reduced likelihood of recovery (Table 9.1). Most remain chronically infected and experience several possible outcomes, but every year about 1% of adult-onset carriers will spontaneously lose HBsAg and seroconvert to anti-HBs. In contrast, 90% of babies who have been infected perinatally or within the first 5 years of life become HBV carriers and have little chance of spontaneous recovery during their lifetime.

Table 9.1 Patterns of the principal HBV markers in acute and chronic hepatitis B

	Acute	Chronic
HBsAg	Positive, disappears	Positive, persists
IgM anti-HBc	Positive, high	Low or negative
Total anti-HBc	Positive	Positive
HBeAg/anti-HBe	Ag positive with seroconversion to Ab	HBeAg or anti-HBe
HBV DNA	Positive, disappears	High or low, persistent
Anti-HBs	Appears upon recovery	Usually negative

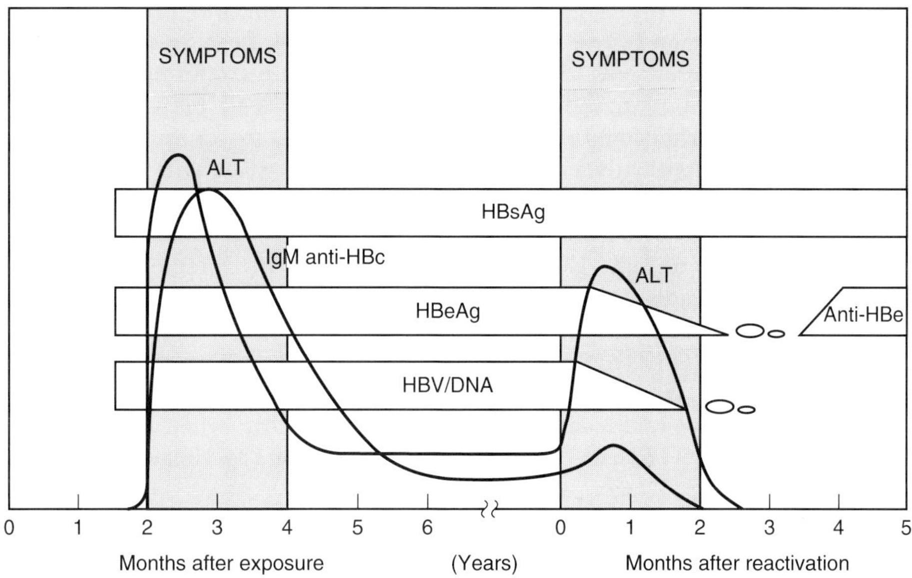

Fig. 9.2 Serological profile of hepatitis B markers in acute hepatitis B progressing to chronicity, followed years later by termination of the replicative phase.

The serological pattern of HBV markers in chronic hepatitis B is depicted in Figure 9.2. After the acute phase, the marker pattern becomes distinguished as a rather stable one; IgM anti-HBc declines slowly, but markers of viral replication – HBeAg and HBV DNA – remain detectable, with anti-HBe and anti-HBs usually undetectable. Elevated ALT values indicate ongoing active hepatitis. Some carriers will have persistently active hepatitis and will progress to cirrhosis and possibly hepatocellular carcinoma (Hoofnagle et al 1987), but the complexities of chronic HBV infection preclude simple prognosis, as discussed later. At unpredictable intervals after the acute phase, many patients become asymptomatic carriers. That is, while HBsAg and anti-HBc persist, ALT levels return to near normal and seroconversion from HBeAg to anti-HBe occurs. HBV DNA declines or is undetectable, but patients remain infectious. This transition from the active to asymptomatic chronic infection can occur directly after the acute phase or it may happen years later, often following a flare-up of symptoms and a brief increase in ALT levels. Occasionally asymptomatic carriers may also experience a return to active hepatitis and reappearance of HBeAg and HBV DNA.

A few chronic carriers have serum levels of HBsAg below detectable limits. While asymptomatic carriers appear to be in an inactive state of hepatitis they remain at significantly increased risk of cirrhosis and hepatocellular carcinoma.

SEROLOGICAL TESTS

HBsAg

The discovery of the Australia antigen and its association with hepatitis (Blumberg 1964, Sutnick et al 1968, Okochi & Murakami 1968, Prince 1968) was a major advance in the laboratory diagnosis of viral hepatitis. The Australia antigen, or hepatitis B surface antigen (HBsAg), could be detected in about two-thirds of patients with acute and chronic disease by simple assay procedures such as agar-gel diffusion (AGD) or counterimmunoelectrophoresis (Gerety et al 1978). It was subsequently found that most of the remaining one-third of patients with hepatitis B also have serum HBsAg but that tests with significantly greater sensitivity are necessary to detect it. In 1972 a modified radioimmunoassay (RIA), called a 'sandwich' RIA, was developed by Overby et al (1973) to detect HBsAg. This diagnostic test has a sensitivity 10 000 times that of AGD and can detect less than 0.5 ng HBsAg per ml of serum. Sandwich assays use anti-HBs that are bound to a plastic bead or microtitre well to capture HBsAg from the specimen and a second labelled anti-HBs reagent to identify the captured antigen. Sandwich assays have remained the methodologies of choice for detecting HBsAg because of their long history of high sensitivity and specificity. In the past decade, enzyme sandwich immunoassays (EIAs) have largely replaced RIAs; recent modified EIAs have employed microparticles (MEIAs) and computerized instrumentation to produce very rapid and completely automated MEIAs for HBsAg (Decker 1991, Eble et al 1991). Table 9.2 compares the features of RIA, EIA and MEIA methods for HBsAg. MEIAs have also been developed to detect the other hepatitis antigen and antibody markers described in this chapter, and their performance characteristics are similar to those for the HBsAg test. Despite the high performance of the current tests for HBsAg, transfusion-associated hepatitis B is still occasionally reported in the USA and elsewhere (Polesky & Hanson 1989, Hoofnagle 1990, Kojima et al 1991). This suggests that some subjects are infected with HBV but have concentrations of HBsAg below levels of detection.

Hepatitis B surface antigen is a non-infectious protein particle of about 22 nm in diameter that can be visualized by electron microscopy (Bayer et al 1968). It is a complexed particle with 100 copies of similar glycosylated protein molecules 27 kD in size, some with additional pre-S sequences of amino acids. The antigenicity of the 22-nm particle is significantly different from that of the 27 kD protein, because many of the epitopes of the particle are conformational. Electron micrographs of purified preparations reveal that the antigen exists in serum occasionally in tubular and complete virion structures, and from this it is proposed that the hepatic expression of the 22-nm particle is the manifestation of a defect in synthesis of the complete virion such that the number of particles is one million-fold more than the virus itself. In rare cases, the amount of HBsAg can reach 1 mg per ml of serum. Viraemia also is uncommonly high during acute and some chronic hepatitis, when the virion concentration is estimated at 10^5–10^8 per ml.

Anti-HBs

HBsAg elicits antibody responses that are directed primarily against conformational epitopes, and their appearance in serum represents a typical convalescent response in cases of self-limited infections. Antibodies are formed against several antigenic sites of HBsAg, and are all generally designated anti-HBs. Some of these are unique to specific viral strains, but all wild strains of HBV contain a common immunological determinant, *a*. Anti-HBs/*a* is the most prominent antibody in convalescent sera or in vaccinees. HBV strains are characterized by a set of subtype epitopes, *d* and *y*, which are mutually exclusive in a strain, and by a second set of epitopes, *w* and *r*, also exclusive of each other (LeBouvier 1971, Bancroft et al 1972, Soulier & Courouce-Pauty 1973). Thus, the most prominent strains of HBV are *adw*, *ayw*, *adr* and *ayr*. Anti-HBs is detected in

Table 9.2 Performance characteristics of three types of immunoassays for detecting HBsAg

	Radioimmunoassay (RIA)	Enzyme immunoassay (EIA)	Microparticle enzyme immunoassay (MEIA)
Signal readout	Radioactivity	Colour	Fluorescence
Sensitivity (ng HBsAg per ml)	<0.5	<0.5	<0.5
Time of assay	3 h	3 h	45 min
Reproducibility, coefficient of variation (%)	15	10–15	3–5
Dynamic range (ng/ml)	0.2–50	0.2–15	0.2–500
Automation	None	Semi-automated	Automated

most laboratories by another sandwich-type RIA, EIA or MEIA in which HBsAgs from mixtures of strains of HBV are affixed to a solid phase and also are labelled with enzyme or ^{125}I (Mimms et al 1989, Ostrow et al 1991). The two or more active arms of the antibody form the binding link between the solid-phase antigen and the labelled probe antigen. The specific antibodies that are detected would normally depend upon the antigens selected for reagents, but since the prominent antibody in serum of most patients is anti-HBs/*a* reagent antigen selection is less important than reagent purity and test conditions, which influence sensitivity and specificity.

In patients recovering from acute hepatitis B, seroconversion to anti-HBs occurs shortly after disappearance of HBsAg. There may be subjects who have an extended period between loss of antigenaemia and appearance of anti-HBs, and this period is referred to as the 'core window' (Hoofnagle et al 1973), that is a time when antibodies to hepatitis B core proteins are the only serological indicators of the HBV infection. This core window has been known to last for a few days to several months. In an HBV infection, humoral anti-HBs indicates lifelong immunity to reinfection by hepatitis B. In recipients of vaccines prepared from purified native or recombinant HBsAg, the immune response that results is not usually as strong as responses to infection, and vaccine-induced antibody titres do not persist as long but decline predictably after the final inoculations (Hilleman et al 1981). Nonetheless, the efficacy of these vaccines against infection proves that humoral anti-HBs and/or related immunocellular responses to these surface antigens provide a major protective mechanism.

An anti-HBs response is induced in most vaccinees, but the response is variable. Semi-quantitative values of anti-HBs have been determined in several ways with the detection assays, and values are usually expressed in millinternational units per ml (mIU/ml) for consistency. A certain percentage of responders will lose all detectable antibody after a few years, and these subjects can be predicted by their anti-HBs titres shortly after completing their vaccinations. In light of these losses of antibody activity after vaccination, some consider it prudent to revaccinate low antibody-positive subjects after 5 years, even though we do not yet know if there is direct correlation between the level of detectable anti-HBs and protective immunity.

There are no accepted differences in virulence between the strains of HBV, but the strains induce antibodies to their subtype antigens that are sometimes detected. These type-specific antibodies probably offer immune protection, but only against the strain to which they are directed. It is known that some HBsAg carriers are simultaneously positive for anti-HBs and that the coexisting antibodies are usually directed at epitopes of a strain of HBV other than the one that is infecting the patient (Koziol et al 1976, LeBouvier et al 1976, Tabor et al 1977, Courouce-Pauty et al 1979). The origin of these antibodies is unknown, but their presence is believed by some to correlate with the degree of viral replication.

Anti-Pre-S

Pre-S proteins are polypeptides that are frequently associated with HBsAg in that they are attached to some of the 27-kD basic proteins that make up the 22-nm HBsAg particle (Neurath et al 1984, Wong et al 1985). A pre-S2 peptide of 55 amino acids is attached proximal to the 5' end; another 108–119 amino acid peptide, pre-S1, may also be attached at the 5' end of pre-S2. Extensive biological study has been devoted to the association of these regions as specific receptors for the hepatocyte and to its relationship with polymerized human serum albumin (pHSA). Antibodies directed against pre-S2, pre-S1, and pHSA occur early in infection, but expectations that detection of these antibodies would provide new diagnostic information in managing the patient remain unmet. Also, it is clear that anti-pre-S antibodies are not essential for immune protection, because neither the native nor recombinant HBsAg vaccine contains these peptides. Studies continue to determine if antibodies to pre-S can supplement the immune protective efficacy of the vaccines. We also must be assured that these additions to the vaccines will not also induce an adverse autoimmune reaction, possibly because of their relationship to host antigens (Hellstrom & Sylvan 1986). To date, licensed commercial tests for anti-pre-S antibodies are not available for such studies.

Anti-HBc

The viral core of HBV is composed of nucleic acid, DNA polymerase and an antigenic nucleoprotein. The core is synthesized in relatively few hepatocytes within the infected liver and is assembled in the nucleus of the hepatocyte to form a structure that is 27 nm in diameter. The core is subsequently encapsulated with a shell of HBsAg to make the virion. Hepatitis B core antigen (HBcAg) is not directly detectable in serum because of the encapsulating HBsAg and because any exposed HBcAg would react with circulating antibody, thus blocking its detection. However, HBcAg can be identified by immunofluorescent techniques in liver biopsy specimens, and the histochemical detection of this antigen is often used as a marker of viral replication. HBcAg can be isolated for serological assay procedures from virions, 'Dane particles' (Dane et al 1970), biochemically purified from serum and from which HBsAg has been chemically removed. Most tests now employ recombinant antigens. The conventional commercial anti-HBc immunoassays in use are based on the principle of competition of the test antibody and a standardized probe anti-HBc labelled with enzyme or ^{125}I for HBcAg, which is bound to a solid phase (Overby & Ling 1976). If a serum specimen is negative for anti-HBc, the labelled probe will bind to the solid phase and an elevated signal will be produced (high c.p.m. or colour), whereas an antibody-positive specimen blocks the signal. In these tests cut-off values are selected to differentiate between positive and negative values. A value that is about half-way between the negative control and a positive specimen producing complete blocking is most frequently selected for a cut-off. Anti-HBc is perhaps the most serologically prominent marker of HBV exposure. The antigen is very immunogenic, and as a result anti-HBc titres are somewhat proportional to viral replication and are induced early during active infection. The antibody appears after the appearance of HBsAg but often before ALT elevations, and it persists in serum throughout disease and recovery (Hoofnagle et al 1973). It may persist in recovered patients even after anti-HBs is no longer detectable. The titres of anti-HBc vary considerably among subjects, and subjects with a history of infection and recovery years earlier generally have much lower activity than do patients with an ongoing chronic infection. The earliest anti-HBc in acute disease is predominantly IgM class antibody (Fig. 9.1), though lower titres of IgG and IgA class anti-HBc are present concurrently. The titre and percentage of IgG anti-HBc continue to rise during early convalescence. There is little evidence, however, that anti-HBc offers any immune protection.

Because of its persistence, anti-HBc is used as an epidemiological marker. In some countries anti-HBc testing is used as a surrogate test of donor blood in order to identify units that are of increased risk of transmitting non-A, non-B hepatitis (NANBH), AIDS and cryptic HBV. In the USA, where the efficacy of such surrogate testing has been studied extensively, the relationship between NANBH and AIDS is attributed to the occurrence of common risk factors for acquiring HBV and for NANBH and HIV. Before the discovery of HCV and the development of a screening test for it, anti-HBc screening of donor blood was estimated to be able to reduce the incidence of post-transfusion NANBH in the USA by up to 40% (Stevens et al 1984, Koziol et al 1986). About 50% of HIV-positive subjects are also anti-HBc positive (Jullien et al 1988, Dodd et al 1991), and it is presumed that they were positive for anti-HBc prior to their infection with HIV. By this reasoning, anti-HBc screening would detect about half of pre-seroconverters of HIV-infected donors. Anti-HBc has a more direct role in HBV detection. Despite the use of highly sensitive tests for HBsAg, transfusion-associated hepatitis B remains a problem in some regions. Studies show that cryptic HBV infections exist in subjects whose only marker of HBV is a high titre of anti-HBc (Hoofnagle et al 1978, Katchaki et al 1978, Lander et al 1978, Lai et al 1989). USA blood banks implemented donor screening for anti-HBc and ALT in 1986, and the subsequent marked decline in reported cases of post-transfusion HBV has been attributed to this testing. The US

Food and Drug Administration (FDA) recently announced its intention to licence the anti-HBc test for donor screening specifically to reduce the incidence of post-transfusion HBV (Dodd et al 1991).

IgM anti-HBc

IgM anti-HBc testing has been applied for the differential diagnosis of acute disease. Methods for detecting class-specific antibody are based on a different test principle than described above (Gerlich et al 1980, Chau et al 1983). The tests employ an IgM capture technique wherein a portion of the serum specimen IgM is captured by antibodies that are attached to a solid phase and are directed against human IgM. The captured IgM antibodies are then sequentially exposed in incubations with HBcAg particles and with labelled anti-HBc. The method is inherently very sensitive, but many commercial companies with tests of this type have intentionally reduced its sensitivity in order to make it capable of distinguishing acute from chronic disease. Without this desensitization IgM anti-HBc would be detectable in some patients for years after their acute infection. One method of desensitization is by elevating the cut-off to a point at which specimen values are positive in most patients for 3–6 months after acute disease. Specimens that give values that are negative but not within the normal range can still be recognized (Gerlich et al 1986, Eble et al 1991), and in some cases of chronic hepatitis B patients have persistently elevated negatives.

In the core window of the acute stage, i.e. between the loss of serum HBsAg and appearance of anti-HBs, IgM anti-HBc can have particular diagnostic utility, especially if the patient experiences an early clearance of HBsAg prior to serological testing for the illness. It has been estimated that as many as 10% of acute hepatitis B infections would have been inapparent if HBsAg were the only seromarker tested for in acute disease (Gerlich et al 1980, Gitnick 1983).

With rare exceptions, a negative test result for anti-HBc IgM excludes a diagnosis of acute hepatitis B. Patients who are chronic HBsAg carriers but who also have underlying HDV or HCV acute infections can thus be distinguished from patients whose acute infection is caused by HBV.

HBeAg/Anti-HBe

HBeAg is a non-structural protein of HBV (Magnius & Espmark 1972). The antigen has amino acid sequences that are essentially identical to a protein that goes to make the HBcAg particle; HBeAg is a smaller protein (16 kD) than HBcAg and it exists in a monomeric form, whereas HBcAg proteins are part of a multimeric 27-nm particle with conformational antigenic sites. The specific function of HBeAg or its relationship to pathogenesis of liver disease is unknown.

HBeAg in serum can be detected by a sandwich immunoassay format similar to that for HBsAg. The antigen is captured by antibody affixed to a solid phase and is then detected with a second labelled antibody (Mushahwar & Overby 1981). The signal produced is directly proportional to the amount of HBeAg in the specimen. An indirect assay procedure is used to detect anti-HBe, using the same kit reagent provided for HBeAg; however, for anti-HBe detection, the unknown sample is mixed with an equal volume of standardized HBeAg-positive serum of predetermined quantity, and the mixture is incubated with the solid-phase antibody. The amount of HBeAg that binds to the solid phase is detected with the second labelled antibody. In this test, a significant reduction in the expected signal indicates the presence of anti-HBe in the test specimen. Serum concentrations of HBeAg and anti-HBe are typically low, and, unlike anti-HBc or anti-HBs, when a patient develops anti-HBe in recovery the antibody will probably be gone in a few months to a year.

HBeAg has been used as a marker of viral replication and an index that correlates with infectiousness of the patient and severity of the disease. Patients presenting with acute disease generally have strong reactivity for HBeAg at the time of maximum ALT, and it has been shown that HBeAg can be first detected at about the time HBsAg begins to be detected in serum (Mushahwar et al 1978). Reactivity declines as the acute phase runs its course, and it becomes undetectable before HBsAg is cleared. The seroconversion to anti-HBe may actually precede loss of HBeAg, but usually there is a small lag time between the two markers. As with HBsAg, persistence of HBeAg has been found to imply progression to chronicity; the persistence of HBeAg for more than 12 weeks indicates chronicity, whereas early seroconversion to anti-HBe signals recovery. In chronic hepatitis B HBeAg usually parallels other indicators of viral replication, such as HBV DNA. Its association with infectiousness has been demonstrated in studies of vertical transmission: perinatal infections are much more likely in babies born to HBeAg-positive carrier mothers than in babies born to anti-HBe-positive carrier mothers (Okada et al 1976, Beasley et al 1977).

The diagnostic interpretation of the patterns of HBeAg and anti-HBe in acute and chronic hepatitis B has recently undergone a significant re-evaluation as a result of the identification of HBV mutants. Some patients with active replication and severe infections do not produce serum HBeAg: quantitative hybridization analyses of HBV DNA had demonstrated that individuals with anti-HBe may in fact have very high amounts of HBV DNA in blood (Kuhns et al 1988). Subsequently, it was discovered that these subjects had a variant of HBV, in which the DNA had a single change of one base pair at position 1896 in the pre-core region (Carman et al 1990), just upstream of the HBcAg initiation site, and this change converted the triplet codon at that site into a 'stop' codon. Therefore, the synthesis of the precursor of HBeAg – and hence the production of HBeAg – does not occur. However, synthesis of HBcAg and the complete and infectious virion is unimpaired. Reports have also suggested that the HBV mutants cause the severe hepatitis and the frequent occurrence of fulminant disease (Carman et al 1991, Omata et al 1991). If this is the case, it will have to be reconciled with the premise that HBV, mutated or not, is a non-cytopathic virus (Eddleston 1988, Thomas 1991). In fact, many patients with this mutant form of HBV have mild disease, and other patients with HBV mutants who develop fulminant disease, do so only late in their illness (Shafritz 1991). Also characteristic of fulminant disease, whether caused by wild-type or mutant HBV, is the lack of significant amounts of virus in the patient's serum.

The HBV mutant story and consequently the proper interpretation of HBeAg and anti-HBe patterns remain to be clarified. There are no specific direct and easy analyses for them, and nucleic acid sequencing in research facilities provides the only reliable detection tool. However, accurate measures of viral replication such as HBV DNA coupled with the HBeAg – anti-HBe profile provide indirect serological evidence for a mutant. These mutants appear to be more common in the Mediterranean countries and the Far East than in Northern Europe and the USA (Seeff 1988).

In summary, there are four patterns of HBeAg – anti HBe: (a) persistent HBeAg with chronic active hepatitis B; (b) persistent HBeAg but without evidence of liver disease; (c) loss of HBeAg and seroconversion to anti-HBe accompanied by cessation of active liver disease; and (d) anti-HBe and chronic liver disease.

HBV DNA

Viral nucleic acid values in serum now form an important part of the serological profile of viral infections. They are the most direct measure of hepatitis B virus and its replication to date, and molecular hybridization with DNA probes is the most specific of the new tools of molecular biology. These methods are several orders of magnitude more sensitive than the best immunoassays, and amplification methods such as the polymerase chain reaction (PCR) increase sensitivity many fold more, down to several molecules. However, for DNA probe tests to be comparable in terms of detectability and diagnostic utility to antigen or antibody tests, a significant increase in sensitivity is essential, because HBV DNA concentration in serum is much less than the concentrations of antigens and antibodies.

HBV contains a circular and partially double-stranded DNA of 3200 bp within the nucleocapsid (Gerber & Thung 1985). The capsid also contains viral DNA polymerase, which is capable of filling in the single-stranded portion of the

DNA. HBV DNA in serum is primarily encapsulated within the virion, and the amount of serum DNA is believed to be directly related to the rate of replication within liver cells. DNA polymerase measurements have also been used as an indirect measure of virus replication and, though the correlation with HBV DNA is very close, methods of polymerase measurement are complex. Furthermore, the sensitivity and detectability of DNA polymerase are affected by sample storage and handling, while HBV DNA is more stable. The utility of HBV DNA in diagnostic evaluations has been limited by the practicality of the procedures. Most clinical research studies have relief upon research laboratories to perform determinations with their techniques, and interlaboratory comparisons of quantitative data at best are difficult. The principle of direct molecular hybridization is to prepare a radiolabelled segment of HBV DNA and use it to hybridize with the complementary DNA sequences of HBV in the test specimen (Bonino et al 1981, Scotto et al 1983). The virions in the serum specimen are extracted and solubilized with solvents to release DNA, and the nucleic acid is placed on a nitrocellulose membrane filter, to which it will adhere. The membrane with the DNA is exposed to the radiolabelled DNA probe. After a suitable time the excess probe is thoroughly washed away, and the membrane is exposed to X-ray-sensitive film for autoradiography, typically for 3–5 days. When the film is developed, the intensity of the darkened spots on the film can be estimated visually or with densitometry by comparison with standards. Many performance characteristics of the procedures depend on the quality of the probes. They are usually produced by molecular cloning or by chemical synthesis. The cloned probes are several hundred to a thousand nucleotides in length and usually possess considerably higher sensitivity and specificity than the smaller (20–40 nucleotide) synthetic oligomers. The probe preparation and test methodology appear to be similar in many laboratories, but despite this the detectability limits for five published HBV DNA procedures varied 1000-fold (Overby 1985). Some commercial hybridization procedures employing solution hybridization techniques have recently become available (Kuhns et al 1988, 1989). They offer several ease-of-use features and provide for interlaboratory consistency. The detectability of a method developed in our laboratory is similar to the membrane-type procedures while providing for high interlaboratory reproducibility. It is a three-step procedure including: solubilization of the virion to release HBV DNA; hybridization in solution with ^{125}I-labelled, cloned DNA probe; and separation of reaction product from unreacted probe by gel filtration in small disposable columns. The void volume eluate from the column is counted in a gamma scintillation counter, and DNA is quantified by comparing values with a standardized DNA-positive control. Detectability has been estimated to be 0.15 pg per test or 4×10^5 genomes per ml, and test values are linear between 0.15 and 200 pg, or three orders of magnitude.

Serum HBV DNA has been detected in patients prior to the onset of their acute hepatitis B and before ALT elevations have developed (Moestrup et al 1985). Levels decline rapidly at or near maximum elevation of ALT and seroconversion to anti-HBe. This is similar to HBV DNA and ALT changes that occur in chronic patients treated with alpha interferon (IFN-α). It is also consistent with the observations of marked loss of HBV DNA in patients with fulminant hepatitis B (Trepo et al 1976, Brechot et al 1984), and implies that immune factors damage the liver while clearing the virus. At present, HBV DNA values have had little application in managing patients with acute infection because the antigen and antibody profiles provide sufficient diagnostic and prognostic information. However, HBV DNA can be a useful tool for evaluating patients in the chronic stages or in patients with unusual conditions in acute infection. The quantity of HBV DNA in a patient's serum has been used, in part, to define a 'replicative' or 'non-replicative' state (Hoofnagle et al 1987, Schalm et al 1990). Patients in the replicative state are characterized by high levels of HBV DNA, DNA polymerase and ALT, and usually HBe antigenaemia, while in patients with a non-replicative state HBV DNA and DNA polymerase are not detectable by unamplified tests, ALT values are normal and HBeAg is negative. In the latter patients liver HBV DNA may be found in biopsy specimens as DNA that is integrated into the liver cell genome. Normal ALT values also indicate histological remission and may signify that the patient is approaching seroconversion from HBsAg to anti-HBs.

DNA is a strong predictor of HBV transmissibility. Tassapoulis et al (1987) recently showed that HBV DNA-positive carriers are more than five times more likely to transmit infection to their heterosexual partners than DNA-negative carriers. These data are similar to reports showing that HBeAg-positive carriers are more likely to infect their sexual partners or, in the case of HBeAg-positive mothers, their infants, and it is expected that HBV DNA presence and HBeAg positivity should correlate well. Seeff (1988) combined all available data from three studies from Europe, Africa, the Middle East, the Far East, Australia and the USA. Of 1171 HBeAg-positive carriers, 87% were HBV DNA positive, while of 1362 anti-HBe-positive carriers, only 20% were HBV DNA positive. On close scrutiny of the data, it appeared that the anti-HBe positives who were also HBV DNA positive were more likely to come from the Mediterranean area and the Far East than from northern Europe and the USA. These are the regions from which precore HBV mutants are more commonly reported. Since the mutants in these patients are not making HBeAg, this is to be expected.

One should be cautious not to extend quantitative interpretations too far. The two phases, replicative and non-replicative chronic hepatitis B, tend to overlap when two markers of replication are used to define them (Berris et al 1987). Kuhns et al (1988) evaluated the relationship between HBV DNA and HBeAg or anti-HBe among US and French carriers and found that most HBeAg-positive carriers had more HBV DNA than anti-HBe-positive carriers; however, among a subgroup of anti-HBe carriers who had HBV DNA detectable by hybridization, 8% had DNA levels indistinguishable from 65% of the HBeAg carriers.

HISTOLOGICAL CLASSIFICATION OF CHRONIC HEPATITIS

Some patients with chronic hepatitis B will recover spontaneously, while others will develop a severe and progressive liver disease. Still others will develop a silent disease that may or may not progress slowly. Efforts to classify the chronic carrier according to his current stage and to his prognosis have been the subject of decades of study, and because of the availability of new therapeutic options a better classification which predicts prognosis remains a priority.

Most hepatologists recognize that the use of symptoms in staging patients with chronic hepatitis is unreliable. The majority of patients are asymptomatic, and the presence or absence of symptoms fails to differentiate mild and progressive disease until patients are in advanced stages (Hoofnagle et al 1987). The accepted standard of current classification is the histological interpretation of a liver biopsy specimen. The examination of tissue sections of the healthy carrier reveals minimal evidence of cellular damage, sometimes 'ground-glass' hepatocytes (Hadziyannis et al 1973), while the tissues of patients with chronic active hepatitis (CAH) reveal extensive destruction, piecemeal necrosis, usually accompanied by infiltration of mononuclear cells, with and without cirrhosis (Bianchi et al 1983). Patients with less severe disease have minimal hepatocyte necrosis and the inflammatory infiltrate is limited to the portal tracts. This condition is classified as chronic persistent hepatitis (CPH). Histological classification has limitations, and these limitations have become more prominent with the emergence of therapeutic opportunities. Biopsies are, after all, unpopular with patients, especially if they have no symptoms. The interpretations of the stages may be clear in biopsies of some patients, but CAH and CPH are two ends of a spectrum of inflammatory reaction, and CPH may progress to CAH. Progressive changes are not easily predicted based on a specimen taken at a single time. CPH can be a misleading concept in that it implies that there are no changes occurring, and it is therefore not a serious condition. Improvements in classification or perhaps new classifications are being sought; in fact, many hepatologists have altered their classification of patients to reflect the stage of HBV replication as well as liver damage.

The information provided by classification aids in decisions regarding therapeutic options and in monitoring therapy responses. If the ultimate goal of therapy is to eradicate the virus and to eliminate inflammatory and fibrotic processes in the liver, criteria for the stages of chronic hepatitis B should include both quantitative information on the rate of virus replication, and information on parameters that assess liver inflammation and fibrosis.

The markers of HBV replication which are the best indices of viral load in the liver are the patient's serum HBV DNA levels, the presence of HBeAg and HBsAg in serum, and the presence of HBcAg in the hepatocyte itself. Many studies show that liver HBcAg has the best correlation with active liver disease of all viral markers (Seeff 1988), but since serum HBV DNA is universally associated with liver HBcAg it provides a more accessible marker. Of most practical use are quantitative serum HBV DNA values. Until recently the replicative state of chronic hepatitis B was defined serologically according to the presence of detectable HBV DNA and of HBeAg, while the non-replicative state was identified when HBV DNA was not detected and anti-HBe was present instead of HBeAg.

The degree of viral replication depends on a quantitative assessment of HBV DNA and to a lesser extent on HBe antigen. The first efforts to use viral replication in disease classification relied on data generated with non-amplified blot or solution hybridization methods, having sensitivities of about 10^5 copies of HBV DNA per ml, and which were relatively easy to quantify. Classification was based on DNA levels within the detectable range of the methods. Chronically infected patients with undetectable HBV DNA generally have less liver damage than those with high levels. However, newer amplification methods such as the polymerase chain reaction (PCR) (Kaneko et al 1989) have sensitivities of such great magnitudes that they can detect HBV DNA in nearly all patients who are silent carriers and who have minimal liver disease, but at present the amplification methods are poorly quantifiable. Because of the relatively high levels of HBV DNA in most patients who are candidates for IFN therapy, it seems that PCR will supplement conventional hybridization methods by verifying the completeness of viral clearance after therapy or recovery. For amplification methods to achieve their full potential as a diagnostic tool they will need significant improvements in quantification, specificity and ease of use.

Another observation that needs to be considered in a serological classification of chronic hepatitis is the occasional discordance between HBV DNA levels and HBeAg. Some of these discordances probably result from pre-core HBV mutants. This possibility is included in the classifying categories proposed in Table 9.3.

There is good evidence that hepatitis B virus of itself is not directly cytopathic. Periods of viraemia (with high HBV DNA) occur in subjects prior to acute symptoms and also in chronic carriers but in either case without evidence of liver damage. There are abundant other data suggesting that the hepatitis results from host-induced immune destruction of liver-infected hepatocytes (Schalm et al 1990, Thomas 1991) and the onset of hepatocyte destruction coincides with the appearance of immunological reactivity to HBV.

Liver inflammation and associated hepatocyte destruction are usually assessed by alanine aminotransferase (ALT), aspartate aminotransferase (AST) or similar hepatocyte-associated enzymes. While not specific for liver damage, these enzymes are the diagnostic hallmark for acute liver inflammation. ALT, the most widely used enzyme, is less reliable in chronic disease, mainly because of its lack of sensitivity. There is not clear acceptance as to what is an abnormal elevation of ALT, but, even so, chronic patients have periods of normal ALT followed by periods of marked elevations (Davis et al 1984, Perrillo et al 1984), or other irregular fluctuations. Despite such limitations, these enzymes are the best indicators of inflammation and abnormal liver pathology that we have available.

Table 9.3 defines the seven most common patterns of replication and inflammation and their relation to a state of active disease that would be expected histologically. Some patterns differ only quantitatively with regard to HBV DNA or ALT elevation, but these patterns are especially relevant to predicting response to IFN

Table 9.3 Seven frequent patterns of markers of replication and inflammation in chronic hepatitis B and their relation to active disease

	I	II	III	IV	V	VI	VII
HBV DNA (pg)	>200	>200	<100	Und	Und	>200	<100
HBeAg	++	++	++	–	–	–	–
Anti-HBe	–	–	–	+	+	+	+
ALT	+++	+/0	+++	++	0	+++	+++
Disease state	Active CAH	Mild CPH	Active or reactive CPH–CAH	Reactive or recovered (CPH)	Inactive CPH	Active CAH	Active CPH–CAH
Predicted response to IFN	Poor	Weak	Good	Good	–	Poor	Good
Other note						(? emergence of mutant)	

Und, undetected.

(see below). The first three patterns are characterized by the presence of HBeAg and HBV DNA, but are distinguished from one another by either different levels of ALT or different ranges of HBV DNA. The last four patterns are those in patients without HBeAg, and some have no HBV DNA detectable by hybridization, or else their ALT and HBV DNA levels differ. Pattern V is the most common in patients with anti-HBe, but patterns VI and VII are more frequently seen in patients from geographical regions where precore mutants occur. Histological studies that have examined the hepatocellular damage relative to these serological patterns indicate a unified picture of replicative serum HBV DNA, ALT and particularly cytoplasmic HBcAg where immunoperoxidase methods have been used to measure this in the nucleus and cytoplasm.

HBV SEROLOGY DURING THERAPY FOR CHRONIC HEPATITIS B

Recombinant interferons have significant but variable efficacy in the treatment of chronic hepatitis B. In the most detailed reports, 40–50% of patients treated for 4 months experienced HBeAg seroconversion, and one-third lost HBsAg (Perrillo et al 1990). Because IFN acts in part through its influence on the immune system, some trials have used corticosteroids with IFN in attempts to modulate the immune reaction, thereby increasing efficacy (Perrillo et al 1988). It is also clear that the probability of successful therapy depends on the criteria of selection of patients for IFN treatment. For instance, patients who acquired their HBV infection as children are poor responders, as are male homosexuals and patients with several other underlying factors (Table 9.4). Serum markers of viral replication have been used in research evaluations of the response to IFN, and levels of these markers prior to treatment have also been found to predict who will be responders.

Figure 9.3 depicts a serological profile of the changes in markers of viral replication and inflammation in a chronic B responder who has been treated with prednisone for 6 weeks, followed by steroid withdrawal prior to IFN treatent for 12 weeks (Kuhns et al 1989, Perrillo 1991). During prednisone treatment, ALT values decline but HBV DNA values increase. This increase in DNA is modest but does not occur in non-responders. When prednisone is terminated there follows a rebound in ALT values that is more prominent in responders than non-responders; HBV DNA

Table 9.4 Factors influencing response to IFN

Favourable	Unfavourable
HBV DNA <100 pg/ml	>200 pg/ml
Adult-acquired HBV	Acquired perinatally
Elevated ALT	Normal ALT
No underlying HIV, HDV, HCV, other disease	Underlying HIV, HDV, HCV
HBeAg	Anti-HBe
Female	Male, homosexual
(IgM HBc)	Significant decompensated cirrhosis

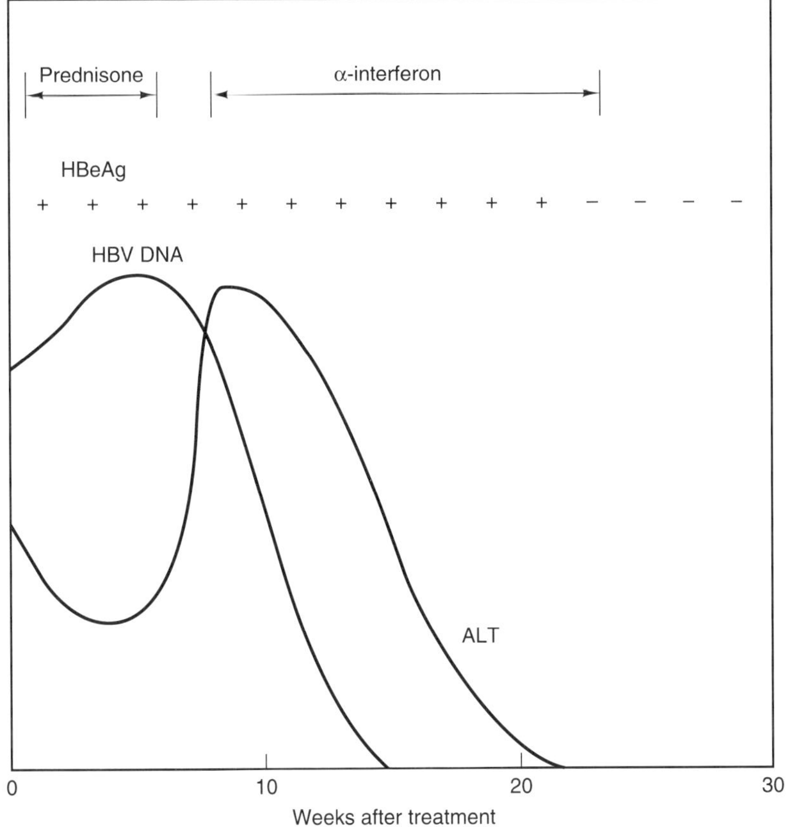

Fig. 9.3 Serological profile of changes in HBV markers of viral replication and inflammation in a patient responding to treatment with prednisone and alpha interferon (Kuhns et al 1989).

values usually start to drop in responder patients even before administration of IFN, with an average 60% decline, but non-responders experience no such drop. When IFN is administered, HBV DNA in responders becomes undetectable by hybridization tests within several weeks, and HBeAg seroconversion occurs about 12 weeks later. Non-responders on the other hand seldom lose HBV DNA, though there may be a transient decline in quantitative values, and they will have no HBeAg seroconversion. Some patients do not have HBeAg as a replicative marker to be used to monitor progress. The only useful markers for this would be HBV DNA and ALT. Table 9.3 indicates the likelihood of response to IFN of chronic B patients with the seven patterns described before. The single most predictive replicating marker of response is an HBV DNA value of less than 100 pg/ml. Patients with viral DNA less than 100 pg/ml and with elevated ALT values have an excellent probability of a favourable response to IFN, but patients with HBV DNA greater than 200 pg/ml have been reported to fare no better with IFN than the untreated control patients (Perrillo et al 1990).

The end point of successful therapy is the cessation of inflammation, absence of HBV DNA and seroconversions of HBeAg and HBsAg with appearance of anti-HBs. Some patients meet all of these criteria, but most do not. Patients who remain negative for HBV DNA and in whom no nucleic acid is detected by PCR are likely to have a good prognosis regardless of lack of changes in other HBV markers. Likewise, patients with normal ALT values but with markers of active viral replication statistically are poor responders.

They are subjects who, for some reason, have an inherently weak immune defence against HBV so that IFN can do little to modulate it.

The presumed consequence of predicting who are responders is that the clinician will treat some chronic hepatitis B patients with IFN and not others. In practice, this may be hard to do. It is eventually desirable to treat all patients, particularly those with concurrent infections of HIV and hepatitis D virus (HDV), but also those with asymptomatic non-progressive disease, because they appear to be at an increased risk of cirrhosis, HCC or of superinfection with HDV. Unfortunately, the interferons do not have the degree of efficacy to do this. Nor are the long-term benefits of IFN therapy known. It is important to document if the termination of replication and inflammation have indeed eliminated the risk of cirrhosis and HCC and infectivity. In this regard, other serological markers of fibrosis and immunity may eventually provide important information.

CONCURRENT INFECTION WITH OTHER HEPATIC VIRUSES

Patients with chronic hepatitis B may develop second viral infections, and these other infections often have a noticeable influence on the serological patterns of HBV. Superinfections with hepatitis A have been well documented, and there is a relatively high frequency of simultaneous or superimposed infections with HDV non-A, non-B hepatitis and HIV. These co-infections would be expected considering the similar epidemiologies of the agents. The other hepatitis agents generally induce a viral interference with HBV, resulting in 10-fold reductions in serum HBV DNA and DNA polymerase (Bradley et al 1983, Brotman et al 1983, Harrison et al 1983). The interference of HBV replication by NANBH is also reflected in a modest reduction in serum HBsAg, but studies of patients with concurrent infections with HDV indicate the possibility that diagnosis of hepatitis B could be missed because of low levels of HBsAg (DeCock et al 1985, Krosgaard et al 1987a, Carreda et al 1988). Acute hepatitis A in chronic hepatitis B patients also results in a transient interference of HBV replication (Viola et al 1982). On the other hand, infection with HIV appears to promote replication of HBV in chronic B patients, and HIV-infected subjects who develop acute hepatitis B may experience an extended period of the acute disease (Krogsgaard et al 1987b). These phenomena are undoubtedly caused by the immunocompromised state induced by HIV; HIV patients with chronic hepatitis B also have diminished inflammatory liver processes (Seeff et al 1991). Some HIV-positive patients can have very high levels of HBV DNA (Bhat et al 1990, Vyas & Ulrich 1991) and occasionally have low titres of circulating anti-HBc (Moller et al 1989).

OTHER MARKERS OF POSSIBLE USE IN CHRONIC HEPATITIS B

IgM anti-HBc

This antibody is very prominent in acute hepatitis B, but it also persists at low levels in chronic hepatitis. Most diagnostic tests are intentionally desensitized so that specimens with these lower levels give signals below the cut-off of the test. Often the low signals can be recognized as above the range of the negative population. Opinions differ widely regarding the significance and utility of these observations. Some investigators believe that low titres of IgM anti-HBc are evidence of active HBc replication and of disease severity (Sjögren & Hoofnagle 1985, Gerlich et al 1986, Bonino 1991). Recent studies have suggested that signals between 0.2 and 2.0 times the cut-off of one test could be used as an aid to monitor therapy in patients on IFN and that this was particularly helpful in patients with HBeAg negativity (Brunetto et al 1989, Bonino 1991). Smith et al (1992) found a significant correlation between IgM anti-HBc and intrahepatic expression of cytoplasmic HBcAg, but IgM anti-HBc lacked a strong correlation with the histology of various disease categories. Also, in this study, the change in IgM was only weakly related to the response to IFN.

Collagen antigens

Obvious cirrhosis appears as a late stage of liver injury associated with chronic active hepatitis B;

cirrhosis only becomes evident after an extended period of aberrant collagen metabolism. Collagen synthesis (fibrogenesis and fibrolysis) is not a process limited to the liver; however, abnormal levels of serum collagen metabolites in the context of chronic liver disease are likely to be liver related. Efforts to find serum indicators of hepatic fibrosis have led to the identification of several collagen antigens that are diagnostic candidates. Type III collagen is found at low levels in normal liver, while total collagen content in cirrhotic liver may be increased to over 10 times these levels (Schuppan et al 1986, Hayesaka et al 1990). A heterogeneous propeptide from the amino-terminal end of collagen III, PIIINP, has been detected at high concentrations in sera of patients with chronic active hepatitis (McCoullough et al 1987), and persistent elevations are claimed to be superior to ALT in differentiating CAH from CPH while predicting the development of fibrogenic liver disease (Schuppan 1991). Type IV collagen is the main component of all basement membranes. The amino- and carboxy-terminal domains of collagen IV are cleaved by proteolysis, and, as with PIIINP, significant elevations of serum PIVNP and PIVCP are believed to occur only in liver disease. Patients with CPH have normal levels of PIVCP and can easily be distinguished from patients with CAH, but unlike serum PIIINP the highest amount of PIVCP is found in liver cirrhosis. Commercial tests for these metabolites of collagen have been or are being developed, and the markers can then be subjected to an evaluation for their practical diagnostic utility. They can also be used to monitor new drugs to control fibrinogenesis.

Autoantibodies

Patients with autoimmune hepatitis (AIH) develop antibodies and specific T-cell responses to liver-specific proteins (Rizzetto et al 1973), and the titres of some of these antibodies correlate with severity of disease and response to therapy (Manns 1989, McFarlane & Eddleston 1990). Antibody levels have been used in some instances to monitor disease progression in AIH patients. Some of these autoantibodies to liver proteins also appear in patients with acute and chronic viral hepatitis B. A liver-specific membrane lipoprotein, LSP, is a relatively crude macromolecular preparation derived from normal heptocytes and probably contains multiple antigens against which these antibodies are directed. Asialoglycoprotein receptor (ASGP-R) is a major antigenic component of LSP (McFarlane et al 1986). It is also liver specific and is located on the membrane of the hepatocyte. Data indicate that immune reactions against ASGP-R induce liver pathology of type I AIH (Wen et al 1990). In hepatitis B, however, the specificity of anti-LSP and anti-ASGP-R may differ from that in AIH, and there is no evidence that they are associated with pathology in HBV infection. McFarlane et al (1986) have detected these circulating antibodies in the majority of patients with acute hepatitis B, and titres decline and disappear upon recovery. Of more interest, the antibodies were found in the majority of patients with CAH-B but not in patients with CPH. If the correlation of antibody with disease activity is confirmed, these markers would be an aid in staging chronic hepatitis B.

Infrequent serological patterns in HBV

Patterns in the combinations of serological markers described above are generally well recognized. Unique patterns occur occasionally in patients and blood donors for reasons that are not clear, and these findings often cause difficulties in interpretation. The unique patterns are seen more often in certain geographical locations and occur more in blood donors than in patients.

HBsAg without anti-HBc

Specimens that are reactive for HBsAg but negative for anti-HBc are rare even though they may be frequently reported (Coursaget et al 1987, Tobias & Miller 1988, Zanetti et al 1988, Echevarria et al 1991). Because HBsAg is the earliest marker to appear in acute infection, even prior to symptoms, it can be the only HBV marker of infection at that time. Later bleedings will reveal IgM anti-HBc and total anti-HBc even if the patient has only a subclinical infection. Other explanations have been considered to account for the HBsAg-only findings. A putative HBV-2 agent has been proposed for this observation in patients from specific geographical regions. Studies of the molecular sequences of HBV DNA sometimes detect variations in the core and pre-core regions, but it remains problematic whether the base changes that are detected can explain the lack of immune response to core antigen in these patients. Several reports of HBsAg-only reactions come from studies of patients who are immunosuppressed or who also have other viral infections. This suggests that the delay in the appearance or absence of anti-HBc is, in part, secondary to an immune suppressive state (Brown et al 1992).

HBsAg and anti-HBs

In the majority of patients, anti-HBs seroconversion occurs during recovery but sometimes takes months to appear after clearance of HBsAg. Codetection of HBsAg and anti-HBs has been observed in occasional patients recovering from acute hepatitis B, and it has been found in up to 30% of patients with various stages of chronic hepatitis (Shiels et al 1987). The ability to find both of these markers is dependent to some extent on the sensitivities of the two tests, but is more frequent in CAH than in asymptomatic carriers (Tsang et al 1986). The subtype of the coexisting antibody is usually unrelated to the subtype of the HBsAg in the specimen, and the more common anti-HBs/*a* is seldom found. Most or all of the latter antibody would probably be bound in an immune complex with HBsAg and therefore would not be detected. The co-occurrence of antigen and antibody is also an indication that the immune response to viral envelope is being activated in these patients, and this has been proposed as evidence of a greater degree of inflammatory activity in such patients.

The presence of HBsAg and anti-HBs in serum of a patient may occasionally be evidence of an HBV 'escape mutant'. Studies of African and Italian children who had received hepatitis B vaccine revealed that some were subsequently positive for both HBsAg and anti-HBs. The HBV DNA from an Italian child was sequenced by Carman et al (1990), who found a mutation in the S gene that resulted in the loss of reactivity for the HBsAg/*a* epitope. Since vaccines induce a predominantly anti-HBs/*a*, response it is understandable how the antigen and antibody could coexist.

Anti-HBc alone

The occurrence of an isolated anti-HBc reaction is frequently found among blood donors in countries where anti-HBc testing is used as a surrogate in donor screening. Some of these reactions, particularly those with weak signals, are known to be false; the non-specific activity is associated with an IgM-like component in the test specimen (Chau et al 1991, Robertson et al 1991). However, others positive for anti-HBc only are specific. These are found in donors and patients who have previous exposure to HBV and in whom HBsAg, anti-HBs and anti-HBe have disappeared or are below levels of detection. A small subset of patients have high titres of anti-HBc and can be shown to have HBV DNA that is detectable by PCR methods (Kroes et al 1991). A subgroup of HDV-infected HBV carriers has been reported to have only anti-HBc and anti-HDV as serological evidence of infection. In rare cases, donor blood positive for anti-HBc only has been linked to post-transfusion hepatitis B (Hoofnagle et al 1978, Katchaki et al 1978, Lander et al 1978, Lai et al 1989). Such donors are probable carriers of cryptic HBV, and a work-up of them as patients using HBV DNA, ALT, anti-HBs and anti-HBe can help to identify them (Parkinson et al 1990).

Anti-HBs alone

Anti-HBs-only reactivity is expected and usually found in sera of subjects who have responded to active immunization with HBsAg vaccine. Occasionally, such reactivity appears sporadically in unvaccinated patients, and it may be the result of natural immunization without infection, or occur in cases where HBsAg and anti-HBc did not develop or where antigen and anti-HBc have disappeared. In several cases anti-HBs reactivity is false. Apparent false reactions have been found in animal sera and in humans (Hoofnagle et al

1983, Kessler et al 1985). These reactions result from IgM-like substances that are not protective; subjects with these reactivities respond with normal rather than anamnestic reactions if they are given HBsAg vaccines. Consequently it is prudent to treat unvaccinated subjects who are anti-HBs only as unprotected and to vaccinate them.

REFERENCES

Bancroft W H, Mundon F K, Russell P K 1972 Detection of additional antigenic determinants of hepatitis B antigen. Journal of Immunology 109: 842–848

Bayer M E, Blumberg B S, Werner B 1968 Particles associated with Australia antigen in the sera of patients with leukaemia, Down's syndrome and hepatitis. Nature 218: 1057

Beasley R P, Trepo C, Stevens C E, Szmuness W 1977 The e antigen and vertical transmission of hepatitis B surface antigen. American Journal of Epidemiology 105: 94–98

Berris B, Sampliner R E, Sooknanan R, Feinman S V 1987 Hepatitis B virus DNA in asymptomatic HBsAg carriers: comparison with HBeAg/anti-HBe status. Journal of Medical Virology 23: 233–239

Bhat R A, Ulrich P P, Vyas G N 1990 Molecular characterization of a new variant of hepatitis B virus in a persistently infected homosexual man. Hepatology 11: 271–276

Bianchi L, Gudet F G 1983 Histo- and immunopathology of viral hepatitis. In: Dienhardt F, Deinhardt J (eds). Viral hepatitis: laboratory and clinical science. Marcel Dekker, New York, pp 335–382

Blumberg B S 1964 Polymorphisms of serum proteins in the development of isoprecipitins in transfused patients. Bulletin of the New York Academy of Medicine 40: 377

Bonino F 1991 Chronic viral hepatitis. From clinical trials to the therapeutic decision in the individual patient. Journal of Hepatology 13: 527–530

Bonino F, Hoyer B, Nelson J et al 1981 Hepatitis B virus DNA in the sera of HBsAg carriers: a marker of active hepatitis B virus replication in the liver. Hepatology 1: 386–391

Bradley D W, Maynard J E, McCaustland K A et al 1983 Non-A, non-B hepatitis in chimpanzees: interference with acute hepatitis A virus and chronic hepatitis B virus infections. Journal of Medical Virology 11: 207–213

Brechot C, Bernuau J, Thiers V et al 1984 Multiplication of hepatitis B virus in fulminant hepatitis. British Medical Journal 288: 270–271

Brotman B, Prince A M, Huima T et al 1983 Interference between non-A, non-B and hepatitis B virus infection in chimpanzees. Journal of Medical Virology 11: 191–205

Brown J L, Carman W F, Thomas H C 1992 The clinical significance of molecular variation within the hepatitis B virus genome. Hepatology 15: 144–148

Brunetto M R, Oliveri F, Rocca G et al 1989 Natural course and response to interferon of chronic type B hepatitis, accompanied by antibody to hepatitis B e antigen. Hepatology 10: 198

Carman W, Zanetti A, Karayiannis P et al 1990 Vaccine induced escape mutant of hepatitis B virus. Lancet 336: 325–329

Carman W F, Fagan E A, Hadziyannis S et al 1991 Association of a pre-core genomic variant of hepatitis B virus with fulminant hepatitis. Hepatology 14: 219–222

Carreda F, Antinori S, Pastecchia P et al 1988 A possible misdiagnosis in patients presenting with acute HBsAg-negative hepatitis: The role of hepatitis delta virus. Infection 16: 358–359

Chau K H, Hargie M P, Decker R H et al 1983 Serodiagnosis of recent hepatitis B infection by IgM class anti HBc. Hepatology 3: 142–149

Chau K H, Chun E H L, Decker R H, Brodsky J P 1991 Improvements in specificity of competitive anti-HBc ELISA by treating serum samples with reducing agents. In: Hollinger F B, Lemon S M, Margolis H (eds) Viral hepatitis and liver disease. Williams & Wilkins, Baltimore, pp 297–301

Courouce-Pauty A, Dronet J, Kleinknecht D 1979 Simultaneous occurrence of hepatitis B surface antigen and antibody to hepatitis B surface antigen of different subtypes. Journal of Infectious Disease 140: 975–978

Coursaget P, Yvonnet B, Bourdil C et al 1987 HBsAg positive reactivity in man not due to hepatitis B virus. Lancet ii: 1354–1358

Dane D S, Cameron C H, Briggs M 1970 Virus-like particles in the serum of patients with Australia antigen positive hepatitis. Lancet i: 695–698

Davis G L, Hoofnagle J H, Waggoner J G 1984 Spontaneous reactivation of chronic type B hepatitis. Gastroenterology 86: 230–235

Decker R H 1991 New diagnostic technologies: automation of immunoassays for hepatitis markers and solution hybridization for HBV DNA. In: Hollinger F B, Lemon S M and Margolis H (eds) Viral hepatitis and liver disease. Williams & Wilkins, Baltimore, pp 795–798

De Cock K M, Govindarajan S, Redeker A G 1985 Acute delta hepatitis without circulating HBsAg. Gut 26: 212–214

Dodd R Y, Popovsky M A et al 1991 Antibodies to hepatitis B core antigen and the infectivity of the blood supply. Transfusion 31: 443–449

Eble K, Clemens J, Krenc C et al 1991 Differential diagnosis of acute viral hepatitis using rapid, fully automated immunoassays. Journal of Medical Virology 33: 139–150

Echevarria J M, Leon P, Domingo C J et al 1991 Characterization of HBV2 like infections in Spain. Journal of Medical Virology 33: 240–247

Eddleston A L W F 1988 Immunological aspects of hepatitis B infection. In: Zuckerman A J (ed) Viral hepatitis and liver disease. Alan R. Liss, New York, pp 603–605

Gerber M A, Thung S N 1985 Biology of disease. Molecular and cellular pathology of hepatitis B. Laboratory Investigation 52: 572–590

Gerety R J, Tabor E, Hoofnagle J H et al 1978 Tests for HBV-associated antigens and antibodies. In: Vyas G N, Cohen S N, Schmid R (eds) Viral hepatitis. Franklin Institute Press, Philadelphia, pp 121–138

Gerlich W H, Luer W, Thomssen R et al 1980 Diagnosis of acute and inapparent hepatitis B virus infections by measurement of IgM antibody to hepatitis B core antigen. Journal of Infectious Disease 142: 95–101

Gerlich W, Uy F, Lambrecht F, Thomssen R 1986 Cutoff values of immunoglobulin M antibody against viral core antigen or differentiation of acute, chronic and post hepatitis B infections. Journal of Clinical Microbiology 24: 288–293

Gitnick G, 1983 Immunoglobulin M hepatitis B core antibody: To titer or not to titer? To use or not to use? Gastroenterology 84: 653–655

Hadziyannis S, Gerber M A, Vissoulis C et al 1973 Cytoplasmic hepatitis B antigen in 'ground-glass' hepatocytes of carriers. Archives of Pathology 96: 327–330

Harrison T J, Tsiquaye K N, Zuckerman A J 1983 Assay of HBV DNA in the plasma of HBV-carrier chimpanzees superinfected with non-A, non-B hepatitis. Journal of Medical Virology 11: 179–189

Hayasaka A, Schuppan D, Ohnishi K et al 1990 Serum concentrations of the carboxyterminal cross-linking domain of procollagen type IV (NC1) and the aminoterminal propeptide of procollagen III (PIIIP) in chronic liver diseases. Journal of Hepatology 10: 17–22

Hellstrom U, Sylvan S 1986 Should pre S coded peptides be used in hepatitis B vaccines? Lancet i: 389–390

Hilleman M R, Bunyak E B, McAleer W S, McLean A A 1981 Human hepatitis B vaccine. In: Krugman S, Sherlock S (eds) Proceedings of the European Symposium on Hepatitis B. Rahway, N S, Merck, Sharp & Dohme, pp 120–139

Hoofnagle J 1990 Post transfusion hepatitis B. Transfusion 30: 384–386

Hoofnagle J H, Gerety R J, Barker L F 1973 Antibody to hepatitis-B virus core in man. Lancet ii: 869–873

Hoofnagle J H, Seeff L B, Bales Z B, Zimmerman H J 1978 Type B hepatitis after transfusion with blood containing antibody to hepatitis B core antigen. New England Journal of Medicine 298: 1379–83

Hoofnagle J H, Schafer D F, Ferenci P et al 1983 Antibody to hepatitis B surface antigen in nonprimate animal species. Gastroenterology 84: 1478–1482

Hoofnagle J H, Shafritz D A, Popper H 1987 Chronic Type B hepatitis and the 'healthy' HBsAg carrier state. Hepatology 7: 758–763

Jullien A M, Courouce A M, Richard D et al 1988 Transmission of HIV by blood from seronegative donors. Lancet ii: 1248–1249

Kaneko S, Feinstone S M, Miller R H 1989 Rapid and sensitive method for the detection of serum hepatitis B virus DNA using the polymerase chain reaction technique. Journal of Clinical Microbiology 27: 1930–1933

Katchaki J N, Brouwer R, Siem T H 1978 Anti-Hbc and blood infectivity. New England Journal of Medicine 298: 1421–1422

Kessler H A, Harris A A, Payne J A et al 1985 Antibodies to hepatitis B surface antigen as the sole hepatitis B marker in hospital personnel. Annals of Internal Medicine 103: 21–26

Kojima M, Shimizu M, Tsuchimochi T et al 1991 Post-transfusion fulminant hepatitis B associated with pre-core defective HBV mutants. Vox Sanguinis 60: 34–39

Koziol D E, Alter J H, Kirchner J P, Holland P V 1976 The development of HBsAg-positive hepatitis despite the previous existence of antibody to HBsAg. Journal of Immunology 117: 2260–2262

Koziol D E, Holland P V, Alling D W et al 1986 Antibody to hepatitis B core antigen as a paradoxical marker for non-A, non-B hepatitis agents in donated blood. Annals of Internal Medicine 104: 488–495

Kroes A C M, Quint W G V, Heijtink R A 1991 Significance of isolated hepatitis B core antibodies detected by enzyme immunoassay in a high risk population. Journal of Medical Virology 35: 96–100

Krogsgaard K, Kryger P, Aldershvile J et al 1987a Delta infection and suppression of hepatitis B virus replication in chronic HBsAg carriers. Hepatology 7: 42–45

Krogsgaard K, Lindhardt B O, Nielsen J O 1987b The influence of HTLV-III infection on the natural history of hepatitis B virus infection in male homosexual HBsAg carriers. Hepatology 7: 37–41

Kuhns M C, McNamara A I, Cabal C et al 1988 A new assay for the quantitative detection of hepatitis B viral DNA in human serum. Zuckerman A J (ed). Viral hepatitis and liver disease. Alan R. Liss, New York, pp 258–262

Kuhns M C, McNamara A L, Perrillo R P et al 1989 Quantitation of hepatitis B viral DNA by solution hybridization: comparison with DNA polymerase and hepatitis B e antigen during antiviral therapy. Journal of Medical Virology 27: 274–281

Lai M E, Farci P, Figus A et al 1989 Hepatitis B virus DNA in the serum of Sardinian blood donors negative for the hepatitis B surface antigen. Blood 73: 17–19

Lander J J, Gitnick L G L, Gelb L H, Aach R D 1978 Anticore antibody screening of transfused blood. Vox Sanguinis 34: 77–80

LeBouvier G L 1971 The heterogenicity of Australia antigen. Journal of Infectious Disease 123: 671

LeBouvier G L, Capper R A, Williams A E, Pelletir M, Katz A J 1976 Concurrently circulating hepatitis B surface antigen and heterotypic anti HBs antibody. Journal of Immunology 117: 2262–2264

Magnius L O, Espmark J A 1972 New specifications in Australia antigen positive sera distinct from LeBouvier determinants. Journal of Immunology 109: 1017–1021

McCullough A J, Stassen W N, Wiesner R H, Czaja A J 1987 Serum type III procollagen peptide concentrations in severe chronic active hepatitis: relationship to cirrhosis and disease activity. Hepatology 7: 49–54

McFarlane B M, McSorley O G, Vergani D et al 1986 Serum autoantibodies reacting with the hepatic asialoglycoprotein receptor (hepatic lectin) in acute and chronic liver disorders. Journal of Hepatology 3: 196–205

McFarlane I G, Eddleston A L W F 1990 Chronic active hepatitis. In: Targan S R, Shanahan F (eds) Immunology and immunopathology of the liver and gastrointestinal tract. Igaku-Shoin, New York, pp 281–304

Manns M 1989 Autoantibodies and antigens in liver diseases – updated. Journal of Hepatology 9: 272–280

Mimms L, Goetze A, Swanson S et al 1989 Second generation assays for the detection of antibody to HBsAg using recombinant DNA derived HBsAg. Journal of Virological Methods 25: 211–232

Moestrup T, Hanssan B G, Widell A et al 1985 Hepatitis B virus DNA in the serum of patients followed up longitudinally with acute and chronic hepatitis B. Journal of Medical Virology 17: 337–344

Moller B, Hopf U, Stemerowitz R et al 1989 HBcAg expressed on the surface of circulating Dane particles in patients with hepatitis B virus infection without evidence of anti HBc formation. Hepatology 10: 179–185

Mushahwar I K, Overby L R 1981 An enzyme immunoassay for hepatitis B e-antigen and antibody. Journal of Virological Methods 3: 89–97

Mushahwar I K, Overby L R, Frosner G et al 1978 Prevalence of hepatitis B e-antigen and its antibody as detected by radioimmunoassays. Journal of Medical Virology 2: 77–87

Neurath A R, Kent S B H, Strick N et al 1984 Location and chemical synthesis of a pre-S gene coded immunodominant epitope of hepatitis B virus. Science 224: 392–395

Okada K, Kamiyama I, Inomata M 1976 e Antigen and anti-e in the serum of asymptomatic carrier mothers as indicators of positive and negative transmission of hepatitis B virus to their infants. New England Journal of Medicine 294: 746–749

Okochi K, Murakami S 1968 Observations on Australia antigen in Japanese. Vox Sang. 15: 374–386

Omata M, Ehata T, Yokosuka O et al 1991 Mutations in the pre core region of hepatitis B virus DNA in patients with fulminant and severe hepatitis. New England Journal of Medicine 324: 1699–1704

Ostrow D H, Edwards B, Kimes D et al 1991 Quantitation of hepatitis B surface antibody by an automated microparticle enzyme immunoassay Journal of Virological Methods 32: 265–276

Overby L R, 1985 Serology of liver diseases. In: Gitnick G (ed) Current hepatology 6, Year Book Medical Publishers, Chicago, pp 49–85

Overby L R, Ling C M 1976 Radioimmunoassay for anti core as evidence for exposure to hepatitis B virus. Rush Presbyterian St. Lukes Medical Bulletin 15: 83–92

Overby L R, Miller J P, Smith I D et al 1973 Radioimmunoassay of hepatitis B virus-associated (Australia) antigen employing ^{125}l antibody. Vox Sanguinis 24: 102–113

Parkinson A J, McMahon B J, Hall D, Ritter D, Fitzgergerald M A 1990 Comparison of enzyme immunoassay with radioimmunoassay for the detection of antibody to hepatitis B core antigen as the only marker of hepatitis B infection in a population with a high prevalence of hepatitis B. Journal of Medical Virology 30: 253–257

Perrillo R P, 1991 Treatment of chronic hepatitis B. In: Hollinger F B, Lemon S M, Margolis H (eds) Viral hepatitis and liver disease. Williams & Wilkins, Baltimore, pp 616–622

Perrillo R P, 1992 Chronic hepatitis. In: Gitnick G, LaBrecque D R, Moody F G (eds) Diseases of the liver and biliary tract, Mosby-Year Book, St Louis, pp 299–310

Perrillo R P, Campbell C R, Sanders G E et al 1984 Spontaneous clearance and reactivation of hepatitis B virus infection among male homosexuals with chronic type B hepatitis. Annals of Internal Medicine 100: 43–46

Perrillo R P, Regenstein F G, Peters M G et al 1988 Prednisone withdrawal followed by recombinant alpha interferon in the treatment of chronic type B hepatitis. A randomized, controlled trial. Annals of Internal Medicine 109: 95–100

Perrillo R P, Schiff E R, Davis G L et al 1990 A randomized, controlled trial of interferon alfa-2b alone and after prednisone withdrawal in the treatment of chronic hepatitis B. New England Journal of Medicine 323: 295–301

Polesky H F, Hanson M R 1989 Transfusion-associated hepatitis C virus (non A, non B) infection. Archives of Pathology and Laboratory Medicine 113: 232–235

Prince A M 1968 An antigen detected in the blood during the incubation period of serum hepatitis. Proceedings of the National Academy of Sciences of the USA 60: 814–821

Rizzetto M, Swana G, Doniach D 1973 Microsomal antibodies in active chronic hepatitis and other disorders. Clinical and Experimental Immunology 15: 331–344

Robertson E F, Weare J A, Randell R et al 1991 Characterization of a reduction-sensitive factor from human plasma responsible for apparent false activity in competitive assays for antibody to hepatitis B core antigen. Journal of Clinical Microbiology 29: 605–610

Schalm S W, Thomas H C, Hadzyannis 1990 Chronic hepatitis B. Progress in Liver Disease 9: 443–462

Schuppan D 1991 Connective tissue polypeptides in serum as parameters to monitor antifibrotic treatment in hepatic fibrogenesis. Journal of Hepatology 13: 517–525

Schuppan D, Besser M, Schwarting R, Hahn E G 1986 Radioimmunoassay for the carboxyterminal cross-linking domain of type IV (basement membrane) procollagen in body fluids. Journal of Clinical Investigation 78: 241–248

Scotto J, Hadchouel M, Hery C et al 1983 Detection of hepatitis B virus DNA in serum by a simple spot hybridization technique: Comparison with results for other viral markers. Hepatology 3: 279–284

Seeff L B 1988 The golden standard serologic marker for hepatitis B virus infectivity. Hepatology 8: 1711–1719

Seeff L B, Ishak K G, Gerber M 1991 Unresolved clinical issues and histopathologic and immunopathologic aspects of chronic active hepatitis B and C. In: Hollinger F B, Lemon S M, Margolis H (eds) Viral hepatitis and liver disease. Williams & Wilkins, Baltimore, pp 805–813

Shafritz D A 1991 Variants of hepatitis B virus associated with fulminant hepatitis liver disease. New England Journal of Medicine 324: 1737–1939

Shiels M T, Taswell H F, Czaja A J et al 1987 Frequency and significance of concurrent hepatitis B surface antigen and antibody in acute and chronic hepatitis B. Gastroenterology 93: 675–680

Sjögren M, Hoofnagle J H 1988 Immunoglobulin M antibody to hepaitis B core antigen in patients with chronic type B Hepatitis. Gastroenterology 89: 252–258

Smith H M, Lau J Y N, Davies S E et al 1992 Significance of serum IgM anti HBc in chronic hepatitis B virus infection. Journal of Medical Virology 36: 16–20

Soulier J P, Courouce-Pauty A M 1973 New determinants of hepatitis B antigen (Au or HB antigen). Vox Sanguinis 25: 212–234

Stevens C E, Aach R D, Hollinger F B et al 1984 Hepatitis B virus antibody in blood donors and the occurrence of non-A, non-B hepatitis in transfusion recipients. An analysis of the transfusion-transmitted viruses study. Annals of Internal Medicine 101: 733–738

Sutnick A I, London W T, Gerstly B J et al 1968 Anicteric hepatitis associated with Australia antigen. Journal of the American Medical Association 205: 670–674

Tabor E, Gerety R J, Smallwood L A, Barker L F 1977 Coincident hepatitis B surface antigen and antibodies of different subtypes in human serum. Journal of Immunology 118: 369–370

Tassapoulos N C, Papaevangelou G J, Roumeliotou-Karayannis A et al 1987 Detection of hepatitis B virus DNA in asymptomatic hepatitis B surface antigen carriers: relation to sexual transmission. American Journal of Epidemiology 126: 587–591

Thomas H C 1991 Pathogenesis of chronic HBV infection and mechanisms of action of antiviral compounds. In:

Hollinger F B, Lemon S M, Margolis H (eds) Viral hepatitis and liver disease. Williams and Wilkins, Baltimore, pp 612–615

Tobias M, Miller J 1988 Hepatitis B virus type 2 in New Zealand. New Zealand Medical Journal 101: 519–520

Trepo C G, Robert D, Motin J et al 1976 Hepatitis B antigen (HBsAg) and/or antibodies (anti HBs and anti HBc) in fulminant hepatitis: Pathologic and prognostic significance. Gut 17: 10–13

Tsang T K, Blei A T, O'Reilly D J, Decker R 1986 Clinical significance of concurrent hepatitis B surface antigen and antibody positivity. Digestive Diseases and Sciences 31: 620–624

Viola L A, Barrison I G, Coleman J C, Murray-Lyon I M 1982 The clinical course of acute type A hepatitis in chronic HBsAg carriers – a report of three cases. Postgraduate Medical Journal 58: 80–81

Vyas G N, Ulrich P P 1991 Molecular characterization of genetic variants of hepatitis B virus. In: Hollinger F B, Lemon S M, Margolis H (eds) Viral hepatitis and liver disease. Williams & Wilkins, Baltimore, pp 135–148

Wen L, Peakman M, Lobo-Yeo A et al 1990 T-cell directed hepatocyte damage in autoimmune chronic active hepatitis. Lancet 336: 1527–1530

Wong D T, Nath N, Sninsky N N 1985 Identification of hepatitis B virus polypeptides encoded by the entire pre S open reading frame. Journal of Virology 55: 223–231

Zanetti A, Tanzi E, Manzillo G et al 1988 Hepatitis B variants in Europe. Lancet ii: 1132–1133

10. Pathogenesis and treatment of chronic infection

Meron R. Jacyna Howard C. Thomas

Many subjects infected with HBV will develop a clinical or subclinical self-limiting acute hepatitis, with spontaneous clearance of hepatocytes supporting HBV replication within a few weeks of infection. No specific antiviral therapy is required for this group of patients, most of whom recover completely without adverse effect. However some individuals infected with HBV will develop a chronic infection, and this group run the major risk of developing cirrhosis and liver cell cancer. On a worldwide basis, more than 250 million people are estimated to suffer from chronic HBV infection, and 50% of these can be expected to die prematurely, either as a result of chronic inflammatory liver disease or the development of hepatocellular carcinoma (Beasley et al 1981a).

Thus chronic HBV infection is a major cause of morbidity and mortality. The age at which an individual is infected determines the likelihood of a chronic infection developing (Fig. 10.1). 98% of babies born to mothers with chronic replicative HBV infection (usually, but not invariably, HBe antigen positive) become infected, and 95% of these will develop a persistent infection (Beasley et al 1981b). However, only 10% of adults infected with HBV develop chronic infection. The reasons for the development of chronic HBV infection and the options for treatment will be explored.

ACUTE HEPATITIS B INFECTION

Successful recovery from HBV infection is dependent on the integrated activities of the patients' interferon and immune systems. In acute infection, it is the cellular arm of the immune system that recognizes HBV-infected hepatocytes and destroys them. The humoral (antibody) response to epitopes on the lipid–protein coat that envelops the virus is believed to be responsible for protective immunity against reinfection. The components of these normal immune defence mechanisms will be first described. However, persistent HBV infection arises when the virus exploits primary defects in these defences or neutralizes essential components of the hosts' interferon and immune systems. Thus the various viral and host factors that may permit chronic HBV infection to be established will also be examined.

Cellular immunity

The existence of a period of viraemia without liver damage in the prodromal phase of acute infection (Lok et al 1988a) and of carriers with high-level HBV replication without liver damage (Chu et al 1985) suggests that HBV itself is probably not directly cytopathic. In acute hepatitis, liver damage coincides with the appearance of immunoglobulin M (IgM) anti-hepatitis B core (HBc) (Lok et al 1988a), suggesting that the hepatitis associated with HBV infection is caused by immune lysis of infected hepatocytes, an essential part of the recovery process. Analysis of the acute inflammatory infiltrate demonstrates the presence of non-specific killer (NK) and cytotoxic T cells (Eggink et al 1982). NK cells differentiate from pre-NK cells during interferon stimulation. Increased NK functional activity has been demonstrated in the blood of patients with early acute HBV infection (Chemello et al 1986), and

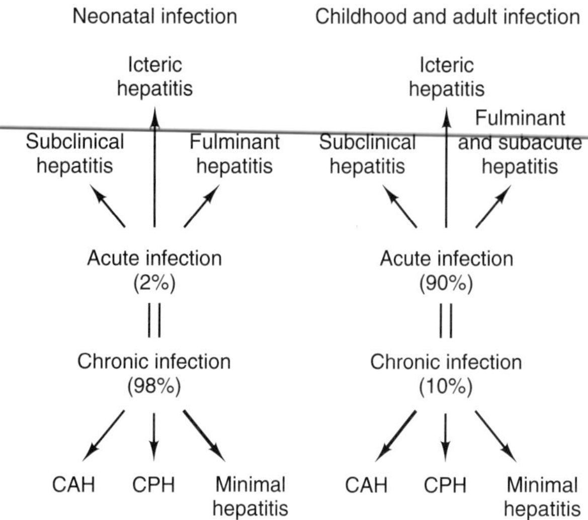

Fig. 10.1 Natural history of hepatitis B virus (HBV) infection after neonatal or adult exposure. CPH, chronic persistent hepatitis; CAH, chronic active hepatitis.

it is probable that this is induced by alpha interferon, which has been demonstrated in the serum of chimpanzees during the prodromal phase of acute HBV infection (Pignatelli et al 1986). The presence of circulating alpha interferon at the onset of viraemia might also explain the fever and malaise that most patients report 2–3 weeks before they develop dark urine, pale stools and icterus. Viral antigens are present on the surface of the hepatocyte (Gudat et al 1975) and it is probable that these, and viral peptides associated with the class I major histocompatability complex (MHC) glycoproteins (Pignatelli et al 1986), make the cell a target for antibody and cytotoxic T-cell lysis (Doherty & Zinkernagel 1975, Schlicht et al 1989, Penna et al 1991).

Studies in patients with chronic HBV infection suggest that the nucleocapsid antigens (HBc and HBe) are an important target for cytotoxicity (Eddleston et al 1982, Pignatelli et al 1987). Whereas antibodies are often directed to conformational epitopes – this is true of the HBc epitope (Waters et al 1986) – helper and cytotoxic T cells usually recognize epitopes on short linear peptides produced by degradation of viral proteins within the antigen-presenting cells (in the case of helper T cells) and in the infected host cell (in the case of cytotoxic T cells). In the case of cytotoxic T cells, the linear viral peptides are physically associated with the MHC class I glycoprotein antigens, and the MHC–virus peptide complex is the signal that the T cell responds to, and initiates the death of the infected cell. Uninfected hepatocytes usually express very little MHC class I glycoprotein (Thomas et al 1982), but in the early stage of acute HBV infection, after the production of alpha interferon, MHC expression on hepatocytes increases and coincidentally transaminase levels rise (Fig. 10.2). Interferon also activates several intracellular enzymes, including 2', 5'-oligoadenylate synthetase (2,5-OAS), endonucleases and a protein kinase, which inhibit viral protein synthesis by either destroying the mRNA or inhibiting translation. These interferon-induced changes would be expected to produce an antiviral state in uninfected regenerating liver cells, preventing reinfection during the lysis of infected hepatocytes.

Humoral immunity

Virus-neutralizing antibodies are directed to epitopes on the envelope of the virus. This is composed of three polypeptides, each with the same carboxy terminus. These are designated the large, middle and small envelope proteins and arise from the 'S' and 'pre-S' genes of HBV. The amino-terminal 120 amino acid region of the large protein, which is not present in the middle and small proteins, is designated pre-S1. This hydrophilic area is myristilated, and recent data indicate that the region aa 21–47 is capable of binding to the membrane of the hepatocyte (Neurath et al 1986) and is therefore probably involved in virus uptake.

The antibodies found in convalescent serum bind predominantly to the epitopes of the HBs gene-encoded region (Machida et al 1983), the carboxy-terminal region that is present in all the envelope proteins. A hydrophilic region of this polypeptide, amino acids 124–147, forms two loops via intramolecular disulphide bridges, and these are the binding region for the majority (more than 80%) of the antigen-binding capacity of convalescent sera. Using monoclonal antibodies binding to these regions, it has been possible to

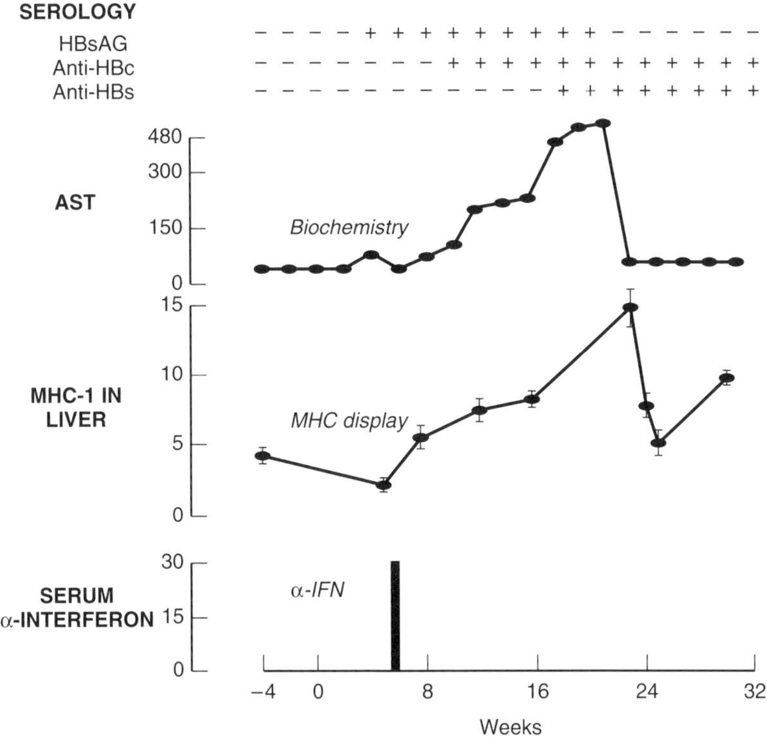

Fig. 10.2 Acute HBV infection in the chimpanzee. Markers of virus infection appear early, coinciding with a detectable pulse of circulating alpha interferon. This is followed by enhanced display of MHC class I antigen on hepatocytes. Liver damage, as indicated by rising serum AST levels, coincides with the first appearance of host humoral immunity to HBV (anti-HBc). AST, aspartate aminotransferase (SGOT).

show that antibody to the region aa 124–137, when administered to chimpanzees, will prevent infection (Iwarson et al 1985). Antibodies to this region, as well as to other epitopes on the S gene-encoded polypeptide, are present in the serum of patients convalescent from HBV infection and in normal subjects immunized with plasma-derived and recombinant DNA-produced HBs vaccine (Ishihara et al 1987).

Although patients recovered from HBV or vaccinated with HBs antigen are protected from further infection, there has been considerable debate on the importance of antibodies to the middle and large pre-S2 and pre-S1-bearing polypeptides. During natural infection, antibodies to pre-S1 and pre-S2 appear before antibodies to the HBs region (Brown et al 1984, Iwarson et al 1985). If, as has been postulated (Neurath et al 1986), the pre-S1 region is important for binding of HBV to the hepatocyte during infection, antibodies to this region would be virus neutralizing and therefore their presence may be important in preventing entry of HBV particles into uninfected hepatocytes. Interference with the production of anti-envelope antibodies thus may be expected to lead to protracted HBV infection, and this is seen in agammaglobulinaemic patients who, when exposed, frequently develop chronic HBV infection.

FACTORS LEADING TO HBV PERSISTENCE

The reasons why certain individuals develop chronic infection, rather than a transient acute infection, may relate to specific viral factors or host factors.

Viral factors

Secretion of HBe antigen. Hepatitis e antigen (HBeAg) is a low molecular weight soluble protein that is part of the nucleocapsid pre-core/core gene (C) product of HBV. When the full pre-core/core gene is translated, a secretory protein is produced. The pre-core-encoded region functions as a signal peptide (Ou et al 1986, Roosinck et al 1986), directing this protein to the cell membrane, ultimately to be secreted from the cell. This protein takes up a conformation that displays the HBe epitopes. When translation of the nucleocapsid open reading frame starts at the second AUG codon, the HBc protein is produced. This, probably because of the absence of the pre-core-encoded signal sequence and the presence of the carboxy-terminal nucleophilic sequence, is not secreted and assembles around HBV RNA–DNA complexes to form virus nucleocapsids.

The pre-core region of the genome is not necessary for the production of infectious virus particles (Chang et al 1987). Its continued presence within the small genome of the virus therefore probably confers some biological advantage by altering the virus to host relationship. The only known function conferred on the infected cell by the presence of this pre-core region is the ability to secrete soluble HBe antigen (Ou et al 1986), and it is likely that secretion of this antigen into the blood alters the immune response favourably for the virus. Some patients with chronic HBV viraemia do not have HBe antigen detectable in the serum, and this group of patients have a more severe and rapidly progressive liver disease (Bonino et al 1986, Chu et al 1985). The reason for this failure to produce HBe antigen is a mutation occurring in the pre-core region of the HBV genome (position 1896), resulting in a novel stop codon that prematurely terminates translation (Carman et al 1989). Thus it may be postulated that HBe antigen in some way may reduce the cytotoxic T-cell response against infected hepatocytes (possibly by inducing immune tolerance against nucleocapsid-derived peptides displayed on the cell surface (Milich et al 1990)) and thus reduces the degree of hepatic inflammation, lessening the risk of death of the host and elimination of the virus (both of which are disadvantageous to the virus). In this way a protracted infection is more likely; a healthy host with persistent infection is more likely to spread the virus to other individuals than a sick host with severe liver disease.

HBeAg may play an important role in the high rate of development of chronic hepatitis B infection in children born to mothers who are HBeAg positive. Almost every child born to an HBeAg-positive mother becomes infected with HBV, and 90% develop a chronic carrier state (Beasley et al 1981b, Chu et al 1985). It has been shown that HBeAg crosses the human placenta (Lin et al 1987), and a recent study (using a transgenic mouse model) has demonstrated that in utero exposure to HBeAg leads to a significant period of neonatal T-cell tolerance to HBeAg and HBcAg in non-transgenic offspring of HBeAg-expressing transgenic female mice (Milich et al 1990). This immunological tolerance may play an important role in the development of a chronic carrier state in neonates.

Secretion of HBs antigen. In addition to secreting soluble nucleocapsid proteins into the serum, the virus also secretes surplus surface (envelope) protein (HBs) into the blood. This excess HBs can be seen in the serum by electron microscopy as 22 nm-sized particles (Fig. 10.1). These particles may confer a biological advantage on the virus, as they will 'divert' antibody to HBs (anti-HBs) away from intact whole virus particles, and thus reduce the chances of virus neutralization by these anti-envelope antibodies. Recent studies have shown that large quantities of murine monoclonal anti-HBs can overcome the 'antibody-diverting' effect of non-infectious HBsAg particles and can shut off HBV replication in agammaglobulinaemic chronic HBV carriers, presumably by stopping infection of regenerating hepatocytes by virus neutralization in the interstitial space (Lever et al 1990).

HBV integration. It is now clear that HBV DNA becomes covalently integrated into the hepatocyte genome at some time during the chronic infection (Brechot et al 1981, Shafritz et al 1981). The continuous secretion of the viral coat protein (HBsAg) in the absence of active viral replication probably represents a phase of infection in which the viral DNA has become integrated into the host DNA, so that some of the viral genes are transcribed and translated as though they were hepatocyte DNA. This integration event may be involved (late in the infection) in the malignant transformation of hepatocytes (Shafritz & Kew 1981). The cells containing integrated sequences must evade the immune elimination processes, and probably do so by not expressing HBc and HBe antigens (the putative targets for cytotoxic T cells) (Thomas 1982). Since the preferred site for integration on the viral genome is in the promoter region of the HBV core gene (Dejean et al 1985), this transcription unit is destroyed during the integration process and thus no nucleocapsid antigens are produced. HBsAg, however, continues to be expressed in these cells because this gene is intact in the integrated viral sequence (Dejean et al 1985). As long as the cell is not recognized by cytotoxic T cells as being infected, integration of the virus will result in viral persistence. Whether HBV integrates or not is dependent on the duration of infection and is usually found if infection has been present for 2 or more years. Studies of attempts to eliminate HBV infection using interferon therapy have indicated that patients who have had chronic infection for many years, and who have integrated HBV DNA, are much less likely to clear HBs antigen than patients with a short period of chronicity and in whom integration is not found (Caselmann et al 1989). In individuals who have 'cleared' replicating virus (HBV DNA, HBV DNA polymerase and HBeAg all negative) and have no evidence of liver disease, reactivation of infection (presumably from integrated HBV) has sometimes been seen when immunosuppressive therapy or acquired immune dysfunction occurs (Hoofnagle et al 1982, Davis et al 1984).

HBV mutants. The pre-core variant of HBV, resulting from a point mutation at nucleotide position 1896, has already been described (Carman et al 1989). This results in a failure to produce HBeAg. Studies have also indicated that there may be more than one type of HBV present in a chronically infected individual. For example, mixed infections of 'wild-type' and pre-core mutant HBV have been described in chronically infected patients (Carman et al 1989). There are also descriptions of pre-core and core mutant HBV present in HBeAg-positive patients with chronic hepatitis, but not in HBeAg asymptomatic individuals (Wakita et al 1991). These data are consistent with the hypothesis that variants of HBV are selected by the immune response, particularly in patients with severe hepatitis.

Host factors

Deficient production of interferon. Alpha interferon production during the early phase of acute HBV infection is believed to be important for successful resolution (Pignatelli et al 1986). Studies of peripheral blood mononuclear cells (PBMCs) taken from patients with acute (Levin & Hahn 1982) and chronic (Kato et al 1982, Abb et al 1985, Ikeda et al 1986a) HBV infection has revealed that the production of alpha interferon is subnormal. It is possible that this reduced production of interferon is directly attributable to HBV infection of the PBMCs (Laure et al 1987), and suppression of interferon production in cells by the core region of the HBV genome has been shown (Twu et al 1988). However, as reduced interferon production is also seen in lymphocytes taken from patients with resolving acute HBV infection (Levin & Hahn 1982), it is unlikely that interferon deficiency is the cause of most cases of persistent HBV infection. This is further supported by studies showing that alpha interferon therapy results in clearance of HBV infection in only about a third of treated patients (Jacyna & Thomas 1990). If persistence of infection was due to deficient interferon production by PBMCs in all cases, then we could expect to see much higher seroconversion rates with alpha interferon therapy.

Deficient response to interferon. In acute HBV infection, alpha interferon is responsible for the initial increase in MHC class I antigen display on hepatocyte membranes and the activation of the 2,5-OAS, endonuclease and protein kinase systems, which result in an effective antiviral state within the liver. However, in chronic HBV-infected subjects there is evidence of abnormal activation of hepatocytes by interferon: levels of 2,5-OAS are only minimally elevated (Ikeda et al

1986b) and MHC class I proteins are present only in very low density on these infected hepatocytes (Montano et al 1982, Ikeda et al 1986b). In the PBMCs of patients with chronic active HBV hepatitis, there is a similar lack of increase in MHC class I expression and 2,5-OAS enzyme activation compared with uninfected subjects (Poitrine et al 1985). These abnormal responses to interferon seem to be acquired as a direct result of infection with HBV. In vitro transfection of HBV into cells in tissue culture makes them specifically unresponsive to interferon; they remain susceptible to lysis by Sindbis virus and MHC class I induction does not occur (Onji et al 1989). MHC class I display is believed to be important for recognition and elimination of HBV-infected hepatocytes by cytotoxic T cells, and the decreased MHC expression, in addition to the reduced 2,5-OAS activation, may increase the likelihood of persistent HBV infection.

It is possible that this abnormal cellular response to interferon is directly attributable to the virus itself, but the exact mechanism by which the virus might achieve this is not clear. One hypothesis is that it may be due to the presence of a short nucleotide sequence at the beginning of the core gene of the virus (Thomas et al 1986). The nucleotide sequence of this region shows a striking homology to a consensus sequence within the host genome that is 'upstream' from genes induced by interferon in mammalian cells (Friedman & Stark 1985). The interferon-induced secondary messenger binds to this site, and the presence of multiple homologous consensus sequences on episomal or integrated HBV DNA might compete for this messenger. Another possible mechanism of interference is by the HBV replicative enzyme (HBV DNA polymerase). One study has shown that cells transfected with the HBV DNA polymerase gene, produce polymerase protein and become unresponsive to the effects of alpha interferon (Foster et al 1991). In this study, transfection with other HBV genes did not affect the cellular response to interferon.

Antibody to nucleocapsid antigens. The first host-induced immunological marker of HBV infection is antibody to the core protein (anti-HBc), which appears shortly after the time HBsAg is first detected in the serum (Hoofnagle 1974). Anti-HBc is not a neutralizing antibody, and high titres of anti-HBc in the absence of HBsAg or anti-HBs may indicate the presence of continuing replication of HBV in the liver and infective HBV particles in the serum (Hoofnagle 1978). Cytotoxic T cells sensitized to nucleocapsid-derived peptides displayed on the hepatocyte membrane recognize and destroy HBV-infected hepatocytes (Eddleston et al 1982, Pignatelli et al 1987). However it has been shown that anti-HBc and anti-HBe block cytotoxic T-cell killing of HBV-infected hepatocytes (Mondelli et al 1982, Brown et al 1984, Pignatelli et al 1987). This blocking effect may be the result of simple steric hindrance if the B- and cytotoxic T-cell epitopes are displayed close to each other on the cell membrane (Pignatelli et al 1987). Thus circulating anti-HBc may modulate T-cell-mediated lysis of infected cells (Trevisan et al 1982) and, by analogy with chronic measles infection of the central nervous system (Fujinam & Oldstone 1981), may be one mechanism leading to viral persistence. Consistent with this hypothesis is the observation that some adult patients progressing from acute to chronic infection produce anti-HBc before those that clear the virus (Lok et al 1988a) and injection of monoclonal anti-HBc and anti-HBe with the virus produce prolonged viraemia (Pignatelli et al 1987).

Of babies born to HBe antigen-positive mothers, 90% become infected, and more than 90% of these develop a chronic infection (Beasley et al 1981b). It has been speculated that the active transport of maternal IgG anti-HBc via placental Fc receptors contributes to the persistence of HBV-infected cells in the child's liver (Alexander & Eddleston 1986a, Pignatelli et al 1987) which, together with the immaturity of the neonatal immune system (Nash 1985), results in chronic infection. IgG antibodies have been shown to modulate viral proteins from the membrane of infected cells (Joseph et al 1975, Perrin et al 1976), a process that would prevent recognition by potentially lytic antibodies. Usually the epitopes recognized by antibodies and cytotoxic T cells are different. In the case of HBV-infected hepatocytes, anti-HBc and anti-HBe will inhibit the lysis of infected hepatocytes by T cells, suggesting that the epitopes recognized by these antibodies and cytotoxic T cells are the same, or displayed near to each other on the cell membrane. Further confirmation of these findings comes from studies showing that murine monoclonal anti-HBc and anti-HBe, when injected into chimpanzees along with an infectious inoculum of HBV, results in a protracted infection lasting 12–18 months (Pignatelli et al 1987).

Abnormalities of lymphocyte function. It is thought that lymphocyte function is broadly deranged in chronic HBV carriers (Alexander & Eddleston 1986b), and many studies measuring suppressor cell function in both acute and chronic HBV infection have been performed (reviewed by Dienstag 1984). Although the results are inconsistent, it does appear that there is a defect in suppressor cell function in both acute and chronic HBV infection as compared with control patients. Further studies of T4/T8 ratios also indicate a reduced ratio in acute and chronic HBV infection (Dienstag 1984). These findings suggest a virus-induced alteration in lymphocyte function in both acutely and chronically infected persons, but do not specifically incline an individual towards HBV persistence. Interleukin 1 production by monocytes from patients with chronic HBV infection with liver disease is also increased, and this correlates with the severity of fibrosis found within the liver (Anastassakos et al 1988). However, once cirrhosis supervenes, interleukin 1 production is significantly reduced compared with normal (Kakumu et al 1988a) and this is probably because of a serum inhibitor found in these patients with advanced disease. However, this defect is not specific for HBV infection, and also HBV carriers without liver disease have normal interleukin production. Defects in B-lymphocyte secretion of antibody in chronic HBV infection have also been described, and are believed to be a physiological response of anti-HBs-secreting B lymphocytes to marked excess of circulating HbsAg (Dusheiko et al 1983). The importance of these various lymphocyte abnormalities in terms of the likelihood of developing chronic HBV infection is still not known.

Serum factors. In addition to the described defect in interleukin production in most patients with liver disease (Anastassakos et al 1988, Kakumu et al 1988a), studies have also suggested that HBV carriers may secrete specific serum factors that predispose to viral persistence. Recent studies have shown that the T cells of the majority of chronic HBV carriers produce a secreted soluble factor (TSF) that selectively suppresses the production of anti-HBs by the B lymphocytes of the patient (Yamauchi et al 1988). Other serum factors which are claimed to adversely alter lymphocyte function have also been described (Berg et al 1982), but these are less specific and are not believed to play a primary role in HBV chronicity (Dienstag 1984).

Anti-idiotype response. One important method of immunoregulatory control is achieved by synthesis of antibodies against the variable region of antibodies. These antibodies, known as anti-idiotypes, can either enhance or, more commonly, limit the immune response. One recent study looking at anti-idiotype antibodies in HBV infection showed that 70–80% of patients with persistent infection had these antibodies (Ibarra et al 1988). Individuals who subsequently cleared the HBV infection were less likely to have the anti-idiotype antibodies and, if they had the antibodies, they were of a lower titre than patients who did not clear the infection (Ibarra et al 1988). These data suggest that anti-idiotypic modulation of the immune response against the virus may be important in predicting viral persistence.

Gender and hormonal factors. Following exposure in adulthood, the likelihood of remaining chronically infected is greater in males than in females. The reasons for this difference are not known, although it may be speculated that they are hormonal in origin. There is a glucocorticoid-responsive element in the genome of HBV (Tur-Kaspa et al 1986), and other studies have indicated that HBsAg gene expression is regulated by sex steroids and glucocorticoids (Farza et al 1987). In addition, HBs antigen is cleared more slowly in male inbred mice than female mice of the same genotype (Craxi et al 1982), suggesting that phagocytic cells in males do not 'see' the viral protein as readily as females.

ANTIVIRAL THERAPY FOR CHRONIC HBV INFECTION

As will be obvious from the preceding text, the precise reason(s) for the development of chronic HBV infection have still not been clearly elucidated. Regardless of the cause, it is clear that chronic HBV infection frequently causes hepatic injury and is a major cause of morbidity and mortality, and thus much attention has been paid to possible antiviral remedies. At present, antiviral therapy is indicated for patients with chronic HBV infection who have active viral replication within the liver – usually, but not invariably, HBeAg positive – and who also have biochemical and/or histological evidence of liver cell injury. The relationship between active HBV replication and liver cell damage has been well described (Realdi et al 1980, Hoofnagle et al 1981, Liaw et al 1983) and the goal of antiviral therapy is permanent elimination of hepatocytes supporting HBV replication. Several studies have now shown that spontaneous disappearance of HBeAg from the serum and development of anti-HBe results in a biochemical and histological remission in the majority of infected individuals (Realdi et al 1980, Hoofnagle et al 1981, Liaw et al 1983). Similarly, loss of HBeAg produced by antiviral therapy using alpha interferon has also been shown to produce immediate (Brook et al 1989a) and long-lasting histological improvements (Perillo & Brunt 1991). Loss of HBeAg is also associated with loss of markers of viral replication, that is HBV DNA and DNA polymerase. Thus the goal of antiviral therapy in HBeAg-positive patients is loss of HBe antigen. However, 5% of HBeAg-negative patients will still continue to have hepatic inflammatory disease (Fattovich et al 1986), sometimes severe (Wu et al 1988). Loss of HBsAg, although desirable, is not essential in terms of ameliorating infectivity and hepatic inflammation. As there is a natural rate of spontaneous seroconversion from HBeAg to anti-HBe, varying from 5 to 16% per annum (Viola et al 1981, Fattovich et al 1986), studies evaluating antiviral therapies should include a matched but untreated control group. Unfortunately many antiviral studies have not been performed in this way, making interpretation of results difficult. In patients with chronic HBV infection with active viral replication but negative for HBeAg (pre-core mutant viraemia), assessment of the antiviral effect has to be made by direct measurement of HBV DNA and/or DNA polymerase.

Chronic HBe antigen-positive HBV infection

Patients with HBeAg-positive chronic HBV infection are potentially infectious (HBV DNA and DNA polymerase positive) and have chronic hepatitis of variable severity.

Single-agent studies

Adenine arabinoside and adenine arabinoside monophosphate. The purine analogue, adenine arabinoside (ARA-A), is a potent inhibitor of DNA polymerase activity. The clinical usefulness of ARA-A is limited by its poor aqueous solubility, which results in it having to be given by intravenous (i.v.) infusion. A controlled study of i.v. ARA-A has shown that a 10-day course produces HBe to anti-HBe seroconversion rates of 40% (Bassendine et al 1981). Most clinical trials on ARA-A have focused on its highly water-soluble derivative, adenine arabinoside monophosphate (ARA-AMP), which can be given by intramuscular injection. Six recent controlled studies of ARA-AMP are summarized in Table 10.1. As can be seen, there are wide variations in response rates, as low as 5% in some studies (Perillo et al 1985) and as high as 80% in others (Trepo et al 1986). The most likely reason for this variation is heterogeneity in the populations being studied: the highest seroconversion rates are seen in heterosexuals and the lowest in male homosexuals (Novick et al 1984). The major problem with ARA-AMP is its toxicity, and many patients develop painful sensory peripheral neuropathies and severe myalgias. Some of these side-effects may cause long-standing disability, as a result of which ARA-AMP has recently been withdrawn for use as a single agent in chronic HBeAg HBV infection. Ways of reducing the

Table 10.1 Controlled trials of treatment of HBeAg-positive chronic HBV infection with ARA-AMP

Regimen	Loss of HBeAg		Reference
	Untreated	Treated	
10 mg kg^{-1} day^{-1} for 4–8 weeks (one cycle)	2/10 (20%)	1/10 (10%)	Yokosuka et al 1985
10 mg kg^{-1} day^{-1} for 5 days, 5 mg kg^{-1} day^{-1} for remaining 23 days (one cycle)	2/9 (26%)	10/18 (55%)	Trepo et al 1984
As above, one cycle	2/10 (20%)	4/10 (40%)	Hoofnagle et al 1984
As above, one cycle	0 (0%)	6/15 (40%)	Weller et al 1985
As above, two cycles	1/17 (5%)	1/18 (5%)	Perillo et al 1985
As above, three cycles	4/27 (14%)	2/22 (9%)	Garcia et al 1987

toxicity of ARA-AMP are to limit the duration of treatment to less than 28 days (Lok et al 1984) and to conjugate ARA-AMP with lactosaminated albumin, a neoglycoprotein that specifically penetrates hepatocytes. This allows a much lower dose (a third to a sixth) of ARA-AMP to be used, with a resultant reduction in toxicity. In an uncontrolled pilot study, this compound given i.v. to five subjects with chronic HBe-positive HBV infection resulted in seroconversion in three of the patients and no side-effects were observed (Fiume et al 1987). There seems to be no doubt that ARA-A and its derivatives inhibit hepatitis B viral replication and may be successful in some patients in producing a seroconversion response, but the poor results in other patient groups (particularly homosexuals) and the toxicity of ARA-A and ARA-AMP restrict their usefulness. Further studies of short courses of ARA-AMP (to rapidly reduce HBV replication) preceding other types of therapy (including immune modulation) and more work on the lactosaminated albumin ARA-AMP derivative, are needed.

Acyclovir. Acyclovir, which is used to treat herpes infections, has also been tried in chronic HBeAg positive HBV infection. Given intravenously over 7 days, it causes a reduction in DNA polymerase (Smith et al 1981) and HBV DNA levels (Weller et al 1983). However, only one small controlled study has been performed (Table 10.2). Acyclovir, if given rapidly intravenously, is nephrotoxic and attempts to give it orally are limited by its poor absorption from the gut. The prodrug of acyclovir, 6-deoxyacyclovir, is essentially completely absorbed when taken orally. Only one pilot study has been performed with this agent with disappointing results and no seroconversions (Weller et al 1986). As a single agent, acyclovir and its derivatives are not a valid option.

Type I interferons (alpha and beta). The exact mechanism of action of interferons in chronic HBV infection is unknown, and there are conflicting data from various studies. However, several changes in the immune system and in the infected hepatocyte are believed to be important (Fig. 10.3). An increase in MHC class I protein display in the hepatocyte (which enhances the recognition of HBV-infected hepatocytes by cytotoxic T cells) occurs within 24 h of starting therapy (Pignatelli et al 1986). However, other studies have shown that MHC class I expression correlates poorly with response to interferon (Paul et al 1991). Intracellular levels of 2',5'-oligoadenylate synthetase (an interferon-inducible

Table 10.2 Controlled trials of treatment of HBeAg-positive chronic HBV infection with acyclovir

Regimen	Loss of HBeAg		Reference
	Untreated	Treated	
45 mg kg^{-1} day^{-1} i.v. for 28 days	1/15 (6%)	4/15 (26%)	Alexander et al 1987a

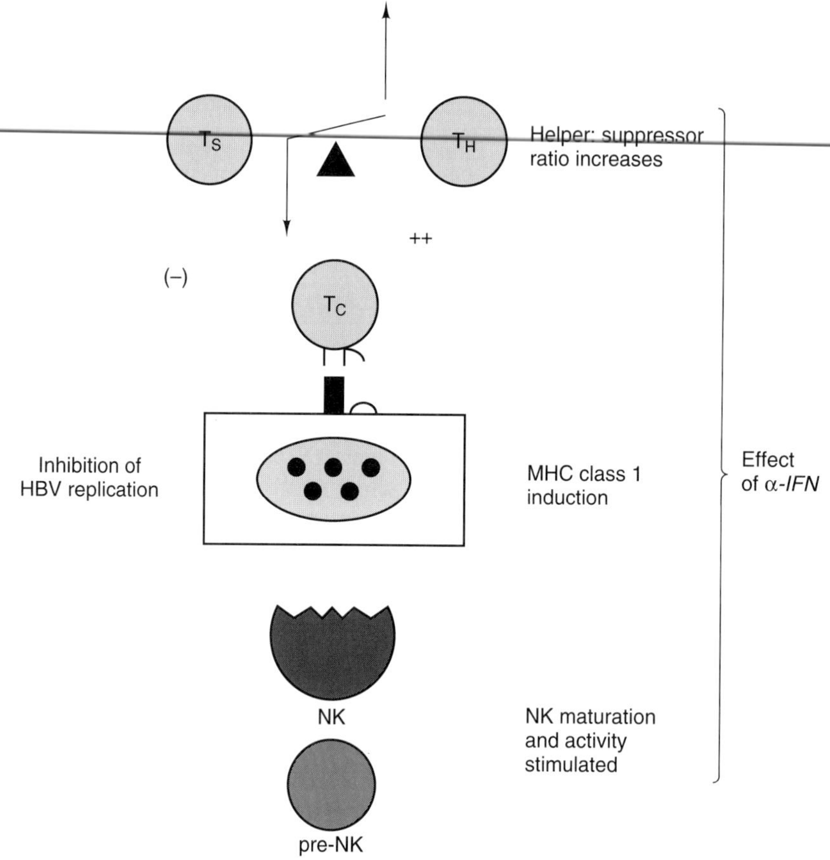

Fig. 10.3 Changes occurring during alpha interferon therapy. There is enhanced MHC class I display on hepatocytes, facilitating recognition of virus-infected cells by the cellular immune mechanisms of the host. HBV replication is inhibited by the intracellular activation of 2', 5'-oligoadenylate synthetase, which produces oligoadenylates that activate an endogenous ribonuclease leading to cleavage of viral RNA. Stimulation of NK cells and an increase in the T-helper/suppressor lymphocyte ratio also occurs.

enzyme that activates intracellular ribonucleases which cleave viral mRNA) become elevated (Fujisawa et al 1987). An increase in the helper/suppressor T-lymphocyte ratio occurs at 6–8 weeks in those subjects who successfully undergo HBe to anti-HBe seroconversion (Dooley et al 1986). Within the liver, during interferon therapy there is an increase in the number of HLA-DR-positive lymphocytes and natural killer cells (Yoo et al 1990). Changes in humoral immunity also occur, and patients who respond to therapy either have IgM anti-HBc present before treatment or develop it during the course of therapy (Chen et al 1989). The net effect of these antiviral and immunostimulatory changes can be seen in patients who respond to interferon therapy (Fig. 10.4). There is an early fall in serum HBV DNA and DNA polymerase levels followed by a delayed 'seroconversion hepatitis', during which transaminase levels rise and loss of HBeAg occurs.

Alpha interferon, mainly derived from monocytes and transformed B lymphocytes, was initially obtained from buffy coat leucocytes, but most recent studies have used lymphoblastoid (obtained from a stimulated lymphoblastoid cell line) or recombinant (alpha-2a or alpha-2b interferons). The interferons are usually administered thrice weekly by deep subcutaneous or intramuscular injection. The main side-effects are fever, chills and myalgia, which occur for a few

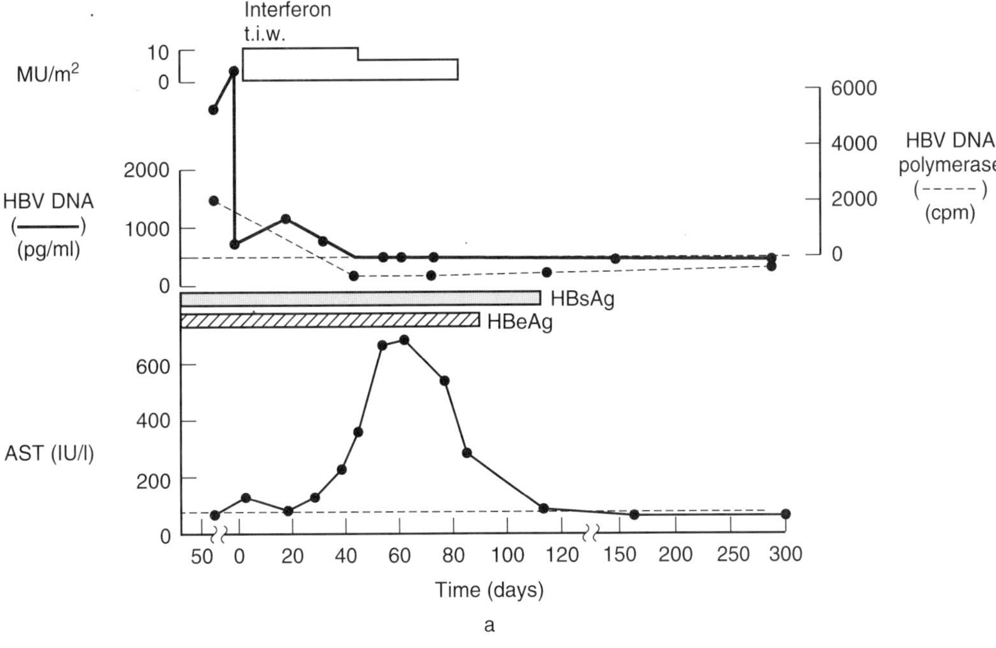

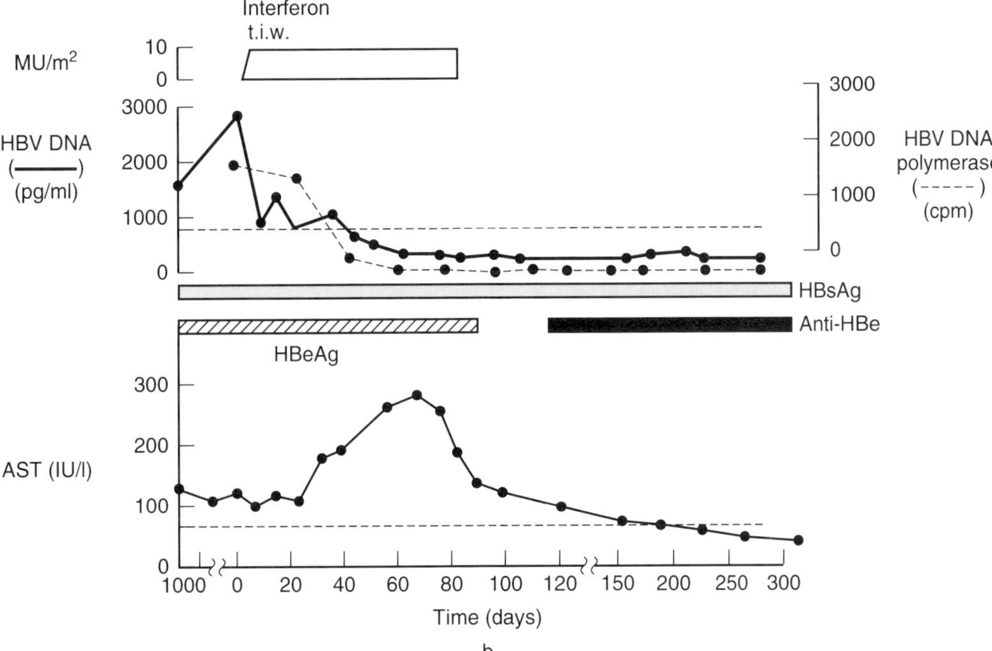

Fig. 10.4 (a) Complete response; inhibition of HBV replication and clearance of HBsAg. (b) Incomplete response; inhibition of HBV replication only. Loss of HBsAg may occur much (several years) later. In both cases note the delayed rise in AST levels which is believed to represent immune-mediated hepatocyte lysis.

Table 10.3 Controlled trial of treatment of HBeAg-positive chronic HBV infection with leucocyte interferon

Regimen	Loss of HBeAg: Untreated	Treated	Reference
<12 MU daily for 6 weeks	4/10 (40%)	2/10 (20%)	Schalm & Heijtink 1982

MU = million units

hours after the initial injections are given. These side-effects are generally well tolerated by most patients and reduce in intensity with time, although a minority of patients may find them unacceptable and require dosage reductions.

Leucocyte alpha interferon. One randomized controlled study of human leucocyte alpha interferon in chronic HBeAg HBV infection (Table 10.3) showed that low doses for 6 weeks produced no short- or long-term response.

Lymphoblastoid alpha interferon. Several controlled studies of human lymphoblastoid alpha interferon in chronic HBeAg HBV infection have been published and are summarized in Table 10.4. Seroconversion (HBeAg loss, usually with development of anti-HBe) rates vary widely, but overall about one-third of patients will respond with loss of HBeAg, and one-third of these responders (i.e. about 10% of those treated) will also immediately lose circulating HBsAg. However, loss of HBsAg can occur many years after HBeAg loss, and further long-term follow-up studies are required in order to determine the final proportion of responders who will lose both viral markers. One of the largest lymphoblastoid alpha interferon studies, a multicentre study from Italy, showed very promising early results – a very high rate of HBeAg loss (88%) in the first 18 patients recruited (Barbara et al 1986). However, the latest data on 66 patients enrolled to this study have shown a more modest overall seroconversion rate of 50% (Mazzella et al 1988). Another study comparing 3 months of lymphoblastoid interferon with ARA-AMP therapy similarly indicated a 45% seroconversion rate for the interferon-treated patients (Lok et al 1985). Further studies reveal that 6 months of therapy may be no better than only 3 months' therapy (Scully et al 1987), and also that thrice-weekly injections for 3 months are more effective and better tolerated than daily injections for 1 month. The factors that predict a response to lymphoblastoid alpha interferon are the same as for recombinant alpha interferon (discussed below).

Recombinant alpha interferon. Results from several controlled trials indicate that recombinant alpha interferon used alone will induce loss of e antigen in about a third of patients (Table 10.5). Again, about 40% of patients will respond with HBeAg loss, and 10% with loss of both HBsAG and HBeAg. Again, loss of HBsAg may occur many years after HBeAg loss; one study has suggested that the majority will lose HBsAg if followed up for long enough (Korenman et al

Table 10.4 Controlled trials of treatment of HBeAg-positive chronic HBV infection with lymphoblastoid interferon

Regimen	Loss of HBeAg: Untreated	Treated	Reference
2.5–7.5 MU/m^2 daily for 28 days	0/16 (0%)	2/14 (14%)	Anderson et al 1986
5–10 MU/m^2 t.i.w for 3 months	1/24 (4%)	12/37 (32%)	Brook et al 1989b
2.5–5.0 MU/M^2 daily for 1 month, then t.i.w. for 5 months	2/9 (22%)	8/9 (88%)	Barbara et al 1986
10 MU/m^2 t.i.w. for 6 months	0/23 (0%)	6/23 (26%)	Alexander et al 1987b

MU = million units

Table 10.5 Controlled trials of treatment of HBeAg-positive chronic HBV infection with recombinant human alpha interferon

Regimen	Loss of HBeAg		Reference
	Untreated	Treated	
5–10 MU/m² every day for 4 months	2/14 (14%)	10/31 (32%)	Hoofnagle et al 1985
2.5–10 MU/m² t.i.w. for 3–6 months	0/9 (0%)	6/32 (19%)	McDonald et al 1987
2.5–5 MU/m² t.i.w. for 3 months	0/23 (0%)	7/37 (19%)	Dusheiko et al 1988
2.5–10 MU/m² t.i.w. for 3–6 months	0/15 (0%)	7/45 (16%)	Lok et al 1988b
2.5–10 MU/m² t.i.w. for 3–6 months	1/6 (17%)	6/18 (33%)	Perez et al 1988
5 MU/m² day or 10 MU/m² t.i.w. for 4 months	1/14 (7%)	10/31 (32%)	Hoofnagle et al 1988
5 MU daily for 4 months	3/43 (7%)	15/41 (37%)	Perillo et al 1990
2.5–10 MU/m² t.i.w. for 6 months	2/7 (28%)	9/23 (39%)	Williams et al 1990
10 MU t.i.w. for 4 months	3/36 (8%)	6/39 (15%)	Lok et al 1992

MU = million units

1991). Increasing the dose of interferon from 2.5 to 10 million units (MU) per m^2 does not result in an increase in response rates (Williams et al 1990). Although loss of HBeAg is associated with loss of serum HBV DNA and DNA polymerase, trace amounts of HBV DNA can still be detected by sensitive amplification methods – the polymerase chain reaction (Korenman et al 1991). This raises the spectre that reactivation of HBV may occur at some time in the future. This does occur in a small minority of patients (<5%), usually within the first 6 months, but longer term follow-up of interferon responders beyond 4 years indicates that loss of HBeAg and serum HBV DNA is generally maintained (Korenman et al 1991).

One study has looked at recombinant alpha interferon following hepatic transplantation in patients with chronic HBV infection (Wright et al 1992). Several patients responded to this therapy. Although the immunostimulatory effects of interferon make graft rejection with this form of treatment a theoretical possibility, this was not seen. These results are very encouraging and further studies are awaited with interest.

Factors predicting response to interferon. A review of the possible factors that might predict a seroconversion response (loss of HBeAg) indicates that high serum transaminases, marked hepatic inflammatory activity, the presence of serum IgM anti-HBc and low serum HBV DNA (Brook et al 1989c, d, Chen et al 1989, Perillo et al 1990) are predictive of a response. Homosexual males seem less responsive than heterosexuals, in particular those who are anti-HIV antibody positive (McDonald et al 1987). Chinese chronic carriers, particularly children, show a very poor response (Lai et al 1987, Lok et al 1988b, c, 1990, 1992), whereas Caucasian heterosexual carriers (who usually acquire their infection in adulthood) respond the best (Brook et al 1989c). The reason for this poor response is that, unlike Caucasian patients, most Chinese patients (particularly children) have normal transaminase levels (Lok & Lai 1988). However, in Chinese patients with elevated transaminase levels, the response rate is the same as for Caucasian patients (Lok et al 1992). Many Chinese carriers have been infected from birth, and it is possible that this induces an immune tolerance that results in a lesser immune reaction against the virus. Another possibility is that Chinese patients are more likely to develop antibodies against interferon. One study has indicated that antibodies against recombinant alpha-2a interferon develop in about 25% of patients overall, and may reduce the chances of successful seroconversion, particularly if they appear whilst the patient is still HBV DNA positive (Porres et al 1989). One study (Lok et al 1990) has suggested that these antibodies are much more likely to develop in Chinese patients (39%) than Caucasian individuals (14%).

Beta interferon. Beta interferon, obtained from fibroblasts, is produced by recombinant DNA technology. An uncontrolled study from Japan using 3–6 MU/M^2 given daily by intravenous infusion suggested a rate of e antigen loss of about 35% (Suzuki et al 1986). However, a preliminary small controlled study from Germany indicated that, as a single agent, beta interferon does not contribute significantly to clinical improvement in chronic HBV infection (Muller et al 1982).

Type II interferon (gamma). Gamma interferon has powerful immunomodulatory effects, but is not as powerful an antiviral agent as type I interferons. One study has shown that gamma interferon produces immunomodulatory effects and slight reductions in HBV DNA polymerase activity but no seroconversions after 8 weeks' therapy with 0.05–1 mU daily (Lisker-Melman et al 1988). Another study comparing gamma interferon with alpha interferon indicates that side-effects are greater, antiviral effects are less and overall response rates lower for gamma interferon (Kakumu et al 1991). As a single agent, gamma interferon may have clinical value, although it appears unlikely that it will be better than type I interferons. Combination studies with type I interferons may be more promising.

Interleukin 2. Again, no controlled studies using this agent in chronic hepatitis B have been published. In an uncontrolled pilot study DNA polymerase levels fell in some treated individuals and HBe antigen to antibody seroconversion was observed in 3 out of 10 treated patients at 1 year (Kakumu et al 1988b). Without a control group these data are encouraging but difficult to interpret.

Combination therapies

Although it is believed that the liver damage in chronic hepatitis B infection is immunologically mediated (Dienstag et al 1982), immunosuppressive therapy in the form of corticosteroid therapy alone has largely been abandoned. The immune system cannot be safely suppressed to a degree that prevents liver damage, and several studies have now shown that, particularly in patients with more advanced liver disease, serious hepatic decompensation may occur when the steroids are withdrawn (Nair et al 1985, Hoofnagle et al 1986). However, a short course of steroids can provide a 'rebound' immunostimulatory effect when the steroids are stopped which, in combination with other antiviral and immunomodulatory therapies, may provide a useful approach, particularly in chronic carriers who have acquired their infection at birth.

Prednisolone withdrawal (priming) and alpha interferon. In a small uncontrolled study on five patients pretreated with steroids followed by interferon three (60%) of the patients seroconverted (Omata et al 1985). However, the results of several controlled studies suggest that seroconversion rates are no higher for this regimen than after interferon alone (Table 10.6). This lack of a significantly increased response rate with prednisolone priming is disappointing, and it is suggested that this regimen only be used in those patients who fail to respond to interferon alone. An interesting finding in one prednisolone priming study was that three anti-HIV antibody-positive patients were treated and two seroconverted (Perillo et al 1988). Both of these patients had normal CD4 to CD8 ratios, and this indicates that anti-HIV positivity per se should not be used as a predictor of treatment failure. However, patients with serious hepatic disease must be excluded from this type of therapy.

Prednisolone priming and adenine arabinoside. Two controlled studies of prednisolone pretreatment followed by ARA-A have been performed (Table 10.7). The seroconversion rates are encouraging, but once again the toxicity of ARA-A and ARA-AMP is the limiting factor.

Acyclovir and interferon. A pilot uncontrolled study has shown that this combination may be better than either agent alone (Schalm et al 1986). One small controlled study on acyclovir plus interferon in chronic hepatitis B infection has been performed (DeMan et al 1988). In this study, 40% of 18 patients treated with lymphoblastoid interferon and oral deoxyacyclovir for 4 months seroconverted from e to anti-e, compared with 0% of 18 patients in the control group. Interferon alone may seroconvert up to 60% and, as no comparison with an identical treatment period of interferon alone was performed, interpretation is difficult. A further case report from the Netherlands has also suggested that the combination of acyclovir and interferon may also be useful in HBV-associated glomerulonephritis (DeMan et al 1989).

Table 10.6 Controlled trials of treatment for HBeAg-positive chronic HBV infection with prednisolone pretreatment followed by interferon

	Loss of HBeAg		
Regimen	Untreated	Treated	Reference
20–60 mg prednisolone for 6 weeks, IFN 5 MU/m^2/day	4/21 (19%)	8/18 (44%)	Omata et al 1985
20–60 mg prednisolone for 6 weeks, 5 MU IFN daily for 4 months	3/43 (7%)	16/44 (36%)	Perillo et al 1990
20–60 mg prednisolone for 6 weeks, IFN 5 MU daily for 4 months	2/14 (14%)	6/15 (40%)	Fevery et al 1990
20–60 mg prednisolone for 6 weeks, IFN 10 MU t.i.w. for 4 months	1/18 (6%)	10/17 (59%)	Perez et al 1990
0.2–0.6 mg/kg prednisolone for 6 weeks, IFN 5 MU t.i.w. for 4 months	0/30 (0%)	4/31 (13%)	Lai et al 1991
15–45 mg prednisolone for 6 weeks, 10 MU IFN t.i.w. for 4 months	3/36 (8%)	9/40 (23%)	Lok et al 1992

MU = million units

Interferon and adenine arabinoside. One study of a 6-month combination of ARA-AMP (given twice daily every other month) and leucocyte interferon (given twice daily, alternating every other month with ARA-AMP) in 13 patients showed no benefit of the combination compared with placebo alone (Garcia et al 1987). Many of the patients in this study suffered considerable neuromuscular toxicity, but the cumulative dose of ARA-AMP used in this study was large, and the interferon was administered twice daily, rather than thrice weekly. Tailored regimens that utilize a shorter course of lactosaminated albuminated ARA-AMP (Fiume et al 1987) pretreatment (to reduce HBV-DNA levels) followed by thrice-weekly interferon may be more successful and less toxic.

Type I and type II interferons. Two studies on the combination of alpha and gamma interferons have been performed (Carreno et al 1987, Di Bisceglie et al 1990). Although a therapeutic effect was seen in one of these studies (Carreno et al 1987), the other study did not suggest any benefit from the combination, and gamma interferon alone had minimal inhibitory activity on viral replication, did not show any additive or synergistic effects when added to alpha interferon and contributed greatly to side-effects (Di Bisceglie et al 1990).

In a pilot controlled study of beta and gamma interferons in combination (Table 10.8), 50% of the treated patients successfully lost HBV infection. No comparison with either of the interferons alone was undertaken, and further studies are needed to evaluate these preliminary results.

HBeAg-negative (pre-core mutant) chronic HBV infection

The majority of anti-HBe-positive patients with

Table 10.7 Controlled trials of treatment of HBeAg-positive chronic HBV infection with prednisolone pretreatment followed by ARA-A or ARA-AMP

	Loss of HBeAg		
Regimen	Untreated	Treated	Reference
40 mg/day prednisolone for 4 weeks, ARA-A 10 mg/kg for 4–8 weeks	2/10 (20%)	6/9 (55%)	Yokosuka et al 1985
40 mg/day prednisolone for 8 weeks, ARA-AMP 10 mg/kg for 5 days then 5 mg/kg for 23 days	1/17 (6%)	8/11 (73%)	Perillo et al 1985

Table 10.8 Controlled trial of treatment of HBeAg-positive chronic HBV infection with combination beta and gamma interferon

	Loss of HBeAg		
Regimen	Untreated	Treated	Reference
3 MU IFN-β daily and 1 MU-IFN-γ for 23 days	1/10 (10%)	5/10 (50%)	Caselmann et al 1989

chronic HBs antigenaemia have no evidence of inflammatory liver disease (serum transaminases and liver histology are normal). However, a minority of patients are HBe antigen negative and have seroconverted to anti-HBe, yet remain viraemic and frequently have a more severe and rapidly progressive liver disease (Chu et al 1985, Bonino et al 1986). This disease is caused by a mutant virus that has a novel translational stop codon in the pre-core/core gene of HBV (Carman et al 1989). Hepatocytes infected with this mutant virus cannot secrete HBe antigen.

Several controlled trials using alpha interferon in HBeAg-negative patients with continuing viraemia due to replication of the mutant HBV have been undertaken (Table 10.9). This type of hepatitis responds in much the same way as HBeAg-positive disease, with response rates varying between 25 and 65%. The biochemical profile of response is different from HBeAg-positive chronic HBV; instead of the delayed 'seroconversion hepatitis', there is instead a rapid and steady fall in serum transaminase levels in responding patients. Reactivation of HBV replication may also be more common than in HBeAg-positive carriers (Hadziyannis et al 1990).

CONCLUSIONS

Despite intensive study, it is still not exactly clear why some patients develop chronic HBV infection and which of the many viral and host factors described are the most important in terms of viral persistence. HBV persistence appears multifactorial, and it is likely that many different reasons may combine to explain why some patients develop the chronic carrier state. For example, in neonates, immaturity of the immune system and transplacental transfer of viral HBeAg and maternal anti-HBc may be important, whilst in adults the quantitative and qualitative interferon abnormalities may be more crucial. The recent description of HBV mutants that may modify disease pathogenicity will undoubtedly further increase our understanding of the mechanisms of HBV persistence.

Because of the morbidity of this virus, several different antiviral therapies have been utilized. At present, lymphoblastoid or recombinant alpha interferons appear to be the best choice, and offer up to a 40% chance of HBe antigen seroconversion (elimination of replicating virus) in patients with evidence of active hepatic inflammation (raised serum transaminases and active hepatitis on liver

Table 10.9 Controlled trials of treatment of HBeAg-negative chronic HBV infection with recombinant or lymphoblastoid alpha interferon

	Loss of HBeAg		
Regimen	Untreated	Treated	Reference
9 MU t.i.w. recombinant IFN for 16 weeks	0/12 (0%)	3/12 (25%)	Brunetto et al 1989
3 MU t.i.w. recombinant IFN for 14–16 weeks	2/18 (11%)	11/17 (65%)	Hadziyannis et al 1990
5 MU/M^2 t.i.w. lymphoblastoid IFN for 6 months	5/30 (17%)	16/30 (53%)	Fattovich et al 1992

biopsy). However, in patients with minimal liver inflammation, response to alpha interferon alone is poor. Higher seroconversion rates may be obtained in this group of patients with combination therapies, in particular those utilizing a pretreatment period with prednisolone. Unfortunately this latter group of patients – infected since birth – constitute by far the largest proportion of chronic carriers (mostly from China and South-East Asia). Further studies of newer single agents and also of different combination regimens are required.

REFERENCES

Abb J, Zachoval R, Eisenberg J et al 1985 Production of interferon alpha and interferon gamma by peripheral blood leucocytes from patients with chronic hepatitis B infection. Journal of Medical Virology 16: 171–176

Alexander G J M, Eddleston ALWF 1986a Does maternal antibody to core antigen prevent recognition of transplacental transmission of hepatitis B virus? Lancet i: 296–297

Alexander G J M, Eddleston AWLF 1986b Immunology of acute and chronic hepatitis. In: Triger DR (ed) Immunology of the gastrointestinal system. John Wright, Bristol pp 176–205

Alexander G J M, Fagan E A, Hegarty J E et al 1987a Controlled clinical trial of acyclovir in chronic hepatitis B virus infection. Journal of Medical Virology 21: 81–87

Alexander G J M, Brahm J, Fagan E A et al 1987b Loss of HBsAg with interferon therapy in chronic HBV infection. Lancet ii: 66–69

Anastassakos C, Alexander G J M, Wolstencroft R A et al 1988 Interleukin 1 and interleukin 2 activity in chronic hepatitis B virus infection. Gastroenterology 94: 999–1005

Anderson M G, Harrison T J, Alexander G J M et al 1986 Randomised controlled trial of lymphoblastoid interferon for chronic active hepatitis B. Journal of Hepatology 3 (suppl. 2): S225–S227

Barbara L, Mazzella G, Baraldini M et al 1986 A randomized controlled trial with human lymphoblastoid interferon vs no therapy in chronic hepatitis B infection. Journal of Hepatology 3 (suppl. 2): S235–238

Bassendine M F, Chadwick R G, Salmeron J et al 1981 Adenine arabinoside therapy in HBsAg-positive chronic liver disease: a controlled study. Gastroenterology 80: 1016–1021

Beasley R P, Hwang L, Lin C et al 1981a Hepatocellular carcinoma and hepatitis B virus: a prospective study of 22 700 men in Taiwan. Lancet ii: 1129–1132

Beasley R P, Hwang L Y, Lin C C et al 1981b Hepatitis B immune globulin (HBIG) in the interruption of perinatal transmission of hepatitis B carrier state. Lancet ii: 388–393

Berg P A, Crattig N, Crauer W 1982 Immunoregulatory serum factors in acute and chronic hepatitis. Liver 2: 275–278

Bonino F, Rosina F, Rizetto M et al 1986 Chronic hepatitis in HBsAg carriers with serum HBV DNA and anti-HBe. Gastroenterology 90: 1268–1273

Brechot C, Scotto J, Charnay P et al 1981 Detection of hepatitis B virus DNA in liver and serum. A direct appraisal of the chronic carrier state. Lancet ii: 765–767

Brook M G, Petrovic L, McDonald J A et al 1989a. Histological improvement after anti-viral treatment for chronic hepatitis B infection. Journal of Hepatology 8: 218–225

Brook M G, Chan G, Yap I et al 1989b. Randomised controlled trial of treatment with lymphoblastoid alpha-interferon in caucasian males with chronic hepatitis B virus infection. British Medical Journal 299: 652–656

Brook M G, Karayiannis P, Thomas H C 1989c Which patients with chronic hepatitis B virus infection will respond to alpha-interferon therapy? A statistical analysis of predictive factors. Hepatology 10: 761–763

Brook M G, McDonald J A, Karayiannis P et al 1989d. Randomised controlled trial of interferon-alfa 2A for the treatment of chronic hepatitis B virus infection: factors that influence response. Gut: 1116–1122

Brown S E, Howard C R, Zuckerman A J et al 1984 Affinity of antibody responses in man to hepatitis B vaccine determined with synthetic peptides. Lancet i: 184–187

Brunetto M R, Oliveri F, Rocca G et al 1989 Natural course and response to interferon of chronic hepatitis B accompanied by antibody to hepatitis Be antigen. Hepatology 10: 198–203

Carman W F, Jacyna M R, Hadziyannis S et al 1989 Mutation preventing formation of hepatitis B e antigen in patients with chronic hepatitis B infection. Lancet ii: 588–591

Carreno V, Mora I 1987 Combination of recombinant interferons alpha and gamma in treatment of chronic hepatitis B. Lancet ii: 1086–1087

Caselmann W H, Eisenberg J, Hofschneider P H et al 1989 Beta and gamma interferon in chronic active hepatitis B: a pilot trial of short-term combination therapy. Gastroenterology 96: 449–455

Chang C, Enders G, Sprengel R et al 1987 Expression of the pre-core region of an avian hepatitis B virus is not required for viral replication. Journal of Virology 61: 3322–3325

Chemello L, Mondelli M, Bortolotti M et al 1986 Natural killer cell activation in patients with acute viral hepatitis. Clinical and Experimental Immunology 64: 59–64

Chen G, Karayiannis P, McGarvey M J et al 1989 Subclasses of anti-HBe in chronic HBV carriers: changes during treatment with interferon and predictors of response. Gut 30: 1123–1128

Chu C M, Karayiannis P, Fowler M J F et al 1985. Natural studies of chronic HBV infection in Taiwan: studies of HBV-DNA in serum. Hepatology 5: 431–434

Craxi A, Montano L, Goodall A et al 1982 Genetic and sex-linked factors influencing HBs antigen clearance. Journal of Medical Virology 9: 117–123

Davis G L, Hoofnagle J H, Waggoner J G 1984 Spontaneous reactivation of chronic hepatitis B infection. Gastroenterology 86: 230–235

Dejean A 1985 Specific hepatitis B virus integration in hepatocellular carcinoma DNA through a viral 11-base-pair

direct repeat. Proceedings of the National Academy of Sciences of the USA 81: 5350–5358
De Man R A, Schalm S W, Heijtink R A et al 1988 Long-term follow-up of antiviral combination therapy in chronic hepatitis B. American Journal of Medicine 85 (suppl. 2A): 150–154
De Man R A, Schalm S W, Van Der Heijden L et al 1989 Improvement of hepatitis B associated glomerulonephritis after antiviral combination therapy. Journal of Hepatology 8: 367–372
Di Bisceglie A M, Rustgi V K, Kassianides C et al 1990 Therapy of chronic hepatitis B with recombinant human alpha and gamma interferons. Hepatology 11: 266–270
Dienstag J L 1984. Immunologic mechanisms in chronic viral hepatitis. In: Vyas G N, Dienstag J L, Hoofnagle J H (eds) Viral hepatitis and liver disease. Grune & Stratton, London, pp 135–166
Dienstag J L, Bhan A K, Klingenstein R J et al 1982 Immunopathogenesis of liver disease associated with hepatitis B. In: Szmuness W, Alter H J, Maynard J E (eds) Viral hepatitis. Franklin Institute Press, Philadelphia, pp 221–236
Doherty P C, Zinkernagel R M A 1975 Biological role for the major histocompatability antigen. Lancet i: 1405–1409
Dooley J S, Davis G L, Peters M et al 1986 Pilot study of recombinant human alpha interferon for chronic type B hepatitis. Gastroenterology 90: 150–157
Dusheiko G M, Hoofnagle J H, Cooksley W G et al 1983 Synthesis of antibodies to hepatitis B virus by cultured lymphocytes from chronic hepatitis B surface antigen carriers. Journal of Clinical Investigation 71: 1104–1113
Dusheiko G M, Kassianides C, Song E et al 1988 Loss of hepatitis B surface antigen in three controlled trials of recombinant alpha-interferon for treatment of chronic hepatitis B. In: Zuckerman A J (ed) Viral hepatitis and liver disease. Alan R. Liss, New York, pp 844–847
Eddleston AWLF, Mondelli M, Mieli-Vergani G et al 1982 Lymphocyte cytotoxicity to autologous hepatocytes in chronic hepatitis B infection. Hepatology 2: 122S–127S
Eggink H F, Houthhoff H J, Huitema S et al 1982 Cellular and humoral immune reactions in chronic liver disease. Lymphocyte subsets in liver biopsies of patients with untreated idiopathic autoimmune hepatitis, chronic active hepatitis B and primary biliary cirrhosis. Clinical and Experimental Immunology 50: 17–24
Farza H, Salman A, Hadchouel M et al 1987 Hepatitis B surface antigen gene expression is regulated by sex steroids and glucocorticoids in transgenic mice. Proceedings of the National Academy of Sciences of the USA 84: 1187–1191
Fattovitch G, Rugge M, Brollo L et al 1986 Clinical, virologic and histologic outcome following seroconversion from HBeAg to anti-HBe in chronic hepatitis type B. Hepatology 6: 167–172
Fattovich G, Farci P, Rugge M et al 1992 A randomized controlled trial of lymphoblastoid interferon-alfa in patients with chronic hepatitis B lacking HBeAg. Hepatology 15: 584–589
Fevery J, Elwaut A, Michielsen P et al 1990 Efficacy of interferon alfa-2b with or without prednisolone withdrawal in the treatment of chronic viral hepatitis B. A prospective double-blind Belgian–Dutch study. Journal of Hepatology 11: S108–S112
Fiume L, Cerenzia M R T, Bonino F et al 1987 Inhibition of hepatitis B virus replication by vidaribine monophosphate conjugated with lactosaminated serum albumin. Lancet ii: 13–15
Foster G R, Ackrill A M, Goldin R D et al 1991 Expression of the terminal protein region of hepatitis B virus inhibits cellular responses to interferons alpha and gamma and double-stranded RNA. Proceedings of the National Academy of Sciences of the USA 88: 2888–2892
Friedman R L, Stark G R 1985 Interferon induced transcription of HLA and metallothionein genes containing homologous upstream sequences. Nature 314: 637–639
Fujinam R S, Oldstone MBA 1981 Alterations in expression of measles virus polypeptides by antibody: molecular events in antibody induced antigenic modulation. Journal of Immunology 125: 78–85
Fujisawa K, Yamzaki K, Kawase H et al 1987 Interferon therapy for chronic viral hepatitis and the use of peripheral lymphocytic 2',5'-oligoadenylate synthetase. In: Zuckerman A J (ed) Viral hepatitis and liver disease. Alan R. Liss, New York, pp 834–839
Garcia G, Smith C I, Weissberg J I et al 1987 Adenine arabinoside monophosphate (vidarabine) in combination with human leukocyte interferon in the treatment of chronic hepatitis B. Annals of Internal Medicine 107: 278–285
Gudat F, Bianchi L, Sonnaband W et al 1975 Pattern of core and surface expression in liver tissue reflects state of immune response in hepatitis B. Journal of Laboratory Investigation 32: 1–9
Hadziyannis S, Bramou T, Makris A et al 1990 Interferon-alfa2b treatment of HBeAg negative/serum HBV-DNA positive chronic active hepatitis type B. Journal of Hepatology 11: S133–S136
Hoofnagle J H 1974 Antibody to hepatitis B core antigen; A sensitive indicator of hepatitis B virus replication. New England Journal of Medicine 290: 1336–1339
Hoofnagle J H 1978 Type B hepatitis after transfusion with blood containing antibody to hepatitis B core antigen. New England Journal of Medicine 298: 1379–1385
Hoofnagle J H, Dusheiko G M, Seef L B et al 1981 Seroconversion from hepatitis B e antigen to antibody in chronic type B hepatitis. Annals of Internal Medicine 94: 744–748
Hoofnagle J H, Dusheiko G M, Schafer D F et al 1982 Reactivation of chronic hepatitis B virus infection by cancer chemotherapy. Annals of Internal Medicine 96: 447–449
Hoofnagle J H, Hanson R G, Minuk G Y et al 1984 Randomized controlled trial of adenine arabinoside monophosphate for chronic type B hepatitis. Gastroenterology 86: 150–157
Hoofnagle J H, Peter M, Mullen K D et al 1985 Randomised controlled trial of a four month course of recombinant alpha interferon in patients with chronic type B hepatitis. Hepatology 5: 1033–1039
Hoofnagle J H, Davis G L, Pappas C et al 1986 A short course of prednisolone in chronic type B hepatitis: report of a randomised, double blind, placebo controlled trial. Annals of Internal Medicine 104: 12–17
Hoofnagle J H, Peters M, Mullen K D et al 1988 Randomized, controlled trial of recombinant human alpha-interferon in patients with chronic hepatitis-B. Gastroenterology 95: 1318–1325
Ibarra M Z, Mora I, Quiroga J A et al 1988 IgG and IgM

autoantiidiotype antibodies against antibody to HBsAg in chronic hepatitis B. Hepatology 8: 775–780

Ikeda T, Lever A M L, Thomas H C 1986a Evidence for a deficiency of interferon production in patients with chronic HBV acquired in adult life. Hepatology 6: 962–965

Ikeda T, Pignatelli M, Lever A M L et al 1986b Relationship of HLA protein display to activation of 2–5A synthetase in HBe antigen or anti-HBe positive chronic HBV infection. Gut 27: 1498–1501

Ishihara K, Waters J, Pignatelli M et al 1987 Charaterisation of the polymerised and monomeric human serum albumin binding sites on hepatitis B surface antigen. Journal of Medical Virology 21: 89–95

Iwarson S, Tabor E, Thomas H C et al 1985 Neutralisation of hepatitis B virus infectivity by a murine monoclonal antibody: An experimental study in the chimpanzee. Journal of Medical Virology 16: 89–96

Jacyna M R, Thomas H C 1990 Antiviral therapy in hepatitis B infection. British Medical Bulletin 46: 368–382

Joseph B S, Cooper N R, Oldstone M B A 1975 Immunologic injury of cultured cells infected with measles virus: Role of IgG antibody and the alternate pathway of complement. Journal of Experimental Medicine 141: 761–774

Kakumu S, Tahara H, Fuji A et al 1988a Interleukin 1 production by peripheral blood monocytes from patients with chronic liver disease and effect of sera on interleukin 1 production. Journal of Clinical and Laboratory Immunology 26: 113–119

Kakumu S, Fuji A, Yoshioka K et al 1988b. Pilot study of recombinant human interleukin 2 for chronic type B hepatitis. Hepatology 8:487–492

Kakumu S, Ishikawa T, Mizokami M et al 1991 Treatment with human gamma interferon of chronic hepatitis B: comparative study with alpha interferon. Journal of Medical Virology 35: 32–37

Kato Y, Nakagawa H, Kobayashi K 1982 Interferon production by peripheral lymphocytes in HBsAg positive liver disease. Hepatology 2: 789–790

Korenman J, Baker B, Waggoner J et al 1991 Long-term remissions of chronic hepatitis B after alpha-interferon therapy. Annals of Internal Medicine 114: 629–634

Lai C-L, Lok A S F, Lin H J et al 1987 Placebo-controlled trial of recombinant alpha interferon in chinese HBsAg carrier children. Lancet ii: 877–880

Lai C-L, Lau J Y-N, Flok A S et al 1991 Effect of recombinant alpha-interferon with or without prednisolone priming in Chinese HBsAg carrier children. Quarterly Journal of Medicine 78: 155–163

Laure F, Chatenoud L, Pasquinelli C et al 1987 Frequent lymphocyte infection by hepatitis B virus in haemophiliacs British Journal of Haematology 65: 181–185

Lever A M L, Thomas H C 1986 Treatment of chronic hepatitis B infection. Clinics in Tropical Medicine and Communicable Diseases 1: 377–393

Lever A M L, Waters J, Brook M G et al 1990 Monoclonal antibody to HBsAg for chronic hepatitis B virus infection with hypogammaglobulinaemia. Lancet 335: 1529–1530

Levin S, Hahn T 1982 Interferon system in acute viral hepatitis. Lancet i: 592–594

Liaw Y F, Chu C M, Su I J et al 1983 Clinical and histological events preceding hepatitis B e antigen seroconversion in chronic type B hepatitis. Gastroenterology 84: 216–219

Lin H H, Lee T Y, Chen D S et al 1987 Transplacental leakage of HBeAg positive maternal blood as the most likely route in causing intrauterine infection with hepatitis B virus. Journal of Pediatrics iii: 877–881

Lisker-Melman M, Peters M, Ambrus J L et al 1988 Effect of recombinant human gamma interferon therapy on immune function in patients with chronic type B hepatitis. In: Zuckerman A J (ed) Viral hepatitis and liver disease. Alan R Liss, New York, pp 868–871

Lok ASF, Lai C L 1988 A longitudinal follow-up of asymptomatic hepatitis B surface antigen positive CHinese children. Hepatology 80: 1130–1133

Lok A S F, Wilson L A, Thomas H C 1984 Neurotoxicity associated with adenosine arabinoside monophosphate in the treatment of chronic hepatitis B virus infection. Journal of Antimicrobial Chemotherapy 14: 93–99

Lok A S F, Novick D M, Karayiannis P et al 1985 A randomised study of the effect of adenine arabinoside 5'-monophosphate (short or long course) and lymphoblastoid interferon on hepatitis B replication. Hepatology 5: 1132–1138

Lok A S F, Karayiannis P, Jowett T et al 1988a Studies of HBV replication during acute hepatitis followed by recovery and acute hepatitis progressing to chronic disease. Journal of Hepatology 51: 671–679

Lok A S F, Lai C L, Wu P C et al 1988b A randomized controlled trial of recombinant alpha-2 interferon in Chinese patients with chronic hepatitis B virus infection. In: Zuckerman A J (ed) Viral hepatitis and liver disease. Alan R. Liss, New York, pp 848–853

Lok A S F, Lai C-L, Wu P-C et al 1988c Long-term follow up in a randomised controlled trial of recombinant alpha-interferon in Chinese patients with chronic hepatitis B infection. Lancet ii: 298–302

Lok A S F, Lai C-L Leung E K-Y 1990 Interferon antibodies may negate the antiviral effects of recombinant alpha-interferon treatment in patients with chronic hepatitis B virus infection. Hepatology 12: 1266–1270

Lok A S F, WU P-C, Lai C-L et al 1992 A controlled trial of interferon with or without prednisolone priming for chronic hepatitis B. Gastroenterology 102: 2091–2097

McDonald J A, Caruso L, Karayiannis P et al 1987 Diminished reponsiveness of male homosexual chronic hepatitis B carriers with HTLV-III antibodies to recombinant alpha-interferon. Hepatology 7: 719–723

Machida A, Kishimoto S, Ohruma H et al 1983 A hepatitis B surface antigen polypeptide (p 31) with the receptor for polymerised human as well as chimpanzee albumin. Gastroenterology 85: 268–274

Mazzella G, Saracco G, Rizetto M et al 1988 Human lymphoblastoid interferon for the treatment of chronic hepatitis B. American Journal of Medicine 85 (suppl. 2A): 141–142

Milich D R, Jones J E, Hughes J L et al 1990 Is a function of the secreted hepatitis B e antigen to induce immunologic tolerance in utero? Proceedings of the National Academy of Sciences of the USA 87: 6599–6603

Mondelli M, Mieli-Vergani G, Alberti A et al 1982 Specificity of T lymphocyte cytotoxicity to autologous hepatocytes in chronic hepatitis B virus infection; evidence that T cells are directed against HBV antigen expressed on hepatocytes. Journal of Immunology 129: 2773–2778

Montano L, Miescher G C et al 1982 Hepatitis B virus and HLA display in the liver during chronic hepatitis B virus infection. Hepatology 2:557–561

Muller R, Deinhardt F, Hofschneider P H et al 1982 Long-term treatment with human fibroblast interferon in chronic hepatitis B infection. In: Szmuness W, Alter H J, Maynard J E (eds) Viral hepatitis. Franklin Institute Press, Philadelphia, p 648

Nair P V, Tong M J, Stevenson D et al 1985 Effects of short-term high dose prednisone treatment of patients with HBsAg-positive chronic active hepatitis. Liver 5: 8–12

Nash AA 1985 Tolerance and suppression in virus disease. British Medical Bulletin 41: 41–45

Neurath A R, Kent S B H, Strick N et al 1986 Identification and chemical synthesis of a host receptor binding site on hepatitis B virus. Cell 46: 429–436

Novick D M, Lok A S F, Thomas et al 1984 Diminished responsiveness of homosexual men to antiviral therapy with HBsAg positive chronic liver disease. Journal of Hepatology 1: 29–35

Omata M, Imazeki F, Yokosuka O et al 1985 Recombinant leukocyte A interferon treatment in patients with chronic hepatitis B virus infection. Pharmacokinetics, tolerance and biologic effects. Gastroenterology 88: 870–880

Onji M, Lever A M L, Saito I, Thomas H C 1989 Defective response to interferons in cells transfected with the hepatitis B genome. Hepatology 9: 92–96

Ou J, Lauk O, Rutter W 1986 Hepatitis B gene function: The pre-core region targets the core antigen to cellular membranes and causes the secretion of the HBe antigen. Proceedings of the National Academy of Sciences of the USA 83: 1578–1582

Paul R G, Roodman S T, Campbell C R et al 1991 HLA class I antigen expression as a measure of response to antiviral therapy of chronic hepatitis B. Hepatology 13: 820–825

Perez V, Tanno H, Fay T et al 1988 Treatment of chronic active hepatitis B with recombinant interferon alpha A. In: Zuckerman A J Viral hepatitis and liver disease. Alan R. Liss, New York, pp 851–854

Perez V, Tanno H, Villamil F et al 1990 Recombinant interferon alfa-2b following prednisolone withdrawal in the treatment of chronic type B hepatitis. Journal of Hepatology 11: S113–S117

Perillo R P, Brunt E M 1991 Hepatic histologic and immunohistochemical changes in chronic hepatitis B after prolonged clearance of hepatitis B e antigen and hepatitis B surface antigen. Annals of Internal Medicine 115: 113–115

Perillo R, Regenstein F, Bodicky C et al 1985 Comparative efficacy of adenine arabinoside 5'-monophosphate and prednisolone withdrawal followed by adenine arabinoside 5'-monophosphate in the treatment of chronic active hepatitis type B. Gastroenterology 88: 780–786

Perillo R, Regenstein F G, Peters M et al 1988 Prednisone withdrawal followed by recombinant alpha interferon in the treatment of chronic hepatitis B. Annals of Internal Medicine 109: 95–100

Perillo R P, Schiff E R, Davis G L et al 1990 A randomised controlled trial of interferon alfa-2b alone and after prednisolone withdrawal for the treatment of chronic hepatitis B. New England Journal of Medicine 323: 295–301

Perrin L H, Joseph B S, Cooper N R et al 1976 Mechanisms of injury of virus infected cells by antiviral antibody and complement: participation of IgG, F(ab) and the alternate complement pathway. Journal of Experimental Medicine 143: 1027–1041

Pignatelli M, Waters J, Lever A M L et al 1986 HLA class I antigens on hepatocyte membrane: Increased expression during acute hepatitis and interferon therapy of chronic hepatitis B. Hepatology 6: 349–353

Pignatelli M, Waters J, Lever A M L et al 1987 Cytotoxic T-cell responses to the nucleocapsid proteins of HBV in chronic hepatitis. Journal of Hepatology 4: 15–21

Poitrine A, Chousterman S, Chousterman M et al 1985 Lack of in vivo activation of the interferon system in HBsAg positive chronic active liver disease. Hepatology 5: 171–174

Porres J C, Carreno V, Ruiz M et al 1989 Interferon antibodies in patients with chronic HBV infection treated with recombinant interferon. Journal of Hepatology 8: 351–357

Realdi G, Alberti A, Rugge M et al 1980 Seroconversion from hepatitis Be antigen to anti-HBe in chronic hepatitis B virus infection. Gastroenterolgy 79: 195–199

Roosinck M, Jamcel S, Loukin S et al 1986 Expression of hepatitis B viral core region in mammalian cells. Molecular and Cell Biology 6: 1393–1400

Schalm S W, Heijtink R A 1982 Spontaneous disappearance of viral replication and liver cell inflammation in HBsAg-positive chronic active hepatitis; results of a placebo vs. interferon trial. Hepatology 2: 791–794

Schalm S W, Heijtink R A, Van Buuren H R et al 1986 Acyclovir enhances the antiviral effect of interferon in chronic hepatitis B. Lancet ii: 358–360

Schlicht H-J, Schaller H 1989 The secretory core protein of HBV is expressed on the cell surface. Journal of Virology 63: 5399–5404

Scully L J, Shein R, Karayiannis P et al 1987 Lymphoblastoid interferon therapy of chronic hepatitis B infection: a comparison of 12 vs. 24 weeks of thrice weekly treatment. Hepatology 5: 51–58

Shafritz D A, Kew M 1981 Identification of integrated hepatitis B virus sequences in human hepatocellular carcinoma. Hepatology 1: 1–8

Shafritz D, Shouval D, Sherman H I et al 1981. Integration of hepatitis B virus DNA into the genome of liver cells in chronic liver disease and hepatocellular carcinoma. New England Journal of Medicine 305: 1067–1073

Smith C I, Scullard G H, Gregory P B et al 1981 Preliminary studies of acyclovir in chronic hepatitis B. American Journal of Medicine 73: 267–270

Suzuki H, Ichida F, Fujisawa K et al 1986 Long term follow-up of HBe antigen positive chronic hepatitis treated with human interferon beta. Hepatology 6: 776–781

Thomas H C 1982 Immunological mechanisms in chronic hepatitis B virus infection. Hepatology 2: 116S–119S

Thomas H C, Shipton U, Montano L 1982 The HLA system: its relevance to the pathogenesis of liver disease. Progress in Liver Disease 7: 517–527

Thomas H C, Pignatelli M, Lever A M L et al 1986 Homology between HBV-DNA and a sequence regulating the interferon-induced antiviral system. Journal of Medical Virology 19: 63–69

Trepo C, Hantz O, Ouzan D et al 1984 Therapeutic efficacy of ARA-AMP in symptomatic, HBeAg positive CAH: a randomized placebo controlled study. Hepatology 4: 1055–1061

Trepo C, Ouzan D, Fontagnes T et al 1986 Therapeutic activity of vidaribine in symptomatic chronic active hepatitis related to HBV. Journal of Hepatology 3 (suppl. 2): S97–S105

Trevisan A, Realdi G, Alberti A et al 1982 Core-antigen specific immunoglobulin G bound to the liver cell membrane in chronic hepatitis B. Gastroenterology 82: 218–222

Tur-Kaspa R, Burk R, Shaul Y et al 1986 Hepatitis B virus DNA contains a glucocorticoid-responsive element. Proceedings of the National Academy of Science of the USA 83: 1627–1631

Twu J S, Lee C H, Lin P M et al 1988 Hepatitis B virus suppresses expression of human beta-interferon. Proceedings of the National Academy of Science USA 85: 252–256

Viola L A, Barrison I G, Coleman J C et al 1981 Natural history of liver disease in chronic hepatitis B surface antigen carriers: a survey of 100 patients from Great Britain. Lancet ii: 1156–1159

Wakita T, Kakumu S, Shibata M et al 1991 Detection of pre-C and core region mutants of hepatitis B virus in chronic hepatitis B virus carriers. Journal of Clinical Investigation 88: 1793–1801

Waters J A, Jowett T P, Thomas H C 1986 Identification of dominant epitopes of the nucleocapsid (HBc) of the hepatitis B virus. Journal of Medical Virology 19: 79–86

Williams S J, Craig P I, Cooksley W G E et al 1990 Randomised controlled trial of recombinant human inteferon-alpha for chronic active hepatitis B. Australian and New Zealand Journal of Medicine 20: 9–19

Weller I V D, Carreno V, Fowler M J F et al 1983 Acyclovir in hepatitis B antigen-positive chronic liver disease; inhibition of viral replication and transient renal impairment with IV bolus administration. Journal of Antimicrobial Chemotherapy 11: 223–231

Weller I V D, Lok A S F, Sherlock S et al 1985 Randomised controlled trial of adenine arabinoside 5'-monophosphate in chronic hepatitis virus infection. Gut 26: 745–751

Weller I V D, Tedder R S, Karayiannis P et al 1986 A pilot study of B W A515U (6-deoxyacyclovir) in chronic hepatitis B infection. Journal of Hepatology 3 (suppl. 2): S119–S122

Wright H I, Gavaler J S, Van Theil T 1992 Preliminary experience with alpha-2b-interferon therapy of viral hepatitis in liver allograft recipients. Transplantation 53: 121–124

Wu J C, Lee S D, Tsay S H et al 1988 Symptomatic anti-HBe positive chronic hepatitis B in Taiwan with special reference to persistent HBV replication and HDV superinfection. Journal of Medical Virology 25: 141–148

Yamauchi K, Nakanishi T, Chiou S S et al 1988 Suppression of hepatitis B antibody synthesis by factor made by T cells from chronic hepatitis B carriers. Lancet i: 324–326

Yokosuka O, Omata M, Imazeki F et al 1985 Combination of short term prednisolone and adenine arabinoside in the treatment of chronic hepatitis B. Gastroenterology 89: 246–251

Yoo Y K, Gavaler J B, Chen K et al 1990 The effect of recombinant interferon-alfa on lymphocyte subpopulations and HLA-DR expression on liver tissue of HBV-positive individuals. Clinical and Experimental Immunology 82: 338–343

UPDATE

- A cytotoxic T lymphocyte (CTL) epitope located between HBcAg residues 141 and 151 that completely overlaps a critical domain in the viral nucleocapsid protein that is essential for its nuclear localization and genome packaging functions as well as processing of the pre-core protein has been reported. The CTL response to this epitope is dually restricted by the HLA-A31 and HLA-Aw68 alleles, which, unexpectedly, appear to use a common binding motif based on the results of alanine substitution and competition analysis, and the binding properties of these two alleles predicted from their known primary sequence, and from the three-dimensional structure of HLA-Aw68. The CTL response to this epitope is polyclonal during acute viral hepatitis, since these two restriction elements can present the HBcAg 141–151 epitope to independent CTL clones derived from a single patient; and the CTL response is multispecific, since HLA-A2-restricted and HLA-Aw68-restricted CTL responses to HBcAg 18–27 and HBcAg 141–151, respectively, have been identified to coexist in another patient. The foregoing argue against the emergence of CTL escape mutants as a significant problem during HBV infection, especially at this locus, where mutations might be incompatible with viral replication. These findings do suggest an association between the HBV-specific CTL response and viral clearance, and they have implications for the design of immunotherapeutic strategies to terminate HBV infection in chronically infected patients (Missale et al 1993).
- REFERENCE

Missale G, Redeker A, Person J et al 1993 HLA-A31- and HLA-Aw68-restricted cytotoxic T cell responses to a single hepatitis B virus nucleocapsid epitope during acute viral hepatitis. Journal of Experimental Medicine 177, 3: 751–762

11. Liver transplantation

Didier Samuel Patrick Marcellin Henri Bismuth
Jean-Pierre Benhamou

Liver transplantation is now a well-developed procedure and is presently the best available treatment for end-stage liver disease. Patients with chronic liver disease due to hepatitis B virus (HBV) infection represent a major group of candidates for liver transplantation (Bismuth et al 1987, Starzl et al 1989). However, after liver transplantation, there is a risk of HBV reinfection of the transplanted liver and, as a consequence, a risk of development of acute or chronic liver disease, leading to graft failure, death or retransplantation (Demetris et al 1986). It appears that the risk of HBV reinfection is very high in patients with detectable HBV replication before liver transplantation. Therefore, the indication for liver transplantation in HBsAg-positive patients, especially in those with HBV replication, remains controversial (Van Thiel et al 1984).

In this chapter, we will discuss the indications for liver transplantation for HBV-related liver disease, the mechanisms involved in HBV reinfection after liver transplantation, methods for prevention of HBV reinfection, and new developments in prevention and treatment of HBV reinfection. Only liver transplantation for HBV-related liver disease in the absence of hepatitis D virus infection will be considered in this chapter; liver transplantation for hepatitis D virus infection-related liver disease is considered in Chapter 22.

INDICATIONS FOR LIVER TRANSPLANTATION FOR HBV-RELATED LIVER DISEASE

The indications for liver transplantation for HBV-related liver disease are broadly similar to those for other diseases. Uncontrolled or poorly controlled ascites, spontaneous bacterial peritonitis, recurrent gastrointestinal bleeding and episodes of encephalopathy, associated with low albumin and prothrombin levels and high serum bilirubin level, are valid indicators of the severity of cirrhosis and, therefore, liver transplantation. There are some specific features of the prognosis of HBV-related chronic liver disease: the disease is frequently progressive in patients in whom HBV replication persists; active disease is suggested by a high level of serum transaminase and, at histological examination, hepatocyte necrosis and infiltration with inflammatory cells. In contrast to other chronic liver diseases, e.g. primary biliary cirrhosis, the prognosis for HBV-related cirrhosis can be difficult to assess, because the course of the disease can be dramatically altered by some events: (a) cessation of HBV replication, either spontaneously or after antiviral treatment, as indicated by the disappearance of HBV DNA from the serum and seroconversion from HBeAg to anti-HBe; (b) HBV reactivation, as indicated by the reappearance of HBV DNA and HBeAg in the serum (Davis & Hoofnagle 1987). Therefore, HBV-related chronic liver disease can either deteriorate to irreversible liver disease, or it can deteriorate transiently, with aggravation during HBeAg/Ab conversion, followed by a dramatic improvement.

RESULTS OF LIVER TRANSPLANTATION FOR HBV-RELATED LIVER DISEASE

Background

The overall risk of HBV reinfection after liver transplantation is up to 80% if no attempt is made to prevent it (Freeman et al 1991, Lake & Wright 1991, Rizzetto et al 1991, Todo et al 1991). In most cases, the reappearance of HBsAg is associated with the development of acute hepatitis (Demetris et al 1990). As for immunosuppressed patients, reappearance of HBsAg is associated with the reappearance of HBV DNA in serum and is followed, in most cases, by chronic infection with HBV. In a few cases, HBV reinfection induces fulminant liver failure, leading either to death or to emergency retransplantation (Demetris et al 1990).

The mechanism of HBV reinfection after liver transplantation is a subject for debate. Three main hypotheses have been postulated: (1) an immediate infection of the graft due to circulating HBV particules during or shortly after liver transplantation; (2) a reinfection of the graft due to the replication and shedding of HBV from extrahepatic sites; (3) a combination of the two. We believe that the second mechanism is involved, at least partly, in the reinfection of the grafted liver. HBV has been demonstrated in some extrahepatic sites, such as mononuclear cells, bone marrow, kidneys and pancreas (Dejean et al 1984). HBV replication has been demonstrated in peripheral blood mononuclear cells from chronically infected patients (Yoffee et al 1986, Hadchouel et al 1988). A replicative form of HBV has also been detected in peripheral blood mononuclear cells from liver-transplanted patients, but not in the serum, which suggests that peripheral blood mononuclear cells are involved in the mechanism of HBV reinfection of the grafted liver (Zignego et al 1988, Feray et al 1990, Yoffee & Muller 1991). In 11 patients HBsAg positive before liver tranplantation, who became HBsAg negative after liver transplantion while receiving anti-HBs immunoglobulins, HBV could be detected with PCR both in serum and peripheral blood mononuclear cells, but not in the grafted liver (Feray et al 1990).

Grafted liver lesions due to HBV reinfection

HBV reinfection of the grafted liver has the following characteristics:

1. After the reappearance of HBsAg in serum, there is a high risk of development of lesions of the grafted liver (Demetris et al 1990, Samuel et al 1991, O'Grady et al 1992).
2. In most cases, the reappearance of HBsAg is associated with the development of acute hepatitis and leads to chronic active hepatitis
3. The rapid development, within 12 months after reappearance of HBsAg, of cirrhosis of the grafted liver can be observed.

The particularly severe course of the disease of the grafted liver is likely to be related to post-transplant immunosuppressive treatment, which enhances HBV replication (Nagington et al 1977, Tur Kaspa & Laub 1990). However, we believe that mechanisms other than immunosuppression may be involved: in immunosuppressed patients affected by HBV-related liver disease (in the absence of liver transplantation) and in patients with HBV-related liver disease having received a kidney transplant, a rapidly severe course of the liver lesion is relatively uncommon (Degos et al 1988, Huang et al 1990).

Some authors have emphasized that, in patients with HBV reinfection after liver transplantation, HBV DNA and HBsAg levels are very high and have suggested that HBV could be directly cytopathic for hepatocytes in this situation (Demetris et al 1990, Lau et al 1992). Large amounts of HBsAg and HBeAg have been demonstrated in the cytoplasm and HBcAg in the nuclei of hepatocytes. The histological features of HBV-related lesions of the grafted liver are a paucity of inflammatory infiltrate, the rapid development of fibrosis and a frequent cholestasis associated with hepatocyte necrosis.

The King's College group in London has described an unusual clinical pathological pattern in some patients, with a particularly poor prognosis, termed fibrosing cholestatic hepatitis (Davies et al 1991). The histological features are extensive periportal fibrosis, canalicular and cellular cholestasis, enlargement of hepatocytes associated with extensive cytoplasmic HBsAg expression, variable degrees of HBcAg and HBeAg cytoplasmic expression and HBcAg and HBeAg nuclear expression; these features are different from those of the usual pattern of HBV-related lesions of the grafted liver, which are characterized by a high expression of HBcAg in nuclei without diffuse, extensive expression of HBsAg. Davies et al (1991) postulated that the widespread presence of HBsAg in patients with fibrosing cholestatic hepatitis suggests a non-immunologically mediated mechanism for hepatocyte damage. Demetris et al (1990) noted a gradual increase of HBsAg expression, both cytoplasmic and nuclear, in patients with HBV reinfection; they emphasized that, in some patients, degeneration of hepatocytes was associated with marked viral expression, but not inflammation; this supports the concept that HBV, in some circumstances, is directly cytopathic. It is noteworthy that, although high levels of HBsAg and HBcAg in the liver were observed in patients with fibrosing cholestatic hepatitis, the level of HBsAg in serum is not different from that in non-transplanted patients with HBV-related liver disease and from that in transplanted patients with HBV reinfection in the absence of fibrosing cholestatic hepatitis (Lau et al 1992). HBV has been shown to be directly cytopathic in transgenic mice models and HBV-transfected HepG2 cell lines (Chisari et al 1987, Roingeard et al 1990). Patients who become and remain serum HBsAg negative after liver transplantation usually show histologically normal liver and no HBV markers in the grafted liver, which emphasizes the importance of preventing HBsAg from reappearing in the serum of patients after liver transplantation (Feray et al 1990, Samuel et al 1991).

ANTI-HBs PASSIVE IMMUNOPROPHYLAXIS

Polyclonal anti-HBs immunoglobulins

The use of anti-HBs immunoglobulins (hepatitis B immunoglobulin, HBIG) to prevent HBV reinfection after liver transplantation was first reported in a patient receiving HBIG at the anhepatic phase and on day 6 post transplantation (Johnson et al 1978). The patient became HBsAg negative after the injection on day 6. The aim of this treatment was to neutralize HBV circulating particles during the anhepatic and post-transplant period. Subsequent reports have shown that, after administration of HBIG in this way, most patients either remained HBsAg positive or became HBsAg positive again in a short time (Lauchart et al 1987a, Todo et al 1991, O'Grady 1992). However, even this short term administration of HBIG seemed to delay the reappearance of HBsAg after liver transplantation (Mora et al 1990).

In Hannover, Germany, very high doses of HBIG were given during the first 6 days post transplantation, in order to neutralize HBsAg. Further HBIG was given iteratively until the sixth month post transplantation, if serum anti-HBs titre was <100 IU/l. All patients became HBs negative after liver transplantation; HBsAg reappeared only in those in whom HBV replication was detectable prior to liver transplantation (Lauchart et al 1987b). In another report by the same group, HBsAg reappeared in some patients after discontinuation of HBIG at 6–12 months post transplantation. We have used the same protocol of administration of HBIG as that proposed by the Hannover group, but without discontinuation of HBIG at 6 months post-transplantation. From June 1986 to September 1989, 40 patients transplanted for post-hepatitis B cirrhosis and 17 patients transplanted for fulminant hepatitis B have received 10 000 units of HBIG during the anhepatic phase, then 10 000 units every day for the first 6 post-operative days; then the titre of anti-HBs in serum was assessed weekly and 10 000 IU was readministered when the titre was <100 IU/l (Samuel et al 1991). The 2-year rate of HBsAg reappearance was much higher in patients with post-hepatitis B cirrhosis (59%) than in those with fulminant hepatitis B (0%). Furthermore, the 2-year rate of HBV reinfection was significantly higher in patients with post-hepatitis B cirrhosis who were serum HBV DNA positive than in those who were HBV DNA negative prior to liver transplantation (96% and 29% respectively). However, there was no correlation between the 2-year rate of HBV reinfection and the serum HBeAg status prior to transplantation: 63% in HBeAg-negative and 55% in HBeAg-positive patients. In patients treated by the Hannover group in whom HBIG administration was discontinued at 6–12 months post-transplantation, the rate of HBV reinfection was 88% in the patients who were HBV DNA positive and 28% in those who were HBV DNA negative prior to transplantation. Interestingly, in some patients given HBIG for 6–12 months, HBsAg reappeared in serum immediately to several months after the discontinuation of the treatment. It should be emphasized that, in these patients, HBsAg always reappeared within 18 months post-transplantation; this observation is consistent with our experience that HBsAg never reappeared over 24 months after liver transplantation in any of our patients.

In patients with fulminant hepatitis B, the risk of HBV reinfection can easily be controlled by HBIG. In our patients transplanted for fulminant hepatitis B and receiving long term HBIG, the rate of HBV reinfection was 0%. In contrast, in the series of Todo et al (1991), HBV reinfection developed in seven of the eight patients transplanted for fulminant hepatitis B who had not received HBIG; likewise, HBV reinfection affected all three of our patients with fulminant hepatitis B who had not received HBIG. It should be noted that HBV reinfection appeared to be less severe in patients transplanted for fulminant hepatitis B than in those transplanted for post-hepatitis B cirrhosis (Todo et al 1991).

The role of pre-transplantation HBV replicative status in post-transplantation HBV reinfection was demonstrated in a study from Pittsburgh, USA, on patients receiving no long-term HBIG: eight of 45 patients who were anti-HBe positive, but none of those who were HBeAg positive, cleared HBsAg after transplantation (Todo et al 1991). In contrast, in a study from King's, HBV reinfection developed after transplantation in 7 out of 9 non-replicative patients and in all 10 replicative patients (O'Grady et al 1992). In our experience and in Hannover, the pre-transplant HBV DNA level, as assessed by direct hybridization, was the best predictor of HBV reinfection after liver transplantation.

Although this conclusion is not based on controlled studies, it is clear that long-term administration of HBIG reduces the rate of HBV reinfection after liver transplantation in HBV DNA-negative patients with post-hepatitis B cirrhosis and in patients with fulminant hepatitis B, but not in HBV DNA-positive patients with post-hepatitis B cirrhosis. The overall rate of HBV reinfection after transplantation in different series of patients with post-hepatitis B cirrhosis is set out in Table 11.1. The rate of HBV reinfection according to the pre-transplantation HBV replicative status is set out in Tables 11.2 and 11.3.

Monoclonal anti-HBs immunoprophylaxis

The high cost of polyclonal HBIG, the need for its long-term administration and its poor results in HBV DNA-positive patients prompted the use of monoclonal anti-HBs. To our knowledge, seven patients have been treated with murine monoclonal anti-HBs; HBsAg has reappeared in four patients at 0, 143, 186, and 230 days post transplantation (Fung et al 1991). A case of HBV reinfection after liver transplantation due to an

Table 11.1 Overall rate of HBV reinfection after liver transplantation for post-hepatitic B cirrhosis

References	Number of patients	Preventive treatment	Rate of HBV reinfection (%)
Samuel et al 1991	40	Long-term anti-HBIG*	59†
Muller et al 1991	23	6–12 months anti-HBIG	57
Todo et al 1991	38	None or IFN† or short-term anti-HBIG	82
Hopf et al 1992	7	Short-term anti-HBIG or long-term anti-HBIG+IFN	71
O'Grady et al 1992	20	None or short-term anti-HBIG	90

*Anti-HBIG, anti-HBs immunoglobulins.
†2-year actuarial rate.
‡IFN, recombinant alpha interferon.

Table 11.2 Rate of HBV reinfection after liver transplantation for HBV replicative post-hepatitis B cirrhosis

References	Number of patients	Preventive treatment	Rate of HBV reinfection (%)
Samuel et al 1991	16	Long-term HBIG*	96†
Muller et al 1991	9	6–12 months HBIG	89
O'Grady et al 1992	11	None or short-term HBIG	100

*HBIG, anti-HBs immunoglobulins.
†2-year actuarial rate.

Table 11.3 Rate of HBV reinfection after liver transplantation for HBV non-replicative post-hepatitis B cirrhosis

References	Number of patients	Preventive treatment	Rate of HBV reinfection (%)
Samuel et al 1991	24	Long-term HBIG*	29†
Muller et al 1991	14	6–12 months HBIG	28
O'Grady et al 1992	9	None or short-term HBIG	78

*Anti-HBIG, anti-HBs immunoglobulins.
†2-year actuarial rate.

HBV mutant has been reported (MacMahon et al 1991); the mutation could be secondary to the monoclonal anti-HBs being too selective against one epitope. In future, it will be necessary to use humanized monoclonal anti-HBs against selected epitopes, thereby avoiding the emergence of mutants.

ANTI-HBs VACCINATION

Active anti-HBV immunization has been tried in liver transplantation either alone or in combination with administration of HBIG. Various protocols have been proposed: four successive administrations of HBIG vaccine or a single high dose of vaccine. In our experience, high doses (four times the recommended dose) of an HBV vaccine containing the pre-S2 protein have given disappointing results, since no anti-HBs response was obtained. Results from other centres are similarly disappointing (Lauchart et al 1987b), while others are encouraging (Colledan et al 1987), which makes it difficult to draw any definite conclusion about the efficacy of HBV vaccination in preventing HBV reinfection.

ANTIVIRAL TREATMENT

Two antiviral drugs have a significant effect on HBV replication: ARA-A or ARA-AMP and recombinant alpha interferon. These drugs have been used for the prevention and for the treatment of HBV reinfection after liver transplantation.

Prior to liver transplantation

The aim of antiviral treatment before liver transplantation is to stop HBV replication and thus reduce the risk of HBV reinfection after liver transplantation.

ARA-A and ARA-AMP

These are potent antiviral agents acting directly on HBV replication without an immunostimulating effect. Adverse effects include neutropenia, myalgias and peripheral neuropathy. These drugs are given either intravenously (ARA-A) or intramuscularly (ARA-AMP) (Lok et al 1985, Marcellin et al 1989). Treatment cannot last more than 6 weeks because of the risk of adverse effects. The potentially poor tolerance and logistical considerations may be responsible for the absence of reports describing the use and results of ARA-A or ARA-AMP before liver transplantation.

Recombinant alpha interferon

Recombinant alpha interferon (IFN) is an antiviral and immunostimulating agent. IFN has been mainly used in patients with chronic active hepatitis B or compensated cirrhosis B and HBV replication (Davis 1991): IFN stops HBV replication as assessed by serum HBV DNA clearance and HBeAg to anti-HBe seroconversion in 30–50% of these patients. The predictors of a good response to IFN are: Caucasian origin, HBV infection during adolescence or adulthood, non-immunosuppressed status and no co-infection with HIV. Those for a poor response are: Asiatic origin, HBV infection at birth or in the perinatal period, and immunodepression (Brook et al 1989, Perrillo 1990). Furthermore, IFN is more effective in patients with low level of HBV DNA and with high level of transaminases, and in those with the wild type of HBV. IFN is usually given at a dose of 3–10 MU three times a week, subcutaneously. Adverse effects include neutropenia, thrombocytopenia, flu-like symptoms, psychiatric disturbances and thyroid disorders.

The experience with IFN in patients with decompensated cirrhosis, neutropenia and thrombocytopenia (such as candidates for liver transplantation) is limited (Di Bisceglie 1989). Aggravation of liver function, which frequently accompanies HBeAg to anti-HBe seroconversion, could be poorly tolerated in patients with severe cirrhosis. IFN could be given in patients waiting for liver transplant, and an urgent transplantation must be considered if severe deterioration of liver function occurs.

We treated with IFN 23 patients with post-hepatitis B cirrhosis who were candidates for liver transplantation, regardless of their HBV replication status, i.e. HBV DNA positive or negative. It was considered that some patients who are HBV DNA negative (by direct hybridization) may have a low level of HBV replication and thus might benefit from this treatment. Patients were given IFN at a dosage of 3 MU three times a week for at least 2 months prior to transplantation; after liver transplantation, all these patients received long-term HBIG. Patients with a bacterial infection, a bilirubin level >50 μmol/l, a platelet count <80 000/mm^3 or a white blood cell count <1500/mm^3 were excluded. Tolerance to IFN was relatively good; in only eight of the 23 patients the dosage was reduced from 3 to 1.5 MU because of neutropenia and/or thrombocytopenia; in one patient, the treatment was discontinued because of a spontaneous bacterial peritonitis. The treatment was transiently interrupted in two patients because of hepatic encephalopathy. At the start of the treatment, eight patients were HBV DNA positive and 15 patients were HBV DNA negative. Of the former, seven became HBV DNA-negative before liver transplantation; five of these were transplanted and two removed from the waiting list because of a dramatic improvement in liver function; one remained HBV DNA positive. HBV reinfection took place in four out of five (80%) HBV DNA-positive transplanted patients and in three of 12 (25%) HBV DNA-negative transplanted patients (Marcellin et al 1991). Thus, the rate of HBV reinfection was not clearly different from that observed in patients receiving long-term HBIG alone without pre-transplantation IFN treatment.

After liver transplantation

ARA-A or ARA-AMP

We treated 21 patients with HBV reinfection after liver transplantation with ARA-AMP. Doses of 10 mg/kg/day were given for 5 days, followed by 10 mg/day intramuscularly for 21 days. Tolerance was relatively good, the main adverse effects being asthenia and transient myalgias. A marked antiviral effect was observed, but this effect was transient (Marcellin et al 1990). At the end of the treatment, all patients remained HBsAg positive and 5 out of 21 became HBV DNA negative; after the end of the treatment, HBV DNA reappeared in all the patients who became HBV DNA negative at the end of the treatment. A second course of ARA-AMP was administered in six patients: three became HBV DNA negative but remained HBsAg positive.

Recombinant alpha interferon

IFN has been reported to cause acute rejection of renal transplants and therefore has been used very cautiously, either for the prevention or for the treatment of HBV reinfection after liver transplantation. In one patient receiving no HBIG, disappointing results were reported for its use for preventing HBV reinfection (Lavine et al 1991). However, in two patients receiving long-term HBIG and IFN, HBV reinfection did not develop (Hopf et al 1991). IFN has also been used for the treatment of HBV reinfection after liver transplantation with no effect on HBV replication (Hopf et al 1991). In 13 patients with HBV reinfection after liver transplantation treated with IFN at a dose of 3 MU three times a week for 6 months, the transaminase level did not change and HBsAg remained present; the effect on HBV DNA level was not reported in this series (Wright et al 1992).

CONCLUSION

The prevalence of HBV reinfection after liver transplantation is higher in patients with post-hepatitis B cirrhosis than in fulminant hepatitis B and is related to the HBV replication status before liver transplantation. Long-term administration of HBIG after liver transplantation is the best available method to prevent HBV reinfection, reducing the reinfection rate to less than 30% in HBV DNA-negative patients with post-hepatitis B cirrhosis and to 0% in patients with fulminant hepatitis B. IFN prior to liver transplantation does not reduce the rate of HBV reinfection; however, longer periods of administration of IFN need to be assessed.

New protocols for prevention and treatment of HBV infection will need to be evaluated in the future. Human monoclonal anti-HBs immunoglobulins, new antiviral agents and combinations of antiviral agents before and after liver transplantation may further reduce the rate of HBV reinfection after liver transplantation.

REFERENCES

Bismuth H, Castaing D, Ericson B G et al 1987 Hepatic transplantation in Europe. First report of the European liver transplant registry. Lancet ii, 674–676

Brook M G, Karayannis P, Thomas H C 1989 Which patients with chronic hepatitis B virus infection will respond to alpha interferon therapy? A statistical analysis of predictive factors. Hepatology 10: 761–763

Colledan M, Gislon M, Doglia M et al 1987 liver transplantation in patients with B viral hepatitis and delta infection. Transplantation Proceedings 19: 4073–4076

Chisari F V, Filippi P, Buras J et al 1987 Structural and pathological effects of synthesis of hepatitis B virus large envelope polypeptide in transgenic mice. Proceedings of the National Academy of Science of the USA 84: 6909–6913

Davies S E, Portmann B C, O'Grady J G, Aldis P M, Chaggar K, Alexander G M, Williams R 1991 Hepatic histologic findings after transplantation for chronic hepatitis B virus infection, including a unique pattern of fibrosing cholestatic hepatitis. Hepatology 13: 150–157

Davis G L 1991 Treatment of chronic hepatitis B. Hepatology 14: 567–569

Davis G L, Hoofnagle J J H 1987 Reactivation of chronic hepatits B virus infection. Gastroenterology 92: 2028–2031

Degos F, Lugassy C, Degott C et al 1988 Hepatitis B virus and hepatitis B related viral infection in renal transplant recipients. A prospective study of 90 patients. Gastroenterology 94: 151–156

Dejean A, Lugassy C, Zafrani S, Tiollais P, Brechot C 1984 Detection of hepatitis B virus DNA in pancreas, kidney and skin of two human carriers of the virus. Journal of Genetic Virology 65: 651–655

Demetris A J, Jaffe R, Sheahan D G et al 1986 Recurrent hepatitis B in liver allograft recipients. Differentiation between viral hepatitis B and rejection. American Journal of Pathology 125: 161–172

Demetris A J, Todo S, Van Thiel DH et al 1990 Evolution of hepatitis B virus liver disease after hepatic replacement. Practical and theoretical considerations. American Journal of Pathology 137: 667–676

Di Bisceglie A M 1989 Interferon therapy of complicated hepatitis B virus infection. Seminars in Liver Diseases 9: 254–258

Feray C, Zignego A L, Samuel D et al 1990 Persistent hepatitis B virus infection of mononuclear cells without concommitent liver infection: the liver transplantation model. Transplantation 49: 1155–1158

Freeman R B, Sanchez H, Lewis W D et al 1991 Serologic and DNA follow-up data from HBsAg-positive patients treated with orthotopic liver transplantation. Transplantation 51: 793–797

Fung J, Ostberg L, Shapiro R, Todo S, Demetris A, Starzl

T E 1991 Human monoclonal antibody against hepatitis B surface antigen in preventing recurrent hepatitis B following liver transplantation. In: Hollinger F B, Lemon S M, Margolis H S (eds) Viral hepatitis and liver disease. Williams & Wilkins, Baltimore, p 651

Hadchouel M, Pasquinelli C, Fournier J G, Hugon R N, Scotto J, Bernard O, Brechot C 1988 Journal of Medical Virology 24: 27–32

Hopf U, Neuhaus P, Lobeck H et al 1991 Follow-up of recurrent hepatitis B and delta infection in liver allograft recipients after treatment with recombinant interferon alpha. Journal of Hepatology 13: 339–346

Huang C C, Lai M K, M T 1990 Hepatitis B liver disease in cyclosporine-treated renal allograft recipients. Transplantation 49: 540–544

Johnson P J, Wansbrough-Jones M H, Portmann B, Eddleston A L W F, Williams R, D'a Maycock W, Calne R Y 1978 Familial HBsAg positive hepatoma: treatment with orthotopic liver transplantation and specific immunoglobulin. British Medical Journal 1: 216

Lake J R, Wright T L 1991 Liver transplantation for patients with hepatitis B: what have we learned from our results? Hepatology 13: 796–799

Lau J Y N, Bain V G, Davies S E, O'Grady J G, Alberti A, Alexander G J M, Williams R 1992 High-level expression of hepatitis B viral antigens in fibrosing cholestatic hepatitis. Gastroenterology 102: 956–962

Lauchart W, Muller R, Pichlmayr R 1987a Immunoprophylaxis of hepatitis B virus reinfection in recipients of human liver allografts. Transplantation Proceedings 19: 2387–2389

Lauchart W, Muller R, Pichlmayr R 1987b Long-term immunoprophylaxis of hepatitis B virus (HBV) reinfection in recipients of human liver allografts. Transplantation Proceedings 19: 4051–4053

Lavine J E, Lake J R, Ascher NL, Ferrel L D, Ganem D, Wright TL 1991 Persistent hepatitis B virus following interferon alpha therapy and liver transplantation. Gastroenterology 100: 263–267

Lok A S F, Novick D M, Karayannis P, Dunk A A, Sherlock S, Thomas H C 1985 A randomized study of the effects of adenine arabinoside 5' monophosphate (short or long courses) and lymphoblastoid interferon on hepatitis B virus replication. Hepatology 5: 1132–1138

MacMahon G, MacCarthy L A, Dottavio D, Östberg L 1991 Surface antigen and polymerase gene variation in hepatitis B virus isolates from a monoclonal antibody-treated liver transplant patient. In: Hollinger FB, Lemon S M, Margolis H S (eds) Viral hepatitis and liver disease Williams and Wilkins, Baltimore, pp 219–221

Marcellin P, Ouzan D, Degos F et al 1989 Randomized controlled trial of adenine arabinoside 5' monophosphate in chronic active hepatitis B: comparison of the efficacy in heterosexual and homosexual patients. Hepatology 10: 328–331

Marcellin P, Samuel D, Loriot M A, Areias J, Bismuth H, Benhamou J P 1990 Anti-viral effect of adenine arabinoside monophosphate (ARA-AMP) in patients with recurrence of hepatitis B virus (HBV) infection after liver transplantation (abstract). Hepatology 12: 966

Marcellin P, Samuel D, Areias J, Gigou M, Benhamou J P, Bismuth H 1991 Effect of pretransplant alpha recombinant interferon treatment on HBV reinfection in patients with cirrhosis B (abstract). Hepatology 14: 71A

Mora N, Klintmaln GB, Poplawski S et al 1990 Recurrence of hepatitis B after liver transplantation: does hepatitis B immunoglobulin modify recurrent disease? Transplantation Proceedings 22: 1549–1550

Muller R, Gubernatis G, Farle M et al 1991 Liver transplantation in HBs antigen (HBsAg) carriers. Prevention of hepatitis B virus (HBV) recurrence by passive immunisation. Journal of Hepatology 13: 90–96

Nagington J, Cossart Y E, Cohen B J 1977 Reactivation of hepatitis B after transplantation operations. Lancet i: 558–560

O'Grady J G, Smith H M, Davies S E et al 1992 Hepatitis B reinfection after orthotopic liver transplantation. Serological and clinical implications. Journal of Hepatology 14: 104–111

Perrillo R P 1990 Factors influencing response to interferon in chronic hepatitis B: implications for asian and western populations. Hepatology 12: 1434–1435

Rizzetto M, Recchia S, Salizzoni M 1991 Liver transplantation in carriers of the HBsAg. Journal of Hepatology 13: 5–7

Roingeard P, Romet-Lemonne J L, Leturcq D, Goudeau A, Essex M 1990 Hepatitis B virus core antigen (HBcAg) accumulation in an HBV nonproducer clone of HepG2-transfected cells is associated with cytopathic effect. Virology 179: 113–120

Samuel D, Bismuth A, Mathieu D et al 1991 Passive immunoprophylaxis after liver transplantation in HBsAg-positive patients. Lancet 337: 813–815

Starzl T E, Demetris A J, Van Thiel D 1989 Liver transplantation (second of two parts). New England Journal of Medicine 321: 1092–1099

Todo S, Demetris A J, Van Thiel D, Teperman L, Fung J, Starzl T E 1991 Orthotopic liver transplantation for patients with hepatitis B virus related liver disease. Hepatology 13: 619–626

Tur-Kaspa R, Laub O 1990 Corticosteroids stimulate hepatitis B virus DNA, mRNA and protein production in a stable expression system. Journal of Hepatology 11: 34–36

Van Thiel D H, Shade R R, Gavaler J S, Shaw B W Jr, Iwatzuki S, Starzl T E 1984 Medical aspects of liver transplantation. Hepatology 4: 79 S-83S

Wright HI, Gavaler J S, Van Thiel D H 1992 Preliminary experience with alpha 2b interferon therapy of viral hepatitis in liver allograft recipients. Transplantation 53: 121–124

Yoffee B, Noonan CA, Melnick J L, Hollinger F B 1986 Hepatitis B virus DNA in mononuclear cells and analysis of cell subsets for the presence of replicative intermediates of viral DNA. Journal of Infectious Diseases 153: 471–477

Yoffee B, Müller R 1991 Liver transplantation in patients with HBV infection: implications of extrahepatic HBV infection. In: Hollinger F B, Lemon S M, Margolis H S (eds) Viral hepatitis and liver disease. Williams and Wilkins, Baltimore, pp 813–819

Zignego A L, Samuel D, Gugenheim J et al 1988 Hepatitis B virus replication and mononuclear blood cells infection after liver transplantation. In: Zuckerman A J (ed) Viral hepatitis and liver disease. Alan R. Liss, New York, 808–809

12. Prevention

Arie J. Zuckerman Jane N. Zuckerman Tim J. Harrison

PREVENTION AND CONTROL OF HEPATITIS A

Passive immunization

Control of hepatitis A infection is difficult. Since faecal shedding of the virus is at its highest during the late incubation period and the prodromal phase of the illness, strict isolation of cases is not a useful control measure. Spread of hepatitis A is reduced by simple hygienic measures and the sanitary disposal of excreta.

Normal human immunoglobulin, containing at least 100 international units (IU)/ml anti-hepatitis A antibody, given intramuscularly before exposure to the virus or early during the incubation period will prevent or attenuate a clinical illness. The dosage should be at least 2 IU of anti-hepatitis A antibody per kg body weight, but in special cases such as pregnancy or in patients with liver disease this dosage may be doubled (Table 12.1). Immunoglobulin does not always prevent infection and excretion of hepatitis A virus, and inapparent or subclinical hepatitis may develop. The efficacy of passive immunization is based on the presence of hepatitis A antibody in the immunoglobulin, but the minimum titre of antibody required for protection has not yet been established. Immunoglobulin is used most commonly for close personal contacts of patients with hepatitis A and for those exposed to contaminated food. Immunoglobulin has also been used effectively for controlling outbreaks in institutions such as homes for the mentally handicapped and in nursery schools. Prophylaxis with immunoglobulin is recommended for people without hepatitis A antibody visiting highly endemic areas. After a period of 6 months the administration of immunoglobulin for travellers should be repeated, unless it has been demonstrated that the recipient has developed hepatitis A antibodies.

Hepatitis A vaccines

In cases of high prevalence, most children have antibodies to hepatitis A virus by the age of 3, and such infections are generally asymptomatic. Infections acquired later in life are of increasing clinical severity. Less than 10% of cases of acute hepatitis A in children up to the age of 6 are icteric, but this increases to 40–50% in the 6–14 age group and to 70–80% in adults. Of 115 551 cases of hepatitis A in the USA between 1983 and 1987, only 9% of the cases, but more than 70% of the fatalities, were in those aged over 49. It is important, therefore, to protect those at risk because of personal contact with infected

Table 12.1 Passive immunization with normal immunoglobulin for travellers to highly endemic areas

Body weight (kg)	Period of stay <3 months	Period of stay >3 months
<25	50 IU anti-HAV (0.5 ml)	100 IU anti-HAV (1.0 ml)
25–30	100 IU anti-HAV (1.0 ml)	250 IU anti-HAV (2.5 ml)
<50	200 IU anti-HAV (2.0 ml)	500 IU anti-HAV (5.0 ml)

individuals or because of travel to highly endemic areas. Other groups at risk of hepatitis A infection include staff and residents of institutions for the mentally handicapped, day-care centres for children, active male homosexuals, narcotic drug abusers, sewage workers, health care workers, military personnel and certain low socioeconomic groups in defined community settings. In some developing countries, the incidence of clinical hepatitis A is increasing as improvements in socioeconomic conditions result in infection later in life and strategies for immunization are yet to be agreed.

Killed hepatitis A vaccines

The foundations for a hepatitis A vaccine were laid in 1975 by Provost and Hilleman, who demonstrated that formalin-inactivated virus extracted from the liver of infected marmosets induced protective antibodies in susceptible marmosets on challenge with live virus. In the following year, Provost & Hilleman (1979) cultivated hepatitis A virus, after serial passage in marmosets, in a cloned line of fetal rhesus monkey kidney cells (FRhK6), thereby opening the way to the production of hepatitis A vaccines. It was subsequently demonstrated by several groups that prior adaptation in marmosets was not a prerequisite to growth of the virus in cell cultures and various strains of virus have been isolated directly from clinical material using several cell lines, including human diploid fibroblasts, and various techniques have been employed to increase the yield of virus in cell culture. Safety and immunogenicity studies of formalin-inactivated hepatitis A vaccines with an adjuvant have now been completed, and the vaccine was licensed in several countries at the end of 1992. Other preparations are under clinical trial.

Live attenuated hepatitis A vaccines

The major advantages of live attenuated vaccines (namely the Sabin type of oral poliomyelitis vaccines) include the ease of administration on a large scale by the oral route, relatively low cost – since the virus vaccine strain replicates in the gut – the production of both local immunity in the gut and humoral immunity, thereby mimicking natural infection, and also longer term protection. Disadvantages include the potential for reversion towards virulence, interference with the vaccine strain by other viruses in the gut, relative instability of the vaccine and shedding of the virus strain in the faeces for prolonged periods.

The most extensively studied live attenuated hepatitis A vaccines are based on the CR326 and HM175 strains of the virus attenuated by prolonged passage in cell culture.

Two variants of the CR326 strain have been investigated after passage in marmoset liver in FRhK6, MRC5 and WI-38 cells. Inoculation of susceptible marmosets demonstrated sero-conversion and protection on challenge. Biochemical evidence of liver damage did not occur in susceptible chimpanzees, although a number had histological evidence of mild hepatitis with the F variant and the vaccine virus was shed in the faeces for about 12 weeks prior to sero-conversion. There was no evidence of reversion towards virulence. Studies in human volunteers indicated incomplete attenuation of the F variant, but better results were obtained with the F1 variant without elevation of liver enzymes (Ellis & Provost 1989).

Studies with the HM175 strain, which was isolated and passaged in African green monkey kidney cells, showed that this strain was not fully attenuated for marmosets, although it did not induce liver damage on challenge. Further passages and adaptation of HM175 revealed some evidence of virus replication in the liver of chimpanzees and minimal shedding of the virus into faeces. Other studies are in progress in non-human primates.

As with vaccine strains of polioviruses, attenuation may be associated with mutations in the 5' non-coding region of the genome which affect secondary structure. There is also evidence that mutations in the region of the genome encoding the non-structural polypeptides may be important for adaptation to cell culture and attenuation. However, markers of attenuation of HAV have not been identified, and reversion to virulence may also be a problem. On the other hand, there is also concern that 'over attenuated' viruses may not be sufficiently immunogenic.

Current candidate live attenuated hepatitis A vaccines require administration by injection. Preparations that may be suitable for oral administration are not available so far.

PREVENTION AND CONTROL OF HEPATITIS B

Passive immunization

Hepatitis B immunoglobulin is prepared from pooled plasma with a high titre of hepatitis B surface antibody and may confer temporary passive immunity under certain defined conditions. The major indication for the administration of hepatitis B immunoglobulin is a single acute exposure to hepatitis B virus, such as occurs when blood containing surface antigen is inoculated, ingested or splashed onto mucous membranes and the conjunctiva. The optimal dose has not been established, but doses in the range 250–500 IU have been used effectively. It should be administered as early as possible after exposure and preferably within 48 h, usually 3 ml (containing 200 IU of anti-HBs per ml) in adults. It should not be administered after 7 days following exposure. It is generally recommended that two doses of hepatitis B immunoglobulin should be given 30 days apart.

Results with the use of hepatitis B immunoglobulin for prophylaxis in babies at risk of infection with hepatitis B virus are encouraging if the immunoglobulin is given as soon as possible after birth or within 12 h of birth, and the chance of the baby developing the persistent carrier state is reduced by about 70%. More recent studies using combined passive and active immunization indicate an efficacy approaching 90%. The dose of hepatitis B immunoglobulin recommended in the newborn is 1–2 ml (200 IU of anti-HBs per ml).

Active immunization

Immunization against hepatitis B is required for groups that are at an increased risk of acquiring this infection. These groups include individuals requiring repeated transfusions of blood or blood products, prolonged in-patient treatment, patients who require frequent tissue penetration or need repeated access to the circulation, patients with natural or acquired immune deficiency and patients with malignant diseases. Viral hepatitis is an occupational hazard among health care personnel and the staff of institutions for the mentally retarded and in some semiclosed institutions. High rates of infection with hepatitis B occur in narcotic drug addicts and drug abusers, homosexuals and prostitutes. Individuals working in high endemic areas are also at an increased risk of infections. Women in areas of the world where the carrier state in that group is high are another segment of the population requiring immunization in view of the increased risk of transmission of the infections to their offspring. Young infants, children and susceptible persons living in certain tropical and subtropical areas where present socioeconomic conditions are poor and the prevalence of hepatitis B is high should also be immunized.

The failure to grow hepatitis B virus in tissue culture has directed attention to the use of other preparations for active immunization. Since immunization with hepatitis B surface antigen leads to the production of protective surface antibody, purified 22-nm spherical surface antigen particles have been developed as vaccines. These vaccines have been prepared from the plasma of symptomless carriers. Trials on protective efficacy in high-risk groups have demonstrated the value of the vaccines and their safety. There is no risk of transmission of the acquired immune deficiency syndrome (AIDS) or any other infection by vaccines derived from plasma which meet the WHO Requirements of 1981, 1983 and 1987. Local reactions reported after immunization have been minor, occurring in less than 20% of immunized individuals, and consisted of slight swelling and reddening at the site of inoculation. Temperature elevations of up to 38°C were observed in only a few individuals.

Site of injection for vaccination

Hepatitis B vaccination should be given in the upper arm or the anterolateral aspect of the thigh and not in the buttock. There are over 100 reports of unexpectedly low antibody seroconversion rates after hepatitis B vaccination using injection into the buttock. In one centre in the USA a low antibody response was noted in 54% of healthy adult health care personnel. Many studies have since shown that the antibody response rate was significantly higher in centres using deltoid injection than centres using the buttock. On the basis of antibody tests after vaccination, the Advisory Committee on Immunization Practices of the Centers of Disease Control, USA, recommended that the arm be used as the site of hepatitis B vaccination in adults, as has the Department of Health in the UK.

A comprehensive study in the USA by Shaw et al (1989) showed that participants who received the vaccine in the deltoid had antibody titres that were up to 17 times higher than those of subjects who received the injections into the buttock. Furthermore, those who were injected in the buttock were 2–4 times more likely to fail to reach a minimum antibody level of 10 mIU/ml after vaccination. Recent reports have also implicated buttock injection as a possible factor in a failure of rabies post-exposure prophylaxis using a human diploid cell rabies vaccine (Baer & Fishbein 1987).

The injection of vaccine into deep fat in the buttocks is likely with needles shorter than 5 cm, and there is a lack of phagocytic or antigen-presenting cells in layers of fat. Another factor may involve the rapidity with which antigen becomes available to the circulation from deposition in fat, leading to delay in processing by macrophages and eventually presentation to T and B cells. An additional factor may be denaturation by enzymes of antigen that has remained in fat for hours or days. The importance of these factors is supported by the finding at the Royal Free Hospital, London, and elsewhere that thicker skin fold is associated with a lowered antibody response (Cockcroft et al 1990).

These observations have important public health implications, well illustrated by the estimate that about 20% of subjects immunized against hepatitis B via the buttock in the USA by March 1985 (about 60 000 people) failed to attain a minimum level of antibody of 10 mIU/ml and were therefore not protected.

Hepatitis B surface antibody titres should be measured in all individuals who have been immunized against hepatitis B by injection into the buttocks, and when this is not possible a complete course of three injections of vaccine should be administered into the deltoid muscle or the anterolateral aspect of the thigh, the only acceptable sites for hepatitis B immunization (Zuckerman et al 1992).

Indications for immunization against hepatitis B

The current indications for the use of hepatitis B vaccines in low prevalence areas are summarized below, although these recommendations are under revision. The recommendations for immunization against this infection in intermediate- and high-prevalance regions also include universal immunization of infants (Zuckerman 1984, Deinhardt & Zuckerman 1985). Many countries, including the USA and Italy, introduced universal immunization for infants in 1992, and it is expected that most countries will implement this policy by 1996.

Current policy

1. All health care personnel in frequent contact with blood or needles and groups at the highest risk in this category include:
   - 1.1 Personnel, including teaching and training staff, directly involved over a period of time in patient care in residential institutions for the mentally handicapped where there is a known high risk of hepatitis.
   - 1.2 Personnel directly involved in patient care over a period of time, working in units giving treatment to those known to be at high risk of hepatitis B infection.
   - 1.3 Personnel directly involved in patient care working in haemodialysis, haemophilia, and other centres regularly performing maintenance treatment of patients with blood or blood products.
   - 1.4 Laboratory workers regularly exposed to increased risk from infected material.
   - 1.5 Health care personnel on secondment to work in areas of the world where there is a high prevalance of hepatitis B infection, if

they are to be directly involved in patient care.

1.6 Dentists and ancilliary dental personnel with direct patient contact.

2. Patients:

2.1 Patients on first entry into those residential institutions for the mentally handicapped where there is a known high incidence of hepatitis B.

2.2 Patients treated by maintenance haemodialysis.

2.3 Patients before major surgery who are likely to require a large number of blood transfusions and/or treatment with blood products.

3. Contacts of patients with hepatitis B:

3.1 The spouses and other sexual contacts of patients with acute hepatitis B or carriers of hepatitis B virus, and other family members in close contact.

4. Other indications for immunization:

4.1 Infants born to mothers who are persistent carriers of hepatitis B surface antigen (HBsAg) or are HBsAg positive as a result of recent infection, particularly if hepatitis B e antigen is detectable or HBV-positive mothers without antibody to e antigen (anti-HBe). The optimum timing for immunoglobulin to be given at a contralateral site is immediately at birth or within 12 h.

4.2 Health care workers who are accidentally pricked with needles used for patients with hepatitis B. The vaccine may be used alone or in combination with hepatitis B immunoglobulin as an alternative to passive immunization with hepatitis B immunoglobulin only. Studies on the efficacy of these different schedules of immunization are nearing completion.

5. Immediate protection:

5.1 Infants born to carrier mothers: Whenever immediate protection is required, as, for example, for infants born to HBsAg-positive mothers (see 4.1) or following transfer of an individual into a 'high-risk' setting or after accidental inoculation, active immunization with the vaccine should be combined with simultaneous administration of hepatitis B immunoglobulin at a different site. It has been shown that passive immunization with up to 3 ml (200 IU of anti-HBs per ml) of hepatitis B immunoglobulin does not interfere with an active immune response. A single dose of hepatitis B immunoglobulin (usually 3 ml for adults; 1–2 ml for the newborn) is sufficient for healthy individuals. If infection has already occurred at the time of the first immunization, virus multiplication is unlikely to be inhibited completely, but severe illness and, most importantly, the development of the carrier state of HBV may be prevented in many individuals, particularly in infants born to carrier mothers.

6. The immune response to the current hepatitis B vaccines is poorer in immunocompromised patients and in the elderly. For example, only about 60% of patients undergoing treatment by maintenance haemodialysis develop anti-HBs. It is suggested therefore that patients with chronic renal damage be immunized as soon as it appears likely that they will ultimately require treatment by maintenance haemodialysis or receive renal transplant. Consideration should be given to the use of blood from healthy immunized donors with high titres of anti-HBs for the routine haemodialysis of such patients who respond poorly to immunization against hepatitis B.

7. Other groups at risk of hepatitis B include the following:

7.1 Individuals who frequently change sexual partners, particularly promiscuous male homosexuals and prostitutes.

7.2 Intravenous drug abusers.

7.3 Staff at reception centres for refugees and immigrants from areas of the world where hepatitis B is very common, such as South-East Asia.

7.4 Although they are at 'lower risk', consideration should also be given to long-term prisoners and staff of custodial institutions, ambulance and rescue services and selected police personnel.

7.5 Military personnel are included in some countries.

Developing new hepatitis B immunization strategies

There is now strong support for the introduction of universal antenatal screening to identify hepatitis B carrier mothers and the vaccination of their babies. It is important that any other strategies do not interfere with the delivery of vaccine to this group. Immunization of this group will have the greatest impact in reducing the number of new hepatitis B carriers. For children outside this group it is difficult to estimate the lifetime risk of acquiring a hepatitis infection.

There are four main approaches:

1. Continue vaccination of the 'high-risk' babies as defined above.
2. Vaccinate all infants.
3. Vaccinate all adolescents.
4. Vaccinate everybody.

Vaccination of adolescents

This approach delivers vaccination at a time close to the time when 'risk behaviour' would expose adolescents to infection. Vaccination could be delivered as part of a wider package on health education in general, to include sex education, risk of AIDS, dangers of drug abuse, smoking, benefits of a healthy diet and lifestyle.

The problems with this approach are as follows:

- Persuading parents to accept vaccination of the children against a sexually transmitted disease, a problem they may not wish to address at that time.
- Ensuring a full course of three doses is given.
- Evaluating and monitoring vaccine cover. The systems for monitoring uptake of vaccine in this age group may not operate efficiently.

Vaccination of infants

The advantages of this approach are:

- It is known that vaccination can be delivered to babies.
- Parents will accept vaccination against hepatitis B along with other childhood vaccinations without reference to sexual behaviour.

The disadvantages of this approach are:

- It is not known whether immunity will last until exposure in later life. This may become less of a problem as more people are vaccinated and thus the chance of exposure to infection is reduced.
- The introduction of another childhood vaccination may reduce the uptake of other childhood vaccinations. This problem would be avoided if hepatitis B vaccine could be delivered in a combined vaccine containing DPT (diphtheria, polio, tetanus), and this proposal may have to await the production and evaluation of a suitable vaccine.

Vaccination of infants is preferable to vaccination of adolescents, as there are sufficient mechanisms to ensure, monitor and evaluate cover. A booster dose could be given in early adolescence combined with a health education package. A rolling programme could be introduced, giving priority to urban areas.

Polypeptide vaccines

Hepatitis B polypeptide vaccines containing specific hepatitis B antigenic determinants of the major non-glycosylated peptide I of the surface antigen with a molecular weight of 22–24 000 and its glycosylated form, a polypeptide with a molecular weight in the range 22–24 000, have been prepared in micellar form (Skelly et al 1981, Young et al 1982). The individual polypeptides of the surface antigen are immunogenic, and the purified 24 000 (designated as p24) and 27 000 (gp27) molecular weight polypeptides are effective antigens. Clinical trials of the polypeptide micelle vaccine are in progress (Hollinger et al 1986).

Production of hepatitis B vaccines by rDNA techniques

Recombinant DNA techniques have been used for expressing hepatitis B surface antigen and core antigen in prokaryotic cells (*Escherichia coli* and *Bacillus subtilis*) and in eukaryotic cells, such as mutant mouse LM cells, HeLa cells, COS cells, CHO cells and yeast cells (*Saccharomyces cerevisiae*).

Recombinant yeast hepatitis B vaccines have undergone extensive evaluation by clinical trials. The results indicated that this vaccine is safe, antigenic and free from side-effects (apart from minor local reactions in a proportion of recipients). The immunogenicity is similar, in general terms, to that of the plasma-derived vaccine. Recombinant yeast hepatitis B vaccines are now being used in many countries. A vaccine based on HBsAg expressed in mammalian (CHO) cells is in use in the People's Republic of China.

The emergence of variants of HBV that are not neutralized by vaccine-induced anti-HBs, as described above, is of major concern (see Ch. 7). Horizontal spread of these viruses has not yet been reported but remains a possibility. If the number of potential variants is limited it may be possible to include these in future formulations of hepatitis B vaccine. It seems that the mutation affecting amino acid residue 145 (glycine to arginine) is the most common, but variants with other changes are being investigated.

Hepatitis B vaccines containing pre-S epitopes

A disadvantage of plasma-derived and recombinant hepatitis B vaccines containing only the major protein of HBsAg (without pre-S sequences) is the lack of immune responsiveness of a minority of vaccinees. The identification of an immunodominant domain in the pre-S2 region of HBsAg (Neurath et al 1984) and the observation that mice which were immunologically non-responsive to the major protein of HBsAg made antibodies to a synthetic peptide corresponding to this epitope (Neurath et al 1985, Milich et al 1985) stimulated interest in incorporation of pre-S sequences in hepatitis B vaccines. Itoh et al (1986) demonstrated that a synthetic peptide encompassing 19 amino acids from the pre-S2 region, when coupled to keyhole limpet haemocyanin, elicited a protective antibody response when administered to chimpanzees. The middle (pre-S2+S) and large (pre-S1+pre-S2-S) forms of HBsAg have been expressed in yeast using constitutive and inducible promoters respectively (Ellis et al 1988, Kniskern et al 1988). The former preparation has been evaluated for safety and immunogenicity (Miskovsky et al 1991). A vaccine containing all three (large, middle and major) forms of HBsAg, synthesized in Chinese hamster ovary (CHO) cells, has been tested in Singapore. The preparation proved safe and immunogenic with a rapid antibody response in 96% of the recipients (Yap et al 1992).

Hybrid virus vaccines

Potential live vaccines using recombinant vaccinia viruses have been constructed for hepatitis B, and also for herpes simplex, rabies and other viruses. Foreign viral DNA is introduced into the vaccinia virus genome by construction of chimaeric genes and homologous recombination in cells, since the large size of the genome of vaccinia virus (185 000 bp) precludes gene insertion in vitro. A chimaeric gene consisting of vaccinia virus promoter sequences ligated to the coding sequence for the desired foreign protein is flanked by vaccinia virus DNA in a plasmid vector.

The recloned vaccinia virus containing hepatitis B surface antigen sequences has been used successfully for 'priming' experimental animals. At present, however, there is no accepted laboratory marker of attenuation or virulence of vaccinia virus for man, either in the host directly inoculated with the virus or after several passages in the same species. Alterations in the genome of vaccinia virus that are concomitant with the selection of recombinants may alter the virulence of the virus. Changes in host range or tissue tropism of vaccinia viruses may occur as a result of their genetic modification, and these could be caused by changes in the virus envelope as a result of the incorporation of gene products of the foreign viral genes inserted into the vaccinia virus.

The advantages of a vaccinia virus recombinant as a vaccine include low cost, ease of administration by multiple pressure or by the scratch technique, vaccine stability, long shelf-life and the possible use of polyvalent antigens. The known adverse reactions with vaccinia virus vaccines are well documented, and their incidence and severity must be carefully weighed against the adverse reactions associated with existing vaccines which a new recombinant vaccine might replace. There are also reports of spread of current strains of vaccinia virus to contacts, and this may present difficulties. Other recombinant viruses as vectors are being explored, and in particular the oral adenovirus vaccines, which have been in use for some 20 years (reviewed by Zuckerman 1990).

Novel hepatitis B vaccines using hybrid particles

More recent developments include the use of the envelope proteins of hepatitis B virus (hepatitis B surface antigen) in a particulate form by expressing the proteins in mammalian cells. In-phase insertions of another virus (poliomyelitis virus type I) of variable length and sequence were made in different regions of the S gene of hepatitis B virus. The envelope proteins carrying the surface antigen and the insert are assembled with cellular lipids in the cultured mammalian cells after transfection. The inserted polio neutralization peptide was found to be exposed on the surface of the hybrid envelope particles and induced neutralizing antibodies against poliovirus in mice immunized experimentally. This approach may also be useful for studying the biological activity of other peptides incorporated into the surface of an organized multimolecular complex. The expression and secretion of hybrid envelope particles by established cell lines may thus provide an efficient system for the production of potential new vaccines.

Another potentially excellent carrier vehicle for human and veterinary vaccines in addition to hepatitis B is the use of the core particles of hepatitis B virus. The advantage of the core structure as a particle includes its ability to induce antibody with approximately 100-fold greater efficiency than the surface antigen particle and an ability to augment T-helper cell function. The feasibility of this approach was recently demonstrated with synthetic and biosynthetic peptides of foot and mouth disease virus (FMDV) after fusion to hepatitis B core (Clarke et al 1987).

Chemically synthesized hepatitis B vaccines

The development of chemically synthesized polypeptide vaccines offers many advantages in attaining the ultimate goal of producing chemically uniform, safe and cheap viral immunogens to replace many current vaccines, which often contain large quantities of irrelevant microbial antigenic determinants, proteins and other material additional to the essential immunogen required for the induction of a protective antibody (Zuckerman 1973, 1990). The preparation of antibodies against viral proteins using fragments of chemically synthesized peptides mimicking viral amino acid sequences is now a possible and attractive alternative approach in immunoprophylaxis (Lerner et al 1981).

Successful mimicking of determinants of HBsAg using chemically synthesized peptides in linear and cyclical forms has been reported by several groups of investigators. Peptides have been synthesized which retain biological function and appropriate secondary structure, even though they have a limited sequence homology with the natural peptide or are much smaller.

Various other studies also confirm that selected overlapping peptides corresponding to relevant epitopes of hepatitis B surface antigen may be useful as synthetic vaccines when combined with adjuvants; antisera to these peptides cross-react with the native surface antigen particles, and protective immunity has been demonstrated in limited experimental studies.

Enhancement of the immunogenicity of the pre-S region of hepatitis B surface antigen has been demonstrated in mice, using chemically synthesized amino acid residues. The immune response to the pre-S2 region has been shown to be regulated by H-2-linked genes, which are distinct from those that regulate the response to the S region. It was also demonstrated that immunization of a 'non-responder' murine strain with particles that contain both S and pre-S2 can circumvent non-responsiveness. More recently, a protein sequence that mediates the attachment of hepatitis B virus to human hepatoma cells was identified. A synthetic peptide analogue, which is recognized by both cell receptors and viral antibodies, elicited antibodies reacting with the virus. Such a preparation may elicit protective antibodies by blocking the attachment of virus to the cells.

However, designing proteins with the correct tertiary structure and with functional activities is exceedingly difficult, since it is not possible to predict the tertiary structure of a protein from its amino acid sequence alone. X-ray crystallography and interactive computer graphics are essential and available tools. The first step is to obtain a highly purified protein which can be crystallized to diffraction quality. The electron density of the crystal can then be calculated and, since crystallography provides information on the non-hydrogen atoms in proteins, it is possible to build a scaffold model for fitting the known amino acid sequence into this structure. The model can then be refined by using sets to test coordinates to improve the density map. More recent techniques using synchrotron X-ray sources may allow the collection of structural information from protein in solution.

Two-dimensional proton nuclear magnetic resonance techniques, which assign peaks to specific protons in the protein, are now available, and the results can be converted to a set of coordinates for the molecule. An alternative approach is to develop comprehensive algorithms to simulate the mechanisms that determine protein structures coupled with establishing libraries of protein database. Another approach is to design synthetic proteins based on the natural folding patterns of the α-helix configuration and the β-pleated sheet. However, there are as yet no proven principles for de novo protein design, although it is equally clear that significant advances are being made in the construction of secondary patterns of proteins.

Nevertheless, there are several reports which show that the modification of peptides based on secondary struture predictions and model building is now feasible. Peptides have been synthesized which retain biological function and appropriate secondary structure, even though they have a limited sequence homology with the natural peptide or are much smaller. For example, studies with hormones have shown that it is possible to stabilize a turn by cyclization of the molecule, either by introducing a disulphide bond or by designing a cyclic peptide. Synthetic peptides may therefore be employed in due course as vaccines, although mixtures of more than one of the peptides may be required. Of the many questions that remain to be answered, the critical issues are whether antibodies induced by synthetic immunogens will be protective and whether protective immunity will persist. Some of the carrier proteins and some of the adjuvants that have linked to the synthetic molecules cannot be used in man, and it is therefore essential to find acceptable and safe material for covalent linkage, or, alternatively, to synthesize sequences that do not require linkage. But the prospect of multivalent chemically synthetic vaccines against a variety of microbial agents is within reach.

REFERENCES

Baer G M, Fishbein D R 1987 Rabies post-exposure prophylaxis. New England Journal of Medicine 316: 1270–1271

Clarke B E, Newton S E, Carrol A R et al 1987 Improved immunogenicity of a peptide epitope after fusion to hepatitis B core protein. Nature 330: 381–384

Cockcroft A, Soper P, Insail C, Kennard Y, Chapman S, Gooch C, Griffiths P 1990 Antibody response after hepatitis B immunisation in health care workers. British Journal of Industrial Medicine 47: 199–202

Deinhardt F D, Zuckerman A J 1985 Immunization against hepatitis B: report on a WHO meeting on Viral Hepatitis in Europe. Journal of Medical Virology 17: 209–217

Ellis R W, Provost P J 1989 Hepatitis B and A vaccines. In: Zuckerman A J (ed) Recent developments in prophylactic immunization. Kluwer Academic Publishers, Dordecht, pp 181–209

Ellis R W, Kniskern P J, Hagopian A et al 1988 Preparation and testing of a recombinant-derived hepatitis B vaccine consisting of pre-S2 + S polypeptides. In: Zuckerman A J (ed.) Viral hepatitis and liver disease. Alan R. Liss, New York, pp 1079–1086

Hollinger F B, Trois C, Heiberg D, Sanchez V, Dreesman G R, Melnick J L 1986 Response to hepatitis B polypeptide vaccine in micelle form in a young adult population. Journal of Medical Virology 19: 229–240

Itoh Y, Takai E, Ohnuma H et al 1986 A synthetic peptide vaccine involving the product of the pre-S(2) region of hepatitis B virus DNA: protective efficacy in chimpanzees. Proceedings of the National Academy of Science of the USA 83: 9174–9178

Kniskern P J, Hagopian A, Burke P et al 1988 A candidate vaccine for hepatitis B containing the complete viral surface protein. Hepatology 8: 82–87

Lerner R A, Green N, Alexander H, Liu F T, Sutcliffe G, Shinnick T M 1981 Chemically synthesized peptides predicted from the nucleotide sequence of hepatitis B virus genome elicit antibodies reactive with the native envelope protein of Dane particles. Proceedings of the National Academy of Science of the USA 78: 3403–3407

Milich D R, Thornton G B, Neurath A R, Kent S B, Michel M L, Tiollais P, Chisari F V 1985 Enhanced immunogenicity of the pre-S region of hepatitis B surface antigen. Science 228: 1195–1199

Miskovsky E, Gershman K, Clements M L et al 1991 Comparative safety and immunogenicity of yeast recombinant hepatitis B vaccines containing S-antigens and pre-S2-S antigens. Vaccine 9: 346–350

Neurath A R, Kent S B H, Strick N 1984 Location and chemical synthesis of a pre-S gene coded immunodominant epitope of hepatitis B virus. Science 224: 392–395

Neurath A R, Kent S B, Strick N, Stark D, Sproul P 1985 Genetic restriction of immune responsiveness to synthetic peptides corresponding to sequences in the pre-S region of the hepatitis B virus (HBV) envelope gene. Journal of Medical Virology 17: 119–125

Provost P J, Hilleman M R 1975 An inactivated hepatitis A virus vaccine prepared from infected marmoset liver. Proceedings of the Society for Experimental Biology and Medicine 159: 201–213

Provost P J, Hilleman M R 1979 Preparation of human hepatitis A virus in cell culture *in vitro*. Proceedings of the Society for Experimental Biology and Medicine 160: 213–221

Shaw F E Jr, Guess I J A, Roets J M et al 1989 Effect of anatomic site, age and smoking on the immune response to hepatitis B vaccination. Vaccine 7: 425–430

Skelly J, Howard C R, Zuckerman A J 1981 Hepatitis B polypeptide vaccine in micelle form. Nature 290: 51–54

Yap L, Guan R, Chan S H 1992 Recombinant DNA hepatitis B vaccine containing pre-S components of the HBV coat protein – a preliminary study on immunogenicity. Vaccine 10: 439–442

Young P, Vaudin M, Dixon J, Zuckerman A J 1982 Preparation of hepatitis B polypeptide micelles from human carrier plasma. Journal of Virological Methods 4: 177–185

Zuckerman A J 1973 Synthetic hepatitis B vaccine. Nature 241: 499

Zuckerman A J 1984 Who should be immunised against hepatitis B? British Medical Journal 289: 1243–1244

Zuckerman A J 1990 Immunization against hepatitis B. British Medical Bulletin 46: 383–398

Zuckerman J N, Cockcroft A, Zuckerman A J 1992 Site of injection for vaccination. British Medical Journal 305: 1158

UPDATE

- Schodel et al (1993) review and extend data on the use of hepatitis B virus (HBV) core (HBcAg) particles as a carrier moiety for B-cell epitopes of the HBV envelope proteins. Virus-neutralizing epitopes of the HBV pre-S region were inserted at the N-terminus, the N-terminus through a pre-core linker sequence, the C-terminus and an internal position of HBcAg by genetic engineering in *Escherichia coli*. The hybrid HBc/pre-S proteins were purified and their antigenicity and immunogenicity analysed. All purified HBc/pre-S particles were particulate. Pre-S epitopes inserted at the N-terminus through a precore polylinker, the truncated C-terminus and at the internal position between HBcA amino acids 75 and 81 were accessible on the particle surface. N-terminal fusions required the presence of the linker sequence to become surface accessible and immunogenic. Fusions to the N- and C-termini of HBcAg did not interfere with HBcAg antigenicity and immunogenicity. In contrast, insertion at the internal site abrogated recognition of HBcAg by 5 out of 6 monoclonal antibodies and diminished recognition by human polyclonal anti-HBc antibodies as well as HBcAg immunogenicity. A pre-S (2) sequence fused to the C-terminus of HBcAg was surface accessible and weakly immunogenic. Pre-S(1) sequences fused to the N-terminus through a pre-core linker were surface accessible and highly immunogenic. The same sequence fused to the core methionine was not surface accessible or immunogenic. Insertion of the same pre-S(1) sequence at an internal position of HBcAg resulted in the most efficient anti-pre-S(1) antibody response.

- REFERENCE

Schodel F, Peterson D, Hughes J, Milich D R 1993 A virulent Salmonella expressing hybrid hepatitis B virus core/pre-S genes for oral vaccination. Vaccine 11, 2: 143–148

SECTION 3

Hepatitis C virus

13. Structure and molecular virology

Michael Houghton Jang Han George Kuo Qui-Lim Choo Amy J. Weiner

THE RELATIONSHIP BETWEEN HCV AND THE FLAVIVIRIDAE FAMILY

The genome of the hepatitis C virus (HCV) comprises a positive-stranded RNA molecule of about 9500 nucleotides (nt) (Choo et al 1989) containing a long translational open reading frame (ORF) that could encode a large polypeptide of approximately 3000 amino acids (aa) beginning with the first in-frame methionine codon (Kato et al 1990, Choo et al 1991a, Takamizawa et al 1991). The 5' terminus of the RNA genome has substantial primary sequence identity with the corresponding region of the pestivirus genomes (Takeuchi et al 1990, Han et al 1991, Choo et al 1991a), and a region of the encoded polypeptide exhibits significant sequence identity with nucleoside triphosphate (NTP)-binding helicases encoded by the pestiviruses and to a lesser extent, the flaviviruses (Miller & Purcell 1990, Choo et al 1991a, b). Protease and replicase sequence motifs conserved among the pestiviruses and flaviviruses are also present within the HCV-encoded polyprotein, which along with the more extensively conserved helicase sequence are all similarly colinear among the three types of viral polyproteins (Choo et al 1991a). Although these are the only regions of HCV exhibiting significant primary sequence identity with the pestiviruses and flaviviruses, the hydropathicity of the HCV-encoded polypeptide is remarkably similar to that of the flaviviruses and, to a lesser extent, to that of the pestiviruses, thus indicating similarities in their basic structures and functions (Choo et al 1991a). In combination, these features indicate that, while HCV is a novel agent, it is most closely related to both the animal pestiviruses (e.g. bovine viral diarrhoea virus and hog cholera virus) and to the human flaviviruses (e.g. yellow fever virus and Dengue fever virus) and therefore deserves classification within the same Flaviviridae family but as a separate genus (Fig. 13.1). The observed relationship between HCV and the well-characterized pestiviruses and flaviviruses is most valuable not only in helping to define the genetic organization of HCV but also in stimulating comparisons and studies of virus–host interactions. It has been established that HCV is the major aetiological agent associated with post-transfusion non-A, non-B hepatitis (NANBH) as well as being a major cause of sporadic NANBH (Kuo et al 1989, Aach et al 1991, Okochi et al 1991, Alter

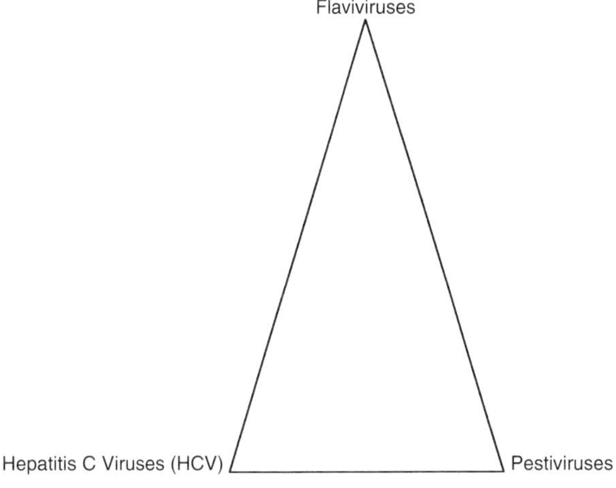

Fig. 13.1 The Flaviviridae family. The isosceles nature of the triangle is used to indicate the three separate genera of the Flaviviridae family as well as the closer evolutionary relationship between HCV and the pestiviruses evident from the level of primary sequence identity at both the nucleotide and amino acid level.

et al 1992, Donahue et al 1992). While not replicating through a DNA intermediate and being unable to integrate into the host genome (Choo et al 1989), HCV causes chronic infection in at least 50% of cases (Dienstag & Alter 1986, Alter et al 1992), which then predisposes to the sequential development of cirrhosis and primary hepatocellular carcinoma (Kiyosawa et al 1990). Current knowledge concerning the interactions of the pestiviruses and flaviviruses with their animal and human hosts is likely to provide some insight into the mechanisms of HCV persistence and pathogenicity.

THE STRUCTURE AND PROCESSING OF THE HCV-ENCODED POLYPROTEIN PRECURSOR

A large ORF extends throughout most of the HCV RNA genomic sequence that could encode a polypeptide of between 3010 and 3033 amino acids depending on the source of viral isolate (Kato et al 1990, Choo et al 1991a, Inchauspe et al 1991, Okamoto et al 1991, Takamizawa et al 1991, Chen et al 1992, Okamoto et al 1992a). As in the case of the pestiviral and flaviviral relatives, it appears that this large HCV ORF encodes a polyprotein precursor that is processed co- and post-translationally to yield a variety of structural (virion) and non-structural (NS) proteins. Structural proteins appear to be processed from the N-terminal region of the HCV polyprotein precursor, beginning with a presumed RNA-binding nucleocapsid polypeptide of basic charge (C; 17–22 kDa) followed by two glycoproteins [E1 (32–35 kDa) and E2/NS1 (68–72 kDa); Fig. 13.2]. These proteins have been identified in in vitro translations of HCV RNA transcribed in vitro from cDNA clones (Hijikata et al 1991a, Houghton 1992) and also from mammalian cells (Harada et al 1991, Kohara et al 1992, Kumar et al 1992, Matsuura et al 1992, Spaete et al 1992) and insect cells (Matsuura et al 1992) transfected with HCV cDNA. By aligning the HCV polyprotein with that of the pestiviruses, the HCV E1 and E2/NS1 glycoproteins appear to correlate with two of the three known envelope glycoproteins of the pestiviruses, bovine viral diarrhoea virus and hog cholera virus and thus are likely to be envelope glycoproteins themselves (Choo et al 1991a).

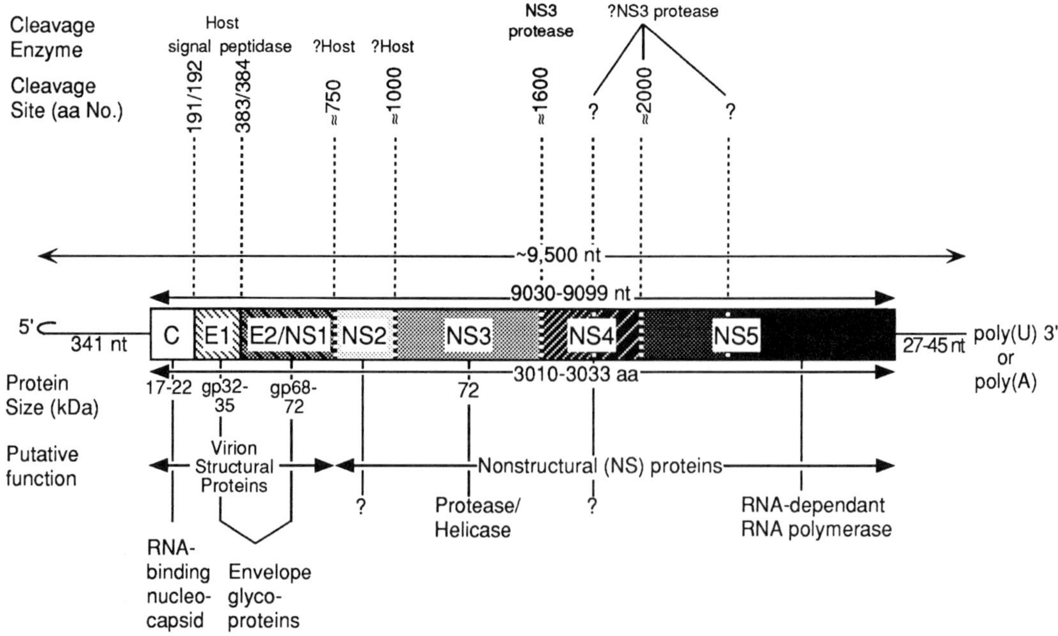

Fig. 13.2 Schematic organization of the HCV genome and encoded proteins.

While the flaviviral counterpart of the HCV E1 glycoprotein is also known to be an envelope protein, the equivalent of the HCV E2/NS1 glycoprotein is a secreted and glycosylated *non-*structural protein (NS1, Rice et al 1986). However, the HCV E2/NS1 moiety is not secreted from mammalian cells transfected with the full-length gene (Spaete et al 1992), suggesting that it probably does not have the same function as the flaviviral NS1. In addition, since HCV is more related to the pestiviruses than to the flaviviruses at the primary sequence level (Miller & Purcell 1990, Choo et al 1991a, Han et al 1991), our working hypothesis is that both HCV glycoproteins are likely to be constituents of the virion envelope.

The processing of the putative structural region of the HCV polyprotein is similar to that of the related flaviviruses and pestiviruses in being mediated at least in part by the host signal peptidase, otherwise known as signalase (Rice et al 1986, Nowak et al 1989, Ruiz-Linares et al 1989, Chambers et al 1990a, Thiel et al 1991, Wiskerchen et al 1991a). Experiments involving in vitro translation of RNA transcribed in vitro from cloned HCV cDNA indicate that internal signal sequences upstream of the E1 and E2/NS1 protein domains direct the precursor polyprotein to the endoplasmic reticulum (ER), where translocation into the lumen and signal cleavage takes place (Hijikata et al 1991a, Houghton 1992). The addition of high-mannose carbohydrate chains, which contribute approximately one-half the mass of each glycoprotein species, occurs within the lumen (Hijikata et al 1991a, Houghton 1992, Spaete et al 1992). The translocated E1 and E2/NS1 glycoproteins are not released as soluble entities into the interior of the ER lumen but appear to remain anchored inside the lumen (Hijikata et al 1991a, Spaete et al 1992). In the case of E2/NS1, this glycoprotein can be released from the ER and secreted through the Golgi apparatus into the cell medium by truncating the hydrophobic C-terminus by gene deletion in vitro (Spaete et al 1992). The C-terminal region of the E1 domain is also very hydrophobic and would terminate apparently with the hydrophobic E2/NS1 signal sequence cleaved by signal peptidase upon translocation into the lumen (Fig. 13.3). Thus, this E2/NS1 signal sequence may serve at

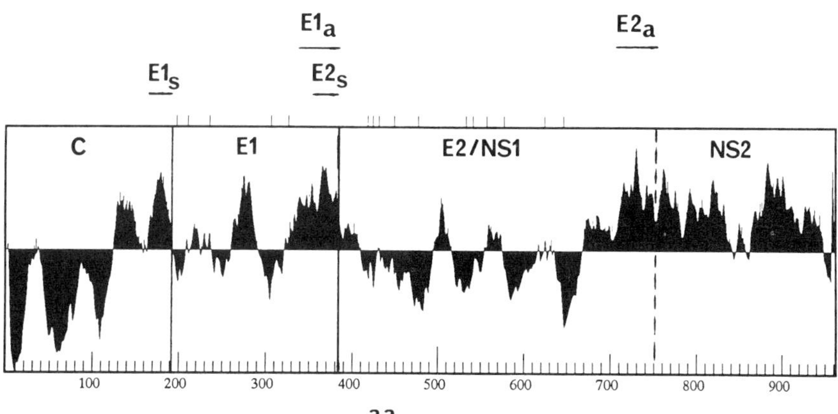

Fig. 13.3 Hydropathicity profile of the N-terminal structural region of the polyprotein encoded by the HCV-1 genome (Choo et al 1991a). Hydrophobic (above the horizontal) and hydrophilic domains (below the horizontal) within the putative nucleocapsid (C), envelope glycoproteins (E1 and E2/NS1) and part of non-structural protein 2 (NS2) are shown along with the regions corresponding to the N-terminal, internal signal sequences (s) and C-terminal membrane anchor sequences (a) of E1 and E2/NS1. The boundaries of C/E1 (aa 191/192) and E1/E2 (NS1) (aa 383/384) established from sequence (Hijikata et al 1991a) and mutation (Houghton 1992) analyses of in vitro RNA translations are shown by solid vertical lines, while the approximate boundary of E2(NS1)/NS2 is notated by the broken vertical (Hijikata et al 1991a, Houghton et al 1992). The locations of potential N-glycosylation sites within E1 (five sites) and E2/NS1 (11 sites) are indicated by short verticals.

least in part as the E1 anchor in a manner very reminiscent of the flaviviral envelope proteins (Nowak et al 1989, Ruiz-Linares et al 1989, Chambers et al 1990a). Similarly, the signal peptidase cleavage between C and E1 would result in the attachment of the hydrophobic E1 signal sequence to the C-terminus of the C protein (Hijikata et al 1991a, Houghton 1992), as also observed in the processing of the flaviviral polyprotein (Nowak et al 1989, Ruiz-Linares et al 1989, Chambers et al 1990a). In in vitro translation experiments, the signalase-processed HCV C protein has been found attached to the cytosol side of the ER, in contrast to the location of the processed E1 and E2/NS1 glycoproteins within the lumen (Hijikata et al 1991a). Thus, following signalase cleavage, the E1 signal sequence may act at least in part to retain the upstream C protein attached to the ER in an analogous manner to that of the flaviviruses (Nowak et al 1989, Ruiz-Linares et al 1989, Chambers et al 1990a). A further cleavage mediated by a flaviviral protease located within non-structural protein 3 (NS3) may serve to cleave off the C-terminal anchor region of the flaviviral nucleocapsid protein (Nowak et al 1989, Ruiz-Linares et al 1989, Chambers et al 1990b, Preugschat et al 1990, Chambers et al 1991). In contrast, the processing of the pestiviral nucleocapsid protein from the polyprotein precursor is mediated in part by an autocatalytic protease located at the extreme N-terminus of the viral polyprotein (Thiel et al 1991, Wiskerchen et al 1991a). It is presently unknown if a similar situation exists for HCV. Flaviviruses do not bud from the plasma membrane (Murphy 1980) but may assemble within vesicles budded from vacuoles within the ER (Leary & Blair 1980, Ishak et al 1988). Those factors governing the assembly, release and maturation of HCV virions remain important topics for future investigations. Systems described recently for potential propagation of HCV in vitro may prove valuable in such investigations (Jacob et al 1991, Shimizu et al 1992).

The organization of the putative non-structural (NS) protein region of HCV appears also to closely resemble that of the flaviviruses and pestiviruses. Small amino acid sequence motifs conserved among proteases, helicases and replicases are colinear in all three types of viral-encoded-polyproteins (Choo et al 1991a, b) and, despite the absence of extensive, overall primary sequence homologies in this region, the hydropathicity profiles of all three viral NS regions are similar, particularly for HCV and the flaviviruses (Choo et al 1991a). Distinctive protein domains characteristic of the flaviviral NS2, 3, 4 and 5 domains can be discerned within the HCV polyprotein (Choo et al 1991a) and are thus named similarly (Fig. 13.2), but experimental data concerning the direct characterization and function of HCV NS proteins are not yet available. However, the N-terminus of the NS3 domain contains primary sequence motifs conserved among trypsin-like serine proteases (Choo et al 1991a, Houghton et al 1991a). Extensive work on the flaviviral and equivalent pestiviral NS3 protease has shown that this viral enzyme mediates many of the cleavages that release the individual NS proteins from the precursor (Preugschat et al 1990, Chambers et al 1990b, 1991, Falgout et al 1991, Wiskerchen & Collett 1991b). Very recent data also indicate a similar function for the HCV NS3 domain (M R Eckart et al, unpublished). The NS3 region also contains a region immediately downstream of the protease domain that has significant sequence identity with NTP-binding helicases of diverse viral and cellular origin (Choo et al 1991a, Houghton et al 1991a). Helicases are capable of unwinding RNA templates and can be operational during replication, translation and splicing of RNA (Koonin 1991). Since it is probable that HCV replicates in the cytoplasm (like its flaviviral and pestiviral relatives), and not in the nucleus where splicing enzymes are localized, it is probable that the HCV helicase is involved in aspects of RNA replication and/or translation.

The large NS5 domain existing at the C-terminus of the polyprotein (Fig. 13.2) has primary sequence motifs conserved among all viral RNA-dependent polymerases, and so it is assumed that this replicase activity represents at least one of its functions (Choo et al 1991a). However, this domain (which is cleaved into two products in the case of pestiviruses) (Wiskerchen & Collett 1991b) is very large (~1000 aa) and is likely to have multiple functions (Choo et al 1991a). Both the NS2 and NS4 domains are very hydrophobic and are each cleaved into two subspecies in the case of the flaviviruses (Chambers et al 1990a).

NS2b is required for activity of the flaviviral NS3 protease (Preugschat et al 1990, Chambers et al 1991, Falgout et al 1991), whereas the pestiviral NS3-like protease does not seem to require the upstream protein for activity (Wiskerchen & Collett 1991b). Preliminary data suggest that, like the pestiviruses, the NS3/NS4 cleavage mediated by the HCV NS3 protease also does not require the upstream NS2 domain (M R Eckart et al, unpublished).

HETEROGENEITY OF THE HCV GENOME

The region encoding the viral polyprotein precursor

As observed for other RNA viruses, there is a substantial fluidity of the HCV genome resulting from an error-prone replicase and the absence of repair mechanisms that operate during DNA replication. This means that, even in a single infected individual, the HCV genome does not exist as a homogeneous species. Rather, it exists as a quasispecies distribution of closely related but nevertheless heterogeneous genomes (Martell et al 1992). In addition, the process of host selection and adaptation of a rapidly mutating genome has led to the evolution of many distinct (yet still fluid) HCV genotypes. Several different HCV genotypes can be distinguished according to the actual degree of nucleotide and amino acid relatedness (Cha et al 1992, Chan et al 1992, Mori et al 1992) and it is likely that many others will be uncovered in the future. Rigorous phylogenetic analyses of the 5' terminal RNA sequence upstream of the large ORF have indicated the existence of three main HCV types: 1, 2 and 3 (Chan et al 1992). However, when extended to the more variable NS3 and NS5 sequence of the ORF itself, HCV types 1 and 2 can each be divided into subtypes a and b (Chan et al 1992; see Fig. 13.4). According to this nomenclature, HCV genotypes 1a and 1b correspond to the previously named HCV groups I and II (Houghton et al 1991b). A very recent analysis of new HCV sequences indicates the existence of at least a fourth HCV type (Simmonds et al 1993). Sequence and genotyping studies indicate that the quite closely related subtypes, HCV-1a and HCV-1b, may predominate in the USA and

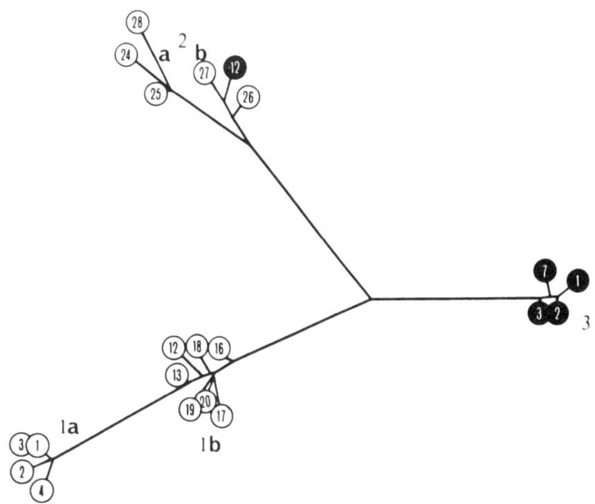

Fig. 13.4 Phylogenetic analysis of HCV RNA sequences within the NS5 region. (Reprinted with permission from Chan et al 1992, courtesy of the Society of General Microbiology.)

Japan, respectively, although less common types also occur in both countries (Takeuchi et al 1989, Enomoto et al 1990, Houghton et al 1991b, Kato et al 1991, Tsukiyama-Kohara et al 1991, Cha et al 1992, Chan et al 1992, Mori et al 1992, Okamoto et al 1992c, Takada et al 1992). In the Netherlands, preliminary sequence data indicate that 1b genotypes may predominate (Cuypers et al 1991), and elsewhere in Europe viruses belonging to the 1a and 1b subtypes have been commonly observed (Kremsdorf et al 1991, Weiner et al 1991, Chan et al 1992, Cha et al 1992, Kumar et al 1992, Martell et al 1992). HCV type 3 has been shown to occur frequently in Scotland along with type 1 viruses (McOmish et al 1993). Type 4 HCV appears to predominate in Egypt and Zaire (Simmonds et al 1993), and yet additional genotypes may be present in Thailand (Mori et al 1992) and South Africa (Cha et al 1992). This substantial heterogeneity has many potentially important ramifications. Firstly, virus–host interactions may vary depending on the infecting HCV genotype, which could lead to important differences in pathogenicity and the progression of disease. Very preliminary data raise the possibility that the severity of hepatitis may be related to the infecting HCV type (Pozzato et al 1991, McOmish et al 1993). Initial studies have also suggested that patient sensitivity to interferon treatment may depend on the infecting genotype. In a preliminary study involving a small number of Italian patients, infections by apparently HCV-1b (or group II) genotypes were found to respond less well relative to non-1b viruses (Pozzato et al 1991). In a larger Japanese study, patients infected with type 1 (mostly 1b presumably) genotypes were also found to be less sensitive to alpha interferon therapy than patients infected with other HCV types (Yoshioka et al 1992). In this same study, those patients infected with HCV type 1 were also found to have pretreatment viral RNA titres – 1–2 orders of magnitude higher than patients infected with other HCV genotypes – suggesting that sensitivity to interferon may be inversely related to viral titre (Yoshioka et al 1992). Further work is required to confirm and extend these important findings.

The presence of a large number of diverse HCV genotypes also raises several important issues related to the diagnosis and control of HCV infection. The second-generation anti-HCV screening assays (van der Poel et al 1991, Chien et al 1992) now utilize a combination of recombinant capture antigens derived from the three most conserved polypeptide regions, C, NS3 and NS4 (Okamoto et al 1992a), and these have been used to detect all of the diverse HCV genotypes reported to date (Takeuchi et al 1989, Enomoto et al 1990, Cuypers et al 1991, Houghton et al 1991b, Kato et al 1991, Tsukiyama-Kohara et al 1991, Weiner et al 1991, Cha et al 1992, Chan et al 1992, Mori et al 1992, Okamoto et al 1992c, Takada et al 1992, McOmish et al 1993, Simmonds et al 1993). However, infections by HCV type 3 genotypes have been reported to generate weakly cross-reacting anti-NS4 antibodies (McOmish et al 1993). HCV type 1 and 2 infections can be serotyped through the use of specific C peptides (Machida et al 1992), and rigorous genotyping is feasible through the use of type-specific polymerase chain reaction (PCR) assay primers and/or restriction fragment length polymorphism (RFLP) analyses (Okamoto et al 1992c, McOmish et al 1993, Simmonds et al 1993).

Considerable differences exist in the two putative envelope glycoproteins, with up to 49% (E1) and 30% (E2) divergence, approximately, at the amino acid level, between HCV types 1 and 2 (groups I, II, III and IV in Okamoto et al 1992a). There are also differences in the number of potential N-glycosylation sites in both putative envelope glycoproteins between different HCV genotypes that may affect protein conformation and immunogenicity (Kato et al 1990, Choo et al 1991a). Consequently, it is possible that virus-neutralizing antibodies may not be cross-reactive against all HCV types, thus raising the possible requirement for a multi-subunit vaccine to effect global protection against HCV infection.

While the average rate of change of the HCV genome within a single persisently infected individual has been estimated to be $1\text{–}2 \times 10^{-3}$ nt changes per site per year (Ogata et al 1991, Okamoto et al 1992b, Abe et al 1992), there is a much higher rate of change at the extreme 5' terminus of the gene encoding the N-terminus of the E2/NS1 glycoprotein (Ogata et al 1991, Abe et al 1992, Okamoto et al 1992b, Weiner et al 1992a, Kumar et al 1993). This E2 hypervariable region (E2HV) spanning aa 384–414 appears to be the most variable region of the HCV polyprotein and is different in virtually every isolate studied so far (Hijikata et al 1991b, Weiner et al 1991). A number of distinct antibody-binding epitopes have been mapped to this region and in one chronically-infected patient, the emergence of an E2HV variant has been documented, suggesting that escape mutants in this E2HV region may play an important role in the development of chronicity (Weiner et al 1992b). The lack of patient response to interferon therapy has also been correlated with heterogeneity of the E2HV region (Okada et al 1991), which is consistent with the hypothesis that persistence of HCV is attributable to E2HV escape mutants (Weiner et al 1992b). Another small region in E2/NS1 (HVR2) just downstream of E2HV also shows significant variation which, although less than that seen in E2HV, may also reflect the consequences of immune pressure (Hijikata et al 1991b).

The 5' terminal leader of HCV genomic RNA

A 5' leader sequence of 341 nt precedes the presumed initiator methionine codon of the large

ORF encoding the polyprotein precursor (Kato et al 1990, Choo et al 1991a, Han et al 1991, Inchauspe et al 1991, Okamoto et al 1991, Takamizawa et al 1991, Chen et al 1992, Okamoto et al 1992a). This is the only region of the HCV genetic sequence that shows substantial nucleotide sequence identity with other known viral genomes, exhibiting approximately 50% identity with the 5' leaders of animal pestiviral RNA genomes (Takeuchi et al 1990, Choo et al 1991a, Han et al 1991). This striking sequence conservation occurs mainly in four regions of the leader and indicates that the leader plays a highly important role in some aspect(s) of viral translation, replication and/or assembly (Han et al 1991). This region is highly conserved among different HCV isolates from around the world, showing at least 90% sequence identity between 81 different HCV isolates (Bukh et al 1992a). This sequence conservation varies throughout the 5' leader, with the 65 nt immediately upstream of the presumed polyprotein initiator codon being completely invariant except for the –2 nt (Bukh et al 1992a), which contains one of the main regions of homology with the pestiviral leaders (Han et al 1991, Bukh et al 1992a). Together with another region further upstream that also shows particular conservation with the pestiviral leaders, these regions represent ideal sequences from which to design PCR primers to amplify and detect otherwise diverse HCV RNA species (Okamoto et al 1990, Han et al 1991, Bukh et al 1992a, b, Weiner et al 1992a, Simmonds et al 1993).

The HCV 5' leader contains up to five very small ORFs (each beginning with a methionine codon), some of which are conserved among different HCV isolates (Bukh et al 1992a). Intriguingly, these ORF conservations may imply active translational functions of great importance to some aspect of the viral lifecycle. Data derived from in vitro translations indicate that ribosomes initiate translation internally within the 5' leader sequence of an HCV-1b (or group II) genotype (Tsukiyama-Kohara et al 1992). Also, a secondary structure model for the 5' HCV leader predicts the existence of a large, conserved stem–loop structure (Brown et al 1992; domain III in Fig. 13.5) within the region thought to be

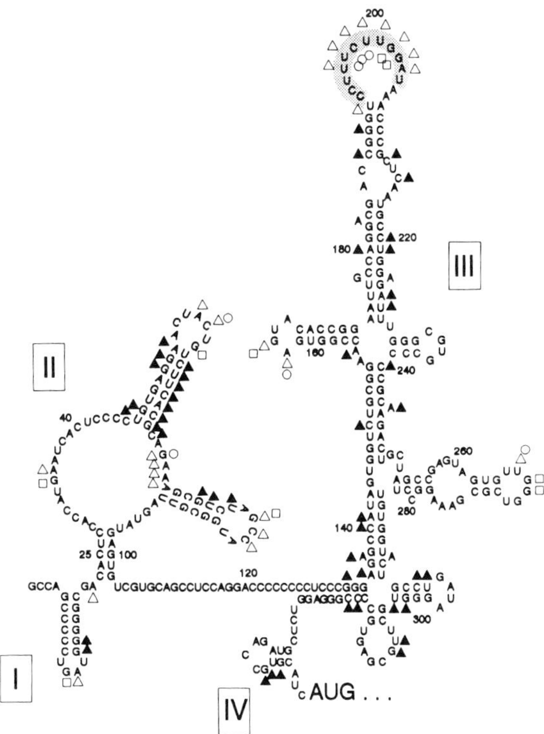

Fig. 13.5 Proposed secondary structure of the 5' HCV RNA leader. Sites of nuclease cleavages are indicated by symbols adjacent to individual nucleotides: □, T_1; ○, T_2; △, S_1 (single-strand specific); and ▲, V_1 (double-strand specific). The pyrmidine-rich tract within the apical loop of domain III, which is complementary to 18S ribosomal RNA, is indicated by a shaded background (Reprinted with permission from Brown et al 1992, courtesy of Oxford University Press.)

essential for internal ribosome initiation in vitro (Tsukiyama-Kohara et al 1992). This model also resembles that of picornaviral leaders (in which ribosomes are known to initiate internally) in exhibiting extensive secondary structure, pyrimidine-rich tracts and regions complementary to 18S ribosomal RNA (Brown et al 1992, Fig. 13.5). However, experimental data derived from transfection of an HCV-1a (or group I) 5' leader placed upstream of a reporter gene appear to be inconsistent with an internal ribosomal entry site (Yoo et al 1992). Translational activity was inhibited by superinfection of transfected cells with poliovirus, which normally stimulates cap-independent internal initiation (Yoo et al 1992). Also, when placed in between two reporter genes, the 5' leader sequence failed to stimulate transla-

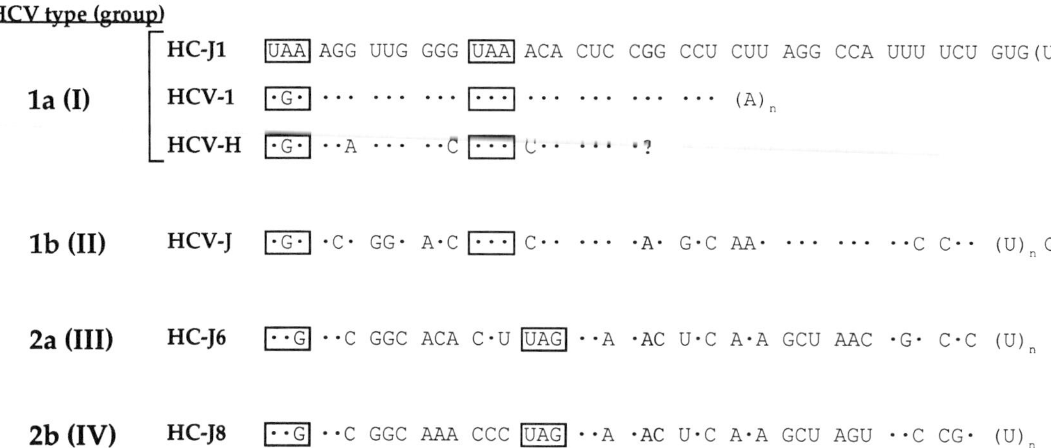

Fig. 13.6 Comparison of 3' untranslated genomic RNA sequences derived from HCV isolates HC-J1 (Okamoto et al 1991), HCV-1 (Han et al 1991), HCV-H (Inchauspe et al 1991), HCV-J (Kato et al 1990), HC-J6 (Okamoto et al 1991) and HC-J8 (Okamoto et al 1992a). Sequence identity with HCV-J1 is indicated by a dot. Boxes denote in-frame stop codons that terminate translation of the viral polyprotein precursor. The HCV isolates are segregated into named types (Chan et al 1992, Simmonds et al 1993) or groups (Houghton et al 1991b, Okamoto et al 1992a) based on phylogenetic analyses.

tion of the downstream RNA, again inconsistent with internal ribosome entry (Yoo et al 1992). Further work is therefore necessary to resolve this issue.

The 3' untranslated region

A very short untranslated region is located downstream of the stop codon terminating the large ORF encoding the viral polyprotein (Fig. 13.6). A second in frame stop codon is situated just downstream of the first one, which exists presumably to ensure termination of translation of the viral polyprotein precursor. This 3' untranslated leader consists of between only 27 and 45 nt depending on the particular viral isolate and is followed by a 3' terminal, homopolymeric tail consisting of poly(rU) in all isolates except in the case of the HCV-1 isolate, which appears to terminate with a poly(rA) tail (Han et al 1991; Fig. 13.6). Although the 3' untranslated, heteronucleotide sequence varies considerably among different isolates (Fig. 13.6), theoretical stem–loop secondary structures appear to be conserved that could be important for the binding and/or priming of the replicase enzyme (or other factors) during genome replication (Han & Houghton 1992). However, the observed sequence variation in this region may result in different priming efficiencies and viral copy numbers, which could conceivably be at least partially responsible for potential differences in viral pathogenicity (Pozzato et al 1991, McOmish et al 1993) and interferon sensitivity (Pozzato et al 1991, Yoshioka et al 1992).

REFERENCES

Aach R D, Stevens C E, Hollinger F B et al 1991 Hepatitis C virus infection in post-transfusion hepatitis. New England Journal of Medicine 325: 1325–1329

Abe K, Inchauspe G, Fujisawa K 1992 Genomic characterization and mutation rate of hepatitis C virus isolated from a patient who contracted hepatitis during an epidemic of non-A, non-B hepatitis in Japan. Journal of General Virology 73: 2725–2729

Alter M J, Margolis H S, Krawczynski K et al 1992 The natural history of community-acquired hepatitis C in the United States. New England Journal of Medicine 327: 1899–1905

Brown E A, Zhang H, Ping L-H, Lemon S M 1992 Secondary structure of the 5' nontranslated regions of hepatitis C virus and pestivirus genomic RNAs. Nucleic Acids Research 20: 5041–5045

Bukh J, Purcell R H, Miller R H 1992a Sequence analysis of the 5' noncoding region of hepatitis C virus. Proceedings of the National Academy of Sciences of the USA 89: 4942–4946

Bukh J, Purcell R H, Miller R H 1992b Importance of primer selection for the detection of hepatitis C virus RNA with the polymerase chain reaction assay. Proceedings of the National Academy of Sciences of the USA 89: 187–192

Cha T-A, Beall E, Irvine B et al 1992 At least five related, but distinct, hepatitis C viral genotypes exist. Proceedings of the National Academy of Sciences of the USA 89: 7144–7148

Chambers T J, McCourt D W, Rice C M 1990a Production of yellow fever virus proteins in infected cells: Identification of discrete polyprotein species and analysis of cleavage kinetics using region-specific polyclonal antisera. Virology 177: 159–174

Chambers T J, Weir R C, Grakoui A et al 1990b Evidence that the N-terminal domain of nonstructural protein NS3 from yellow fever virus is a serine protease responsible for site specific cleavages in the viral polyprotein. Proceedings of the National Academy of Sciences of the USA 87: 8898–8902

Chambers T J, Grakoui A, Rice C M 1991 Processing of the yellow fever virus nonstructural polyprotein: a catalytically active NS3 proteinase domain and NS2B are required for cleavages at dibasic sites. Journal of Virology 65: 6042–6050

Chan S-W, McOmish F, Holmes E C et al 1992 Analysis of a new hepatitis C virus type and its phylogenetic relationship to existing variants. Journal of General Virology 73: 1131–1141

Chen P-J, Lin M-H, Tai K-F, Liu P-C, Lin C-J, Chen D-S 1992 The Taiwanese hepatitis C virus genome: sequence determination and mapping the 5' termini of viral genomic and antigenomic RNA. Virology 188: 102–113

Chien D Y, Choo Q-L, Tabrizi A et al 1992 Diagnosis of hepatitis C virus (HCV) infection using an immunodominant chimeric polyprotein to capture circulating antibodies: re-evaluation of the role of HCV in liver disease. Proceedings of the National Academy of Sciences of the USA 89: 10011–10015

Choo Q-L, Kuo G, Weiner A J, Overby L R, Bradley D W, Houghton M 1989 Isolation of a cDNA clone derived from a blood-borne non-A, non-B viral hepatitis genome. Science 244: 359–362

Choo Q-L, Richman K H, Han J et al 1991a Genetic organization and diversity of the hepatitis C virus. Proceedings of the National Academy of Sciences of the USA 88: 2451–2455

Choo Q-L, Han J, Weiner A J et al 1991b Hepatitis C virus is a distant relative of the flaviviruses and pestiviruses. In: Viral hepatitis C, D and E (Proceedings of the International Meeting on Non-A, Non-B Hepatitis, Tokyo, Japan). Elsevier Science Publishers, Amsterdam, pp 47–52

Cuypers H T M, Winkel I N, Van der Poel et al 1991 Analysis of genomic variability of hepatitis C virus. Hepatology 13: S15–S19

Dienstag J L, Alter H J 1986 Non-A, non-B hepatitis: evolving epidemiologic and clinical perspective. In: Seminars in Liver Disease. Thieme, New York, pp 67–81

Donahue J G, Muñoz A, Ness P M et al 1992 The declining risk of post-transfusion hepatitis C virus infection. New England Journal of Medicine 327: 369–373

Enomoto N, Takada A, Nakao T, Date T 1990 There are two major types of hepatitis C virus in Japan. Biochemistry Biophysics Research Communications 170: 1021–1025

Falgout B, Pethel M, Zhang Y-M, Lai C-J 1991 Both nonstructural proteins NS2B and NS3 are required for the proteolytic processing of Dengue virus nonstructural proteins. Journal of Virology 65: 2467–2475

Han J H, Houghton M 1992 Group specific sequences and conserved secondary structures at the 3' end of HCV genome and its implication for viral replication. Nucleic Acids Research 20: 3520

Han J H, Shyamala V, Richman K H et al 1991 Characterization of the terminal regions of hepatitis C viral RNA: identification of conserved sequences in the 5' untranslated region and poly(A) tails at the 3' end. Proceedings of the National Academy of Sciences of the USA 88: 1711–1715

Harada S, Watanabe Y, Takeuchi K et al 1991 Expression of processed core protein of hepatitis C virus in mammalian cells. Journal of Virology 65: 3015–3021

Hijikata M, Kato N, Ootsuyama Y, Nakagawa M, Shimotohno K 1991a Gene mapping of the putative structural region of the hepatitis C virus genome by in vitro processing analysis. Proceedings of the National Academy of Sciences of the USA 88: 5547–5551

Hijikata M, Kato N, Ootsuyama Y, Nakagawa M, Ohkoshi S, Shimotohno K 1991b Hypervariable regions in the putative glycoprotein of hepatitis C virus. Biochemistry Biophysics Research Communications 175: 220–228

Houghton M 1992 Heterogeneity of the HCV genome: importance for control of the disease. In: Hepatitis C virus: scientific and clinical status. Advanced Therapeutic Communications, New Jersey, pp 8–9

Houghton M, Richman K, Han J et al 1991a Hepatitis C virus (HCV): A relative of the pestiviruses and flaviviruses. In: Hollinger F B, Lemon S M, Margolis H (eds) Viral hepatitis and liver disease (Proceedings of the 1990 International Symposium on Viral Hepatitis and Liver Disease). Williams & Wilkins, Baltimore, pp 328–333

Houghton M, Weiner A, Han J, Kuo G, Choo Q-L 1991b Molecular biology of the hepatitis C viruses: implications for diagnosis, development and control of viral disease. Hepatology 14: 381–388

Inchauspe G, Zebedee S L, Lee D-H, Sugitani M, Nasoff M S, Prince A M 1991 Genomic structure of the human prototype strain H of hepatitis C virus: Comparison with American and Japanese isolates. Proceedings of the National Academy of Sciences of the USA 88: 10292–10296

Ishak R, Tovey D G, Howard C R 1988 Morphogenesis of yellow fever virus 17 D in infected cell cultures. Journal of General Virology 69: 325–335

Jacob J R, Sureau C, Burk K H, Eichberg J W, Dreesman G R, Landford R E 1990 In vitro replication of non-A, non-B hepatitis virus. In: Hollinger F B, Lemon S M, Margolis H (eds) Viral hepatitis and liver disease (Proceedings of the 1990 International Symposium on Viral Hepatitis and Liver Disease). Williams & Wilkins, Baltimore, pp 387–392

Kato N, Hijikata M, Ootsuyama Y et al 1990 Molecular cloning of the human hepatitis C virus genome from Japanese patients with non-A, non-B hepatitis. Proceedings of the National Academy of Sciences of the USA 87: 9524–9528

Kato N, Ootsuyama Y, Ohkoshi S et al 1991 Distribution of plural HCV types in Japan. Biochemistry Biophysics Research Communications 181: 279–285

Kiyosawa K, Tanaka E, Sodeyama T et al 1990 Transition of antibody to hepatitis C virus from chronic hepatitis to hepatocellular carcinoma. Japan Journal of Cancer Research 81: 1089–1091

Kohara M, Tsukiyama-Kohara K, Maki N et al 1992 Expression and characterization of glycoprotein gp35 of hepatitis C virus using recombinant vaccinia virus. Journal of General Virology 73: 2313–2318

Koonin E V 1991 Similarities in RNA helicases. Nature 352: 290

Kremsdorf D, Porchon C, Kim J P, Reyes G R, Bréchot C 1991 Partial nucleotide sequence analysis of a French hepatitis C virus: implications for HCV genetic variability in the E2/NS1 protein. Journal of General Virology 72: 2557–2561

Kumar U, Cheng D, Thomas H C, Monjardino J 1992 Cloning and sequencing of the structural region and expression of putative core gene of hepatitis C virus from a British case of chronic sporadic hepatitis. Journal of General Virology 73: 1521–1525

Kumar U, Brown J, Monjardino J, Thomas H C 1993 Sequence variation in the large envelope glycoprotein(E2/NS1) of the hepatitic virus during chronic infection. Journal of Infectious Diseases 167: 726–730

Kuo G, Choo Q-L, Alter H J et al 1989 An assay for circulating antibodies to a major etiologic virus of human non-A, non-B hepatitis. Science 244: 362–364

Leary K R, Blair C D 1980 Sequential events in the morphogenesis of Japanese encephalitis virus. Journal of Ultrastructural Research 72: 123

Machida A, Ohnuma H, Tsuda F et al 1992 Two distinct subtypes of hepatitis C virus defined by antibodies directed to the putative core protein. Hepatology 16: 886–891

McOmish F, Chan S-W, Dow B C et al 1993 Detection of three types of hepatitis C virus in blood donors: Investigation of type-specific differences in serologic reactivity and rate of alanine aminotransferase abnormalities. Transfusion 33: 7–13

Martell M, Esteban J I, Quer J et al 1992 Hepatitis C virus (HCV) circulates as a population of different but closely related genomes: quasispecies nature of HCV genome distribution. Journal of Virology 66: 3225–3229

Matsuura Y, Harada S, Suzuki R et al 1992 Expression of processed envelope protein of hepatitis C virus in mammalian and insect cells. Journal of Virology 66: 1425–1431

Miller R H, Purcell R H 1990 Hepatitis C virus shares amino acid sequence similarity with pestiviruses and flaviviruses as well as members of two plant virus supergroups. Proceedings of the National Academy of Sciences of the USA 87: 2057–2061

Mori S, Kato N, Yagyu A et al 1992 A new type of hepatitis C virus in patients in Thailand. Biochemistry and Biophysics Research Communications 183: 334–342

Murphy F A 1980 Togavirus morphology and morphogenesis. In: The togaviruses. Academic Press, New York, pp 241–316

Nowak T, Färber P M, Wengler G, Wengler G 1989 Analyses of the terminal sequences of West Nile Virus structural proteins and of the *in vitro* translation of these proteins allow the proposal of a complete scheme of the proteolytic cleavages involved in their synthesis. Virology 169: 365–376

Ogata N, Alter H J, Miller R H, Purcell R H 1991 Nucleotide sequence and mutation rate of the H strain of hepatitis C virus. Proceedings of the National Academy of Sciences of the USA 88: 3392–3396

Okada S I, Akahane Y, Suzuki H, Okamoto H, Mishiro S 1992 The degree of variability in the amino terminal region of the E2/NS1 protein of hepatitis C virus correlates with responsiveness to interferon therapy in viremic patients. Hepatology 16: 619–624

Okamoto H, Okada S, Sugiyama Y et al 1990 The 5'-terminal sequence of the hepatitis C virus genome. Japanese Journal of Experimental Medicine 60: 167–177

Okamoto H, Okada S, Sugiyama Y et al 1991 Nucleotide sequence of the genomic RNA of hepatitis C virus isolated from a human carrier: comparison with reported isolates for conserved and divergent regions. Journal of General Virology 72: 2697–2704

Okamoto H, Kurai K, Okada S-I et al 1992a Full-length sequence of a hepatitis C virus genome having poor homology to reported isolates: comparative study of four distinct genotypes. Virology 188: 331–341

Okamoto H, Kojima M, Okada S-I et al 1992b Genetic drift of hepatitis C virus during an 8.2-year infection in a chimpanzee: variability and stability. Virology 190: 894–899

Okamoto H, Sugiyama Y, Okada S et al 1992c Typing hepatitis C virus by polymerase chain reaction with type-specific primers: application to clinical surveys and tracing infectious sources. Journal of General Virology 73: 673–679

Okochi K, Inaba S, Tokunaga K et al 1991 Effect of screening for hepatitis C virus antibody and hepatitis B core antibody on incidence of post-transfusion hepatitis. Lancet 338: 1040–1041

Pozzato G, Moretti M, Franzin F et al 1991 Severity of liver disease with different hepatitis C viral clones. Lancet 338: 509

Preugschat F, Yao C-W, Strauss J H 1990 In vitro processing of Dengue virus type 2 nonstructural proteins NS2A, NS2B, and NS3. Journal of Virology 64: 4364–4374

Rice C M, Strauss E G, Strauss J H 1986 Structure of the flavivirus genome. In: Schlesinger S, Schlesinger M J (eds) The togaviridae and flaviviridae. Plenum Press, New York, pp 279–326

Ruiz-Linares A, Cahour A, Desprès P, Girard M, Bouloy M 1989 Processing of yellow fever virus polyprotein: Role of cellular proteases in maturation of the structural proteins. Journal of Virology 63: 4199–4209

Shimizu Y K, Iwamoto A, Hijikata M, Purcell R H, Yoshikura H 1992 Evidence for *in vitro* replication of hepatitis C virus genome in a human T-cell line. Proceedings of the National Academy of Sciences of the USA 89: 5477–5481

Simmonds P, McOmish F, Yap P L et al 1993 Sequence variability in the 5' non-coding region of hepatitis C virus: identification of a new virus type and restrictions on sequence diversity. Journal of General Virology 74: 661–668

Spaete R R, Alexander D, Rugroden M E et al 1992 Characterization of the hepatitis C virus E2/NS1 gene product expressed in mammalian cells. Virology 188: 819–830

Takada N, Takase S, Takada A, Date T 1992 HCV genotypes in different countries. Lancet 339: 808

Takamizawa A, Mori C, Fuke I et al 1991 Structure and organization of the hepatitis C virus genome isolated from human carriers. Journal of Virology 65: 1105–1113

Takeuchi K, Boonmar S, Katayama T et al 1989 A cDNA fragment of hepatitis C virus isolated from an implicated donor of post-transfusion non-A, non-B hepatitis in Japan. Nucleic Acids Research 24: 10367–10372

Takeuchi K, Kubo Y, Boonmar S et al 1990 The putative nucleocapsid and envelope protein genes of hepatitis C virus determined by comparison of the nucleotide sequences of two isolates derived from an experimentally infected chimpanzee and healthy human carriers. Journal of General Virology 71: 3027–3033

Thiel H-J, Stark R, Weiland E, Rumenapf T, Meyers G 1991 Hog cholera virus: Molecular composition of virions from a pestivirus. Journal of Virology 65: 4705–4712

Tsukiyama-Kohara K, Kohara M, Yamaguchi K et al 1991 A second group of hepatitis C virus. Virus Genes 5: 243–254

Tsukiyama-Kohara K, Iiauka N, Kohara M, Nomoto A 1992 Internal ribosome entry site within hepatitis C virus RNA. Journal of Virology 66: 1476–1483

van der Poel C L, Cuypers H T M, Reesink H W et al 1991 Confirmation of hepatitis C virus infection by new four-antigen recombinant immunoblot assay. Lancet 337: 317–319

Weiner A J, Brauer M J, Rosenblatt J et al 1991 Variable and hypervariable domains are found in the regions of HCV corresponding to the flavivirus envelope and NS1 proteins and the pestivirus envelope glycoproteins. Virology 180: 842–848

Weiner A J, Shyamala V, Hall J E, Houghton M, Han J 1992a PCR: Application of polymerase chain reaction to hepatitis C virus research and diagnostics. In: Beeker Y, Darai G (eds) Frontiers in virology: diagnosis of human viruses by polymerase chain reaction technology. Springer-Verlag, Heidelberg, pp 86–100

Weiner A J, Geysen H M, Christopherson C et al 1992b Evidence for immune selection of Hepatitis C Virus (HCV) putative envelope glycoprotein variants: Potential role in chronic HCV infections. Proceedings of the National Academy of Sciences of the USA 89: 3468–3472

Wiskerchen M, Belzer S K, Collett M S 1991a Pestivirus gene expression: The first protein product of the bovine viral diarrhea virus large open reading frame, p20, possesses proteolytic activity. Journal of Virology 65: 4508–4514

Wiskerchen M, Collett M S 1991b Pestivirus gene expression: Protein p80 of bovine viral diarrhea virus is a proteinase involved in polyprotein processing. Virology 184: 341–350

Yoshioka K, Kakaumu S, Wakita T et al 1992 Detection of hepatitis C virus by polymerase chain reaction and response to interferon-α therapy: relationship to genotypes of hepatitis C virus. Hepatology 16: 293–299

Yoo B J, Spaete R R, Geballe A P, Selby M, Houghton M, Han J H 1992 5' End-dependent translation initiation of hepatitis C viral RNA and the presence of putative positive and negative translational control elements within the 5' untranslated region. Virology 191: 889–899

UPDATE

- To test the role of the 5' untranslated region (UTR) in controlling the expression of the HCV polyprotein, Yoo et al (1992) fused full-length or deleted versions of the 5' UTR of HCV-1 RNA to chloramphenicol acetyl transferase (CAT) mRNA to monitor CAT activity in vivo. They found:
  1. the full-length 5' UTR of HCV-1 RNA is translationally inactive while 5' deletions which mimic a 5' subgenomic RNA detected in vivo are active
  2. an efficient *cis*-acting element which represses translation is found at the 5' terminus
  3. a putative element which enhances translation is found near the 3' terminus of the 5' UTR
  4. additional *cis*-acting elements including small open reading frames (ORFs) upstream from the putative enhancer element downregulate translation. No evidence supported the existence of an internal ribosome entry site in the 5' UTR of HCV-1 RNA. These data suggest that HCV may employ a distinctive translation control strategy such as the generation of subgenomic viral mRNA in infected cells. Translational control of HCV might be responsible for some of the characteristic pathobiology seen in viral infection.
- In a study by Grakoui et al (1993), a cDNA clone encompassing the long open reading frame of the HCV H strain (3011 amino acid residues) has been assembled and sequenced. This clone and various truncated derivatives were used in vaccinia virus transient-expression assays to map HCV-encoded polypeptides and to study HCV polyprotein processing. HCV polyproteins and cleavage products were identified by using convalescent human sera and a panel of region-specific polyclonal rabbit antisera. Similar results were obtained for several mammalian cell lines examined, including the human HepGa hepatoma line. The data

indicate that at least nine polypeptides are produced by cleavage of the HCV H strain polyprotein. Putative structural proteins, located in the N-terminal one-fourth of the polyprotein, include the capsid protein C (21 kDa) followed by two possible virion envelope proteins, E (31 kDa) and E2 (70 kDa), which are heavily modified by N-linked glycosylation. The remainder of the polyprotein probably encodes nonstructural proteins including NS2 (23 kDa), NS3 (70 kDa), NS4A (8 kDa), NS4B (27 kDa), NS5A (58 kDa), and NS5B (68 kDa). An 82- to 88-kDa glycoprotein which reacted with both E2 and NS2-specific HCV antisera was also identified (called E2-NS2). Preliminary results suggest that a fraction of E1 is associated with E2 and E2-NS2 via disulphide linkages.

• REFERENCES

Grakoui A, Wychowski C, Lin C, Feinstone S M, Rice C M 1993 Expression and identification of hepatitis C virus polyprotein cleavage products. Journal of Virology 67, 3: 1385–1395

Yoo B J, Spaete R R, Geballe A P, Selby M, Houghton M, Han J H 1992 5' end-dependent translation initiation of hepatitis C viral RNA and the presence of putative positive and negative translational control elements within the 5' untranslated region. Virology 191, 2: 889–899

14. Natural history and experimental models

Patrizia Farci   Robert H. Purcell

Viral hepatitis has been recognized since ancient times, but it was only in the early 1940s, through transmission studies in volunteers, that direct evidence for the viral aetiology of hepatitis was obtained for the first time (Havens 1947,1963, reviewed by McCallum et al 1951). Subsequently, more than two decades elapsed before the first aetiological agent of human hepatitis was identified. In an era that encompassed major discoveries in clinical virology, the aetiological agents of hepatitis remained among the most difficult to study. The major hindrances to their identification were the lack of suitable animal models and the inability to isolate and propagate the hepatitis viruses in vitro. Despite several attempts to transmit hepatitis to non-human primates, the results were inconclusive and what progress was achieved came from experimental transmission studies in human volunteers. These studies, conducted by McCallum in the early 1940s in England (McCallum & Bauer 1944, McCallum 1947) and by Krugman in the late 1950s and early 1960s at the Willowbrook State School in New York (Krugman et al 1967, 1971, Krugman & Giles 1973), provided the best evidence for the existence of two antigenically distinct forms of viral hepatitis, as well as important information about the modes of transmission and the physicochemical properties of the hepatitis viruses. Of the two forms of hepatitis, one, termed 'infectious hepatitis' or hepatitis A, had a short incubation period (2–6 weeks) and was primarily transmitted by the faecal–oral route. The other, termed 'serum hepatitis' or hepatitis B, was predominantly transmitted through the parenteral route and was characterized by a long incubation period (6 weeks to 6 months). However, the essential breakthrough in hepatitis research was not achieved until 1963, when Blumberg, while investigating the polymorphism of human serum proteins, discovered the 'Australia antigen' (Blumberg et al 1965). The new antigen was eventually associated with viral hepatitis (Blumberg et al 1967), but was subsequently shown to be more specifically an incomplete form of the envelope of hepatitis B virus (HBV) and for this reason designated hepatitis B surface antigen (HBsAg) (Prince 1968, Giles et al 1969). This discovery galvanized the scientific community and provided the impetus for a great ferment in hepatitis research around the world. The identification and characterization of HBsAg permitted the development of sensitive and specific serological tests with which to identify infection with HBV. The body of knowledge gathered from the application of such tests was fundamental not only to the study of the natural history of HBV infection, but also for the subsequent discovery of the other hepatitis viruses. In fact, serological screening of transfusion-associated hepatitis (TAH) demonstrated that only a proportion of such cases were associated with detectable HBsAg in serum (Gocke et al 1970, 1972, Okochi et al 1970, Holland et al 1973). Despite the introduction of progressively more sensitive tests for the detection of HBsAg and the universal screening of blood donors, which virtually eradicated type B TAH (Goldfield et al 1975, Hollinger et al 1975), TAH per se did not disappear. With the discovery of hepatitis A virus (HAV) in 1973 and the development of serological assays for this virus (Feinstone et al 1973), it was possible to demonstrate that the newly discovered agent was not the cause of non-B TAH (Feinstone et al 1975). Thus, in 1975, the existence of a third type of hepatitis was recognized and named 'non-A, non-B (NANB) hepatitis,' under the assumption that specific tests for it would soon be forthcoming. In retrospect, there were clues for the existence of additional forms of hepatitis, besides hepatitis A and B, long before the discovery of NANB hepatitis. These clues included the clinical observation of more than two episodes of acute hepatitis in drug addicts and haemophiliacs (Mosley et al 1977, Hruby & Schauf 1978), an incubation period intermediate between hepatitis A and B (Mosley 1975) and the high rate of chronicity in non-B TAH (Dienstag 1983a, HJ Alter 1989).

The development of animal model systems has provided an invaluable resource for the study of human viral hepatitis (Purcell 1992). Although the first attempts to transmit this disease to non-human primates date back to the 1950s (Evans 1954), the potential value of a laboratory animal model was not clearly recognized until the early 1970s, when the first successful transmission of HBV infection to chimpanzees was reported (Maynard et al 1972). In retrospect, it now appears that many of the failures in transmitting hepatitis to non-human primates were due to the fact that many animals were already immune to the challenge virus. It was not until sensitive serological tests for identifying infections with HAV and HBV became available that consistent success could be achieved.

Non-human primates have played an important role in furthering our understanding of hepatitis A and B, but their use became widespread only after the discovery of the two causative agents, HAV and HBV (Purcell 1992). In contrast, much of our understanding of NANB hepatitis, as well as the discovery of its major causative agent, hepatitis C virus (HCV) (Choo et al 1989), came from studies in chimpanzees. The first proof that NANB hepatitis was indeed an infectious disease caused by a transmissible agent came from almost simultaneous independent reports of successful transmission of human NANB hepatitis to chimpanzees (HJ Alter et al 1978b, Hollinger et al 1978, Tabor et al 1978a), and the demonstration of serial transmission to other animals (Tabor et al 1978b, 1979a, Bradley et al 1979). Chimpanzees were essential to the demonstration that the transmissible agent was filterable (Prince et al 1978) and had a lipid-containing envelope (Feinstone et al 1983). Moreover, chimpanzees also provided an in vivo system for the biological amplification of the putative virus in order to obtain sufficient material for attempts at identification. However, more than 15 years elapsed between the first rigorous description of the disease and the discovery of the aetiological agent (Choo et al 1989). The first specific serological assay for HCV infection was not developed until 1989 (Kuo et al 1989). This resulted from the partial cloning of the HCV genome following its recovery from plasma of an experimentally infected chimpanzee.

In this chapter, we review the role that non-human primate models have played before and after the discovery of the aetiological agent of NANB hepatitis.

THE CHIMPANZEE AS A MODEL FOR THE STUDY OF NANB HEPATITIS IN THE PRE-HCV ERA

Prospective studies of TAH conducted in the USA (Aach et al 1978, HJ Alter et al 1978a, Seeff et al 1978) and in Europe (Sugg et al 1976, Frey-Wettstein 1977) in the 1960s and 1970s were instrumental in defining the natural history of NANB hepatitis. As a result of these studies, it became clear that NANB hepatitis was the most common and important complication of transfusion therapy, accounting for the majority of cases of TAH. Even more importantly, prospective studies demonstrated that NANB hepatitis had a remarkable propensity to progress to chronicity (reviewed by Dienstag 1983a, HJ Alter et al 1987, 1989). Moreover, besides the transfusion-associated form of NANB hepatitis, it was found that a significant proportion of cases, classified as sporadic, community-acquired NANB hepatitis, were not associated with identifiable percutaneous exposure (MJ Alter et al 1982, 1990). Thus, like HBV, both a parenteral and a putative non-parenteral route were identified for the transmission of NANB hepatitis.

The discovery of NANB hepatitis led to a concerted effort to identify the causative agent.

Numerous immunological and serological tests were developed, but none was sufficiently reliable, reproducible or specific to be accepted as a serological marker of NANB hepatitis (Dienstag 1983b). In this setting, the development of a suitable animal model for NANB hepatitis represented an important breakthrough (Tabor & Gerety 1982). The animal model was crucial to defining the nature of the causative agent, evaluating suspected epidemiological risk factors and potential sources of infection, and reproducing the natural history of the disease. In addition, the chimpanzee was useful for evaluating the effectiveness of viral inactivation procedures.

Among the potential animal models, chimpanzees were identified as the most promising candidates, because they were the only available non-human primates reproducibly susceptible to both hepatitis A and hepatitis B (Tabor et al 1983). The suitability of chimpanzees for hepatitis research stemmed from the close phylogenetic relationship between chimpanzees and humans, as indicated by their high degree of genetic relatedness and similarities in the immune responses and host–pathogen interactions to a variety of human agents (Purcell 1992). The similarity between humans and chimpanzees also had practical applications, such as the ability to use the same reagents to detect proteins of the two species. Indeed, the chimpanzee has proven to be an excellent animal model for NANB hepatitis, since the course of primary infection, the acute phase of the disease, the development of the host immune response and the long-term sequelae of HCV infection in chimpanzees mimic very accurately the clinical and immunological observations in humans. The host range of NANB hepatitis is remarkably limited (Tabor 1989). Attempts to transmit the disease to other non-human primate species with inocula of proven infectivity yielded negative or equivocal results. Only the marmoset emerged as a potentially susceptible species (Feinstone et al 1981, Karayiannis et al 1983, Watanabe et al 1987), although the variability in the results obtained with marmosets has considerably limited the value of this animal model and has raised questions about their susceptibility.

Clinical features of NANB hepatitis in chimpanzees

Conclusive evidence that the different epidemiological forms of NANB hepatitis are associated with a transmissible agent(s) was provided by the successful transmission of NANB hepatitis to chimpanzees. Serum or plasma from different sources was used to inoculate the animals. Sources included patients with acute or chronic post-transfusion or community-acquired hepatitis or blood donors implicated in the transmission of hepatitis, as well as concentrates of coagulation factors VIII and IX and fibrinogen (reviewed by Dienstag 1983b). Following the first experiments in 1978, several laboratories around the world promptly reproduced the transmission of NANB hepatitis to chimpanzees. Between 1978 and 1980, using a variety of inocula, 152 animals were inoculated, 110 of which (70%) developed acute hepatitis. The success rate reached 100% in domestically raised chimpanzees that were inoculated with pedigreed infectious inocula (Tabor 1981).

The clinical features of NANB hepatitis in chimpanzees closely reproduce those seen in humans (Dienstag 1983b). The incubation period, defined as the time between inoculation and first increase in the alanine aminotransferase (ALT) levels, has ranged from 2 to 20 weeks, with a mean of approximately 7–8 weeks. The acute disease is relatively mild, with peak ALT levels ranging from 100 to 600 IU, and, as seen in humans, both monophasic and biphasic ALT patterns can be observed. The incubation period and the severity of acute hepatitis are unrelated to the amount of the inoculum or to the route of administration. Moreover, there is no correlation between the severity of the disease and the number of passages in serial transmission studies.

A question raised by the clinical studies of NANB hepatitis was the observation of discrete short and long incubation periods. The short incubation period, as brief as 4 days, was predominantly seen in haemophiliacs following therapy with factor VIII concentrates (Hruby & Schauf 1978, Bamber et al 1981a, b), whereas the long incubation period (7–8 weeks) was a regular feature of classical TAH. Based on these observations, some authors hypothesized the existence of two distinct transmissible agents. These speculations, however, were not always supported by transmission studies of viruses from factor VIII concentrates to chimpanzees (Bradley et al 1979, Feinstone et al 1981). The incubation period and the clinical and histological characteristics of the disease in the chimpanzees were indistinguishable from those observed in animals developing NANB hepatitis after exposure to viruses associated with long-incubation-period hepatitis.

The development of chronic hepatitis, a hallmark of NANB hepatitis, is also a common sequela in chimpanzees. Long-term follow-up of experimentally infected animals demonstrated that NANB hepatitis progressed to chronicity in more than 50% of the cases, a rate similar to that reported in humans. Several patterns of ALT elevations were seen in chronically infected chimpanzees. Interestingly, the fluctuating profile of the ALT levels, which is the most characteristic feature of chronic NANB hepatitis in humans, has also been observed in chimpanzees. Other patterns include persistent elevations of ALT or recrudescence of the disease several years after the first acute episode (Bradley et al 1981, 1991, Tabor et al 1983).

Ultrastructural features

Shimizu et al (1979) described two different types of ultrastructural alterations in liver cells of chimpanzees inoculated with plasma obtained from two different patients, one with chronic (strain F) and one with acute (strain H) NANB hepatitis. These consisted of peculiar tubular or circular structures within the cytoplasm of hepatocytes in animals receiving strain F, whereas those infected with strain H showed clusters of intranuclear particles, 20–27 nm in diameter. Such distinct types of ultrastructural abnormalities were detected during the acute phase, at the time of peak serum ALT elevation. At that time, cytoplasmic and nuclear structures were thought to be mutually exclusive in individual animals, thus providing support to epidemiological data (Mosley et al 1977) that there could be more than one NANB hepatitis agent. Cytoplasmic tubular structures were also reported by Jackson et al (1979) in the liver of experimentally infected chimpanzees with acute NANB hepatitis. The observation by Shimizu et al (1979) was extended by Tsiquaye et al (1980), who associated the nuclear changes with the short-incubation type of NANB hepatitis and the cytoplasmic changes with the long-incubation type of NANB hepatitis. Studies conducted in humans confirmed the initial observations in chimpanzees, although in humans nuclear and cytoplasmic changes were not found to be mutually exclusive (Busachi et al 1981, De Wolf-Peeters et al 1981, Marciano-Cabral et al 1981). Coexistence of the nuclear and cytoplasmic alterations was subsequently reported also in experimentally infected chimpanzees (Burk et al 1981, Tsiquaye et al 1981). Pfeiffer et al (1980) extended the morphological spectrum of ultrastructural alterations observed in hepatocytes of chimpanzees during NANB hepatitis. These authors distinguished four types of cytoplasmic changes and observed that some of them were already present during the incubation period. Type I, appearing first (4–6 weeks post inoculation) were defined as sponge-like inclusions composed of a dense matrix and irregularly arranged membranes; type II structures, attaching curved membranes that develop by close apposition of two cisternae of the smooth endoplasmic reticulum, were detected at week 8; type III, which include the cytoplasmic changes previously described (Jackson et al 1979, Shimizu et al 1979, Tsiquaye et al 1980) and consist of double-walled cylinders with a total diameter between 150 and 300 nm, were detected at week 10; type IV, which include microtubular aggregates usually in the vicinity of the areas containing type III structures, were detected at week 10. Additional studies in chimpanzees confirmed these findings (Schaff et al 1984) and provided evidence that persistent ultrastructural alterations in the liver of chimpanzees may be associated with chronic NANB infection (Bradley et al 1983a, Brotman et al 1983). The significance of the cytoplasmic and nuclear structures associated with NANB hepatitis is still unknown. None of these structures was observed in the liver of chimpanzees with hepatitis A or B. In contrast, characteristic cytoplasmic tubular structures analogous to those observed in NANB hepatitis were detected in chimpanzees infected with HDV (Kamimura et al 1983, Canese et al 1984). However, the same alterations were observed also in lymphocytes of patients with acquired immunodeficiency syndrome (AIDS) (Sidhu et al 1983, Kostianovsky et al 1984). Similarly, nuclear changes of the type described in NANB hepatitis were found in preinoculation liver biopsies of chimpanzees, suggesting also that these alterations are not specific for NANB hepatitis (Bradley et al 1980, Schaff et al 1984). In addition, analogous abnormalities were observed in malignant fibrous histiocytoma (Talka et al 1982), as well as in other pathological conditions (reviewed by Dienstag 1983b). Subsequently, Feinstone et al (1981) showed that the chimpanzees originally identified as having only nuclear or cytoplasmic structures actually had both simultaneously, thereby laying to rest the hypothesis of mutual exclusiveness.

Crystalline structures containing 25–30 nm particles were visualized in the cytoplasm of endothelial or Kupffer cells in acute-phase liver biopsies from chimpanzees with NANB hepatitis (Bradley et al 1980, De Vos et al 1981, McCaul et al 1982). However, the same crystalline structures have also been seen in a chimpanzee infected with HAV (Bradley et al 1980), as well as in uninfected chimpanzees (De Vos et al 1981, Schaff et al 1984).

At present, it is unknown whether the structures visualized by electron microscopy in NANB hepatitis are of viral or cellular origin. Shimizu et al (1985) have produced monoclonal antibodies which recognize a seemingly cellular antigen present in post-inoculation but not preinoculation liver biopsies from animals with experimental NANB or type D hepatitis. Using immunoelectron microscopy, this antigen was shown to react with clusters of cytoplasmic microtubular structures. Recent data indicate that analogous structures may be induced in response to cytokines such as interferon, most likely released as a consequence of the viral infection (Bockus et al 1988). In fact, treatment of chimpanzees with an interferon inducer has been shown to evoke intrahepatic expression of the antigen recognized by the monoclonal antibodies of Shimizu & Purcell (1989).

Infectivity studies in chimpanzees

In the absence of any reliable serological tests, the chimpanzee model was instrumental in establishing the duration of viraemia in NANB hepatitis virus infection. Successful transmission from sequential serum samples obtained at various times during the course of acute NANB hepatitis to additional chimpanzees demonstrated that the infectious agent was present in serum as early as 12 days prior to the first ALT elevation (Hollinger et al 1978) and persisted at least until week 13 after inoculation (1 week after the peak ALT level) (Tabor et al 1979a). Serological re-evaluation of serial subinoculation studies conducted in volunteers in 1969 documented that viraemia appeared within the first week after inoculation (Dienstag et al 1981). Although the persistence of elevated ALT levels following the acute episode suggested that the disease had progressed to chronicity, it was only through transmission studies in chimpanzees that conclusive proof of the persistence of the NANB agent in blood, in both humans and chimpanzees, could be obtained (Tabor et al 1978b, 1979a, Bradley 1979). In addition, successful transmission of NANB hepatitis from blood donors or chimpanzees with normal ALT levels provided definitive evidence for the existence of asymptomatic chronic carriers (Tabor et al 1980). Evidence was obtained in chimpanzees that a patient was continuously infectious in chimpanzees for 6½ years after the onset of acute hepatitis, even at times when the ALT levels were within normal limits (Tabor et al 1980).

The availability of the chimpanzee model permitted determination of infectivity titres of sera containing NANB hepatitis (Feinstone et al 1981, Tabor et al 1983). End-point titres of infectivity, defined as the greatest dilution of the inocula at which 50% of the animals became infected, were determined for several clinical samples implicated in the transmission of the disease. The results of these titration studies showed that the end-point infectivity titre of NANB hepatitis is generally very low, ranging from 10^0 to $10^{2.5}$ 50% chimpanzee infectious doses (CID_{50}) per ml; only two inocula among those reported to date had a high infectivity titre ($10^{6.5}$/ml each) (Feinstone et al 1981, Bradley et al 1991). Thus, the infectivity of NANB hepatitis viruses in serum is markedly lower than that commonly observed in HBV (10^8) (Tabor et al 1983) and HDV infection (10^{11}) (Ponzetto et al 1987). This feature of NANB hepatitis may help to explain the difficulties initially encountered in transmission studies, before the introduction of pedigreed inocula, as well as the difficulty encountered in attempting to identify the causative agent.

PHYSICOCHEMICAL PROPERTIES OF THE NANB AGENT

Most of the physicochemical properties of the putative agent of NANB hepatitis have been determined in experiments utilizing the chimpanzee. Both in humans and in experimentally infected chimpanzees, studies of serum and liver biopsies by electron microscopy failed to identify virus-like particles specific for NANB hepatitis. This failure most likely stemmed from the low infectivity titres of virus in clinical materials. The absence of any serological assays and the inability to grow the virus in vitro further hampered the characterization of the causative agent by in vitro methods. Infectivity studies in chimpanzees demonstrated that the agent was stable at pH 8.0, but could be inactivated by formalin at a concentration of 1:1000 at 37°C for 96 h (Tabor & Gerety 1980) or 1:2000 at 37°C for 72 h (Yoshizawa et al 1982). Infectivity could be abolished by heating at 100°C for 5 min (Yoshizawa et al 1982) or at 60°C for 10 h (Tabor & Gerety 1982). Complete inactivation of the agent was also achieved by heating at 60°C for 30 h after lyophilization (Purcell et al 1985), a system that has been widely employed for the treatment of pooled coagulation factors for transfusion. The agent is sensitive to a combination of beta-propionolactone and ultraviolet light (Heinrich et al 1982, Prince et al 1985). Inactivation by exposure to lipid solvents, such as chloroform, indicated that the agent contained essential lipids, presumably in an envelope (Feinstone et al 1983, Bradley et al 1983b). Only an isolated report by Bradley et al (1983b) demonstrated the existence of a chloroform-resistant agent of NANB hepatitis, in addition to the common chloroform-sensitive agent.

To determine the size of the NANB agent, several studies were undertaken by filtration through membranes of defined pore size. Infectivity was retained after filtration through 220-, 80- (Bradley et al 1985) and 50-nm filters (He et al 1987), but was removed by a 30-nm filter (He et al 1987, Yuasa et al 1991).

The results of the biochemical and physical analyses suggested that the NANB agent was a small virus, with a diameter of 30–60 nm, coated by a lipid-containing envelope. These properties further suggested that the NANB virus could belong to the togavirus–flavivirus group, the hepadnavirus family, the HDV-like agents or a previously unrecognized category of virus. That the NANB agent was not related to hepadnavirus or to HDV was subsequently suggested by nucleic acid hybridization studies (Fowler et al 1983, Weiner et al 1987). Some authors had even proposed that the agent could be a retrovirus, based on the occasional detection of reverse transcriptase activity in the serum of infected patients (Seto et al 1984). However, in subsequent studies with pedigreed sera, these data were not reproduced in other laboratories (Khan & Hollinger 1986). Moreover, given the estimated size of the NANB hepatitis virus, the hypothesis that it was a retrovirus seemed highly unlikely.

THE ROLE OF THE ANIMAL MODEL IN THE DISCOVERY OF HEPATITIS C VIRUS

The pathway leading to the identification of the causative agent of NANB hepatitis has been long and tortuous. In retrospect, the length of this process can be explained by the low levels of infectivity and by the weak and delayed humoral immune response of the host (Purcell 1993). For these reasons, attempts using conventional virological methods produced only deep frustration for many years. Instead, it was through an unconventional approach, taking advantage of the increasingly refined techniques of molecular biology, that success was eventually achieved.

Again, the availability of the chimpanzee model was critical for the discovery of HCV, because it represented the only suitable source for the biological amplification of the putative agent. It was from a chronically infected chimpanzee that large amounts of pooled plasma with an unusually high titre of infectivity (10^6) were obtained for the molecular cloning of the viral genome (Choo et al 1989). Litres of plasma were pelleted to concentrate the virus particles, total RNA was extracted from the pellet and retrotranscribed into cDNA. More than 1 000 000 colonies in a lambda gt11 expression system were screened with serum from a chronically infected patient, who served as a source of antiviral antibodies. A single positive clone that expressed a virus-specific immunogenic peptide was finally identified. This clone, designated 5-1-1, was used to identify a larger clone (C100-3) encoding a single open reading frame that was expressed in yeast as a fusion protein with superoxide dismutase. By using overlapping clones, the entire sequence of the HCV genome was subsequently obtained. Thus, HCV represents the first virus in the history of virology that has been characterized primarily by molecular means before it was visualized by electron microscopy or isolated in culture.

The hepatitis C virus has a single-stranded positive-sense RNA genome that contains a single open reading frame encoding a large polyprotein of approximately 3000 amino acids and two untranslated regions of approximately 340 and 50 nucleotides at the 5' end and 3' end respectively (Choo et al 1991). Comparative analysis of the viral nucleotide sequence reveals that HCV is not closely related to any known agent, but shares biophysical and genetic characteristics with the Flaviviridae family of viruses. The HCV genome is organized in a manner similar to that of the flaviviruses and pestiviruses and is more closely related to pestiviruses (Miller & Purcell 1990). The large open reading frame initially was thought to include a 5' structural region encoding the nucleocapsid and the envelope-like protein, and a 3' non-structural region containing five non-structural proteins designated NSI–NS5. However, the NS1 protein of HCV, initially thought to be a non-structural protein analogous to NS1 of flaviviruses, is now believed to be a second envelope protein analogous to the envelope protein gp53/55 of pestiviruses and has been named E2/NS1 (Houghton et al 1991). The recent discovery of a hypervariable region within this gene, similar to the third hypervariable domain in the envelope of human immunodeficiency virus (HIV) (Benn et al 1985), further suggests that it may encode for a second envelope-like protein. This region has the highest degree of genetic heterogeneity, possibly resulting from the continuous immune pressure of the host (Hijikata et al 1991, Weiner et al 1991).

The cloning and sequencing of the HCV genome and the development of serological assays for antibodies to HCV have transformed the diagnosis of NANB hepatitis from one merely based on exclusion into that of a specific disease, hepatitis C. The application of this assay to clinical practice has finally provided the best evidence that HCV is the major aetiological agent of post-transfusion NANB hepatitis (Alter et al 1989, Esteban et al 1990, Aach et al 1991) as well as of community-acquired NANB hepatitis (Alter 1991).

The diagnosis of hepatitis C is routinely based on indirect markers of HCV infection such as the humoral response of the infected host, measured by solid-phase enzyme immunoassay (EIA) (Kuo et al 1989). The first-generation EIA, based on the recombinant C100-3 antigen expressed in yeast, contains amino acid sequences derived from the NS3 and NS4 non-structural gene products of HCV. The second-generation EIA includes, in addition to C100-3 antigen, two epitopes derived from the structural nucleocapsid (core) region and the NS3 gene. Several EIAs that measure antibodies to sequences from the 5' end of the NS5 gene product, to the envelope protein (E1) or to the E2/NS1 region have been developed. These three tests are not yet commercially available and their application has been limited to experimental studies.

Currently, tests to detect HCV antigenaemia are also limited to experimental assays. The absence of such tests has hampered progress in understanding the natural history of this infection. Detection of nucleic acid sequences with the polymerase chain reaction (PCR) or other nucleic acid-based techniques is the only practical method currently available to detect viraemia in the course of infection with HCV (Garson et al 1990, Weiner et al 1990). A sensitive assay such as PCR is particularly crucial in the identification of HCV infection, in which low levels of viraemia, as demonstrated by experimental studies in chimpanzees, appear to be the rule. The animal model has been fundamental to evaluating the sensitivity of the PCR technique. By analysing 10-fold serial dilutions of a reference plasma (strain H) whose infectivity was $10^{6.5}$ CID_{50}/ml, PCR assays were capable of detecting HCV with a sensitivity greater than infectivity titrations in chimpanzees (Cristiano et al 1991, Farci et al 1991, Bukh et al 1992).

THE CONTRIBUTION OF THE ANIMAL MODEL TO THE STUDY OF THE NATURAL HISTORY OF HCV INFECTION

Chimpanzees have represented a valuable resource for the study of the natural history of HCV infection, because they have provided a unique model in which to reproduce, under carefully controlled experimental conditions, the disease observed in humans. The extensive clinical and experimental studies of NANB hepatitis conducted before the discovery of HCV had raised many questions that were difficult to address in the absence of specific diagnostic markers. Following the discovery of HCV, antibody assays, as well as sensitive assays such as PCR for detecting the HCV genome, became available to investigators. These advances provided an opportunity to re-evaluate the early studies of experimental transmission in chimpanzees. The animal model has represented an optimal source of controlled clinical material for studying the kinetics of viral replication, the host immune response and the relationship between viraemia and antibody response during the entire course of acute and chronic HCV infection.

Primary HCV infection in chimpanzees is characterized by the early appearance of HCV viraemia (Figs 14.1 and 14.2), which in most cases becomes detectable within 1 week after inoculation (range: <1–5 weeks), long before other markers can be detected (Shimizu et al 1990, Farci et al 1991, Abe et al 1992, Beach et al 1992, Farci et al 1992a, Hilfenhaus et al 1992, Shindo et al 1992). In two chimpanzees, in which serum and liver specimens were obtained daily during the first week of infection, HCV RNA in serum was documented as early as 3–4 days after inoculation (Shimizu et al 1990). That viral replication is an early event in experimental HCV infection was further confirmed by the detection of HCV RNA in the liver of chimpanzees, by in situ hybridization, 2 days after infection (Negro et al 1992). This finding supports the concept that the early appearance of viraemia reflects de novo viral replication, rather than passive transfer of the virus from the inoculum. The detection of serum HCV RNA precedes the appearance in the hepatocytes of the ultrastructural changes (Shimizu et al 1990, Schlauder et al 1991) and the cytoplasmic antigen recognized by monoclonal antibody 48–1 (Shimizu et al 1990). Intrahepatic HCV antigens, as detected by direct immunofluorescence, were found in the cytoplasm of hepatocytes in the early phase of acute hepatitis, prior to the appearance of the antibody response (Krawczynski et al 1992).

Evidence of hepatitis was found on average 7–10 weeks after inoculation, although low-level elevations of liver enzyme values often occurred earlier, within the first 1–3 weeks after exposure to HCV (HJ Alter et al 1978b, Feinstone et al 1981). This pattern resembles that observed in humans and is believed to result directly from HCV infection. The infectivity titre of the inoculum does not appear to correlate with the severity of hepatitis, as measured by the ALT levels (Feinstone et al 1982, Bradley et al 1990).

In self-limiting HCV infection of chimpanzees, the viraemia is transient and lasts for a variable period of time, ranging from 10 to 38 weeks (Abe et al 1992, Farci et al 1992a, Hilfenhaus et al 1992). During the incubation period, HCV RNA is persistently detectable in serum (Shimizu et al 1990, Farci et al 1991, 1992a, Abe et al 1992, Hilfenhaus et al 1992), although during the early stage of infection in some animals PCR-positive samples are separated by periods in which no viral RNA can be detected prior to the ALT peak (Beach et al 1992).

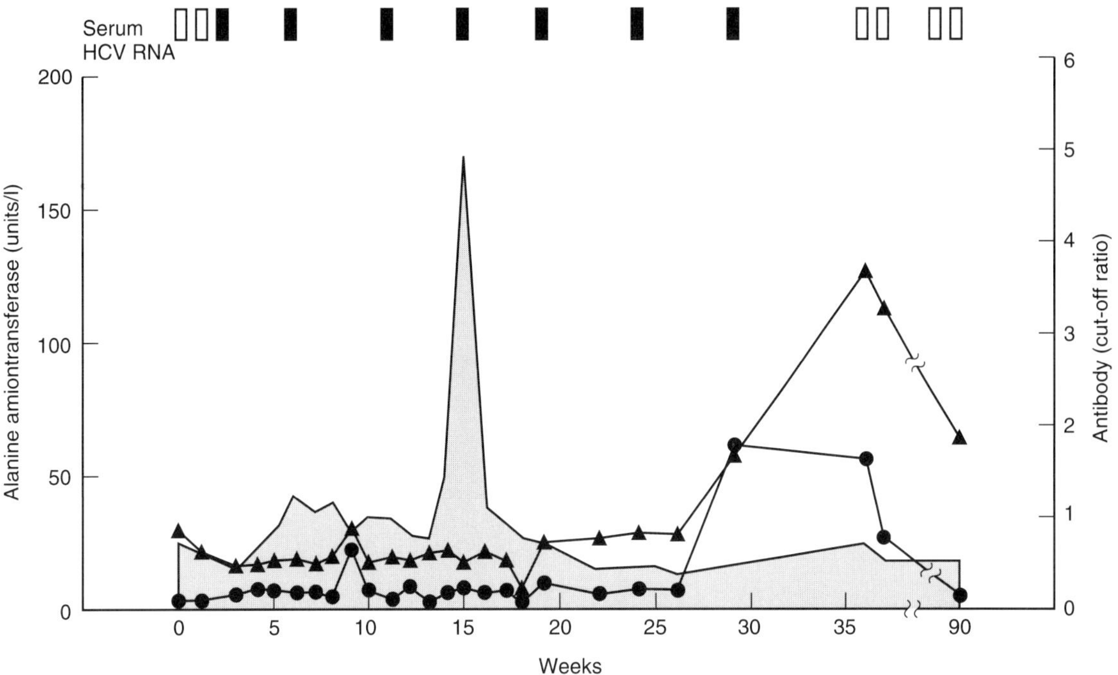

Fig. 14.1 Pattern of antibody response to hepatitis C virus (HCV) in chimpanzee 105 with transient HCV viraema. The animal was inoculated with antihaemophilic factor (factor VIII, lot A) implicated in the transmission of NANB hepatitis to haemophiliacs (Craske et al 1975, Hruby & Schauf 1978). Open bars indicate negative assays for serum HCV RNA by PCR, and solid bars positive assays. The grey area indicates the values of serum alanine aminotransferase. First-generation anti-HCV assay is indicated by circles, second-generation anti-HCV assay is indicated by triangles. Cut-off ratio represents the ratio between the absorbance value for the test sample and that for the assay cut-off; values above 1 were considered positive. (This figure was reproduced with modifications from P Farci 1992 The natural history of infection with hepatitis C virus (HCV) in chimpanzees: comparison of serologic responses measured with first and second generation assays and relationship to HCV viraemia, Journal of Infectious Diseases, 165: 1006–1011, with the permission of the publisher.)

The humoral antibody response to primary HCV infection is usually delayed with respect to the clinical onset of the disease. There is a time interval ranging from a few weeks to several months between inoculation and antibody seroconversion, and the length of this interval is extremely variable and dependent on the antibody being measured. Antibodies directed to the nucleocapsid protein (anti-core) of HCV are usually the first to appear and can be detected immediately before or coincident with the major ALT peak, although there is an extreme variability in individual chimpanzees (Abe et al 1992, Farci et al 1992a). Antibodies to the NS3 non-structural protein (clone 33c) appear coincident with or shortly after antibodies to core (Farci et al 1992a). In other studies, however, anti-33c antibodies were the first to become detectable (Beach et al 1992, Hilfenhaus et al 1992). Antibodies to C100-3 (part of the NS4 non-structural protein, which was used to develop the first-generation EIA) are usually the last to appear, on average 10–15 weeks after the major peak of ALT activity (Farci et al 1991, Lanford et al 1991, Beach et al 1992, Hilfenhaus et al 1992, Abe et al 1992, Farci et al 1992a). Anti-C100-3 usually appears soon after the clearance of serum HCV RNA in parallel with the resolution of the acute phase. The shortest interval from the onset of hepatitis has been observed using the second-generation assay, which combines in a single test the three previously mentioned antigens (C100-3, core and 33c) (Beach et al 1992, Hilfenhaus et al 1992, Farci et al 1992a).

Besides the variations observed in the detection of antibodies directed to different HCV antigens,

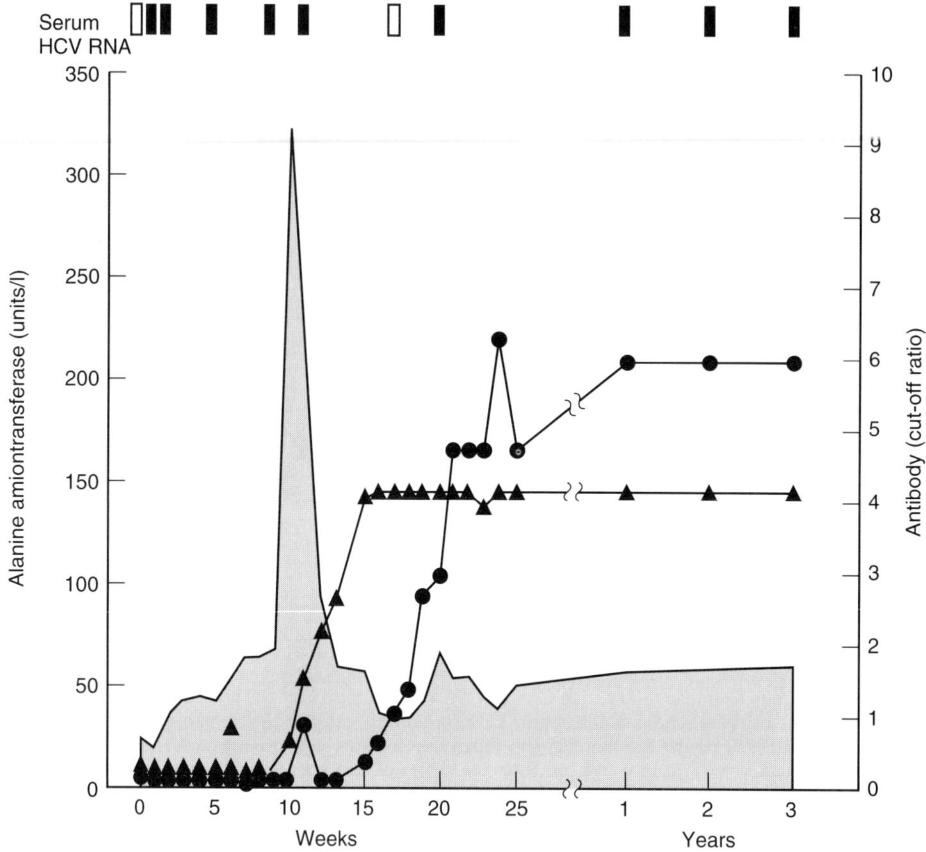

Fig. 14.2 Pattern of antibody response to hepatitis C virus (HCV) in chimpanzee 51 with chronic HCV infection and persistent HCV viraemia. The animal was inoculated with serum from a patient with chronic post-transfusion hepatitis (strain F), fifth passage in chimpanzees. Open bars indicate negative assays for serum HCV RNA by PCR, and solid bars positive assays. The grey area indicates the values of serum alanine aminotransferase. First-generation anti-HCV assay is indicated by circles, second-generation anti-HCV assay is indicated by triangles. Cut-off ratio represents the ratio between the absorbance value for the test sample and that for the assay cut-off; values above 1 were considered positive. (This figure was reproduced with modifications from P Farci 1992 The natural history of infection with hepatitis C virus (HCV) in chimpanzees: comparison of serologic responses measured with first and second generation assays and relationship to HCV viraemia, Journal of Infectious Diseases 165: 1006–1011, with the permission of the publisher.)

variations in the interval to seroconversion among individual chimpanzees also reflect intrinsic differences in the immune response of chimpanzees. This variability involves not only the time of seroconversion, but also the pattern of antibody response in individual cases. In some animals, HCV infection is associated with the appearance of an isolated anti-core response, whereas in others seroconversion is limited to anti-C100-3 (Abe et al 1992). In other reports the antibody response was limited to anti-33c and anti-C100-3 (Beach et al 1992, Hilfenhaus et al 1992). The importance of individual variability is emphasized by the observation that the same inoculum can induce different patterns of antibody response in different chimpanzees (Bradley et al 1990). The introduction of the second-generation assay has diminished the variability in the humoral response observed with the single assays and has narrowed the length of the seronegative window (Figs 14.1, 14.2 and 14.3) to an average of 5–8 weeks (Beach et al 1992, Farci et al 1992a, Hilfenhaus

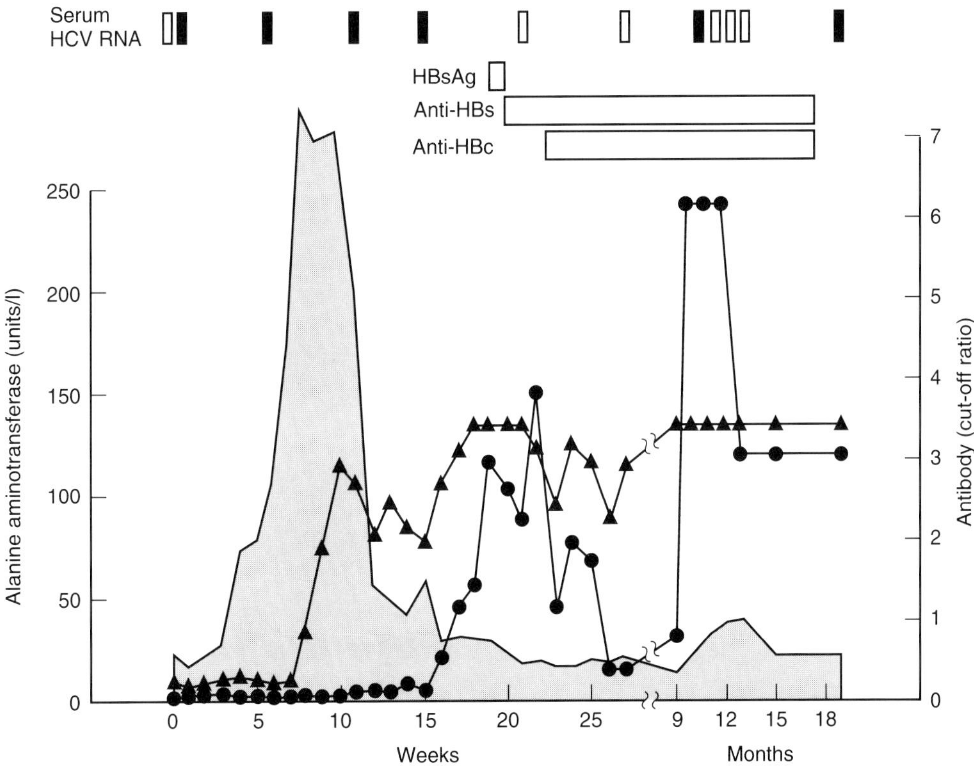

Fig. 14.3 Pattern of antibody response to hepatitis C virus (HCV) in chimpanzee 888 with chronic HCV infection and persistent HCV viraemia. The animal was inoculated with antihaemophilic factor (factor VIII, lot B) implicated in the transmission of NANB hepatitis to haemophiliacs (Craske et al 1975, Hruby & Schauf 1978). Open bars indicate negative assays for serum HCV RNA by PCR, and solid bars positive assays. The grey area indicates the values of serum alanine aminotransferase. First-generation anti-HCV assay is indicated by circles, second-generation anti-HCV assay is indicated by triangles. Cut-off ratio represents the ratio between the absorbance value for the test sample and that for the assay cut-off; values above 1 were considered positive. Horizontal bars indicate the time during which serum was positive for hepatitis B surface antigen (HBsAg), for antibody to HBsAg (anti-HBs) and for antibody to hepatitis B core antigen (anti-HBc). (This figure was reproduced with modifications from P Farci 1992 The natural history of infection with hepatitis C virus (HCV) in chimpanzees: comparison of serologic responses measured with first and second generation assays and relationship to HCV viraemia, Journal of Infectious Diseases 165: 1006–1011, with the permission of the publisher.)

et al 1992). Moreover, it has considerably increased the sensitivity of the assay, as evidenced by the identification of cases that would not be diagnosed as HCV infection because of the absence of antibodies detectable by first generation assay (anti-C100-3) (Fig. 14.4) (Farci et al 1992a). This notwithstanding, variability in the time of seroconversion has been observed also with the second-generation assay.

The biological reasons for the variable immune response observed in primary HCV infection are unclear at present. Analysis of a large series of chimpanzees has shown that there is no correlation between the first appearance of HCV viraemia and the time of antibody seroconversion (Abe et al 1992, Farci et al 1992a, Hilfenhaus et al 1992), or between the infectivity titre and the time of seroconversion (Bradley et al 1990, Abe et al 1992, Purcell unpublished data). During the early phase of acute hepatitis, data obtained both from the animal model and from humans failed to identify any virological or serological markers that may be of value in predicting the outcome of HCV infection. The initial antibody pattern showed no significant difference between animals that developed chronic HCV infection and those

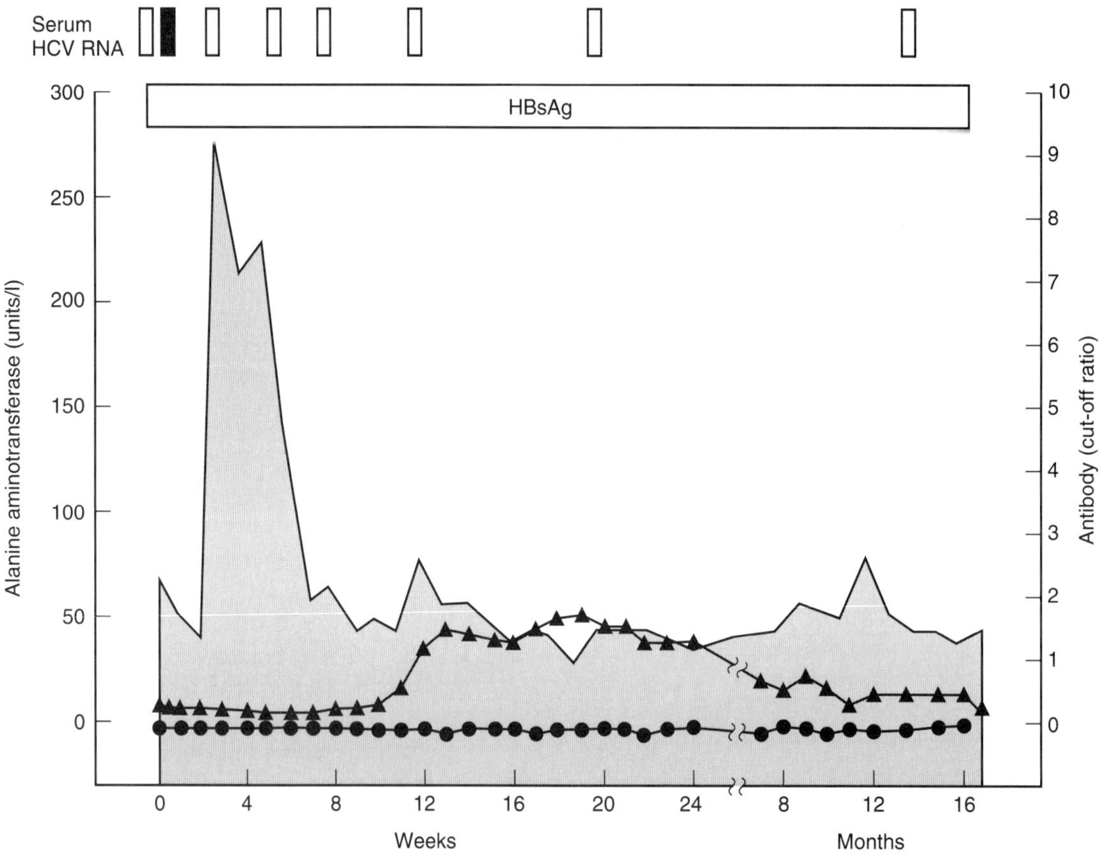

Fig. 14.4 Pattern of antibody response and HCV viraemia in chimpanzee 904, which was inoculated with serum from a patient with acute post-transfusion hepatitis (strain H). The animal was a chronic carrier of hepatitis B surface antigen (HBsAg) at the time of inoculation. Open bars indicate negative assays for serum HCV RNA by PCR, and solid bars positive assays. The grey area indicates the values of serum alanine aminotransferase. First-generation anti-HCV assay is indicated by circles, second-generation anti-HCV assay is indicated by triangles. Cut-off ratio represents the ratio between the absorbance value for the test sample and that for the assay cut-off; values above 1 were considered positive. The horizontal bar indicates the time during which serum was positive for hepatitis B surface antigen (HBsAg).

that cleared the viraemia (Hilfenhaus et al 1992). Thus, the detection of serum HCV RNA is the only currently available test that may provide important prognostic information on the outcome of the disease. Sustained clearance of HCV RNA correlates with resolution of the disease, whereas persistence of detectable HCV RNA predicts progression to chronicity (Farci et al 1991). However, the lack of detectable HCV RNA by PCR does not necessarily exclude the presence of tiny amounts of infectious virus (Beach et al 1992). HCV RNA is also the crucial marker for establishing an early diagnosis of primary HCV infection. In fact, although the introduction of second-generation antibody assays has considerably narrowed the seronegative window and increased the sensitivity of the test, there is still a prolonged interval (on average 13 weeks) between the first detection of HCV RNA and antibody seroconversion (Farci et al 1992a). This seronegative window has not been further narrowed by the introduction of tests for IgM class antibodies against different HCV antigens (Beach et al 1992). In infected chimpanzees, the IgM response rates were lower than those of IgG, appeared usually concomitant with the IgG and were of shorter duration. However, IgM appeared to be a good marker of primary infection, since neither boosting nor re-exacerbation of the ALT levels in the chronic phase elicited a secondary IgM response (Beach et al 1992). With the antibody assays so far available, there is still a serologically silent period, during which HCV RNA, as detected by PCR, is the only marker that permits early diagnosis of primary infection and identification of potentially infectious individuals who would be missed by conventional antibody testing (Farci et al 1991, Schlauder et al 1991, Abe et al 1992, Beach et al 1992, Farci et al 1992a, Hilfenhaus et al 1992). However, the value of the PCR assay to predict infectivity is not absolute, especially in view of the fact that the volumes of plasma tested by PCR are usually lower than those used for experimental inoculation in chimpanzees. In this respect, Beach et al (1992) reported successful transmission of HCV infection with 17-ml and 100-ml samples of two inocula that were negative for HCV RNA when 50-μl samples were tested by PCR.

The duration and the patterns of the antibody response vary according to the type of antibody analysed and, in some cases, are strictly dependent upon the outcome of HCV infection. Of major clinical relevance is the fact that, in most patients with transient HCV viraemia, antibodies to certain non-structural proteins, such as anti-C100, disappear after an extremely variable period that may range from 1 week to several months (Abe et al 1992, Beach et al 1992, Farci et al 1992a). Similarly, anti-NS5 seroconversion occurs late in the course of the acute disease, often during the convalescence phase, and then the antibodies disappear following the clearance of HCV viraemia (Farci et al 1992b). In contrast, antibodies directed against a structural protein, the nucleocapsid, or core, do not seem to be influenced by the outcome of HCV infection, since they remain persistently detectable in chimpanzees even after recovery (Abe et al 1992, Farci et al 1992a, b). These observations indicate that antibodies to specific non-structural proteins, such as anti-C100-3 and anti-NS5, parallel more closely the pattern of HCV viraemia, and therefore seem to be indirect markers of infectivity (Figs 14.3 and 14.5).

As in humans, experimental NANB hepatitis in chimpanzees progresses to chronicity in more than 50% of the cases (Bradley et al 1981, Tabor et al 1983, Burk et al 1984, Bradley et al 1991). The virological and serological profiles of chronic HCV infection differ from those seen in acute hepatitis. In chronic HCV infection, HCV viraemia usually follows two main patterns: persistent or intermittent (Figs 14.2 and 14.3) (Abe et al 1992, Beach et al 1992, Farci et al 1992a, Hilfenhaus et al 1992). In contrast to the variable, delayed and weak antibody response seen in acute hepatitis, the serological pattern in chronic HCV infection is more sustained and consistent. The pattern of persistent viraemia is associated with antibodies against structural and non-structural proteins, both of which increase in parallel with the progression of the hepatitis and persist at high titres as the disease continues (Fig. 14.2) (Farci et al 1992b). The pattern of continuous viraemia for up to 10 years, seen in one chimpanzee (Schlauder et al 1991), resembles the pattern seen in chronically infected humans, in whom HCV viraemia has been documented for up to 14 years (Farci et al 1991). In chimpanzees with intermittent viraemia, the antibody profiles may differ from those observed in animals with continuous viraemia. Antibodies to non-structural protein, such as anti-C100, may exhibit a fluctuating profile that closely parallels the pattern of viraemia (Farci et al 1992a, b). In contrast, antibodies to structural proteins, such as anti-core, remain persistently detectable in chimpanzees with either transient or persistent viraemia (Abe et al 1992, Farci et al 1992a, b). Thus, in the presence of such fluctuating HCV viraemia, only antibodies against structural proteins are continuously able to identify HCV infection. As noted above, however, these antibodies are not useful in differentiating between resolved and active HCV infection because they persist regardless of the pattern of HCV viraemia. Thus, in the absence of any test to detect HCV antigenaemia, the detection of HCV RNA in serum still represents the only available tool for identifying with certainty an ongoing HCV infection. No correlation is observed between the pattern of HCV viraemia and the ALT profile during long-term follow-up (Farci et al 1991, Beach et al 1992, Farci et al 1992a). Persistent

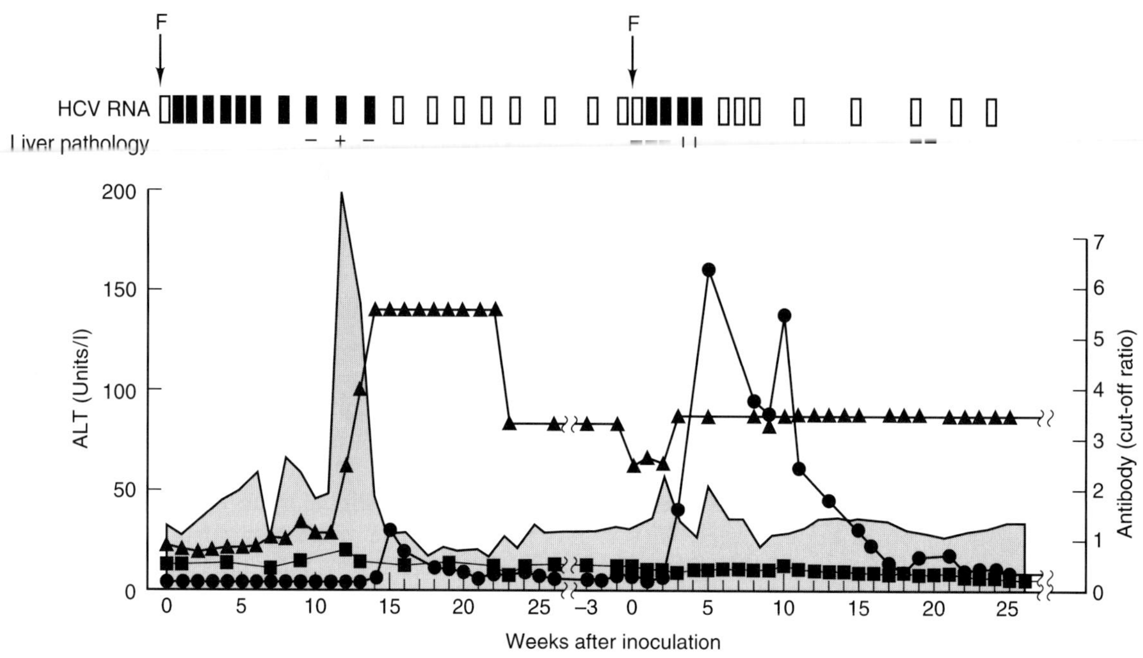

a

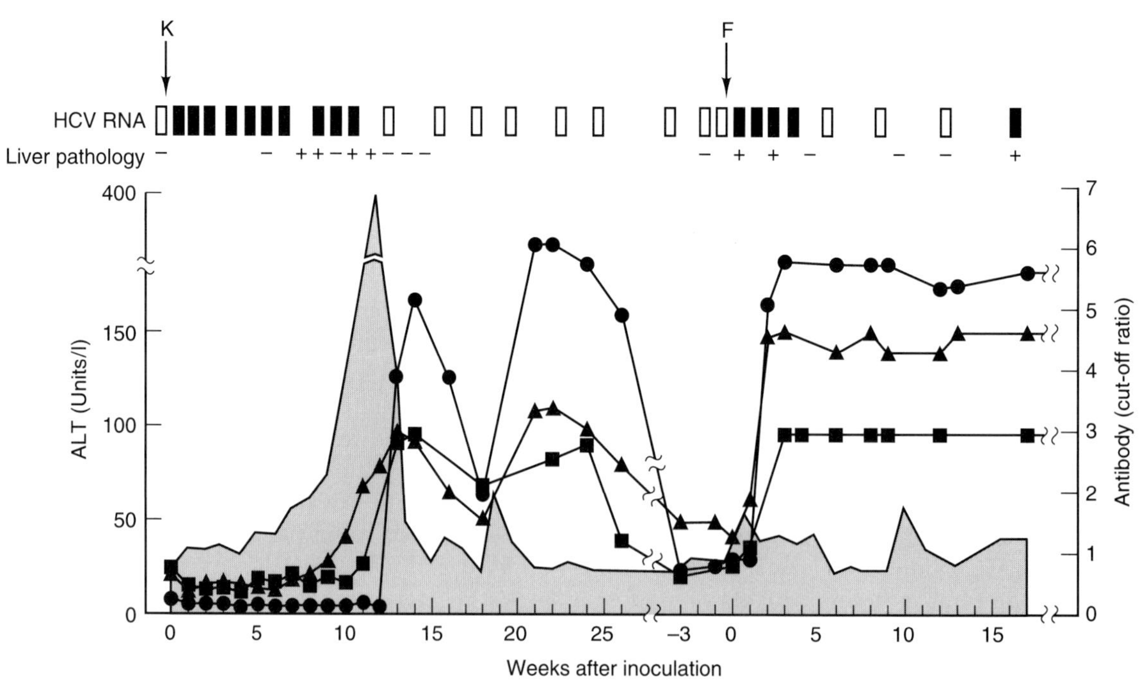

b

Fig. 14.5 Course of HCV infection in chimpanzee 963 rechallenged with the homologous HCV strain (a) and in chimpanzee 793 with a heterologous HCV strain (b). The grey areas indicate the values of serum ALT. The arrows indicate the time of challenge and the strain used for inoculation. Open bars indicate negative assays for serum HCV RNA by PCR, and solid bars positive assays. Liver pathology indicates necroinflammatory changes rated as negative or positive. First-generation anti-HCV assay is indicated by circles, second generation anti-HCV assay is indicated by triangles, and squares indicate anti-NS5. Cut-off ratio represents the ratio between the absorbance value for the test sample and that for the assay cut-off; values above 1 were considered positive. This figure was reproduced with modifications from P. Farci 1992 Lack of protective immunity against reinfection with hepatitis C virus, Science, 258: 135, with the permission of the publisher; copyright 1992 by the AAAS.)

viraemia may be associated with the characteristic ALT fluctuations, or with mild, nearly normal ALT values. This disparity between HCV RNA and ALT levels indicates that HCV replication is not always associated with serious liver damage, for reasons that are not understood. In both humans and chimpanzees the absence of ALT elevations for extended periods of time does not exclude the presence of circulating viral RNA and does not imply recovery from disease (Beach et al 1992). These clinical features complicate the definition of acute self-limiting hepatitis and suggest that caution should be used in the diagnosis of resolution of HCV infection.

HCV AND FULMINANT HEPATITIS

The contribution of NANB hepatitis to the aetiology of fulminant hepatitis is the object of intensive investigation, now that specific and sensitive tools for the diagnosis of HCV infection have become available. Before the discovery of HCV, the role of putative NANB agents in fulminant hepatitis was difficult to establish, as diagnosis was merely based on exclusion criteria (reviewed by Dienstag 1983a). In such studies, NANB hepatitis accounted for 27–44% of all cases of fulminant hepatitis. However, these values probably overestimate the true incidence, since cases of drug toxicity or fulminant hepatitis B with undetectable HBsAg could be included in this group. In contrast, prospective studies of post-transfusion NANB hepatitis suggest that fulminant NANB hepatitis is a rare event (Lee et al 1991, Dasarathy et al 1992). In a large series of patients prospectively followed at the NIH, only one case out of several hundred developed fulminant hepatitis (Esteban et al 1993). With the discovery of HCV, it has become possible to investigate more accurately the contribution of NANB hepatitis to fulminant hepatitis. The evidence thus far accumulated suggests that the association between HCV and fulminant hepatitis differs markedly according to the geographic area considered. In several studies conducted in Japan, HCV infection, as determined by antibody seropositivity or by the presence of viraemia, was documented in a high proportion of patients, ranging from 50% to more than 90% (Muto et al 1990, Yanagi et al 1991, Yoshiba et al 1991a, b, Akbar et al 1992, Kikuchi et al 1992). In contrast, studies conducted in the USA and in Europe demonstrated a very low prevalence of HCV infection in fulminant hepatitis in these areas (Liang et al 1991, Sallie et al 1991, Wright et al 1991, Munoz et al 1992). These discrepancies are likely to reflect geographic differences in the epidemiology of HCV. Alternatively, HCV may go unrecognized because factors, such as the timing of sampling or improper handling and storage of the clinical specimens, may result in damage to HCV virions with possible loss of detectable HCV RNA, but this is unlikely.

Attempts were made to transmit hepatitis to chimpanzees from plasma of patients with fulminant hepatitis not related to hepatitis A or B, but no disease could be transmitted (Feinstone et al 1981). Recently, using a small amount of serum from a patient with fulminant hepatitis whose serum was positive for HCV RNA (Munoz et al 1992), HCV was successfully transmitted to a chimpanzee (P Farci & R H Purcell, unpublished data). The animal developed an acute hepatitis characterized by unusually high levels of ALT values (peak ALT: 744 U/1) and developed anti-HCV. These data represent the first experimental transmission of HCV from a patient with fulminant hepatitis and provide additional evidence for an aetiological role of HCV in the development of fulminant hepatitis.

In this clinical setting, the chimpanzee animal model has again been a valuable instrument for establishing the role of hepatitis viruses in human disease. Moreover, it will be important in the search for yet unidentified hepatitis viruses that may be implicated in the aetiology of non-A, non-B, non-C, fulminant hepatitis.

INTERACTIONS AMONG HEPATITIS VIRUSES IN CHIMPANZEES

The chimpanzee animal model has been instrumental in documenting the phenomenon of viral interference in vivo between hepatotropic viruses. This notion has emerged from the observation that simultaneous or sequential infection of chimpanzees with more than one hepatitis virus could alter the course of infection. Several experimental studies have documented that, in chimpanzees with chronic NANB hepatitis, superinfection with HAV or HBV is associated with a significantly attenuated acute hepatitis (Bradley et al 1983a, 1987, Brotman et al 1983). Conversely, chronic HBV infection does not appear to interfere with the clinical expression of acute hepatitis caused by superinfection with other hepatitis viruses. Instead, superinfection with other hepatitis viruses consistently causes a suppression of HBV replication (Bradley et al 1983a, Harrison et al 1983, Tsiquaye et al 1983, Dienes et al 1990). The most striking example of such an effect is superinfection of chronic HBV carriers with hepatitis delta virus, a unique RNA virus that requires the helper function of HBV for infection (Rizzetto et al 1986). Similarly, superinfection of chronic HBV carriers with HAV results in the transient suppression of serum HBV DNA, usually not associated with variations in the titre of HBsAg (Tsiquaye et al 1984), whereas superinfection with NANB virus does interfere with HBV synthesis, as evidenced by suppression of both HBV DNA and HBsAg serum levels (Bradley et al 1983a, Harrison et al 1983, Tsiquaye et al 1983, Dienes et al 1990).

The effect of chronic HBV infection on the replication of HCV was unknown until recently. Using PCR, it has been possible to re-evaluate this aspect in sera from previous experimental studies in chimpanzees (Farci et al 1992a). One chimpanzee, a chronic carrier of HBsAg, was inoculated with HCV-positive serum from a patient with post-transfusion NANB hepatitis. In this animal, serum HCV RNA was detected within 1 week after inoculation, preceding the clinical onset by 2 weeks (ALT peak of 280 U/l), and remained detectable for only 1 week (Fig. 14.4). This unusual pattern of HCV viraemia may be the consequence of an inhibitory effect of HBV infection on HCV replication. The animal developed a transient anti-HCV antibody response detected by the second-generation assay, but failed to develop antibodies to C100-3. It is likely that the short duration of HCV viraemia was responsible for the weak humoral immune response. The animal remained HBsAg positive throughout the study. Replication of HBV was depressed during superinfection of this chimpanzee with HCV (Dienes et al 1990). Thus, there may be a reciprocal inhibition of replication in dual infections by HBV and HCV. Although the short duration of HCV viraemia in this animal did not seem to influence the clinical picture of the acute episode, the acute disease occurred significantly earlier than usual (week 3 after inoculation). Another chimpanzee was inoculated with a commercial source of factor VIII containing both HBV and HCV (Fig. 14.3). This animal developed acute NANB hepatitis that progressed to chronicity. Serum HCV RNA appeared 1 week after inoculation, remained positive during the acute phase and then fluctuated from positive to negative. Nineteen weeks after inoculation and approximately coincident with the disappearance of serum HCV RNA, the chimpanzee became transiently HBsAg positive (for 1 week). One week later, anti-HBs and anti-HBc became detectable. Liver enzymes remained normal at the time of the appearance of these markers of HBV infection. The delay observed in the incubation period of hepatitis B may result from an inhibitory effect of HCV on HBV replication. This observation is consistent with other studies that documented that co-infection of chimpanzees with inocula containing both HBV and HCV may delay the onset of acute HBV infection (Purcell et al 1985).

HCV AND HEPATOCELLULAR CARCINOMA

The aetiological role of HBV in the development of hepatocellular carcinoma has been well established by epidemiological studies (Beasley et al 1981, Beasley 1988) as well as by studies of experimental carcinogenesis in the woodchuck animal model (Gerin et al 1989). Virtually 100% of woodchucks chronically infected with woodchuck hepatitis virus (WHV), a member of the family Hepadnaviridae, and antigenically and structurally related to HBV (Summers 1981), developed liver cancer within approximately 4 years after infection (Popper et al 1987, Korba et al 1989). The risk of hepatocellular carcinoma (HCC) in chronic WHV infection is similar to that calculated by Beasley (1982) for chronic HBV infection: over 40% of HBsAg carriers are predicted to die of HCC or some other form of liver disease.

The association of HCV with liver cancer is not yet as well established as for HBV (Purcell 1989). Such an association has been hard to document because of the absence, until recently, of serological tests specific for HCV. The propensity of acute NANB hepatitis to progress to chronicity in at least 50% of prospectively followed patients and the development of cirrhosis in 20% of such cases make HCV a likely candidate as a cause of long-term sequelae in infected patients (Realdi et al 1982, H J Alter et al 1989). Before the discovery of HCV, several studies supported the epidemiological, clinical and histological evidence of an association between chronic NANB hepatitis and liver cancer (Resnick et al 1983, Gilliam et al 1984, Kiyosawa et al 1984, Okuda et al 1992). With the advent of HCV serology and PCR, there is growing evidence that HCV may be aetiologically associated with non-HBV HCC. In several studies, patients with liver cancer without evidence of infection with HBV were found to have a high prevalence of antibodies to HCV (60–80%) compared with the general population (approximately 1%) (Bruix et al 1989, Colombo et al 1989, Kew et al 1989, Kiyosawa et al 1990, Saito et al 1990, Tanaka et al 1991). Studies of HCV RNA by PCR in such patients have yelded similar results (Yoneyama et al 1990, Chou et al 1991, Lok et al 1992, Ruiz et al 1992, Bukh et al 1993a).

At present, there are no useful animal models for the study of HCV-associated hepatocarcinogenesis. Chimpanzees can be readily infected with HCV, resulting in either acute or chronic infection, but hepatocellular carcinoma has been thus far reported only in one chimpanzee experimentally infected with serum obtained from a patient with chronic NANB hepatitis (Linke et al 1987). The animal had developed acute NANB hepatitis that progressed to chronicity. HCC was diagnosed 7 years after the initial inoculation. A homogenate of liver obtained from this animal at autopsy transmitted NANB hepatitis to another chimpanzee. HCC, however, was independently found in two other chimpanzees in the same facility, and no association with HCV infection could be established in these animals, thus weakening the association between HCV infection and HCC in the first animal (Muchmore & Krawczynsky 1990). Indeed, many chimpanzees chronically infected with HBV or HCV have been followed for over 18 and 12 years, respectively, without detecting HCC (Purcell 1989). If HCV is carcinogenic for chimpanzees, the incubation period must be similar to that seen in humans. This is not surprising since the lifespan of chimpanzees is only slightly less than that of humans. The long-term observation of chimpanzees following experimental hepatitis C may eventually help to clarify the issue of the putative role of HCV in the aetiology of HCC.

Evidence for more than one NANB hepatitis agent and immunity to HCV

Shortly after NANB hepatitis was identified, clinical and experimental data suggesting the existence of more than one NANB hepatitis agent accumulated (Dienstag et al 1991). The clinical evidence was based on the sequential occurrence of multiple, distinct episodes of acute NANB hepatitis in individuals, such as haemophiliacs (Craske et al 1978, Hruby & Schauf 1978), drug-addicts (Mosley et al 1977, Norkrans et al 1980) or haemodialyzed patients (Galbraith et al 1979, Ware et al 1979), who were repeatedly exposed to blood or its derivatives. Another clinical finding that lends more credence to this hypothesis was the observation, as noted above, of two distinct forms of NANB hepatitis: one characterized by a short (1–3 weeks) and one by a long (7–9 weeks) incubation period. The former occurs more frequently in haemophiliacs (Hruby & Schauf 1978, Bamber et al 1981a, b). Additional evidence for the existence of more than one NANB virus came from cross-challenge studies in chimpanzees. These studies documented a clinical pattern similar to that seen in humans and characterized by multiple bouts of acute hepatitis in single animals infected with different inocula (Bradley et al 1979, Tsiquaye & Zuckerman 1979, Hollinger et al 1980, Yoshizawa et al 1981, Burk et al 1984, Tabor et al 1984).

Despite multiple lines of evidence suggesting the existence of at least two agents of NANB hepatitis, other observations in experimentally infected chimpanzees argue against this hypothesis. The availability of an animal model permitting the repetition of experiments under carefully controlled conditions generated data that generally failed to confirm the existence of multiple NANB hepatitis agents. The short incubation period seen in haemophiliacs did not always 'breed true' in chimpanzees infected with factor VIII concentrate preparations previously implicated in the transmission of such forms of NANB hepatitis (Bradley et al 1979, Feinstone et al 1981). Similarly, most cross-challenge studies in chimpanzees failed to induce a second episode of acute hepatitis (Tabor et al 1979b, Bradley et al 1980, Feinstone et al 1981). To further complicate the picture, recurrent episodes of hepatitis were also seen in chimpanzees that were not rechallenged (Bradley et al 1980), as well as in animals rechallenged with the same inoculum

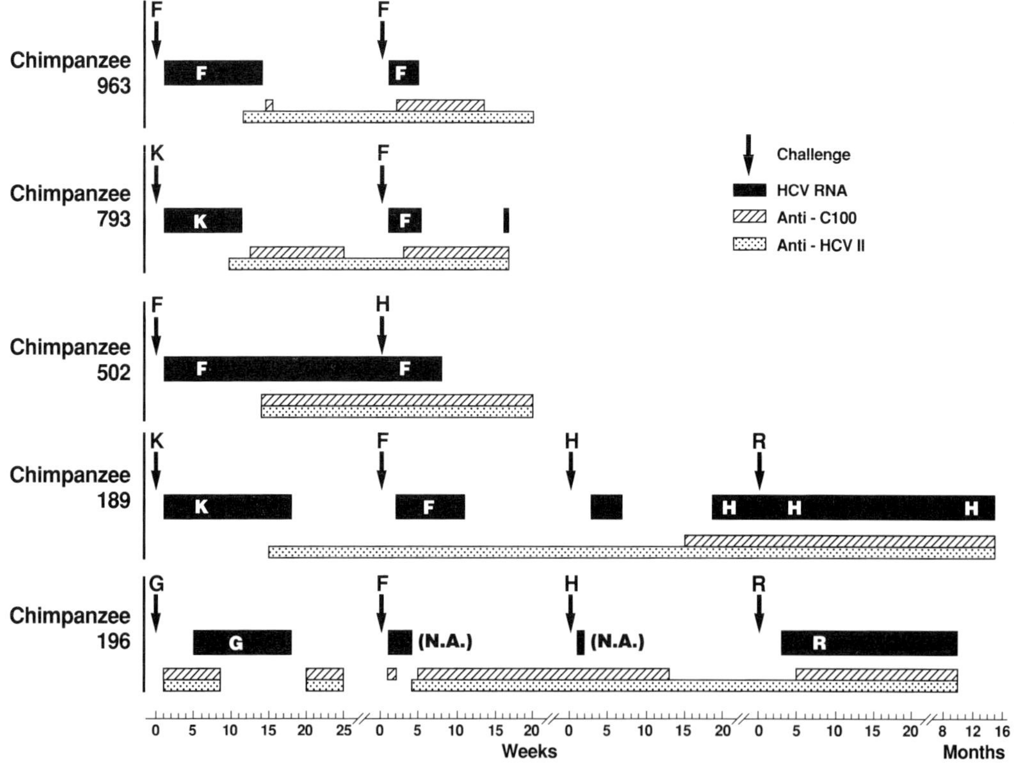

Fig. 14.6 Patterns of HCV viraemia and serological responses in multiple cross-challenge studies in chimpanzees; the numbers of animals are indicated to the left. HCV viraemia was determined weekly or biweekly for the first 20 weeks after each virus challenge and then every 4 weeks throughout the observation period. Antibodies to HCV were tested weekly or biweekly. The arrows indicate the time of challenge with the HCV strains used for inoculation. HCV RNA is indicated by the filled boxes, first-generation anti-HCV is indicated by the diagonal shading, second-generation anti-HCV is indicated by the stippled shading. In chimpanzee 196, antibodies to HCV detected by first- and second-generation assays appeared in the first sample tested, 1 week after inoculation, which reflects passive transfer of antibodies by the large (75-ml) inoculum. Passively transferred antibodies became undetectable 8 weeks later, and seroconversion occurred 20 weeks after inoculation. None of the animals developed detectable concentrations of antibodies to E2/NS1 during the multiple cross-challenge studies. The letters in the PCR (HCV RNA) bar indicate the strain identified by sequencing after challenge (there was not sufficient serum available from chimpanzee 196 for PCR amplification of the E2/NS1 region after the second and third challenges); NA, not available. (This figure was reproduced with modifications from P Farci 1992 Lack of protective immunity against reinfection with hepatitis C virus, Science, 258: 135, with the permission of the publisher; copyright 1992 by the AAAS.)

(Brotman et al 1985, Eder et al 1988). Thus, explanations other than the existence of multiple NANB hepatitis agents could account for these observations.

Extensive seroepidemiological studies have conclusively shown that HCV is the major cause of NANB hepatitis, and that, if other agents exist, they account for only a minority of such cases. Therefore, the cause of recurrent NANB hepatitis must be explained in other ways, such as the existence of different HCV serotypes, the spontaneous generation of neutralization escape mutants or the failure of the host to mount an effective immune response, leading to reactivation or reinfection with the same virus. These unanswered questions can now be explored with new sensitive and specific techniques, such as PCR. To investigate whether primary infection with HCV elicits protective immunity against reinfection with homologous or heterologous strains of virus, cross-challenge studies in chimpanzees were re-evaluated (Farci et al 1992b). The patterns of viraemia and antibody response were studied in five chimpanzees sequentially inoculated over a 3-year period with different HCV strains of proven infectivity, obtained from individual patients included in the NIH prospective study of post-transfusion NANB hepatitis. Three chimpanzees were challenged twice and two were challenged four times (Fig. 14.6). The animals were followed for a mean period of 32 months (range 12–51 months). One chimpanzee was rechallenged with the homologous inoculum, while the remaining four were rechallenged with heterologous inocula. Following the first virus challenge, all animals developed acute NANB hepatitis. Viraemia was transient in four animals, but became chronic in one. All chimpanzees seroconverted to HCV, as measured by first- or second-generation antibody assays. In contrast, none of the animals developed detectable antibodies directed to the E2/NS1 glycoprotein, and only two had detectable antibodies to the NS5 gene product (anti-NS5). Each rechallenge of a convalescent chimpanzee, negative for serum HCV RNA at the time of reinoculation, resulted in the reappearance, within 1–3 weeks, of serum HCV RNA (Fig. 14.6), as detected by PCR with primers derived from the non-coding region (Han et al 1991, Bukh et al 1992). The duration of the viraemia during rechallenge was shorter (range 1–10 weeks) than that seen during primary infection (range 11–17 weeks), although the risk of developing a chronic HCV infection was not lower than after primary infection (Fig. 14.6). The recurrence of viraemia was always associated with reappearance of antibodies against the non-structural proteins C100-3 or NS5, an indication that viral replication had recurred (Figs 14.6 and 14.6). The reappearance of viraemia was associated with histopathological evidence of acute hepatitis, although the serum ALT levels during rechallenge never reached the values observed during primary HCV infection. Sequencing of the hypervariable region demonstrated that the recurrence of viraemia was not due to reactivation of the original challenge strain, but to infection with the rechallenge HCV strain (Fig. 14.5). By contrast, the rechallenge virus could not be detected in the serum of chimpanzees persistently infected with the original challenge HCV. Thus they apparently resisted superinfection with another strain of HCV, suggesting that viral interference, a mechanism recognized in other types of viral hepatitis, may also play a role in this setting. However, other mechanisms such as the presence of neutralizing antibodies, or technical impediments to detecting both viruses simultaneously, could also be involved. In one chimpanzee, sequencing data provided evidence for the generation of variant viruses with mutations in the hypervariable region encoding a putative envelope protein, suggesting the emergence of viruses that may escape neutralization by the host's immune system. Reinfection occurred several times in a chimpanzee rechallenged with four different HCV strains, and also occurred in a chimpanzee rechallenged with the homologous inoculum. That chimpanzees lack immunity to reinfection with HCV has also been hypothesized by Prince et al (1992), who reported the reappearance of HCV viraemia in chimpanzees rechallenged with the homologous or a heterologous virus.

The data obtained from the animal model may provide a key to interpreting the multiple episodes of transfusion-associated hepatitis with short incubation period that have been described in individual haemophiliacs and other subjects at risk of repeated exposure to HCV. The short incubation period observed in chimpanzees repeatedly exposed to HCV suggests a similar aetiology for the multiple attacks of short incubation hepatitis seen in haemophiliacs.

The mechanisms responsible for the lack of protective immunity against reinfection with HCV are at present unknown. We can postulate that either genetic variability at selected neutralization epitopes or insufficient protective immunity may be involved. Regarding the first hypothesis, several studies have documented that HCV, like most RNA viruses, is subjected to a high rate of genetic variation that is not uniformly distributed in the viral genome. The highest degree of genetic heterogeneity has been identified within two regions presumably coding for the envelope proteins (E1, NS1/E2) (Hijkata et al 1991, Weiner et al 1991). Ogata et al (1991) have sequenced HCV isolates obtained from an individual patient during the acute hepatitis phase and after 13 years of follow-up. Their analysis, based on 50% of the HCV genome, showed a mutation rate of 1.92×10^{-3} base substitutions per site per year. A similar study was recently conducted by Okamoto et al (1992) in a chimpanzee experimentally infected with HCV. Sequence analysis of the complete genome of two isolates obtained during the acute phase and 8.2 years later demonstrated a mutation rate of 1.44×10^{-3} per site per year. These data suggest that, although it is possible that neutralization escape mutants may emerge, this mechanism is not sufficient to explain the lack of protective immunity against HCV. Two lines of evidence indicate that HCV infection does not elicit an effective neutralizing immune response. First, as discussed above, a chimpanzee was reinfected with the homologous HCV strain and the virus isolated after reinfection had no mutations in the hypervariable region. Second, recent experiments performed in our laboratory (Farci et al 1992c) suggest that little or no neutralizing antibodies to HCV were present in the plasma of a patient chronically infected with HCV for 13 years. This plasma, containing antibodies to both structural (core, E1, E2) and non-structural proteins (NS3, NS4, NS5) of HCV, was used to attempt to neutralize the homologous strain of HCV in vitro. The mixture was then evaluated for residual infectivity by i.v. inoculation of seronegative chimpanzees. Following the virus challenge, the animals developed early viraemia, as well as biochemical and histopathological evidence of acute hepatitis. Albeit preliminary, these data suggest that HCV does not elicit an effective neutralizing immune response. This could also explain why the immune response against HCV during persistent infection fails to mediate resolution of the disease in 50% of cases. Alternatively, it is possible that HCV does elicit protective neutralizing antibodies, but that a putative second factor(s) (e.g. blocking antibodies) abrogates their protective effect, as previously reported for retroviruses (Massey & Schochetman 1981, Homsy et al 1989).

The high endemicity of HCV infection throughout the world and its high rate of progression to chronicity indicate that prevention is a high priority in the control of NANB hepatitis. However, the apparent absence of neutralizing antibodies, together with the observation of the lack of protective immunity against homologous rechallenge in convalescent chimpanzees, and the high degree of genetic heterogeneity of HCV, raise concerns regarding the feasibility of developing effective HCV vaccines. Further understanding of the mechanisms of protective immunity against HCV is needed to devise effective strategies for vaccine development.

THE FUTURE

It is likely that chimpanzees will continue to play an important role in research on hepatitis C. In the absence of useful cell culture systems in which to propagate HCV, the chimpanzee will continue to provide a means of biologically amplifying rare or interesting strains of HCV. Furthermore, emerging information about the genetic heterogeneity of HCV strains indicates that some may be so different as to represent entirely different serotypes (Bukh et al 1993b). If this is true, chimpanzees provide the only means at present of detecting new serotypes, by demonstrating second cases of hepatitis C in rechallenged chimpanzees. Cross-challenge studies to date (see above) have probably utilized HCV strains representing relatively closely related genetic groups. As noted, rechallenge with such HCV strains has resulted in reinfection but minimal hepatitis. Cross-challenge with widely divergent strains of HCV might reveal complete absence of cross-protection.

A major role for chimpanzees will undoubtedly be in attempts at vaccine development. Preliminary attempts at vaccinating chimpanzees with recombinant HCV structural proteins yielded results similar to those obtained by cross-challenge: diminished hepatitis but failure to protect against infection or chronicity (M Houghton 1992, personal communication). However, it is not yet clear which antibodies, if any, are capable of neutralizing HCV, and in vitro neutralization experiments followed by assay of residual infectivity by inoculation of chimpanzees will continue to be useful in attempts to identify such antibodies.

REFERENCES

Aach R D, Lander J J, Sherman L A et al 1978 Transfusion-transmitted viruses: interim analysis of hepatitis among transfused and nontransfused patients. In: Vyas G N, Cohen S N, Shmid R (eds) Viral hepatitis. Franklin Institute Press, Philadelphia, pp 383–396

Aach R D, Stevens C E, Hollinger F B et al 1991 Hepatitis C virus infection in post-transfusion hepatitis. New England Journal of Medicine 325: 1325–1329

Abe K, Inchauspe G, Shikata T, Prince A M 1992 Three different patterns of hepatitis C virus infection in chimpanzees. Hepatology 15: 690–695

Akbar S M, Onji M, Ohta Y 1992 Estimation of IgG subclasses of anti-HCV (C100-3) in non-A, non-B fulminant, acute and chronic hepatitis and its significance. Gastroenterologica Japanica 27: 514–520

Alter H J 1987 You'll wonder where the yellow went: a 15-year retrospective of posttransfusion hepatitis. In Moore S B (ed.) Transfusion-transmitted viral diseases. American Association of Blood Banks, Arlington, pp 53–86

Alter H J 1989 Chronic consequences of non-A, non-B hepatitis. In: Seeff L B, Lewis J H (eds) Current prospective in hepatology. Plenum Publishing, New York, pp 83–97

Alter H J, Purcell R H, Feinstone S M, Holland P V, Morrow A G 1978a Non-A/non-B hepatitis: a review and interim report of an ongoing prospective study. In: Vyas G N, Cohen S N, Schmid R (eds) Viral Hepatitis. Franklin Institute Press, Philadelphia, pp 359–381

Alter H J, Purcell R H, Holland P V, Popper H 1978b Transmissible agent in 'non-A, non-B' hepatitis. Lancet i: 459–463

Alter H J, Purcell R H, Shih J W et al 1989 Detection of antibody to hepatitis C virus in prospectively followed transfusion recipients with acute and chronic non-A, non-B hepatitis. New England Journal of Medicine 321: 1494–1500

Alter M J 1991 Epidemiology of community-acquired hepatitis C. In Hollinger F B, Lemon S M, Margolis H (eds) Viral hepatitis and liver disease. William & Wilkins, Baltimore, pp 410–413

Alter M J, Gerety J, Smallwood L A et al 1982 Sporadic non-A, non-B hepatitis: frequency and epidemiology in an urban US population. Journal of Infectious Diseases 145: 886–893

Alter M J, Hadler S C, Judson F N et al 1990 Risk factors for acute non-A, non-B hepatitis in the United States and association with hepatitis C virus infection. Journal of the American Medical Association 264: 2231–2235

Bamber M, Murray A, Kernoff P B, Thomas H 1981a Short incubation non-A, non-B hepatitis transmitted by factor VIII concentrates in patients with congenital coagulation disorders: a preliminary report of an antigen/antibody system. Medical Laboratory Sciences 38: 373–378

Bamber M, Murray A, Arborgh B A et al 1981b Short incubation non-A, non-B hepatitis transmitted by factor VIII concentrates in patients with congenital coagulation disorders. Gut 22: 854–859

Beach M J, Meeks E L, Mimms L T et al 1992 Temporal relationships of hepatitis C virus RNA and antibody responses following experimental infection of chimpanzees. Journal of Medical Virology 36: 226–237

Beasley R P 1982 Hepatitis B virus as the etiologic agent in hepatocellular carcinoma – epidemiologic considerations. Hepatology 2: 21S-26S

Beasley R P 1988 Hepatitis B virus: the major etiology of hepatocellular carcinoma. Cancer 61: 1942–1956

Beasley R P, Hwang L Y, Lin C C et al 1981 Hepatocellular carcinoma and hepatitis B virus: a prospective study of 22,707 men in Taiwan. Lancet ii: 1006–1008

Benn S, Rutledge R, Folks T, Gold J et al 1985 Genomic heterogeneity of AIDS retroviral isolates from North America and Zaire. Science 230: 949–951

Blumberg B S, Alter H J, Visnich S 1965 A new antigen in leukemia serum. Journal of the American Medical Association 66: 924–931

Blumberg B S, Gerstley B J S, Hungerford D A, London W T, Sutnick A 1967 A serum antigen (Australia antigen) in Down's Syndrome, leukemia and hepatitis. Annals of Internal Medicine 66: 924–931

Bockus D, Remington F, Luu J Y, Bean M, Hammar S 1988 Induction of cylindrical confronting cisternae (AIDS inclusions) in Daudi lymphoblastoid cells by recombinant alpha-interferon. Human Pathology 19: 78–82

Bradley D W, Cook E H, Maynard J E et al 1979 Experimental infection of chimpanzees with antihemophilic (factor VIII) materials: recovery of virus-like particles associated with non-A, non-B hepatitis. Journal of Medical Virology 3: 253–269

Bradley D W, Maynard J E, Cook E H et al 1980 Non-A/non-B hepatitis in experimentally infected chimpanzees: cross-challenge and electron microscopic studies. Journal of Medical Virology 6: 185–201

Bradley D W, Maynard J E, Popper H et al 1981 Persistent non-A, non-B hepatitis in experimentally infected chimpanzees. Journal of Infectious Diseases 143: 210–218

Bradley D W, Maynard J E, McCaustland K A, Murphy B L, Cook E H, Ebert J W 1983a Non-A, non-B hepatitis in chimpanzees: interference with acute hepatitis A virus and chronic hepatitis B virus infections. Journal of Medical Virology 11: 207–213

Bradley D W, Maynard J E, Popper H et al 1983b Posttransfusion non-A, non-B hepatitis: physicochemical properties of two distinct agents. Journal of Infectious Diseases 148: 254–265

Bradley D W, McCaustland K A, Cook E H et al 1985 Posttransfusion non-A, non-B hepatitis in chimpanzees: physicochemical evidence that the tubule-forming agent is a small, enveloped virus. Gastroenterology 88: 773–779

Bradley D W, Krawczynski K, Humphrey C D, McCaustland K A 1987 Biochemically silent posttransfusion non-A, non-B hepatitis interferes with superinfection by hepatitis A virus. Intervirology 27(2): 86–90

Bradley D W, Krawczynski K, Ebert J W et al 1990 Parenterally transmitted non-A, non-B hepatitis: virus-specific antibody response patterns in hepatitis C virus-infected chimpanzees. Gastroenterology 99: 1054–1060

Bradley D W, Krawcynski K, Beach M, Purdy M 1991 Non-A, non-B hepatitis: toward the discovery of hepatitis C and E viruses. Seminars in Liver Disease 11: 128–146

Brotman B, Prince A M, Huima T, Richardson L, van den Ende M C, Pfeifer U 1983 Interference between non-A, non-B and hepatitis B virus infection in chimpanzees. Journal of Medical Virology 11: 191–205

Brotman B, Prince A M, Huima T 1985 Non-A, non-B hepatitis virus: is there more than a single blood-borne strain? Journal of Infectious Diseases 151: 618–625

Bruix J, Barrera J M, Calvet X et al 1989 Prevalence of antibodies to hepatitis C virus in Spanish patients with hepatocellular carcinoma and hepatic cirrhosis. Lancet ii: 1004–1006

Bukh J, Purcell R H, Miller R H 1992 Importance of primer selection for the detection of hepatitis C virus RNA with the polymerase chain reaction assay. Proceedings of the National Academy of Sciences of the USA 89: 187–191

Bukh J, Miller R H, Kew M C, Purcell, R H 1993a Hepatitis C virus RNA in southern African blacks with hepatocellular carcinoma. Proceedings of the National Academy of Sciences of the USA 90(5): 1848–1851

Bukh J, Purcell R H, Miller R H 1993b At least 12 genotypes of hepatitis C virus predicted by sequence analysis of the putative E1 gene of isolates collected worldwide. Proceedings of the National Academy of Sciences of the USA 90: 8234–8238

Burk K H, Cabral G A, Dreesman G R, Peters R L, Alter H J 1981 Ultrastructural changes and virus-like particles localized in liver hepatocytes of chimpanzees infected with non-A, non-B hepatitis. Journal of Medical Virology 7: 1–19

Burk K H, Dreesman G R, Cabral G A, Peters R L 1984 Long-term sequelae of non-A, non-B hepatitis in experimentally infected chimpanzees.Hepatology 4: 808–816

Busachi C A, Realdi G, Alberti A, Badiali de Georgi L, Tremolada F 1981 Ultrastructural changes in the liver of patients with chronic non-A, non-B hepatitis. Journal of Medical Virology 7: 205–212

Canese M G, Rizzetto M, Novara R, London W T, Purcell R H 1984 Experimental infection of chimpanzees with the HBsAg-associated delta (δ) agent: an ultrastructural study. Journal of Medical Virology 13: 63–72

Choo Q L, Kuo G, Weiner A J, Overby L R, Bradley D W, Houghton M 1989 Isolation of a cDNA clone derived from a blood-borne non-A, non-B hepatitis genome. Science 244: 359–362

Choo Q L, Richman K H, Han J H et al 1991 Genetic organization and diversity of the hepatitis C virus. Proceedings of the National Academy of Sciences of the USA 88: 2451–2455

Chou W H, Yoneyama T, Takeuchi K, Harada H, Saito I, Miyamura T 1991 Discrimination of hepatitis C virus in liver tissues from different patients with hepatocellular carcinoma by direct nucleotide sequencing of amplified cDNA of the viral genome. Journal of Clinical Microbiology 29: 2860–2864

Colombo M, Kuo G, Choo Q L et al 1989 Prevalence of antibodies to hepatitis C virus in Italian patients with hepatocellular carcinoma. Lancet ii: 1006–1008

Craske J, Dilling N, Stern D 1975 An outbreak of hepatitis associated with intravenous injection of factor-VIII concentrate. Lancet ii: 221–223

Craske J, Spooner R J D, Vandervelde E M 1978 Evidence for existence of at least two types of factor-VIII-associated non-B transfusion hepatitis (letter). Lancet ii: 1051–1052

Cristiano K, Di Bisceglie A M, Hoofnagle J H, Feinstone S M 1991 Hepatitis C viral RNA in serum of patients with chronic non-A, non-B hepatitis: detection by the polymerase chain reaction using multiple primer sets. Hepatology 14: 51–55

Dasarathy S, Misra S C, Acharya S K, Irshad M et al 1992 Prospective controlled study of post-transfusion hepatitis after cardiac surgery in a large referral hospital in India. Liver 12(3): 116–120

DeVos R, DeWolf-Peeters C, Desmet V, DeGroote G, Desmyter J 1981 Crystalline arrays and non-A, non-B hepatitis. Lancet i: 1364

DeWolf-Peeters C, DeVos R, Desmet V et al 1981 Human non-A, non-B hepatitis: ultrastructural alterations in hepatocytes. Liver 1: 50–55

Dienes H P, Purcell R H, Popper H, Ponzetto A 1990 The significance of infections with two types of viral hepatitis demonstrated by histologic features in chimpanzees. Journal of Hepatology 10: 77–84

Dienstag J L 1983a Non-A, non-B hepatitis. I. Recognition, epidemiology, and clinical features. Gastroenterology 85: 439–462

Dienstag J L 1983b Non-A, non-B hepatitis. II. Experimental transmission, putative virus agents and markers, and prevention. Gastroenterology 85: 743–768

Dienstag J L, Krotoski W A, Howard W A et al 1981 Non-A, non-B hepatitis after experimental transmission of malaria by blood inoculation. Journal of Infectious Diseases 143: 200–209

Dienstag J, Katkov W, Cooly H 1991 Evidence for non-A, non-B hepatitis agents besides hepatitis C virus. In: Hollinger F B, Lemon S M, Margolis H (eds) Viral hepatitis and lives disease. Williams & Wilkins, Baltimore, pp 349–356

Eder G, Bianchi L, Gudat F 1988 Transmission of non-A, non-B hepatitis to chimpanzees: a second and third episode caused by the same inoculum. In Zuckerman A J (ed.) Viral hepatitis and liver disease. Alan R. Liss, New York, 550–552

Esteban J I, Gonzalez A, Hernandez J M et al 1990 Evaluation of antibodies to hepatitis C virus in a study of transfusion-associated hepatitis. New England Journal of Medicine 323: 1107–1112

Esteban J I, Genesca J, Alter H J 1993 Hepatitis C: molecular biology, pathogenesis, epidemiology, clinical features and prevention. In: Boyer J L, Ockner R K (eds) Progress in Liver Diseases 10 (in press)

Evans A S 1954 Attempts to transmit the virus of human hepatitis to primates other than man. Symposium on the Laboratory Propagation and Detection of the Agent of Hepatitis. Publication No. 322. National Academy of Sciences–National Research Council, Washington DC, pp 58–68

Farci P, Alter H J, Wong D, Miller R H, Shih J W, Jett B, Purcell R H 1991 A long-term study of hepatitis C virus replication in non-A, non-B hepatitis. New England Journal of Medicine 325: 98–104

Farci P, London W T, Wong D C, Dawson G J, Vallari D S, Engle R, Purcell R H 1992a The natural history of infection with hepatitis C virus (HCV) in chimpanzees: comparison of serologic responses measured with first- and second-generation assays and relationship to HCV viremia. Journal of Infectious Diseases 165: 1006–1011

Farci P, Alter H J, Govindarajan S et al 1992b Lack of protective immunity against reinfection with hepatitis C virus. Science 258: 135–140

Farci P, Alter H J, Wong D, Ogata N, Miller R, Shapiro M, Purcell R 1992c Attempts to neutralize hepatitis C virus (HCV) in vitro with plasma from a chronically infected patient: evaluation in chimpanzees. Hepatology 16: 105a

Feinstone S M, Kapikian A Z, Purcell R H 1973 Hepatitis A detection by immune electron microscopy of a virus-like antigen associated with acute illness. Science 182: 1026–1028

Feinstone S M, Kapikian A Z, Purcell R H, Alter H J, Holland P V 1975 Transfusion-associated hepatitis not due to viral hepatitis type A or B. New England Journal of Medicine 292: 767–770

Feinstone S M, Alter H J, Dienes H P et al 1981 Non-A, non-B hepatitis in chimpanzees and marmosets. Journal of Infectious Diseases 144(4): 588–598

Feinstone S M, Alter H J, Dienes H P et al 1982 Studies of non-A, non-B hepatitis in chimpanzees and marmosets. In: Szmuness W, Alter H J, Maynard J E (eds) Viral hepatitis: 1981 International Symposium. The Franklin Institute Press, Philadelphia, pp 295–304

Feinstone S M, Mihalik K B, Kamimura T et al 1983 Inactivation of hepatitis B virus and non-A, non-B hepatitis by chloroform. Infection and Immunity 41: 816–821

Fowler M J F, Monjardino J, Weller I V et al 1983 Failure to detect nucleic acid homology between some non-A, non-B viruses and hepatitis B virus DNA. Journal of Medical Virology 12: 205–213

Frey-Wettstein 1977 How frequent is post-transfusion hepatitis after the introduction of 3rd generation donor screening for hepatitis B? What is the probable nature? Vox Sanguinis 32: 352–353

Galbraith R M, Dienstag J L, Purcell R H, Gower P H, Zuckerman A J, Williams R 1979 Non-A, non-B hepatitis associated with chronic liver disease in a hemodialysis unit. Lancet i: 951–953

Garson J A, Tedder R S, Briggs M et al 1990 Detection of hepatitis C viral sequences in blood donations by 'nested' polymerase chain reaction and prediction of infectivity. Lancet 335: 1419–1422

Gerin J L, Cote, J P, Korba, B E, Tennant B C 1989 Hepadnavirus-induced liver cancer in woodchucks. Cancer Detection and Prevention 14: 227–229

Giles J P, McCollum R W, Berndtson L W Jr 1969 Viral hepatitis: relation of Australia/SH antigen to the Willowbrook MS-2 strain. New England Journal of Medicine 281: 119–122

Gilliam J H, Geisinger K R, Richter J E 1984 Primary hepatocellular carcinoma after chronic non-A, non-B post-transfusion hepatitis. Annals of Internal Medicine 101: 794–795

Gocke D J 1972 A prospective study of posttransfusion hepatitis: the role of the Australia antigen. Journal of the American Medical Association 219: 1165–1170

Gocke D J, Greenberg H B, Kavey N B 1970 Correlation of Australia antigen with posttransfusion hepatitis. Journal of the American Medical Association 212: 877–879

Goldfield M, Black H C, Bill J, Srihongse S, Pizzuti W 1975 The consequences of administering blood pretested for HBsAg by third generation techniques: a progress report. American Journal of the Medical Sciences 270: 335–342

Han J H, Shyamala V, Richman K H et al 1991 Characterization of the terminal regions of hepatitis C viral RNA: identification of conserved sequences in the 5' untranslated region and poly A tails at the 3' end. Proceedings of the National Academy of Sciences of the USA 88: 1711–1715

Harrison T J, Tsiquaye K N, Zuckerman A J 1983 Assay of HBV DNA in the plasma of HBV-carrier chimpanzees superinfected with non-A, non-B hepatitis. Journal of Virological Methods 6: 295–302

Havens W P Jr 1947 The etiology of infectious hepatitis. Journal of the American Medical Association 134: 653–655

Havens W P Jr 1963 Viral hepatitis. Postgraduate Medical Journal 39: 212–223

He L F, Alling D, Popkin T, Shapiro M, Alter H J, Purcell R H 1987 Non-A, non-B hepatitis virus: determination of size by filtration. Journal of Infectious Diseases 156: 636–640

Heinrich D, Kotitschke R, Berthold H 1982 Clinical evaluation of the hepatitis safety of a β-propiolactone/ ultraviolet treated factor IX concentrate (PPSB). Thrombosis Research 28: 75–83

Hijikata M, Kato N, Ootsuyama Y, Nakegawa M, Ohkoshi S, Shimotohno K 1991 Hypervariable regions in the putative glycoprotein of hepatitis C virus. Biochemical and Biophysical Research Communications 175: 220–228

Hilfenhaus J, Krupka U, Nowak T et al 1992 Follow-up of hepatitis C virus infection in chimpanzees: determination of

viraemia and specific humoral immune response. Journal of General Virology 73: 1015–1019
Holland P V, Alter H J, Purcell R H, Walsh J J, Morrow A G, Schmidt P J 1973 The infectivity of blood containing the Australia antigen. In: Prier J E, Friedman H (eds) Australia antigen. University Press, Baltimore, pp 191–203
Hollinger F B, Dreesman G R, Fields H, Melnick J L 1975 HBcAg, anti-HBc, and DNA polymerase activity in transfused recipients followed prospectively. American Journal of the Medical Sciences 270: 343–348
Hollinger F B, Gitnick G L, Aach R D et al 1978 Non-A, non-B hepatitis transmission in chimpanzees: a project of the Transfusion-Transmitted Viruses Study Group. Intervirology 10: 60–68
Hollinger F B, Mosley J W, Szmuness W, Aach R D, Peters S L, Stevens C E 1980 Transfusion-transmitted viruses study: experimental evidence for two non-A, non-B hepatitis agents. Journal of Infectious Diseases 142: 400–407
Homsy J, Meyer M, Tateno M, Clarkson S, Levy J A 1989 The Fc and not CD4 receptor mediates antibody enhancement of HIV infection in human cells. Science 244: 1357–1360
Houghton M, Weiner A, Han J, Choo QL 1991 Molecular biology of the hepatitis C viruses: implications for diagnosis, development, and control of viral disease. Hepatology 14: 381– 391
Hruby M A, Schauf V 1978 Transfusion-related short-incubation hepatitis in hemophilic patients. Journal of the American Medical Association 240: 1355–1357
Jackson D R, Tabor E, Gerety R J 1979 Acute non-A, non-B hepatitis: specific ultrastructural alterations in endoplasmic reticulum of infected hepatocytes. Lancet i: 1249–1250
Kamimura T, Bonino F, Ponzetto A, Feinstone M S, Gerin J L, Purcell R H 1983 Cytoplasmic tubular structures in liver of HBsAg carrier chimpanzees infected with delta-agent and comparison with cytoplasmic structures in non-A, non-B hepatitis. Hepatology 3: 631–637
Karayiannis P, Scheuer P J, Bamber M et al 1983 Experimental infection of tamarins with human non-A, non-B hepatitis virus. Journal of Medical Virology 11: 251–256
Kew M C, Houghton M, Choo Q L, Kuo G 1990 Hepatitis C virus antibodies in southern African blacks with hepatocellular carcinoma. Lancet 335: 873–874
Khan N, Hollinger F B 1986 Non-A, non-B hepatitis agent. Lancet i: 41
Kikuchi T, Onji M, Michitaka K et al 1992 Anti-HCV immunoglobulin M antibody in patients with hepatitis C. Third Department of Internal Medicine, Ehime University School of Medicine, Japan. Journal of Gastroenterology Hepatologica 7: 246–248
Kiyosawa K, Akahane Y, Nagata A, Furate S 1984 Hepatocellular carcinoma after non-A, non-B posttransfusion hepatitis. American Journal of Gastroenterology 79: 777–781
Kiyosawa K, Sodeyama T, Tanaka E et al 1990 Interrelationship of blood transfusion, non-A, non-B hepatitis and hepatocellular carcinoma: analysis by detection of antibody to hepatitis C virus. Hepatology 12: 671–675
Korba B E, Wells F, Baldwin B et al 1989 Hepatocellular carcinoma in woodchuck hepatitis virus-infected woodchucks: presence of viral DNA in tumor tissue from chronic carriers and animals serologically recovered from acute infections. Hepatology 9: 461–470
Kostianovsky M, Kang Y H, Grimley P M 1984 Abnormal cytoplasmic inclusions in acquired immunodeficiency syndrome (AIDS). AIDS Research 1: 181
Krawczynski K, Beach M J, Bradley D W et al 1992 Hepatitis C virus antigen in hepatocytes: immunomorphologic detection and identification. Gastroenterology 103: 622–629
Krugman S, Giles J P 1973 Viral hepatitis, type B (MS-2-strain): further observations on natural history and prevention. New England Journal of Medicine 288: 755–760
Krugman S, Giles J P, Hammond J 1967 Infectious hepatitis. Evidence for two distinctive clinical epidemiological and immunological types of infection. Journal of the American Medical Association 200: 365–373
Krugman S, Giles J P, Hammond J 1971 Viral hepatitis type B (MS-2 strain). Studies on active immunization. Journal of the American Medical Association 217: 41–45
Kuo G, Choo Q-L, Alter H J et al 1989 An assay for circulating antibodies to a major etiologic virus of human non-A, non-B hepatitis. Science 244: 362–364
Lanford R E, Noivall L, Barbosa L H, Eichberg J W 1991 Evaluation of a chimpanzee colony for antibodies to hepatitis C virus. Journal of Medical Virology 34: 148–153
Lee S D, Tsai Y T, Hwang S J, Wu J C et al 1991 A prospective study of post-transfusion non-A, non-B hepatitis (type C) following cardiovascular surgery in Taiwan. Journal of Medical Virology 33: 188–192
Liang T J, Jeffers L, Findor A et al 1991 Lack of evidence for hepatitis C virus infection in non-A, non-B fulminant and late-onset hepatic failure. Hepatology 14: 129A
Linke H K, Miller M F, Peterson D A et al 1987 Documentation of non-A, non-B hepatitis in a chimpanzee with hepatocellular carcinoma. In: Robinson W, Koike K, Will H (eds) Hepadna viruses. Alan R. Liss, New York, pp 357–370
Lok A S F, Cheung R, Chan R, Liu V 1992 Hepatitis C viremia in patients with hepatitis C virus infection. Hepatology 15: 1007–1012
MacCallum F O 1947 Homologous serum hepatitis. Lancet ii: 691–692
MacCallum F O, Bauer D J 1944 Homologous serum jaundice transmission experiments with human volunteers. Lancet i: 622–627
MacCallum F O, McFarlan A M, Miles J A R, Pollock M R, Wilson C 1951 Infective hepatitis. Studies in East Anglia during the period 1943–47. Special Reports *Ser* Medical Research Council 273
McCaul T F, Tsiquaye K N, Tovey G, Hames C, Zuckerman A J 1982 Application of electron microscopy to the study of structural changes in liver in non-A, non-B hepatitis. Journal of Virological Methods 4: 87–106
Marciano-Cabral F, Rublee K L, Carithers R L Jr, Galen E A, Sobieski T J, Cabral G A 1981 Chronic non-A, non-B hepatitis: ultrastructural and serologic studies. Hepatology 1: 575–582
Massey R J, Schochetman G 1981 Viral epitopes and monoclonal antibodies: isolation of blocking antibodies that inhibit virus neutralization Science 213: 447–449
Maynard J E, Berquist K R, Krushak D H, Purcell R H 1972 Experimental infection of chimpanzees with the virus of hepatitis B. Nature 237: 514–515
Miller R H, Purcell R H 1990 Hepatitis C virus shares amino

acid sequence similarity with pestiviruses and flaviviruses as well as members of two plant virus supergroups. Proceedings of the National Academy of Sciences of the USA 87: 2057–2061
Mosley J W 1975 The epidemiology of viral hepatitis: an overview. The American Journal of Medical Science 270: 253–270
Mosley J W, Redeker A G, Feinstone S M, Purcell R H 1977 Multiple hepatitis viruses in multiple attacks of acute viral hepatitis. New England Journal of Medicine 296: 75–78
Muchmore E, Socha W W, Krawczynski C 1990 Hepatocellular carcinoma in chimpanzees. In: Sung J L, Chen D S (eds) Proceedings of Viral hepatitis and hepatocellular carcinoma. Excerpta Medica. Current Clinical Practice Series 57
Munoz S J, Farci P, Martin P, Purcell R H 1992 Frequency of hepatitis C virus RNA in serum of patients with fulminant non-A, non-B hepatitis. 5th National Forum on AIDS, Hepatitis, and other Blood-Borne Diseases, Atlanta, Georgia, March 29–April 1, P21: 39 (abstract)
Muto Y, Sugihara J, Ohnishi H, Moriwaki H, Nishioka K 1990 Anti-hepatitis C virus antibody prevails in fulminant hepatic failure. Gastroenterologia Japonica 25: 32–35
Negro F, Pacchioni D, Shimizu Y, Miller R H, Bussolati G, Purcell R H, Bonino F 1992 Detection of intrahepatic replication of hepatitis C virus RNA by in situ hybridization and comparison with histopathology. Proceedings of the National Academy of Sciences of the USA 89: 2247–2251
Norkrans G, Frosner G, Hermodsson S, Iwarson S 1980 Multiple hepatitis attacks in drug addicts. Journal of the American Medical Association 243: 1056–1058
Ogata N, Alter H J, Miller R H, Purcell R H 1991 Nucleotide sequence and mutation rate of the H strain of hepatitis C virus. Proceedings of the National Academy of Sciences of the USA 8: 3392–3396
Okamoto H, Kojima M, Okada S I et al 1992 Genetic drift of hepatitis C virus during an 8.2-year infection in a chimpanzee: variability and stability. Virology 190: 894–899
Okochi K, Murakami S, Ninomiya K, Kaneko M 1970 Australia antigen, transfusion and hepatitis. Vox Sanguinis 18: 289–300
Okuda K 1992 Hepatocellular carcinoma: recent progress. Hepatology 15: 948–963
Pfeifer U, Thomssen R, Legler K, Bottcher U, Gerlich W, Weinmann O, Klinge O 1980 Experimental non-A, non-B hepatitis: four types of cytoplasmic alteration in hepatocytes of infected chimpanzees. Virchows Archiv B Cell Pathology 33: 233–243
Ponzetto A, Hoyer B H, Popper H, Engle R, Purcell R H, Gerin J L 1987 Titration of the infectivity of hepatitis D virus in chimpanzees. Journal of Infectious Diseases 156: 72–78
Popper H, Roth L, Purcell R H, Tennant B C, Gerin J L 1987 Hepatocarcinogenicity of the woodchuck hepatitis virus. Proceedings of the National Academy of Sciences of the USA 84: 866–870
Prince A M 1968 An antigen detected in the blood during the incubation period of serum hepatitis. Proceedings of the National Academy of Sciences of the USA 60: 814
Prince A M, Brotman B, van den Ende M C, Richardson L, Kellner A 1978 Non-A, -non-B hepatitis: identification of a virus-specific antigen and antibody: a preliminary report. In: Vyas G N, Cohen S N, Schmid R (eds) Viral hepatitis. Franklin Institute Press, Philadelphia, pp 633–640
Prince A M, Stephen W, Dichtelmuller H, Brotman B, Huima T 1985 Inactivation of the Hutchinson strain of non-A, non-B hepatitis virus by combined use of β-propiolactone and ultraviolet irradiation. Journal of Medical Virology 16: 199–125
Prince A M, Brotman B, Huima T, Pascual D, Jaffery M, Inchauspe G 1992 Immunity in hepatitis C infection. Journal of Infectious Diseases 165: 438–443
Purcell R H 1989 Does non-A, non-B hepatitis cause hepatocellular carcinoma? Cancer Detection and Prevention 14: 203–207
Purcell R H 1992 Primates and hepatitis research. In: Erwin J, Landon J C (eds) Chimpanzee conservation and public health: environments for the future. Diagnon Corporation/Bioqual, Rockville, pp 15–20
Purcell R H 1993 Hepatitis C virus. In: Webster R G, Granoff A (eds) Encyclopedia of Virology. W B Saunders, Philadelphia (in press)
Purcell R H, Gerin J L, Popper H et al 1985 Hepatitis B virus, hepatitis non-A, non-B virus and hepatitis delta virus in lyophilized antihemophilic factor: relative sensitivity to heat. Hepatology 5: 1091–1099
Realdi G, Alberti A, Rugge M et al 1982 Long term follow-up of acute and chronic non-A, non-B posttransfusion hepatitis: evidence of progression to liver cirrhosis. Gut 23: 270–275
Resnick R H, Stone K, Antonioli D 1983 Primary hepatocellular carcinoma following non-A, non-B posttransfusion hepatitis. Digestive Diseases and Sciences 28: 908–11
Rizzetto M, Ponzetto A, Bonino F, Purcell R H 1986 Superimposed delta hepatitis and the effect on viral replication on chronic hepatitis B. Proceedings of International Symposium on Anti-Viral Agents in Chronic Hepatitis B virus Infection, November 11–12, London, England. Journal of Hepatology 3: S35–S41
Ruiz J, Sangro B, Cuende J I et al 1992 Hepatitis B and C viral infections in patients with hepatocellular carcinoma. Hepatology 16: 637–641
Saito I, Miyamura T, Ohbayashi A et al 1990 Hepatitis C virus infection is associated with the development of hepatocellular carcinoma. Proceedings of the National Academy of Sciences of the USA 87: 6547–6549
Sallie R, Tibbs C, Silva A E, Sheron N, Eddlestone A, Williams R 1991 Detection of hepatitis 'E' but not 'C' in sera of patients with fulminant NANB hepatitis. Hepatology 14: 68A
Schlauder G G, Leverenz G J, Amann C W, Lesniewski R R, Peterson D A 1991 Detection of the hepatitis C virus genome in acute and chronic experimental infection in chimpanzees. Journal of Clinical Microbiology 29: 2175–2179
Seto B, Coleman W G, Iwarson S et al 1984 Detection of reverse transcriptase activity in association with non-A, non-B hepatitis agent(s). Lancet ii: 941–942
Seeff L B, Wright E C, Zimmerman H J et al 1978 Post-transfusion hepatitis, 1973–1975: a Veterans Administration cooperative study. In: Vyas G N, Cohen S N, Schmid R (eds) Viral hepatitis. Franklin Institute Press, Philadelphia, pp 219–242
Schaff Z, Tabor E, Jackson D R, Gerety R J 1984 Ultrastructural alterations in serial liver biopsy specimens from chimpanzees experimentally infected with a human non-A, non-B hepatitis agent. Virchows Archiv B Cell Pathology 45: 301–312

Shimizu Y, Purcell R H 1989 Cytoplasmic antigen in hepatocytes of chimpanzees infected with non-A, non-B hepatitis virus or hepatitis delta virus: relationship to interferon. Hepatology 10: 764–768

Shimizu Y K, Feinstone S M, Purcell R H, Alter H J, London W T 1979 Non-A, non-B hepatitis: ultrastructural evidence for two agents in experimentally infected chimpanzees. Science 205: 197–200

Shimizu Y K, Omura M, Abe K et al 1985 Production of antibody associated with non-A, non-B hepatitis in a chimpanzee lympoblastoid cell line established by a vitro transformation with Epstein-Barr virus. Proceedings of the National Academy of Sciences of the USA 82: 2138–2142

Shimizu Y K, Weiner A J, Rosenblatt J et al 1990 Early events in hepatitis C virus infection of chimpanzees. Proceedings of the National Academy of Sciences of the USA 87: 6441–6444

Shindo M, Di Bisceglie A M, Biswas R, Mihalik K, Feinstone S M 1992 Hepatitis C virus replication during acute infection in the chimpanzee. Journal of Infectious Diseases 166: 424–427

Sidhu G S, Stahl R E, El-Sadr W, Zolla-Pazner S 1983 Ultrastructural markers of AIDS. Lancet i: 990–991

Sugg U, Frosner G G, Schneider W, Stunkat R 1976 Hepatitishaufgheit nach transfusion von HBsAg negativem und anti-HBs positivem. Blut Klinische Wschr 53: 1133–1136

Summers J 1981 Three recently described animal virus models for human hepatitis B virus. Hepatology 1: 179–183

Tabor E, Gerety R J, Drucker J A et al 1978a Transmission of non-A, non-B hepatitis from man to chimpanzee. Lancet i: 463–466

Tabor E, Gerety R J, Drucker J A et al 1978b Experimental transmission and passage of human non-A, non-B hepatitis in chimpanzees. In: Vyas G N, Cohen S N, Schmid R (eds) Viral hepatitis. Franklin Institute Press, Philadelphia, 419–421

Tabor E, April M, Seeff L B et al 1979a Acute non-A, non-B hepatitis: prolonged presence of the infectious agent in blood. Gastroenterology 76: 680–684

Tabor E, April M, Seeff L B, Gerety R J 1979b Acquired immunity to human non-A, non-B hepatitis: cross-challenge of chimpanzees with three infectious human sera. Journal of Infectious Diseases 40: 789–793

Tabor E, Seeff L B, Gerety R J 1980 Chronic non-A, non-B hepatitis carrier state: transmissible agent documented in one patient over a six-year period. New England Journal of Medicine 303: 139–143

Tabor E, Gerety R J 1980 Inactivation of an agent of human non-A, non-B hepatitis by formalin. Journal of Infectious Diseases 142: 677–770

Tabor E 1981 Development and application of the chimpanzee animal model for human non-A, non-B hepatitis. In Gerety R J (ed.) Non-A, non-B hepatitis. Academic Press, New York, pp 189–206

Tabor E, Gerety R J 1982 The chimpanzee animal model for non-A, non-B hepatitis: new applications. In: Szmuness W, Alter H J, Maynard J E (eds) Viral hepatitis: 1981 international symposium. Franklin Institute Press, Philadelphia, 305–317

Tabor E, Purcell R H, Gerety R J 1983 Primate animal models and titered inocula for the study of human hepatitis A, hepatitis B, and non-A, non-B hepatitis. Journal of Medical Primatology 1: 305–318

Tabor E, Snoy P, Jackson D R, Schaff Z, Blatt PM, Gerety R J 1984 Additional evidence for more than one agent of human non-A, non-B hepatitis: transmission and passage studies in chimpanzees. Transfusion 24: 224–230

Tabor E 1989 Nonhuman primate models for non-A, non-B hepatitis. Cancer Detection and Prevention 14: 221–225

Tanaka K, Hirohata T, Koga S et al 1991 Hepatitis C and hepatitis B in the etiology of hepatocellular carcinoma in the Japanese population. Cancer Research 51: 2842–2847

Tralka S T, Yee C, Trich T J, Costa J, Dienes H P 1982 Unusual intranuclear inclusions in malignant fibrous histiocytoma: presence in primary tumor, metastases, and xenografts. Ultrastructural Pathology 3: 161–167

Tsiquaye K N, Zuckerman A J 1979 New human hepatitis virus. Lancet i: 1135–1136

Tsiquaye K N, Bird R G, Tovey G, Wyke J, Williams R, Zuckerman A J 1980 Further evidence of cellular changes associated with non-A, non-B hepatitis. Journal of Medical Virology 5: 63–71

Tsiquaye K N, Amini S, Kessler H, Bird R G, Tovey G, Zuckerman A J 1981 Ultrastructural changes in the liver in experimental non-A, non-B hepatitis. British Journal of Experimental Pathology 62: 41–51

Tsiquaye K N, Portmann B, Tovey G et al 1983 Non-A, non-B hepatitis in persistent carriers of hepatitis B virus. Journal of Medical Virology 11: 179–189

Tsiquaye K N, Harrison T J, Portmann B et al 1984 Acute hepatitis A infection in hepatitis B chimpanzee carriers. Hepatology 4: 504–509

Ware A J, Luby J P, Hollinger F B et al 1979 Etiology of liver disease in renal-transplant patients. Annals of Internal Medicine 91: 364–371

Watanabe T, Katagiri J, Kajima H et al 1987 Studies on transmission of human non-A, non-B hepatitis to marmosets. Journal of Medical Virology 22: 143–146

Weiner A J, Wang-K S, Choo Q-L et al 1987 Hepatitis delta cDNA clones: undetectable hybridization to nucleic acids from infectious non-A, non-B hepatitis materials and hepatitis B DNA. Journal of Medical Virology 21: 239–247

Weiner A J, Kuo G, Bradley D W et al 1990 Detection of hepatitis C viral sequences in non-A, non-B hepatitis. Lancet 335: 1–3

Weiner A J, Brauer M J, Rosenblatt J et al 1991 Variable and hypervariable domains are found in the regions of HCV corresponding to the flavivirus envelope and NS1 proteins and the pestivirus envelope glycoproteins. Virology 180: 842–848

Wright T L, Hsu H, Donegan E et al 1991 Hepatitis C virus not found in fulminant non-A, non-B hepatitis. Annals of Internal Medicine 115: 111–112

Yanagi M, Kaneko S, Unoura M et al 1991 Hepatitis C virus in fulminant liver failure. New England Journal of Medicine 324: 1895

Yoneyama T, Takeuchi K, Watanabe Y et al 1990 Detection of hepatitis C virus cDNA sequence by the polymerase chain reaction in hepatocellular carcinoma tissues. Japanese Journal of Medical Science and Biology 43: 89–94

Yoshiba M, Sekiyama K, Sugata F, Okamoto H, Mayumi M 1991a Persistence of HCV replication in non-A, non-B fulminant viral hepatitis. Gastroenterologia Japonica 26: 235

Yoshiba M, Sekiyama K, Sugata F, Okamoto H 1991b Diagnosis of type C fulminant hepatitis by the detection of antibodies to the putative core proteins of hepatitis C virus. Gastroenterologia Japonica 26: 234

Yoshizawa H, Itoh Y, Iwarkiri S et al 1981 Demonstration of two different types of non-A, non-B hepatitis by reinjection and cross-challenge studies in chimpanzees. Gastroenterology 81: 107–113

Yoshizawa H, Itoh Y, Iwarkiri S et al 1982 Non-A, non-B (type 1) hepatitis agent capable of inducing tubular ultrastructures in the hepatocyte cytoplasm of chimpanzees: inactivation of formalin and heat. Gastroenterology 82: 502–506

Yuasa T, Ishikawa G, Manabe S, Sekiguchi S, Takeuchi K, Miyamura T 1991 The particle size of hepatitis C virus estimated by filtration through microporous regenerated celullose fiber. Journal of General Virology 72: 2021–2024

15. Liver cancer

Kunio Okuda

The establishment of an epidemiological and an aetiological association between hepatocellular carcinoma (HCC) and hepatitis B virus (HBV) led to the general belief that, along with aflatoxins, HBV infection was the major aetiogical factor in hepatocarcinogenesis. Hepatitis C virus (HCV) was then discovered and it appeared to be a further aetiological factor in HCC, but with a different geographical prevalence from HBV. Whilst there is genetic and epidemiological evidence that HCV has infected man for thousands of years, data from Japan suggest that the causative role of HCV in HCC is relatively new: in Japan there has been a sharp increase in the incidence of HCC in the post-war period, and this is attributed to HCV.

The molecular mechanisms involved in HCV-associated HCC probably differ from those in HBV-associated HCC. Reverse transcription of viral RNA to DNA does not occur with HCV, and hence no integration of viral genomic sequences into the host chromosomal DNA is possible. However, the strength of the association between HCV infection and hepatocarcinogenesis indicates that HCV not only is the cause of post-hepatitis cirrhosis, which in itself is a preneoplastic state, but expedites hepatocarcinogenesis by an unknown mechanism.

Unlike HBV, HCV infection appears to be more prevalent in industrialized countries than in developing countries, which may be partly because of the earlier medical use of needles and more frequent blood transfusions in the former, and there is no evidence that HCV transmission increases with poor sanitary conditions. In Japan at least, sporadic HCV infections outnumber transfusion-associated infections and the mode of transmission remains an enigma.

Since biochemical diagnosis of chronic hepatitis became possible, a high prevalence of chronic non-A, non-B hepatitis has been recorded in the adult population in Japan, and the prevalence of non-A, non-B hepatitis is now nearly synonymous with HCV incidence. Chronic hepatitis C frequently progresses to cirrhosis and then at a high rate to HCC; the incidence of HCC in men has more than doubled over the past 15 years in Japan, posing a major public health problem. Unlike HBsAg, the carrier rate of HCV does not vary greatly between countries, yet the incidence of HCV fluctuates widely across regions. Japan has perhaps the highest incidence of HCV-associated HCC, and may well serve as a target for epidemiological study.

CURRENT STATUS OF HCV-ASSOCIATED HEPATOCELLULAR CARCINOMA IN JAPAN

Japan had a low incidence of HCC up until around 1970 (Munoz & Linsell 1982). An increase in the number of HCC patients was then noted, and a significant number of these patients had undergone surgery for pulmonary tuberculosis after the Second World War when tuberculosis was rampant among the poorly nourished population. Such surgical operations require many units of blood. It then became apparent that this trend was not confined to a particular hospital or area but was a phenomenon throughout the country.

When HBsAg was first identified by insensitive methods in Japan some 25 years ago, it was found that nearly half of HCC cases were positive. The positivity for HBsAg among HCC cases slowly declined thereafter, but it took a decade to prove that the trend was real. Starting in 1968, and bi-annually from 1978, the Liver Cancer Study Group of Japan surveyed HBsAg positivity among authentic cases of HCC. It was 40.7% in 1968–77 (Okuda 1980) and has since declined steadily to the latest figure of 18.2% (Liver Cancer Study Group of Japan 1984, 1986, 1987, 1988, 1991). It was also noted from several cancer registries that HCC incidence was increasing sharply, particularly among men (Okuda et al 1987). According to the Osaka Cancer Registry it was $15.8/10^5$ per year in 1969–71 and rose steadily to the 1984–86 figure of $40.9/10^5$ per year (I Fujimoto, personal communication), i.e. the increase was more than two fold in 15 years. The vital statistics published yearly by the Ministry of Health and Welfare show the same trend (Statistics & Information Department 1990). If the HBsAg positivity rate (as determined by the Liver Cancer Study Group from several thousand HCC cases every 2 years) is compared with the number of deaths due to liver cancer in Japan, and used to calculate the number of HBsAg-positive and HBsAg-negative patients dying from cancer, the number of deaths in HBsAg-positive patients has been constant over this period; the increase is attributable solely to HBsAg-negative patients (Fig. 15.1). It now seems that the majority of HBsAg-negative patients have HCV infection. In other words, chronic HCV infection is the cause of the recent sharp rise in HCC incidence. The increase among women has not been dramatic and lags somewhat behind that in men.

The decreasing HBsAg positivity among patients with HCC led to the suggestion of an aetiological relationship between chronic non-A, non-B hepatitis/cirrhosis and HCC (Iwama et al 1982). This was subsequently confirmed throughout Japan. It was also found that a considerable proportion of HBsAg-negative HCC patients had had a blood transfusion. The reported frequency of past transfusion varies from 20% to 40% among non-A, non-B HCC patients (Kiyosawa & Furuta 1991), whereas it is much lower among HBsAg-positive subjects (Table 15.1). The time interval from blood transfusion to diagnosis of

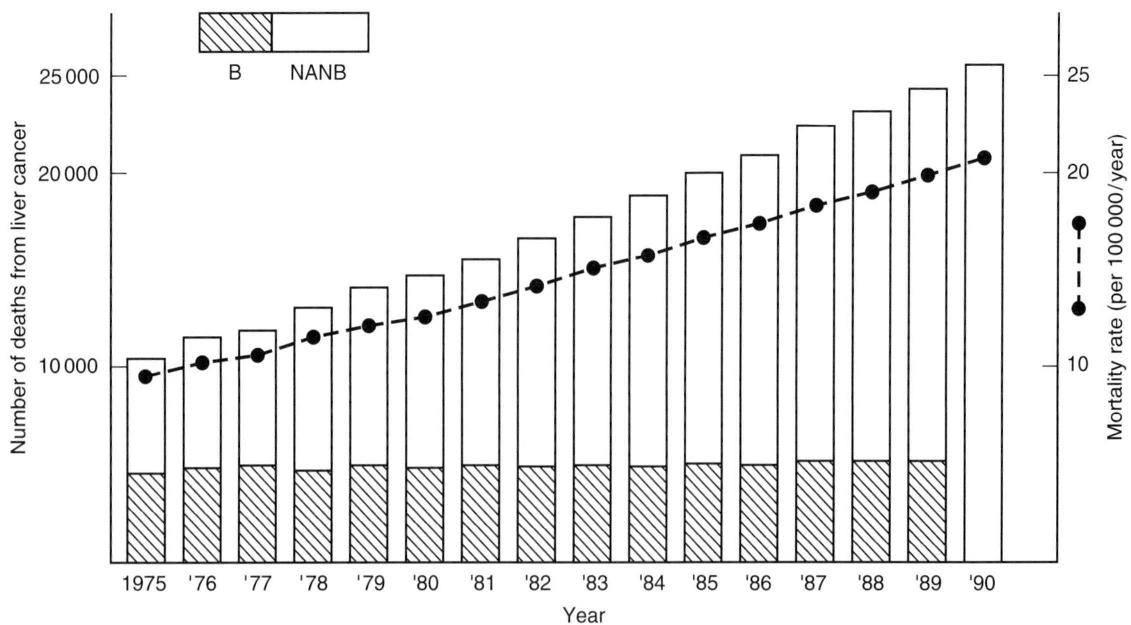

Fig. 15.1 Time trends in liver cancer mortality in Japan. Relation between HBsAg-positive and -negative (non-A, non-B) patients based on vital statistics for Japan 1989 (Statistics & Information Department 1990). The number of deaths of HBsAg-positive patients (shaded) was calculated from HBsAg positivity rates among HCC patients published by the Liver Cancer Study Group of Japan. Note that the number of deaths related to HBV is unchanged in the past 15 years, while deaths of patients with non-A, non-B hepatitis have more than tripled.

Table 15.1 Prevalence of a history of blood transfusion before diagnosis of chronic liver disease (From Kiyusawa and Furuta 1991, with permission)

Disease	No. of cases	Percentage with history of blood transfusion
Type C		
Chronic hepatitis	200	49.0
Cirrhosis	106	42.5
HCC	80	38.8
Type B		
Chronic hepatitis	242	2.9
Cirrhosis	110	5.5
HCC	64	4.7
Type non-B, non-C		
Chronic hepatitis	62	45.2
Cirrhosis	53	26.2
HCC	25	20

HCC ranges from 20 to 40 years, averaging about 30 years (Kiyosawa et al 1990) (Figs 15.2 and 15.3).

There is now considerable evidence that non-A, non-B hepatitis transmitted by blood transfusion has been common over recent years. Before the introduction of the volunteer blood donation system in 1965, blood was purchased from 'professional' donors, and up to 80% of patients who had undergone a major operation requiring many units of blood developed post-transfusion hepatitis (T Tobe, personal communication). At the National Tokyo Sanitorium, where many lung operations are carried out, the frequency of post-transfusion hepatitis in 1963–64 was 51%, and this dropped to 16% in 1968–72 when all blood

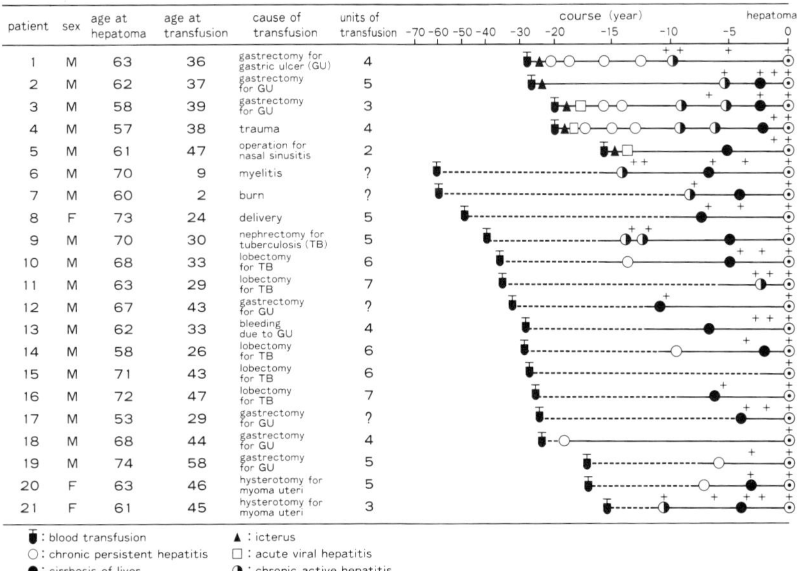

Fig. 15.2 The clinical course of patients who had acquired chronic liver disease due to HCV transmitted by blood transfusion and eventually developed HCC (From Kiyosawa et al 1990, with permission.)

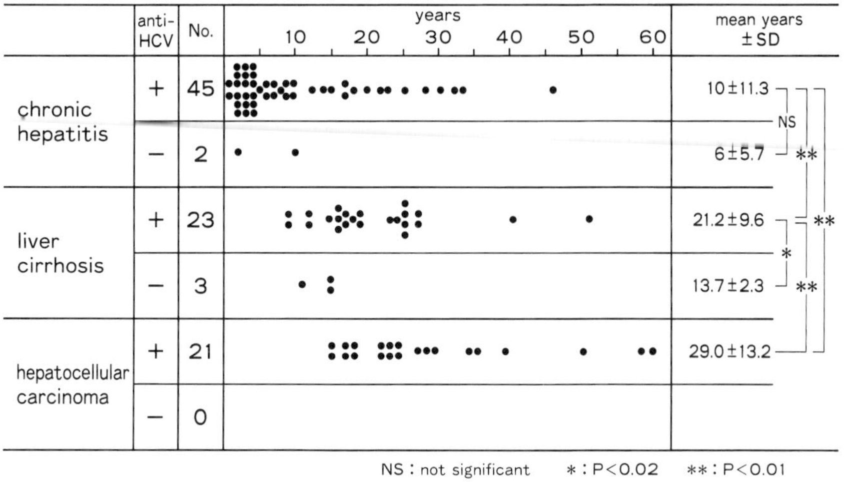

	anti-HCV	No.	years	mean years ±SD
chronic hepatitis	+	45		10±11.3
	−	2		6±5.7
liver cirrhosis	+	23		21.2±9.6
	−	3		13.7±2.3
hepatocellular carcinoma	+	21		29.0±13.2
	−	0		

NS : not significant * : P<0.02 ** : P<0.01

Fig. 15.3 Interval in years between blood transfusion and the diagnosis of chronic hepatitis, cirrhosis and HCC in patients who had acquired chronic HCV infection (from Kiyosawa et al 1990, with permission.)

was donated by volunteers. After the introduction of testing for HBsAg, HBV transmission was nearly eliminated, yet the frequency of post-transfusion hepatitis at this and other hospitals remained at between 5.2% and 26% until very recently (Katayama 1990) (Table 15.2).

Non-A, non-B hepatitis, regardless of its mode of transmission, frequently develops into chronicity in developed countries and, although spontaneous regression occurs in a limited number of patients, the majority develop cirrhosis in 20–25 years; liver histology looks deceivingly benign until a certain point in the clinical course, but it eventually evolves into chronic active hepatitis progressing to cirrhosis. Furthermore, HCC is an extremely common sequele in such patients. With the advent of real-time ultrasound, small HCCs can be detected in patients with cirrhosis, and the frequency with which HCC is detected in such patients is alarmingly high. The yearly detection rate for HCC among patients with cirrhosis has been reported at 6–25%, depending on serology (Oka et al 1990).

The availability of the C100-3 test showed the

Table 15.2 Frequency of post-blood transfusion non-A, non-B hepatitis in Japan

	Hospital								
Period	A	B	C	D	E	F	G	H	I
1976–80	18.4%	14.5%	16.7%					11.3%	
	(143/779)	(47/324)	(13/78)					(16/162)	
1981–85	14.5%	16.1%	13.7%	21.9%	13.9%	20.4%		14.7%	
	(102/703)	(41/254)	(35/256)	(91/416)	(11/79)	(37/181)		(97/658)	
1986–88	5.2%	15.0%	18.6%	26.0%	18.0%	7.7%	15.9%	14.5%	10.9%
	(16/306)	(16/107)	(24/129)	(246/958)	(9/50)	(15/194)	(65/408)	(25/173)	(26/238)

A, National Sendai; B, National Tokyo Sanatorium; C, Hyogo-Ken Rehabilitation Center; D, Kyushu University Central Lab.; E, National Nagasaki Med. Center; F, Nagasaki Univ. Cardiovascular Surgery; G, Osaka Adult Dis. Center; H, National Hospital Med. Center; I, Tokyo Women's Med. College Cardiovascular Center (From Katayama 1990 with permission.)

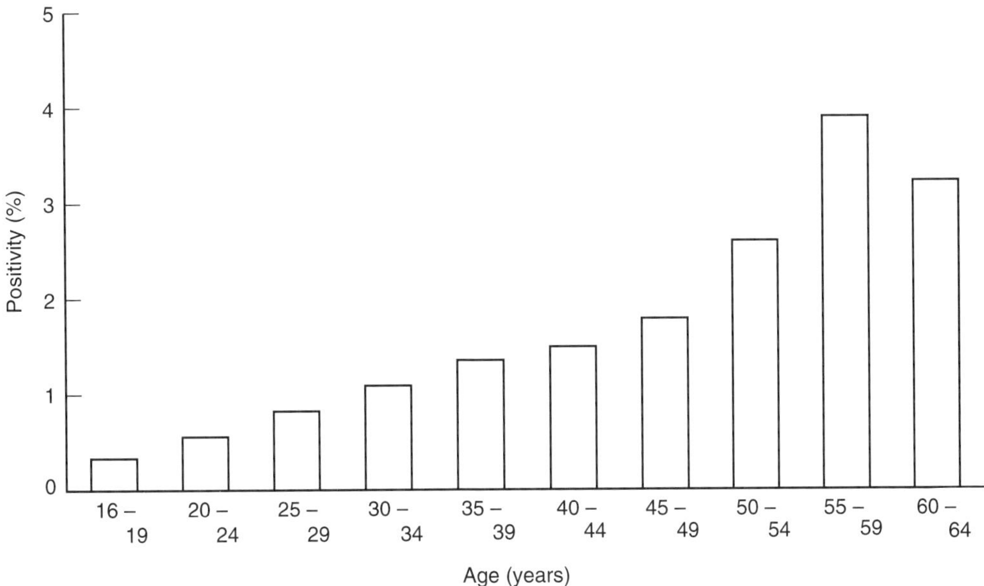

Fig. 15.4 Frequency of positive tests for C100–3 antibody in relation to age among 132 725 blood donors in Japan (From Yoshizawa 1991 with permission.)

HCV carrier rate among blood donors in Japan to be about 1% nationwide, that it increases with age, particularly after age 50 years (Yoshizawa 1991) (Fig. 15.4), and that the majority of patients with chronic non-A, non-B liver disease have HCV infection (Kobayashi et al 1991) (Table 15.3). The positivity of HCV antibodes among those with chronic non-A, non-B disease acquired by transfusion is higher than among those in whom the disease is not associated with transfusion, suggesting that yet another type of viral hepatitis accounts for the difference. Several reports suggest a correlation between the level of HCV antibodies and the size of a skin tattoo. A number of villages and areas have been found to have an extremely high incidence of HCV antibody positivity, particularly among the elderly. In one area in Saga, where chronic liver disease is prevalent in adults, the antibody positivity was 15% in the over-50 age group (Setoguchi et al 1991), in one village in Shinshu it was 37.2% in the over-35s (Kiyosawa & Tanaka 1991), and in a study in the Gifu area 482 out of 1060 (45.4%) villagers over the age of 30 were positive for

Table 15.3 Positivity rate for C100–3 antibody test among Japanese patients with chronic liver disease

		Positive for C100–3	
Diagnosis	Number of patients	Number	Per cent
Chronic persistent hepatitis	43	32	74.4
Chronic active hepatitis 2A	544	414	76.1
Chronic active hepatitis 2B	342	249	72.8
Liver cirrhosis	410	282	68.8
Hepatocellular carcinoma	240	177	73.4*
Total	1619	1154	71.3

*For males alone, this is 80.7%.
From Kobayashi et al (1991) with permission.

either C100-3 or core protein (CP)-9 or CP-10 antibody (Okamoto et al 1992). The village in the last study was divided into three zones: zone A had a crude HCC incidence of $49/10^5$ per year among those aged over 30 and C100-3 seropositivity of 27.8%, whereas in zones B and C the values were $19/10^5$ per year and 16.8% and $0/10^5$ per year and 8.2% respectively. However, in this high-incidence area there was no evidence of a high exposure of the residents to therapies involving needle punctures (Tokita et al 1992 a,b), e.g. acupuncture or school vaccination programmes. The number of HCV particles circulating in the blood is much smaller than for HBV, reducing the chance of infection through needles, but some patients do show high virus levels in the blood and are more infective.

The recent sharp increase in HCV associated HCC in Japan, and perhaps also in Italy, suggests that among the aged it is an iatrogenic phenomenon (Okuda 1991). The prevalence of HCV antibodies is almost zero in those aged under 15 years (Tanaka et al 1992) and the introduction of disposable needles (1970, widely available 1975) coincides with the birth of this generation which is free of HCV infection.

EPIDEMIOLOGY OF HCV-ASSOCIATED HEPATOCELLULAR CARCINOMA

Shortly after the introduction of the C100-3 antibody test, high antibody positivity among HCC patients was found worldwide, as had been anticipated from earlier case reports of patients who had had post-transfusion non-A, non-B hepatitis and were found to have developed HCC on follow-up (Resnick et al 1983, Kiyosawa et al 1984). Also, the majority of cases of cryptogenic chronic hepatitis in the USA have been found to be caused by HCV infection (Feffers et al 1992).

The first reported epidemiological study of HCC and HCV infection in Milan found 86 of 132 cases (65%) with HCV antibodies (Colombo et al 1989). This report was quickly followed by similar observations in other parts of Italy (Simonetti 1989, Chiaramonte et al 1990, Caporaso et al 1991, Levrero et al 1991), Spain (Bruix et al 1989), France (Nalpas et al 1991), Japan (Kiyosawa et al 1990, Nishioka et al 1991, Tanaka et al 1991) and the USA (Hasan et al 1990) (Table 15.4). Reports from less industrialized countries gave lower figures for anti-HCV positivity (Kew et al 1990, Han et al 1991, Kaklamani et al 1991, Oon et al 1991, Al Karawi et al 1992). Yet compared with the control values in blood donors (< 1%), the differences are highly significant, clearly indicating a role for HCV infection in HCC. These countries are well known for their high HBsAg positivity in HCC, but the results do not suggest mutual exclusion (Table 15.5).

Colombo et al (1989) emphasized the more frequent coexistence of anti-HBc with anti-HCV in patients with HCC than in patients with chronic non-B hepatitis, suggesting an indirect role for past HBV infection. Although the results in Japan do not confirm this link (Table 15.6), a Greek study showed a four-fold higher relative risk in anti-HCV positive subjects with HBsAg compared with those negative for HBsAg (Kaklamani et al 1991). Previous HBV and current HCV infection may have a synergistic effect in hepatocarcinogenesis because integration of HBV DNA is demonstrable in some patients negative for HBsAg (Brechot et al 1981) and the development of carcinogenesis is a multistep process. Past infection with HBV may serve as one of the hepatocarcinogenetic steps, regardless of serological status. In areas where HBV infection is endemic, it may be the major aetiological factor, yet a positivity rate of about 30% among HCC patients in South Africa (Kew et al 1990) and Taiwan (Chen et al 1990, Tsai et al 1991) is very significant, and a role for HCV infection cannot be overlooked. The positivity figures vary somewhat in reports from certain countries, e.g. France (Decreux et al 1990, Nalpas et al 1991, Zarski et al 1991) and the USA (Hasan et al 1990, Yu et al 1990), but this may be the result of either small numbers of cases or false positives. With the second-generation tests, false positive C100-3 tests will be eliminated and lower figures are expected, although this is not borne out by some recent studies. In one study in Japan, a positivity rate of 85.2% in 27 HCC cases was revised to 100% with the Abbott's second-generation test (Matsumoto et al 1992). A considerable proportion of patients with non-A, non-

Table 15.4 Prevalence of anti-HCV among patients with hepatocellular carcinoma in selected countries

Area/country	Reference	Anti-HCV positivity of HCC (%) (no./total)	Control value (%)
Milan/Italy	Colombo et al 1989	65 (86/132)	0.87[1]
Padua/Italy	Simonetti et al 1989	76 (152/200)	
Milan/Italy	Sbolli et al 1990	59 (46/78)	
Rome, Padua/Italy	Levrero et al 1991	58 (97/167)	
Naples/Italy	Caporaso et al 1991	72 (63/88)	
Le Kremlin Bicetre/France	Ducreux et al 1990	28 (21/74)	0.68[2]
Paris/France	Nalpas et al 1991	58 (32/55)	
Paris/France	Zarski et al 1991	20 (8/40)	
Barcelona/Spain	Bruix et al 1989	75 (72/96)	0.5
Tokyo/Japan	Saito et al 1990	55 (138/253)	1.3[3]
Matsumoto/Japan	Kiyosawa et al 1990	73 (61/83)	
Niigata/Japan	Ohkoshi et al 1990	58 (58/100)	
Kyushu/Japan	Tanaka et al 1991	68 (62/91)	
Whole of Japan	Nishioka et al 1991	76 (80/105)*	
Athens/Greece	Kaklamani et al 1991	39 (72/185)**	
Miami/USA	Hasan et al 1990	53 (31/59)	0.5[4]–1.4[5]
Los Angeles//USA	Yu et al 1990	29 (15/51)	
Johannesburg/S. Africa	Kew et al 1990	29 (110/380)	0.7
Taipei/Taiwan	Chen et al 1990	33 (22/66)	0.95
Kaohsiung/Taiwan	Tsai et al 1991	26 (71/270)	0
Riyadh/Saudi Arabia	Al Karawi et al 1992	26 (11/42)	1.5
Thailand	Boonmar et al 1990	6 (3/47)	2.6
Singapore	Oon et al 1991	15 (7/47)	0
Pusan/Korea	Han et al 1991	13 (15/118)	1.3
New Delhi/India	Ramesh et al 1992	15 (8/53)	

Positivity among blood donors: *HBsAg-negative cases only; **strongly positive cases only.
1 = Sirchia et al (1989); 2 = Janot et al (1989); 3 = Watanabe et al (1990); 4 = Hasan et al (1990); 5 = Stevens et al (1990).

B disease who are negative for C100-3 have HCV in their serum when tested by the polymerase chain reaction (PCR) (Hagiwara et al 1992, Kato et al 1990, Okamoto et al 1991). Blood transfusion is the best-documented mode of HCV transmission, and in 11 801 haemophiliacs given transfusions in western countries 10 cases of HCC were reported; this frequency is more

Table 15.5 Relationship of anti-HCV to HBsAg status in hepatocellular carcinoma

Reference	Country	Anti-HCV positivity (%) (no. of cases)	
		HBsAg positive	HBsAg negative
Colombo et al 1989	Italy	54 (22/41)	70 (64/91)
Sbolli et al 1990	Italy	13 (1/8)	72 (43/60)
Nalpas et al 1991	France	75 (9/12)	57 (20/35)
Bruix et al 1989	Spain	56 (5/9)	82 (72/87)
Hasan et al 1990	USA	14 (4/28)	53 (31/59
Yu et al 1990	USA	45 (10/22)	17 (5/29)
Kaklamani et al 1991	Greece	51 (43/85)*	29 (29/100)*
Kew et al 1990	S. Africa	24 (44/184)	45 (49/110)
Kiyosawa et al 1990	Japan	35 (10/28)	94 (51/54)
Ohkoshi et al 1990	Japan	19 (8/42)	86 (50/58)
Nishioka et al 1991	Japan	16 (11/75)	76 (80/105)
Chen et al 1990	Taiwan	17 (7/42)	63 (15/24)
Tsai et al 1991	Taiwan	16 (29/184)	55 (47/86)

* Strongly positive cases only.

Table 15.6 Frequency of co-positivity for anti-HBc and anti-HCV in HBsAg-negative HCC patients

Reference	Country	Frequency of positivity for anti-HBc and anti-HCV	
		Hepatocellular carcinoma (%)	Chronic hepatitis (%)
Colombo et al 1989	Italy	54 (49/91)	19
Levrero et al 1991	Italy	42 (48/114)	
Sbolli et al 1990	Italy	22 (13/60)	
Ohkoshi et al 1990	Japan	23 (13/56)	
Saito et al 1990	Japan	< 23 (46/202)*	

* Anti-HBs and anti-HBc combined.

than 30 times the background. All 10 patients had cirrhosis, five being positive for HBsAg and four for anti-HCV (Colombo et al 1991). In Mediterranean areas, statistical analysis by multiple regression has indicated that age, male sex and anti-HCV positivity are the only risk factors significantly correlated with the development of HCC in cirrhotic patients (Caporaso et al 1991).

Although HCC is a frequent complication in most types of cirrhosis, primary biliary cirrhosis (PBC) is considered to be an exception. In a large series of autopsies in Los Angeles, not a single case was seen (Edmondson & Peters 1982, Edmonson & Craig 1987). The first report of an association between PBC and HCC appeared in 1979 in the UK (Krasner et al 1979), and was followed by several other reports (Melia et al 1984, Gluskin et al 1985, Sakaeda et al 1986). In the Japanese Annual Autopsy Registries from 1977 to 1987, 319 cases of PBC were recorded, and 13 of these had complicating HCC (4.1%). In this survey, not a single case of HCC in PBC was recorded up to the end of 1982 (Nakanuma et al 1990). HCC began to appear among PBC patients in 1983, and HCC was seen thereafter on a yearly basis. It seems that PBC complicated by HCC is a recent phenomenon and it would be of interest to know whether those PBC patients who had developed HCC had HCV infection. Anti-HCV-positive patients have recently been reported in the literature (Hata et al 1992). Suzuki et al (1991) clinically diagnosed four cases of HCC among 53 PBC patients; all were in Scheuer's stage IV and HCC constituted 22% of the advanced PBC cases. Three had a history of blood transfusion, although they were C100-3 negative. It will be of interest to determine the extent to which HCV infection is involved in other types of cirrhosis, such as Wilson's disease, which is known to be complicated by HCC.

ALCOHOL, HCV INFECTION AND HEPATOCELLULAR CARCINOMA

Although the study by Caporaso et al (1991) did not suggest alcohol as an aetiological factor, a study in France showed that 41% of drinkers with cirrhosis and HCC had anti-HCV compared with 26% of those without HCC (Poynard et al 1991). The role of HCV infection in alcoholics who develop HCC has been disputed in Europe (Bode et al 1991). Among Japanese patients who are heavy drinkers, the role of HCV in hepatocarcinogenesis appears to be unequivocal. In one study, 14 of 18 alcoholic cirrhotic patients (75%) were positive for anti-HCV (Ishii et al 1990), and in another study heavy drinkers who had chronic hepatitis, cirrhosis and HCC all had high levels of anti-HCV antibodies (Table 15.7).

The liver histology of patients in Japan with alcoholic liver disease differs from that of similar patients in western countries; changes compatible with chronic viral hepatitis are seen more frequently and can be explained by superimposed HCV infection in heavy drinkers developing liver disease. Interestingly, alcoholics without liver disease have a very low rate of anti-HCV antibodies. Ethanol is not a carcinogen, but a number of epidemiological studies suggest an indirect role for it in the development of hepatocarcinogenesis (Bassendine 1986), and in

Table 15.7 Positivity for HCV antibodies among heavy drinkers in Japan

Histological diagnosis	No. of patients	Age (± SD)	Anti-HCV (%)	
			ELISA	RIBA
Fatty liver	10	35.5 ± 8.5	0 (0)	0 (0)
Alcoholic fibrosis	22	49.6 ± 9.5	1 (4.5)	0 (0)
Alcoholic hepatitis	3	32.3 ± 1.5	0 (0)	0 (0)
Chronic hepatitis	15	49.8 ± 11.8	11 (73.3)	8 (53.3)
Liver cirrhosis	39	49.1 ±8.9	18 (46.2)	14 (35.9)
Hepatocellular carcinoma	24	60.2 ± 7.3	20 (83.3)	14 (58.3)
Alcoholism	121	53.0 ± 10.4	6 (5.0)	5 (4.2)

ELISA, enzyme-linked: immunosorbent assay; RIBA, recombinant immunoblot assay.
From Shimizu et al (1991) with permission.

a rodent chemical carcinogenesis model it acts as a promoter (Takada et al 1986). Ohnishi et al (1982) found the average age of HBsAg-positive alcoholic cirrhotic patients in whom HCC had developed to be 10 years younger than comparable non-drinking patients with HCC.

CHARACTERISTICS OF HCV-ASSOCIATED HEPATOCELLULAR CARCINOMA

Is HCV-associated HCC any different from HCC associated with HBV and other types of cirrhosis? In a study comparing the gross pathology of HBV-seronegative and -seropositive HCCs, the expanding type was found in 82% of the former and only 36.8% of the latter, while the other multinodular/spreading types were more frequent in the latter (58% *vs.* 18%) (H Okuda et al 1984, K Okuda et al 1984). It is the general consensus among Japanese hepatologists that HCC detected by clinical follow-up and imaging when it is still small, and is growing slowly, but the underlying cirrhosis will be quite advanced, a contraindication to surgical intervention in many instances. In an early study it was found that fewer highly cirrhotic livers with HCC were positive for HBsAg compared with ordinary cirrhotic livers with HCC (Okuda et al 1982). Differences between HCV- and HBV-associated HCC would not be surprising as the carcinogenic molecular processes involved in the two may well differ.

In Japan, at least, it is established that the majority of juvenile patients with HCC are positive for HBsAg, presumably acquired from the mother (Furuta et al 1990). HCV infection is very uncommon before 15 years of age and hepatocarcinogenesis due to HCV infection is perhaps a late event compared with HBV-related HCC; the age of HCV-associated HCC cases is expected to be higher, but data are not yet available. HBsAg-positive HCC patients are generally younger than HBsAg negative patients (MacNab et al 1976, Fisher et al 1976, Akagi et al 1982, Okuda et al 1982), and the majority of the latter are now known to have HCV infection.

GLOBAL SPREAD OF HCV AS AN AETIOLOGICAL FACTOR FOR HCC

Unlike hepatitis A virus (HAV), there is no evidence that HCV is transmitted by the faecal–oral route. In developing countries where people live in poor sanitary conditions, exposure to HAV occurs at a young age and most acquire antibodies by about the age of 15. Blood-borne HBV is highly contagious, and transmission through wounds in childhood is common in South African blacks, but the carrier rate for HCV among them is low (Kew et al 1990). Unlike honeymoon hepatitis B, HCV infection is a relatively late event among spouses. These observations are compatible with the experimental demonstration of a low infectivity for HCV. It thus appears that prior to the widespread use of needles and blood transfusions HCV existed with humans in a non-proliferative fashion.

Acute hepatitis following blood transfusion used to be referred to as 'serum hepatitis', and probably consisted of HBV and HCV infections, at least.

The mandatory vaccination of children for certain diseases, e.g. smallpox, and transfusions with blood purchased from 'professional' donors contributed to the recent sudden spread of HCV infection in some industrialized countries. In Japan, and possibly also in Italy, the timing of the increase in post-transfusion hepatitis and in HCC incidence is compatible with such a view. Differences in HCC incidence among industrialized countries are probably due to variation in the prevalence of hepatocarcinogenic factors, which are still poorly recognized.

SUMMARY AND PERSPECTIVE

Epidemiological data suggest that HCC associated with HCV infection has been increasing in industrialized countries more than in developing countries, but the prospect for a reduction in HCV-related HCC is promising. Since a considerable proportion of patients with chronic hepatitis C do respond to treatment, the development of cirrhosis and then hepatocarcinogenesis in cirrhotics may be preventable in some responding patients. The transmission of HCV by blood transfusion is now largely preventable, and acute hepatitis C may be prevented from becoming chronic (Omata et al 1991). With the elucidation of the mechanism whereby HCV infection predisposes to hepatocarcinogenesis and its mode of transmission, other than through blood transfusion and needle punctures, better control of chronic HCV-related liver disease may be expected in the near future.

REFERENCES

Akagi G, Furuyu K, Otsuka H 1982 Hepatitis B antigen in the liver in hepatocellular carcinoma in Shikoku, Japan. Cancer 49: 678–682

Al Karawi M A, Shariq S, Mohamed ARES, Saeed A A, Ahmed AMMM 1992 Hepatitis C virus infection in chronic liver disease and hepatocellular carcinoma in Saudi Arabia. Journal of Gastroenterology and Hepatology 7: 237–239

Bassendine M F 1986 Alcohol: a major risk factor for hepatocellular carcinoma? Journal of Hepatology 2: 513–519

Bode J C, Biermann J, Kohse K P, Walker S, Bode C 1991 High incidence of antibodies to hepatitis C virus in alcoholic cirrhosis: fact or fiction? Alcohol and Alcoholism 26: 111–114

Boonmar S, Pojanagaroon B, Watanabe Y, Tanaka Y, Saito I, Miyamura T 1990 Prevalence of hepatitis C virus antibody among healthy blood donors and non-A, non-B hepatitis patients in Thailand. Japanese Journal of Medical Science and Biology 43: 29–36

Brechot C M, Hadchouel M, Scott J et al 1981 State of hepatitis B virus DNA in hepatocytes of patients with hepatitis B surface antigen-positive and -negative liver diseases. Proceedings of the National Academy of Sciences of the USA 78: 3906–3910

Bruix J, Barrera J M, Calvet X et al 1989 Prevalence of antibodies to hepatitis C virus in Spanish patients with hepatocellular carcinoma and hepatic cirrhosis. Lancet ii: 1004–1006

Caporaso N, Romano M, Marmo R et al 1991 Hepatitis C infection is an additive risk factor for development of hepatocellular carcinoma in patients with cirrhosis. Journal of Hepatology 12: 367–371

Chen D S, Kuo G C, Sung J L et al 1990 Hepatitis C virus infection in an area hyperendemic for hepatitis B and chronic liver disease: the Taiwan experience. Journal of Infectious Diseases 162: 817–822

Chiaramonte M, Farinati T, Gagiuoli S et al 1990 Antibody to hepatitis C virus in hepatocellular carcinoma. Lancet 335: 301–302

Colombo M, Kuo M, Choo Q L et al 1989 Prevalence of antibodies to hepatitis C virus in Italian patients with hepatocellular carcinoma. Lancet ii: 1006–1008

Colombo M, Mannucci P M, Brettler D B et al 1991 Hepatocellular carcinoma in hemophilia. American Journal of Hematology 37: 243–246

Ducreux M, Buffet C, Dussaix E et al 1990 Antibody to hepatitis C virus in hepatocellular carcinoma. Lancet 335: 301

Edmondson H A, Craig J R 1987 Neoplasms of the liver. In: Schiff L, Schiff E R (eds) Diseases of the liver, 6th edn. Lippincott, Philadelphia, p 1125

Edmondson H A, Peters R L 1982 Neoplasms of the liver. In: Schiff L, Schiff E R (eds) Diseases of the liver, 5th edn. Lippincott, Philadelphia, p 1120

Feffers L J, Hasan F, De Medina M et al 1992 Prevalence of antibodies to hepatitis C virus among patients with cryptogenic chronic hepatitis and cirrhosis. Hepatology 15: 187–190

Fisher R L, Scheuer P J, Sherlock S 1976 Primary liver cell carcinoma in the presence or absence of hepatitis B antigen. Cancer 38: 901–905

Furuta T, Kanematsu T, Matsumata T et al 1990 Clinicopathologic features of hepatocellular carcinoma in young patients. Cancer 66: 2395–2398

Gluskin L E, Guariglia P, Payne J A, Banner B F, Economou P 1985 Hepatocellular carcinoma in a patient with precirrhotic primary liver cirrhosis. Journal of Clinical Gastroenterology 7: 441–444

Hagiwara H, Hayashi N, Mita E et al 1992 Detection of hepatitis C virus RNA in chronic non-A, non-B liver disease. Gastroenterology 102: 692–694

Han B H, Koo J Y, Park B C 1991 Prevalence of hepatitis B and C viral markers in Korean patients with hepatocellular carcinoma (abstract). Proceedings of the 3rd International Symposium on Viral Hepatitis and Hepatocellular Carcinoma. Taipei, Gastroenterological Society of the Rupublic of China, Taipei, p 158

Hasan F, Jeffers L J, Madina M et al 1990 Hepatitis C-associated hepatocellular carcinoma. Hepatology 12: 589–591

Hata K, Nagayama S, Hatakeyama S et al 1992 A case of hepatocellular carcinoma in primary biliary cirrhosis positive for anti-HCV. Acta Hepatol Jpn 33: 167–173

Ishii J, Sata M, Kumashiro R et al 1990 Studies on anti-HCV in hepatocellular carcinoma with alcoholic cirrhosis. Acta Hepatologica Japonica 31: 1181–1185 (in Japanese)

Iwama S, Ohnishi K, Nakajima Y et al 1982 A clinical study of hepatocellular carcinoma (HCC) in relation to hepatitis B seromarkers: implication of non-A, non-B hepatitis (NANB) (abstract). Hepatology 2: 117

Janot C, Courouce A M, Maneiz M 1989 Antibodies to hepatitis C virus in French blood donors. Lancet ii: 796–797

Kaklamani E, Trichopoulos D, Tzonou A et al 1991 Hepatitis B and C viruses and their interaction in the origin of hepatocellular carcinoma. Journal of the American Medical Association 265: 1974–1976

Katayama T 1990 The incidence of posttransfusion hepatitis. Kan-Tan-Sui 20: 15–20 (in Japenese)

Kato N, Yokosuka O, Omata M, Hosoda K, Ohto M 1990 Detection of hepatitis C ribonucleic acid in the serum by amplification with polymerase chain reaction. Journal of Clinical Investigation 86: 1764–1767

Kew M C, Houghton M, Choo Q L, Kuo G 1990 Hepatitis C virus antibodies in southern African blacks with hepatocellular carcinoma. Lancet i: 873–874

Kiyosawa K, Furuta S 1991 Review of hepatitis C in Japan. Journal of Gastroenterology and Hepatology 6: 381–391

Kiyosawa K, Akahane Y, Nagata A, Furuta S 1984 Hepatocellular carcinoma after non-A, non-B posttransfusion hepatitis. American Journal of Gastroenterology 79: 777–781

Kiyosawa K, Sodeyama T, Tanaka E et al 1990 Interrelationship of blood transfusion, non-A, non-B hepatitis and hepatocellular carcinoma: analysis by detection of antibody to hepatitis C virus. Hepatology 12: 671–675

Kiyosaka K, Tanaka E 1991 Route of HCV infection – blood transfusion unrelated infection. Acta Hepatologica Japonica 32: 219–220

Kobayashi M, Kumada H, Arase Y et al 1991 Positive rate of C-100 antibody and changes of long term follow up cases of chronic liver disease. Acta Hepatologica Japonica 32: 683–687

Krasner N, Johnson P J, Neuberger H, Zaman S, Portmann B C, William R 1979 Hepatocellular carcinoma in primary biliary cirrhosis: report of four cases. Gut 20: 255–258

Levrero M, Tagger A, Balsano C et al 1991 Antibodies to hepatitis C virus in patients with hepatocellular carcinoma. Journal of Hepatology 12: 60–63

Liver Cancer Study Group of Japan 1984 Primary liver cancer in Japan. Cancer 54: 1747–1755

Liver Cancer Study Group of Japan 1986 Primary liver cancer in Japan Seventh report. Acta Hepatologica Japonica 27: 1161–1169 (in Japanese)

Liver Cancer Study Group of Japan 1987 Primary liver cancer in Japan. Sixth report. Cancer 60: 1400–1411

Liver Cancer Study Group of Japan 1988 Primary liver cancer in Japan. Eighth report. Acta Hepatologica Japonica 29: 1619–1626 (in Japanese)

Liver Cancer Study Group of Japan 1991 Primary liver cancer in Japan. Ninth report. Acta Hepatologica Japonica 32: 1138–1147 (in Japanese)

MacNab G M, Urbanowicz J M, Geddes E W, Kew M C 1976 Hepatitis B surface antigen and antibody in Bantu patients with primary hepatocellular cancer. British Journal of Cancer 33: 544–548

Matsumoto A, Tanaka E, Nakatsuji Y, Kiyosawa K, Furuta S 1992 Prevalence of type C hepatitis in patients with chronic liver disease determined with second-generation HCV antibody. Igakuno Ayumi 160: 523–524 (in Japanese)

Malia W M, Johnson P J, Neuberger H, Zaman S, Portman B C, William H 1984 Hepatocellular carcinoma in primary biliary cirrhosis: detection by fetoprotein estimation. Gastroenterology 87: 660–663

Munoz N, Linsell A 1982 Epidemiology of primary liver cancer. In: Correa P, Haenszel W (eds) Epidemiology of cancer of the digestive tract. Martinus Nijhoff, Hague, pp 161–195

Nakanuma Y, Terada T, Doishita K, Miwa A 1990 Hepatocellular carcinoma in primary biliary cirrhosis: an autopsy study. Hepatology 11: 1010–1016

Nalpas B, Driss F, Pol S et al 1991 Association between HCV and HBV infection in hepatocellular carcinoma and alcoholic liver disease. Journal of Hepatology 12: 70–74

Nishioka K, Watanabe J, Furuta S et al 1991 A high prevalence of antibody to the hepatitis C virus in patients with hepatocellular carcinoma in Japan. Cancer 67: 429–433

Ohkoshi S, Kojima H, Tawaraya H et al 1990 Prevalence of antibody against non-A, non-B hepatitis virus in Japanese patients with hepatocellular carcinoma. Japanese Journal of Cancer Research 81: 550–553

Ohnishi K, Iida S, Iwama S et al 1982 The effect of chronic habitual alcohol intake on the development of liver cirrhosis and hepatocellular carcinoma: relation to hepatitis B surface antigen carriage. Cancer 49: 672–677

Oka H, Kurioka N, Kim K et al 1990 Prospective study of early detection of hepatocellular carcinoma in patients with cirrhosis. Hepatology 12: 680–687

Okamoto H, Okada S, Sugiyama Y et al 1991 Detection of hepatitis C virus RNA by a two-stage polymerase chain reaction with two pairs of primers deduced from the 5'-noncoding region. Japanese Journal of Experimental Medicine 60: 215–222

Okamoto H, Tsuda F, Machida A et al 1992 Antibodies against synthetic oligopeptides deduced from the putative core gene for the diagnosis of hepatitis C virus infection. Hepatology 15: 180–186

Okuda H, Obata H, Motoike Y, Hisamitsu T 1984 Clinicopathological features of hepatocellular carcinoma – comparison of hepatitis B seropositive and seronegative patients. Hepatogastroenterology 31: 64–68

Okuda K, Liver Cancer Study Group of Japan 1980 Primary liver cancers in Japan. Cancer 45: 2663–2669

Okuda K 1991 Hepatitis C virus and hepatocellular carcinoma. In: Tabor E, DiBisceglie A M, Purcell R H (eds) Etiology, pathology, and treatment of hepatocellular carcinoma in North America. Portofolio Publishing, Woodlands, pp 119–126

Okuda K, Nakashima T, Sakamoto K et al 1982 Hepatocellular carcinoma arising in noncirrhotic and highly cirrhotic livers: a comparative study of histopathology and frequency of hepatitis B markers. Cancer 49: 450–455

Okuda K, Peters R L, Simson I W 1984 Gross anatomic features of hepatocellular carcinoma from three disparate geographic areas. Proposal of new classification. Cancer 54: 2165–2173

Okuda K, Fujimoto I, Hanai A, Urano Y 1987 Changing incidence of hepatocellular carcinoma in Japan. Cancer Research 47: 4967–4972

Omata M, Yokosuka O, Takano S et al 1991 Resolution of acute hepatitis C after therapy with natural beta interferon. Lancet 338: 914–915

Oon C J, Chia S C, Fock K M 1991 Prevalence of hepatitis C in liver diseases and in a random population in Singapore (abstract) Proceedings of the 3rd International Symposium on Viral Hepatitis and Hepatocellular Carcinoma, Taipei. Gastroenterological Society of the Republic of China, Taipei, p 141

Poynard T, Aubert A, Lazizi Y et al 1991 Independent risk factors for hepatocellular carcinoma in French drinkers. Hepatology 13: 896–901

Ramesh R, Muhshi A, Panda S K 1992 Prevalence of hepatitis C virus antibodies in chronic liver disease and hepatocellular carcinoma patients in India. Journal of Gastroenterology and Hepatology 7: 393–395

Resnick R H, Stone K, Antonioli D 1983 Primary hepatocellular carcinoma after non-A, non-B posttransfusion hepatitis. Digestive Diseases and Science 28: 908–911

Saito I, Miyamura T, Ohbayashi A et al 1990 Hepatitis C virus infection is associated with the development of hepatocellular carcinoma. Proceedings of the National Academy of Sciences of the USA 87: 6547–6549

Sakaeda H, Saibara T, Fujikawa M et al 1986 A case of an 80-year-old man with primary biliary cirrhosis complicated with primary hepatocellular carcinoma. Acta Hepatologica Japonica 27: 497–503

Sbolli G, Zanotti A R, Tanzi E et al 1990 Serum antibodies to hepatitis C virus in Italian patients with hepatocellular carcinoma. Journal of Medical Virology 30: 230–232

Setoguchi Y, Yamamoto K, Ozaki I et al 1991 Prevalence of chronic liver diseases and anti-HCV antibodies in different districts of Saga. Gastroenterologica Japonica 26: 157–161

Shimizu S, Kiyosawa K, Sodeyama T, Tanaka E, Nakano M 1991 High prevalence of antibody to hepatitis C virus in heavy drinkers with chronic liver diseases in Japan. Journal of Gastroenterology and Hepatology 7: 30–35

Simonetti R G, Cottone M, Craxi A et al 1989 Prevalence of antibodies to hepatitis C virus in hepatocellular carcinoma. Lancet ii: 1338

Sirchia G, Bellobuono A, Giovanetti A, Marconi M 1989 Antibodies to hepatitis C virus in Italian blood donors. Lancet ii: 797

Statistics & Information Department 1990 Vital statistics 1989 Japan, Vol. 1. Minister's Secretariat, Ministry of Health and Welfare, pp 252–254

Stevens G, Taylor R E, Pincyck J et al 1990 Epidemiology of hepatitis C virus: a preliminary study in volunteer blood donors. Journal of the American Medical Association 263: 49–53

Suzuki K, Yamasaki K, Sato S 1991 Hepatocellular carcinoma complicating primary biliary cirrhosis – frequency and etiologic considerations (abstract). Acta Hepatologic Japonica 32: suppl 50

Takada A, Nei J, Takase S, Matsuda Y 1986 Effects of ethanol on experimental hepatocarcinogenesis. Hepatology 6: 65–72

Tanaka K, Hirohata T, Koga S et al 1991 Hepatitis C and hepatitis B in the etiology of hepatocellular carcinoma in the Japanese population. Cancer Research 51: 2842–2847

Tanaka E, Sodeyama T, Yoshizawa K et al 1992 Prevalence of hepatitis C virus related C100-3 antibody in school children in Matsumoto area. Acta Hepatologica Japonica 32: 205–206

Tokita H, Shimizu M, Kojima M et al 1992a Seroepidemiological survey of hepatitis C virus related anti C100-3, anti CP-9 and CP-10 and anti GOR antibodies in an endemic area for non-A, non-B hepatitis. Acta Hepatologica Japonica 32: 1093–1110

Tokita H, Shimizu M, Kojima M, Tsuda F 1992b High incidence of hepatocellular carcinoma in the endemic area for hepatitis C virus. Acta Hepatologica Japonica 32: 193–194

Tsai J F, Jeng J E, Chang W Y et al 1991 Relationship of hepatitis C virus infection to clinical manifestation in patients with chronic liver disease (abstract). Proceedings of the 3rd International Symposium on Viral Hepatitis and Hepatocellular Carcinoma, Taipei. Gastroenterological Society of the Republic of China, Taipei, p 123

Watanabe J, Minegishi K, Mitsumori T et al 1990 Prevalence of anti-HCV antibody in blood donors in the Tokyo areas. Vox Sanguinis 59: 86–88

Yoshizawa K 1991 Seroepidemiology of hepatitis C. In: Tsujii T (ed.) Western liver forum, Iji Shuppan, Tokyo, pp 72–85

Yu M C, Tong M J, Coursaget P et al 1990 Prevalence of hepatitis B and C viral markers in black and white patients with hepatocellular carcinoma in the United States. Journal of the National Cancer Institute 82: 1038–1041

Zarski J P, Lunel F, Dardelet D et al 1991 Hepatitis C virus and hepatocellular carcinoma in France: detection of antibodies using two second generation assays. Journal of Hepatology 13: 376–377

UPDATE

- It has recently been shown that certain areas of the HCV RNA sequence have marked heterogeneity, and this virus is now divided into at least four major subtypes. Type II which constitutes about 70% of HCV infection in Japan is more resistant to interferon therapy, and although not yet clearly shown, it may be more frequently responsible for hepatocarcinogenesis in Japan.
- In several reported isolated villages where the HCV carrier rate is extremely high, it is now attributed to an iatrogenic transmission in the past through the needle/syringe by a careless practitioner in the village.

16. Diagnosis

David Brown Geoffrey Dusheiko

It became clear in the early 1970s that an agent other than the viruses that cause hepatitis A or B is responsible for the majority of cases of post-transfusion hepatitis (Feinstone et al 1975). This disease was given the enigmatic name non-A, non-B hepatitis (NANBH) and was diagnosed on the basis of clinical and biochemical symptoms, patient history and the exclusion of other possible viral causes. Not all patients thought to have NANBH had a history of blood transfusion or parenteral exposure, and were therefore said to have sporadic or community-acquired NANBH. The two illnesses appeared to follow the same course, with approximately 50% of cases developing chronic disease and a significant number progressing to chronic active hepatitis and cirrhosis.

Many attempts were made to identify the aetiological agent(s) responsible for NANBH, but none of the claims was reproducible (Dienstag 1983a, b). However, the transmission of NANBH to chimpanzees provided important impetus to this research, (H J Alter et al 1978, Tabor et al 1978) and eventually led to the seminal discovery in 1988 of the virus associated with most cases of post-transfusion and community-acquired NANBH. The nucleic acid extracted from the plasma of an animal with an ostensibly high infectious titre was used to produce a cDNA library in an expression vector, which was extensively screened with the serum of a patient with chronic NANBH. Eventually, a clone termed 5-1-1, which contained an NANB-specific sequence was identified (Choo et al 1989). This provided the basis for characterization of the virus now known as hepatitis C virus (HCV), which has been proven to be the major cause of both sporadic and transfusion-acquired NANBH (Choo et al 1990). It has also allowed the develpoement of reagents and methodologies essential for diagnosis of HCV infection.

HCV may cause acute disease, which can be severe or asymptomatic and unnoticed. The acute disease may resolve completely, but unfortunately hepatitis C has a disturbing propensity to lead to chronic hepatitis. In turn, chronic hepatitis C may lead to mild illness, which may be asymptomatic for decades and not progressive. The disease will not be detected in these patients unless screening for hepatitis C is undertaken. Some patients have prolonged remissions, only to relapse later. In some of these patients the disease resolves; in others, the disease is inexorably progressive, and persistent life-long infection leads progressively to chronic active hepatitis, cirrhosis, portal hypertension and even hepatocellular carcinoma.

Sensitive and specific markers of hepatitis C infection are now available. The hepatitis C markers used in diagnosis still rely on either recombinantly cloned antigens or DNA technology, and in some circumstances the diagnosis remains difficult.

MOLECULAR VIROLOGY OF HCV: IMPLICATIONS FOR DIAGNOSIS

All indications are that HCV is an enveloped RNA virus of 30–80 nm in size (Bradley et al 1983, Feinstone et al 1983, Yuasa et al 1991). The complete nucleotide sequence of the HCV genome has now been determined in a number of isolates and shown to be a positive-stranded RNA of approximately 9400 nucleotides (Kato et al 1990a, Choo et al 1991, Okamoto et al 1991, Takamizawa et al 1991). This consists of one long open reading frame encoding a polyprotein of 3010–3033 amino acids, which is cleaved into functionally distinct polypeptides either during or after translation. Analysis of the sequence of the HCV genome and its polyprotein shows it to have similar organization to pestiviruses and flaviviruses of the family Flaviviridae (Miller & Purcell 1990). In common with the Flaviviridae the nucleocapsid and envelope proteins are encoded at the 5' end of the genome, while the non-structural elements are downstream of these with the viral replicase at the carboxy terminus (Houghton et al 1991). A major difference between flaviviruses and pestiviruses is found in the region following the envelope domain which in pestiviruses encodes gp53, a second envelope glycoprotein (Collett et al 1989), but in the flaviviruses encodes a secreted but non-structural protein called NS1 (Chambers et al 1990). The function of the 73-kDa glycoprotein product of this region in HCV is unknown and is therefore termed E2/NS1.

The total or partial nucleotide sequences obtained from the considerable number of isolates to date indicate that they may be divided into at least three different subgroups based upon nucleotide and deduced amino acid homology (Enomoto et al 1990, Houghton et al 1991, Inchauspe et al 1991). It is also noted that even within the subgroups there are regions of moderate and hypervariability, especially in the E1 and E2/NS1 domains (Takeuchi et al 1990a, b, Kremsdorf et al 1991, Weiner et al 1991). These regions, especially those in the envelope glycoprotein(s), may be important antigenic sites and variability will have implications in diagnostic screening, immunoprophylaxis and perhaps persistence of infection.

At either end of the viral genome, upstream of the polyprotein initiation codon and downstream of the stop codon, are found short untranslated regions (Kato et al 1990a, Choo et al 1991, Takamizawa et al 1991). The 5' untranslated region consists of approximately 340 nucleotides, is highly conserved between isolates, contains several potential small open reading frames and probably plays an important role in replication (Okamoto et al 1991a, Han et al 1991). The 3' region, which has proved more difficult to analyse, consists of 27–55 nucleotides and shows greater heterogeneity than the 5' end (Kato et al 1991, Takamizawa et al 1991). Although there have been reports of a 3' polyadenylated tail, this does not seem to be a consistent finding (Han et al 1991).

The cloning of the HCV genome has facilitated the production of a panel of recombinant antigens produced in yeast and *Escherichia coli*, on which are based the now widely used immunodiagnostic assays for the detection of antibody to HCV (Kuo et al 1989). Sequence data have also allowed the production of synthetic peptides for use in similar immunoassays (Hosein et al 1991, D Brown et al 1992).

ANTIBODIES TO HCV

HCV probably circulates in the serum at a concentration of between 10^2 and 5×10^7 particles per millilitre (Ulrich et al 1990, Bradley & Maynard 1986, Simmonds et al 1990), and so far it has proved impossible to detect viral antigens by conventional methods. Therefore, the detection of antibodies to HCV has become important as an indication of past or present infection. Most of the early epidemiological and diagnostic studies were carried out using the so-called first-generation enzyme-linked immunosorbent assay (ELISA) based on antibody capture. This assay detected antibodies to C100-3, a 363 amino acid fusion polypeptide representing part of the NS4 region of the HCV genome, constructed from three overlapping clones identified with the aid of 5-1-1 and expressed in yeast with superoxide dismutase (Kuo et al 1989). The presence of antibody to C100-3 proved a good marker for infection with HCV in both post-transfusion and sporadic NANBH (H J Alter et al 1989, Esteban et al 1989, M J Alter et al 1990, Hopf et al 1990, Miyamura et al 1990). Seropositivity was also shown to be associated with chronic infections and correlated with infectivity in blood donations (Esteban et al 1990, Miyamura et al 1990, Van der Poel et al 1990, Tanaka et al 1991).

It soon became evident that there were problems with the specificity of the assay, especially when screening low-risk groups such as blood donors, in whom there was a substantial risk of false positivity (McFarlane et al 1990, Housset et al 1991). This was possibly because of the non-specific binding of IgG or immune complexes to the solid phase (McFarlane et al 1990, Aceti et al 1990). False-positive results were also common in patients with hypergammaglobulinaemia, and in stored tropical samples (Ellis et al 1990, McFarlane et al 1990).

The assay also lacked sensitivity in that anti-C100-3 was not present in the sera of all individuals with past or present HCV infection (Van der Poel et al 1991a, Marcellin et al 1991) or during the early clinical phase of the illness and can take up to 1 year after elevation of transaminases to become detectable (H J Alter et al 1989) Anti-C100-3 also disappears fairly rapidly after the resolution of HCV infection but may persist throughout chronic disease (E Tanaka et al 1991).

The deficiencies in the first-generation assays were responsible for the development of second-generation tests, which incorporated two extra HCV-derived recombinant proteins, which increased the sensitivity of the assay (Aach et al 1991, McHutchison et al 1992). The first of these (C22-3) represents the majority of the 22-kDa nucleocapsid protein, the amino terminus of which encodes an immunodominant epitope (Nasoff et al 1991). Antibodies to C22–3 are an earlier finding and occur more frequently than those to C100-3 during the course of HCV infection (Muraiso et al 1990, Chiba et al 1991, Harada et al 1991, Dourakis et al 1992, Katayama et al 1992, McHutchison et al 1992). They have been detected in blood donations involved in transmission of HCV and in the serum of patients with NANB hepatitis, both of which were found previously to be anti-C100-3 negative (Chiba et al 1991). The reasons for this are probably conservation of amino acid sequence in this region together with greater immunogenicity of the core peptide. It has also been suggested that detection of antibodies to C22-3 alone is a more common finding in sporadic than parenterally acquired NANB hepatitis (J Brown et al 1992). Anti-C22-3 antibodies are probably not neutralizing antibodies in that they are found throughout chronic infection (McHutchison et al 1992).

A protein derived from the NS3 and NS4 regions (C200), or a smaller fragment of it (C33c) from NS3 alone, is also included in the second-generation assays. The C200 protein is the product of a large cloned fragment, combining both the C33c and C100-3 regions. Antibodies to C200 are also likely to be more common than those to C100-3, presumably as a result of reactivity to epitopes in the C33c fragment (Van der Poel et al 1991b, McHutchison et al 1992). Overall, the second-generation ELISA shows enhanced sensitivity when compared with the first generation, although it is doubtful if specificity is altered, especially when used to test low-risk groups.

The detection of antibodies to the E1 and E2/NS1 glycoproteins has proven elusive, probably because of the sequence heterogeneity found in these regions. If, as in the case of flaviviruses and pestiviruses, they are found to be neutralizing (Schlesinger et al 1986, Donis et al 1988, Weiland et al 1990, van-Zijl et al 1991), their detection would be of major importance as a measure of recovery from and immunity to HCV infection.

IgM responses to HCV C100-3 antigen have been investigated in acute and chronic disease. Detectable levels have been found early as 4 weeks after inoculation but can last up to 2 years in individuals with chronic infection (Quiroga et al 1991). Such antibodies are therefore of doubtful significance in distinguishing between the two clinical courses but may have some predictive value regarding progression to chronicity. It is to be hoped that future generations of immunoassays will enable us to distinguish current and resolved infection, acquired immunity and perhaps even between the putative HCV subgroups.

The format of the second-generation assay is the same as the first-generation assay and therefore has the same risk of false positives. The danger of lack of specificity has therefore necessitated the development of supplemental assays for the confirmation of positive results.

Supplementary tests for antibody to HCV

Methods employed to confirm results obtained by ELISA should ideally be of equal sensitivity and specificity, use a different assay format and utilize different antigens. Most of the supplementary tests used at present fulfil at least two of these criteria. The most widely used method is the recombinant immunoblot assay (RIBA, Chiron Corporation, CA, USA), in which recombinant antigens of HCV are coated in bands on nitrocellulose strips, which are then incubated with serum at a dilution of 1:50. Individual reactivities are detected with peroxidase-labelled anti-IgG and 4-chloro-1-naphthol as substrate. The first-generation RIBA used C100-3 and 5-1-1 antigens produced in *E. coli* to coat the strips, while the second-generation tests (RIBA4) added bands coated with C22-3 and C33c, also produced in *E.coli*. Samples are regarded as confirmed positive if antibodies to two or more of the HCV proteins are present and indeterminate if only one antibody is found. The value of RIBA in excluding false-positive results has been extensively demonstrated, as has correlation between RIBA positivity and viraemia (Ebeling et al 1990, Van der Poel et al 1991c), the latter potentially facilitating the discrimination between infective and non-infective blood donations. However, care should be taken when applying the results of RIBA tests because not all positive samples are necessarily infectious. Also, indeterminate and negative donations have been proven to transmit infection and contain detectable viral genome (Bellobuono et al 1990, Zanetti et al 1990).

Neutralization assays have also been used to confirm positive results obtained by ELISA. This method uses the initial immunosorbent assay with and without the addition of another recombinant HCV antigen whose only difference is that it has been produced differently. Confirmation of positivity is justified when the initial result is neutralized by the second antigen, proving specificity for the viral antigen.

The usefulness of synthetic peptides as antigens in the immunodiagnosis of HIV infection, for which they were shown to produce assays with good sensitivity and specificity, led to the production of similar peptides using the deduced amino acid sequence of HCV. These have found some use in primary screening for antibodies and confirmation of positive ELISA results using a variety of assay formats.

DETECTION OF VIRAL GENOME

In the absence of a direct assay for antigenaemia, the detection of the viral genome is necessary for diagnosis of HCV infection, but as mentioned previously virus numbers are usually too low for direct detection of HCV RNA by conventional nucleic acid hybridization techniques. Fortunately, the polymerase chain reaction (PCR) has provided a sensitive and specific assay for HCV RNA in the blood and other tissues (Weiner et al 1990, Kato et al 1990b). The procedure involves extraction of nucleic acids present in the sample and reverse transcription of the RNA with the aid of random or antigenomic primers to produce a single-stranded cDNA, which is then amplified using HCV-specific primers in a PCR. Using this method, HCV RNA can be detected in the majority of anti-HCV-positive patients with NANB hepatitis and also in a proportion of those who are antibody negative. It is possible that the latter findings represent false-positive results, but they more likely identify individuals who have failed to raise antibodies detectable by current immunoassays. Similarily, the absence of HCV RNA in anti-HCV-positive individuals indicates resolution of infection, a negative phase of intermittent viraemia or false reactivity in the immunoassay.

Owing to nucleotide sequence heterogeneity, the selection of PCR primers has great effect on the sensitivity of the assay, with differences seen in the rate of detection when primers are chosen from the various regions of the genome. As would be expected, the least sensitive assays use primers representing areas with the greatest heterogeneity, such as the envelope and NS5 regions (Cristiano et al 1991), while dramatic improvement in detection can be obtained using primer sequences derived from the highly conserved 5' untranslated region (Garson et al 1990a, Okamoto et al 1990b). The high specificity in the PCR is ensured by rigorous selection of primers to rule out cross-reactivity with other known sequences together with hybridization of the product with an HCV-specific probe. Sensitivity is maximized by using double or nested PCR, which can detect as little as one molecule of cDNA (Simmonds et al 1990). The second reaction also acts as a liquid hybridization step, thus increasing specificity and avoiding the need for another hybridization step, which is time-consuming and unlikely to increase sensitivity. Single-round PCR does require hybridization with labelled probe and is probably equally sensitive as the nested reaction.

It must also be borne in mind that sample handling can have dramatic effects on the results obtained from PCR of HCV, and to ensure maximum sensitivity specimens should ideally be processed immediately and frozen in aliquots to prevent repeated freezing and thawing. It has been reported that prolonged storage of serum or blood at room temperature can result in a thousandfold reduction in detectable viral RNA, with freeze–thawing also having a significant effect (Busch & Wilber 1992). This could have profound effects on quantification of HCV RNA and its detection in samples with low virus numbers. As with all PCR technology rigorous precautions (Kwok & Higuchi 1989) need to be employed to prevent cross-contamination with negative controls included at each step. Successful reactions are able to detect less than one chimpanzee infectious dose (Farci et al 1991), a unit that has as yet not been quantified in terms of number of virus particles. Others using limiting dilution assays have defined the sensitivity of the reverse transcription, nested PCR for HCV as 4×10^3 virus particles per ml (Simmonds et al 1990).

Apart from primer selection, other factors important in determining sensitivity appear to be yield of nucleic acid from the extraction step and the efficiency of the reverse transcription, which may be below 5% (Zhang et al 1991). It has been suggested that designing primers to amplify very short sequences (<100 nt) of viral genome further enhances sensitivity (Garson et al 1991).

HCV RNA appears in the blood long before other markers and often within days of infection, and at present is the only definitive test for diagnosis of HCV infection (Garson et al 1990b, Shimizu et al 1990, Farci et al 1991). Three possible patterns of viraemia that have clinical relevance have been identified; there may be a transient viraemia accompanying an acute resolving hepatitis, persistent viraemia with progression to chronicity and intermittent viraemia characterized by an initial loss of HCV RNA but which recurs after some months.

In hepatitis B infection, HBV DNA has been detected by PCR many years after clinical and biochemical resolution of disease, and thus low levels of viral genome detected by a technique as sensitive as PCR may be of doubtful significance (Carman et al 1991, Xu et al 1992) either clinically or as an infectivity risk. A similar situation may exist in HCV infection, and the results of PCR tests should be assessed in combination with all available clinical, biochemical and pathological information. To this end, the detection of negative-stranded intermediates in the serum or other tissues may be of help in identifying active viral replication (Fong et al 1991b, Takehara et al 1992). Testing for such intermediates will also be of use in identifying sites of replication, and also perhaps evaluation of response to antiviral therapy (Fong et al 1991a).

Methods for quantification have until now been based on dilution analysis and suggest that titres of HCV RNA in the serum, while not corresponding to degree of liver injury, may correlate with clinical and biochemical parameters (Shindo et al 1991a). More accurate methods of HCV RNA quantification are being developed, and it is to be hoped that these will be of use in monitoring clinical course and response to antiviral therapy (Chung et al 1991, Shindo et al 1991b).

The sequencing of PCR products enables information on genome diversity between isolates to be rapidly gathered, and may provide the basis for a genotypic classification of HCV (Simmonds et al 1990). This will be especially important if, as has been suggested, the clinical outcome and response to treatment are determined by the infecting subtype (Takada et al 1992). The development of methods for subtyping, using tools such as type-specific probes, is already under way (Nakao et al 1991, Takada et al 1992).

Detection of HCV in the tissues

There has been a report of visualization of appropriate-sized viral particles isolated from infected sera (Abe et al 1989). However, examination of tissues has failed to identify similar particles, and it is probable that most ultrastructural changes seen by electron microscopy are non-specific (Shimizu et al 1989). Therefore, the development of histological markers of infection would be an aid to diagnosis, although work in this field has not advanced at the pace of other forms of detection. Using immunohistochemical techniques with mono- and polyclonal antibodies to HCV proteins, several groups have detected evidence of HCV infection in liver tissue (Infantolino et al 1990, Hiramatsu et al 1991, Yap et al 1991), and it appears that the presence of virus-specific antigen in the cytoplasm is a very early finding in the course of infection with HCV (Shimizu et al 1991). With the aid of in situ hybridization, several groups claim to have detected the HCV genome in infected liver tissue (Haruna et al 1991, Negro et al 1992, Lamas et al 1992) but the methodologies are not easy to perform or interpret and will await confirmation. The finding that HCV RNA can be successfully amplified from fixed, paraffin-embedded material (Goeser et al 1992) also opens up the vast wealth of archived material to research and retrospective study.

Table 16.1 Groups for consideration of HCV testing

Persons with signs and symptoms of hepatitis	
Patients with chronic hepatitis, cirrhosis or hepatocellular carcinoma	
Persons with unexplained increases in serum ALT or AST	
Intravenous drug abusers, or those with a history of past drug abuse	
Transfusion recipients: patients with malignancies or thalassaemia	
Recipients of blood products: haemophilia, Von Willebrand's disease, other coagulopathies	
Hypogammaglobulinaemics	
Plasmapheresed patients	
Sexually promiscuous people and prostitutes	
Occupational exposure:	Medical, dental and laboratory health care workers, those with needlestick injuries or those routinely exposed to blood products
Spouse or sexual partner of HCV-infected person	
Haemodialysis patients	
Liver, bone marrow or kidney transplant recipients	
Inmates of custodial institutions	
Infants of anti-HCV positive mothers	

CLINICAL DIAGNOSIS OF ACUTE AND CHRONIC HCV INFECTION

The clinical manifestations of the viral hepatitides are similar, so that clinical diagnosis of viral hepatitis frequently relies on an epidemiological history and serological confirmation. Many persons with chronic hepatitis C have silent, asymptomatic disease, and the diagnosis requires the clinician to measure serum aminotransferases and antibody to HCV. The epidemiology of hepatitis C can now be studied more readily. A full discussion of hepatitis C associated with blood transfusions and blood products is discussed elsewhere in this volume, and therefore only the salient features of the epidemiology of the disease relating to diagnosis are given here.

A number of groups of individuals at higher risk of HCV infection have been recognized. These groups are summarized in Table 16.1.

Population studies of hepatitis C

The prevalence of type C hepatitis in blood donors has how been ascertained in many countries. The positive immunoassay rate ranges from 0.18 to 1.4%. In most western countries, the prevalence ranges from 0.3 to 0.7%; in Japan and southern Europe from 0.9 to 1.2%. A higher prevalence has been found in southern Italy and eastern Europe than in northern Europe (Rassam & Dusheiko 1991). A higher prevalence has also been found in the Middle East and Africa; for example, in South Africa up to 4.2% of men are anti-HCV positive (Coursaget et al 1990, Ellis et al 1990). The prevalence in paid donors is also higher (10–15%). As mentioned earlier, the ELISA tests are poorly specific in low-risk blood donors, and only 20–60% of donors have a positive supplemental test (RIBA 2) (Barbara & Contreras 1991, Dawson et al 1991).

Hepatitis C in at-risk populations

Although the precise mode of acquisition of hepatitis C is often uncertain, hepatitis C is known to be transmitted by parenteral, or inapparent parenteral, contact routes. Transmission by blood transfusion and blood products including factor VII, factor IX, fibrinogen and cryoglobulin has been unequivocally documented. A number of studies in chimpanzees have documented serial passage of NANB hepatitis (now known to be HCV) using sera derived from blood donors implicated in cases of NANB post-transfusion hepatitis (H J Alter et al 1978).

The highest prevalences worldwide are found in haemophiliacs, 50–90% of whom are anti-HCV positive, depending upon age, the duration of infection, factor VIII requirement and the source of factor VIII (Schramm et al 1989). The high prevalence in haemophiliacs reflects the frequent use of factor VIII, which is derived from thousands of donors. A form of NANB hepatitis with a short incubation period (4–19 days) reported in haemophiliacs probably reflects a shortened incubation period due to infusion of a large inoculum of hepatitis C (Hruby & Schauf 1978). Haemophiliacs may also be HCV RNA positive without detectable anti-HCV, particularly if also infected with human immunodeficiency virus (HIV) (Simmonds et al 1990). Human immunoglobulin is generally regarded as a safe product, but there are occasional reports of transmission by inadequately prepared intravenous immunoglobulin batches (Lever et al 1984).

The prevalence of anti-HCV is high in multiply transfused patients with thalassaemia major, but varies geographically according to the source of the blood administered to patients (Wonke et al 1990).

The prevalence in intravenous drug users is extremely high (70–92%), because of repeated exposure to carriers of HCV through shared, contaminated needles. Community-based outbreaks of NANB hepatitis due to intravenous drug use have been identified (Morbidity and Mortality Weekly Reports 1989).

Several other groups have been shown to be at risk. These include haemodialysed patients, particularly in endemic areas such as the Middle East or Japan (Oguchi et al 1990). The disease has been transmitted by coagulum pyelolithotomy, in which the coagulum is prepared from a mixture of cryoprecipitate, thrombin and calcium chloride (McVary et al 1989). Anti-HCV is apparently also common in transplant patients requiring frequent blood transfusions, including renal, liver and bone marrow transplant recipients (Baur et al 1991, Ponz et al 1991, Poterucha et al 1991). Liver transplantation is a relatively common therapeutic necessity for patients with cirrhosis due to hepatitis C, and recurrent hepatitis C disease is apparently common in these patients after transplantation. In all these groups, previously positive patients may lose antibody after the procedure as a result of immunosuppression (Read et al 1991a). The role of immunosuppression in the expression of liver disease caused by HCV remains to be determined (Read et al 1991b), but it is apparent that some immunosuppressed patients, although seronegative for anti-HCV, are HCV RNA positive in serum. Hepatitis C has also been transmitted by organ transplantation, and this may cause severe post-organ transplantation liver disease (Pereira et al 1991).

Transmission after needle stick injury may also occur. Nosocomial or occupational exposure is being evaluated. Health care workers appear to be at relatively low risk (Hofmann & Kunz 1990, Polywka & Laufs 1991). However, there are well-documented instances of needlestick transmission of HCV, and of NANB hepatitis after surgery, or even hospitalization without transfusion (Giusti et al 1987).

Community-acquired hepatitis C

The disease is prevalent in many parts of the world where transmission cannot be explained by blood transfusion or intravenous drug abuse, and careful investigation of patients does not always uncover a source of infection. In many patients, geographic origin from an area of relatively high endemicity is the only risk factor that can be invoked. The precise mechanism of transmission of most cases of community-acquired disease is uncertain, but transmission by close person-to-person contact from carriers of HCV is the most plausible method of transmission in these societies. Transmission by insect vectors remains only a speculative possibility. It can also be speculated that in some countries the disease is spread by intramuscular injection or operations without adequate sterilization or disposable equipment (Dull 1961). In the USA, the proportion of patients with type C hepatitis with a history of blood transfusion has declined in the past 7 years, whereas in contrast the proportion with a history of parenteral drug use has increased. In approximately 40% of patients the source is unknown (M J Alter 1991a, b). The advent of serological testing has shown that most community-acquired NANB hepatitis is also due to hepatitis C. A substantial proportion of acute community-acquired cases remain unclassified, and PCR to detect

HCV RNA remains, the only diagnostic test to exclude another virus.

Fulminant hepatitis is more common in sporadic NANB hepatitis. Although most cases of NANB fulminant hepatitis in Japan are due to hepatitis C, the same may not be true in the West, where an as yet unidentified virus may be important.

Sexual transmission of hepatitis C

Sexual transmission seems certainly possible, albeit a relatively inefficient and infrequent means of contagion. Anti-HCV has been found in 11% of sexual partners of anti-HCV-positive intravenous drug abusers, and may correlate with the presence of HIV (Tor et al 1990). The overall HCV infection rate is also higher in sexually promiscuous groups than in voluntary blood donors. Significantly more homosexual than heterosexual subjects attending a sexually transmitted disease clinic were found to be positive for anti-HCV, and the prevalence of anti-HCV correlates with the lifetime number of sexually transmitted diseases (Tedder et al 1991). The prevalence of anti-HCV is usually higher in sexually promiscuous patients who admit to intravenous drug abuse. Other studies, however, have not found a high prevalence of sexual transmission in partners of anti-HCV-positive haemophiliacs (Schulman & Grillner 1990).

HCV RNA has been detected in saliva (or saliva containing blood), and transmission of HCV by this means and by a human bite have been reported (Dusheiko et al 1990, Abe & Inchauspe 1991, Wang et al 1991). Dentists in New York, particularly those practising oral surgery, have a higher prevalence of anti-HCV antibody than blood donors (Klein et al 1991).

Intrafamilial transmission of hepatitis C

The role of intrafamilial transmission requires clarification. Although household transmission appears to be relatively infrequent, the true attack rate may be underestimated, since the prevalence of HCV infection in family members is based on the current diagnostic tests, which usually reflect chronic infection rather than resolved disease. In Japan, up to 8% of family members of an index patient with HCV were found to be anti-HCV positive, but no specific relative could be linked to HCV positivity, making it difficult to identify the route of infection (Kiyosawa et al 1991).

Maternal-infant transmission of hepatitis C

Mother-to-infant transmission has been observed, but appears to be relatively uncommon. The importance of this route remains controversial. Children born to anti-HCV-positive mothers acquire passively transferred antibodies that are transiently present in serum and disappear within 7–11 months (Wejstal et al 1990). Active production of antibody and abnormal serum aminotransferases have subsequently been observed (Giovannini et al 1990). However, a disturbing finding has been the detection of persistent HCV RNA in serum in the absence of anti-HCV in newborn babies delivered by women who were anti-HCV positive, suggesting silent transmission of HCV (Thaler et al 1991).

DIAGNOSIS OF ACUTE HEPATITIS C

The mean incubation period of hepatitis C is 6–12 weeks. However, with a large inoculum, such as following administration of factor VIII, the incubation period is reduced to 4 weeks or less (Bamber et al 1981, Lim et al 1991). The typical clinical pattern is not dissimilar to other forms of viral hepatitis, and cannot reliably be distinguised solely by clinical findings or routine biochemical tests.

The acute course of HCV infection is clinically mild, and the peak serum alanine aminotransferase (ALT) elevations are less than those encountered in acute hepatitis A or B. Only 25% of patients are icteric, and subclinical disease is common; such patients may first present decades later with sequelae such as cirrhosis or hepatocellular carcinoma (HCC). If the disease is at all apparent, the onset is insidious with non-specific symptoms or no symptoms; malaise, anorexia, nausea and sometimes right upper quadrant pain may be present. If icterus develops, fatigue and anorexia usually worsen. Jaundice can last for a few days to a few months, but is usually restricted to less than a month. Some pruritis and steatorrhoea may occur, as well as mild (2–5 kg) weight loss.

Fatigue usually abates after the jaundice resolves, but may persist for several months. The physical signs of acute hepatitis C are also unremarkable. Hepatomegaly and splenomegaly are found in only a small percentage of patients.

During the early clinical phase the serum ALT levels may fluctuate, and may become normal or near normal, making the determination of true convalescence difficult. The serum alkaline phosphatase is slightly elevated, but less so than ALT. Arthritis, rashes and neurological syndromes have been reported.

A slightly elevated white cell count may be found, with large atypical lymphocytes. In rare cases, agranulocytosis or aplastic anaemia develops during NANB viral hepatitis, but most cases are not apparently attributable to hepatitis C (Perrillo et al 1981, Zeldis et al 1983, Tzakis et al 1988, Pol et al 1990).

The prothrombin time may be prolonged, related to severity and extent of hepatocyte necrosis. Severe or fulminant hepatitis C is rare, but may occur. The diagnosis of such cases requires confirmation by HCV RNA testing.

Serological diagnosis: acute hepatitis C

Figure 16.1 represents what is thought to be a typical serological response in acute resolving hepatitis C virus infection. Anti-C100-3 appears in the circulation after a mean interval of 15 weeks from the acute illness and first elevations of the aminotransferases (Lee et al 1991). Although roughly one-third of seroconversions take place early in the acute phase of the disease, sometimes as early as 2 weeks (Lim et al 1991), seroconversion can be delayed for a year or longer. The average time from transfusion to seroconversion is of the order of 11–12 weeks with the first-generation tests and 7–8 weeks with the second-generation tests, anti-C33 or anti-C22 not infrequently appearing a week or two earlier than anti-C100-3. Antibodies to HCV are found in a varying proportion of patients with acute sporadic NANB

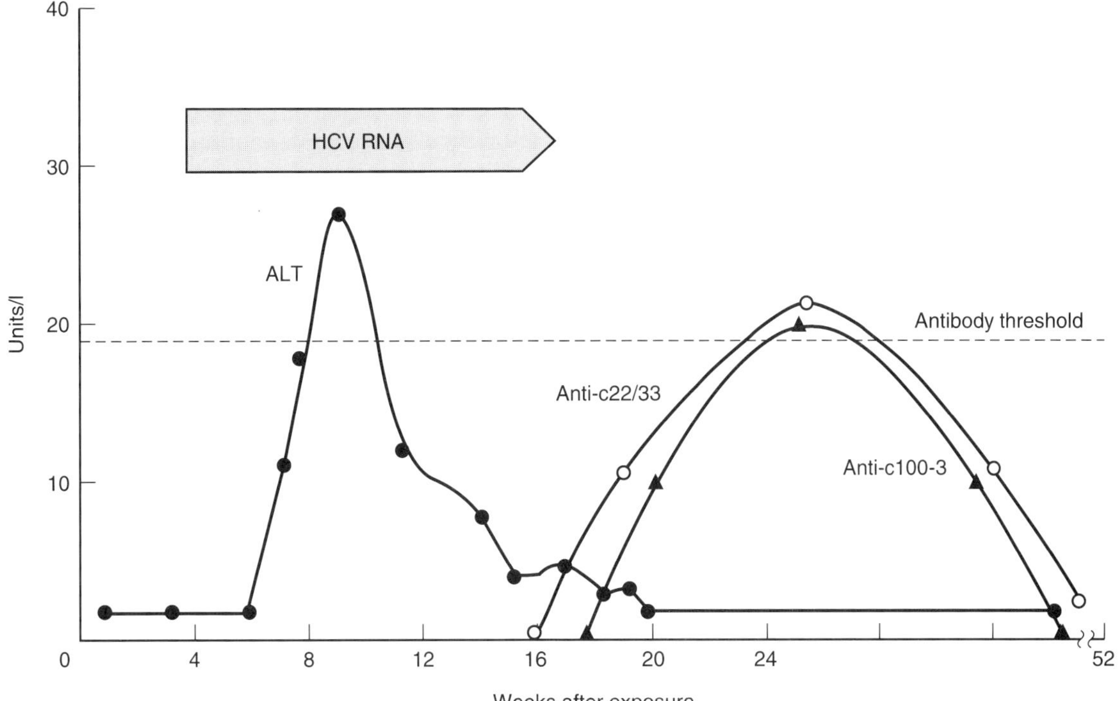

Fig. 16.1 A stylized depiction of the serological course in acute resolving HCV infection. In some patients, antibodies to HCV proteins are demonstrable. It is unclear whether all individuals mount a humoral immune response detectable by current immunoassays.

hepatitis depending upon the geographic location, mode of acquisition of hepatitis and severity of the disease. Seroconversion occurs much less frequently, and in lower titre, in acute self-limiting infections compared with those that progress to become chronic (H J Alter et al 1989, M J Alter & Sampliner 1989, Nishioka et al 1991). However, a substantial proportion of patients with sporadically acquired NANB patients remain anti-HCV seronegative, and it will be important to define whether these patients represent HCV infection with poor serological response or infection due to other unclassified NANB agents.

The acute disease is often silent, and may resolve completely with clearance of HCV RNA from serum. A suitable immunodiagnostic test for resolved infection and immunity is not available, but antibodies to the envelope region are being sought.

Post-transfusion hepatitis C

Serological testing now indicates that seroconversion to anti-HCV occurs in 85–100% of patients with chronic post-transfusion NANB hepatitis (Esteban et al 1990). In studies of post-transfusion hepatitis in Spain, seroconversion to anti-C100-3 occurred 6–8 weeks after transfusion in 38%, 20–26 weeks after transfusion in 56% and 38–52 weeks after transfusion in 6% (Esteban et al 1989). In some patients a very early appearance of anti-HCV may be due to passively acquired antibody from the donor blood.

Retrospective studies have shown a higher prevalence of anti-HCV at onset in those developing chronic disease (83%) than those who recover from post-transfusion hepatitis (Bortolotti et al 1991). Anti-HCV persists for years and even decades in chronic hepatitis C, but may decline in titre or disappear with resolution.

During the early phase of primary HCV infection, serum HCV RNA is the only diagnostic marker of infection, and RNA testing therefore remains the only means of diagnosis in seronegative patients. Unfortunately, the test is only available in research laboratories. Serum HCV RNA has been detected within 1–3 weeks of transfusion in patients with hepatitis C, and usually lasts less than 4 months in patients with acute self-limiting hepatitis C but may persist for decades in patients with chronic disease (M J Alter et al 1990, Farci et al 1991).

Histological features

Liver biopsy is not a usual investigation in acute viral hepatitis unless the diagnosis is in question. The histological features of acute hepatitis C are similar to those seen in hepatitis A or B, except for more marked sinusoidal cell activation. The distinction from evolving chronic hepatitis C can be difficult. The major pathological features are those of acute hepatitis: liver cell swelling, acidophil body formation, cholestasis and infiltration of sinusoids by lymphocytes are the main abnormalities but the appearances vary according to the timing of the biopsy, the severity and the clinical outcome.

The inflammatory infiltrate is composed of lymphocytes, macrophages and plasma cells. Pale cells (ballooning degeneration) are noted. Cells with acidophilic cytoplasm (acidophilic cells) are seen and are an often important hallmark of acute hepatitis.

Subacute hepatitic necrosis or fulminant hepatitis is characterized by extensive hepatic necrosis. The organ may shrink as a result of extensive necrosis. The different causes of acute hepatitis are difficult to separate morphologically. In acute hepatitis A, periportal inflammation and necrosis and perivenular cholestasis are prominent. In acute hepatitis B, HBsAg can rarely be found histochemically. Staining for HBcAg is usually associated with active viral replication and is more commonly seen in chronic hepatitis B. Predictions of chronicity of a case of hepatitis C cannot usually be made from the biopsy appearance. In early infection striking lymphocytic portal reaction occurs, and the extensive lobular changes of chronic infection make the distinction between acute and chronic infection quite difficult.

DIAGNOSIS OF CHRONIC HEPATITIS C

The clinical and epidemiological features of transfusion-associated and sporadic NANB hepatitis have been well documented, despite the fact that the disease previously required identification by prospective biochemical monitoring.

The majority of cases will not have been preceded by an episode of clinically apparent, icteric hepatitis, and most hepatitis C carriers are unaware of their disease and their potential infectivity. Between 50 and 75% of patients with type C post-transfusion hepatitis continue to have abnormal serum aminotransferase levels after 12 months and chronic hepatitis histologically (Lee et al 1991). The risk of chronic infection after sporadic hepatitis C is probably similar.

Most patients with chronic hepatitis C are asymptomatic or only mildly symptomatic. In symptomatic patients, fatigue is the most common complaint, and is variously described as lack of energy, increased need for sleep or fatiguability. Many patients do not give a history of acute hepatitis or jaundice. Physical findings are generally mild and variable and there may be no abnormalities. With more severe disease, spider angiomata and hepatosplenomegaly may be found. Serum aminotransferases decline from the peak values encountered in the acute phase of the disease, but typically remain increased by two- to eightfold. The serum ALT concentrations may fluctuate over time and may even intermittently be normal. Many patients have a sustained elevation of the serum aminotransferases. The relationship between HCV RNA in serum and serum aminotransferases is complex, and although most patients with raised serum ALT are HCV RNA positive the converse is not always true.

The spectrum of chronic disease varies. Most patients appear to have an indolent, only slowly progressive course with little increase in mortality after 20 years. However, cirrhosis develops in approximately 20% of patients with chronic disease within 10 years, although the cirrhosis may remain indolent and only slowly progressive for a prolonged period (Berman et al 1979, Koretz et al 1980, Mattsson 1989, Patel et al 1991). The disease is not necessarily benign however, and rapidly progressive cirrhosis can occur. Older age at infection, concomitant alcohol abuse and concurrent HBV or HIV infection or other illness may be important aggravating co-factors. With the development of cirrhosis, weakness, wasting, oedema and ascites become more common. Older patients may present with complications of cirrhosis, or even HCC. With progressive disease, the laboratory values become progressively more abnormal. The finding of aspartate aminotransferases (AST) greater than ALT, low albumin and prolonged prothrombin time suggest cirrhosis. Low levels of autoantibodies may also become detectable.

Serological diagnosis: chronic hepatitis C

Figure 16.2 represents a typical serological response in chronic hepatitis C virus infection. Anti-HCV antibodies persist in the majority of patients with chronic post-transfusion NANB hepatitis, with serological testing showing a high prevalence of anti-HCV in patients with chronic active hepatitis and/or cirrhosis considered to be due to NANB hepatitis (H J Alter et al 1989). The majority (75–95%) of patients with post-transfusion chronic NANB hepatitis in the USA and Europe are positive for anti-HCV. The disease in many patients with chronic NANB hepatitis may or may not be associated with a history of blood transfusion. The prevalence varies according to the background endemicity of hepatitis C in the population (Pohjanpelto et al 1991). Tests for anti-HCV are now important in establishing a diagnosis of what was formerly considered cryptogenic cirrhosis (J Brown et al 1992).

In studies in chimpanzees, anti-HCV (i.e. anti-C100-3) was not neutralizing, in that primates with high levels of this antibody were also shown to have high titres of circulating hepatitis C virus (Bradley et al 1990). The development and maintenance of current diagnostic antibodies to hepatitis C virus therefore appears to reflect concomitant virus replication and consequently a high potential for infectivity.

A proportion of patients may improve spontaneously, but the number of patients who do so is unclear. These patients lose antibody after follow-up of at least 5 years and usually develop normal serum aminotransferases (E Tanaka et al 1991). Other patients may show a decline in anti-HCV titre with time (H J Alter et al 1989).

HCV RNA usually persists in patients with abnormal serum aminotransferases and anti-HCV. However, HCV RNA, and hence viraemia, can also be found in patients with normal liver function tests. Isolates of HCV in individual patients may

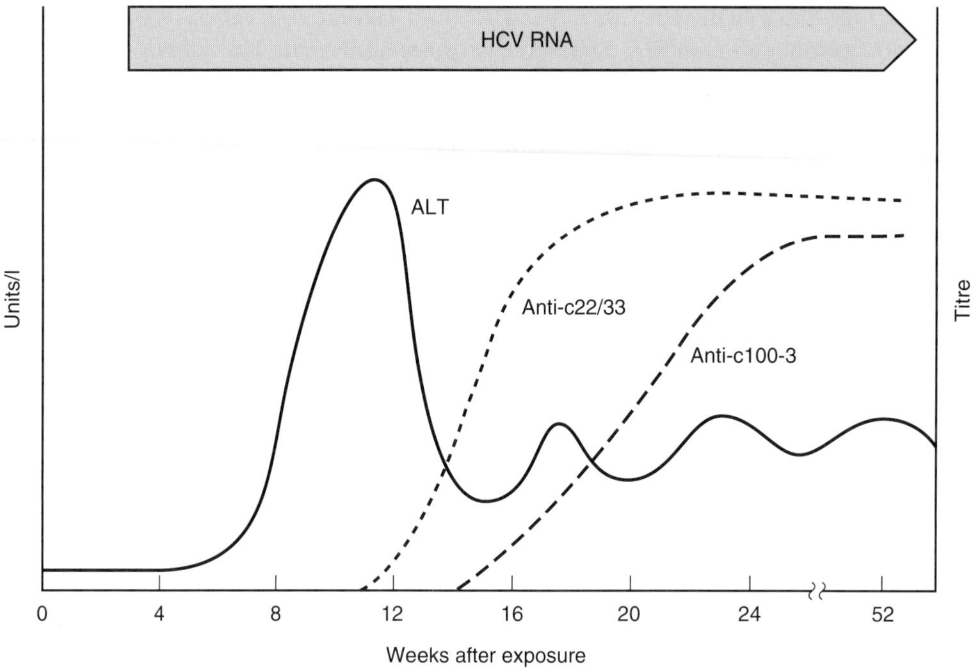

Fig. 16.2 A stylized depiction of the serological course in chronic hepatitis C infection.

show nucleotide substitutions with time, suggesting that the HCV RNA mutates at a rate similar to other RNA viruses (Ogata et al 1991). Preliminary but unconfirmed reports have suggested the HCV antigens can be detected in liver biopsy preparations in chronic carriers (discussed above).

Histological features

Three main pathological forms of chronic hepatitis, chronic active hepatitis, chronic persistent hepatitis and chronic lobular hepatitis, occur in hepatitis C. These terms refer to certain defining morphological features that may have prognostic implications. However, these diagnoses are not separate entities and do not take into account the dynamic process of chronic hepatitis over time. Nonetheless, these definitions are in widespread use. Typically patients with chronic hepatitis C have relatively mild chronic hepatitis histologically. Lymphoid follicles in the portal tracts, bile duct damage, lobular activity including acidophilic cells and lymphocytes in sinusoids and fatty change are the most common features. The single most characteristic feature is the lymphoid follicle, ranging from loose aggregates of lymphocytes to well-defined structures with germinal centres (Scheuer et al 1992). Although follicles are not restricted to hepatitis C, they are often pointers that alert the pathologist of the possibility of HCV infection.

Mild chronic hepatitis C may persist for many years without evidence of progression to severe chronic hepatitis. The patient's health remains good (Wejstal et al 1987, Vucelic et al 1988). In more severe chronic hepatitis C, several patterns of necrosis are seen, including spotty focal necrosis or confluent and bridging necrosis. This may link either portal veins or the terminal hepatic venules. Hepatic venules linking portal tracts, known as central portal bridging, may represent more severe lesions with a strong likelihood of developing cirrhosis. In patients with long-standing chronic hepatitis, fibrotic change and progression to cirrhosis may occur.

It is not easy to project the prognosis for patients seen at one point in time (Lai et al 1991). Episodes of hepatic necrosis may progress at variable rates to cirrhosis, and conversely the lesion may revert in some patients to inactive hepatitis. Cirrhosis develops after chronic hepatitis rather than following massive hepatic necrosis and may develop in patients with mild histological pattern. The mechanism for this transition is not known, but it may occur after repeated attacks of lobular necrosis associated with piecemeal necrosis. However, a relationship between histological exarcerbations and episodic clinical course is not proven.

The morphological features of cirrhosis due to hepatitis C are not specific to the disease; in the early stages, lymphoid aggregates may be seen.

Interestingly, routine screening of blood donors for anti-HCV indicates that a significant proportion of asymptomatic anti-HCV positive blood donors indeed have progressive liver disease. Several histological studies in asymptomatic anti-HCV positive donors have shown that 45–62% have chronic active hepatitis and 7–15% have active cirrhosis (Alberti et al 1991). Progression to hepatocellular carcinoma is also well documented and, despite the indolent and slowly progressive nature of the disease in many, it is apparent from serological testing for anti-HCV that HCV is a leading cause of morbidity from liver disease in the western world.

Treatment with alpha interferon may result in a reduction in the disease activity, particularly the lobular hepatitis.

ASSOCIATION OF OTHER DISEASES WITH HCV

Hepatitis B and HIV

HCV may cause disease concurrently with hepatitis B, particularly in risk groups such as haemophiliacs and drug abusers, or where these diseases are endemic in the same environment. The combination may cause aggravated disease (Fattovich et al 1991, Fong et al 1991b). Likewise, in drug abusers and haemophiliacs, HIV and HCV may coexist and cause severe, accelerated liver disease.

Autoimmune hepatitis

There are conflicting reports regarding the occurrence of hepatitis C antibodies in patients with autoimmune liver disease. Clearly ELISA for anti-HCV is prone to false-positive results in patients with high concentrations of immunoglobulins in serum (McFarlane et al 1990). These false-reactive anti-HCV antibodies in patients with anti-smooth muscle antibody may actually disappear with immunosuppressive treatment as globulin levels decrease (Schvarcz et al 1990). However, Italian patients with autoimmune chronic active hepatitis appear to have a high frequency of genuine exposure to HCV, whereas seropositivity in English patients usually represents a false-positive result. It is therefore not certain whether anti-HCV in patients with chronic active hepatitis represents persistent anti-HCV from earlier disease, whether the autoimmune disease in induced by HCV (Lenzi et al 1991) or whether autoantibodies in autoimmune hepatitis patients cross-react with HCV-related antigens (Onji et al 1991). In Japan, 80% of patients with chronic NANB hepatitis have circulating antibodies to a pentadecapeptide (Gor), an epitope of normal hepatocytes; this phenomenon may represent an autoimmune response peculiar to type C hepatitis (Mishiro et al 1990).

Up to 50% of patients with type II autoimmune hepatitis (anti-liver kidney microsomal (LKM) antibody positive) are anti-HCV positive, and anti-HCV and anti-LKM in association may also represent another example of molecular mimicry. Anti-HCV-positive patients with anti-LKM autoimmune chronic active hepatitis are usually male, older, and have lower titres of anti-LKM, than patients without anti-HCV. The target antigen of antibodies to LKM is a portion of the cytochrome P450 II D6 molecule; anti-LKM is not directed to a C100-3 epitope, but some sequence homology between HCV and cytochrome P450 may exist (Manns et al 1991). This association has some therapeutic implications, as the autoimmune disease is responsive to corticosteroids and may be aggravated by alpha interferon. It is preferable to confirm HCV viraemia in these patients by PCR.

Alcoholic liver disease

In several countries, a higher prevalence of anti-HCV has been found in patients with alcoholic liver disease. The prevalence of hepatitis C antibodies correlates with the severity of liver injury, and is higher in patients with cirrhosis than those with only fatty change (Pares et al 1990). The relationship is a complex one (Mendenhall et al 1991), which apparently reflects in part the higher rate of transfusions in alcoholics with decompensated liver disease and a common environmental risk.

Hepatocellular carcinoma

Serological analysis of patients with HCC has shown a high prevalence of anti-HCV in patients with hepatocellular carcinoma. Several case–control studies in Europe have suggested that up to 70% of male patients with HCC are anti-HCV positive (Bruix et al 1989, K Tanaka et al 1991). The highest prevalence of HCV in HCC is found in Italian, Japanese and Spanish patients; the prevalence is lower in Chinese and African patients, in whom the disease is more commonly associated with chronic hepatitis B. Since HCV is an RNA virus, it is believed that chronic HCV infection induces necroinflammatory change that progresses to cirrhosis and eventual malignant transformation (Levrero et al 1991), rather than an insertional oncogenic event. In Japan, at least, a history of transfusion has been documented in 42% of anti-HCV-positive patients with HCC. The mean interval between the date of transfusion and the diagnosis of cirrhosis and HCC is usually long, 21 and 29 years respectively (Kiyosawa et al 1990).

Non-hepatic disease

NANB hepatitis has been thought to be associated with aplastic anaemia (Pol et al 1990). Suprisingly, cryoglobulinaemia has also been associated with hepatitis C, with up to 54% of patients with mixed cryoglobulinaemia having been found anti-HCV positive (verified by RIBA). The role of HCV in the pathogenesis of this disease is unknown (Durand et al 1991, Ferri et al 1991). Recently, Sjögren's syndrome has been found in a high proportion of patients with chronic hepatitis C (Haddad et al 1992).

REFERENCES

Aach R D, Stevens C E, Hollinger B F et al 1991 Hepatitis C virus infection in post-transfusion hepatitis. An analysis with first and second-generation assays. New England Journal of Medicine 325: 1325–1329

Abe K, Inchauspe G 1991 Transmission of hepatitis C by saliva. Lancet 337: 248

Abe K, Kurata T, Shikata T 1989 Non-A, Non-B hepatitis: visualisation of virus-like particles from chimpanzee and human sera. Archives of Virology 104: 351–355

Aceti A, Taliani G, De Bac C, Sebastiani A 1990 Anti-HCV false positivity in malaria. Lancet 336: 1442–1443

Alberti A, Chemello L, Cavaletto D et al 1991 Antibody to hepatitis C virus and liver disease in volunteer blood donors. Annals of Internal Medicine 114: 1010–1012

Alter H J, Purcell R H, Holland P V, Popper H 1978 Transmissible agent in non-A, non-B hepatitis. Lancet i: 459–463

Alter H J, Purcell R H, Shih J W, Melpolder J C, Houghton M, Choo Q–L, Kuo G 1989 Detection of antibody to hepatitis C virus in prospectively followed transfusion recipients with acute and chronic non-A, non-B hepatitis. New England Journal of Medicine 321: 1494–1500

Alter M J 1991a Inapparent transmission of hepatitis C: footprints in the sand. Hepatology 14: 389–391

Alter M J 1991b Hepatitis C: A sleeping giant. American Journal of Medicine 91 (suppl. 3B): 112S–115S

Alter M J, Sampliner R E 1989: Hepatitis C: and miles to go before we sleep (editorial). New England Journal of Medicine 321: 1538–1540

Alter M J, Hadler S C, Judson F N et al 1990 Risk factors for acute non-A, non-B hepatitis in the United States and association with hepatitis C virus infection. Journal of the American Medical Association 462: 2231–2235

Bamber M, Murray A, Arborgh BAM et al 1981 Short incubation non-A, non-B hepatitis transmitted by factor VIII concentrates in patients with congenital coagulation disorders. Gut 22: 854–859

Barbara J A, Contreras M 1991 Non-A, non-B hepatitis and the anti-HCV assay. Vox Sanguinis 60: 1–7

Baur P, Daniel V, Pomer S, Scheurlen H, Opelz G, Roelcke D 1991 Hepatitis C-virus (HCV) antibodies in patients after kidney transplantation. Annals of Hematology 62: 68–73

Bellobuono A, Mozzi F, Petrini G, Zanella A, Sirchia G 1990 Infectivity of blood that is immunoblot intermediate reactive on hepatitis C virus antibody testing (letter). Lancet 336: 309

Berman M, Alter H J, Ishak K G, Purcell R H, Jones E A 1979 The chronic sequelae of non-A, non-B hepatitis. Annals of Internal Medicine 91: 1–6

Bortolotti F, Tagger A, Cadrobbi P, Crivellaro C, Pregliasco F, Ribero M L, Alberti A 1991 Antibodies to hepatitis C virus in community-acquired acute non-A, non-B hepatitis. Journal of Hepatology 12: 176–180

Bradley D W, Maynard J E 1986 Etiology and natural history of post-transfusion and enterically-transmitted non-A, non-B hepatitis. Seminars on Liver Disease 6: 56–66

Bradley D W, Maynard J E, Popper H et al 1983

Posttransfusion non-A, non-B hepatitis: physicochemical properties of two distinct agents. Journal of Infectious Diseases 148: 254–265
Bradley D W, Krawczynski K, Ebert J W, McCaustland K A, Choo Q–L, Houghton M A, Kuo G 1990 Parenterally transmitted non-A, non-B hepatitis: virus-specific antibody response patterns in hepatitis C virus-infected chimpanzees. Gastroenterology 99: 1054–1060
Brown D, Powell L, Morris A et al 1992 Improved diagnosis of chronic hepatitis C infection by detection of antibody to multiple epitopes: confirmation by antibody to synthetic oligopeptides. Journal of Medical Virology 38: 167–171
Brown J, Dourakis S, Karayiannis P T et al 1992 Seroprevalence of hepatitis C virus nucleocapsid antibodies in patients with cryptogenic chronic liver disease. Hepatology 15: 175–179
Bruix J, Barrera J M, Calvet X et al 1989 Prevalence of antibodies to hepatitis C virus in Spanish patients with hepatocellular carcinoma and hepatic cirrhosis. Lancet ii: 1004–1006
Busch M P, Wilber J C 1992 Hepatitis C virus replication. New England Journal of Medicine 326: 64–65
Carman W F, Dourakis S, Karayiannis P, Crossey M, Drobner R, Thomas H C 1991 Incidence of hepatitis B viraemia, detected using the polymerase chain reaction, after successful therapy of hepatitis B virus carriers with interferon-α. Journal of Medical Virology 34: 114–118
Chambers T J, Hahn C S, Galler R, Rice C M 1990 Flavivirus genome organization, expression and replication. Annual Review of Microbiology 44: 649–688
Chiba J, Ohba H, Matsuura Y et al 1991 Serodiagnosis of hepatitis C virus (HCV) infection with an HCV core protein molecularly expressed by a recombinant baculovirus. Proceedings of the National Academy of Sciences of the USA 88: 4641–4645
Choo Q L, Kuo G, Weiner A J, Overby L R, Bradley D W, Houghton M 1989 Isolation of a cDNA clone derived from a blood-borne non-A, non-B viral hepatitis genome. Science 244: 359–362
Choo Q L, Weiner A J, Overby L R, Kuo G, Houghton M, Bradley D W 1990 Hepatitis C virus: the major causative agent of viral non-A, non-B hepatitis. British Medical Bulletin 46: 423–441
Choo Q L, Richman K H, Han J H et al 1991 Genetic organization and diversity of the hepatitis C virus. Proceedings of the National Academy of Sciences of the USA 88: 2451–2455
Chung R T, Dienstag J L, Kaplan L M 1991 Precise quantitation of hepatitis C RNA using a competitive polymerase chain reaction: correlation of clinical course with levels of circulating RNA. Hepatology 14: 65A
Collett M S, Moennig V, Horzinek M C 1989 Recent advances in pestivirus research. Journal of General Virology 70: 253–266
Coursaget P, Bourdil C, Kastally R et al 1990 Prevalence of hepatitis C virus infection in Africa: anti-HCV antibodies in the general population and in patients suffering from cirrhosis or primary liver cancer. Research in Virology 141: 449–454
Cristiano K, Di Bisceglie A M, Hoofnagle J H, Feinstone S M 1991 Hepatitis C viral RNA in serum of patients with chronic non-A, non B hepatitis: detection by the polymerase chain reaction using multiple primer sets. Hepatology 14: 51–55
Dawson G J, Lesniewski R R, Stewart J L et al 1991 Detection of antibodies to hepatitis C virus in U.S. blood donors. Journal of Clinical Microbiology 29: 551–556
Dienstag J L 1983a Non-A, non-B hepatitis. I. Recognition, epidemiology, and clinical features. Gastroenterology 85: 439–462
Dienstag J L 1983b Non-A, non-B hepatitis. II. Experimental transmission, putative virus agents and markers, and prevention. Gastroenterology 85: 743–768
Donis R O, Corapi W, Dubovi E J 1988 Neutralizing monoclonal antibodies to bovine viral diarrhoea virus bind to the 56K to 58K glycoprotein. Journal of General Virology 69: 77–86
Dourakis S, Brown J, Kumar U et al 1992 Serological response and detection of viraemia in acute hepatitis C virus infection. Journal of Hepatology 14: 370–376
Dull H B 1961 Syringe transmitted hepatitis: a recent epidemic in historic perspective. Journal of the American Medical Association 176: 413–418
Durand J M, Lefevre P, Harle J R, Boucrat J, Vitvitski L, Soubeyrand J 1991 Cutaneous vasculitis and cryoglobulinaemia type II associated with hepatitis C virus infection. Lancet 337: 499–500
Dusheiko G M, Smith M, Scheuer P J 1990 Hepatitis C transmitted by a human bite. Lancet 336: 503–504
Ebeling F, Naukkarinen R, Leikola J 1990 Recombinant immunoblot assay for hepatitis C virus antibody as predictor of infectivity (letter). Lancet 335: 982–983
Ellis L A, Brown D, Conradie J D et al 1990 Prevalence of hepatitis C in South Africa: detection of anti-HCV in recent and stored serum. Journal of Medical Virology 32: 249–251
Enomoto N, Takada A, Nakao T, Date T 1990 There are two major types of hepatitis C virus in Japan. Biochemical and Biophysical Research Communications 170: 1021–1025
Esteban J L, Esteban R, Viladomiu L et al 1989 Hepatitis C virus antibodies among risk groups in Spain. Lancet ii: 294–297
Esteban J L, Gonzalez A, Hernandez J M et al 1990 Evaluation of antibodies to hepatitis C virus in a study of transfusion-associated hepatitis. New England Journal of Medicine 323: 1107–1112
Farci P, Alter H J, Wong D, Miller R H, Shih J W, Jett B, Purcell R H 1991 A long-term study of hepatitis C virus replication in non-A, non-B hepatitis. New England Journal of Medicine 325: 98–104
Fattovich G, Tagger A, Brollo L et al 1991 Hepatitis C virus infection in chronic hepatitis B virus carriers. Journal of Infectious Diseases 163: 400–402
Feinstone S M, Kapikian A Z, Purcell R H, Alter H J, Holland P V 1975 Transfusion associated hepatitis not due to viral hepatitis type A or B. New England Journal of Medicine 292: 767–770
Feinstone S M, Mihalik K B, Kamimura T, Alter H J, London W T, Purcell R H 1983 Inactivation of hepatitis B virus and non-A, non-B hepatitis by chloroform. Infection and Immunity 41: 816–821
Ferri C, Greco F, Longombardo G et al 1991 Antibodies to hepatitis C virus in patients with mixed cryoglobulinemia. Arthritis and Rheumatism 34: 1606–1610
Fong T-L, Shindo M, Feinstone S M, Hoofnagle, J H, Di Bisceglie A M 1991a Detection of replicative intermediates of hepatitis C viral RNA in liver and serum of patients with chronic hepatitis C. Journal of Clinical Investigation 88: 1058–1060
Fong T–L, Di Bisceglie A M, Waggoner J G, Banks S M, Hoofnagle J H 1991b The significance of antibody to

hepatitis C virus in patients with chronic hepatitis B. Hepatology 14: 64–67

Garson J A, Ring C, Tuke P, Tedder R S 1990a Enhanced detection by PCR of hepatitis C virus RNA. Lancet 336: 878–879

Garson J A, Tuke P W, Makris M, Briggs M, Machin S J, Preston F E, Tedder R S 1990b Demonstration of viraemia patterns in haemophiliacs treated with hepatitis-C-virus-contaminated factor VIII concentrates. Lancet 336: 1022–1025

Garson J A, Ring C J A, Tuke P W 1991 Improvement of HCV genome detection with 'short' PCR products. Lancet 338: 1466–1467

Giovannini M, Tagger A, Ribero M L et al 1990 Maternal-infant transmission of hepatitis C virus and HIV infections: a possible interaction (letter). Lancet 335: 1166

Giusti G, Galanti B, Gaeta G B, Gallo C 1987 Etiological, clinical and laboratory data of post-transfusion hepatitis: a retrospective study of 379 cases from 53 Italian hospital. Infection 15: 111–114

Goeser T, Müller H, Padron G, Pfaff E, Hoffman W J, Kommerell B, Theilmann L 1992 Hepatitis C virus replication. New England Journal of Medicine 326: 65

Haddad J, Deny P, Munz-Gotheil C et al 1992 Lymphocytic sialadenitis of Sjögren's syndrome associated with chronic hepatitis C virus liver disease. Lancet 339: 321–323

Han J H, Shyamala V, Richman K H et al 1991 Characterization of the terminal regions of hepatitis C viral RNA: identification of conserved sequences in the 5' untranslated region and poly (A) tails at the 3' end. Proceedings of the National Academy of Sciences of the USA 88: 1711–1715

Harada S, Watanabe Y, Takeuchi K et al 1991 Expression of processed core protein of hepatitis C virus in mammalian cells. Journal of Virology 65: 3015–3021

Haruna Y, Hayashi N, Hiramatsu N, Kashahara A, Fusamoto H, Kamada T 1991 Detection of hepatitis C virus RNA in liver tissue by in situ hybridisation techniques. Hepatology 14: 125A

Hiramatsu N, Hayashi N, Haruna Y et al 1991 Detection of hepatitis C virus (HCV) infected hepatocytes in chronic liver disease. Hepatology 14: 66A

Hofmann H, Kunz C 1990 Low risk of health care workers for infection with hepatitis C virus. Infection 18: 286–288

Hopf U, Moller B, Kuther D, Stemerowicz R et al 1990 Long-term follow-up of posttransfusion and sporadic chronic hepatitis non-A, non-B and frequency of circulating antibodies to hepatitis C virus (HCV). Journal of Hepatology 10: 69–76

Hosein B, Fang C T, Popovsky M A, Ye J, Zhang M, Wang C Y 1991 Improved serodiagnosis of hepatitis C virus infection with synthetic peptide antigen from capsid protein. Proceedings of the National Academy of Sciences of the USA 88: 3647–3651

Houghton M, Weiner A, Han J, Kuo G, Choo Q-L 1991 Molecular biology of the hepatitis C viruses: Implications for diagnosis, development and control of viral disease. Hepatology 14: 381–388

Housset C, Hirschauer C, Degos F 1991 False-positive anti-HCV in biliary cirrhosis (letter). Annals of Internal Medicine 114: 252

Hruby M A, Schauf V 1978 Transfusion related short incubation hepatitis in hemophiliac patients. Journal of the American Medical Association 240: 1355–1357

Inchauspe G, Zebedee S, Lee D-H, Sugitani M, Nasoff M, Prince A M 1991 Genomic structure of the human prototype strain H of hepatitis C virus: comparison with American and Japanese isolates. Proceedings of the National Academy of Sciences of the USA 88: 10292–10296

Infantolino D, Bonino F, Zanetti A R, Lesniewski R R, Barbazza R, Chiaramonte M 1990 Localization of hepatitis C virus (HCV) antigen by immunochemistry on fixed-embedded liver tissue. Italian Journal of Gastroenterology 22: 198–199

Katayama T, Mazda T, Kikuchi S et al 1992 Improved serodiagnosis of non-A non-B hepatitis by an assay detecting antibody to hepatitis C virus core antigen. Hepatology 15: 391–394

Kato N, Hijikata M, Ootsuyama Y, Nakagawa M, Ohkoshi S, Sugimura T, Shimotohno K 1990a Molecular cloning of the human hepatitis C virus genome from Japanese patients with non-A, non-B hepatitis. Proceedings of the National Academy of Science of the USA 87: 9524–9528

Kato N, Yokosuka O, Omata M, Hosoda K, Ohto M 1990b Detection of hepatitis C virus ribonucleic acid in the serum by amplification with polymerase chain reaction. Journal ofClinical Investigation 86: 1764–1767

Kato N, Hijikata M, Nakagawa M, Ootsuyama Y, Muraiso K, Ohkoshi S, Shimotohno K 1991 Molecular structure of the Japanese hepatitis C viral genome. FEBS Letters 280: 325–328

Kiyosawa K, Sodeyama T, Tanaka E et al 1990 Interrelationship of blood transfusion, non-A, non-B hepatitis and hepatocellular carcinoma: analysis by detection of antibody to hepatitis C virus. Hepatology 12: 671–675

Kiyosawa K, Sodeyama T, Tanaka E et al 1991 Intrafamiliar transmission of hepatitis C virus in Japan. Journal of Medical Virology 33: 114–116

Klein R S, Freeman K, Taylor P E, Stevens C E 1991 Occupational risk for hepatitis C virus infection among New York City dentists. Lancet 338: 1539–1542

Koretz R L, Stone O, Gitnick G L 1980 The long term course of non-A, non-B post-transfusion hepatitis. Gastroenterology 79: 893–898

Kremsdorf D, Porchon C, Kim J P, Reyes G R, Bréchot C 1991 Partial nucleotide sequence analysis of a French hepatitis C virus: Implications for HCV genetic variability in the E2/NS1 protein. Journal of General Virology 72: 2557–2561

Kuo G, Choo Q L, Alter H J et al 1989 An assay for circulating antibodies to a major etiologic virus of human non-A, non-B hepatitis. Science 244: 362–364

Kowk S, Higuchi R 1989 Avoiding false positives with PCR (published erratum appears in Nature 1989 Jun 8: 339(6224): 490). Nature 339: 237–238

Lai E C S, Ng I O L, You K T, Fan S T, Mok F P T, Tan E S Y, Wong J 1991 Hepatic resection for small hepatocellular carcinoma: The Queen Mary Hospital experience. World Journal of Surgery 15: 654–659

Lamas E, Baccarini P, Housset C, Kremsdorf D, Bréchot C 1992 Detection of hepatitis C virus (HCV) RNA sequences in liver tissue by in situ hybridisation. Journal of Hepatology 16: 219–223

Lee S-D, Hwang S-J, Lu R-H, Lai K-H, Tsai Y-T, Lo K-J 1991 Antibodies to hepatitis C virus in prospectively followed patients with posttransfusion hepatitis. Journal of Infectious Diseases 163: 1354–1357

Lenzi M, Johnson P J, McFarlane I G et al 1991 Antibodies to hepatitis C virus in autoimmune liver disease: evidence for geographical heterogeneity. Lancet 338: 277–280

Lever A M L, Webster A D B, Brown D, Thomas H C 1984 Non-A, non-B hepatitis occurring in agammaglobulinaemic patients after intravenous immunoglobulin. Lancet ii: 1062–1064
Levrero M, Tagger A, Balsano C et al 1991 Antibodies to hepatitis C virus in patients with hepatocellular carcinoma. Journal of Hepatology 12: 60–63
Lim S G, Lee C A, Charman H, Tilsed G, Griffiths P D, Kernoff P B A 1991 Hepatitis C antibody assay in a longitudinal study of haemophiliacs. British Journal of Haematology 78: 398–402
McFarlane I G, Smih H M, Johnson P J, Bray G P, Vergani D, Williams R 1990 Hepatitis C virus antibodies in chronic active hepatitis: pathogenetic factor or false-positive result? Lancet 335: 754–757
McHutchison J G, Person J L, Govindarajan S et al 1992 Improved detection of hepatitis C virus antibodies in high-risk populations. Hepatology 15: 19–25
McVary K T, O'Conor V J 1989 Transmission of nonA/nonB hepatitis during coagulation pyelolithotomy. Journal of Urology 141: 923–925
Manns M P, Griffin K J, Sullivan K F, Johnson E F 1991 L K M-1 autoantibodies recognize a short linear sequence in P450IID6, a cytochrome P-450 monooxygenase. Journal of Clinical Investigation 88: 1370–1378
Marcellin P, Martinot-Peignoux M, Boyer N, Pouteau M, Aumont P, Erlinger S, Benhamou J-P 1991 Second generation (RIBA) test in diagnosis of chronic hepatitis C. Lancet 337: 551–552
Mattsson L 1989 Chronic non-A, non-B hepatitis with special reference to the transfusion-associated form. Scandinavian Journal of Infectious Diseases suppl. 59: 1–55
Mendenhall C L, Seeff L, Diehl A M, Ghosn S J et al 1991 Antibodies to hepatitis B virus and hepatitis C virus in alcoholic hepatitis and cirrhosis: Their prevalence and clinical relevance. Hepatology 14: 581–589
Miller R H, Purcell R H 1990 Hepatitis C virus shares amino acid sequence similarity with pestiviruses and flaviviruses as well as members of two plant virus supergroups. Proceedings of the National Academy of Sciences of the USA 87: 2057–2061
Mishiro S, Hoshi Y, Takeda K et al 1990 Non-A, non-B hepatitis specific antibodies directed at host-derived epitope: implication for an autoimmune process. Lancet 336: 1400–1403
Miyamura T, Saito I, Katayama T et al 1990 Detection of antibody against antigen expressed by molecularly cloned hepatitis C virus cDNA: application to diagnosis and blood screening for posttransfusion hepatitis. Proceedings of the National Academy of Sciences of the USA 87: 983–987
Morbidity and Mortality Weekly Reports 1989 Non-A, non-B hepatitis-Illinois. Morbidity and Mortality Weekly Reports 38: 529–531
Muraiso K, Hijikata M, Ohkoshi S, Cho M J, Kikuchi M, Kato N, Shimotohno K 1990 A structural protein of hepatitis C virus expressed in E. coli facilitates accurate detection of hepatitis C virus. Biochemical and Biophysical Research Communications 172: 511–516
Nakao T, Enomoto N, Takada N, Takada A, Date T 1991 Typing of hepatitis C virus genomes by restriction fragment length polymorphism. Journal of General Virology 72: 2105–2112
Nasoff M S, Zebedee S L, Inchauspé G, Prince A M 1991 Identification of an immunodominant epitope within the capsid protein of hepatitis C virus. Proceedings of the National Academy of Sciences of the USA 88: 5462–5466
Negro F, Pacchioni D, Shimizu Y, Miller R H, Bussolati G, Purcell R H, Bonino F 1992 Detection of intrahepatic replication of hepatitis C virus RNA by in situ hybridisation and comparison with histopathology. Proceedings of the National Academy of Sciences of the USA 89: 2247–2251
Ogata N, Alter H J, Miller R H, Purcell R H 1991 Nucleotide sequence and mutation rate of the H strain of hepatitis C virus. Proceedings of the National Academy of Sciences of the USA 88: 3392–3396
Oguchi H, Terashima M, Tokunaga S et al 1990 Prevalence of anti-HCV in patients on long-term hemodialysis. Nippon Jinzo Gakkai Shi 32: 313–317
Okamoto H, Okada S, Sugiyama Y et al 1990a The 5'-terminal sequence of the hepatitis C virus genome. Japanese Journal of Experimental Medicine 60: 167–177
Okamoto H, Okada S, Sugiyama Y et al 1990b Detection of hepatitis C virus RNA by a two-stage polymerase chain reaction with two pairs of primers deduced from the 5'-noncoding region. Japanese Journal of Experimental Medicine 60: 215–222
Okamoto H, Okada S, Sugiyama Y et al 1991 Nucleotide sequence of the genomic RNA of hepatitis C virus isolated from a human carrier: Comparison with reported isolates for conserved and divergent regions. Journal of General Virology 72: 2697–2704
Onji M, Kikuchi T, Michitaka K, Saito I, Miyamura T, Ohta Y 1991 Detection of hepatitis C virus antibody in patients with autoimmune hepatitis and other chronic liver diseases. Gastroenterologica Japonica 26: 182–186
Pares A, Barrera J M, Caballeria J et al 1990 Hepatitis C virus antibodies in chronic alcoholic patients: association with severity of liver injury. Hepatology 12: 1295–1299
Patel A, Sherlock S, Dusheiko G, Scheuer P J, Ellis L A, Ashrafzadeh P 1991 Clinical course and histological correlations in post-transfusion hepatitis C: The Royal Free Hospital experience. European Journal of Gastroenterology and Hepatology 3: 491–495
Pereira B J G, Milford E L, Kirkman R L, Levey A S 1991 Transmission of hepatitis C virus by organ transplantation. New England Journal of Medicine 325: 454–460
Perrillo R P, Pohl D A, Roodman S T, Tsai C C 1981 Acute non-A, non-B hepatitis with serum sickness-like syndrome and aplastic anaemia. Journal of the American Medical Association 245: 494–496
Pohjanpelto P, Tallgren M, Farkkila M et al 1991 Low prevalence of hepatitis C antibodies in chronic liver disease in Finland. Scandinavian Journal of Infectious Diseases 23: 139–142
Pol S, Driss F, Devergie A, Bréchot C, Berthelot P, Gluckman E 1990 Is hepatitis C virus involved in hepatitis-associated aplastic anemia? Annals of Internl Medicine 113: 435–437
Polywka S, Laufs R 1991 Hepatitis C virus antibodies among different groups at risk and patients with suspected non-A, non-B hepatitis. Infection 19: 81–84
Ponz E, Campistol J M, Barrera J M, Gil C, Pinto J, Andreu J, Bruguera M 1991 Hepatitis C virus antibodies in patients on hemodialysis and after kidney transplantation. Transplant Proceedings 23: 1371–1372
Poterucha J J, Rakela J, Ludwig J, Taswell H F, Wiesner R H 1991 Hepatitis C antibodies in patients with chronic hepatitis of unknown etiology after orthotopic liver transplantation. Transplant Proceedings 23: 1495–1497
Quiroga J A, Campillo M L, Catillo I, Bartolomé J, Porres

J C, Carreño V 1991 IgM antibody to hepatitis C virus in acute and chronic hepatitis C. Hepatology 14: 38–43
Rassam S W, Dusheiko G M 1991 Epidemiology and transmission of hepatitis C infection. European Journal of Gastroenterology 3: 585–591
Read A E, Donegan E, Lake J et al 1991a Hepatitis C in patients undergoing liver transplantation. Annals of Internal Medicine 114: 282–284
Read A E, Donegan E, Lake J et al 1991b Hepatitis C in liver transplant recipients. Transplant Proceedings 23: 1504–1505
Scheuer P J, Ashrafzadeh P, Sherlock S, Brown D, Dusheiko G M 1992 The pathology of hepatitis C. Hepatology 15: 567–571
Schlesinger J J, Brandriss M W, Cropp C B, Monath T P 1986 Protection against yellow fever in monkeys by immunization with yellow fever virus nonstructural protein NS1. Journal of Virology 60: 1153–1155
Schramm W, Roggendorf M, Rommel F et al 1989 Prevalence of antibodies to hepatitis C virus (HCV) in haemophiliacs. Blut 59: 390–392
Schulman S, Grillner L 1990 Antibodies against hepatitis C in a population of Swedish haemophiliacs and heterosexual partners. Scandinavian Journal of Infectious Diseases 22: 393–397
Schvarcz R, von-Sydow M, Weiland O 1990 Autoimmune chronic active hepatitis: changing reactivity for antibodies to hepatitis C virus after immunosuppressive treatment. Scandinavian Journal of Gastroenterology 25: 1175–1180
Shimizu Y K, Purcell R H 1989 Cytoplasmic antigen in hepatocytes of chimpanzees infected with non-A, non-B hepatitis virus or hepatitis delta virus: relationship to interferon. Hepatology 10: 764–768
Shimizu Y K, Weiner A J, Rosenblatt J et al 1990 Early events in hepatitis C virus infection of chimpanzees. Proceedings of the National Academy of Sciences of the USA 87: 6441–6444
Shimizu, Y K, Weiner, A J, Rosenblatt, J et al 1991 Early events in hepatitis C virus infection in chimpanzees. In: Hollinger F B, Lemon S M, Margolis H S (eds) Viral hepatitis and liver disease. Williams & Wilkins, Baltimore, pp 393–396
Shindo M, Di-Bisceglie A M, Cheung L, Shih J W, Cristiano K, Feinstone S M, Hoofnagle J H 1991a Decrease in serum hepatitis C viral RNA during alpha-interferon therapy for chronic hepatitis C. Annals of Internal Medicine 115: 700–704
Shindo M, Di Bisceglie A M, Silver J, Limjoco T, Hoofnagle J H, Feinstone S M 1991b Quantitation of hepatitis C virus RNA in serum using the polymerase chain reaction and a colorimetric enzyme detection system. Hepatology 14: 64A
Simmonds P, Zhang L Q, Watson H G et al 1990 Hepatitis C quantification and sequencing in blood products, haemophiliacs, and drug users. Lancet 336: 1469–1472
Tabor E, Gerety R J, Drucker J A et al 1978 Transmission of non-A, non-B hepatitis from man to chimpanzee. Lancet i: 463–466
Takada N, Takase S, Enomoto N, Takada A, Date T 1992 Clinical backgrounds of the patients having different types of hepatitis C virus genomes. Journal of Hepatology 14: 35–40
Takamizawa A, Mori C, Fuke I et al 1991 Structure and organization of the hepatitis C virus genome isolated from human carriers. Journal of Virology 65: 1105–1113
Takehara T, Hayashi N, Mita E et al 1992 Detection of the minus strand of hepatitis C virus RNA by reverse transcription and polymerase chain reaction: Implications for hepatitis C virus replication in infected tissue. Hepatology 15: 387–390
Takeuchi K, Kubo Y, Boonmar S et al 1990a The putative nucleocapsid and envelope protein genes of hepatitis C virus determined by comparison of the nucleotide sequences of two isolates derived from an experimentally infected chimpanzee and healthy human carriers. Journal of General Virology 71: 3027–3033
Takeuchi K, Kubo Y, Boonmar S et al 1990b Nucleotide sequence of core and envelope genes of the hepatitis C virus genome derived directly from human healthy carriers. Nucleic Acids Research 18: 4626
Tanaka E, Kiyosawa K, Sodeyama T et al 1991 Significance of antibody to hepatitis C virus in Japanese patients with viral hepatitis: relationship between anti-HCV antibody and the prognosis of non-A, non-B post-transfusion hepatitis. Journal of Medical Virology 33: 117–122
Tanaka K, Hirohata T, Koga S et al 1991 Hepatitis C and hepatitis B in the etiology of hepatocellular carcinoma in the Japanese population. Cancer Research 51: 2842–2847
Tedder R S, Gilson R J, Briggs M et al 1991 Hepatitis C virus: evidence for sexual transmission. British Medical Journal 302: 1299–1302
Thaler M M, Park C-K, Landers D V et al 1991 Vertical transmission of hepatitis C virus. Lancet 338: 17–18
Tor J, Llibre J M, Carbonell M et al 1990 Sexual transmission of hepatitis C virus and its relation with hepatitis B virus and HIV. British Medical Journal 301: 1130–1133
Tzakis A G, Arditi M, Whitington P F et al 1988 Aplastic anemia complicating orthotopic liver transplantation for non-A, non-B hepatitis. New England Journal of Medicine 319: 393–396
Ulrich P P, Romeo J M, Lane P K, Kelly I, Daniel L J, Vyas G N 1990 Detection, semiquantitation, and genetic variation in hepatitis C virus sequences amplified from the plasma of blood donors with elevated alanine aminotransferase. Journal of Clinical Investigation 86: 1609–1614
Van der Poel C L, Reesink H W, Schaasberg W, Leentvaar-Kuypers A, Bakker E, Exel-Oehlers P J, Lelie P N 1990 Infectivety of blood seropositive for hepatitis C virus antibodies. Lancet 335: 558–560
Van der Poel C, Cuypers H, Reesink H et al 1991a Risk factors in hepatitis C virus-infected blood donors. Transfusion 31: 777–779
Van der Poel C L, Reesink H W, Mauser-Bunschoten E P et al 1991b Prevalence of anti-HCV antibodies confirmed by recombinant immunoblot in different population subsets in The Netherlands. Vox Sanguinis 61: 30–36
Van der Poel C L, Cuypers H T M, Reesink H W et al 1991c Confirmation of hepatitis C virus infection by new four-antigen recombinant immunoblot assay. Lancet 337: 317–319
van-Zijl M, Wensvoort G, de-Kluyver E et al 1991 Live attenuated pseudorabies virus expressing envelope glycoprotein E1 of hog cholera virus protects swine against both pseudorabies and hog cholera. Journal of Virology 65: 2761–2765
Vucelic B, Hadzic N, Dubravcic D 1988 Chronic persistent hepatitis. Long term prospective study on the natural course of the disease. Scandinavian Journal of Gastroenterology 23: 551–554
Wang J-T, Wang T-H, Lin J-T, Sheu J-C, Lin S-M,

Chen D-S 1991 Hepatitis C virus RNA in saliva of patients with post-transfusion hepatitis C infection. Lancet 337–48
Weiland E, Stark R, Haas B, Rumenapf T, Meyers G, Thiel H J 1990 Pestivirus glycoprotein which induces neutralizing antibodies forms part of a disulfide-linked heterodimer. Journal of Virology 64: 3563–3569
Weiner A J, Kuo G, Bradley D W et al 1990 Detection of hepatitis C viral sequences in non-A, non-B hepatitis. Lancet 335: 13
Weiner A J, Brauer M J, Rosenblatt J et al 1991 Variable and hypervariable domains are found in the regions of HCV corresponding to the flavivirus envelope and NS1 proteins and the pestivirus envelope glycoproteins. Virology 180:842–848
Wejstal R, Lindberg J, Lundin P, Norkrans G 1987 Chronic non-A, non-B hepatitis. A long-term follow-up study in 49 patients. Scandinavian Journal of Gastroenterology 22: 1115–1122
Wejstal R, Hermodsson S, Iwarson S, Norkrans G 1990 Mother to infant transmission of hepatitis C virus infection. Journal of Medical Virology 30: 178–180
Wonke B, Hoffbrand A V, Brown D, Dusheiko G 1990 Antibody to hepatitis C virus in multiply transfused patients with thalassaemia major. Journal of Clinical Pathology 43: 638–640
Xu J, Brown D, Harrison T, Lin Y, Dushieko G 1992 Absence of hepatitis B virus pre-core mutants in patients with chronic hepatitis B responding to alpha interferon. Hepatology 15: 1002–1006
Yap S H, Willems M, Van Den Ord J, Habets W, Middledorp J M, Hellings J-A, Nevens F et al 1991 Detection of HCV antigen by immunohistochemical staining: a histological marker of HCV infection. Hepatology 14: 67A
Yuasa T, Ishikawa G, Manabe S, Sekiguchi S, Takeuchi K, Miyamura T 1991 The particle size of hepatitis C virus estimated by filtration through microporous regenerated cellulose fibre. Journal of General Virology 72: 2021–2024
Zanetti A R, Tanzi E, Zehender G et al 1990 Hepatitis C virus RNA in symptomless donors implicated in post-transfusion non-A, non-B hepatitis (letter). Lancet 336: 448
Zeldis J B, Dienstag J L, Gale R P 1983 Aplastic anemia and hepatitis. American Journal of Medicine 74: 64–68
Zhang L Q, Simmonds P, Ludlam C A, Brown A J 1991 Detection, quantification and sequencing of HIV-1 from the plasma of seropositive individuals and from factor VIII concentrates. AIDS 5: 675–681

UPDATE

- *Serology*. The detection of antibodies to additional recombinant proteins and synthetic peptides, especially those representative of NS5 and envelope regions, has been a feature of recent work. Increased sensitivity and better serologic profile has been obtained by the addition of further antigens to new and prototype third-generation assays. It is to be hoped that these can be improved to a stage where the serologic data obtained will be of use in identifying viraemia and predicting prognosis or response to treatment.

- *Genotypes*. It is now clear that there are at least six clearly defined subgroups or genotypes of HCV. The recognition of these will be important for optimal diagnostic testing especially if, as has been suggested, the infecting genotype can affect serologic response. As with serologic profile, there is a growing body of evidence suggesting that genotyping may be of value as a prognostic indicator or in predicting response to treatment. At the moment however, the pressing need is for standardization of nomenclature and methodologies for genotyping of HCV.

17. Treatment

Jay H. Hoofnagle

Chronic hepatitis C ranks as one of the most important causes of chronic liver disease, cirrhosis and hepatocellular carcinoma. The recent identification of the hepatitis C virus (HCV) (Choo et al 1989) and development of immunoassays for detection of specific antibody (anti-HCV) (Kuo et al 1989) have provided the means of accurate assessment of the role of hepatitis C in causing morbidity and mortality from liver disease. In most developed countries of the world, chronic hepatitis C is second only to alcohol as a cause of end-stage liver disease and is now a major indication for liver transplantation. Typically, chronic hepatitis C is a prolonged and insidious disease marked by persistent elevations in serum aminotransferases and HCV RNA in serum. As such, this disease warrants a specific and effective therapy. At present, however, the treatment of chronic hepatitis C is problematical and unsatisfactory. The only agent of proven benefit is alpha interferon.

TRIALS OF ALPHA INTERFERON

Pilot studies of alpha interferon were begun before the identification of HCV, but nevertheless demonstrated that therapy was followed by marked improvements in serum aminotransferases in up to 70% of patients (Hoofnagle et al 1987). Subsequently, multiple randomized controlled trials have documented that a 6 month course of alpha interferon in doses of 2–5 million units (MU) thrice weekly leads to a remission in disease in approximately 50% of patients (Davis et al 1989, Di Bisceglie et al 1989, Jacyna et al 1989, Weiland et al 1989, Ferenci et al 1990, Gomez-Rubio et al 1990, Realdi et al 1990, Saracco et al 1990, Causse et al 1991, Marcellin et al 1991, Alberti et al 1992, Craxi et al 1992). These remissions were marked by a fall in serum aminotransferases into the normal range and improvement in liver histology, particularly the degree of hepatocellular necrosis and inflammation. Retrospective analyses demonstrated that this decrease in aminotransferase activities was accompanied by a fall in HCV RNA levels in blood and that most patients who developed normal aminotransferases on therapy became HCV RNA negative (Shindo et al 1991, 1992a).

Unfortunately, most studies of alpha interferon in chronic hepatitis C found a very high relapse rate once therapy was stopped. This relapse was accompanied by a return of serum HCV RNA and progressive liver injury. Thus, in most studies the rate of long-term responses to alpha interferon has been only 10–25% (Davis et al 1989, Di Bisceglie et al 1989, Marcellin et al 1990). Preliminary results from two European trials provide conflicting result on whether higher doses and more prolonged courses of interferon result in appreciably higher long-term response rates (Alberti et al 1992, Craxi et al 1992).

RECOMMENDATIONS

Alpha interferon is currently licensed for use in chronic hepatitis C. Patients should have well-compensated chronic hepatitis C with persistently raised serum aminotransferase activities, chronic hepatitis by liver biopsy and serological or epidemiological evidence of HCV infection (anti-HCV or a history of exposure to blood before the onset of hepatitis).

The recommended regimen of alpha interferon is 3 MU given either subcutaneously or intramuscularly three times weekly for 6 months (24 weeks). Actually, the optimal dose and duration of therapy are controversial, with some investigators recommending higher doses (5 MU three times weekly) for more prolonged periods (12 months or 48 weeks).

Initial evaluation

Therapy should not be started until a firm diagnosis of chronic hepatitis C is made. Chronic hepatitis C can be diagnosed on the basis of finding persistent elevations of aminotransferases, anti-HCV in serum and liver histology compatible with chronic hepatitis. Patients should have elevations in serum aminotransferases for at least 6 months, or for a shorter period if it is clear from the history that the disease has been long-standing. A liver biopsy is necessary to document that chronic hepatitis is present, to assess the severity of hepatocellular injury and fibrosis and to help rule out other diagnoses such as alcoholic liver disease, haemochromatosis and sclerosing cholangitis. Patients should have firm serological or epidemiological evidence of hepatitis C. Current assays for anti-HCV are somewhat problematical. A small percentage (5–10%) of patients with chronic HCV infection will test negative for anti-HCV, even by second-generation enzyme immunoassays (false-negative results) (Kuo et al 1989, Shindo et al 1991). Furthermore, a proportion of patients with other forms of liver disease will test positive for anti-HCV (false-positive results) (McFarlane et al 1990, Alter 1991). With future improvements in assays for anti-HCV these problems will lessen. At present, some form of confirmatory testing in needed to verify the diagnosis. Thus, the presence of a compatible history or epidemiological features (exposure to blood or blood products), the finding of HCV RNA in serum (Wiener et al 1990, Farci et al 1991, Shindo et al 1991) or HCV antigen in liver (Krawczynski et al 1992), or the application of confirmatory assays for anti-HCV such as Western blot or neutralization (Van del Poel et al 1991), are valuable in confirming the diagnosis.

Starting therapy

Alpha interferon is usually given as a subcutaneous injection three time weekly. Patients need to be carefully trained in how to measure and administer the injection and how to dispose correctly of all materials. Most adolescents and adults can be trained to self-administer interferon.

Alpha interferon therapy can be started on an outpatient basis but patients should be warned that there is frequently a period of fever and chills, malaise, body aches and nausea that begins 4–8 h after the injection and lasts for 4–12 h. This influenza-like syndrome is common and is most severe with the initial dose of interferon. The severity of the reaction lessens with each subsequent injection and often disappears. Most patients find that taking acetaminophen at the time of the injection or a few hours thereafter is helpful in preventing or lessening the symptoms.

Side-effects

Alpha interferon has many side-effects, but most are self-limiting and tolerable, and almost all are rapidly and fully reversible when the drug is stopped (Renault & Hoofnagle 1989). Furthermore, most side-effects are dose related and can be ameliorated with modification of the dosage. A thorough discussion of side-effects often makes patients and physicians wary of therapy. However, it should be stressed that in the typical doses of 3 MU three times weekly alpha interferon is well tolerated by most patients. Indeed, a percentage of patients with chronic hepatitis C feel better during interferon therapy than before. The fear of interferon's side-effects should not cause avoidance of therapy. Treatment can be started and if side-effects are truly intolerable, interferon can be stopped early. In randomized trials of alpha interferon, only 3–10% of patients were not able to tolerate the full 6 months of treatment (Davis et al 1989, Marcellin et al 1990).

As discussed above, an influenza-like syndrome of fever (to 39°C), chills, anorexia, nausea, myalgia, sleep disturbance and fatigue occurs in almost all patients 4–8 h after the initial injection of alpha interferon. This syndrome lessens with subsequent injections, but some degree of chronic or intermittent fatigue, muscle aches and feverishness persists in many patients with prolonged therapy at doses of 3–5 MU three times weekly. Fatigue is the most common, troublesome side-effect; it is typically intermittent, variable and somewhat unpredictable. Muscle and back aches, headaches, poor appetite, nausea, gastrointestinal upset and diarrhoea are also common; and some patients lose weight while receiving interferon. About 20% of patients experience hair loss during interferon therapy, but normal hair growth resumes soon after interferon is stopped. Patients may also complain of mental torpor, and increased need for sleep, a reduction in mental concentration and attention span and difficulty with short-term memory.

Psychological side-effects of alpha interferon include depression, mood swings, irritability and anxiety. These psychiatric side-effects occur in 10–20% of patients and are the most common reason for discontinuing therapy early (Renault & Hoofnagle 1989). All of these side-effects are partially alleviated by reducing the dose of interferon. Others are helped by psychological counselling or even steady encouragement by the physician. In patients who complain of irritability and depression, small doses of methylphenidate (15–30 mg twice daily) can be of benefit in allowing continuation of therapy at the appropriate dose.

Alpha interferon also has myelosuppressive effects. In doses of 3–5 MU three times weekly, white blood cells and platelet counts decrease by 25–50%, usually within 2 weeks of starting therapy. The haematocrit also falls during the 6-month course of interferon, but usually by only 5–10%. Some patients are more susceptible to the myelosuppressive effects of interferon, particularly those who have pre-existing bone marrow compromise. Patients generally tolerate the myelosuppression of interferon very well, and problems with severe infections, bleeding or anaemia are rare without the presence of other predisposing factors.

Serious side-effects of alpha interferon therapy are uncommon but need to be discussed with the patient and remembered by the physician who is monitoring therapy. These adverse effects include induction of autoimmunity and autoimmune diseases, increased susceptibility to infections and severe psychiatric syndromes. Retrospective testing reveals that more than half of patients treated for 6 months with alpha interferon develop serological autoimmune reactions, such as antithyroid or antinuclear autoantibodies (Mayet et al 1989). Approximately 2% of patients will also develop autoimmune disease, most typically autoimmune thyroid disease – either hyper- or hypothyroidism (Lisker-Melman et al 1992). There have been individual case reports of other autoimmune conditions developing during interferon therapy such as haemolytic anaemia, granulocytopenia, thrombocytopenic purpura, type 1 diabetes and autoimmune hepatitis. Most but not all of these autoimmune conditions eventually resolved after therapy was stopped.

Susceptibility to bacterial infections is perhaps the most important serious side-effect of therapy. Bacterial infections are particularly common among patients with cirrhosis or with a history of recurrent bacterial infections (urinary tract infections, bronchitis, sinusitis). Patients who develop fever after the first week of interferon therapy should be carefully evaluated for a bacterial infection.

Finally, severe psychiatric complications develop in a small proportion of patients receiving interferon, particularly if they have had previous central nervous system trauma or dysfunction. Cases of severe psychotic reactions, paranoid ideation, deep depression, anxiety or panic attacks and attempted suicide have been reported in patients during interferon treatment (Renault & Hoofnagle 1989). These reactions should lead to immediate discontinuation of treatment. Other rare, poorly documented, severe side-effects of alpha interferon therapy include acute allergic reactions, acute cardiac failure, acute renal failure and seizures.

Monitoring

Patients should be seen, questioned about side-effects and have blood tested for serum aminotransferases and blood counts every 1–4 weeks while on therapy. The frequency of the visits should be based upon the severity of the liver disease and the degree of side-effects experienced. Follow-up should be for at least 6 months after stopping therapy to assess whether the response obtained is sustained. Follow-up liver biopsies are not needed unless retreatment is considered.

In hepatitis C, serum aminotransferases generally decrease during interferon therapy. Indeed, a worsening of serum aminotransferases is a reason for early discontinuation of therapy. Several cases of acute exacerbation of hepatitis C with alpha interferon therapy have been reported, and some of these have been severe and even life-threatening (Papo et al 1992, Shindo et al 1992b). The cause of the exacerbations was unclear; some patients were found to have autoimmune hepatitis rather than hepatitis C as initially suspected.

RESPONSE TO TREATMENT

Definition of response

Responses to alpha interferon therapy in chronic hepatitis C can be grouped into four patterns. Approximately 25% of all patients have a *sustained beneficial response* (Fig. 17.1). In these patients, aminotransferases begin to fall within the first months of treatment and are often normal by 2–3 months. Simultaneous testing for HCV RNA in serum reveals that the fall in aminotransferases is accompanied by a loss of this marker of viraemia. Aminotransferases remain normal and HCV RNA undetectable even after therapy is stopped. Late relapses can occur but are not common and have been reported only in patients who had HCV RNA in serum despite normal aminotransferases.

Another 25% of patients with chronic hepatitis C have a complete response while on alpha interferon but promptly *relapse* when the medication is stopped (Fig. 17.2). These patients may become negative for HCV RNA on treatment, but redevelop this viral marker when interferon is stopped and aminotransferases rise. Disease activity eventually returns to the original level in these individuals, but some amelioration of disease has been reported in a percentage of these patients. Retreatment is often considered in these patients, but should only be undertaken if the alpha interferon therapy was well tolerated and if an altered regimen is given, using either a higher dose or a more prolonged course.

A third group consists of about 25% of patients with chronic hepatitis C who have *a partial or transient response* only. In some patients, serum aminotransferases decrease but do not become normal (Fig. 17.3: partial response). In others, serum aminotransferases become normal only

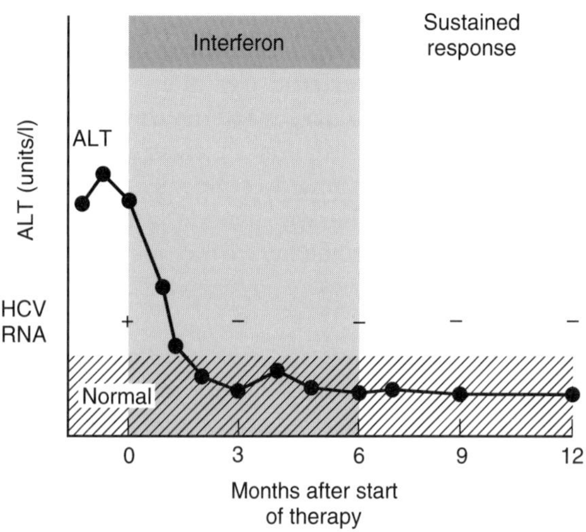

Fig. 17.1 A sustained complete response to alpha interferon in a patient with chronic hepatitis C. Abbreviations: HCV RNA, hepatitis C virus RNA by polymerase chain reaction; ALT, alanine aminotransferase.

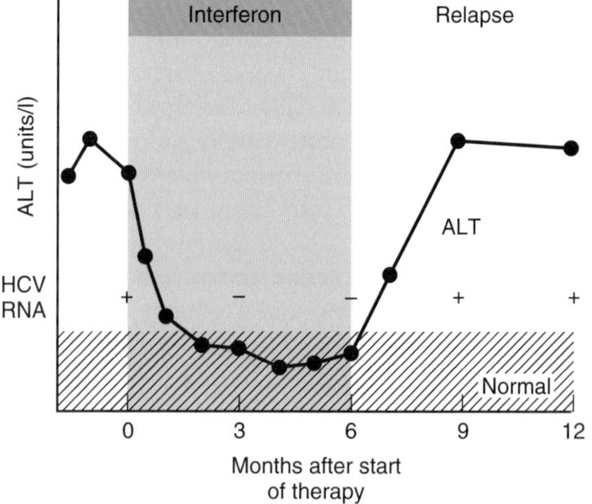

Fig. 17.2 A transient complete response to alpha interferon with relapse when therapy was stopped in a patient with chronic hepatitis C.

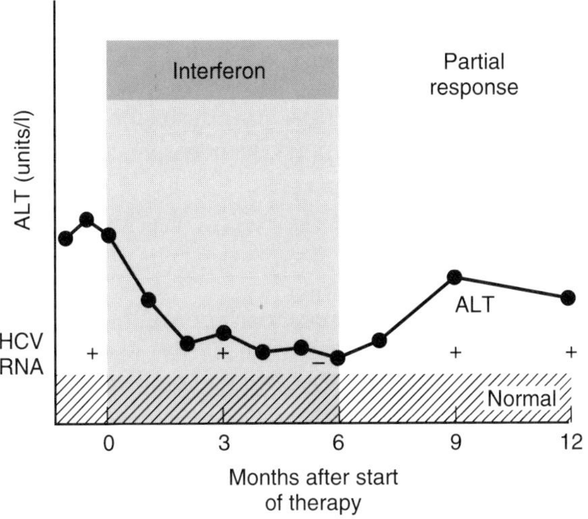

Fig. 17.3 A partial response to alpha interferon with improvement but not normalization of serum aminotransferases.

transiently and then rise despite continuation of treatment (Fig. 17.4: breakthrough). Such patients may manifest a fall of aminotransferases into the normal range if the dose of interferon is increased. Unfortunately, not all patients will be able to tolerate the increase in side-effects that usually accompanies the higher dose. Most of these patients do not have a sustained amelioration of disease activity with treatment.

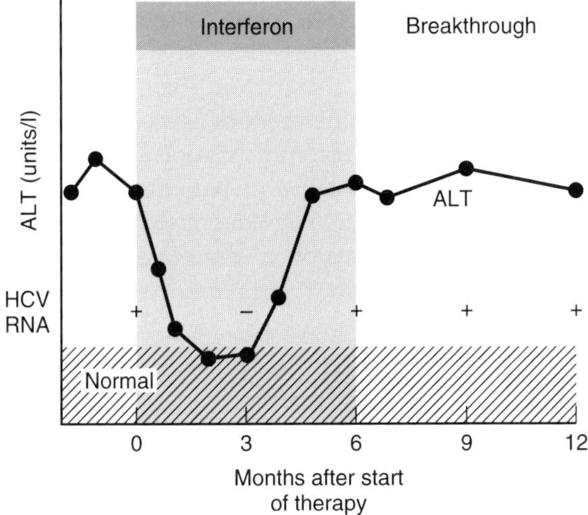

Fig. 17.4 A transient complete response to alpha interferon with a break-through despite continuation of therapy in a patient with chronic hepatitis C.

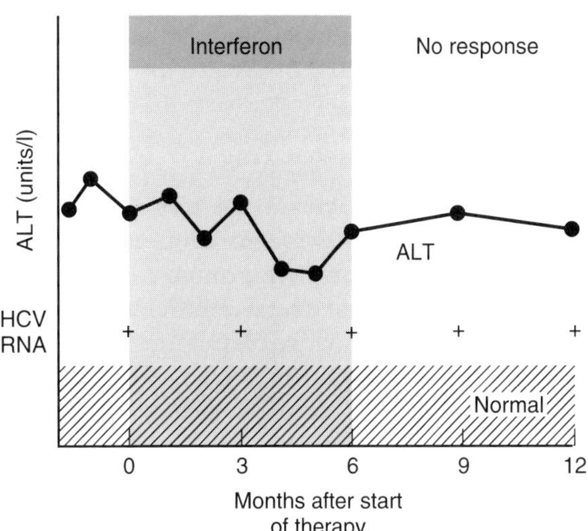

Fig. 17.5 No response to alpha interferon therapy in a patient with chronic hepatitis C.

A final 25% of patients with chronic hepatitis C have *no response* to alpha interferon therapy at all (Fig. 17.5). In these patients serum aminotransferase activities remain elevated and serum HCV RNA is present during treatment. The cause of these patients' resistance to interferon effects is unclear. Treatment should be stopped early – after 2–3 months – in these patients, and they should not be given higher doses or repeated courses.

Predictors of response

Unfortunately, there are no reliable features that predict which patient is likely to respond to treatment, nor are there reliable features that can predict when a sustained response has occurred before therapy is stopped (Davis et al 1989, Camma et al 1992). A few clinical features appear to be weak predictors of the type of response to alpha interferon. Thus, patients who manifest a breakthrough in disease activity on therapy are usually those with severe disease and high initial levels of serum aminotransferases (an elevation of greater than 10-fold) (Di Bisceglie et al 1989). Patients who manifest no response at all tend to be those with advanced disease and cirrhosis (Marcellin et al 1990, Camma et al 1992). The profile of a patient who is most likely to have a long-term beneficial response to treatment is someone with mild to moderate hepatitis C with a relatively short history of chronic disease.

Increasing the response rate

Most attempts to increase the response rate in chronic hepatitis C have focused on using higher doses of interferon or more prolonged periods of treatment. At present there is little information regarding the advisability of retreatment or use of higher doses of alpha interferon. Pilot studies have assessed other antiviral agents in chronic hepatitis C that might be used alone or in combination with alpha interferon. The most promising agent is ribavirin, a nucleoside analogue that has been reported to reduce serum aminotransferase levels in a high proportion of patients with chronic hepatitis C (Reichard et al 1991, Di Bisceglie et al 1992). Unfortunately, the improvements in aminotransferases have not been matched by improvements in liver histology or serological markers. The possible role of a combination of ribavirin with interferon awaits further investigations.

Obviously, advances in understanding of the HCV on a molecular basis and development of cell culture systems for HCV replication would aid in screening and assessing antiviral compounds for this disease (Houghton et al 1991). In the absence of such a system, use of agents that have activity against other flaviviruses in cell culture would be appropriate.

Patients with atypical forms of chronic hepatitis C

The current recommendations for alpha interferon therapy are for patients with typical, well-compensated chronic hepatitis C. The criteria for selecting patients eliminates some patients who may deserve treatment, such as patients with acute hepatitis C, those with advanced cirrhosis, those with normal serum aminotransferase levels, patients who are anti-HCV negative and those who are immunosuppressed.

Acute hepatitis C

Acute hepatitis C represents approximately 25% of sporadic hepatitis in the USA and western countries. The disease can be severe and prolonged, although it is rarely fulminant. Most importantly, however, acute hepatitis C commonly progresses to chronic hepatitis C with persistence of the viraemia and persistence of the hepatocellular injury (Alter 1991). For these reasons, therapies of acute hepatitis C have focused on prevention of chronic disease rather than amelioration of the acute disease. Indeed, it seems logical that early intervention in acute hepatitis C is warranted to prevent chronicity and the injury of chronic hepatitis.

There have been three prospective controlled trials of alpha interferon therapy of acute (post-transfusion) hepatitis C (Table 17.1) (Alberti et al 1991, Omata et al 1991, Viladomiu et al 1992). All three studies were small, but all demonstrated a decreased rate of chronicity in treated patients. Unfortunately, cases of chronic hepatitis C still occurred despite treatment. Whether therapy during the acute phase offered any benefit over delaying therapy to the chronic phase was not evaluated. While all three studies suggested benefit for alpha interferon therapy, in practice it should not be used for routine cases of acute hepatitis C. The reasons for this recommendation are several.

First, as many as 50% of patients with acute hepatitis C recover spontaneously and alpha interferon would thus be an unnecessary expense

Table 17.1 Alpha interferon therapy of acute hepatitis C: three trials

Reference	Normal ALT at 12 months		
	No. treated	Interferon (%)	Placebo (%)
Omata et al 1991	20	64	11
Alberti et al 1991	22	57	37
Viladomiu et al 1992	28	53	31

and burden for these patients. Furthermore, the trials done in acute hepatitis C concerned cases of post-transfusion hepatitis only, which has become an exceedingly rare cause of hepatitis C as a result of routine testing of blood donations. Finally, the diagnosis of acute hepatitis C is very problematic at present; anti-HCV is rarely present in serum until late in the disease or in convalescence so that early diagnosis to facilitate early treatment is usually not possible (Alter et al 1989).

Thus, alpha interferon should not be used in routine cases of acute hepatitis C. Therapy can, however, be considered in acute cases in which it becomes clear that the disease is not resolving normally. Thus, if serum aminotransferases remain elevated for more than 2 months after onset of illness, therapy is appropriate, especially since interferon is well tolerated during acute hepatitis and can result in prompt improvement in serum aminotransferases. The optimal dose and duration of therapy is not known; it is reasonable to use the same regimen recommended for chronic hepatitis C: 3 MU thrice weekly for 6 months.

Patients with decompensated liver disease

Patients with advanced chronic hepatitis C and clinically apparent cirrhosis can respond to alpha interferon treatment (Martin et al 1989). These patients, however, have troublesome side-effects from interferon, such as severe fatigue, weight loss, anorexia, bacterial infections and psychological changes. Treatment should be reserved for those patients with early or mildly decompensated cirrhosis. For more advanced cases, liver transplantation offers the only possibility for a sustained improvement in health. Thus, patients with clinically apparent cirrhosis due to chronic hepatitis C should be treated only by physicians with experience in using interferon and in caring for patients with severe liver disease. Patients should be carefully monitored for adverse side-effects, particularly bacterial infections.

Patients with normal aminotransferases

Patients with chronic HCV infection have various degrees of liver injury. Many patients with this infection will have no elevations in serum aminotransferases. Some of these may have a degree of chronic hepatitis by liver biopsy. These patients are often detected when they have donated blood and been found to be anti-HCV positive. At present, one would not recommend treatment of patients with chronic hepatitis C who have normal or near-normal serum aminotransferase activities. Chronic HCV infection can be benign and not associated with progressive liver injury (Di Bisceglie et al 1991). These patients should be followed and treated only if biochemical evidence of disease becomes manifest.

Children with chronic hepatitis C

There have been few reports of therapy of chronic hepatitis C in children (Ruiz-Moreno et al 1992). However, there is no reason to believe that children would be either more or less susceptible to interferon treatment, and treatment is recommended in doses of 3 MU/m^2 (up to 3 MU total dose) three times weekly for 6 months. The criteria for treatment should be the same as those for adults. Most small children tolerate interferon therapy very well with no side-effects except for moderate degrees of hair loss that is reversed within 3–6 months after therapy is completed.

Patients with atypical serological patterns

Some patients with chronic hepatitis C test negative for anti-HCV, and some of these may not have clear-cut evidence of exposure to hepatitis C. The diagnosis can be established by research assays such as those for anti-HCV by immunoblotting or for HCV RNA by reverse transcription–polymerase chain reaction (Farci et al 1991, Shindo et al 1991). These patients can be treated, but only if there is clear-cut evidence of HCV infection. There is need for caution because patients with autoimmune hepatitis who are mistakenly thought to have hepatitis C can exhibit a worsening of the hepatitis with interferon treatment (Papo et al 1992, Shindo et al 1992b). Autoimmune hepatitis is typically associated with the presence of hyperglobulinaemia and autoantibodies such as antinuclear antibody (ANA) and smooth muscle antibodies (SMA). However, 10–20% of adults with chronic hepatitis C have ANA or SMA or both reactivities and may, nevertheless, respond well to alpha interferon (Di Bisceglie et al 1989, 1991).

Immunosuppressed patients

Patients with immune deficiencies or those receiving immunosuppressive medications are frequently infected with HCV and represent a difficult group of patients to manage. Chronic hepatitis C is common among oncology patients, renal dialysis patients, patients with human immunodeficiency virus (HIV) infection and patients who have received a solid organ transplant. Furthermore, the immunosuppression itself may worsen the underlying liver disease (Martin et al 1989, 1991, Pereira et al 1991).

There have been no prospective, controlled trials of therapy of chronic hepatitis C in immunosuppressed patients. Small uncontrolled trials of therapy of patients who have both HCV and HIV infection suggest that interferon may ameliorate the chronic hepatitis (Boyer et al 1992). Furthermore, preliminary reports of therapy of patients with recurrent hepatitis C after liver transplantation suggest that alpha interferon can suppress viral replication and improve serum aminotransferases even in the face of large doses of immunosuppressive medications (H I Wright et al 1992, T L Wright et al 1992). The safety and relative benefit of interferon therapy in these situations is still unclear and warrants further study. At the present time, immunosuppressed patients should probably not receive therapy outside of prospective controlled trials.

Patients who do not respond to interferon

At present there is no information to suggest that non-responder patients benefit from a repeat course of alpha interferon. These patients are excellent candidates for future trials of other antiviral agents. Patients who have no response to alpha interferon should also be carefully evaluated for the possibility of having another form of liver disease, perhaps unrelated to their HCV infection, such as autoimmune (McFarlane et al 1990) or alcoholic hepatitis (Mendenhall et al 1991).

Patients who respond to alpha interferon initially but relapse when therapy is stopped can occasionally benefit from higher doses given for a more prolonged period (Shindo et al 1992a). Other patients may benefit from long-term remission. However, these uses of alpha interferon must be considered experimental and only used if the response to treatment is clear cut, the underlying disease severe, and the interferon well tolerated.

CONCLUSIONS

Alpha interferon is effective as therapy for patients with well-compensated chronic hepatitis C. The recommended treatment regimen is 3 MU given subcutaneously three times weekly for 6 months. Side-effects can limit treatment, and some patients, especially those with advanced disease or other significant medical illnesses, cannot tolerate therapy. Most importantly, however, alpha interferon induces long-term remissions in disease in only 10–25% of patients. In view of these shortcomings, new approaches to therapy of chronic hepatitis C are needed. The most promising approaches are combinations with other antiviral agents. With the recent characterization of the HCV and the development of in vitro and in vivo methods to study viral replication and pathogenesis, the possibilities for significant breakthroughs in therapies of acute and chronic hepatitis C are great.

REFERENCES

Alberti A, Chemello L, Benvegnu L, Belussi F, Tagger A, Roul A 1991 Pilot study of interferon alpha-2a therapy in preventing chronic evolution of acute hepatitis C. In: Hollinger F B, Lemon S M, Margolis H (eds) Viral hepatitis and liver disease. Williams & Wilkins, Baltimore, pp 656–658

Alberti A, Chemello G, Diodati et al 1992 Treatment of chronic hepatitis C with different regimens of interferon alpha-2a. Hepatology (abstract) 16: 75A

Alter H J 1991 Descartes before the horse: I clone, therefore I am: the hepatitis C virus in current perspective. Annals of Internal Medicine 115: 644–648

Alter H J, Purcell R H, Shih J W, Melpolder J C, Houghton M, Choo Q–L, Kuo G 1989 Detection of antibody to hepatitis C virus in prospectively followed transfusion recipients with acute and chronic non-A, non-B hepatitis. New England Journal of Medicine 321: 1494–1499

Boyer N, Marcellin P, Degott C et al 1992 Recombinant interferon-alpha for chronic hepatitis C in patients positive for antibody to human immunodeficiency virus. Journal of Infectious Diseases 165: 723–724

Camma C, Craxi A, Tine F et al 1992 Predictors of response to alpha-interferon in chronic hepatitis C: a multivariate analysis on 361 treated patients (abstract). Hepatology 16: 131A

Causse X, Godinot H, Chevallier M et al 1991 Comparison of 1 or 3 MU of interferon alfa-2b and placebo in patients with chronic non-A, non-B hepatitis. Gastroenterology 101: 497–502

Choo Q–L, Kuo G, Weiner A J, Overby L R, Bradley D W, Houghton M 1989 Isolation of a cDNA clone derived from a blood-borne non-A, non-B viral hepatitis genome. Science 244: 359–363

Craxi A, Di Marco V, Lo Iacono O et al 1992 Lymphoblastoid alpha interferon for post-transfusion chronic hepatitis C: a randomized trial of 6 vs. 12 months treatment (abstract). Journal of Hepatology 16: 58

Davis G L, Balart L A, Schiff E R et al 1989 Treatment of chronic hepatitis C with recombinant interferon alfa: a multicenter randomized, controlled trial. New England Journal of Medicine 321: 1501–1506

Di Bisceglie A M, Martin P, Kassianides C et al 1989 Recombinant interferon alfa therapy for chronic hepatitis C: a randomized, double-blind, placebo-controlled trial. New England Journal of Medicine 321: 1506–1510

Di Bisceglie A M, Goodman Z D, Ishak K G, Hoofnagle J H, Melpolder J J, Alter H J 1991 Long-term clinical and histopathological follow-up of chronic posttransfusion hepatitis. Hepatology 14: 969–973

Di Bisceglie A M, Shindo M, Fong T–L et al 1992 A pilot study of ribavirin therapy for chronic hepatitis C. Hepatology 16: 649–654

Farci P, Alter H J, Wong D, Miller R H, Shih J W, Gett B, Purcell R H 1991 A long-term study of hepatitis C virus replication in non-A, non-B hepatitis. New England Journal of Medicine 325: 98–104

Ferenci P, Vogel W, Pristautz H et al 1990 One-year treatment of chronic non-A, non-B hepatitis with interferon alfa-2b. Journal of Hepatology 11: S50–S56

Gomez-Rubio M, Porres J C, Castillo I, Quiroga J A, Moreno A, Carreno V 1990 Prolonged treatment (18 months) of chronic hepatitis C with recombinant alpha-interferon in comparison with a control group. Journal of Hepatology 11: S63–S67

Hoofnagle J H, Mullen K D, Jones D B et al 1987 Treatment of chronic non-A, non-B hepatitis with recombinant human alpha interferon. A preliminary report. New England Journal of Medicine 315: 1575–1578

Houghton M, Weiner A, Han J, Kuo G, Choo Q L 1991 Molecular biology of the hepatitis C viruses: implications for diagnosis, development and control of viral disease. Hepatology 14: 381–388

Jacyna M R, Brooks M G, Loke R H T, Main J, Murray-Lyons I M, Thomas H C 1989 Randomised controlled trial of interferon alpha (lymphoblastoid interferon) in chronic non-A, non-B hepatitis. British Medical Journal 298: 80–82

Krawczynski K, Beach M J, Bradley D W et al 1992 Hepatitis C virus antigen in hepatocytes: immunomorphologic detection and identification. Gastroenterology 102: 622–629

Kuo G, Choo Q–L, Alter H J et al 1989 An assay for circulating antibodies to a major etiologic virus of human non-A, non-B hepatitis. Science 244: 359–364

Lisker-Melman M, Di Bisceglie A M, Usala S J, Weintraub B, Murray L M, Hoofnagle J H 1992 Development of thyroid disease during therapy of chronic viral hepatitis with interferon alfa. Gastroenterology 102: 2155–2160

McFarlane I G, Smith H M, Johnson P J, Bray G P, Vergani D, Williams R 1990 Hepatitis C virus antibodies in chronic active hepatitis: pathogenic factor or false-positive result? Lancet 335: 754–757

Marcellin P, Boyer N, Giostra E et al 1991 Recombinant human alpha-interferon in patients with chronic non-A, non-B hepatitis: a multicenter randomized controlled trial from France. Hepatology 13: 393–397

Martin P, Di Bisceglie A M, Kassianides C, Lisker-Melman M, Hoofnagle J H 1989 Rapidly progressive non-A, non-B hepatitis in patients with human immunodeficiency virus infection. Gastroenterology 97: 1559–1561

Martin P, Munoz S J, Di Bisceglie A M et al 1991 Recurrence of hepatitis C infection following orthotopic liver transplantation. Hepatology 13: 719–721

Mayet W–J, Hess G, Gerken G, Rossol S, Voth R, Manns M, Meyer zum Buschenfelde K–H 1989 Treatment of chronic type B hepatitis with recombinant alpha interferon induces autoantibodies not specific for autoimmune chronic hepatitis. Hepatology 10: 24–28

Mendenhall C L, Seeff L, Diehl A M et al 1991 Antibodies to hepatitis C virus in alcoholic hepatitis and cirrhosis: their prevalence and clinical relevance.

Omata M, Yokosuka O, Takano S et al 1991 Resolution of acute hepatitis C after therapy with natural beta interferon. Lancet 338: 914–915

Papo T, Marcellin P, Bernuau J, Durand F, Poynard T, Benhamou J–P 1992 Autoimmune chronic hepatitis exacerbated by alpha-interferon. Annals of Internal Medicine 166: 51–53

Pereira B J G, Milford E L, Kirkman R L, Levey A S 1991 Transmission of hepatitis C virus by organ transplantation. New England Journal of Medicine 325: 454–460

Realdi G, Diodata G, Bonetti P, Scaccabarozzi S, Alberti A, Ruol A 1990 Recombinant human interferon alfa-2a in community-acquired non-A, non-B chronic active hepatitis: preliminary results of a randomized, controlled trial. Journal of Hepatology 11: S68–S71

Renault P F, Hoofnagle J H 1989 Side effects of alpha interferon. Seminars in Liver Disease 9: 273–281

Reichard O, Andersson J, Schvarcz R, Weiland O 1991 Ribavirin treatment for chronic hepatitis C. Lancet 337: 1058–1061

Ruiz-Moreno M, Rua M J, Castillo I et al 1992 Treatment of children with chronic hepatitis C with recombinant interferon-alpha: a pilot study. Hepatology 16: 882–885

Saracco G, Rosina F, Torrani Cerenzia M R et al 1990 A randomized controlled trial of interferon alfa-2b as therapy for chronic non-A, non-B hepatitis. Journal of Hepatology 11: S43–S49

Shindo M, Di Bisceglie A M, Cheung L et al 1991 Decrease in serum hepatitis C viral RNA during alpha-interferon therapy for chronic hepatitis C. Annals of Internal Medicine 115: 700–704

Shindo M, Di Bisceglie A M, Hoofnagle J H 1992a Long-

term follow-up patients with chronic hepatitis C treated with alpha interferon. Hepatology 15: 1013–1016
Shindo M, Di Bisceglie A M, Hoofnagle J H 1992b Acute exacerbation of liver disease during alpha interferon therapy for chronic hepatitis C. Gastroenterology 102: 1406–1408
Van der Poel C L, Cuypers H T M, Reesink H W et al 1991 Confirmation of hepatitis C virus infection by new four-antigen recombinant immunoblot assay. Lancet 337: 317–319
Viladomiu L, Genesca J, Esteban J I, et al 1992 Interferon-alpha in acute posttransfusion hepatitis C: a randomized, controlled trial. Hepatology 16: 767–769
Weiland O, Schvarcz R, Wejstal R, Norkrans G, Foberg U, Fryden A 1989 Interferon alpha 2b treatment of chronic post-transfusion non-A, non-B hepatitis: interim results of a randomized controlled open study. Scandinavian Journal of Infectious Diseases 21: 127–132
Weiner A J, Kuo G, Bradley D W et al 1990 Detection of hepatitis C viral sequences in non-A, non-B hepatitis. Lancet 335: 1–3
Wright H I, Gavaler J S, Van Thiel D H 1992 Preliminary experience with alpha-2b interferon therapy of viral hepatitis in liver allograft recipients. Transplantation 53: 121–124
Wright T L, Ferrell L, Lake J et al 1992 Hepatitis C viral RNA in patients on interferon (IFN)-alpha for post-liver transplant (OLTx) hepatitis (abstract). Gastroenterology 102: A910

18. Epidemiology and prevention

Alan D. Kitchen   John A. J. Barbara

Current data suggest that, although hepatitis C virus (HCV) may not be the cause of all cases of non-A, non-B hepatitis (NANBH), it probably accounts for between 75 and 90% of cases of post-transfusion NANBH (PT-NANBH). Furthermore, 60–85% of haemophiliacs, 50–75% of intravenous drug users and 10–20% of haemodialysis patients are, or have been, infected with the virus (Esteban et al 1990, S D Lee et al 1991, Yuki et al 1992). Additionally, there are likely to be cases of HCV infection in individuals outside of these risk groups, which may be associated with unnoticed elevations in transaminase levels because they are otherwise asymptomatic. Although our knowledge of the epidemiology of HCV infection is currently incomplete the new assays have been responsible for rapid progress in the field.

EPIDEMIOLOGY OF HCV INFECTION

Several points should be borne in mind when analysing the reported data concerning HCV infection. Firstly, many of the currently quoted prevalence rates for HCV infection are based on 'first generation' (C100–3) assays (see Ch. 16 for details of anti-HCV assays) and are often therefore likely to be underestimated. Conversely, several reports lack subsequent confirmation of the screening results, leading to considerable overestimation of prevalence rates. The 'second-generation' assays now available are far superior to the original tests (Aach et al 1991, Laurian et al 1992). The use of a range of different antigens on the solid phase (Ch. 16) and also in the improved 'confirmatory' (or supplementary) assays has improved considerably the predictive value of anti-HCV testing, although there is still considerable scope for improvement.

Secondly, as might be expected, there are discrepancies between the prevalence data generated by the use of serological tests and results obtained using the polymerase chain reaction (PCR). The latter detects the presence of viral nucleic acid. HCV infection can lead to a chronic carrier state in a proportion of infected individuals, and this is marked by the presence of HCV RNA usually, but not always, in the presence of anti-HCV (Cuthbertson et al 1991). HCV RNA in the absence of anti-HCV may occur in patients in the viraemic stage early in acute infection, and indeed may be of diagnostic value in identifying such individuals as there may be a delay of several months following infection before seroconversion occurs (see Ch. 14).

There are also a number of individuals in whom anti-HCV is present but HCV RNA cannot (or can no longer) be detected. It is possible that in some individuals the carrier state is not established and detection of anti-HCV simply signals previous (resolved) infection; in this case the antibody might be expected to disappear gradually. Alternatively, if anti-HCV levels are maintained, the carrier state may be established with low-level viral replication in the liver resulting in very low (undetectable) levels of circulating RNA. A further possibility is that viraemia may be intermittent with periods of either no circulating RNA, or very low levels of circulating RNA that again might not be readily detected.

Thirdly, there is evidence that a number of infected individuals 'serorevert', so that anti-HCV may no longer be detectable. In these patients HCV RNA can also no longer be detected. It is possible that this could occur in individuals who do not develop chronic infection, and it may represent clearance of the virus. If this is the case, many instances of seroreversion will not be identified unless long-term monitoring of infected individuals is undertaken. The possibility also remains that some individuals who are 'confirmed' anti-HCV positive by supplementary assays in the absence of PCR reactivity are truly immune. Extensive follow-up studies are required to resolve these various issues.

In an attempt to close the 'window period' between initial HCV infection and the detection of anti-HCV (a period in which HCV RNA may be detected), the value of the detection of IgM anti-HCV has been studied (Clemens et al 1992). The IgM class of antibody to the core of HCV was detected in 13 of 15 PT-NANBH patients. In 9 of the 13 it was detected at the same time, or earlier than, the IgG anti-HCV core response. Late IgM anti-HCV was detectable in a number of patients. Although detection of IgM anti-HCV may be a useful marker of acute infection, it is unlikely to be of value in 'closing' the window period, because it does not appear significantly earlier than IgG anti-HCV.

Transmission of HCV

The transmission of HCV may conveniently be considered in relation to the specific route of infection and the particular groups of individuals at risk of infection.

Although the mechanism of transmission of HCV is likely to be similar to that of HBV, it is clear that there are some significant differences. Current data suggest that in developed countries the sources of HCV infection in infected individuals can be grouped as follows: in approximately 43% of patients the source of transmission is undefined; 35% of patients have a history of intravenous drug use (IVDU); 15% have been directly exposed to the virus; 5% of patients have a history of transfusion; and 2% are health care workers (M J Alter et al 1989, Insight 1992). How representative these figures are is hard to determine as there are so many factors to take into account, not the least of which is the effectiveness of the questioning and the accuracy of the histories volunteered by infected individuals.

Following infection, anti-HCV does not usually appear until relatively late after the onset of hepatitis, at least with first-generation assays, with up to 30% of patients seroconverting during the acute infection, up to 85% seroconverting within 6 months of infection, and up to 99% seroconverting within 1 year (Esteban et al 1989). As mentioned earlier, a few patients do not produce detectable anti-HCV at any time during chronic infection, although serum HCV RNA may be detected; in other patients the lack of detectable anti-HCV may represent earlier, resolved, acute infection. In addition, acute infection may occasionally resolve spontaneously, usually within a year, with the disappearance of anti-HCV and the absence of chronicity. In one analysis, approximately 50% of HCV infections progressed to chronic liver disease, 20% of which subsequently progressed to cirrhosis (Alter 1989).

The route of infection is unclear in a significant proportion of individuals who have been infected with HCV. Furthermore, as yet we have no convenient marker of the level of infectivity of HCV carriers analogous, for example, to the HBeAg/anti-HBe status of HBV carriers. Factors such as elevated liver function tests (LFTs) in HCV carriers may provide some clue as to level of infectivity (Bellobuono et al 1991), but we do not know if the level of infectivity of a carrier decreases, or increases, or even fluctuates, over a period of time. Individuals in whom HCV infection can be shown to have occurred, or may be likely to occur, can be divided into the following general groups:

1. Intravenous drug users.
2. Recipients of blood and blood derivatives.
3. Recipients of organ and tissue transplants.
4. Those infected by undefined routes ('sporadic' or 'community acquired' with no readily identifiable risk factors).
5. Close contacts of individuals infected by one of the other routes.

Transmission by intravenous drug use (IVDU)

Individuals sharing syringes or needles for IVDU are at high risk of infection by parenterally transmitted blood-borne infectious agents. Consequently, the prevalence of anti-HCV in intravenous drug users is high. The reported prevalences range from 48 to 80% in a number of studies performed in developed countries (Esteban et al 1989, Mortimer et al 1989, Roggendorf et al 1989, van der Poel et al 1991). Alter et al (1990) reported a prevalence of 55% in intravenous drug users in the USA when tested within 6 weeks of the onset of illness; however, this figure rose to 94% when these individuals were monitored for extended periods of up to 4 years. Whether this is also the case in other countries is not known, although it has been reported that seroconversion may not occur for ever a year from the point of exposure to HCV (H J Alter et al 1989), at least when using first-generation enzyme-linked immunosorbent assays (ELISAs).

Transmission by blood and blood products

It is clear that transfusion of infected blood and blood products is a particularly efficient route of transmission of HCV, and indeed of other blood-borne infectious agents. There is now clear evidence that approximately 80–90% of cases of PT-NANBH are due to HCV infection (H J Alter et al 1991). Whilst there are a large amount of data concerning both the transmission of HCV through blood and blood products and the prevalence of HCV in blood donors, only 0.5–10% of unscreened blood (red cell or single-donor product) transfusions give rise to PT-NANBH (van der Poel et al 1989, Esteban et al 1990, Aach et al 1991, Contreras et al 1991). Although blood transfusion is an efficient route of transmission, it cannot account for the prevalence and maintenance of HCV in the population; most individuals do not receive a transfusion during their lifetime. However, transfusion can be a significant source of infection in certain patient groups, such as haemophiliacs, who are exposed to large amounts of single donor products or to products derived from large pools of plasma. Prior to current safety practices the majority of patients in these groups showed evidence of transfusion-transmitted HCV infection.

One important aspect of transfusion-transmitted infection is that the actual point of infection can be identified, both in terms of time and of the specific donor(s) implicated as source(s) of the various infectious agents.

Transmission to patients receiving single-donor products As reported above, generally less than 10% of recipients of unscreened transfusions develop PT-NANBH, and the figure is often much lower. In those who do develop PT-NANBH, more than 80% develop HCV infection (Esteban et al 1989, Conover et al 1991); in some studies 100% of the NANBH patients studied developed HCV infection (Lelie et al 1992). Table 18.1 presents data from a number of countries on the incidence of PT-NANBH transmitted by single-donor products and the percentage of these cases subsequently found to be due to HCV infection. Transmission was not linked with age or sex, but was linked to the number of units of blood transfused (Lee et al 1991, Takano et al 1992) and, more specifically, to those units containing HCV-RNA (Farci et al 1991). Not all anti-HCV-positive donations will transmit HCV (Aach et al 1991), but this may in part reflect a lack of specificity of the test in certain studies.

Haemodialysis patients are a well-defined risk group because of the dangers of long-term intensive transfusion therapy. In these patients risk is linked solely to the number of units transfused. Not surprisingly, the prevalence of anti-HCV in these patients is higher in areas with a higher prevalence of HCV infection in the general, and hence donor, population (Nasser et al 1992, Tamura et al 1992). The prevalence of anti-HCV in haemodialysis patients varies widely, from as little as 2.4% in the Netherlands (van der Poel et al 1991) to 20% in Spain (Esteban et al 1989), and as high as 45.5% in Saudi Arabia (Nasser et al 1992) and 47.2% in Taiwan (Sheu et al 1992).

Transmission to patients receiving products derived from large pools of plasma. This group largely comprises haemophilia A and B patients, whose high risk of infection through infected blood products has long been recognized because of their high donor exposure. The effectiveness of virally inactivated factor VIII concentrates will be discussed later in the section concerned with the prevention of HCV infection; however, emerging data do indicate that effectively treated products do not transmit HCV infection

Table 18.1 Reported incidence of PTNANBH and the role of HCV

Country	Incidence of PT-NANBH (%)	PT-NANBH due to HCV (%)	Reference
Germany	NG	79	Roggendorf et al 1989
Japan	23	62	Takano et al 1992
Netherlands	2	78	van der Poel et al 1989
Netherlands	2	100	Lelie et al 1992
Spain	10	88	Esteban et al 1989
Taiwan	13	87	Lee et al 1991
Taiwan	11	80	Wang et al 1992
UK	0.5	50	Contreras et al 1991
USA	NG	88	H J Alter et al 1989
USA	9	91	Aach et al 1991

NG, not given.

(Study Group of UK Haemophilia Centre Directors 1988, C Pereira et al 1991, Pistello et al 1991).

Between 60 and 100% of haemophiliacs who have at any time received untreated products are anti-HCV positive (Roggendorf et al 1989, Schulman & Grillner 1990, Pistello et al 1991, Laurian et al 1992). The high risk of transmission of infectious virus in the uninactivated concentrates was clearly reflected in the report of Simmons et al (1990), who found HCV RNA in all the standard commercial batches of factor VIII tested. Heat-treated concentrates were found not to contain HCV RNA.

As with other risk groups, Pistello et al (1991) found that the transmission of HCV is not related to the age of the patient or the type and severity of haemophilia. The transfused products are the only factors associated with risk of infection; haemophiliacs who had never been treated with clotting factor concentrates were anti-HCV negative. The finding of a small number of haemophiliacs who either do not develop detectable anti-HCV or who serorevert after a period of time (H J Alter et al 1989, Schulman & Grillner 1990) indicates that even in such a high-prevalence population not all infected patients progress to chronic infection; some undergo acute infection with apparent resolution.

Transmission by organ and tissue transplantation

There is now evidence to suggest that HCV infection may be transmitted through organ and tissue transplantation. Post-transplantation liver disease is still an important cause of morbidity and mortality, especially in renal transplant recipients (Braun 1990), in whom NANBH has been considered to be a significant cause (Weir et al 1985, Boyce et al 1988).

In an attempt to define the role of HCV infection in post-transplantation liver disease, B J G Pereira et al (1991) screened a group of 716 organ donors for anti-HCV. Thirteen (1.8%) of these donors were anti-HCV positive. A total of 29 organs (kidney, heart, liver) were given to 29 recipients, 14 of whom (48%) developed NANBH. Eight of the 14 were anti-HCV positive. These results indicated that organ transplantation could transmit HCV.

A case of transmission of HCV by a frozen bone graft was subsequently reported by Eggen & Nordbo (1992) in an interesting sequence of events. Bone substance from a patient undergoing hip replacement (who was subsequently found to be HCV seropositive) was stored frozen for 8 weeks before use in a bone graft to a previously healthy blood donor with no other risk factors. This donor recovered from the operation, subsequently resumed donating but transmitted HCV infection because he had suffered an asymptomatic HCV infection.

Present data on HCV transmission by donated organs and tissues are limited, but it is clear that the screening of potential organ donors for anti-HCV would be beneficial in minimizing any risks of post-transplantation HCV infection.

Transmission by undefined routes

In approximately 40–50% of cases of HCV infection the precise route of infection cannot be defined (M J Alter et al 1989, 1990). In infected individuals with no defined risks, sporadic or community-acquired infection can occur, raising the possibility of less obvious routes of infection.

Sexual transmission

By analogy with HBV, sexual transmission (especially homosexually) seemed a likely mode of spread of HCV. Whilst a number of studies have addressed the question of sexual transmission of HCV, results are somewhat conflicting. However, the weight of evidence does seem to favour some degree of sexual transmission. The presence of anti-HCV has been demonstrated in 11–35% of spouses or sexual partners of HCV-infected patients (M J Alter et al 1989, Akahane et al 1992, Liou et al 1992), the antibody in these individuals correlating with the detection of HCV RNA in the patient's serum. However, the results of other similar studies do not concur with this data. H H Lin et al (1991) did not detect anti-HCV in the spouses of 11 pregnant women; Schulman & Grillner (1990) did not detect anti-HCV in the spouses of 13 HCV-infected haemophiliacs, and Crawford et al (1992) found only one anti-HCV-positive partner amongst the partners of 26 intravenous drug users. If intravenous drug use is the likely cause of HCV infection in one partner, it is often difficult to exclude drug use as a cause of infection in the other partner, if they are also seropositive.

It is not clear whether the conflicting study results are due to differences in the susceptibility of different populations to HCV infection, differences in the level of infectivity in individuals, infection with different strains of HCV that may have different degrees of infectivity, the frequency of sexual contact, the extent of condom use or the number of partners. Riestra & Carcaba (1991) have found a higher prevalence of anti-HCV in homosexual men who have multiple sexual partners, 23.1% for those with more than three partners per week compared with 0% for those with fewer than three partners per week. Sexual transmission in prostitutes (Hyams et al 1992) and individuals with multiple partners may indicate that in some instances the specific risk factor for sexual transmission is the number of partners.

Overall, current data suggest that sexual transmission of HCV does occur to some extent. The importance of this route is uncertain as the efficiency of transmission appears to be low (van Doornum et al 1991, Brettler et al 1992). Transmission is clearly not as efficient as that of HBV infection, and in general there are significant differences in the transmission patterns of the two viruses. This is particularly apparent when the sexual transmission of HCV in homosexual men is studied; the transmission rates of HCV are very low, unlike the high rates of infection with HBV (Esteban et al 1989, Melbye et al 1990). This is noteworthy since sexual transmission of HBV and HIV is more likely to occur during homosexual than during heterosexual intercourse.

Mother to child transmission

From our current knowledge of the routes of transmission of HCV it is likely that vertical transmission from mother to infant, as frequently seen with HBV- or HIV-infected mothers, does occur. If this is indeed the case, this route may play some part in the maintenance of the reservoir of HCV in the population and may contribute to the occurrence of sporadic or community-acquired cases of HCV infection.

Although Reesink et al (1990) demonstrated infection in infants, the infants came from anti-HCV-negative as well as anti-HCV positive mothers, so that mother to child transmission could not be confirmed. Subsequently Thaler et al (1991) did find evidence of transmission; 8 of 10 pregnant women were found to be anti-HCV and HCV RNA positive; HCV RNA was detected in all eight of their infants and persisted during the 2 to 19-month period in which it was possible to follow up the infants. However, several of the reported cases of materno-fetal infection with HCV involve HIV-infected mothers, and this may increase the chances of HCV transmission.

It is not certain whether transmission to the infant occurs in utero by infection via the placenta during the development of the fetus, during birth by direct infection with virus present in the cervical secretions or in the perinatal period through breast milk. All three routes are well documented for methods of mother to child infection of a number of infectious agents, and transmission of HCV may thus be possible by any one (or more) of these routes.

Transmission to non-sexual close contacts

A number of cases of infection through non-sexual household contact have been reported. Kiyosawa et al (1991a) studied the family members of patients with chronic HCV liver disease and found that 15 of 195 (8%) of the family members of anti-HCV-positive patients were anti-HCV positive. This compared with 0 of 100 (0%) of the family members of anti-HCV-negative patients; Bellobuono et al (1991) found that the prevalence of anti-HCV in family members of anti-HCV-positive blood donors was 7.3% compared with 0.62% in the local blood donor population: elevated alanine aminotransferase (ALT) levels in the index case may be associated with an increased risk of transmission. Nishiguchi et al (1992) also reported similar findings: 21% of children of anti-HCV-positive parents were anti-HCV positive, whilst none of the children of anti-HCV-negative parents was anti-HCV positive, but they also showed that transmission occurred when the index patients had a large viral load. The actual route of transmission in all of these cases has still to be determined.

It is possible that horizontal infection may occur as a result of contamination of household items such as eating utensils or toothbrushes, or through the small spillages of blood and body fluids that may occur in the domestic situation. To try to identify potentially infectious body fluids, Liou et al (1992) examined saliva, urine and ascites from seropositive patients with chronic liver disease for the presence of HCV RNA. Wang et al (1992) also investigated the presence of HCV in saliva and examined the saliva from patients with PT HCV for HCV RNA. Both studies found HCV RNA in these body fluids; interestingly both groups found HCV RNA in the saliva of 50% of the patients studied. Liou et al (1992) found HCV RNA in 100% of ascites samples and in 7% of urine samples. Further evidence for the role of saliva in the transmission of HCV was provided by Dusheiko et al (1990), who reported the probable transmission of HCV by a human bite. In all cases the presence of HCV RNA in body fluids correlated with the presence of HCV RNA in serum, and the amount of RNA was less than that present in serum. It is therefore clear that transmission of HCV by body fluids is quite feasible and many cases of household contact may result from transmission in this way. However, the possibility of blood contaminating saliva should be borne in mind.

Increased prevalences of anti-HCV by ELISA-1 in institutions for mentally handicapped children have also been reported (Vranckx 1989), consistent with the possibility of transmission via saliva.

Transmission through non-human vectors

Transmission through non-human vectors, notably arthropods, is a well-defined routed for some infectious agents. Yellow fever virus, the prototype flavivirus, is transmitted by this route. Currently, however, there are no confirmed reports of non-human transmission of HCV.

Transmission to contacts of individuals infected by one of the other routes

Whilst the likely mechanisms of transmission of HCV in this group are as discussed above, we have considered them separately because the specific exposure may not be immediately obvious. In most cases individuals in this group are likely to have been infected by household or personal contact, both sexual and non-sexual, or by occupational contact.

Occupational contact. Some individuals may be at increased risk of infection by a number of infectious agents by the nature of their occupation. In these cases transmission is invariably by exposure to infectious body fluids following direct and close contact with infected individuals. Needlestick injuries in nursing and medical staff are probably the most common cause of occupational exposure in the clinical environment. A number of cases of needlestick transmission of HCV infection have been reported in nursing and medical staff (Schlipkoter et al 1990, Vaglia et al 1990, Cariani et al 1991, Kiyosawa et al 1991b). Although clearly identifying such cases, Kiyosawa et al (1991) pointed out that the actual rate of infection (4 of 110 anti-HCV-positive needlestick victims developed hepatitis and three of the four seroconverted) is quite low when the transmission rate of HCV by transfusion of seropositive blood and the risk of HBV infection following needlestick are considered. The reason for this is probably the generally low virus titre in serum and the consequently small inoculum involved in needlestick injury.

The reports of the probable transmission of HCV by saliva (Dusheiko et al 1990, Liou et al 1992, Wang et al 1992) have been of some concern in dental practice, where the degree of exposure of dental staff to the saliva and blood of patients is high. In a large study in New York dentists, Klein et al (1991) found that the prevalence of anti-HCV in dentists and dental surgeons, having excluded any with any other infection risk, was higher than in control groups, 1.75% of all dentists compared with 0.14% of control, and 9.3% of dental surgeons compared with 0.97% of other dentists were seropositive. Thus dental staff did appear to be at increased risk of HCV infection. A smaller study of dentists in South Wales (Herbert et al 1992) did not produce similar results. None of the dentists in this study had detectable anti-HCV. As with several other questions relating to HCV transmission, further studies are needed to resolve the inconsistencies.

The epidemiology of HCV infection is not fully understood. Although the advent of screening assays for anti-HCV and the use of PCR to demonstrate HCV RNA have generated rapidly a large amount of data, there are still some very large gaps in our understanding of HCV infection. These relate especially to the precise routes of transmission and the mechanisms of maintenance of the reservoir of infection in the general population.

PREVENTION OF HCV INFECTION

General preventive measures

The prevention of the transmission of any infectious agent requires knowledge of the routes of infection to identify the points at which preventive intervention would be most effective. The problems of prevention of transmission of HCV are likely to be similar to those of HIV and HBV, where a number of different routes are involved and a combination of direct and indirect measures are required.

A vaccine to protect against HCV infection is not yet available and may take some time to develop. Passive protection using high-titre specific immunoglobulin is also currently unavailable although the production of such a preparation may be feasible. However, at present the role of specific HCV antibodies in the prevention and control of infection has not been defined.

Currently therefore, prevention of HCV transmission can be achieved only by preventing exposure to the virus. This may either be by indirect means – screening blood and organ donors for evidence of infection – or by direct means – physical prevention of exposure to the virus. The screening of donated blood and organs will ensure that the majority of the blood components and organs are free from HCV and recipients of blood or organs will therefore not be exposed to the virus. Methods to prevent any physical contact with the virus will reduce transmission by some routes, such as parenteral transmission in intravenous drug users, transmission through sexual contact and transmission through occupational contact. Unfortunately, there may also be other routes of transmission (e.g. via saliva) which are harder to prevent.

In the case of HCV infection, prevention can be applied to some, but not all, of the routes of infection identified. On the basis of current figures (H J Alter et al 1989), it is hard to see how transmission could be avoided in the approximately 40% of cases of HCV with an undefined source of transmission.

The methods of prevention of HCV transmission will be considered in relation to the individual routes or categories of transmission:

- blood transfusion
- organ transplantation
- IVDU
- sexual contact
- sporadic/community-acquired infection.

Prevention of transmission by blood transfusion

The prevention of transmission of any infectious agent by transfusion of blood or blood products can be approached in a number of ways. All approaches are directed towards minimizing the exposure of transfusion recipients to the infectious agent. There are four ways of achieving this.

Self-exclusion. Ensuring the safety of donated blood begins with the identification of the 'safe donor'. Safe donors are those who, by virtue of their normal behavioural patterns, are at low risk of parenteral or sexual infections. Potential donors are now provided with sufficient information to be able to decide not to donate if they think they have been exposed to dangerous activities. This system is by no means perfect but it is a vital first stage in maintaining the safety of the blood supply.

Serological screening of donated blood. Transfusion-transmitted infections are largely preventable if the appropriate screening programmes are designed and implemented. As described above, the use of the screening assays themselves should form only one part (albeit a significant part) of an overall strategy for ensuring the safety of transfused blood and its derivatives.

Donors infected by HCV, and therefore potentially at risk of transmitting the virus, are initially identified by the presence of antibodies to the virus in the serum. The primary screening tests performed are thus directed at detecting circulating anti-HCV. In addition to antibody, viral nucleic acid can also be detected in the serum of a number of infected individuals, both in the presence of antibody and occasionally, but importantly, in the absence of (detectable) antibody. Current data suggest that donors with circulating HCV RNA are more likely to transmit HCV through transfusion than those possessing anti-HCV in the absence of RNA (Farci et al 1991). Thus, not all anti-HCV positive donations will transmit infection and, importantly, not all potentially infectious donors will necessarily be detected by current screening tests for anti-HCV. Whilst blood donors cannot be considered to be completely representative of the total population of any country, screening data obtained can give some indication of the prevalence of persistent (and often inapparent) infections in the population. They may thus assist in the design of public health policies for dealing with the spread of such infections.

Primary anti-HCV screening. The effectiveness of blood donor screening to detect infectious agents depends upon the sensitivity and specificity of the primary assays. Sensitivity and specificity are influenced by several factors, one of the more important being the nature of the antigen used. Following the original work of Choo et al (1989) further HCV proteins have been identified and a proposed structure for the complete genome has been constructed (see Ch. 00). Currently most commercial assays are based upon a combination of proteins from one or more of the core, NS3, NS4 and NS5 regions.

The first anti-HCV assay (Ortho Diagnostics) was based upon the non-structural C100-3 protein, the original HCV protein expressed by Choo et al (1989). It was soon realized that the assay lacked both specificity and sensitivity (Bresters et al 1992, Garson et al 1992). A significant number of repeatedly reactive samples were unreactive or indeterminate with the original recombinant immunoblot assay (RIBA). It also became clear that antibodies to the C100-3 protein might not be the first to appear following infection and indeed might not appear at all. Although the data generated by this assay were novel and of great importance to the understanding of the mechanisms of HCV transmission and infection, estimates of prevalence based on its use must be considered as underestimates.

Second-generation assays using more than one antigen were soon developed by a number of commercial companies. As stated above, these assays generally comprise combinations of one or more antigens from the core, NS3, NS4, NS5 regions, either as individual antigens or as fusion proteins. They were found to be far more sensitive and specific than the single-protein (C100-3) first-generation assays (Bresters et al 1992, Garson et al 1992). Importantly the period of time between infection and the detection of antibody was decreased (Lelie et al 1992, van der Poel et al 1992).

The lack of sensitivity of the first-generation assays is shown in Table 18.2, which compares reported anti-HCV prevalence using first- and

Table 18.2 Comparison of the sensitivity of first- and second-generation anti-HCV assays

Group studied	Assay used		Anti-HCV prevalence (%)		Reference
	First generation	Second generation	First generation	Second generation	
PT HCV	Ortho	Abbott	66	80	Wang et al 1992
PT HCV	Ortho	Abbott	81	93	Aach et al 1991
PT HCV	Ortho	Ortho	67	100	van der Poel et al 1992
PT HCV	Ortho	Abbott	78	100	Lelie et al 1992
Haemophiliacs	Abbott	Abbott	59	71	Bresters et al 1992
Organ transplant recipients	Ortho	Abbott	62	69	Pereira et al 1991
NANBH liver disease	Ortho	Ortho	0	69	Yuki et al 1992
HBV carriers	Ortho	Ortho	0	7	Yuki et al 1992
Haemodialysis	Ortho/Abbott	Ortho/Abbott	5	9	Willems et al 1991

second-generation assays in various patient groups. Although reports of prevalence require careful analysis of the methods used for confirmation, data based merely on repeatable reactivity by ELISA are more predictive of infection in high-prevalence populations than in low-prevalence populations such as blood donors.

Table 18.3 shows anti-HCV prevalence in blood donors using second-generation screening ELISAs (ELISA-2). The prevalence rates confirmed by second-generation RIBA are presented where data are available. Despite the limited information based on ELISA-2, the data are likely to be more accurate than reports based on ELISA-1.

Although second-generation assays have undoubtedly improved the efficiency of HCV detection there is still some concern about the suitability of the specific antigens used in the tests. Third generation assays that address such concerns are now available. These assays include a full range of the currently defined antigens but also use combinations of selected immunodominant peptides. It is possible that certain infected individuals who show very low antibody levels or an atypical antibody response, only produce antibody specific to an antigen not included in the assay. Furthermore, the spatial configuration of the antigens may be important in the interaction between antibody and antigen. To provide some degree of tertiary structure in the antigens some manufacturers have fused individual antigens into one or two fusion proteins. However, even with existing assays, a significant reduction in PT-NANBH rates can be achieved. After the

Table 18.3 Prevalence of anti-HCV in blood donors using ELISA-2

Country	Prevalence (%)		Reference
	Primary screen reactive	RIBA-2 positive	
Scotland	0.4	0.12	Follet et al 1991
USA (Kansas)	NG	0.26	Alter H J et al 1991
UK (Multi-centre)	NG	0.05	Garson et al 1992
Scotland	0.35	0.1	Crawford et al 1992
UK (Manchester)	0.3	0.08	Gesinde et al 1992
UK (Cambridge)	0.28	0.06	Allain et al 1992
Egypt	NG	18.3	Saeed et al 1991
Peru	0	0	Hyams et al 1992

NG, not given.

introduction of anti-HBc and anti-HCV donor screening in Japan the PT-NANBH rates fell from 4.9 to 1.0% for 1–10 unit transfusions and from 16.3 to 3.3% for 11–20 unit transfusions (Japanese Red Cross NANBH Research Group 1991).

'Confirmatory' (supplementary) assays. At present *truly* confirmatory assays for HCV serology are not available commercially. Those that are currently available (the Ortho recombinant immunoblot assay, the Abbott HCV supplemental 'Matrix', assay, the Innogenetics Inno-LIA line assay, and the Murex Western blot) make use of essentially the same proteins used in the primary screening assays and are better described as supplementary assays. Although they still have limitations, assays such as RIBA have proved very useful in interpreting the bulk of ELISA-reactive samples. However, one of the more problematical residual problems of tests such as RIBA are the 'indeterminate' samples that, according to test interpretation criteria, cannot be considered positive but are not necessarily negative. A minority of such samples have been found to contain HCV RNA, a marker of viral replication, indicating that these individuals were indeed infected (Follett et al 1991). Interpretation of such results and appropriate counselling of donors is therefore sometimes very difficult.

Polymerase chain reaction (PCR). The polymerase chain reaction (PCR), although still in its infancy, has revolutionized some areas of diagnostic virology. Whilst its high sensitivity can also highlight problems of cross-contamination, it provides the potential for the direct detection of the presence of the infectious agent in any tissue. Using reverse transcriptase (RT) PCR, the RNA genome of HCV can be detected. The judicious use of PCR allows one to monitor the stages of HCV infection and to determine the potential infectivity of different stages. Primers from the conserved 5' non-coding region of the genome have been found to give the best and most consistent PCR results (Han et al 1991); most PCR procedures are now based on 'nested' analysis using a second set of primers internal to the first set to achieve the sensitivity required (Garson et al 1990).

PCR has been used to demonstrate the presence of HCV RNA in blood donors with HCV-specific antibodies, and most RIBA-2-positive samples contain HCV RNA (Claeys et al 1992, Garson et al 1992). In addition, as previously mentioned, PCR has demonstrated the presence of HCV RNA in a minority of the blood donors who produce indeterminate reactions with the supplementary assays (Garson et al 1992) and in a small number of anti-HCV-negative samples (Sugitani et al 1992). This last observation is of concern to blood transfusion services, although the frequency of these donors is unknown but likely to be very low in most donor populations. Currently, PCR is not practical or even possible as a routine screening procedure, not least because of the problem of cross-contamination in a busy mass screening laboratory (Barbara & Garson 1993).

Serum alanine aminotransferase (ALT) measurement. Although it is not appropriate to review here the role of ALT measurement in the laboratory diagnosis of NANBH, HCV infection and ALT elevation do correlate to a certain extent (van der Poel et al 1990, Takano et al 1992). In some instances monitoring ALT levels can indicate the onset of hepatitis before either HCV RNA or anti-HCV can be detected (Aach et al 1991, Lin et al 1992). The limitation is that ALT elevation is not a specific marker of HCV infection. It is a marker of liver damage in general and may occur for a number of reasons. Not all HCV carriers will have raised ALT levels and not all individuals with raised ALT levels will be undergoing HCV infection. ALT elevations by themselves do not prove the occurrence of HCV infection. Furthermore, in prospective studies of transfusion recipients (e.g. Holland, van der Poel et al 1990; or Spain, Barrera et al 1991), anti-HCV screening of donors has clearly been shown to be more predictive of HCV infectivity than detection of elevated ALT levels. Similar considerations apply to the use of anti-HBc as a 'surrogate' marker for NANBH. Anti-HBc as a marker for NANBH is particularly non-specific in areas that are endemic for HBV infection.

Inactivation of infectious agents in blood products. Although blood transfusion services have adopted comprehensive measures to minimize transfusion-transmitted infection, these cannot be totally foolproof. Blood may be donated during the 'window period' of a recent infection or markers of infection may be subliminal. Such events are very rare, but the relative risk is magnified in products made from large pools of plasma if they are not virally inactivated (Cuthbertson et al 1991).

The most important products in this respect are the clotting factor concentrates, factor VIII and factor IX, used to treat haemophilia patients. Treatment of pooled plasma products to inactivate any residual viruses has therefore been introduced worldwide. Most commonly, heat treatment of the prepared concentrates is used. In the UK the freeze-dried factor VIII concentrates are heated at 80°C for 72 h. However, a variety of other effective treatments including solvent/detergent inactivation are also available. These procedures have now been employed successfully for a number of years. Patients who have received only heat-treated or solvent/detergent-treated factor VIII concentrates have not seroconverted, and in groups of patients who have previously received untreated concentrates but who are now receiving treated ones the number of seroconversions has fallen dramatically (C Pereira et al 1991, Pistello et al 1992, Lee 1992).

Another group of pooled plasma products that are generally considered to be free of the risk of transmission of infectious agents are the intravenous (i.v.) and intramuscular (i.m.) immunoglobulins. Over the years these products have proved to be very safe. To date the only virus proven to have been (rarely) transmitted by i.v. but *not* i.m. immunoglobulins is HCV (Ochs et al 1986, Williams et al 1988). Recently Nowak et al (1992) demonstrated the effectiveness of pasteurization and *S*-sulphonation of the immunoglobulin preparations for inactivation of any residual HCV. Both these treatments inactivated HCV and a number of other Flaviviridae that had been artificially added to samples of intermediate product from a production run.

Appropriate use of blood. As discussed earlier, even with an appropriate and effective screening programme, each transfusion always carries a slight residual risk of transmission of an infectious agent. The greater the number of units transfused, the greater the risk that a patient may be exposed to an infectious agent. Blood and its components should only be transfused when absolutely necessary. Likewise, techniques of blood salvage can be applied when appropriate.

Prevention of transmission by organ transplantation

In keeping with blood transfusion policy, organ donors should be screened for evidence of HCV infection prior to transplantation. The situation may arise when both the organ donor and the potential recipient are HCV seropositive. How advisable is the use of an anti-HCV-positive organ for an anti-HCV-positive patient? In this situation it may be appropriate to use the donated organ if both the patient and the donor are chronically infected (HCV RNA present in both), or if the patient is chronically infected (HCV RNA positive) and the donor is HCV RNA negative. If the patient is HCV RNA negative and the donor is chronically infected (HCV RNA positive), reinfection of the patient may then occur with the possibility of chronic infection.

Although a case can be made for not using anti-HCV-positive organs (BJG Pereira et al 1991), many organs are in short supply and this could be considered as being unnecessarily wasteful, especially if specialized laboratory testing is available.

Prevention of transmission by intravenous drug users

HCV infection in intravenous drug users is transmitted parenterally through contaminated syringes and needles. HCV transmission can be minimized by educating intravenous drug users not to reuse or share syringes and needles or any other items involved in drug taking. As a 'minimal' approach, simple techniques for sterilizing such equipment have been suggested for preventing HIV transmission in intravenous drug users. The same suggestion may apply for the prevention of HCV transmission by this route.

Prevention of sexual transmission

Transmission through sexual contact can be minimized by protected sex. The exact risks of sexual transmission have still not been clearly defined (see earlier), and no marker for level of risk of sexual transmission is available. If a couple have had a long-term sexual relationship and there is evidence of HCV infection in only one partner, it may appear unreasonable to advise the adoption of condom use. However, it is not known if levels of infectivity remain stable in HCV carriers, and more studies are needed before fully informed advice on the risks of sexual transmission can be provided.

Prevention of sporadic/community-acquired infection

Unless the likely mechanism of infection is known, prevention of transmission cannot be attempted. In a health care setting, although HCV vaccine and immunoglobulin are not available, existing standard procedures for avoiding needlestick accidents and blood-borne transmission of HBV should also be effective for preventing transmission of HCV.

REFERENCES

Aach, Stevens C E, Hollinger F B et al 1991 Hepatitis C virus infection in post-transfusion hepatitis. An analysis with first- and second-generation assays. New England Journal of Medicine 325: 1325–1329

Akahane Y, Aikawa T, Suagi Y, Tsuda F, Okamoto H, Mishiro S 1992 Transmission of HCV between spouses. Lancet 339: 1059–1060

Allain J-P, Rankin A, Kuhns M C, McNamara A 1992 Clinical importance of HCV confirmatory testing in blood donors. Lancet 339: 1171–1172

Al Nasser M N, Al Mugeiren M A, Asuhaimi S A, Obineche E, Onwabalili J, Ramis S 1992 Seropositivity to hepatitis C virus Saudi haemodialysis patients. Vox Sanguinis 62: 94–97

Alter H J 1989 Chronic consequences of non-A, non-B hepatitis. In: Seeff L B, Lewis J H (eds) Current perspectives in hepatology. Plenum Medical, New York, pp 83–97

Alter H J, Purcell R H, Shih J W, Melpolder J C, Houghton M, Choo Q L, Kuo G 1989 Detection of antibody to hepatitis C virus in prospectively followed transfusion recipients with acute and chronic non-A, non-B hepatitis. New England Journal of Medicine 321: 1494–1500

Alter H J, Tegtmeier G E, Jett B W, Quan S, Shih J W, Bayer W L, Polito A 1991 The use of a recombinant immunoblot assay in the interpretation of anti-hepatitis C virus reactivity among prospectively followed patients, implicated donors, and random donors. Transfusion 31: 771–776

Alter M J, Coleman P J, Alexander W J 1989 Importance of heterosexual activity in the transmission of hepatitis B and non-A, non-B hepatitis. Journal of the American Medical Association 262: 1201–1205

Alter M J, Hadler S C, Judson F N 1990 Risk factors for acute non-A, non-B hepatitis in the United States and association with hepatitis C virus infection. Journal of the American Medical Association 264: 2231–2235

Barbara J A J, Garson J A 1993 Polymerase chain reaction and transfusion microbiology. Vox Sanguine 64: 73–81

Barrerra J M, Bruguera M, Ercilla M G et al 1991 Incience of non-A, non-B hepatitis after screening blood donors for antibodies to hepatitis C virus and surrogate markers. Annals of Internal Medicine 115: 596–600

Bellobuono A, Zanella A, Petrini G, Zanuso F, Mozzi F, Sirchia G 1991 Intrafamilial spread of hepatitis C virus. Transfusion 31: 475

Boyce N W, Holdsworth S R, Hooke D, Thomson N M, Atkins R C 1988 Non hepatitis B associated liver disease in a renal transplant population. American Journal of Kidney Disease 11: 307–312

Braun W E 1990: Long-term complications of renal transplantation. Kidney International 37: 1363–1378

Bresters D, Cuypers H T M, Reesink H W et al 1992 Enhanced sensitivity of a second generation ELISA for antibody to hepatitis C virus. Vox Sanguinis 62: 213–217

Brettler D B, Mannucci P M, Gringeri A et al 1992 The low risk of hepatitis C virus among sexual partners of hepatitis C-infected haemophiliac males: an international, multicenter study. Blood 80: 540–543

Cariani E, Zonaro A, Primi D et al 1991 Detection of HCV RNA and antibodies to HCV after needlestick injury. Lancet 337: 850

Choo Q L, Kuo G, Weiner A J, Overby L R, Bradley D W, Houghton M 1989 Isolation of a cDNA clone derived from a blood-borne non-A, non-B viral hepatitis genome. Science 244: 359–362

Claeys H, Volckaerts A, De Beenhouver H, Vermylen C 1992 Association of hepatitis C virus carrier state with the occurrence of hepatitis C virus core antibodies. Journal of Medical Virology 36: 259–264

Clemens J M, Taskar S, Chau K, Vallari D, Shih JW–K, Alter H J, Schleicher J B, Mimms L T 1992 IgM antibody response in acute hepatitis C viral infection. Blood 79: 169–172

Conover P T, Fang C T, Lam E, Hirschler N V, Jackson J B, Yomtovian R A 1991 Antibodies to hepatitis C virus in autologous blood donors. Transfusion 31: 616–619

Contreras M, Barbara J A J, Anderson C C et al 1991 Low incidence of non-A, non-B post-transfusion hepatitis in London confirmed by hepatitis C virus serology. Lancet 337: 753–757

Crawford R J, Frame W D, Mitchell R 1992 HCV confirmatory testing of blood donors. Lancet 339: 928

Cuthbertson B, Reid K J, Foster P R 1991 Viral

contamination of human plasma and procedures for preventing virus transmission by plasma products. In: Harris J R (ed) Blood separation and plasma fractionation. Wiley–Liss, New York, pp 385–435
Dusheiko G M, Smith M, Scheuer P J 1990 Hepatitis C virus transmitted by human bite. Lancet 336: 503–504
Eggen B M, Nordbo S A 1992 Transmission of HCV by bone graft. New England Journal of Medicine 326: 411
Esteban J I, Esteban J I, Viladomiu L et al 1989 Hepatitis C virus antibodies among risk groups in Spain. Lancet ii: 294–296
Esteban J I, González A, Hernández J M et al 1990 Evaluation of antibodies to hepatitis C virus in a study of transfusion-associated hepatitis. New England Journal of Medicine 323: 1107–1112
Farci P, Alter H J, Wong D, Miller R H, Shih J W, Jett B, Purcell R H 1991 A long-term study of hepatitis C virus replication in non-A, non-B hepatitis. New England Journal of Medicine 325: 98–104
Follett E A C, Dow B C, McOmish F et al 1991 HCV confirmatory testing of blood donors. Lancet 338: 1024
Garson J A, Tedder R S, Briggs M et al 1990 Detection of hepatitis C viral sequences in blood donations by 'nested' polymerase chain reaction and prediction of infectivity. Lancet 335: 1419–1422
Garson J A, Clewley J P, Simmonds P 1992 Hepatitis C viraemia in United Kingdom blood donors. Vox Sanguinis 62: 218–223
Gesinde M O, Love E M, Lee D 1992 HCV confirmatory testing of blood donors. Lancet 339: 928–929
Han J H, Shyamula V, Richman K H et al 1991 Characterization of the terminal regions of hepatitis C viral RNA: identification of conserved sequences in the 5' untranslated region and poly(A) tails at the 3' end. Proceedings of National Academy of Sciences USA 81: 1711–1715
Herbert A–M, Walker D M, Davies K J, Bagg J 1992 Occupationally acquired hepatitis C virus infection. Lancet 339: 305
Hyams K C, Phillips I A, Moran A Y, Tejada A, Wignall F S, Escamilla J 1992 Seroprevalence of HCV in Peru. Journal of Medical Virology 37: 127–131
Insight 1992 In: Infectious Disease Newsletter No. 4. Ortho Diagnostic Systems, pp 3–4
Japanese Red Cross non-A, non-B hepatitis research group 1991 Effect of screening for hepatitis C virus antibody and hepatitis B virus core antibody on incidence of post-transfusion hepatitis. Lancet 338: 1040–1041
Klein R S, Freeman K, Taylor P E, Stevens C E 1991 Occupational risk for hepatitis C virus infection among New York City dentists. Lancet 338: 1539–1542
Kiyosawa K, Sodeyama T, Tanaka E et al 1991a Intrafamilial transmission of hepatitis C virus in Japan. Journal of Medical Virology 33: 114–116
Kiyosawa K, Sodeyama T, Tanaka E et al 1991b Hepatitis C in hospital employees with needlestick injuries. Annals of Internal Medicine 115: 367–369
Laurian Y, Blanc A, Delaney S R, Allain J–P 1992 All exposed hemophiliacs have markers of HCV. Vox Sanguinis 62: 55–56
Lee C A 1992 Haemophilia and the hepatitis C virus. Insight 4: 4–6
Lee S D, Tsai Y T, Hwang S J, Wu J C, Yung C H, Cheng K K, Lo K J 1991 A prospective study of post-transfusion non-A, non-B (type C) hepatitis following cardiovascular surgery in Taiwan. Journal of Medical Virology 33: 188–192
Lelie P N, Cuypers T M, Reesink H W et al 1992 Patterns of serological markers in transfusion-transmitted hepatitis C virus infection using second-generation HCV assays. Journal of Medical Virology 37: 203–209
Lin C K, Chu R, Li K B, Leong S 1992 A study of hepatitis C virus antibodies and serum alanine amino transferase in blood donors in Hong Kong chinese. Vox Sanguinis 62: 98–101
Lin H H, Hsu H Y, Chang M H et al 1991 Low prevalence of hepatitis C virus and infrequent perinatal or spouse infections in pregnant women in Taiwan. Journal of Medical Virology 35: 237–240
Liou T C, Chang T T, Young K C, Lin X Z, Lin C Y, Wu H L 1992 Detection of HCV RNA in saliva, urine, seminal fluid, and ascites. Journal of Medical Virology 37: 197–202
Melbye M, Bigger R J, Wantzin P, Krogsgaard K, Ebbesen P, Becker N G 1990 Sexual transmission of hepatitis C virus: cohort study (1981–1989) among European homosexual men. British Medical Journal 301: 210–212
Mortimer P P, Cohen B J, Littou P A, Vandervelde E M, Bassendine M F, Brind A M, Hambling M H 1989 Hepatitis C antibody. Lancet ii: 798
Nishiguchi S, Kuroki T, Fukuda K et al 1992 Familial clustering of HCV. Lancet 339: 1486
Nowak T, Gregersen J–P, Klockmann U, Cummins L B, Hilfenhaus J 1992 Virus safety of human immunoglobulins: efficient inactivation of hepatitis C and other human pathogenic viruses by the manufacturing procedure. Journal of Medical Virology 36: 209–216
Ochs H D, Fischer S H, Virant F S, Lee M L, Mankarios S, Kingdom H S, Wedgwood R J 1986 Non-A, non-B hepatitis after intravenous immunoglobulin. Lancet i: 322–323
Pereira B J G, Milford E L, Kirkman R L, Levey A S 1991 Transmission of hepatitis C virus by organ transplantation. New England Journal of Medicine 325: 454–460
Pereira C, Lee C A, Dusheiko G 1991 Hepatitis C virus. British Medical Journal 303: 783
Pistello M, Ceccherini-Nelli L, Cecconi N, Bendinelli M, Panicucci 1991 Hepatitis C virus seroprevalence in Italian haemophiliacs injected with virus-inactivated concentrates: five year follow-up and correlation with antibodies to other viruses. Journal of Medical Virology 33: 43–46
Reesink H W, Wong V C W, Ip H M H, van der Poel C L, van Exel-Oehlers P J, Lelie P N 1990 Mother-to-infant transmission and hepatitis C virus. Lancet 335: 1216–1217
Riestra S, Cárcaba V 1991 Hepatitis C virus: evidence for sexual transmission. British Medical Journal 303: 310–311
Roggendorf M, Deinhardt F, Rasshofer R et al 1989 Antibodies to hepatitis C virus. Lancet ii: 324–325
Saeed A A, Al-Admawi A M, Al-Rasheed A, Fairclough D, Bacchus R 1991 Hepatitis C virus infection in Egyptian volunteer blood donors in Riyadh. Lancet: 338: 459–460
SchlipRöter V, Roggendorf M, CholmaRow K, Weise A, Deinhardt F 1991 Transmission of hepatitis C virus (HCV) from a haemodialysis patient to a medical staff member. Scandinavian Journal of Infectious Diseases 22: 757–758
Schulman S, Grillner L 1990 Antibodies against hepatitis C in a population of Swedish haemophiliacs and heterosexual partners. Scandinavian Journal of Infectious Diseases 22: 393–397
Sheu J–C, Lee S–H, Wang J–T, Shih L–N, Wang T–H, Chen D–S 1992 Prevalence of anti-HCV and HCV

viraemia in haemodialysis patients in Taiwan. Journal of Medical Virology 37: 108–112

Simmons P, Zhang L Q, Watson H G et al 1990 Hepatitis C quantification and sequencing in blood products, haemophiliacs, and drug users. Lancet ii: 1469–1472

Study Group of UK Haemophilia Centre Directors on Surveillance of Virus Transmission by Concentrates 1988 Effects of dry heating of coagulation factor concentrates at 80°C for 72 hours on transmission of non-A, non-B hepatitis. Lancet ii: 814–816

Sugitani M, Inchauspé G, Shindo M, Prince A M 1992 Sensitivity of serological assays to identify blood donors with hepatitis C viraemia. Lancet 339: 1018–1019

Takano S, Omata M, Ohto M, Satomura Y 1992 Posttransfusion hepatitis in Japan. Vox Sanguinis 62: 156–164

Tamura I, Koda T, Kobayashi Y, Ichimura H, Kurimura O, Kurimura T 1992 Prevalence of four blood-borne viruses (HBV, HCV, HTLV–1, HIV–1) among haemodialysis patients in Japan. Journal of Medical Virology 36: 271–273

Thaler M M, Park C–K, Landers D V et al 1991 Vertical transmission of hepatitis C virus. Lancet 338: 17–18

Vaglia A, Nicolin R, Puro V, Ippolito G, Bettini C, de Lalla F 1990 Needlestick hepatitis C virus conversion in a surgeon. Lancet 338: 1539–1542

van der Poel C L, Reesink H W, Lelie P N, Leentvaar-Kuypers A, Choo Q–L, Kuo G, Houghton M 1989 Anti-hepatitis C antibodies and non-A, non-B post-transfusion hepatitis in the Netherlands. Lancet ii: 297–298

van der Poel C L, Reesink H W, Mauser-Bunschoten E P et al 1991 Prevalence of anti-HCV antibodies confirmed by recombinant immunoblot in different population subsets in the Netherlands. Vox Sanguinis 61: 30–36

van der Poel C L, Bresters D, Reesink H W et al 1992 Early antihepatitis C virus response with second generation C200/C22 ELISA. Vox Sanguinis 62: 209–212

van Doornum C J J, Hooykaas C, Cuypers M T, van der Linden M M D, Coutinho R A 1991 Prevalence of hepatitis C virus infections among heterosexuals with multiple partners. Journal of Medical Virology 35: 22–27

Vranckx R 1989 Anti-HCV in institutionalised mentally handicapped children. Proceedings of the First International Symposium on Hepatitis C Virus, Rome: 36–37

Wang J–T, Wang T–H, Sheu J–C, Lin J–T, Chen D–S 1992 Hepatitis C RNA in saliva of patients with posttransfusion hepatitis and low efficiency of transmission among spouses. Journal of Medical Virology 36: 28–31

Weir M R, Kirkham R L, Strom T B, Tilney N L 1985 Liver disease in recipients of 8 long-functioning renal allografts. Kidney International 28: 839–844

Williems M, de Jong G, Moshage H, Verresen L, Goubau P, Desmyter J, Yap S H 1991 Surrogate markers are not really useful for identification of HCV carriers in chronic haemodialysis patients. Journal of Medical Virology 35: 303–306

Williams P E, Yap P L, Gillon J, Crawford R J, Galea G, Cuthbertson B 1988 Non-A, non-B hepatitis transmission by intravenous immunoglobulin. Lancet ii: 501

Yuki N, Hayashi N, Hagiwara H, Takehara T, Oshita M, Kasahara A, Fusamoto H, Kamada T 1992 Improved serodiagnosis of chronic hepatitis C in Japan by a second-generation enzyme-linked immunosorbent assay. Journal of Medical Virology 37: 237–240

UPDATE

- Some individuals infected with hepatitis C virus (HCV) experience multiple episodes of acute hepatitis. It is unclear whether these episodes are due to reinfection with HCV or to reactivation of the original virus infection. Markers of viral replication and host immunity were studied in five chimpanzees sequentially inoculated over a period of 3 years with different HCV strains of proven infectivity. Each rechallenge of a convalescent chimpanzee with the same or a different HCV strain resulted in the reappearance of viraemia, which was due to infection with the subsequent challenge virus. The evidence indicates that HCV infection does not elicit protective immunity against reinfection with homologous or heterologous strains, which raises concern for the development of effective vaccines against HCV (Farci et al 1992).
- REFERENCE

Farci P, Alter H J, Govindarajan S et al 1992 Lack of protective immunity against reinfection with hepatitis C virus. Science 258, 5079: 135–140

SECTION 4

Hepatitis D virus

19. Structure and molecular virology

John Monjardino Michael M. C. Lai

Hepatitis delta virus (HDV) was first detected as a new nuclear antigen in the hepatocytes of patients infected with hepatitis B virus (HBV) and was frequently associated with severe acute or chronic hepatitis (Rizzetto et al 1977, Rizzetto & Verme 1985). The antigen was thought to be a previously undescribed HBV-encoded antigen, but later was found to be associated with a new transmissible agent, an RNA-containing virus enveloped by the surface antigen of HBV, HBsAg (Rizzetto et al 1980a). Delta antigen was subsequently shown to be an internal component of the delta virion (Bonino et al 1984), and antibodies against this viral structural protein were detected in patients during infection (Bonino et al 1984). The presence of delta antigen in the nuclei of infected hepatocytes in liver biopsy specimens remains the most reliable test of delta virus infection.

HDV infection has been reported worldwide, with particularly high prevalence rates in the Mediterranean Basin, South America, Middle East, West Africa and certain South Pacific islands (Rizzetto et al 1980b, Ponzetto et al 1985). Transmission of HDV requires either co-infection with HBV or superinfection in individuals who are HBV carriers. Although HDV infection is closely associated with HBV, HDV clearly belongs to a distinct virus group. However, the taxonomic status of HDV has not been decided. The understanding of HDV has undergone a dramatic advancement in recent years. HDV possesses many unique molecular features, the understanding of which will eventually translate into the understanding of the viral pathogenesis and improvements in the diagnosis, treatment and prevention of the disease.

VIRION STRUCTURE

HDV is a small RNA virus consisting of spherical particles of about 36 nm in diameter and with a buoyant density of 1.25 g/cm^3 in caesium chloride (Bonino et al 1981, 1984, 1986). A recent study has reported virus particles of larger diameter (40 nm) and a lower buoyant density of 1.19 g/cm^3 produced from tissue culture infection (Ryu et al 1992). The outer coat of HDV consists of hepatitis B surface antigen (HBsAg), which envelopes the RNA genome and the delta antigen (Rizzetto et al 1980a, Bonino et al 1984). No distinct spikes are seen on the virion surface, and no distinct nucleocapsid core structure can be visualized inside the virion. The HBsAg coat of HDV virion particles consists mostly of the major (small) HBsAg polypeptide with less than 5% middle and large HBsAg components (Bonino et al 1986), a ratio that is different from that of the infectious HBV Dane particles, but more like that of the 22-nm non-infectious HBV particles.

THE GENOME

The RNA genome is approximately 1700 nucleotides long, single-stranded and circular, with a high (60%) G+C content and a high degree (up to 70%) of intramolecular base pairing (Kuo et al 1988a, Makino et al 1987, K S Wang et al 1987, Saldanha et al 1990a, T Kos et al 1991). The last property was clearly demonstrated by electron microscopy, in which native HDV RNA molecules appear as compact rods, but convert to circular molecules under denaturing conditions (A Kos et al 1986) (Fig. 19.1). Because of its

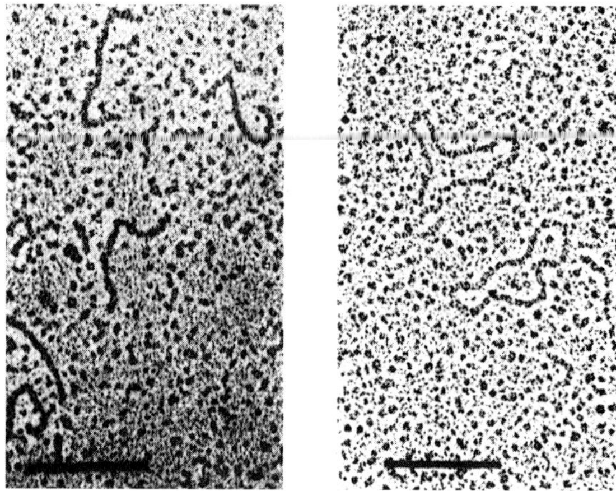

Fig. 19.1 Electron micrograph of HDV RNA: (a) native condition; (b) denatured condition. (From Kos et al 1986 with permission.)

double-strandedness under native conditions, HDV RNA is relatively stable under a variety of manipulations.

Several different HDV isolates obtained directly from human patients' serum or after its passage in chimpanzees or woodchucks have been partially or fully sequenced (A Kos et al 1986, Makino et al 1987, Wang et al 1987, Kuo et al 1988a, Y-C Chao et al 1990, Saldanha et al 1990, T Kos et al 1991, C M Lee et al 1992). The HDV RNA sequences vary in length between 1678 and 1683 nucleotides, with homologies ranging between 82% and 95%. One Japanese isolate exhibits an even higher degree of divergence (up to 25%) (Imazeki et al 1990). Even HDV isolates from patients of the same geographical area show a high degree of differences (YC Chao et al 1991). The RNA genome also exhibits another level of heterogeneity: HDV RNA in any single patient represents a collection of RNA molecules with minor sequence variations (microheterogeneity) (K S Wang et al 1987, Y-C Chao et al 1991, C M Lee et al 1992), and thus each virus population constitutes a virus 'quasi-species' (Eigen & Biebericher 1988). HDV RNA in patients also undergoes continuous evolution throughout the clinical course of disease, with an evolution rate as high as 3×10^{-2} to 3×10^{-3} substitutions per nucleotide per year in some cases (Imazeki et al 1990, C M Lee et al 1992).

For purposes of genomic sequence organization, a *Hind*III restriction site present in the cDNA copy of the prototype chimpanzee-passaged HDV RNA (K S Wang et al 1987) was designated nucleotide 0 (Fig. 19.2). The region between nucleotides 615 and 1350 appears to be highly conserved among isolates, while that between 1 and 615 is more variable (Y-C Chao et al 1990, 1991, C M Lee et al 1992). Sequence comparison with other known viruses shows no significant overall homology.

HDV RNA exhibits a ribozyme activity, i.e. an autocatalytic cleavage and ligation activity (Kuo et al 1988b, Sharmeen et al 1988, 1989, H-N Wu & Lai 1989, H N Wu et al 1989). Cleavage occurs in the absence of protein and requires divalent cations such as Mg^{++}. The cleavage site is located between the U and G at nucleotide 688/689 (in the Makino et al 1987 sequence) (Kuo et al 1988b, H N Wu et al 1989). Sequence requirements for the ribozyme activity have been mapped to a region of no more than 85 nucleotides surrounding the cleavage site (nucleotides 683–767) (Perrotta & Been 1990, H-N Wu & Lai 1990, H N Wu et al 1992). The RNA structural elements required for the catalytic cleavage activity have been partially determined and include at least two stem-and-loop structures (Fig. 19.3) (Perrotta & Been 1991, H N Wu et al 1992). Higher order RNA structures involving a pseudoknot structure have also been proposed (Perrotta & Been 1991). The unique structural and sequence requirements of HDV RNA catalysis indicate that HDV RNA belongs to a novel class of ribozymes, distinct from other known ribozymes, such as the 'hammerhead' or 'hairpin' types (Forster & Symans 1987, Hampel et al 1990). The antigenomic sense RNA also possesses a corresponding catalytic activity with the cleavage site located at nucleotide 903/904 (Sharmeen et al 1988, Kuo et al 1988b). This antigenomic cleavage activity is localized in a region complementary to the genomic ribozyme in the proposed HDV RNA rod form, and shows structural and sequence requirements that are very similar to the genomic ribozyme (Perrotta & Been 1990, 1991).

The circularity, high degree of intramolecular base pairing, and ribozyme activity of HDV RNA, and the mode of replication (see below)

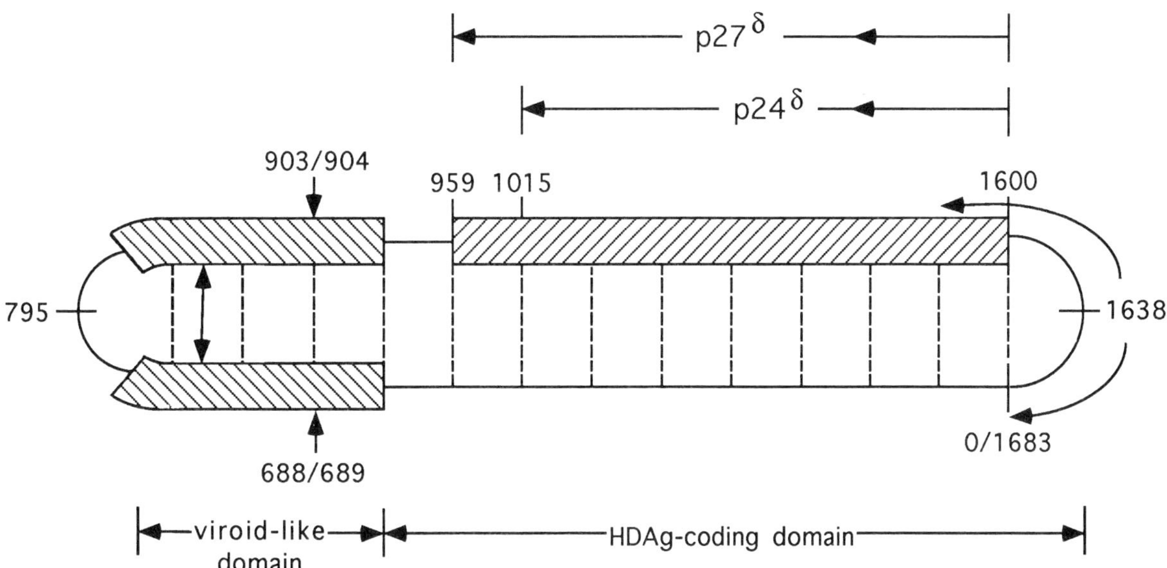

Fig. 19.2 Structure of HDV RNA. The direction of the genomic sense RNA sequence is clockwise, while that of the antigenomic sense RNA is counterclockwise. The HDAg-coding region (▨) is on the antigenomic sense RNA. The dashed lines indicate complementary sequences. (▧) indicates ribozyme domains. 688/689 is the cleavage site for genomic sense RNA, while 903/904 is the cleavage site for antigenomic sense RNA. The numbering of nucleotides is according to Makino et al (1987). (Adapted from Branch et al 1989 with permission.)

suggest a close resemblance to viroids, virusoids or plant satellite RNAs. Viroids are small, single-stranded circular RNAs of about 250–400 nucleotides, which lack any protein component, and yet are capable of self-replication (Riesner & Gross 1985). Virusoids and some plant satellite RNAs are similar to viroids in structure but encapsidated within the structural proteins of helper viruses and may have protein-coding capacity (Francki 1985). They require helper viruses for replication. HDV has features characteristic of all three types of pathogens. Several sequences that are hallmarks of viroids and may be involved in viroid replication (Diener 1986), GAAAC, GAUUUU and a 21-nucleotide-long palindromic sequence, are also conserved in the HDV genome. However, it is not clear whether these sequences are actually involved in HDV RNA replication. In addition, a tertiary RNA structure detectable by UV cross-linking has been demonstrated in both HDV RNA and some of the viroid RNAs (Branch et al 1989). Thus, there could be an evolutionary relationship between HDV RNA and plant viroid-like agents. Indeed, an analysis of the sequence relationship of these RNAs placed HDV RNA in the same evolutionary tree as the plant viroid and virusoid RNA families, most closely related to subterranean clover mottle virus and solanum nodiflorum mottle virus RNA

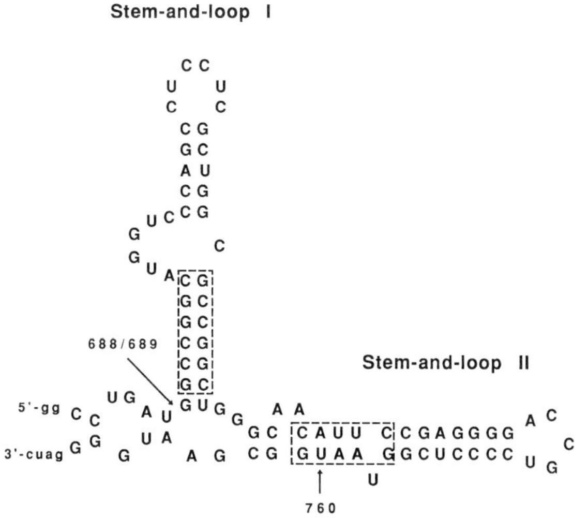

Fig. 19.3 Structure of the minimum HDV RNA ribozyme. The regions boxed with dashed lines require a stem structure regardless of nucleotide sequences. (From H N Wu et al 1992 with permission.)

(Elena et al 1991). On the other hand, HDV RNA is much larger than the typical viroid or virusoid RNAs, and, unlike viroid RNAs, HDV contains at least one functional open reading frame (ORF) that is conserved in all of the HDV isolates.

Although several other ORFs are present on both the genomic and antigenomic strands, they are not strictly conserved among different HDV isolates, and their functional significance is unclear. One of these ORFs could potentially encode a protein related to the terminal protein of HBV (Khudyakov & Makhov 1990), but its existence has not been demonstrated. The only ORF whose function has been established is located on the antigenomic strand and encodes the delta antigen (HDAg). This ORF exists in two sizes, a small and a large form, with coding capacities for 195 and 214 amino acids respectively. The difference between these two ORFs resides in a single base mutation at position 1015. This nucleotide on the antigenomic strand is either A, which leads to a termination codon UAG, or G, giving UGG (Trp), which allows for the read-through of 19 additional amino acids. This nucleotide heterogeneity has been detected in HDV RNA preparations obtained from every patient examined so far (Wang et al 1987, Y-C Chao et al 1990, 1991, C M Lee et al 1992, Xia et al 1990). The generation of this mutation is related to its replication strategy (see below).

Based on the consideration of the biochemical properties and potential functions, the HDV RNA molecule can be divided into two structural domains (Fig. 19.2) (Branch et al 1989). One is the viroid-like domain (roughly from nucleotides 650 to 980), which contains the ribozyme activity and thus is similar to viroids. The other contains the ORF for HDAg on the antigenomic strand. According to this interpretation, one additional region (nucleotides 1–650) is devoid of any known function or structural features. Significantly, this is also the most heterogeneous region among different HDV isolates (Y-C Chao et al 1990, 1991, C M Lee et al 1992). Nevertheless, this region may be involved in the stabilization of HDV RNA through intramolecular complementarity to the HDAg-coding region.

HEPATITIS DELTA ANTIGEN (HDAg)

HDAg is the only known protein encoded by HDV RNA, and is an internal component of HDV virion particles (Rizzetto et al 1980a, Bonino et al 1984). HDAg is usually found in patients' serum or liver in two forms of 27 000 kD and 24 000 kD molecular weight (Bonino et al 1986, Bergmann & Gerin 1986, Pohl et al 1989, Zyzik et al 1987), designated large and small HDAg respectively. These forms are not present in a fixed stoichiometric ratio as expected for structural proteins of a defined regular structure. As indicated above, these two HDAg forms are translated from two RNA species different by a single point mutation. The two protein forms are identical except that the large HDAg has 19 additional amino acids at the C-terminus (Weiner et al 1988). The N-terminal two-thirds of the protein are highly basic, while the C-terminal one-third is relatively uncharged (Chang et al 1988). Both forms are phosphoproteins, with phosphorylation occurring at the serine residues (Chang et al 1988, Hwang eg al 1992), although large HDAg appears to be more heavily phosphorylated (Hwang et al 1992). HDAg is an RNA-binding protein (Lin et al 1990, Macnaughton et al 1990a, M Chao et al 1991, Hwang et al 1992), with particularly high binding affinity for HDV RNA. HDAg–RNA binding in vitro requires a specific HDV RNA structure, but it is not dependent on a strict HDV RNA sequence (Lin et al 1990). One report has suggested that HDAg–RNA binding requires the HDV RNA rod structure (M Chao et al 1991), although some other double-stranded RNAs have been shown not to bind the HDAg (Lin et al 1990). In the virion particles, HDAg is also bound to HDV RNA (Lin et al 1990). This HDAg-RNA interaction is likely to have a role not only in the structural organization of virion particles, but also in HDV RNA replication (see below). In virus-infected cells, HDAg is localized exclusively in the nuclei (Rizzetto et al 1977), although variations are seen in its accumulation in nucleoli, nucleoplasm or diffusely throughout the nuclei (Xia et al 1992). Its presence in the nuclei is consistent with its functional role in HDV RNA replication, which has been shown to take place in the nuclei (Gowans et al 1988).

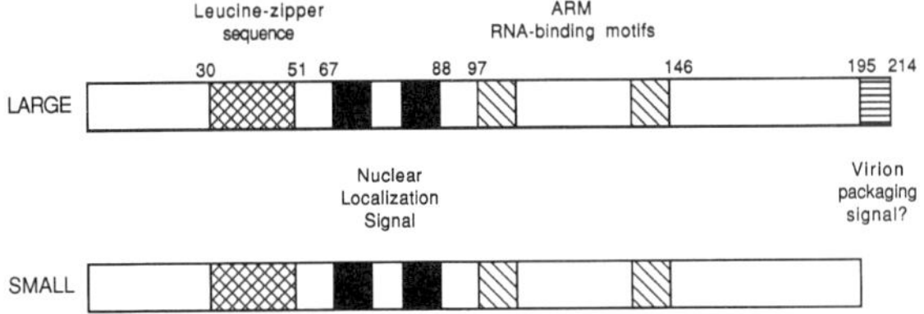

Fig. 19.4 Schematic diagram of the functional domains of hepatitis delta antigen.

Three functional domains have been identified in HDAg (Fig. 19.4). The first is the RNA-binding motif, which is located in the middle one-third of HDAg (Lin et al 1990). This domain consists of two stretches of arginine-rich motif (ARM) (C Z Lee et al 1993), which is characteristic of many RNA-binding proteins, including *tat* and *rev* of human immunodeficiency virus (Lazinski et al 1989). The unusual feature of the RNA-binding sequence in HDAg is that both of the ARM sequences and a spacer sequence of appropriate length are required for specific RNA binding (C Z Lee et al 1993). This property suggests that HDAg may simultaneously bind to two regions of HDV RNA, which is consistent with the requirement for a rod structure in HDAg–RNA binding (M Chao et al 1991). The second domain is a nuclear localization, signal located in the N-terminal one-third of the protein (Xia et al 1992). This domain contains two stretches of basic amino acids, both of which are required for the targeting of HDAg to the nuclei. The third domain is a leucine zipper-like sequence also present in the N-terminal region of the protein (Chen et al 1992, Xia & Lee 1992). This domain is responsible for oligomerization of the protein, which has been demonstrated to occur both in vitro and in vivo (Xia & Lee 1992). The oligomerization of HDAg is required for the various functions of HDAg (see below). The large HDAg has an additional region of functional importance, i.e. the last 19 amino acids at the C-terminus. The final four amino acids constitute a signal for isoprenylation (CXXX, X being any amino acid), and are required for virion assembly (J Glenn & J White, personal communication).

The functions of the two forms of HDAg have been elucidated. The small HDAg is required for HDV RNA replication (Kuo et al 1989), although its precise role has not been determined. The small HDAg can act in trans and thus complement defects of the HDAg-coding region within the HDV RNA (Kuo et al 1989). This trans-acting function requires an intact RNA-binding domain (C Z Lee et al 1993) and the leucine zipper sequence (Xia & Lai 1992). Thus, it appears that the small HDAg forms an oligomer, which binds to HDV RNA to participate in HDV RNA replication. However, HDAg appears not to be required for HDV RNA synthesis per se, since HDV RNA synthesis occurred even in the absence of HDAg in a cell-free nuclear extract (Macnaughton et al 1990b). On the other hand, the large HDAg can suppress HDV RNA replication (M Chao et al 1990) and is required for the assembly or export of virion particles (Chang et al 1992, Ryu et al 1992, Sureau et al 1992). The molecular basis for the different functions of the small and large HDAg is unclear. The presence of additional 19 amino acids at the C-terminus of the large HDAg may confer upon large HDAg the ability to interfere with HDV RNA replication. However, the mutational analysis of these extra amino acids suggested that the inhibitory activity of large HDAg is not a simple function of the extra length of large HDAg or the specific sequence of these 19 amino acids (Glenn & White 1991), but, rather, the alteration of a specific conformation of HDAg. This suggestion is supported by the finding that substitution of a proline residue at the C-terminus has a dramatic effect on the activity of large HDAg (Glenn & White 1991). Furthermore, the inhibitory activity of large HDAg requires an intact leucine zipper sequence, suggesting that the large HDAg complexes with small HDAg to interfere with its activity in HDV RNA replication (Chen et al 1992, Xia & Lai 1992). Thus, the inhibitory activity of the large HDAg is most likely the result of disruption of conformation of the small HDAg complex. This interpretation is also supported by the finding that the N-terminal one-third alone of HDAg can interfere with HDV RNA replication (Xia & Lai 1992). The conformational difference between the small and large HDAg has been demonstrated by the recent isolation of a monoclonal antibody that recognizes only the small HDAg, not the large HDAg (Hwang & M M C Lai 1993).

The second function of large HDAg, i.e. assembly or export of virion particles, appears to involve the last 19 amino acids of large HDAg. Particularly, the last four amino acids with isoprenylation may provide the interaction with HBsAg (Chang et al 1992, Ryu et al 1992, Sureau et al 1992).

Epitope mapping of HDAg has been carried out in several laboratories using either synthetic peptides or truncated forms of the antigen expressed in prokaryotic cells (Bergmann et al 1989, Saldanha et al 1990b, J G Wang et al 1990). Several immunodominant epitopes have been identified.

REPLICATION

The mode of HDV entry into target cells is currently unknown. Since the HDV envelope consists of all three protein species of HBsAg (Bonino et al 1984, 1986), HDV probably utilizes the same cellular receptor as HBV. However, there is a slight difference in host range between HBV and HDV. For instance, HDV can infect woodchucks but HBV cannot (Ponzetto et al 1984, Choi et al 1988, Taylor et al 1988, Dourakis et al 1991); and HDV can infect primary hepatocytes of chimpanzees (Sureau et al 1991) while HBV cannot. Once inside cells, HDV can replicate in the absence of HBV (Kuo et al 1989, Chen et al 1990, Glenn et al 1990).

Replication of HDV RNA occurs in the cell nuclei since both HDAg, detected by immunofluorescence, and HDV RNA, detected by in situ hybridization, have been shown to be localized exclusively to nuclei (Gowans et al 1988, Negro et al 1989a, Dourakis et al 1991). Although HDV infects only hepatocytes in vivo, HDV RNA can replicate in a wide range of cell types, including hepatocytes, fibroblasts and monkey kidney cell lines, upon transfection of HDV RNA or cDNA into those cells (Chen et al 1990, Glenn et al 1990, Macnaughton et al 1990b). However, cell type-specific differences in RNA replication activity have been observed with certain HDV cDNA constructs (T Macnaughton & M M C Lai, unpublished observation).

Replication of HDV RNA is thought to occur via a rolling circle mechanism similar to that described for the replication of viroids (Branch & Robertson 1984). In this model, antigenomic RNA of multiple genomic lengths is synthesized, followed by processing into monomer-size RNAs (Fig. 19.5). The monomer antigenomic RNA is ligated to form a circular RNA and used for a second round of rolling circle replication to generate the monomer genomic sense RNA, thus completing the replication cycle. This model is called the 'double rolling circle mechanism'. An alternative model is that the linear multiple-genomic-length antigenomic RNA may be used directly as template for the synthesis of genomic sense RNA of multiple lengths, which is then cleaved and ligated to form the genomic circular RNA. This model would require only one round of rolling circle replication. The rolling circle model of HDV RNA replication is supported by the detection in HDV-infected chimpanzee and woodchuck livers of replicative-intermediate RNA of both polarities, of two and three times genomic length (Chen et al 1986, Taylor et al 1988, Makino et al 1989). The processing of multiple-length HDV RNA intermediates appears to be carried out by autocatalytic cleavage into molecules of genomic size, which are subsequently converted into circular genomes by self-ligation. Both of

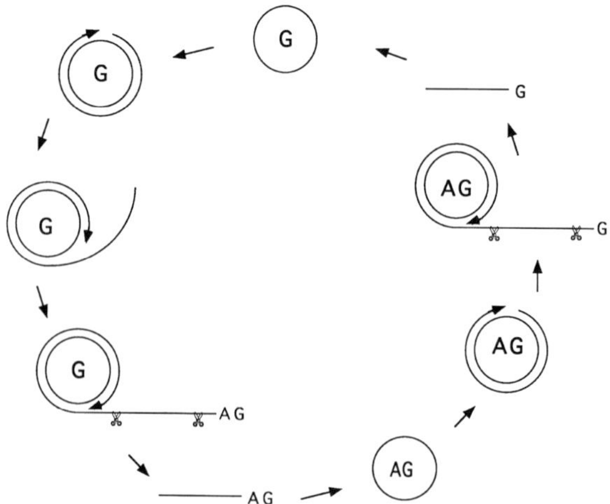

Fig. 19.5 A double rolling circle model for HDV RNA replication. G, genomic sense RNA; AG, antigenomic sense RNA. (Adapted from Branch & Robertson 1984 with permission.)

these autocatalytic activities have been demonstrated in vitro using a small fragment of HDV RNA (Kuo et al 1988b, H-N Wu & Lai 1989, H-N Wu et al 1989). Curiously, the longer HDV RNA was usually cleaved poorly in vitro (Kuo et al 1988b, H-N Wu et al 1989), probably as a result of unfavourable RNA conformation (Perrotta & Been 1990, H-N Wu & Lai 1990). Thus, it is likely that cellular factors may contribute to HDV RNA cleavage in infected cells. The autocatalytic activity of HDV RNA has been demonstrated on both genomic and antigenomic RNA strands. The double rolling circle model appears to be the more likely mechanism, as suggested from studies of cleavage site mutants on either the genomic or antigenomic strands (T Macnaughton & M M C Lai, unpublished observation). These studies also suggested that the cleavage site specificity in vivo is the same as that in vitro in the absence of proteins.

An antigenomic sense 0.8-kb RNA of very low abundance (roughly 60 molecules per cell as compared with 6000 molecules of the antigenomic RNA and 300 000 molecules of the genomic RNA) has also been detected in some infected chimpanzee or woodchuck livers (Chen et al 1986, Hsieh et al 1990). This RNA species contains a poly(A) sequence (Chen et al 1986). The 5'-end of this transcript starts at position 1631 or 1632 (Hsieh et al 1990), which is near the initiation codon of the ORF for HDAg. The 3'-end of the transcript is 76 nucleotides downstream from the termination codon of HDAg and is preceded (15 nucleotides upstream) by an AAUAAA polyadenylation signal. Thus, this RNA is probably the mRNA for the translation of HDAg. Although the genome-length antigenomic sense RNAs are poor templates for translation in vitro (Chang et al 1988), current evidence suggests that they may also be translated into HDAg (T Macnaughton & M M C Lai, unpublished observation). It has been postulated that the 5'-end of the HDAg mRNA also represents the origin of replication for the antigenomic sense RNA (Hsieh et al 1990). Based on this interpretation, RNA replication is thought to start from nucleotide 1631 and terminate at the polyadenylation signal, resulting in the synthesis of the 0.8-kb RNA species. This RNA is used for the translation of HDAg, which, in turn, serves as an anti-terminator protein allowing the subsequent rounds of RNA synthesis to pass beyond the polyadenylation sequence (Hsieh & Taylor 1991). As a result, a multimeric RNA is synthesized (Fig. 19.6). The anti-terminator activity of HDAg has been demonstrated (Hsieh & Taylor 1991). The mechanism of synthesis of the genomic sense RNA has not been explained.

During HDV RNA replication, a specific nucleotide conversion (U → C) occurs at nucleotide 1015 of the genomic sense RNA, changing the termination codon for small HDAg (on the antigenomic strand) to a tryptophan codon and extending the ORF for an additional 19 amino acids (Luo et al 1990). This mutation results in the synthesis of large HDAg, which, in turn, inhibits further HDV RNA replication (M Chao et al 1990b). The mechanism of this specific mutation (RNA editing) is not yet clear; it appears to require a rod-like RNA structure and a specific nucleotide sequence and complementary sequences around the cleavage site. In addition, it occurs on the genomic sense RNA rather than the antigenomic sense RNA (Casey et al 1993).

The enzymology of HDV RNA replication is not yet understood. The observation in HDV cDNA-transfected cells that HDV RNA replication is suppressed by α-amanitin does suggest (as with viroids) the involvement of DNA-dependent RNA polymerase II (Macnaughton et al 1990b, Gowans et al 1991). The question remains as to how RNA polymerase II can utilize an RNA template rather than its normal DNA template. Possibly, HDAg may complex with polymerase II and alter its template specificity. This would explain the requirement of HDV RNA synthesis for HDAg (Kuo et al 1989). However, it is inconsistent with the observation that some HDV RNA synthesis does occur in the absence of HDAg in cell-free lysates (Macnaughton et al 1990b). Alternatively, the rod-shaped structure of HDV RNA may resemble double-stranded DNA, thus enabling RNA polymerase II to transcribe from the RNA template. Indeed, the double-stranded DNA counterpart of the region encompassing the replication origin for the antigenomic strand exhibits a promoter activity for transcription. This promoter does not contain

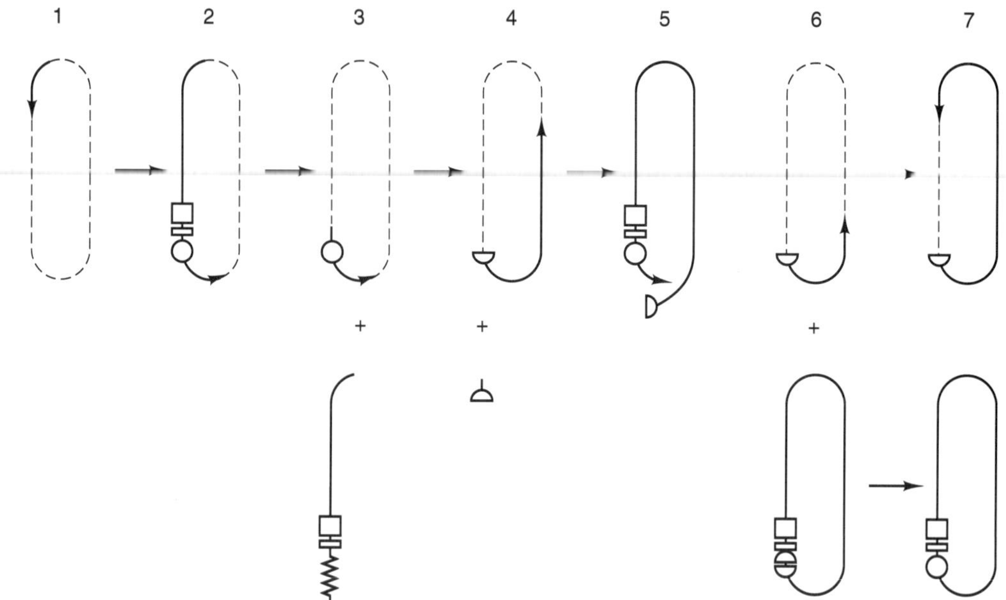

Fig. 19.6 A proposed model for the mechanism of synthesis of antigenomic sense RNA of HDV (see text). (From Hsieh & Taylor 1991 with permission.)

the TATA box typical of the conventional promoters (T Macnaughton & M M C Lai, unpublished). The precise mechanism of HDV RNA transcription remains unclear.

VIRUS ASSEMBLY

Co-transfection studies using HBsAg genes coding for either form of HDAg and HDV cDNAs have shown that the large form, but not the small form, of HDAg is required for packaging HDV particles (Ryu et al 1992, Chang et al 1991, Sureau et al 1992). Furthermore, the small HBsAg alone is sufficient for HDV particle assembly (Ryu et al 1992, Sureau et al 1992), but the presence of large HBsAg (pre-S1) polypeptides in the assembled particles is required for infectivity in primary primate hepatocyte cultures (Sureau et al 1992). Although the small HDAg is not required for HDV particle assembly, it can be packaged into virus particles, probably because of its interaction with large HDAg (Chen et al 1992). The relative ratio of the large and small HDAg in HDV virus particles obtained from infected serum (Weiner et al 1988, Gerlich et al 1987) varies from 0.5 to 10 or higher, suggesting that there is no strict requirement for a fixed ratio between the large and small forms of HDAg in virus particles. Alternatively, there may be a population of virus particles containing exclusively the large form.

The mode of interaction between HDAg and HBsAg is not clear. HDAg is present in the cell nuclei, while HBsAg is localized in the cytoplasm; the cellular location where the interaction between them occurs is not known. A recent study showed that an HDAg mutant with a deletion in the nuclear localization signal could still be packaged into virus particles (Chen et al 1992). The isoprenylation of the large HDAg may allow it to interact with a cellular membrane component that harbours HBsAg. This interaction may be the nucleation point of virus assembly. All other components, such as the small HDAg and HDV RNA, are then incorporated into virus particles through their interaction with either the large HDAg or HBsAg.

HDV RNA is not required for virus particle assembly (Chang et al 1991, Ryu et al 1992, Sureau et al 1992). Its incorporation into virus particles is most likely due to its interaction with either the large or small HDAg. However, only the genomic sense RNA is packaged into virion although the antigenomic sense RNA binds equally well to HDAg (Lin et al 1990, M Chao et al 1991). Thus, other packaging factors are probably involved. The HDAg–HDV RNA interaction has been demonstrated in the assembled virus particles (Lin et al 1990). The observation that no distinct nucleocapsid structure is seen within virus particles may be related to the lack of a defined ratio between large and small HDAg in virions. Large and small HDAg bind to HDV RNA with the same binding affinity (Hwang et al 1992), and the heterodimer and homodimer formation between the large and small HDAg also occur at equal efficiency (Xia & Lai 1992), thus contributing to their non-regulated incorporation into particles.

MOLECULAR BASIS OF VIRAL PATHOGENESIS

Although many questions remain to be answered, current information on the molecular biology and replication of HDV provides clues toward understanding the viral pathogenesis and clinical manifestation of HDV infection. One prediction from such knowledge is that virus spread and reinfection will occur only after replicating genomes (coding for the small HDAg) have undergone the mutation leading to the generation of large HDAg. Once the large HDAg is produced, further HDV RNA replication is inhibited (M Chao et al 1990b). However, as virus particles are released, the accumulated pool of large HDAg in the cells may decrease more rapidly than small HDAg, thus allowing HDV RNA replication to proceed again. Although the kinetics of viral replication and virus release in the infected liver are not precisely known, one would predict a dynamic equilibrium to be attained between inhibition of RNA replication and release of virus particles. Thus, the ratio between the two forms of HDAg at equilibrium may be critical in determining the severity of the lesions and/or the natural course of the disease.

HDV pathogenicity may be determined by certain genetic regions of HDV RNA, but in spite of the sequence heterogeneity found amongst different HDV isolates no correlation has emerged so far between specific genetic changes and viral pathogenicity. In the case of potato spindle tuber viroid, a gradient of increased disease severity has been associated with sequence changes that lead to decreasing thermodynamic stability of the viroid RNA (Hammond & Owens 1987), and viral pathogenicity involves a region termed the pathogenicity modulating sequence (PMS) (Hammond & Owens 1987). The more unstable form of the viroid RNA contains less intramolecular base pairing and is presumably available to interact with some cellular components, leading to the perturbation of cellular functions. It has been noted that a stretch of HDV RNA sequence bears homology to the cellular 7S RNA (Negro et al 1989b, Young & Hicke 1990), which is involved in protein translation and transport, although no evidence is available to suggest that translation of cellular proteins is affected by HDV infection. Alternatively, HDAg itself might be cytotoxic (Macnaughton et al 1990b, Cole et al 1991). The apparent association between high levels of HDAg expressed and cell death in HDV cDNA-transfected cells (Cole et al 1991) suggests a possible cytopathic role for delta antigen. HDAg could potentially bind to certain cellular RNAs because of its RNA-binding properties, or to cellular proteins because of the leucine zipper sequence. Still another possibility is that the pathogenesis of HDV is due to immunopathic attack by cytotoxic T lymphocytes (Negro et al 1988, Chu & Liaw 1989, Ottobrelli et al 1991). This possibility is also suggested by the finding that experimental vaccination of chimpanzees or woodchucks with HDAg exacerbated the illness of subsequent HDV infection (Karayiannis et al 1990). These possibilities remain to be investigated.

An additional curious observation concerning HDV pathogenicity is the transient suppression of HBV replication by HDV superinfection (Arico et al 1985, Hadziyannis et al 1985, Wu et al 1990). This phenomenon has also been observed in experimental transmission of HDV to HBV-infected chimpanzees (Rizzetto et al 1980c, Sureau et al 1989). The suppression has been reported to be mediated by HDAg (J C Wu et al 1991). It is not clear whether the suppression of HBV replication contributes to the pathogenesis of HDV. The understanding of the mechanism of inhibition by HDV may lead to the potential development of therapy for HBV infections.

REFERENCES

Arico S, Aragona M, Rizzetto M, Caredda F et al 1985 Clinical significance of antibody to the hepatitis delta virus in symptomless HBsAg carriers. Lancet ii: 356–358

Bergmann K F, Gerin J L 1986 Antigens of hepatitis delta virus in the liver and serum of human and animals. Journal of Infectious Diseases 154: 702–706

Bergmann K F, Cote P J, Moriarty A, Gerin JL 1989 Hepatitis delta antigen: antigenic structure and humoral immune response. Journal of Immunology 143: 3714–3721

Bonino F, Hoyer B, Ford E, Shih J W-K, Purcell R H, Gerin J L 1981 The δ agent: HBsAg particles with δ antigen and RNA in the serum of an HBV carrier. Hepatology 1: 127–131

Bonino F, Hoyer B, Shih J W K et al 1984 Delta hepatitis agent: structural and antigenic properties of the delta-associated particle. Infection and Immunity 43: 1000–1005

Bonino F, Heerman K H, Rizzetto M, Gerlich W H 1986 Hepatitis delta virus: protein composition of delta antigen and its hepatitis B virus-derived envelope. Journal of Virology 58: 945–950

Branch A D, Robertson H D 1984 A replication cycle for viroids and small infectious RNAs. Science 223: 450–455

Branch A D, Benenfeld B J, Baroudy B M, Wells F V, Gerin J L, Robertson H D 1989 An UV-sensitive RNA structural element in a viroid-like domain of the hepatitis delta virus. Science 243: 649–652

Casey J L, Bergmann K, Brown T L, Gerin J L 1992 Structural requirements for RNA editing in hepatitis δ virus: Evidence for a Uridine-to-cytidine editing mechanism. Proc. Natl. Acad. Sci. 89: 7149–7153

Chao M, Hsieh S-Y, Taylor J 1990b Role of two forms of hepatitis delta virus antigen: evidence for a mechanism of self-limiting genome replication. Journal of Virology 64: 5066–5069

Chao M, Hsieh S-Y, Taylor J 1991 The antigen of hepatitis delta virus: examination of in vitro RNA-binding specificity. Journal of Virology 65: 4057–4062

Chao Y-C, Chang M-F, Gust I, Lai, M M C 1990 Sequence conservation and divergence of hepatitis delta virus RNA. Virology 178: 384–392

Chao Y-C, Lee C-M, Tang H-S, Govindarajan S, Lai M M C 1991 Molecular cloning and characterization of an isolate of hepatitis delta virus from Taiwan. Hepatology 13: 345–352

Chang M-F, Baker S C, Soe L H et al 1988 Human hepatitis delta antigen is a nuclear phosphoprotein with RNA-binding activity. Journal of Virology 62: 2403–2410

Chang F-L, Chen P-J, Tu S-J et al 1991 The large form of hepatitis antigen is crucial for assembly of hepatitis δ virus. Proceedings of the National Academy of Sciences of the USA 88, 8490–8494

Chen P-J, Kalpana J, Goldberg W et al 1986 Structure and replication of the genome of the hepatitis delta virus. Proceedings of the National Academy of Sciences of the USA 83: 8774–8778

Chen P-J, Kuo M Y-P, Chen M-L, Tu S J, Chiu M-N, Wu H L, Hsu H-C, Chen D-S 1990 Continuous expression and replication of the hepatitis δ virus genome in HepG2 hepatoblastoma cells transfected with cloned viral DNA. Proceedings of the National Academy of Sciences of the USA 87: 5253–5257

Chen P-J, Chang F-L, Wang C-J, Lin C-J, Sung S-Y, Chen D-S 1992 Functional study of hepatitis delta virus large antigen in packaging and replication inhibition: role of the amino terminal leucine zipper. Journal of Virology 66: 2853–2859

Choi S-S, Rasshofer R, Roggendorf M 1988 Propagation of woodchuck hepatitis delta virus in primary woodchuck hepatocytes. Virology 167: 451–457

Chu C-M, Liaw Y-F 1989 Studies on the composition of the mononuclear cell infiltrates in liver from patients with chronic active delta hepatitis. Hepatology 10: 911–915

Cole S M, Gowans E J, Macnaughton T B et al 1991 Direct evidence for cytotoxicity associated with expression of hepatitis delta antigen. Hepatology 13: 845–851

Diener T O 1986 Viroid processing: a model involving the central conserved region and hairpin I. Proceedings of the National Academy of Sciences of the USA 83: 58–62

Dourakis S, Karayiannis P, Goldin R, Taylor M, Monjardino J, Thomas H C 1991 An in situ hybridization, molecular biological and immunohistochemical study of hepatitis delta virus in woodchucks. Hepatology 14: 534–539

Eigen M, Biebericher C K 1988 Sequence space and quasispecies distribution. In: Domingo E, Holland J J, Ahlquist P (eds) RNA genetics, Vol. III. CRC Press, Boca Raton, pp 211–245

Elena S F, Dopazo J, Flores R, Diener T O, Moya A 1991 Phylogeny of viroids, viroid-like satellite RNAs and the viroid-like domain of hepatitis δ virus RNA. Proceedings of the National Academy of Sciences of the USA 88: 5631–5634

Forster A C, Symons R H 1987 Self-cleavage of plus and minus RNAs of a virusoid and a structural model for the active sites. Cell 49: 211–220

Francki R I B 1985 Plant virus satellites. Annual Review of Microbiology 39: 151–174

Gerlich W H, Heermann K H, Ponzetto A et al 1987 In: Rizzetto M, Gerin J L, Purcell R H (eds) The hepatitis delta virus and its infection. Alan R. Liss, New York, pp 97–103

Glenn J S, White J M 1991 *trans*-dominant inhibition of human hepatitis delta virus genome replication. Journal of Virology 65: 2357–2361

Glenn J S, Taylor J M, White J M 1990 In vitro synthesized hepatitis delta virus RNA initiates genome replication in culture cells. Journal of Virology 64: 3104–3107

Gowans E J, Baroudy B M, Negro F, Ponzetto A, Purcell R H, Gerin J L 1988 Evidence for replication of hepatitis delta virus RNA in hepatocytes nuclei after in vivo infection. Virology 167: 274–278

Gowans E, Macnaughton T, Jilbert A, Burrell C 1991 Cell culture model systems to study HDV expression, replication and pathogenesis. In: Purcell R H, Rizzetto M, Gerin J L (eds) The hepatitis delta virus. Wiley–Liss, New York, pp 299–308

Hadziyannis S J, Sherman M, Lieberman HM, Shafritz D A 1985 Liver disease activity and hepatitis B virus replication in chronic delta antigen-positive hepatitis B virus carriers. Hepatology 5: 544–547

Hammond R W, Owens R A 1987 Mutational analysis of potato spindle tuber viroid reveals complex relationships between structure and infectivity. Proceedings of the National Academy of Sciences of the USA 84: 3967–3971

Hampel A, Tritz R, Hicks M, Cruz P 1990 'Hairpin' catalytic RNA model: evidence for helices and sequence requirement for substrate RNA. Nucleic Acids Research 18: 299–304

Hsieh S Y, Taylor J M 1991 Regulation of polyadenylation of hepatitis delta virus antigenomic RNA. Journal of Virology 65: 6438–6446

Hsieh S-Y, Chao M, Coates L, Taylor J 1990 Hepatitis delta virus genome replication: a polyadenylated mRNA for delta antigen. Journal of Virology 64: 3192–3198

Hwang S, Lee C-Z, Lai M M C 1992 Hepatitis delta antigen expressed by recombinant baculoviruses: Comparison of biochemical properties and post-translational modification between the large and small forms. Virology 190: 413–422

Hwang S B, Lai M M C 1993 A unique conformation at the carboxyl terminus of the small hepatitis delta antigen revealed by a specific monoclonal antibody. Virology 193: 924–931

Imazeki F, Omato M, Ohto M 1990 Heterogeneity and evolution rates of delta virus RNA sequences. Journal of Virology 64: 5594–5599

Karayiannis P, Saldanha J A, Monjardino J et al 1990 Immunization of woodchucks with recombinant hepatitis dlta antigen does not protect against delta hepatitis infection. Hepatology 12, 1125–1128

Khudyakov Y E, Makhov A M 1990 Amino acid sequence similarity between the terminal protein of hepatitis B virus and predicted hepatitis delta virus gene product. FEBS Letters 262 345–348

Kos A, Dijkema R, Arnberg A C, van der Meide P H, Schellekens H 1986 The hepatitis delta virus possesses a circular RNA. Nature 323: 558–560

Kos T, Molijn A, van Doorn L-J et al 1991 Hepatitis Delta virus cDNA sequence from an acutely HBV-infected chimpanzee: sequence conservation in experimental animals. Journal of Medical Virology 34: 268–279

Kuo M Y-P, Sharmeen L et al 1988a Molecular cloning of hepatitis delta virus RNA from an infected woodchuck liver: sequence structure and application. Journal of Virology 62: 1855–1861

Kuo M Y-P, Sharmeen L, Dieter-Gottleib G, Taylor J 1988b Characterization of self-cleaving RNA sequences on the genome and anti-genome of human hepatitis delta virus. Journal of Virology 62: 4439–4444

Kuo M Y-P, Chao M, Taylor J 1989 Initiation of replication of the human hepatitis delta virus genome from cloned DNA: Role of delta antigen. Journal of Virology 63: 1945–1950

Lazinski D, Grzadziekska E, Das A 1989 Sequence-specific recognition of RNA hairpins by bacteriophage antiterminators requires a conserved arginine-rich motif. Cell 59: 209–218

Lee C-M, Bih F Y, Chao Y-C, Govindarajan S, Lai M M C 1992 Evolution of hepatitis delta virus RNA during chronic infection. Virology 188: 265–273

Lee C-Z, Lin J-H, McKnight K, Lai M M C 1993 RNA-binding of hepatitis delta antigen requires two arginine-rich motifs (ARMs) and is required for hepatitis delta virus RNA replication. Journal of Virology 67: 2221–2229

Lin J-H, Chang M-F, Baker S C et al 1990 Characterization of hepatitis delta antigen: specific binding to hepatitis delta virus RNA. Journal of Virology 64: 4051–4058

Luo G, Chao M, Hsieh S-Y et al 1990 A specific base transition occurs on replicating hepatitis delta virus RNA. Journal of Virology 64: 1021–1027

Macnaughton T B, Gowans E J, Reinboth B, Jilbert A R, Burrell, C J 1990a Stable expression of the small polypeptide of hepatitis delta virus antigen in a eukaryotic cell line. Journal of General Virology 71: 1339–1345

Macnaughton T, Gowans E J, Jilbert A R, Burrell C J 1990b Hepatitis delta virus RNA, protein synthesis and associated cytotoxicity in a stably transfected cell line. Virology 117: 692–698

Makino S, Chang M-F, Shieh C-K et al 1987 Molecular cloning and sequencing of a human hepatitis delta virus RNA. Nature 329, 343–346

Makino S, Chang M-F, Shieh C-K, Kamahora T, Vannier D M, Govindarajan G, Lai M M C 1989 Molecular biology of a human hepatitis delta virus RNA. In: Robinson W, Koike K, Will H (eds) Hepadnaviruses. Alan R. Liss, New York, pp 549–564

Negro F, Bergmann K F, Baroudy B M et al 1988 Chronic hepatitis delta virus (HDV) infection in hepatitis B virus carrier chimpanzees experimentally superinfected with HDV. Journal of Infectious Diseases 158: 151–159

Negro F, Kobra B E, Forzani B et al 1989a Hepatitis delta virus (HDV) and woodchuck hepatitis virus (WHV) nucleic acids in the tissues of HDV-infected chronic WHV carrier woodchucks. Journal of Virology 63: 1612–1618

Negro F, Gerin J L, Purcell R H, Miller R H 1989b Basis of hepatitis delta virus disease. Nature 341: 111

Ottobrelli A, Marzano A, Smedile A et al 1991 Patterns of hepatitis delta virus reinfection and disease in liver transplantation. Gastroenterology 101: 1649–1655

Perrotta A T, Been M D 1990 The self-cleaving domain from the genomic RNA of hepatitis delta virus: sequence requirements and the effects of denaturants. Nucleic Acids Research 18: 6821–6827

Perrotta A T, Been M D 1991 A pseudoknot structure required for efficient self-cleavage of hepatitis delta virus RNA. Nature 350: 434–436

Pohl C, Baroudy B M, Bergmann K F, Cote P J, Purcell R H, Hoffnagel J, Gerin J L 1989 A human monoclonal antibody that recognizes viral polypeptides and in vitro translation products of the genome of the hepatitis D virus. Journal of Infectious Diseases 156: 622–629

Ponzetto A, Cote P J, Popper H et al 1984 Transmission of the hepatitis B-associated delta agent to the eastern woodchuck. Proceedings of the National Academy of Sciences of the USA 81: 2208–2212

Ponzetto A, Forzani B, Parravicini P P, Hele C, Zanetti A, Rizzetto M 1985 Epidemiology of hepatitis delta virus infection. European Journal of Epidemiology 1: 257–263

Riesner D, Gross H J 1985 Viroids. Annual Review of Biochemistry 54: 531–564

Rizzetto M, Verme G 1985 Delta hepatitis: present status. Journal of Hepatology 1: 187–193

Rizzetto M, Canese M G, Arico S et al 1977 Immunofluorescence detection of a new antigen-antibody system (delta/anti-delta) associated to hepatitis B virus in liver and in serum of HBsAg carriers. Gut 18: 997–1003

Rizzetto M, Hoyer B, Canese M G, et al 1980a Delta antigen: the association of delta antigen with hepatitis B surface antigen and ribonucleic acid in the serum of delta infected chimpanzees. Proceedings of the National Academy of Sciences of the USA 77: 6124–6128

Rizzetto M, Purcell R H, Gerin J L 1980b Epidemiology of HBV-associated delta agent: geographical distribution of anti-δ and prevalence in polytransfused HBsAg carriers. Lancet i: 1215–1218

Rizzetto M, Canese M G, Gerin J L, London W T, Sly D L,

Purcell R H 1980c Transmission of the hepatitis B virus-associated delta antigen to chimpanzees. Journal of Infectious Diseases 141: 590–602
Ryu W-S, Bayer M, Taylor J 1992 Assembly of hepatitis delta virus. Journal of Virology 66: 2310–2315
Saldanha J A, Thomas H C, Monjardino J 1990a Cloning and sequencing of RNA of hepatitis delta virus isolated from human serum. Journal of General Virology 71: 1603–1606
Saldanha J, Homer E, Goldin R, Thomas H C and Monjardino J 1990b Cloning and expression of an immunodominant region of hepatitis delta antigen. Journal of General Virology 71: 471–475
Sharmeen L, Kuo M Y-P, Dieter-Gottleib B, Taylor J 1988 Antigenomic RNA of human delta virus can undergo self-cleavage. Journal of Virology 62: 2674–2679
Sharmeen L, Kuo M Y-P, Taylor J 1989 Self-ligating RNA sequences on the antigenome of human hepatitis delta virus. Journal of Virology 63: 1428–1430
Sureau C, Taylor J, Chao M, Eichberg J W, Lanford R E 1989 Cloned hepatitis delta virus cDNA is infectious in the chimpanzee. Journal of Virology 63 4292–4299
Sureau C, Jacob J R, Eichberg J W, Lanford R E 1991 Tissue culture system for infection with human hepatitis delta virus. Journal of Virology 65: 3443–3450
Sureau C, Moriarty A M, Thornton G B, Lanford R 1992 Production of infectious hepatitis delta virus in vitro and neutralization with antibodies directed against hepatitis B virus pre-S antigens. Journal of Virology 66: 1241–1245
Taylor J M, Mason W, Summers J et al 1988 Replication of human hepatitis delta virus in primary cultures and woodchuck hepatocytes. Journal of Virology 62: 2981–2985
Wang J-G, Jansen R W, Brown E, Lemon S 1990 Immunogenic domains of hepatitis delta virus antigen: peptide mapping of epitopes recognized by human and woodchuck antibodies. Journal of Virology 64: 1108–1116
Wang K-S, Choo Q-L, Weiner A J et al 1987 Structure, sequence and expression of the hepatitis delta (δ) viral genome. Nature 328: 456
Weiner A J, Choo Q-L, Wang K-S et al 1988 A single antigenomic open reading frame of the hepatitis delta virus encodes the epitope(s) of both hepatitis delta antigen polypeptides $p24^{\delta}$ and $p27^{\delta}$. Journal of Virology 62: 594–599
Wu H-N, Lai M M C 1989 Reversible cleavage and ligation of hepatitis delta virus RNA. Science 243: 652–654
Wu H-N, Lai M M C 1990 RNA conformational requirements of self-cleavaage of hepatitis delta virus RNA. Molecular and Cellular Biology 10: 5575–5579
Wu H-N, Lin Y-J, Lin F-P et al 1989 Human delta hepatitis virus RNA subfragments contain an autocleavage activity. Proceedings of the National Academy of Sciences of the USA 86: 1831–1835
Wu H-N, Wang Y-J, Hung C-F, Lee H-J, Lai M M C 1992 Sequence and structure of the catalytic RNA of hepatitis delta virus genomic RNA. Journal of Molecular Biology 223: 233–245
Wu J C, Lee S D, Govindarajan S, Kung T W, Ting L P 1990 Correlation of serum delta RNA with clinical course of acute hepatitis delta virus superinfection in Taiwan: a longitudinal study. Journal of Infectious Diseases 161, 1116–1120
Wu J-C, Chen P-J, Kuo M Y P, Lee S-D, Chen D-S, Ting L-P 1991 Production of hepatitis delta virus and suppression of helper hepatitis B virus in a human hepatoma cell line. Journal of Virology 65: 1099–1104
Xia Y-P, Lai M M C 1992 Oligomerization of hepatitis delta antigen is required for the trans-activating and trans-dominant inhibitory activities of the delta antigen. Journal of Virology 66: 6641–6648
Xia Y-P, Chang M-F, Govindarajan S, Lai M M C 1990 Heterogeneity of hepatitis delta antigen. Virology 178: 331–336
Xia Y-P, Yeh C-T, Ou J-H, Lai M M C 1992 Characterization of nuclear targeting signal of hepatitis delta antigen: nuclear transport as a protein complex. Journal of Virology 66: 914–921
Young B, Hicke B 1990 Delta virus as a cleaver. Nature 343: 28
Zyzik E, Ponzetto A, Forzani B, Hele C, Heermann K, Gerlich W H 1987 Proteins of hepatitis virus in serum and liver. In: Robinson W, Koike K, Will H (eds) Hepadnaviruses Alan R. Liss, New York, pp 565–577

UPDATE

- The biological significance of the RNA-binding activity of HDAg was studied by examining the trans-activating activity of the RNA-binding mutants. The plasmids expressing HDAgs with various mutations in the RNA-binding motifs were cotransfected with a replication-defective HDV dimer cDNA construct into COS cells. It was found that all the HDAg mutants which had lost the in vitro RNA-binding activity also lost the ability to complement the defect of HDV RNA replication. It was concluded that the transactivating function of HDAg requires its binding to HDV RNA (Lee et al 1993).
- REFERENCES

Lee C-Z, Lin J-H, McKnight K, Lai M M C 1993 RNA-binding of hepatitis delta antigen requires two arginine-rich motifs (ARMs) and is required for hepatitis delta virus RNA replication. Journal of Virology 67: 2221–2229

20. Natural history

Hari S. Conjeevaram Adrian M. Di Bisceglie

Delta hepatitis is caused by dual infection with the hepatitis delta virus (HDV) and the hepatitis B virus (HBV). When HDV was first discovered, it was recognized that HDV infection is very often associated with severe or progressive liver disease (Rizzetto 1983, Sagnelli et al 1984). While this is often true, it has become apparent more recently that the natural history of HDV infection may vary considerably, from fulminant acute hepatitis to a healthy carrier state (Rizzetto & Durazzo 1991, Hoofnagle 1986, 1989) (Fig. 20.1).

CLINICAL FEATURES

Acute Hepatitis

Two forms of acute delta hepatitis are recognized, depending on whether or not the infected individual is already infected with HBV. The term co-infection is used when both HDV and HBV are acquired at the same time. Superinfection refers to HDV infection occurring in an individual already chronically infected with HBV. These two conditions are contrasted in Table 20.1. The clinical and biochemical features of acute delta hepatitis are generally indistinguishable from those associated with other forms of hepatitis in individual cases, and the diagnosis must usually be made with appropriate serological tests (see Ch. 21).

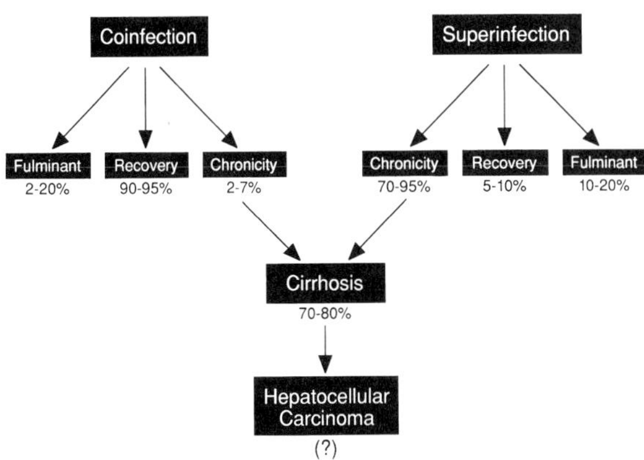

Fig. 20.1 A schematic representation of the possible outcome of co-infection or superinfection with the hepatitis delta virus (Adapted from Hadler et al 1984, Caredda et al 1985, De Cock et al 1986, Buti et al 1987, Lettau et al 1987, Hoofnagle 1989, Lindh et al 1990.)

Acute delta hepatitis tends to be more severe than acute hepatitis B alone and is more likely to result in fulminant hepatitis (Smedile et al 1982, Govindarajan et al 1984) (Table 20.2). In an outbreak of hepatitis associated with intravenous drug use in a community in the USA (Lettau et al 1987), 91% of patients with fulminant hepatitis had anti-HDV in their serum, whereas only 45% of patients with non-fulminant cases had anti-HDV. In the majority of patients with delta co-infection, the disease is self-limiting (Caredda et al 1985, Buti et al 1987, Lindh et al

Table 20.1 Two forms of acute delta hepatitis

Characteristic	Co-infection	Superinfection
HBV infection	Acute	Chronic
HDV infection	Acute	Acute to chronic
Mortality rate	1–2 %	1–5 %
Chronicity rate	2–7 %	70–90 %
HBsAg in serum	+, transient	+, usually persists
IgM anti-HBc	+	–
Anti-HDV	Transient low titre	+, persists, rising
IgM anti-HDV	+, transient	+, usually persists
HDV RNA in serum	+, persists	+, persists

Adapted from Hoofnagle (1986) with permission.

Table 20.2 Severity of acute delta hepatitis: percentage of HBsAg positive acute hepatitis with anti-HDV

Reference	No. tested	Anti-HDV (%)	
		Benign, self-limiting	Fulminant
Smedile et al (1982)	643	19	39
Govindarajan et al (1984)	189	4	34
Lettau et al (1987)	107	45	91

Anti-HDV, antibody to hepatitis delta virus.

1990). Serum aminotransferases return to normal and markers of viraemia (HBsAg, HBV DNA, HDV RNA, IgM anti-HDV) disappear from serum over a period of 2–10 weeks, although IgG anti-HDV may persist for years afterwards. A common feature of delta co-infection is a biphasic pattern to the illness with two separate peaks in serum aminotransferases thought to reflect injury caused by each of the two viruses sequentially (Moestrup et al 1983, Caredda et al 1986, De Cock et al 1986, Lindh et al 1990). The second peak usually follows the initial illness by 2–4 weeks. Relapses associated with the second peak of serum aminotransferase activity may range widely in severity and may occasionally cause liver injury severe enough to result in subacute or fulminant hepatic failure. Caredda et al (1985) found that a biphasic illness occurred in 29% of patients with delta co-infection, compared with 13% with HBV infection alone. Severe relapses resulting in a fulminant course were noted in as many as 20% of patients by Govindarajan et al (1986a), who also noted that in the majority of subjects a significant rise in serum aminotransferases and prothrombin time coincided with the second peak.

Chronicity after delta co-infection occurs in no more than 10% of patients (Buti et al 1987). However, acute delta hepatitis very often becomes chronic following superinfection, (Lin et al 1989), presumably because chronic HBV infection is already established in that individual. With delta superinfection, levels of anti-HDV (both IgM and total) tend to rise more rapidly and to reach higher levels than with delta co-infection. In a study describing the clinical outcome of patients with acute delta hepatitis in Spain, Buti et al (1987) noted that 1 of 42 patients with delta co-infection developed fulminant hepatitis compared with 3 of 17 with delta superinfection. Of 38 patients with delta superinfection from Taiwan, 24 were noted to have prolonged hepatic inflammation, five (20%) developed cirrhosis and two died during a 4-year follow-up period (Wu et al 1990). Acute delta superinfection occurring in patients with pre-existing cirrhosis related to HBV infection may precipitate hepatic decompensation or even death (Liaw et al 1990).

During delta superinfection, HBV replication tends to be suppressed (Rizzetto et al 1980). This is presumed to be related to a competitive interaction between the two viruses, which is poorly understood. The inhibition tends to be transient, but permanent loss of hepatitis B e antigen has been noted to occur in some cases. Interestingly, acute delta superinfection may occasionally result in permanent clearance of HBsAg from serum with complete resolution of liver disease activity (Ichimura et al 1988, Pastore et al 1990).

Chronic delta hepatitis

Chronic delta hepatitis most commonly develops following acute delta superinfection (Caredda et al 1985, Govindarajan et al 1986b, Gerken & Meyer zum Buschenfelde 1991). Patients may present with non-specific features of chronic liver disease such as fatigue and general malaise, although many are asymptomatic until they develop signs or symptoms of advanced liver disease such as ascites, jaundice or bleeding from oesophageal varices. In asymptomatic patients the diagnosis of delta hepatitis is often made coincidentally, at the time of routine examinations for insurance or other purposes. Patients found to have HBsAg in serum may often not be suspected of having delta hepatitis unless this diagnosis is actively and systematically sought (usually by testing for anti-HDV in serum).

Patients with chronic delta hepatitis often have severe or advanced liver disease noted on liver biopsy (Colombo et al 1983, Sagnelli et al 1984, Fattovich et al 1987, Villari et al 1989). In a study from Italy of liver biopsy material from 203 consecutive patients with HBsAg-positive chronic liver disease (Sagnelli et al 1989), those with markers of HDV infection had more severe liver disease than those who did not (30% *vs.* 12%). Patients with HDAg-positive cirrhosis were significantly younger than those with HDAg-negative cirrhosis, suggesting that delta hepatitis has a more rapidly progressive course.

Among 2487 apparently healthy individuals incidentally found to have HBsAg in serum, 112 (5%) had anti-HDV (Arico et al 1985). Those patients with anti-HDV were significantly more likely to have raised serum aminotransferases (38% *vs.* 9%) and significant histological changes on liver biopsy (61% *vs.* 19%) than others in the group.

Rizzetto et al (1983) have followed a cohort of patients with chronic delta hepatitis for many years. Most of their patients had chronic active hepatitis or cirrhosis on initial liver biopsy. On follow-up, a significant proportion of patients developed cirrhosis within less than 5 years. Approximately one-third of patients with established cirrhosis died during the follow-up period (Bonino et al 1991). These authors also noted that immunosuppressive therapy did not seem to have any beneficial effect on the condition.

Chronic delta hepatitis in children appears to follow a progressive course similar to that seen in adults. Farci et al (1985) followed 34 children with chronic delta infection for 2–7 years. During the follow-up period, the hepatitis deteriorated in 38% of the cases and improved in only 9%. In contrast, only 7% of a cohort of 236 patients with delta-negative chronic hepatitis B showed a deterioration of their liver disease, while remission was noted in 55%. Like Rizzetto et al (1983), these authors also noted that the disease was unresponsive to immunosuppressive treatment.

Histopathology

Although certain histological features have been noted in liver samples from patients with delta infection, these features are not specific (Rizzetto et al 1983, Popper et al 1987). It is only with the use of immunostaining for HDAg that a definitive diagnosis of delta hepatitis can be made on liver biopsy. Patients with acute delta hepatitis do not often have liver biopsies done. However, material has been examined from patients dying with fulminant delta hepatitis. An unusual change has been noted in liver samples from such patients in Venezuela. Acute delta hepatitis in tropical countries has been associated with foamy change in hepatocytes due to microvesicular steatosis, in addition to more typical changes of acute hepatitis such as apoptosis and inflammation (Hadler et al 1984, Buitrago et al 1986, Popper et al 1987). An unusual form of eosinophilic degeneration that appears to be distinct from apoptosis has been noted. Clusters of cells showing this change are found in biopsies from patients with chronic delta hepatitis. The presence of 'morula' cells has been said to be specific for delta hepatitis (Buitrago et al 1986).

The changes seen in patients with chronic delta hepatitis are those of chronic hepatitis except that they tend to be severe (Table 20.3) and patients are more likely to have chronic active hepatitis or cirrhosis. Most patients have hepatic HDAg detectable by immunostaining, although often only a few cells are stained. The number of HDAg-containing cells may decrease with time and increasing severity of liver disease.

Factors influencing the outcome of delta hepatitis

It has become apparent that although chronic delta hepatitis tends to run a more severe course than HBV infection alone, there is a great deal of variability in the outcome of HDV infection (Rizzetto & Verme 1985). In fact, individuals who appear to be 'healthy carriers' of HDV have been described (Arico et al 1985, Hadziyannis et al 1991). The reasons for this clinical heterogeneity are uncertain. Several fac tors have been

Table 20.3 Percentage of patients with chronic hepatitis B (HBsAg positive) with markers of delta infection (hepatic HDAg or anti-HDV in serum) according to histological severity of hepatitis

Reference	Total cases	Histological diagnosis				
		NL/NSH (%)	CPH (%)	CLH (%)	CAH (%)	Cirrhosis (%)
Colombo et al 1983	192	0	14	0	32	52
Weller et al 1983	71	0	0	0	11	31
Govindarajan et al 1983	80	0	4	0	32	28
Sagnelli et al 1989	203	0	14	36	46	30

Abbreviations: HDAg, hepatitis delta antigen; anti-HDV, antibody to hepatitis delta virus; NL, normal; NSH, non-specific hepatitis; CPH, chronic persistent hepatitis; CLH, chronic lobular hepatitis; CAH, chronic active hepatitis.

suggested as being important in determining the outcome of HDV infection. One of these is the presence and level of HBV replication (Fig. 20.2). Those patients with evidence of HBV replication (HBV DNA in serum detectable by dot-blot hybridization) tend to have more severe chronic liver disease and progress more rapidly to end-stage liver disease (Smedile et al 1991a–c). The reason for this is not clear but is presumably related to the so-called 'helper function' of HBV, which may permit increased levels of HDV replication.

The mechanism by which HDV infection results in liver injury remains obscure. HDV infection by itself does not seem to be directly cytopathic in experimental models and in the post-transplant situation (Negro & Rizzetto 1991, Smedile et al 1991d). However, patients with chronic HDV infection do have very high intracellular levels of HDV replication, and it is

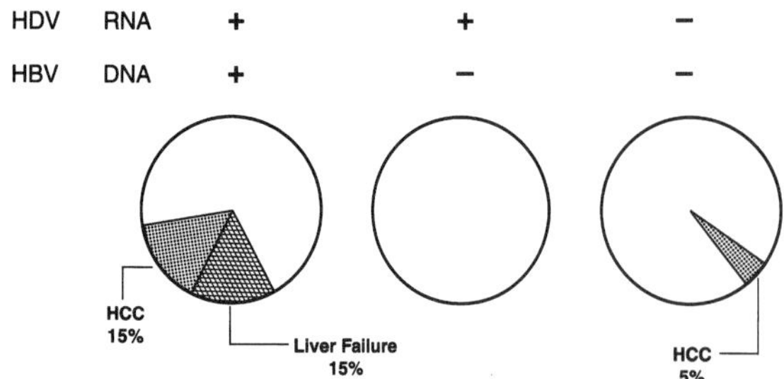

Fig. 20.2 The effect of HBV replication on the outcome of chronic delta hepatitis. Note that patients with evidence of hepatitis B viral replication appear to be more likely to develop cirrhosis and liver failure. HCC, hepatocellular carcinoma. (Adapted from A Smedile 1991b, with permission.)

possible that the load imposed on normal cellular metabolic pathways by viral replication in the hepatocyte may result in cellular injury. One interesting hypothesis is based on the observation that the antigenomic RNA strand of the HDV genome has a high degree of nucleotide homology with 7S ribosomal RNA, suggesting that annealing of the antigenomic HDV RNA to 7S RNA may occur with ribozymic cleavage of the 7S RNA and derangement of smooth endoplasmic reticulum structure and function (Negro et al 1991).

The role of the immune system in pathogenesis of delta hepatitis is uncertain. Portal tracts are infiltrated with chronic inflammatory cells in patients with chronic delta hepatitis, suggesting that the immune system plays some role. However, corticosteroid therapy does not appear to have a beneficial effect on the course of the disease (Rizzetto et al 1983, Colombo et al 1983). Various autoantibodies have been observed in serum of patients with chronic delta hepatitis. The role of these autoantibodies in causing liver injury is unknown (Bonino et al 1991).

Patients with chronic delta hepatitis often do not have the hepatitis B e antigen (HBeAg) detectable in serum, although almost all have HBsAg. This may be related to having low levels of HBV replication or, in some cases, to being infected with the e-minus variant form of HBV. The course of delta hepatitis seems to be somewhat milder in patients who do not have HBeAg (Brunetto et al 1991).

It remains unclear whether patients with HDV infection from various sources have different outcomes. This has been difficult to study as the source of hepatitis differs in each of the large centres studying the disease. Thus, in Italy and Greece, most patients do not give a history of intravenous drug abuse or blood transfusion and their hepatitis is presumed to represent intrafamilial spread. Although many patients from these areas have severe disease, they are perhaps more likely to be 'healthy carriers' of HDV than those who contracted HDV infection following intravenous drug use, possibly because the latter group are exposed to other blood-borne agents such as human immunodeficiency virus (HIV) and HCV. The role of HCV infection in patients with chronic delta hepatitis has not been closely examined. However, patients with HIV infection and delta hepatitis do not appear to have an unusually unfavourable outcome of their liver disease, although they may have higher levels of HBV replication and lower levels of delta antibodies than non-HIV-infected patients (Govindarajan et al 1991). Monno et al (1991), in their study of delta hepatitis patients with and without HIV infection, found no significant difference in liver histology in the two groups. They also noted that the presence of HDAg in liver was similar in all HIV-infected patients irrespective of their CD4 counts.

Hepatocellular carcinoma and HDV

Chronic HBV infection is an important risk factor for the development of hepatocellular carcinoma (HCC). Similar associations have been sought with chronic HDV infection, but have not been clearly demonstrated. For example, in a recent study from Italy, similar proportions of patients with cirrhosis with and without HCC were found to have serological markers of HDV infection (Ponzetto et al 1988). In some parts of the world where HBV-related HCC is very common (such as southern Africa and Taiwan) very few cases of HCC associated with chronic delta hepatitis have been found (Chen et al 1984, Kew et al 1984). It has been suggested that HDV may act as an indirect promoting factor by causing severe liver disease and accelerating the development of cirrhosis (Verme et al 1991). Persistent necroinflammatory changes associated with hepatic regeneration may be expected to enhance the development of HCC in some cases. Oliveri et al (1991) reported that patients with HBsAg and HDV superinfection developed active cirrhosis and HCC at an earlier age than patients with HBsAg alone. The median age for development of HCC was 56 years for patients with chronic hepatitis B or C versus 48 years for patients infected with HBV and HDV, with or without the hepatitis C virus. In the woodchuck animal model, the presence of HDV infection does not seem to either prevent or enhance the development of HCC (Schlipkoter et al 1990). HDAg is not often detected in HCC tissue in patients with chronic delta hepatitis and HCC, whereas it may be found in the surrounding nontumorous liver (Govindarajan et al 1986b).

Unusual forms of delta hepatitis

An unusual form of jaundice associated with sudden onset of fever, black vomit and fulminant hepatic failure has been described in the northern part of South America, particularly the Amazon Basin. This form of hepatitis has been referred to as Labrea hepatitis, black fever and Santa Marta hepatitis (Buitrago et al 1986). A retrospective analysis of liver biopsy material collected from these patients showed that most had evidence of delta hepatitis. These cases showed several striking histological features including the presence of microvesicular steatosis and eosinophilic necrosis. The reason for the unusually severe features of this form of delta hepatitis is unknown.

Spontaneous transient exacerbations of delta hepatitis have been noted in some patients (Govindarajan et al 1989). Whilc this could be accounted for in some cases by an exacerbation of HBV infection, some patients seemed to show a spontaneous rise in levels of HDV replication with an accompanying rise in serum aminotransferases. A similar pattern may be noted, albeit more frequently, in patients with chronic hepatitis C. The possible significance of these fluctuations is not known but they may be associated with episodes of severe necrosis resulting in progressive liver injury.

An unusually benign form of HDV infection has been noted in a community on the island of

Rhodes, Greece (Hadziyannis et al 1991). Among 71 patients with chronic delta hepatitis who had serum aminotransferases estimated or a liver biopsy done, 59% were asymptomatic with normal serum aminotransferase activities and essentially normal liver biopsies. Again, the reason for this variant and its possible geographic distribution are not known.

Occasional cases of chronic delta hepatitis occur with unusual serological markers. Thus, some haemophiliacs with HIV infection and no anti-HDV in serum have been noted to have HDV RNA in serum. Occasional patients have been found to have HDAg in the liver with no anti-HDV in serum (Becherer et al 1991). In the woodchuck animal model of delta hepatitis, an unusual course was noted in one animal who was a carrier of HBV and was inoculated with HDV but did not develop anti-HDV. However, HDV RNA was later found within the liver by Northern blot analysis (Schlipkoter et al 1990).

LESSONS FROM ANIMAL MODELS OF HDV INFECTION

Although HDV infection is not known to occur naturally in animals, certain species have been experimentally infected, and these animal models have been very useful in studying biology of HDV infection (Ponzetto et al 1991). The original series of experiments which determined that the delta antigen was related to a transmissible agent distinct from HBV were done in chimpanzees. Rizzetto et al (1980) showed that chimpanzees who were immune to HBV could not be infected with delta, while those who were susceptible or already infected with HBV could be infected. It was in these studies that it was first noticed that HDV superinfection seemed to have an inhibitory effect on HBV replication. Some of the infected animals who had had no evidence of liver disease previously, despite being chronically infected with HBV, developed significant liver injury following infection with HDV. During the acute phase of delta infection, the occurrence of hepatic injury was closely associated in time with the appearance of HDAg, suggesting a direct pathogenic effect of HDV in hepatocytes. HDV infection often becomes and remains chronic in chimpanzees though the chronically infected state does not appear to be associated with significant hepatic injury (Negro et al 1988). In an interesting experiment, Negro et al (1989) rechallenged chronic HBV carrier chimpanzees with HDV and found that HDV RNA reappeared in serum, suggesting that they may have been reinfected or perhaps had latent HDV infection reactivated in some way.

Animals infected with hepadnaviruses other than hepatitis B have also been innoculated with HDV. Although ducks carrying the duck HBV did not seem to be susceptible to delta infection, woodchucks infected with the woodchuck hepatitis virus readily became infected with HDV and provided a very useful animal model (Ponzetto et al 1984). Chimpanzees are not readily available, are difficult to handle and expensive to keep. However, woodchucks are much more readily available and easier to keep in captivity. HDV infection in woodchucks shows biological and pathological features similar to those seen in humans and may be a useful model to test new antiviral drugs, vaccines and possibly examine new isolates of HDV for pathogenicity.

PREVENTION OF DELTA HEPATITIS

No effective vaccine is available against HDV infection. Obviously, HDV infection can be avoided by preventing HBV infection and thus HBV vaccination would prevent delta hepatitis. However, the individuals most at risk of HDV infection – carriers of HBsAg – would not benefit from HBV vaccination. Patients with chronic HBV infection should be advised that they are at risk from continued intravenous drug abuse or promiscuous sexual behaviour.

Programmes of mass vaccination against HBV are underway in many countries around the world, including some of those where HDV infection is particularly prevalent, such as Pacific islands, some parts of South America, Taiwan, and recently in Romania. Recombinant HDAg is now available and has been used to try and prevent HDV infection in an animal model without success (Karayiannis et al 1990). More recent studies with recombinant vaccinia containing HDV inserts have shown that this method of immunization, which may induce cytotoxic T-cell sensitization, is capable of controlling the level of HDV viraemia (Karayiannis et al 1992).

SUMMARY AND CONCLUSIONS

HDV infection occurs only in individuals already infected with HBV. Acute infection appears to result in severe or fulminant hepatitis more often than HBV alone. Similarly, chronic delta hepatitis very often results in rapid progression of the liver disease to cirrhosis and liver failure. Although HDV infection is generally associated with this more severe and progressive form of hepatitis, it has become apparent that there is a great deal of variability in the outcome and natural history of HDV infection. Factors such as host susceptibility, environmental background and viral features should be examined more closely to determine their impact on the outcome of delta hepatitis.

REFERENCES

Arico S, Rizzetto M, Zanetti A et al 1985 Clinical significance of antibody to the hepatitis delta virus in symptomless HBsAg carriers. Lancet ii: 356–358

Becherer P R, Wang J-G, White G C et al 1991 Hepatitia delta virus infection in hemophiliacs. In: Hollinger F B, Lemon S M, Margolis H S (eds) Viral hepatitis and liver disease. Williams & Wilkins, Baltimore, pp 492–494

Bonino F, Brunetto M R, Negro F 1991 Factors influencing the natural course of HDV hepatitis. In: Gerin J L, Purcell R H, Rizzetto M (eds) The hepatitis delta virus. Wiley–Liss, New York, pp 137–146

Brunetto M R, Oliveri F, Baldi M et al 1991 Does HBeAg minus HBV modify the course of HDV superinfection? In: Gerin J L, Purcell cell, Rizzetto M (eds) The hepatitis delta virus. Wiley–Liss, New York, pp 211–216

Buitrago B, Popper H, Hadler S C et al 1986 Specific histological features of Santa Marta hepatitis: a severe form of hepatitis δ-virus infection in northern South America. Hepatology 6: 1285–1291

Buti M, Esteban R, Jardi R et al 1987 Clinical and serological outcome of acute delta infection. Journal of Hepatology 5: 59–64

Caredda F, Rossi E, d'Arminio Monforte A et al 1985 Hepatitis B virus-associated coinfection and superinfection with δ agent: indistinguishable disease with different outcome. Journal of Infectious Diseases 151: 925–928

Caredda F, Antinori S, Re T et al 1986 Biphasic hepatitis in HBV/HDV coinfected parenteral drug users. Gut 27: 19–22

Chen D-S, Lai M-Y, Sung J-L 1984 Delta agent infection in patients with chronic liver diseases and hepatocellular carcinoma – an infrequent finding in Taiwan. Hepatology 4: 502–504

Colombo M, Cambieri R, Rumi M G et al 1983 Long-term delta superinfection in hepatitis B surface antigen carriers and its relationship to the course of chronic hepatitis. Gastroenterology 85: 235–239

De Cock K M, Govindarajan S, Chin K P, Redeker A G 1986 Delta hepatitis in the Los Angeles area: a report of 126 cases. Annals of Internal Medicine 105: 108–114

Farci P, Barbera C, Navone C et al 1985 Infection with the delta agent in children. Gut 26: 4–7

Fattovich G, Boscaro S, Noventa F et al 1987 Influence of hepatitis delta virus infection on progression to cirrhosis in chronic hepatitis type B. The Journal of Infectious Diseases 155: 931–935

Gerken G, Meyer zum Buschenfelde K-H 1991 Chronic hepatitis delta virus (HDV) infection. Hepato-gastroenterology 38: 29–32

Govindarajan S, Kanel G C, Peters R L 1983 Prevalence of delta-antibody among chronic hepatitis B virus infected patients in Los Angeles area: its correlation with liver biopsy diagnosis. Gastroenterology 85: 160–162

Govindarajan S, Chin K P, Redeker A G, Peters R L 1984 Fulminant B viral hepatitis: role of delta agent. Gastroenterology 86: 1417–1420

Govindarajan S, Valinluck B, Peters L 1986a Relapse of acute B viral hepatitis – role of delta agent. Gut 27: 19–22

Govindarajan S, De Cock K M, Redeker A G 1986b Natural course of delta superinfection in chronic hepatitis B virus-infected patients: Histopathologic study with multiple liver biopsies Hepatology 6: 640–644

Govindarajan S, Smedile A, De Cock K M et al 1989 Study of reactivation of chronic hepatitis delta infection. Journal of Hepatology 9: 204–208

Govindarajan S, Cassidy W, Valinluck B, Redeker A G 1991 Interactions of HDV, HBV and HIV in reactivation of chronic D infection. In: Gerin J L, Purcell R H, Rizzetto M (eds) The hepatitis delta virus. Wiley–Liss, New York, pp 207–210

Hadler S C, De Monzon M, Ponzetto A et al 1984 Delta virus infection and severe hepatitis. Annals of Internal Medicine 100: 339–344

Hadziyannis S J, Papaioannou C, Alexopoulou A 1991 The role of hepatitis delta virus in acute hepatitis and chronic liver disease in Greece. In: Gerin J L, Purcell R H, Rizzetto M (eds) The hepatitis delta virus. Wiley–Liss, New York, pp 51–62

Hoofnagle J H 1986 Type D hepatitis and the hepatitis delta virus. In: Thomas H C, Jones E A (eds) Recent advances in hepatology. Churchill Livingstone, Edinburgh, pp 73–92

Hoofnagle J H 1989 Type D (Delta) Hepatitis. Journal of the American Medical Association 261: 1321–1325

Ichimura H, Tamura I, Tsubakio T et al 1988 Influence of hepatitis delta virus superinfection on the clearance of hepatitis B virus (HBV) markers in HBV carriers in Japan. Journal of Medical Virology 26: 49–55

Karayiannis P, Saldanha J, Monjardino J et al 1990 Immunization of woodchucks with recombinant hepatitis delta agent does not protect against hepatitis delta virus infection. Hepatology 12: 1125–1128

Kew M C, Dusheiko G M, Hadziyannis S J, Patterson A

1984 Does delta infection play a part in the pathogenesis of hepatitis B virus related hepatocellular carcinoma? British Medical Journal 288: 1727
Lettau L A, Mc Carthy J G, Smith M J et al 1987 Outbreak of severe hepatitis due to delta and hepatitis B viruses in parenteral drug abusers and their contacts. New England Journal Medicine 317: 1256–1262
Liaw Y-F, Chen T-J, Chu C-M, Lin H-H 1990 Acute hepatitis delta virus superinfection in patients with liver cirrhosis. Journal of Hepatology 10: 41–45
Lin H-H, Liaw Y-F, Chen T-J et al 1989 Natural course of patients with chronic type B hepatitis following acute hepatitis delta virus superinfection. Liver 9: 129–134
Lindh G, Mattsson L, von Sydow M, Weiland O 1990 Acute hepatitis B and hepatitis D co-infection in the Stockholm region in the 1970s and 1980s. A comparison. Infection 18: 357–360
Moestrup T, Hansson B G, Widell A, Nordenfelt E 1983 Clinical aspects of delta infection. British Medical Journal 286: 87–90
Monno L, Angarano G, Santantonio T et al 1991 Lack of HBV and HDV replicative activity in HBsAg-positive intravenous drug addicts with immune deficiency due to HIV. Journal of Medical Virology 34: 199–205
Negro F, Rizzetto M 1991 Pathobiology of hepatitis delta virus. In: Hollinger F B, Lemon S M, Margolis H S (eds) Viral hepatitis and liver disease. Williams & Wilkins, Baltimore, pp 477–480
Negro F, Bergmann K F, Baroudy B M et al 1988 Chronic hepatitis D virus (HDV) infection in hepatitis B virus carrier chimpanzees experimentally superinfected with HDV. The Journal of Infectious Diseases, 158: 151–159
Negro F, Shapiro M, Satterfield W C et al 1989 Reappearance of Hepatitis D virus (HDV) replication in chronic hepatitis B virus carrier chimpanzees rechallenged with HDV. The Journal of Infectious Diseases 160: 567–571
Negro F, Gerin J L, Purcell R H, Miller R 1991 Sequence homology between HDV RNA and 7SL RNA: Implications for pathogenesis. In: Gerin J L, Purcell R H, Rizzetto M (eds) The hepatitis delta virus. Wiley–Liss, New York, pp 327–333
Oliveri F, Brunetto M R, Baldi M et al 1991 Hepatitis delta virus (HDV) infection and hepatocellular carcinoma (HCV). In: Gerin J L, Purcell R H, Rizzetto M (eds) The hepatitis delta virus. Wiley–Liss, New York, pp 217–222
Pastore G, Monno L, Santantonio T et al 1990 Hepatitis B virus clearance from serum and liver after acute hepatitis delta virus superinfection in chronic HBsAg carriers. Journal of Medical Virology 31: 284–290
Ponzetto A, Cote P J, Popper H et al 1984 Transmission of the hepatitis B virus-associated δ agent to the eastern woodchuck. Proceedings of the National Academy of Sciences of the USA 81: 2208–2212
Ponzetto A, Hele C, Forzani B, Avanzini L, Rizzetto M 1988 Hepatitis delta virus and hepatocellular carcinoma. Gastroenterology 94(5): A583
Ponzetto A, Negro F, Gerin J L, Purcell R H 1991 Experimental hepatitis delta virus infection in the animal model. In: Gerin J L, Purcell Rh, Rizzetto M (eds) The hepatitis delta virus. Wiley–Liss, New York, pp 147–157
Popper H, Buitrago B, Hadler S C et al 1987 Pathology of hepatitis delta infection in the Amazon basin. In: Rizzetto M, Gerin J L, Purcell R H (eds) The Hepatitis delta virus and its infection. Progress in Clinical and Biological Research 234: 121–126
Rizzetto M 1983 The delta agent. Hepatology 5: 729–737
Rizzetto M, Durazzo M 1991 Hepatitis delta virus (HDV) infections. Epidemiological and clinical heterogeneity. Journal of Hepatology 13 (suppl. 4): S116–S118
Rizzetto M, Verme G 1985 Delta hepatitis – present status. Journal of Hepatology 1: 187–193
Rizzetto M, Canese M G, Gerin J L et al 1980 Transmission of the hepatitis B virus-associated delta agent to chimpanzees. Journal of Infectious Diseases 141: 590–602
Rizzetto M, Verme G, Recchia S et al 1983 Chronic hepatitis in carriers of hepatitis B surface antigen, with intrahepatic expression of the delta antigen. Annals of Internal Medicine 98: 437–441
Sagnelli E, Piccinino F, Pasquale G et al 1984 Delta agent infection: an unfavourable event in HBsAg positive chronic hepatitis. Liver 4: 170–175
Sagnelli E, Felaco F M, Filippini P et al 1989 Influence of HDV infection on clinical, biochemical and histological presentation of HBsAg positive chronic hepatitis. Liver 9: 229–234
Schlipkoter U, Ponzetto A, Fuchs K et al 1990 Different outcomes of chronic hepatitis delta virus infection in woodchucks. Liver 10: 291–301
Smedile A, Verme G, Cargnel A et al 1982 Influence of Delta infection on severity of hepatitis B. Lancet ii: 945–947
Smedile A, Rosina F, Saracco G et al 1991a Hepatitis B virus replication modulates pathogenesis of hepatitis D virus in chronic hepatitis D. Hepatology 13: 413–416
Smedile A, Rosina F, Chiaberge E et al 1991b Presence and significance of hepatitis B virus replication in chronic type D hepatitis. In: Gerin J L, Purcell R H, Rizzetto M (eds) The hepatitis delta virus. Wiley–Liss, New York, pp 185–195
Smedile A, Chiaberge E, Rosina F et al 1991c HBV replication influences the course of chronic hepatitis D. In: Hollinger F B, Lemon S M, Margolis H S (eds) Viral hepatitis and liver disease. Williams & Wilkins, Baltimore, pp 480–483
Smedile A, Marzano A, Farci P et al 1991d Liver transplant for viral hepatitis. Recurrence of reinfection. Journal of Hepatology 13 (suppl 4): S134–S137
Verme G, Brunetto M R, Oliveri F et al 1991 Role of Hepatitis delta virus infection in hepatocellular carcinoma. Digestive Diseases and Sciences 36: 1134–1136

Villari D, Raimondo G, Smedile V et al 1989 Hepatitis B-DNA replication and histological patterns in liver biopsy specimens of chronic HBsAg positive patients with and without hepatitis delta virus superinfection. Journal of Clinical Pathology 42: 689–693
Weller IVD, Karayiannis P, Lok A S F et al 1983 The significance of delta agent infection in chronic viral hepatitis B infection in Great Britain. Gut 24: 1061–1063
Wu J-C, Lee S-D, Govindarajan S et al 1990 Sexual transmission of hepatitis D virus infection in Taiwan. Hepatology 11: 1057–1061

21. Epidemiology and diagnosis

Adrian M. Di Bisceglie

EPIDEMIOLOGY OF DELTA HEPATITIS

The hepatitis delta virus (HDV) was first discovered in 1977 by Rizzetto and co-workers in Italy (Rizzetto et al 1977). These investigators found nuclear staining for hepatitis delta antigen (HDAg) predominantly in liver biopsies from patients in southern Italy. However, when an assay for antibody to HDV (anti-HDV) was developed and stored serum samples were tested, evidence of HDV infection was found all around the world (Rizzetto et al 1980).

Although delta hepatitis was only recognized in the late 1970s, it is likely that it has been present for much longer. Testing of old stored serum samples showed that anti-HDV was present in serum samples drawn as long ago as 1971 (Ponzetto et al 1985). A sample of normal human immunoglobulin prepared in the USA during the Second World War was found to have anti-HDV reactivity (Ponzetto et al 1984). Interestingly, liver samples from patients with Santa Marta hepatitis in South America, which had been obtained between 1937 and 1977, showed HDAg staining, confirming that the HDV had been causing human infection for a considerable period (Buitrago et al 1986).

Rizzetto et al (1991) estimated that no fewer than 15 000 000 persons are infected with HDV worldwide (they assumed that approximately 5% of HBsAg carriers are infected with HDV). It is more difficult to determine the number of cases of acute or fulminant hepatitis related to HDV infection as the incidence varies between continents, countries and regions. In the USA it has been estimated that 7500 acute HDV coinfections or superinfections occur annually. There are approximately 70 000 HDV carriers, and up to 1000 persons die from chronic or fulminant HDV infection each year (M Alter 1992, personal communication).

Routes of transmission

The hepatitis delta virus (HDV) is a blood-borne virus and may thus be transmitted by parenteral contact with blood or blood products. Common methods of transmission of HDV infection include intravenous drug abuse, transfusion, sexual contact and nosocomial infection (Table 21.1). In addition, inapparent parenteral spread is probably responsible for spread of HDV infection within families.

HDV infection has been detected among carriers of HBsAg throughout the world to a greater or lesser extent. The distribution of HDV infection is quite uneven, and prevalence rates may vary markedly in adjacent regions or communities (Table 21.2). In general three epidemiological patterns of HDV infection can be identified. These include the endemic pattern (such as occurs in

Table 21.1 Sources and routes of transmission of delta hepatitis

Intravenous drug abuse
Intrafamilial
Transfusion
Nosocomial
haemodialysis
injection, vaccinations
fingerstick device
Sexual contact (homosexual and heterosexual)
Inapparent parenteral spread

Table 21.2 Epidemiology of delta hepatitis: presence of anti-HDV among chronic carriers of HBsAg around the world

Continent	Carriers tested	Anti-HDV positive	
South America	669	51	(7.6%)
North America	940	112	(11.9%)
Asia	1651	179	(10.8%)
Africa	167	1600	(10.4%)
Australia/Oceania	144	9	(6.3%)
Europe			
eastern	1556	56	(3.6%)
northern	587	73	(12.4%)
southern	2697	484	(17.9%)

Adapted from Rizzetto et al (1991) with permission.

southern Italy and Greece), the epidemic pattern (epidemics have been described in the Amazon Basin of Venezuela) and the occurrence of HDV infection among high-risk groups such as intravenous drug users (in developed western countries).

HDV infection appears to be endemic in some populations, particularly in countries around the Mediterranean Sea. In southern Italy up to 23% of HBsAg carriers have anti-HDV, and in Greece up to 27% (Rizzetto et al 1991). Many of the patients in these regions seem to acquire HDV infection early in life, possibly even in childhood. Males tend to be affected more than females. The route of spread of HDV in these poulations is uncertain, as patients often do not seem to have any of the typical risk factors such as intravenous drug use and blood transfusion.

The role of sexual spread in propagating HDV infection is still unclear. HDV infection may be transmitted sexually, although not as readily as hepatitis B. Among homosexual men who are infected with HBV, rates of HDV infection range widely, from 0 (in England) to 40% (Italy) (Mele et al 1988, Goldin et al 1990). However, in most countries, the rate is less than 10% (Hess et al 1986, Bodsworth et al 1989, Weisfuse et al 1989). Many studies of delta hepatitis in homosexual men include individuals with a history of intravenous drug abuse, which is a potential confounding factor. In a study from France that did not include drug users, 6 of 42 homosexual men (14%) were found to have anti-HDV, suggesting that they may have acquired their disease sexually (Pol et al 1989). In the USA, HDV infection appears to be more common among homosexual men living on the west coast than in the midwest or east coast (Solomon et al 1988). In Taiwan, sexual spread of HDV infection has been described among male contacts of female prostitutes infected with HDV (Liaw et al 1990, Wu et al 1990). In endemic areas such as Italy and Greece sexual transmission is unlikely to account for those cases that originate in childhood but may be the cause of cases occurring later in life.

HDV appears to be only rarely transmitted by transfusions of whole blood (less than 1 in 3000 transfusions) despite screening of blood for HBsAg (Rosina et al 1985). However, it represents a major hazard to HBsAg-positive patients such as those with haemophilia treated with clotting factors prepared from large plasma pools. Among a group of HBsAg-positive haemophiliacs in the USA, 34% were found to have anti-HDV, and many of these patients had evidence of severe liver disease (Becherer et al 1991). Other, rarer routes of transmission include via haemodialysis (Lettau et al 1986) and via a spring-loaded fingerstick device (Mendez et al 1991).

Patterns of infection

HDV infection has also been noted to occur in epidemics in some populations. Separate epidemics have been described in the Yupca and Yanomani Indians of Venezuela (Hadler et al 1984, Torres & Mondolfi, 1991). Small-scale outbreaks of HDV infection have also been related to nosocomial transmission, either by haemodialysis (Lettau et al 1986) or during the course of cancer chemotherapy (Ratner 1986). An epidemic of delta hepatitis was described among intravenous drug addicts in Worcester, Massachusetts, in the USA (Lettau et al 1987). An interesting feature of this epidemic was the secondary outbreak of delta hepatitis among the sexual contacts of the drug addicts.

In northern Europe and the USA HDV infection is relatively uncommon, except among high-risk groups such as intravenous drug addicts and multiply transfused patients (e.g. haemophiliacs).

In a multicentre study from Europe, between 31% and 75% of HBsAg-positive drug addicts had markers of delta infection (Raimondo et al 1982). Among a group of 372 addicts in New York, 80 (22%) had anti-HDV (Kreek et al 1990).

Some regions appear to have unexpectedly low rates of HDV infection, often in the face of a high HBsAg carrier rate. An example of this is southern Africa, where the HBsAg carrier rate among blacks may be as high as 15% in some rural areas, but no cases of HDV infection have been noted (Dusheiko et al 1989, Abdool Karim et al 1991). However, further north in Africa delta hepatitis occurs more frequently. In Ethiopia for example, 6% of a group of military recruits were found to have anti-HDV (Rapicetta et al 1988), and in Cameroon 27% of 110 HBsAg-positive individuals also had anti-HDV in serum (Ndumbe 1991).

An unusually high prevalence of HDV infection has been noted in Romania where up to 83% of HBsAg-positive patients have anti-HDV (Tapalaga et al 1986). The reasons for this are not known but may be related to the use of contaminated needles for injections and inoculations and unusual medical practices such as administering whole blood by intramuscular injection.

Some isolated Pacific islands also have unusually high rates of HDV infection. Among 130 HBsAg-positive individuals in Kiribati (an independent republic composed of 26 islands), 90 (69%) had anti-HDV. Although the liver disease among these patients was not well characterized, none of the patients surveyed gave a history of acute hepatitis or jaundice (Tibbs 1989). On the neighbouring Pacific island of Nauru, 23% of HBsAg carriers were found to have anti-HDV (Speed et al 1989).

The epidemiology of HDV infections does seem to be changing in some regions. For example, the rate of HDV infection appears to be declining among individuals living in the Amazon Basin following a large-scale campaign of vaccination against HBV (L C D C Gayotto, personal communication, 1992). Similarly, the rate of new HDV infections has declined markedly in a community studied in Greece, where the most notable change introduced was the use of disposable needles for injections and vaccinations (J Hadziyannis, personal communication, 1992).

Immigration patterns can be expected to have an impact on HDV infection. For example, people migrating from previously communist countries such as Albania or Romania may bring with them HDV infection (E V Tsianos, personal communication, 1992). Southern Africa has been relatively isolated from the rest of Africa until quite recently, but with increasing travel and trade between these regions the pool of HBsAg-positive carriers in southern Africa is at risk of becoming infected with HDV. In the USA, the recent introduction of a policy of universal infant vaccination against HBV may succeed in decreasing the rate of HDV infection in later life.

Summary and conclusions

In summary, the epidemiology of HDV infection varies unpredictably in incidence and pattern from one region to another. The prevalence of delta hepatitis may be decreased by the practice of vaccination against HBV and the introduction of modern aseptic techniques. However, mass migration of individuals may continue to introduce HDV infection to previously unexposed populations.

DIAGNOSIS OF HEPATITIS DELTA VIRUS INFECTION

It is important to be able to recognize hepatitis delta virus (HDV) infection when it is present for several reasons. Firstly, knowing that HDV infection is present in a patient with hepatitis B viral (HBV) infection allows the outcome of that individual's condition to be predicted more accurately. Thus, patients with acute HDV infection are more likely to develop severe or fulminant hepatitis and those with chronic HDV infection are significantly more likely to progress to cirrhosis and liver failure (Hoofnagle 1989). Another reason for determining whether HDV infection is present is that the response of patients with chronic delta hepatitis to antiviral therapy differs significantly from that of patients with chronic hepatitis B. Chronic delta hepatitis may respond to alpha interferon therapy with a transient decline in serum aminotransferase activities and HDV RNA levels (Di Bisceglie et al 1990). In contrast, approximately 30–40% of patients with HBV infection alone have a transient exacerbation of hepatitis during interferon therapy followed by the loss of HBV DNA and hepatitis B e antigen from serum (Hoofnagle 1990). Finally, in patients with end-stage liver disease being evaluated for liver transplantation, it may be important to know whether they have HDV infection as such patients often do quite well after transplantation. HBV infection appears to recur less frequently after liver transplantation in patients with co-existent HDV infection than in patients with HBV infection alone (Marzano et al 1991).

In diagnosing HDV infection, it is important to distinguish between patients with acute HDV and chronic infection. Among those with acute infection, it is similarly important to separate those with delta co-infection from those with delta superinfection, again because the outlook may vary considerably for these two conditions.

A series of serological and histological tests are used in the diagnosis of HDV infection (Table 21.3). Making a complete diagnosis often involves testing for several markers to establish the type and stage of delta infection (Table 21.4).

Clinical features

It may be very difficult to diagnose HDV infection on clinical grounds alone. Patients may present with typical features of acute hepatitis (jaundice, malaise, anorexia) or the disease may go undetected until it presents ultimately with cirrhosis and end-stage liver disease. In patients with acute delta co-infection, a biphasic pattern of disease has been noted with a secondary rise in serum aminotransferase levels (Caredda et al 1986). The epidemiological features of the patient may raise suspicions about delta hepatitis. For example, drug addicts or patients living in endemic areas should be suspected of having delta infection.

Because it is important to recognize HDV infection, and because the clinical features alone are often not helpful, all patients with evidence of HBV infection (hepatitis B surface antigen or IgM antibody to hepatitis B core antigen) should be tested for HDV infection. Even in the face of an initial negative antibody test, if a strong clinical suspicion of HDV infection remains, it may be appropriate to repeat the testing at a later stage when convalescent antibodies may be more readily detectable (Aragona et al 1987).

Hepatic delta antigen

The 'gold standard' of diagnosis of HDV infection remains the detection of HDAg in the liver by immunostaining; other methods of diagnosing HDV infection are always compared to hepatic HDAg. It was the observation of nuclear staining by immunoflourescence that first led to the discovery of the delta agent (Rizzetto et al 1977), and it is still one of the most sensitive, specific and readily available tests for HDV infection. HDAg is detected by immunostaining, using either the immunofluorescence technique (which requires frozen liver tissue) or the immunoperoxidase technique (which may be done on

Table 21.3 Diagnostic tests for hepatitis delta virus infection

Marker	Detection method	Comment
Hepatic HDAg	Immunostaining	'Gold standard' of diagnosis
Serum HDAg	Western blot	Research assay only
	RIA	Useful in acute delta hepatitis
Serum HDV RNA	Northern blot	Most sensitive marker
Hepatic HDV RNA	Northern blot	Research only
	In situ hybridization	Research only
Total anti-HDV	ELISA or RIA	Diagnostic, if detected
IgM anti-HDV	ELISA or RIA	Acute > chronic

RIA, radioimmunoassay; ELISA, enzyme-linked immunosorbent assay.

Table 21.4 Summary of diagnostic tests for HDV infection

Test	Acute delta hepatitis		Chronic delta hepatitis
	Co-infection	Superinfection	
HBsAg	Usually positive	Positive	Positive
HDAg	Transient	Transient/prolonged	Present
anti-HDV (total)	Transient, low titre	Rising titre	High titre
anti-HDV (IgM)	Transient, low titre	Rising titre	Present
HDV RNA	Transient	Transient/prolonged	Present
IgM anti-HBc	Positive	Negative	Negative

either frozen or fixed material) (Recchia et al 1981, Stocklin et al 1981). In most laboratories, the source of antibody to HDAg used for immunostaining has been human plasma or serum. Patients with chronic HDV infection have high titres of anti-HDV in their serum, which reacts specifically with HDAg in nuclei of hepatocytes. Because these patients also have anti-HBc in serum, which may detect nuclear HBcAg and thus be confused with nuclear HDAg, the serum must be sufficiently diluted so that anti-HBc reactivity disappears (this usually occurs at dilutions of >1:200) but reactivity to HDAg remains (at dilutions of up to 1:1 000 000 or more).

Tissue samples are reacted with immunoglobulins prepared from serum with high titres of anti-HDV. Bound antibody may itself be labelled with fluorescein (for direct immunofluorescence) or it may be detected using a secondary antibody (anti-human IgG), which is itself labelled with peroxidase. Using these reagents HDAg is detected as nuclear staining in varying numbers of hepatocytes (Hadziyannis et al 1985). The number of stained nuclei may give some idea of the level of HDV replication occurring within the liver. The amount of HDAg seems to decline with time and increasing disease severity. Thus, in patients with chronic delta hepatitis, only occasional hepatocytes may stain positively and the whole section must be examined carefully before concluding that the stain for HDAg is negative. In contrast, patients with acute delta hepatitis or recurrent HDV infection after liver transplantation often have as many as 50% of hepatocytes stained, suggesting that they have higher levels of HDV replication. Cytoplasmic HDAg staining may be detected in occasional hepatocytes in some cases. In experimental systems, HDAg may be detected in non-hepatocytes that have been transfected with HDV (Gowans et al 1991). However HDAg is not found in non-parenchymal liver cells in infected patients.

More recently, since recombinant HDAg has become available, non-human anti-HDV has been developed by inoculating animals with recombinant HDAg. The animal serum thus provides a ready source of anti-HDV for immunostaining and may avoid some of the problems associated with using human serum as a reagent (such as limitations in supply, working with potentially infectious material and high levels of background staining related to the presence of immunoglobulins adherent to liver tissue. Animal sera containing high titres of anti-HDV are now generally available, and since techniques used to detect hepatic HDAg are quite straightforward and commonly used in surgical pathology laboratories most laboratories should be able to routinely stain liver biopsy samples for HDAg.

HDAg in serum

In addition to being present in the liver, HDAg has also been detected in the serum of infected individuals, although this presents more of a technical challenge. HDAg is readily detectable by Western blot analysis in serum of individuals with both acute and chronic HDV infection (Bergmann & Gerin 1986). For this assay, HDV particles are pelleted by ultracentrifugation through sucrose and then subjected to acrylamide gel electrophoresis. Proteins in the gel are blotted onto nitrocellulose or nylon membranes and HDAg bound to these membranes can be detected by using anti-HDV labelled with radioisotopes, peroxidase or some other suitable reagent. Using this approach, Buti et al (1989) found HDAg in serum of 71% of patients with chronic HDV infection.

Using Western blot analysis, two forms of HDAg can be detected in serum, 24 and 26 kD in size. The production of these two proteins is related to spontaneous mutations that occur in the gene coding for HDAg. Their production in varying proportions is an important factor in regulating the replication of HDV (Chao et al 1991).

Unfortunately the Western blot technique is somewhat cumbersome and technically difficult and requires the use of radioisotopes. Thus other means have been sought to detect HDAg in serum, for example solid-phase immunoassays (radioimmunoassay, RIA; or enzyme-linked immunoassay, EIA) have been extensively evaluated. Results with these assays have been mixed. A study from the USA found that only 26% of patients with acute delta hepatitis had HDAg detectable using a commercially available EIA (Govindarajan et al 1986), whereas a similar study from Ireland found that HDAg could be detected in all patients with acute delta hepatitis using a different EIA system (Shattock & Morgan 1984). A study from Spain evaluated the same assay and found delta antigenaemia in 88% of patients with acute delta hepatitis studied (Buti et al 1989).

These discrepant results may be related to the timing of the blood samples. The method and promptness of diagnosis may also affect the sensitivity of the test being considered. Thus, HDAg is only present for 1–2 weeks in the early phases of HDV infection and thereafter may not be detectable. An alternative explanation for these findings is a significant difference in the sensitivity of the tests used. The amount of HDAg present in serum may also vary with time and the stage of HDV infection. In summary, patients with chronic delta hepatitis usually do not have HDAg detectable in serum by EIA or RIA. And even though assays for detecting HDAg by solid-phase immunoassay have been developed, they are not widely used for the diagnosis of HDV infection.

One possible explanation for the increased sensitivity of Western blot analysis compared with solid-phase immunoassay for detection of HDAg in serum could be the competing effect of anti-HDV in serum. HDAg is a soluble protein that circulates in particulate form enclosed by a coating of HBsAg. If this particle were to be disrupted, for example during processing for EIA or RIA, it is likely that the soluble HDAg would form complexes with anti-HDV in serum. These complexes might precipitate, making HDAg undetectable. Bound anti-HDV might prevent reaction with anti-HDV in the assay. In the Western blot assay, HDV particles are separated from the serum by ultracentrifugation and denatured prior to undergoing gel electrophoresis, thus preventing formation of HDAg-anti-HDV complexes.

Antibody to hepatitis delta virus

The presence of anti-HDV in serum also appears to be a reliable and specific way of diagnosing HDV infection. In addition, testing large numbers of serum samples for the presence of anti-HDV has allowed large-scale epidemiological studies of HDV infection to be carried out. Anti-HDV can be reliably detected by solid-phase immunoassays, including RIA and EIA (Aragona et al 1987). Several assays for anti-HDV are commercially available. These tests generally detect both IgG and IgM antibodies to HDV, although IgM antibodies can be detected separately and may be useful diagnostically (Smedile et al 1982, Shattock et al 1989). Anti-HDV becomes detectable in more than 90% of cases within 1–2 months of acute HDV infection. Thereafter the changes in antibody patterns and titres depend on the type of HDV infection. Thus, in patients with acute delta co-infection, in which the HDV infection is usually transient, anti-HDV titres may be quite low (less than 1:100), or even undetectable in some cases. In such patients, anti-HDV titres may be more easily detectable on subsequent serum samples, and several samples may need to be tested over a few weeks in order to confirm a suspected diagnosis of delta hepatitis. Under these circumstances anti-HDV remains detectable beyond the acute illness, but it remains uncertain how long it may persist. In contrast, in

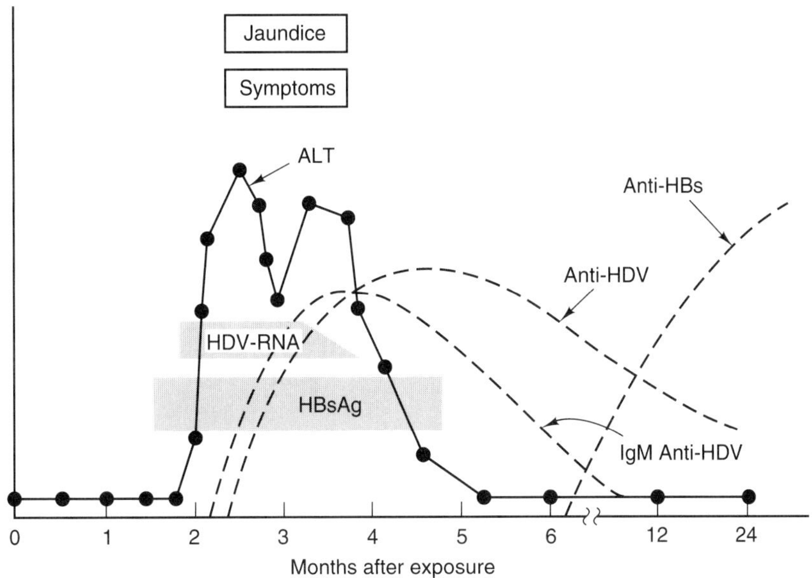

Fig. 21.1 Serological and serum biochemical changes associated with acute delta co-infection. ALT, alanine aminotransferase; HBsAg, hepatitis B surface antigen; anti-HDV, antibody to hepatitis delta virus; anti-HBs, antibody to HBsAg. (Reproduced from Hoofnagle & Di Bisceglie 1991 with permission.)

patients with delta superinfection, in whom the HDV infection usually becomes chronic as they are already chronically infected with HBV, anti-HDV tends to appear sooner and to reach higher titres. This pattern rapidly evolves into that associated with chronic delta hepatitis, in which persistently high titres of anti-HDV may be detected. Titres of total anti-HDV may exceed 1:1 000 000 in patients with chronic delta hepatitis, and titres of more than 1:1000 are considered diagnostic. Liver biopsy with staining for HDAg may only be required for evaluation of severity of

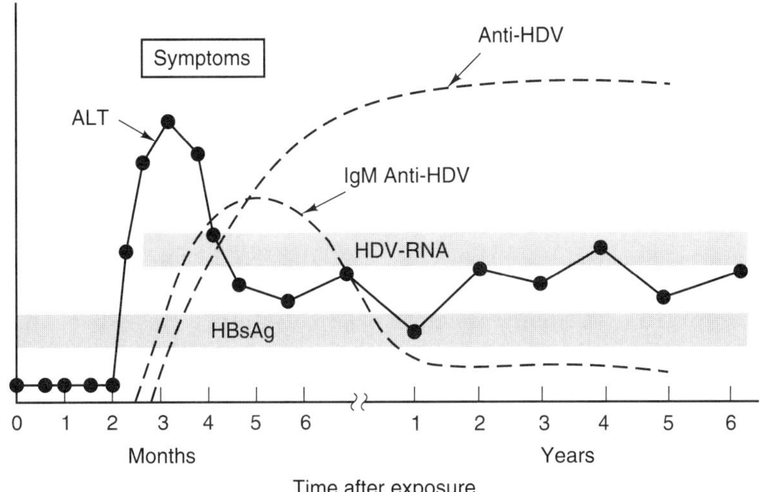

Fig. 21.2 Serological and serum biochemical changes associated with acute delta superinfection (see legend to Fig. 21.1 for abbreviations). (Reproduced from Hoofnagle & Di Bisceglie 1991 with permission.)

hepatic injury associated with HDV infection or in cases in which the diagnosis is in doubt.

The presence of IgM anti-HDV is very useful as it appears to correlate with levels of HDV replication. Thus, during the acute phase of delta hepatitis when viral replication levels are high, titres of IgM anti-HDV may be high. As the hepatitis subsides, so levels of anti-HDV may fall. IgM anti-HDV is transiently present in more than 90% of cases of acute delta co-infection and when found together with rising titres of total anti-HDV confirms the diagnosis. The presence of IgM anti-HDV may persist into the chronic phase of infection and indeed may remain detectable as long as significant levels of viral replication persist (Smedile et al 1982). IgM anti-HDV is thus a useful marker to follow changes associated with antiviral therapy as IgM anti-HDV titres appear to fall when HDV replication is inhibited by treatment with agents such as alpha interferon.

Although the presence of anti-HDV may be a very useful screening test for HDV infection, it may not be totally reliable in immunosuppressed patients, who may not be able to mount an antibody response sufficient to be detected. In patients with acute delta co-infection who have a very strong immune response, anti-HDV may be detected even after they have cleared HBsAg from serum.

Hepatitis delta virus RNA

The HDV has a single-stranded RNA genome approximately 1700 nucleotides in length of negative polarity (Wang et al 1986). HDV RNA can be detected in the serum of individuals infected with HDV, and this forms the basis of a diagnostic test (Smedile et al 1986). Viral particles are first pelleted from serum by ultracentrifugation through serum. RNA is then extracted from this pelleted material. HDV RNA can be specifically detected using techniques of molecular hybridization. Extracted RNA can either be spotted onto nitrocellulose or nylon membranes for dot-blot hybridization or subjected to agarose gel electrophoresis and then transferred to a membrane for subsequent hybridization.

Membranes are then hybridized using radiolabelled probes specific for HDV RNA and exposed to radiographic film. HDV RNA may be detected as spots on the resulting autoradiogram or as bands corresponding to 1700 bp in length by Northern blot hybridization. Earlier assays to detect HDV RNA used only a small fraction of the HDV genome as a probe, resulting in an assay with relatively limited sensitivity. Subsequently, full-length RNA probes were used for detecting HDV RNA and appeared to have greater sensitivity (Table 21.3).

In patients with acute HDV infection, HDV RNA can be detected in as many as 64% of cases within the first week of the disease. HDV viraemia then persists in those patients who go on to develop chronic delta hepatitis (Buti et al 1988).

Among patients with chronic delta hepatitis, more than 80% have HDV RNA detectable in serum using dot-blot or Northern blot hybridization. The amount of HDV RNA circulating may be quantitated by comparing the hybridization signal with that of known amounts of HDV cDNA or RNA. Using this approach combined with chimpanzee infectivity experiments, it has been determined that patients with chronic delta hepatitis may have very high levels of viraemia, often more than 10^{12} virions per ml of serum (Ponzetto et al 1988).

In addition to diagnostic uses, levels of HDV RNA in serum may be useful for monitoring the effect of antiviral therapy. During therapy with alpha interferon, HDV RNA becomes undetectable in those patients who respond with their serum aminotransferase activities falling into the normal range (Di Bisceglie et al 1990). Very often, when interferon therapy is discontinued, the condition appears to relapse and serum aminotransferase activities become elevated and HDV RNA becomes detectable again.

More recently, assays have been developed to detect HDV RNA using the very sensitive polymerase chain (PCR) reaction technique (Negro et al 1991). Although the exact sensitivity of PCR for detecting HDV RNA is not known, it is likely that it will be consistently more sensitive than molecular hybridization. The ability of PCR techniques to detect HDV RNA may be limited by the high degree of internal base pair complementarity of the viral genome. However, the potential clinical and epidemiological implications of these more sensitive assays are not yet apparent.

The HDV RNA detected in serum of infected individuals is of negative polarity. However, in the liver, where HDV replicates, both negatively and positively stranded HDV RNA may be detected by molecular hybridization. Hepatic HDV RNA can be detected in liver biopsy samples either by Northern blot hybridization or by in situ hybridization. HDV RNA can be detected predominantly in the cytoplasm of hepatocytes which stain for HDAg (Gowans et al 1988, Negro et al 1989). In situ hybridization does appear not to be more sensitive or offer any diagnostic advantage over conventional immunostaining for HDAg and is unlikely to have any role in routine diagnosis of chronic HDV infection.

Autoantibodies associated with HDV infection

Several patterns of autoantibodies have been detected in the serum of patients with chronic delta hepatitis. These include antibodies to microsomes of liver and kidney cells, to the basal cell layer and to thymic epithelial cells (Bonino et al 1991). The microsomal autoantibodies are of particular interest, as these may also be detected in type II autoimmune chronic active hepatitis, which is not known to be associated with viral infection. Crivelli et al (1983) studied serum from 81 patients with chronic delta hepatitis and found that 13% had reactivity to cytoplasm of liver and kidney cells (both human and animal) that could not be blocked by serum from a patient with type II autoimmune hepatitis, suggesting that it was a different antibody (referred to as anti-LKM_3). The significance of these autoantibodies remains uncertain but, so far, they do not have any proven role in the pathogenesis of chronic delta hepatitis. However, they may occasionally be the cause of some diagnostic confusion.

Tests for HBV infection

Because HDV infection always occurs in association with HBV infection, evaluating the status of the HBV infection *is* an important part of diagnosing of delta hepatitis. Virtually all patients with HDV infection have HBsAg in serum. The only possible exceptions to this include patients with acute or fulminant hepatitis who clear HBsAg very rapidly from serum. As many as 10–15% of patients with acute hepatitis may not have HBsAg detectable in serum on initial presentation. The presence of IgM antibodies to HBcAg (IgM anti-HBc) in serum may be sufficient to diagnose acute hepatitis B in this group of patients (Tassopoulos et al 1990). IgM anti-HBc is detectable during acute delta co-infection but usually not in association with acute delta superinfection or chronic delta hepatitis.

Patients with chronic HDV infection have HBsAg detectable in serum, but markers of active HBV replication (HBV DNA and HBeAg) are often not present, possibly because of suppression of HBV replication by the HDV. Low levels of IgM anti-HBc not detectable by the usual commercial assays may be useful markers of continuing HBV replication in patients with chronic delta hepatitis. Indeed, evaluation of levels of IgM anti-HBc and IgM anti-HDV may be helpful in determining which of the two viruses is dominant in a particular patient.

Patients with recurrent HDV following liver transplantation may have HDAg detected in the transplanted liver as soon as 1 or 2 weeks after surgery. It is only weeks or months later that HBsAg becomes detectable in serum and liver and HBcAg becomes detectable within the liver.

Summary and conclusions

Selection of the appropriate tests for diagnosing HDV infection should be done in the context of individual patients. Thus, for example, patients with acute hepatitis B who test negative for anti-HDV should be retested if the diagnosis is suspected strongly on clinical grounds. In patients with stable chronic hepatitis, the absence of anti-HDV in a single serum sample would exclude a diagnosis of chronic delta hepatitis. If they are available, tests for HDAg and IgM anti-HDV in serum may be useful supplementary tests. The best test for confirming HDV infection is staining liver biopsy samples for HDAg. The techniques for doing this are relatively simple and widely available. Although HDV RNA is perhaps the most sensitive test for HDV infection, the lack of availability of this assay will probably limit it to research uses. Similarly, the detection of HDAg in serum by Western blot and of HDV RNA in liver by in situ hybridization remain available as research tools only.

REFERENCES

Abdool Karim S S, Windsor I M, Gopal W 1991 Low prevalence of delta hepatitis virus infection among blacks in Natal. South African Medical Journal 80: 193–194

Aragona M, Caredda F, Lavarini C et al 1987 Serological response to the hepatitis delta virus in hepatitis D. Lancet i 478–480

Becherer P R, Wang J-G, White G C et al 1991 Hepatitis delta virus infection in hemophiliacs. In: Hollinger F B, Lemon S M, Margolis H S (eds) Viral hepatitis and liver disease. Williams & Wilkins, Baltimore, pp 492–494

Bergmann K F, Gerin J L 1986 Antigens of hepatitis delta virus in the liver and serum of humans and animals. Journal of Infectious Diseases 514: 702–705

Bodsworth N J, Donovan B, Gold J, Cossart Y E. 1989 Hepatitis delta virus in homosexual men in Sydney. Genitourinary Medicine 65: 235–238

Bonino F, Brunetto M R, Negro F 1991 Factors influencing the natural course of HDV hepatitis. In: Gerin J L, Purcell R H, Rizzetto M (eds) The hepatitis delta virus. Wiley–Liss, New York, pp 137–146

Buitrago B, Popper H, Hadler S C, Thung S N, Gerber M A, Purcell R H, Maynard J E 1986 Specific histologic features of Santa Marta Hepatitis: a severe form of hepatitis δ-virus infection in northern South America. Hepatology 6: 1285–1291

Buti M, Esteban R, Roggendorf M et al 1988 Hepatitis D virus RNA in acute delta infection: serological profile and correlation with other markers of hepatitis D virus infection. Hepatology 8: 1125–1129

Buti M, Esteban R, Jardi R et al 1989 Chronic delta hepatitis: detection of hepatitis delta virus antigen in serum by immunoblot and correlation with other markers of delta viral replication. Hepatology 10: 907–910

Caredda F, Antinori S, Pastecchia C, Moroni M 1986 Biphasic hepatitis in HBV/HDV coinfected parenteral drug abusers (letter). Gut 27: 747

Chao M, Hsieh S-Y, Luo G, Taylor J 1991 The antigen of human hepatitis delta virus: the significance of the two major electrophoretic forms. In: Gerin J L, Purcell R H, Rizzetto M (eds) The hepatitis delta virus. Wiley–Liss, New York, pp 275–282

Crivelli O, Lavarini C, Chiaberge E, Amoroso A et al 1983 Microsomal autoantibodies in chronic infection with the HBsAg associated delta (δ) agent. Clinical and Experimental Immunology 54: 232–238

Di Bisceglie A M, Martin P, Lisker-Melman M et al 1990 Therapy of chronic delta hepatitis with interferon alfa-2b. Journal of Hepatology 11: S151–S154

Dusheiko G M, Brink B A, Conradie J D, Marimuthu T, Sher R 1989 Regional difference of hepatitis B, delta and human immunodeficiency virus infection in southern Africa: A large population survey. American Journal of Epidemiology 129: 138–145

Goldin R, Saldanha J, Thomas H C 1990 Hepatitis delta virus infection in human immunodeficiency virus-positive patients (letter). Hepatology 11: 903

Govindarajan S, Valinluck B, Peters L 1986 Relapse of acute B viral hepatitis – role of delta agent. Gut 27: 19–22

Gowans E J, Baroudy B M, Negro F, Ponzetto A, Purcell R H, Gerin J L 1988 Evidence for replication of hepatitis delta virus RNA in hepatocyte nuclei after in vivo infection. Virology 167: 274–278

Hadler S C, De Monzon M, Ponzetto A et al 1984 Delta virus infection and severe hepatitis. An epidemic in the Yupca Indians of Venezuela. Annals of Internal Medicine 100: 339–344

Hadziyannis S J, Sherman M, Lieberman H M, Shafritz D A 1985 Liver disease activity and hepatitis B virus replication in chronic delta antigen-positive hepatitis B virus carriers. Hepatology 5: 544–547

Hess G, Bienzle U, Slusarczyk, Hansson B G, Meyer Zum Buschenfelde K H 1986 Hepatitis B virus and delta infection in male homosexuals. Liver 6: 13–16

Hoofnagle J H 1989 Type D (delta) hepatitis. Journal of the American Medical Association 261: 1321–1325

Hoofnagle J H 1990 α-interferon therapy of chronic hepatitis B. Current status and recommendations. Journal of Hepatology 11: S100–S107

Hoofnagle J H, Di Bisceglie A M 1991 Serologic diagnosis of acute and chronic viral hepatitis. Seminars on Liver Disease 11: 73–83

Kreek M J, Des Jarlais D C, Trepo C L, Abdul-Quader A, Raghunath J 1990 Contrasting prevalence of delta hepatitis markers in parenteral drug abusers with and without AIDS. Journal of Infectious Diseases 162: 538–541

Lettau L A, Alfred H J, Glew R H et al 1986 Nosocomial transmission of delta hepatitis. Annals of Internal Medicine 104: 631–635

Lettau L A, McCarthy J G, Smith M H et al 1987 Outbreak of severe hepatitis due to delta and hepatitis B viruses in parenteral drug abusers and their contacts. New England Journal of Medicine 317: 1256–1262

Liaw Y-F, Chiu K-W, Chu C-M, Sheen I-S, Huang M-J 1990 Heterosexual transmission of hepatitis delta virus in the general population of an area endemic for hepatitis B virus infection: a prospective study. Journal of Infectious Diseases 162: 1170–1172

Marzano A, Ottobrelli A, David E, Durazzo M, Rizzetto M 1991 Hepatitis delta virus infection and disease: The lesson from the liver transplantation model. In: Gerin J L, Purcell R H, Rizzetto M (eds) The hepatitis delta virus. Wiley-Liss, New York, pp 439–445

Mele A, Franco E, Caprilli F et al 1988 Hepatitis B and delta virus infection among heterosexuals, homosexuals and bisexual men. European Journal of Epidemiology 4: 488–491

Mendez L, Reddy R, Di Prima R A, Jeffers L J, Schiff E R 1991 Fulminant hepatic failure due to acute hepatitis B and delta co-infection: Probable bloodborne transmission associated with a spring-loaded fingerstick device. American Journal of Gastroenterology 86: 895–896

Negro F, Bonino F, Di Bisceglie A, Hoofnagle J H 1989 Intrahepatic markers of hepatitis delta virus infection: A study by in situ hybridization. Hepatology 10: 916–920

Negro F, Emerson S, McRill C et al 1991 A polymerase-chain reaction-based assay for serum HDV RNA. In: Gerin J L, Purcell R H, Rizzetto M (eds) The hepatitis delta virus. Wiley-Liss, New York, pp 173–178

Ndumbe P M 1991 Hepatitis D in Yaounde, Cameroon. APMIS 99: 196–198

Pol S, Debois F, Roingeard P et al 1989 Hepatitis delta virus infection in French male HBsAg-positive homosexuals. Hepatology 10: 342–345

Ponzetto A, Hoofnagle J H, Seeff L B 1984 Antibody to the hepatitis B virus-associated delta-agent in immune serum globulins. Gastroenterology 87: 1213–1216

Ponzetto A, Seeff L B, Buskell-Bales Z et al 1985 Hepatitis B markers in United States drug addicts with special emphasis on the delta hepatitis virus. Hepatology 4: 1111–1115

Ponzetto A, Negro F, Popper H et al 1988 Serial passage of hepatitis delta virus in chronic hepatitis B virus carrier chimpanzees. Hepatology 8: 1655–1661

Raimondo G, Gallo L, Ponzetto A, Smedile A, Balbo A, Rizzetto M 1982 Multicentre study of prevalence of HBV-associated delta infection and liver disease in drug-addicts. Lancet i: 249–251

Rapicetta M, Hailu K, Ponzetto A et al 1988 Delta hepatitis virus infection in Ethiopia. Eur J Epidemiol 4: 185–188

Ratner L 1986 Delta hepatitis outbreak in a group of patients with leukemia (letter). Annals of Internal Medicine 105: 972

Recchia S, Rizzi R, Acquaviva F, Rizzetto M, Tison V, Bonino F, Verme G 1981 Immunoperoxidase staining of the HBV-associated delta antigen in paraffinated liver specimens. Pathologica 73: 773–777

Rizzetto M, Canese M G, Arico S et al 1977 Immunofluorescence detection of a new antigen/antibody system (delta-antidelta) associated with the hepatitis B virus in the liver and in the serum of HBsAg carriers. Gut 18: 997–1003

Rizzetto M, Purcell R H, Gerin J L 1980 Epidemiology of HBV-associated delta agent: geographical distribution of anti-delta and prevalence in poly-transfused HBsAg carriers. Lancet i: 1215–1218

Rizzetto M, Verme G, Recchia S et al 1983 Chronic HBsAg hepatitis with intrahepatic expression of delta antigen: an active and progressive disease unresponsive to immunosuppressive therapy. Annals of Internal Medicine 98: 437–441

Rizzetto M, Ponzetto A, Forzani I 1991 Epidemiology of hepatitis delta virus: overview. In: Gerin J L, Purcell R H, Rizzetto M (eds) The hepatitis delta virus. Wiley–Liss, New York, pp 1–20

Rosina F, Saracco G, Rizzetto M 1985 Risk of post-transfusion infection with the hepatitis delta virus. New England Journal of Medicine 312: 1488–1491

Shattock A G, Morgan B M 1984 Sensitive enzyme immunoassay for the detection of delta antigen and anti-delta, using serum as the delta antigen source. Journal of Medical Virology 13: 73–82

Shattock A G, Morris M, Kinane K, Fagan C 1989 The serology of delta hepatitis and the detection of IgM anti-HD by EIA using serum derived delta antigen. Journal of Virological Methods 23: 233–240

Smedile A, Lavarini C, Crivelli O et al 1982 Radioimmunoassay detection of IgM antibodies to the HDV-associated delta antigen: clinical significane in delta infection. Journal of Medical Virology 9: 131–138

Smedile A, Rizzetto M, Denniston K et al 1986 Type D hepatitis: The clinical significance of hepatitis D virus RNA in serum as detected by a hybridization-based assay. Hepatology 6: 1297–1302

Solomon R E, Kaslow R A, Phair J P et al 1988 Human immunodeficiency virus and hepatitis delta virus in homosexual men. Annals of Internal Medicine 108: 51–54

Speed B R, Dimitrikakis M, Thoma K, Gust I D 1989 Control of HBV and HDV infection in an isolated Pacific island: 1. Pattern of infection. Journal of Medical Virology 29: 13–19

Stocklin E, Gudat F, Krey G et al 1981 δ-antigen in hepatitis B: immunohistology of frozen and paraffin-embedded liver biopsies and relation to HBV infection. Hepatology 1: 238–242

Tapalaga D, Forzani B, Paravacini O, Ponzetto A, Theilmann L 1986 Prevalence of the hepatitis delta virus in Rumania. Hepato-gastroenterology 33: 238–239

Tassopoulos N C, Koutelou M G, Macagno S, Zorbas P, Rizzetto M 1990 Diagnostic significance of IgM antibody to hepatitis delta virus in fulminant hepatitis B. Journal of Medical Virology 30: 174–177

Tibbs C 1989 Delta hepatitis in Kiribati: a Pacific focus. Journal of Medical Virology 29: 130–132

Torres J R, Mondolfi A 1991 Protracted outbreak of severe delta hepatitis: Experince in an isolated Amerindian population of the upper Orinoco basin. Review of Infectious Diseases 13: 52–55

Wang K-S, Choo Q-L, Weiner A J et al 1986 Structure, sequece and expression of the hepatitis delta (δ) viral genome. Science 323: 508–512

Weisfuse I B, Hadler S C, Fields H A et al 1989 Delta hepatitis in homosexual men in the United States. Hepatology 9: 872–874

Wu J-C, Lee S-D, Govindarajan S et al 1990 Sexual transmission of hepatitis D virus infection in Taiwan. Hepatology 11: 1057–1061

22. Treatment

Mario Rizzetto Floriano Rosina

Concomitant infection with an RNA (HDV) and a DNA (HBV) virus may make chronic hepatitis D more difficult to treat than chronic hepatitis B. As for hepatitis B, poor results were obtained in the early 1980s with immunosuppressive and immunostimulant drugs (Arrigoni et al 1983, Rizzetto et al 1983). In the mid-1980s clinical trials indicated that the cytokine interferon (IFN) could inhibit HDV replication and control the associated liver disease in some groups of patients. This effect, however, did not last usually beyond the end of IFN therapy (Farci et al 1989, Rosina & Rizzetto 1989).

CLINICAL TRIALS WITH INTERFERON

On the assumption that more prolonged treatment with interferon might induce a longer remission, and possibly eradicate viral infection, several clinical trials were undertaken in the late 1980s (Tables 22.1 and 22.2).

The trials showed that the rate of response was proportional to the dose of IFN: patients treated with 9 MU responded better than patients treated with 3 MU (Farci 1992); virological and biochemical evidence of relapse was common when IFN was reduced to 3 MU/m^2 after a 4-month course with 5 MU/m^2 (Rosina et al 1991, Gaudin et al 1992). Daily administration of a 5-MU dose reduced the burden of side-effects but also the probability of recovery (Di Bisceglie et al 1990). More complex schedules and combinations of IFN with other antiviral drugs, e.g. acyclovir, were not more successful and again reactivation during follow-up was the rule (Berk et al 1991, Marinucci et al 1991, Cotonat et al 1992).

Histological examination revealed that a significant decrease in hepatic injury and HDAg staining was often seen in patients who had responded to IFN (Kleiner et al 1990, Farci 1992).

Reported side-effects in the above trials can be largely ascribed to IFN (flu-like symptoms, fatigue and weight loss), were seen in almost all treated patients, and the severity of reactions was usually proportional to the IFN dose. Two patients had a severe hepatitic episode while on full-dose IFN (Rosina et al 1991, Marinucci et al 1991): liver–kidney microsomal antibodies were present in the serum of one of these patients (Todros et al 1991). One patient developed hyperthyroidism, one committed suicide during the eleventh month of treatment, and one attempted suicide shortly after the discontinuation of treatment (Gaudin et al 1992).

Analysis of the pretreatment characteristics of patients did not identify any differences between responders and non-responders to IFN with regard to demographic, clinical, serological, biochemical and histological findings.

Many adults and children with HDV infection and active HBV replication cleared HBV DNA and HBeAg from serum and often seroconverted to anti-HBe during interferon therapy; this event occurred without much change in liver chemistry and was not usually followed by return of alanine aminotransferase (ALT) to normal levels (Craxi et al 1990, Rosina et al 1991, Gaudin et al 1992). However, in view of the poor prognosis of patients with active replication of both viruses (Smedile et al 1991), HBV inhibition should be considered a desirable event in the long term.

Although one patient with anti-LKM autoantibodies had a severe bout of hepatitis, which led

Table 22.1 Controlled trials of treatment of chronic HDV hepatitis with alpha interferon

Reference	No. of patients	IFN type and schedule	End of treatment		End of follow-up	
			HDV RNA –ve	ALT normal	HDV RNA –ve	ALT normal
Rosina et al 1989	12	Alpha 2b t.i.w. 5 MU/m^2 x 3 months	4 (33%)	4 (33%)	1 (8%)	1 (8%)
	12	Untreated	2 (17%)	0 (0%)	2 (17%)	0 (0%)
Rosina et al 1991	31	Alpha 2b t.i.w. 5 MU/m^2 x 4 months 3 MU/m^2 x 8 months	14 (45%)	8 (25%)	14 (45%)	1 (3%)
	30	Untreated	8 (27%)	0 (0%)	10 (33%)	0 (0%)
Farci 1992	14	Alpha 2a t.i.w. 9 MU x 12 months	10 (71%)	10 (71%)	0 (0%)	5 (36%)
	14	Alpha 2a t.i.w. 3 MU x 12 months	5 (36%)	4 (28%)	0 (0%)	0 (0%)
	14	Untreated	1 (7%)	1 (7%)	0 (0%)	0 (0%)
Gaudin et al 1992	11	Alpha 2b t.i.w. 5 MU/m^2 x 4 months 3 MU/m^2 x 8 months	7 (66%)	7 (66%)	1 (9%)	1 (9%)
	11	Untreated	4 (36%)	2 (18%)	?	?
Cotonat et al 1992	12	Alpha 2a t.i.w. 18 MU x 6 months 9 MU x 1 month 6 MU x 1 month 3 MU x 4 months	6 (50%)	4 (37%)	0 (0%)	0 (0%)
	14	Alpha 2a daily 3 MU x 12 months	3 (19%)	1 (7%)	0 (0%)	0 (0%)

t.i.w., thrice weekly; ?, data not available.

to interruption of therapy, 10 such patients have in different trials completed cycles of IFN therapy without complications (Todros et al 1991).

While short duration of the disease seems to improve the response to treatment (Marzano et al 1992), a young age may have an adverse influence, as in the case of IFN treatment of chronic hepatitis B. None of the 10 children treated by Craxi et al (1990) improved clinically or histologically after treatment for a year. Studies in drug addicts with multiple blood-borne infections have shown a response in those who are anti-HIV seropositive and in whom immunocompetence is preserved (Taillan et al 1988, Buti et al 1989).

MECHANISM OF ACTION OF IFN

The mechanism of action of IFN in chronic hepatitis D is poorly understood: response to IFN is often characterized by a concomitant reduction in HD viraemia and ALT levels, suggesting a direct, antiviral effect of the cytokine on HDV. However, normal ALT levels can occur and persist despite the presence of active HDV replication (Farci 1992). Furthermore, clearance

Table 22.2 Uncontrolled trials of treatment of chronic HDV hepatitis with alpha interferon

Reference	No. of patients	IFN type and schedule	End of treatment		End of follow-up	
			HDV RNA –ve	ALT normal	HDV RNA –ve	ALT normal
Thomas et al 1987	5	Lymphoblastoid t.i.w. 2.5–7.5 MU/m^2 × 2–12 weeks	4 (80%)	0 (0%)	4 (80%)	0 (0%)
Hoofnagle et al 1987	5	Alpha 2b daily 5 MU x 4 months	3 (60%)	3 (60%)	0 (0%)	0 (0%)
Buti et al 1989	4	Alpha 2a t.i.w. 9 MU x 6 months	3 (75%)	3 (75%)	?	?
Taillan et al 1988	8	Alpha 2b t.i.w. 5 MU x 6 months	?	2 (25%)	?	?
Di Bisceglie et al 1990	12	Alpha 2b daily 5 MU x 4–36 months	5 (42%)	0 (0%)	?	?
Marinucci et al 1991	8	Alpha 2a t.i.w. 6 MU x 12 months 1 month stop 1 MU x 12 months	3 (37%)	1 (12%)	1 (12%)	1 (12%)
Craxi' et al 1990	10	Alpha 2b t.i.w. 5 MU/m^2 x 4 months 3 MU/m^2 x 8 months	7 (70%)	?	2 (20%)	?
Berk et al 1991	10	Lymphoblastoid daily 5 MU x 4 months Acyclovir 2 g daily x 2 weeks × two cycles	?	5 (50%)	?	2 (20%)
Marzano et al 1992	7	Lymphoblastoid t.i.w. 5 MU/m^2 x 4 months 3 MU/m^2 x 8 months	5 (71%)	5 (71%)	3 (43%)	3 (43%)

t.i.w., thrice weekly; ?, data not available.

of serum HBsAg and anti-HBs seroconversion is a common event in patients who maintain the response obtained during treatment (Rosina et al 1990). It is therefore conceivable that IFN activity against HBV may play a crucial role: although HDV infection inhibits HBV replication per se, some degree of HBV replication is required by HDV to exert its pathogenic potential. If HBV replication is suppressed further by IFN, HDV could be cleared itself or enter a non-pathogenetic phase analogous to that observed in the liver transplant model (Ottobrelli et al 1991).

OTHER TREATMENTS

Animal (woodchuck) and cell culture systems (woodchuck hepatocytes) are available to screen antiviral compounds for activity against HDV. Suramin in vitro blocks entry of HDV virions into hepatocytes (Rasshofer et al 1991), but the drug is too toxic for long-term use in humans. Acyclovir, used previously and unsuccessfully as an adjuvant therapy in IFN-treated patients (Berk et al 1991), seems to enhance HDV replication in vitro (Rasshofer et al 1991). Ribavirin, a nucleotide analogue, is effective in HCV chronic hepatitis (Reichard et al 1991) and inhibits HDV replication in cell culture (Rasshofer et al 1991). It was given at 15 mg /kg/day orally for 16 weeks to nine patients but had to be suspended in two of them after 2 weeks, in one case because of haemolytic anaemia and in the other because of intractable itching. No significant virological or biochemical results were seen (Garripoli et al 1993). Similar unfavourable results were found in another small randomized controlled study (Buti et al 1992).

Thymosin fractions or their synthetic analogues represent a possible alternative treatment: experimental evidence in woodchucks and their efficacy in chronic HBV infection point to a possible role for these immunomodulatory compounds in the treatment of HDV hepatitis (Mutchnick et al 1991).

Future possibilities for treatment are suggested by the finding that the HDV RNA sequence has sites with ribozyme activity that may be targets for pharmacological attack. Ribozymes are RNA molecules capable of enzymatic self-cleaving without protein involvement (Cech 1988). A clearer understanding of HDV self-cleavage may lead to strategies for blocking HDV replication, since self-cleavage of genomic and antigenomic HDV RNAs may be an essential component of the viral replication mechanism (Belinsky & Dinter-Gottlieb 1991).

CURRENT THERAPY

Alpha IFN represents the only treatment for chronic hepatitis D. Available data show that patients respond to IFN if adequate doses (i.e. 9–10 MU three times weekly) are administered for a sufficient length of time. Since HDV superinfection runs a chronic course in over 90% of cases, and since early administration of IFN may improve the response rate, treatment should be begun in patients with acute hepatitis progressing to chronicity as soon as the acute phase is over. Patients with no history of overt acute hepatitis and of decompensated liver cirrhosis should be treated as soon as a diagnosis is made.

Unfortunately, in chronic hepatitis D the 'timing' of IFN treatment remains a largely unresolved issue. While parameters predictive of response (low HBV DNA and elevated ALT serum levels, active liver disease at histology) are known in patients with HBV/HBeAg-positive chronic hepatitis, they are still unknown for chronic hepatitis D. Furthermore, whereas in chronic HBV and HCV hepatitis response to IFN occurs within 1–3 months from the beginning of the treatment, in HDV infection response can take up to 10 months. Thus IFN should be administered for at least a year before a patient is regarded as a non-responder.

Another major challenge is deciding when to stop therapy in a patient with a good initial response. Loss of serum HDV RNA and HDAg does not reflect accurately the clearance of the virus, as patients who respond to treatment will lose these serum viral markers but may relapse once the treatment is stopped. Treatment, however, can be safely interrupted if serum HBsAg and/or anti-HD IgM have disappeared (Rosina et al 1991, Marinucci et al 1993). If both these events do not occur within 1 year of effective treatment (i.e. 1 year of undetectable HDV RNA and normal ALT), the therapeutic regimen should be determined by histological and immunohistochemical findings. In patients with no detectable liver HDAg, IFN should be stopped and the patients monitored for a potential relapse. If HDAg is still detectable, but liver histology has improved, IFN should be continued, possibly until it disappears. Careful medical supervision of patients treated for a long time is mandatory for early detection and management of major medical and psychiatric complications.

TRANSPLANTATION

The advent of liver transplantation has given new hope to the poor prognosis for HDV disease. As with other viral disorders, transplantation is aggravated by the risk of reinfection, but this is lower for HDV than for HBV and HCV and the clinical course of recurrent hepatitis is milder than for HBV.

Of 27 patients who were transplanted and who received no or only short-term prophylaxis with anti-HBs, 22 (80%) became reinfected with HDV but only 11 (40%) experienced a recurrence of hepatitis (Ottobrelli et al 1991). A high risk of reinfection (80%) was also reported in 14 untreated transplant recipients with HDV, but again the rate of hepatitis relapse was lower than for transplant recipients with hepatitis B (Reynes et al 1989). 25 of the 27 patients in the first study and all the patients in the second were alive 1–4 years after transplantation.

Of six transplants with recurrent hepatitis D who are being followed up long term at the time of writing, two have a chronic persistent hepatitis, one has a mild lobular hepatitis, one has a chronic active hepatitis and two have developed cirrhosis. Interferon (3–5 MU three times weekly for up to 3 months) has not proved efficacious in these patients. In another seven HDV patients who were transplanted and received short-term prophylaxis, four became reinfected with HBV and HDV; three of these cleared both viruses after an episode of acute hepatitis, whereas one developed cirrhosis 11 months after transplantation (Bettale et al 1992).

The prospect of an uneventful clinical course after transplantation can be improved further by long-term administration of hyperimmune serum against HBsAg. Only 14% of 36 transplant patients with HDV and cirrhosis and 20% of five with fulminant hepatitis given anti-HBs long-term developed recurrent infections in the liver graft after 8–58 months' follow-up (Samuel et al 1991).

Apart from providing another therapeutic option, transplantation is a unique model for studying the biology and pathology of HDV infection. Virological testing has shown that the recurrence of hepatitis D in liver grafts follows two patterns (Ottobrelli et al 1991): disease develops following the simultaneous return of HDV and HBV; or HDV first establishes itself as an autonomous infection and only later does HBV infection recur. In the latter group, patients remain symptom-free until HBV reinfects the graft; invariably, the reactivation of HBV leads to the intrahepatic spread of HDV and to the relapse of the disease. Early HDV reinfection in the absence of HBsAg has also been documented in one of two HDV patients who received an auxiliary liver graft (Ten Kate & Schalm 1991).

Evidence from the transplant model that HDV can establish itself as a subclinical infection independently of an overt HBV infection suggests that HDV is in itself neither pathogenic nor dependent on HBV; cooperation with HBV is only necessary for disease expression. In a number of transplant patients HDV, but not HBV, has recurred and the clinical course has been asymptomatic.

Liver specimens from nine transplant patients with relapsing hepatitis D, for whom an adequate histological follow-up was available, have been examined (David et al 1992). While in four patients a rise in aminotransferase heralding the return of hepatitis D, corresponded with necroinflammation, in five patients the histology corresponded with a syndrome of acute hepatitis (degenerative lesions of the hepatocytes consisting of balloon-like degeneration, micro- and macrosteatosis and eosinophilic changes to the cytoplasm) and inflammation was absent. In contrast to the pattern of recurrent HBV in the former group, which comprised productive HBV infection accompanied by the full battery of HBV markers, the pattern of HBV reinfection seen in the latter patients was atypical; HBV DNA in the serum and HBcAg in the liver were absent. In four of these five patients, HBV infection converted to the typical productive pattern within a few weeks and concurrently the histology changed to the classic necroinflammatory picture of viral hepatitis.

Although the cytopathic changes that accompany acute hepatitis syndrome are also a feature of non-viral liver disorders, e.g. fatty liver in pregnancy (Kaplan 1985), Reye's syndrome (Bove et al 1975), tetracycline and valproic acid toxicity (Zimmerman & Ishak 1982), they are a particular feature of HDV infections of man in temperate climates. Similar degenerative changes were associated with hepatitis D in Indians living in the Amazon Basin (Popper et al 1983). In this setting, the regressive changes characterized early disease but were not observed in those cases that progressed to chronicity. In the patients we have studied, this unusual histological pattern was associated with incomplete HBV synthesis, which presumably resulted from some inhibitory interaction of the HDV replicative cycle on the HBV replicative cycle. We speculate that, as a result of this interaction, the expression of nucleocapsidic HBV antigens is abrogated and the host immune reaction to the virus is abolished; thus, cytopathic changes are related to a direct effect of HDV. In most patients, however, HBV suppression is only transitory; its infection rapidly resumes virulence with expression of the HBcAg and the induction of the usual lymphocytotoxic reaction.

CONCLUSION

Medical treatment of chronic hepatitis D rests at present on alpha interferon, which should be administered at high doses (9–10 MU thrice weekly) to patients with well-compensated liver disease, possibly in the early phases of chronicity. Treatment should be prolonged for at least 1 year: if no response occurs — ALT levels remain elevated and HDV RNA persists — therapy should be stopped; if a response occurs — clearance of HDV RNA and normalization of ALT levels — IFN should be continued possibly until the clearance of HBsAg from serum. Careful medical supervision of treated patients is mandatory for early detection of major medical and psychiatric complications.

Patients with decompensated liver disease should be considered for liver transplantation. As in the case of other viral disorders, transplantation is associated with a high risk of reinfection (80%); this risk, however, is dramatically decreased (16–25%) if adequate protection with hyper-immune serum against HBsAg is given. Furthermore, reinfection is followed by relapse of hepatitis in only half of the cases and the relapsed hepatitis usually runs a mild course.

REFERENCES

Arrigoni A, Ponzetto A, Actis G C, Bonino F 1983 Levamisole and chronic delta hepatitis. Annals of Internal Medicine 98: 1024

Belinsky M, Dinter-Gottlieb G 1991 Characterizing the self cleavage of a 135 nucleotide ribozyme from genomic hepatitis delta virus. In: Gerin J L, Purcell R H, Rizzetto M (eds) The hepatitis delta virus. Wiley–Liss, New York, pp 265–274

Berk L, Man R A, Housset C, Berthelot P, Schalm SW 1991 Interferon combination therapy for chronic hepatitis type D. In: Gerin J L, Purcell R H, Rizzetto M (eds) The hepatitis delta virus. Wiley–Liss, New York, pp 411–420

Bettale G, Alberti A, Belli L S et al 1992 Recurrence of HBV and HDV infection after liver transplantation (OLT). In: Taylor J, Bonino F, Hadziyannis S (eds) Hepatitis delta virus, fourth conference. Wiley–Liss, New York (in press)

Bove K E, McAdams A J, Partin J C, Partin G S, Hug G, Schubert W K 1975 The hepatic lesions in Reye's syndrome. Gastroenterology 69: 695–697

Buti M, Esteban R, Roget M et al 1989 Long term treatment with recombinant alpha 2 interferon in patients with chronic delta hepatitis and human immunodeficiency antibodies. Journal of Hepatology 9: S131

Buti M, Esteban R, Jardi R, Rodriguez F, Arranz J A, Guardia J 1993 Ribavirin therapy in chronic delta hepatitis. In: Taylor J, Bonino F, Hadziyannis S (eds) Hepatitis delta virus: molecular biology, pathogenesis and clinical aspects. Wiley Liss, New York, p 468

Cech T R 1988 Ribozymes and their medical implications. Journal of the American Medical Association 260: 3030–3034

Cotonat T, Madejon A, Carreno V 1992 Treatment of chronic delta hepatitis with IFN: additional information is obtained with PCR technology. In: Taylor J, Bonino F, Hadziyannis S (eds) Hepatitis delta virus, fourth conference. Wiley–Liss, New York (in press)

Craxi' A, Di Marco V, Volpes R et al 1990 Treatment with interferon alpha 2b of chronic HDV hepatitis in children. Journal of Hepatology 11: S175

David E, Rahier J, Pucci A et al 1993 Recurrence of hepatitis D (delta) in liver transplants: histopathological aspects. Gastroenterology 104: 1122–1128

Di Bisceglie A M, Marin P, Lisker-Melman et al 1990 Treatment of chronic delta hepatitis with interferon alpha-2b: pilot study conducted at NIH. Journal of Hepatology 11: S151-S154

Farci P, Karayiannis P, Brook M G et al 1989 Treatment of chronic hepatitis delta virus (HDV) infection with human lymphoblastoid alpha interferon. Quarterly Journal of Medicine 73: 1045–1054

Farci P 1992 Treatment of chronic delta hepatitis with high and low doses of interferon alpha-2a. A randomized controlled trial. In: Taylor J, Bonino F, Hadziyannis S (eds) Hepatitis delta virus: molecular biology, pathogenesis and clinical aspects. Wiley–Liss, New York, p 457

Gaudin J L, Faure P, Codinot H, Gerard F, Trepoc 1992 The French experience of treatment of chronic type D hepatitis with 12 month course of IFN alpha-2b. Results of a randomized double blind, controlled trial. In: Taylor J, Bonino F, Hadziyannis S (eds) Hepatitis delta virus, fourth conference. Wiley–Liss, New York (in press)

Kaplan M M 1985 Current concepts: acute fatty liver of

pregnancy. New England Journal of Medicine 313: 367–370
Kleiner D, Axiotis C A, Lisker-Melman M et al 1990 Treatment of chronic delta hepatitis with interferon alpha-2b: pilot study conducted at NIH. Hepatology 12: 846
Marzano A, Ottobrelli A, Spezia C, Daziano E, Soranzo M L, Rizzetto M 1992 Treatment of early chronic delta hepatitis with lymphoblastoid alpha interferon: a pilot study. Italian Journal of Gastroenterology 24: 119–121
Marinucci G, Hassan G, Di Giacomo C et al 1991 Long term treatment of chronic delta hepatitis with alpha recombinant interferon. In: Gerin J L, Purcell R H, Rizzetto M (eds) The hepatitis delta virus. Wiley–Liss, New York pp 405–410
Marinucci G, Hassan G, Di Giacomo C, Dato A, Barlattani A, Costa F 1993 Prognostic significance of IgM to HDV during interferon therapy. In: Taylor J, Bonino F, Hadziyannis S (eds) Hepatitis delta virus: molecular biology, pathogenesis and clinical aspects. Wiley–Liss, New York p 311–318
Mutchnick M G, Happelman H D, Chung H T et al 1991 Thymosin treatment of chronic hepatitis B: a placebo-controlled pilot trial. Hepatology 14: 409–415
Ottobrelli A, Marzano A, Smedile A et al 1991 Patterns of hepatitis delta virus reinfection and disease in liver transplantation. Gastroenterology 101: 1649–1655
Popper H, Thung S N, Gerber M A et al 1983 Histologic studies of severe delta agent infection in Venezuelan Indians. Hepatology 6: 906–912
Rasshofer R, Choi S-S, Wolfl P, Roggendorf M 1991 Interference of antiviral substances with replication of hepatitis delta virus RNA in primary woodchuck hepatocytes. In: Gerin J L, Purcell R H, Rizzetto M (eds) The hepatitis delta virus. Wiley–Liss, New York pp 223–234
Reichard O, Anderson J, Schvarcz R, Weiland O 1991 Ribavirin treatment for chronic hepatitis C. Lancet 337: 1058–1061
Reynes M, Zignego L, Samuel D et al 1989 Graft hepatitis delta virus reinfection after orthotopic liver transplantation in HDV cirrhosis. Transplant Proceedings 21: 2424–2425
Rizzetto M, Verme G, Recchia S et al 1983 Chronic HBsAg hepatitis with intrahepatic expression of delta antigen. An active and progressive disease unresponsive to immunosuppressive treatment. Annals of Internal Medicine 98: 437–441
Rosina F, Rizzetto M 1989 Treatment of chronic type D (delta) hepatitis with alpha interferon. Seminars in Liver Disease 9: 264–266
Rosina F, Marzano A, Garripoli A et al 1990 Chronic type D hepatitis: clearance of hepatitis B surface antigen during and after treatment with alfa interferon. Hepatology 12: 883
Rosina F, Pintus C, Meschievitz C, Rizzetto M 1991 A randomized controlled trial of a 12 month course of recombinant human interferon alpha in chronic delta (type D) hepatitis: a multicenter Italian study. Hepatology 13: 1052–1056
Samuel D, Bismuth A, Serres C et al 1991 HBV infection after liver transplantation in HBsAg-positive patients: experience with long-term immunoprophylaxis. Transplantation Proceedings 23: 1492–1494
Smedile A, Rosina F, Saracco G et al 1991 Hepatitis B virus replication modulates pathogenesis of hepatitis D virus in chronic hepatitis D. Hepatology 13: 413–416
Taillan B, Fuzibet J G, Vinti H, Pesce A, Cassuto J P, Dujardin P 1988 Interferon and delta hepatitis (letter). Annals of Internal Medicine 109: 760
Ten Kate F J W, Schalm S W 1991 Course of hepatitis delta virus infection in auxiliary liver grafts in patients with delta virus cirrhosis. In: Gerin J L, Purcell R H, Rizzetto M (eds) The hepatitis delta virus. Progress in Clinical and Biological Research 364: 425–437
Todros L, Touscoz G, D'Urso N et al 1991 Hepatitis C virus-related chronic liver disease with autoantibodies to liver–kidney microsomes (LKM). Journal of Hepatology 13: 128–131
Zimmerman H J, Ishak K G 1982 Valproate induced hepatic injury. Analysis of 23 fatal cases. Hepatology 2: 591–597

SECTION 5

Hepatitis E virus

23. Structure and molecular virology

D. W. Bradley K. Krawczynski M. A. Purdy

Hepatitis E virus (HEV) has been characterized and its genome cloned and sequenced (Table 23.1).

PHYSIOCHEMICAL PROPERTIES OF HEV

The virus appears to be extremely labile and will not tolerate exposure to high concentrations of salt, including caesium chloride. Pelleting of the virus from faeces suspension or gradient fractions frequently results in loss or degradation of virus. However, rate-zonal banding of 32–34 nm virus-like particles (VLPs) in linear, preformed sucrose gradients has been found to yield partially purified virus suitable for further immune electron microscopy (IEM) and primate transmission studies (Bradley 1990). The computed sedimentation coefficient of the enterically transmitted non-A, non-B hepatitis (ET-NANBH)-assisted virus is approximately 183S, in contrast to 165S; these particles are presumed to be defective and may lack a complete viral genome. Isopycnic banding of an aliquot of the Telixtac (Mexico) no. 14 faeces suspension in a potassium tartrate/glycerol gradient revealed 32–34 nm VLPs at a buoyant density of 1.29 g/cm^3. These biophysical properties are consistent with the notion that the major agent of hepatitis E is calicivirus-like. Like caliciviruses, the 32–34 nm VLPs described here are also sensitive to freeze-thawing, storage in liquid suspensions at temperatures between -70°C and +8°C, and pelleting from solutions of sucrose or buffer. HAV (HAS-15 strain, partially purified from tissue culture lysates) and HEV contained in the faeces of patients with hepatitis E from Burma, Mexico, Somalia and the former Soviet Union were independently measured by three individuals at the Centers for Disease Control (CDC) in Georgia, USA. HAV and HEV were found to have mean particle diameters of 27.8 nm and 32.2 nm respectively.

Table 23.1 Properties of hepatitis E virus (HEV)

Size	32–34 nm in diameter (80% of virus particles visualized by IEM; 32.2 nm mean diameter; range 27–38 nm)
Morphology	Spherical, non-enveloped particle; spikes and indentations visible on surface of virus
Biophysical properties	Sedimentation coefficient = 183S (defectives, 165S); buoyant density = 1.29 g/cm^3 in potassium tartrate/glycol sensitive to caesium chloride freeze–thawing and pelleting
Genome	Single-stranded, polyadenylated RNA of approx. 7.5 kb; three open reading frames; structural protein encoded at 3' end
In vitro propagation	Unsuccessful (FRhK-4, AGMK, HEK, BSC-1, etc.)
In vivo	No effect on suckling mice inoculated intracerebrally with numerous case stool suspensions (10% w/v)

MOLECULAR CLONING OF THE VIRAL GENOME

Although attempts were made to clone the genome from faecal concentrates or sucrose gradient fractions rich in virus particles, none resulted in a virus-specific clone. Clearly, a high-titre preparation of virus lacking the nucleic acid complexity of faeces or liver was needed. Because virus particles recovered from faeces were also frequently found to be degraded or in the process of degradation, it was concluded that molecular cloning of the virus could not be achieved unless it could be stabilized first, or another, more plentiful, source of virus could be identified. The probable deleterious effects of proteases or other processes on the integrity of HEV during its transit through the small intestine led investigators to look for the virus in the gall bladder bile prior to its discharge into the duodenum. Aspiration of bile from the gall bladders of several HEV-infected cyanomolgus macaques during the early acute phase of disease yielded one sample with a very high virus particle count (>1000 VLPs per electron microscopy grid square). Virus particles contained in gall bladder bile were found to have a diameter of 32–34 nm and were morphologically indistinguishable from those recovered from faeces.

Molecular cloning of the viral genome of the 32–34 nm VLPs described above was carried out by the CDC in collaboration with Genelabs, (Redwood City, CA, USA). A 'plus–minus' (genomic) screening approach was used because of the availability of large amounts of virus in infected bile. This source material also lacked the nucleic acid 'complexity' of either faeces or liver, i.e. the ratio of non-viral to viral nucleic acid was relatively low. Molecular cloning of HEV was approached with the assumption that it has an RNA genome. Molecular clones of HEV were identified by two separate procedures using lambda gt10 and gt11 as cloning and expression vectors respectively. cDNA was prepared from both uninfected and HEV (Burma isolate)-infected bile and inserted into lambda gt10 for 'plus–minus' screening using cDNA probes (from both cDNA libraries) labelled by random priming. Differential hybridization studies, using radiolabelled probes, revealed the presence of several candidate clones derived from infected bile, including ET1.1, the first virus-specific clone to be identified (Reyes et al 1990). ET1.1 was shown to:

1. Hybridize specifically to infected source cDNA.
2. Hybridize specifically to infected liver RNA (to an approximately 7.5-kb polyadenylated molecule).
3. Encode a portion of an RNA-dependent RNA polymerase consensus motif.
4. Be exogenous to both infected and uninfected primate DNA.
5. Have a sequence different from any contained in GenBank.

Clone ET1.1 was also shown specifically to hybridize to cDNAs prepared from HEV-infected faeces collected from outbreak-related cases in Borneo, Mexico, Pakistan, Somalia and the Soviet Union. The cDNAs were prepared by a novel cDNA amplification procedure (SISPA, sequence-independent single-primer amplification) (Reyes & Kim 1992) that permitted the expansion of the limited amount of cDNA originally prepared from the source faeces.

The second approach to HEV clone identification relied on the use of immunoscreening of cDNA libraries (prepared from the faeces of a patient in a Mexican outbreak) prepared in lambda gt11, a highly efficient expression vector. Virus-specific proteins, expressed as β-galactosidase fusion proteins, were identified using convalescent serum from another well-documented case of hepatitis E from a separate outbreak in Mexico. Two of these virus-specific clones, 406.3–2 and 406.4–2, were used to identify additional virus-specific messages of 2.0 and 3.7 kb in poly(A) RNA extracted from HEV-infected macaque liver, indicating the possible presence of subgenomic RNAs required for virus replication. Panelling of expressed proteins against a variety of paired acute- and convalescent-phase human sera from geographically distinct regions of the world, as well as preinoculation, acute-phase, and convalescent-phase sera from infected animals, demonstrated the utility of these expressed proteins to detect both IgM (acute phase) and IgG (generally convalescent phase) anti-HEV antibodies.

GENOMIC ORGANIZATION

Analysis of the entire nucleotide sequence of the HEV Burma isolate has revealed the presence of several consensus sequences, including one associated with a nucleoside triphosphate (NTP)-binding, helicase-like function 5' to the putative RNA-dependent RNA polymerase. These non-structural elements are contained within a single open reading frame (ORF) of approximately 5 kb, 28 nucleotides from the 5' end of the genome. Clone 406.3–2 was contained within a second ORF that extended another 2 kb to a point 68 bases upstream from the poly(A) tail. ORF2 is thought to encode the major structural protein(s) of HEV. The second immunoreactive clone, 406.4–2, was identified within a third ORF (plus 2 frame) that contained only 369 nucleotides. It overlapped ORF1 by one nucleotide and ORF2 by 328 nucleotides. HEV appears to be substantially different from picornaviruses, including HAV, in that it has an RNA genome that encodes for structural and non-structural proteins through the use of discontinuous, partially overlapping ORFs (Fig. 23.1).

The genomes of both Burma and Mexico HEV isolates have now been cloned and completely sequenced; they have been shown to possess the basic genomic features described above. The key elements of the genetic organization and expression strategy of HEV (still tentative, pending sequencing of authentic viral proteins) have now been elucidated and shown to set it apart from other previously defined hepatotropic viruses of man. Studies of the genome of Norwalk virus

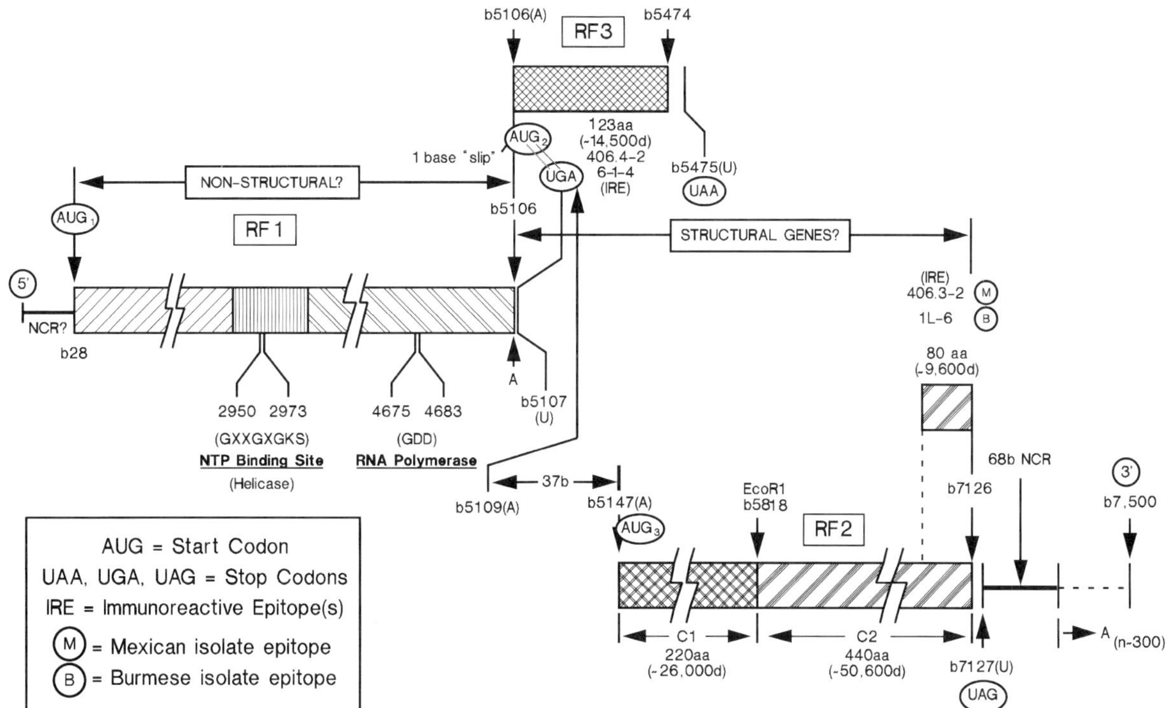

Fig. 23.1 Genetic organization of the HEV genome. The three open reading frames are indicated by RF1, RF2 and RF3. The 3' and 5' non-coding regions (NCRs) are shown as single lines and the 3' poly (A*n*) tail is shown on the right-hand side. The non-structural gene region, RF1, contains consensus sequences for a nucleotide binding site as part of a putative helicase protein and another consensus sequence (GDD) common to all viral RNA-dependent RNA polymerases. The putative structural gene sequence, shown as RF2, encodes the C2 portion of the *trp*E-C2 fusion protein. Note that the three ORFs overlap one another and that the stop codon for RF1 has been cleverly used, by incorporation of a one-base 'slip', to form the start codon for RF3.

Table 23.2 Nucleotide and amino acid differences between HEV isolates from the USSR, Burma and Mexico

Comparison between	NUC	AA	TI	TV	First	Second	Third
T and B	93.7	95.5	52	13	10	5	50
B and M	76.9	90.0	101	101	30	18	154
M and T	76.5	86.8	99	106	30	21	154

Comparisons between geographically distinct HEV isolates from: T = Tashkent, USSR, (outbreak isolate); B = Rangoon, Burma (passaged three times in cynomolgus macaques); M = Telixtac, Mexico (outbreak isolate).
NUC, percentage nucleotide similarity (873 nucleotides); AA, percentage amino acid similarity (291 amino acids); TI, transitions; TV, transversions; first, number of differences at the first codon position; second, number of differences at the second codon position; third, number of differences at the third codon position.

(M K Estes, personal communication) and feline calicivirus (FCV) (Tohya et al 1991) further suggest that HEV may belong to a larger family of single-stranded, polyadenylated RNA viruses that possess two or three separate ORFs with three distinctly different RNA transcripts. This group of viruses is also associated with the presence of two or more 3' subgenomic RNAs (in infected tissues or cultured cells) with sizes ranging between 2 and 4 kb (2.0 and 3.7 HEV).

GENETIC VARIATION

Molecular cloning and sequencing of the Burma, Tashkent and Mexico isolates of HEV have revealed an unexpectedly high degree of sequence divergence between the North American (Mexico) isolate and the Asian isolates (Table 23.2; M Purdy, unpublished data).Computer analysis of nucleotide sequences (869 bases in length) contained within the region encoding the putative RNA-dependent RNA polymerase (RDRP) showed that the Tashkent and Burma isolates share homologies of 93.7% and 95.5% at the nucleotide and amino acid level respectively, whereas these two isolates share only 77% nucleotide and 87–90% amino acid homology with the Mexican isolate. It is worth noting that the ratios of codon changes in the first, second or third position are nearly constant for all three isolates (see Table 23.2). The number of transitions (TI) far outnumbers the number of transversions (TV) when the Tashkent and Burma sequences are compared. By contrast, comparison of either the Tashkent or Burma sequence with that of the Mexico isolate shows that transversions are just as likely to be observed as transitions. These findings clearly indicate that the Mexico isolate is genetically distinct from the 'Asian' isolates, a sign that these viruses probably diverged from each other in the distant past. Cloning and sequencing of other HEV isolates obtained from South America, Central Africa and Borneo, for example, may reveal subtler evolutionary changes at the nucleotide level and provide some insight into the specific nucleotide sequences that are absolutely required for functionality of the deduced proteins.

REFERENCES

Bradley D W 1990 Enterically-transmitted non-A, non-B hepatitis. British Medical Bulletin 46: 442–461

Reyes G R, Kim J P 1992 Sequence independent, single-primer amplification (SISPA) of complex populations. Molecular and Cellular Probes (in press)

Reyes G R, Purdy M A, Kim J P et al 1990 Isolation of a cDNA from the virus responsible for enterically transmitted non-A, non-B hepatitis. Science 247: 1335–1339

Tohya Y, Taniguchi Y, Utagawa E et al 1991 Sequence analysis of the 3' end of feline calicivirus genome. Virology 183: 810–814

UPDATE

- Genetic variation of different HEV strains has been observed and it will be important to determine the extent to which this variation may pose problems in the diagnosis and treatment of HEV infection. To analyse differences at the genetic level between HEV (Mexico; M) and the previously characterized HEV (Burma; B) and HEV (Pakistan; P) isolates, overlapping cDNAs were cloned from samples obtained from an infected human and an experimentally inoculated cynomolgus macaque. These cDNA clones, representing the nearly complete (7185-bp) genome of HEV(M), confirmed an expression strategy for the virus that involves the use of 3 forward open reading frames (ORFs). The HEV (M) strain has an overall 76 and 77% nucleic acid identity with the HEV(B) strain and HEV(P) strain, respectively; however, the degree of sequence variation was not uniform throughout the viral genome. A hypervariable region was identified in ORF1 that exhibited a 58 and 54% nucleic acid sequence and 13% amino acid similarity with the Burma strain and the Pakistan strain, respectively. A large number of the nucleotide differences occurred at the third codon position, with the deduced amino acid sequences similarity of 83, 93, and 87% between HEV(M) and HEV(B) isolates in ORF1, ORF2, and ORF3, respectively, and with 84, 93, and 87% amino acid identities between HEV(M) and HEV(P) isolates in ORF1, ORF2, and ORF3, respectively. The nucleotide sequences derived from the highly conserved regions of HEV genome will be useful in developing polymerase chain reaction-based tests to confirm the viral infection. Knowledge of the extent of the sequence variation encountered with HEV will not only aid in the future development of diagnostic and vaccine reagents but also further our understanding of how HEV strain variation might impact the pathological outcome of infection (Huang et al 1992).
- REFERENCE

Huang C C, Nguyen D, Fernandez J, Yun K Y, Fry K E, Bradley D W, Tam A W 1992 Molecular cloning and sequencing of the Mexico isolate of hepatitis E virus (HEV). Virology 191, 2: 550–558

24. Epidemiology, natural history and experimental models

D. W. Bradley K. Krawczynski M. A. Purdy

A substantial proportion of cases of acute viral hepatitis occurring in young to middle-aged adults in Asia and the Indian subcontinent appear to be caused by an agent that is serologically unrelated to either hepatitis A virus (HAV) or hepatitis B virus (HBV) (Wong et al 1980). This disease has been shown to occur in both epidemic and sporadic, endemic forms and is primarily associated with the ingestion of faecally contaminated drinking water (Tables 24.1 and 24.2). The term enterically transmitted non-A, non-B hepatitis (ET-NANBH) evolved from the water-borne mode of virus transmission and presumed an enteric route of natural infection in humans (Bradley et al 1988a, 1990). This type of hepatitis was first documented in New Delhi, India, in 1955, when 29 000 cases of icteric hepatitis were identified following widespread faecal contamination of the city's drinking water (Viswanathan 1957). A similar epidemic of viral hepatitis occurred between December 1975 and January 1976 in Ahmedabad City, India, again due to contaminated water supplies (Sreenivasan et al 1978). Both outbreaks were thought originally to be caused by HAV, however retrospective serological analysis of paired serum specimens from documented cases revealed that neither HAV nor HBV could be implicated as the aetiological agent (Wong et al 1980). Large epidemics of enterically transmitted viral hepatitis have also been observed in the Kirgiz Republic (former Soviet Union). Between 1955 and 1956 more than 10 800 cases of acute viral hepatitis were documented there in young to middle-aged adults; approximately 18% of infected pregnant women died as a result of acute disease. The epidemiological and clinical features of these outbreaks are remarkably similar to those associated with the 1955–56 New Delhi outbreak. Subsequent outbreaks of epidemic and sporadic NANBH were documented in north India (Tandon et al 1982) and in Kashmir, India (Khuroo et al 1983). Outbreaks of epidemiologically similar cases of hepatitis E have also been reported in South-East Asia, including Burma and Nepal (Kane et al 1984), and were associated with a high mortality rate in infected pregnant women. Between June 1976 and August 1977, more than 20 000 icteric cases occurred in Mandalay, Burma, with a case fatality ratio of 18% in pregnant women (Centers for Disease Control, unpublished data). An epidemic of viral hepatitis involving 10 000 cases in the Kathmandu Valley, Nepal, in 1973 was also reported to be associated with a high mortality rate in infected pregnant women (Kane et al 1984). The occurrence of hepatitis E in Pakistan has been inferred from the observation of cases of disease imported into the USA (De Cock et al 1987).

Table 24.1 Clinical features of ET-NANB hepatitis

1. Self-limiting acute disease resembling hepatitis A
2. Incubation period from 2 to 9 weeks (mean 6 weeks)
3. Most fatal cases occur in infected pregnant women
4. Mild or subclinical forms possible, but not documented
5. Chronic liver disease of persistent viraemia has not been observed

Outbreaks of hepatitis E have also been reported in Africa, including Algeria, Ivory Coast, eastern Sudan, Gambia, Kenya (see below) and Somalia. Between October 1980 and January 1981, more than 780 cases of NANBH were documented in

Table 24.2 Outbreaks of ET-NANB hepatitis

Site	Dates	Number of cases	Source of infection
Indian subcontinent			
India (New Delhi)	1955–56	29 000	Contaminated water
India (Ahmedabad)	1975–76	2 572	Contaminated water
Nepal (Kathmandu Val.)	1973	10 000	Not determined
Nepal (Kathmandu Val.)	1981–82	6 000	Not determined
Pakistan (Karachi)	1985	several cases (five imported to USA)	
South-East Asia			
Burma (Rangoon)	1982–83	399	Contaminated water
Indonesia (Borneo)	1987–88	2 000	Contaminated water
Central Asia			
USSR (Kirgiz Republic)	1955–56	10 812	Not determined
China (Xinjiang Region)	1986–88	119 280	Contaminated water
*Africa**			
Algeria	1980–81	788	Contaminated water
Ivory Coast (Tortiya)	1983–84	623	Not known
Chad	1983–84	38	(?) Contaminated water
Sudan (Eastern)	1985	2 012	Contaminated water
Somalia (refugee camps)	1985–86	2 000	Contaminated water
North America			
Mexico (Huitzililla)	1986	94	Contaminated water
Mexico (Telixtac)	1986	129	Contaminated water

*Outbreaks in Gambia and Nigeria were also reported.

Algeria and linked to the use of faecally contaminated drinking water. Mostly young adults were affected, and nine of nine infected pregnant women died as a direct result of NANBH. A similar number of NANBH cases in Tortiya, Ivory Coast, was observed between 1983 and 1984. Although no precise figure was given, a high mortality rate among infected pregnant women was noted. More recently, large outbreaks of hepatitis E have been documented in Eritrean and Tigrean (Ethiopian) refugees encamped in eastern Sudan (Centers for Disease Control 1987). More than 2000 cases occurred in these refugees between August and September 1985, again as the result of faecally contaminated water. Several thousand cases of hepatitis E were also noted in Ethiopian refugees residing in Tog Wajale and other camps in north-west Somalia (Centers for Disease Control 1987); these accounted for the majority of acute viral hepatitis cases observed in these camps between 1985 and 1986. The mortality rate among hepatitis E-infected pregnant refugee women was greater than 17% and a faecally contaminated environment was again implicated as the vehicle for virus transmission. A similar outbreak of hepatitis E was observed in 1991 in Somalian and Ethiopian refugees in Liboi, Kenya; this outbreak involved more than 1700 clinically apparent (jaundiced) cases (Centers for Disease Control, unpublished results of outbreak investigation; L Polish & E Mast, unpublished data).

However, hepatitis E does not appear to be confined to Asia, the Soviet Union and North Africa. In fact, outbreaks of NANBH associated with faecally contaminated drinking water have been documented in Borneo and in two rural villages located south of Mexico City. More than 90 cases of presumed hepatitis E were recorded in Huitzililla, Mexico, between June and October of 1986. Additional cases of NANBH were seen in Telixtac, Mexico, shortly thereafter. Virological and serological studies of faeces and serum specimens, respectively, obtained from affected persons suggested that the aetiological agent responsible for disease in North America might be similar or identical to that associated with hepatitis E in other regions of the world. As noted above, the only cases seen in the USA have been imported by travellers who have contracted the disease in endemic areas, and no cases of secondary exposure have been reported in the USA. Table 24.2 summarizes a number of representative outbreaks of hepatitis E that have occurred in endemic regions of the world.

UNANSWERED QUESTIONS

In developing countries, more than 50% of acute viral hepatitis appears to be caused by agents other than HAV or HBV. It is assumed that a high proportion of NANBH in these countries is associated with an enterically transmitted agent, because environmental conditions in most endemic areas favour the faecal–oral route of transmission. In this regard, however, the preponderance of clinically apparent ET-NANBH cases in individuals between the ages of 15 and 40 years suggests that infection either occurs subclinically in younger individuals or does not occur at all. The latter presumption is difficult to justify in view of the fact that seroprevalence studies conducted in these countries clearly indicate that nearly all individuals acquire anti-HAV before the age of 10 years. In fact serological studies showed that Sudanese children exposed to HEV during the course of an outbreak acquired antibody to HEV (M Carl, personal communication). Clearly, further studies are needed to identify additional factors involved in the epidemiology and pathogenesis of hepatitis E.

Another important but unexplained observation is the unusually high mortality rate observed in infected pregnant women. Approximately 20% of women with ET-NANBH in their third trimester of pregnancy succumb, in contrast to 0.5–3% of the local or general population suffering from ET-NANBH. The effect of pregnancy on viral hepatitis does not explain this observation, for only negligible mortality is seen in infected pregnant women with other types of viral hepatitis. In this regard, the unexpectedly high mortality rate observed in HEV-infected pregnant women may reflect a unique feature of viral replication or disease pathogenesis in these individuals.

Another notable feature of hepatitis E is the relatively low frequency of clinical disease observed in case contacts, an unusual phenomenon for enterically transmitted agents. For example, among household contacts of hepatitis E patients during the 1981–82 epidemic in Kathmandu Valley, Nepal, clinical illness developed in only 2.4%. This is in sharp contrast to the much higher secondary attack rate of 10–20% observed in household contacts of patients with hepatitis A occurring in the same region. The relative instability of the 32–34 nm virus-like particles (VLPs) described above may account for the decreased secondary transmission of hepatitis E; however, definitive studies of virus stability and infectivity will be required to support or refute this notion.

EXPERIMENTAL PRIMATE MODELS

Transmission of hepatitis E to non-human primates was reported first by Balayan et al (1983). Two cynomolgus macaques ('cynos') were inoculated intravenously with a 10%(w/v) suspension of faeces from a human volunteer that was positive by immune electron microscopy (IEM) for 27–30 nm diameter VLPs. In these animals, elevations in alanine aminotransferase (ALT) activity developed between 24 and 36 days after inoculation; they excreted 27–30 nm VLPs in their preacute-phase faeces and seroconverted, as demonstrated by IEM, acquiring antibody to morphologically similar VLPs in the inoculum. Andjaparidze et al later reported the successful transmission of hepatitis E to African Green monkeys, as well as cynos, using faecal specimens positive by IEM for 27–30 nm VLPs obtained from patients with hepatitis E. Although hepatitis E was serially passaged in these animals, a decreased efficiency of transmission was observed during each successive passage. Intravenous inoculation of four *Saguinus mystax* (tamarins) at the Centers for Disease Control (CDC) with another acute-phase stool suspension obtained in 1982 from a patient with hepatitis E in Nepal resulted in biochemical evidence of liver injury in three;

27–30 nm VLPs were observed in several early acute-phase faeces specimens of one animal studied in detail (Kane et al 1984).

Animal transmission studies have been conducted in cynos, tamarins and chimpanzees using highly characterized inocula. These studies relied on the use of susceptible primate species specifically for the purpose of developing a reliable source of infected faeces and liver tissue. These same studies have provided preinoculation, acute-phase and convalescent-phase sera for use in coded serum panels, in immunofluorescence antibody assays, (see Ch. 25), and in immunoscreening studies of lambda gt11 cDNA libraries. Intravenous inoculation of four tamarins with faeces pool from the 1982–83 Burma outbreak (positive by IEM for 32–34 nm VLPs) caused elevated serum isocitrate dehydrogenase (SICD) activity in three animals, with peak values occurring between 70 and 80 days after inoculation. Three or four cynos inoculated i.v. with the same material developed elevated ALT activity after an average incubation period of 38 days. This HEV isolate was passaged in cynos using preacute-phase faeces suspension from animals exhibiting the highest elevations of ALT activity. The incubation period at each passage level appeared to be shorter, and all animals became infected (Bradley et al 1987). Additional passage of disease in cynos using either liver or faeces resulted in incubation periods as short as 5 days (D Bradley, unpublished data). Intravenous inoculation of four cynos with a partially purified virus preparation (Mexico patients faeces; see Ch. 23 for details) containing a relatively large number of 32–34 nm VLPs resulted in elevated ALT activity after incubation periods of 5, 5, 8 and 12 days. Intravenous inoculation of colony-born chimpanzees with this same inoculum resulted in biochemical evidence of liver disease and histopathology consistent with a diagnosis of viral hepatitis (K Krawczynski & D Bradley, unpublished data). It is interesting to note that inoculation of other chimpanzees with patient-derived stools obtained from hepatitis E outbreaks in geographical areas other than Mexico or containing fewer numbers of 32–34 nm VLPs (or smaller VLPs) demonstrated less severe disease or no disease at all. The faeces used in these studies were derived from cases of hepatitis E occurring in India, the Soviet Union (A Andjaparidze & D Bradley, unpublished data) and Miyanmar (Burma) (D Bradley, unpublished data).

Although reliable and efficient transmission of hepatitis E was demonstrated to cynos, tamarins and chimpanzees with inocula containing 32–34 nm VLPs, VLPs were not consistently recovered with a similar or identical morphology from proven infectious faeces pools. These findings indicated either that HEV was normally present in few numbers in infected stools or that it was so labile that passage through the gut resulted in substantial particle degradation. The latter presumption was favoured in view of the observed instability of virus in stored faeces suspensions and the lack of virus particles in a high percentage of well-documented cases of severe disease. As a result, in order to demonstrate a serological relationship between ET-NANBH in experimentally infected primates and virus particles associated with human disease, numerous patient faeces specimens had to be screened in order to find several that contained sufficient numbers of virus particles to facilitate meaningful IEM studies. The results of one IEM study showed a consistent and specific relationship between hepatitis E in primates (and humans) and 32–34 nm VLPs recovered from patient faeces in Mexico and the former Soviet Union (Bradley et al 1988b). Earlier IEM studies at the Centers for Disease Control relied on the use of paired preinoculation and convalescent-phase sera from experimentally infected primates in order to show a serological relationship between disease and the putative viral agent of hepatitis E. However, because some of the convalescent-phase sera failed to react with reagent virus particles; many of the results were inconsistent or unconvincing. Further studies using faeces containing large numbers of 32–34 nm VLPs revealed that acute-phase sera from both human cases and experimentally infected primates were much more likely to aggregate virus than convalescent-phase sera from the same individuals. This finding was considered to be significant in that it allowed a clear serological relationship to be consistently demonstrated between 32–34 nm VLPs and experimentally induced disease in non-human primates.

REFERENCES

Andjaparidze A, Balayan M S, Sarinau A P, Braginsky D M, Poleschuk V F, Zamyatina N A 1986 Fecal-orally transmitted non-A, non-B hepatitis induced in monkeys. Voprosy virusologii 1: 73–80

Balayan M S, Andjaparidze A G, Savinskya S S, Ketiladze E S, Braginsky D M, Savinov A P, Poleschuk V F 1983 Evidence for a virus in non-A, non-B hepatitis transmitted via the faecal-oral route. Intervirology 20: 23–31

Bradley D W 1990 Enterically-transmitted non-A, non-B hepatitis. British Medical Bulletin 46: 442–461

Bradley D W, Krawczynski K, Cook E H et al 1987 Enterically transmitted non-A, non-B hepatitis: serial passage of disease in cynomolgus macaques and tamarins and recovery of disease-associated 27–34 nm virus-like particles. Proceedings of the National Academy of Sciences of the USA 84: 6277–6281

Bradley D W, Krawczynski K, Cook E H et al 1988a Enterically transmitted non-A, non-B hepatitis: etiology of disease and laboratory studies in nonhuman primates. In Zuckerman A J (ed) Viral hepatitis and liver disease. Alan R. Liss, New York, pp 138–147

Bradley D W, Andjaparidze A, Cook E H et al 1988b Aetiological agent of enterically transmitted non-A, non-B hepatitis. Journal of General Virology 69: 731–738

Centers for Disease Control 1987 Enterically transmitted non-A, non-B hepatitis – East Africa. Morbidity and Mortality Weekly Report 36: 241–244

De Cock K M, Bradley D W, Sandford N L et al 1987 Epidemic non-A, non-B hepatitis in patients from Pakistan. Annals of Internal Medicine 106: 227–230

Kane M A, Bradley D W, Shrestha S M et al 1984 Epidemic non-A, non-B hepatitis in Nepal: recovery of a possible etiologic agent and transmission studies in marmosets. Journal of the American Medical Association 252: 3140–3145

Khuroo S M, Duermeyer W, Zarger S A et al 1983 Acute sporadic non-A/non-B hepatitis in India. American Journal of Epidemiology 118: 360–364

Sreenivasan M A, Banerjee K, Pandya P G et al 1978 Epidemiological investigations of an outbreak of infectious hepatitis in Ahmedabad city during 1975–76. Indian Journal of Medical Research 67: 197–206

Tandon B N, Joshi Y K, Jain S K et al 1982 An epidemic of non-A, non-B hepatitis in North India. Indian Journal of Medical Research 75: 793–744

Viswanathan R 1957 Infectious hepatitis in Delhi (1955–56): a critical study: epidemiology. Indian Journal of Medical Research 45: 1–30

Wong D C, Purcell R H, Sreenivasan M A et al 1980 Epidemic and endemic hepatitis in India: evidence for non-A/non-B hepatitis virus aetiology. Lancet ii: 876–878

25. Diagnosis

D.W. Bradley   K. Krawczynski   M.A. Purdy

The diagnosis of acute hepatitis E is made by serological exclusion complemented by supportive epidemiological circumstances. The laboratory tests currently used for diagnosis of hepatitis E are not generally available. These include:

1. immune electron microscopic (IEM) examination of patient faeces for virus-like particles.
2. a fluorescent antibody-blocking assay for the detection of virus-specific antibodies in patient sera.
3. a Western blot assay for IgM and or IgG anti-HEV.
4. two different PCR (polymerase chain reaction) assays for the detection of HEV RNA (as cDNA) in patient faeces or in acute-phase sera (see below).

Commercial prototype enzyme-linked immunoassay (EIA) tests for IgM and IgG anti-HEV have also been developed but are not widely available for routine diagnosis of suspected cases of hepatitis E.

ELECTRON MICROSCOPIC STUDIES

Although several reports of 27–30 nm virus-like particles (VLPs) associated with hepatitis E have appeared in the literature, independent confirmation of the specificity of these candidate viruses for disease has been complicated by the limited availability of patient-derived faeces specimens and the relative instability of reagent virus. IEM studies at the Centers For Disease Control (CDC) of faeces specimens for VLPs were initiated in 1982 when stools from cases of hepatitis E occurring in Kathmandu Valley, Nepal, were examined using convalescent serum as a source of antibody. One of nine stools was found to be positive for 27–32 nm VLPs; convalescent (but not preinoculation) serum from a tamarin in which NANBH had developed after inoculation with this stool specimen was shown to have antibody against these viruses (Kane et al 1984). This finding suggested that the animal had seroconverted specifically by acquiring antibodies to VLPs contained in the inoculum and indicated further that these particles (or a related particle) might be causally related to disease. Subsequent serological studies with these virus particles were compromised by the diminished number of particles found in stored and freeze–thawed stool suspensions. Faeces from another outbreak of hepatitis E occurring in 1982–83 in Rangoon, Burma (Miyanmar), were available to the CDC through collaboration with the Ministry of Health (Myint). Four of 31 patient-derived faeces specimens were found to be positive by IEM for 27–30 and 32–34 nm VLPs. Both sets of particles appeared to possess surface features that were morphologically similar to those found on the Nepal patient–derived stool particles described above. One perplexing aspect of these studies was the notable discrepancy in the antibody coating of 27–30 and 32–34 nm VLPs; the smaller particles appeared to be minimally reactive with antibody contained in patient sera, whereas the larger virus particles were found to be heavily coated. Unfortunately, the lack of 'pedigreed' serum panels containing preinfection and preinoculation sera from human patients and experimentally infected primates precluded further serological analyses of the unexpectedly large virus particles found in these faeces. In addition, freeze–thawing and/or long-term storage of these stools as 10% (w/v) suspensions was found to result in a complete loss of intact, 32–34 nm VLPs, although some 27–30 nm particles could still be visualized by IEM.

These studies clearly suggest that the larger, 32–34 nm VLP is responsible for all or nearly all cases of hepatitis E. The smaller 27–30 nm VLP found associated with some cases of hepatitis E may either be a degradation product of the larger 'parent' particle or a co-infecting or coexisting virus that is unrelated to the infectious agent. Proteolytic digestion or denaturation of the 32–34 nm virus during its passage through the gut may be responsible for some of the discrepancies in reported particle diameters. Proteolytic degradation of HEV may also account for the unexpectedly low numbers of VLPs found in acute-phase stools.

More extensive IEM studies were performed using faeces obtained from two outbreaks that occurred in the (former) Soviet Union and Mexico. One faeces specimen recovered from a case of hepatitis E in Tashkent (1982–83 epidemic) was found to contain large numbers of 32–34 nm diameter virus particles. These particles reacted specifically with acute-phase and convalescent-phase sera from well-documented cases occurring in other regions of the world, including Burma, Pakistan, Nepal, Somalia, Sudan, Borneo and Mexico (Bradley et al 1988). More convincing evidence for the association between the larger 32–34 nm VLPs and hepatitis E derived from the demonstrated seroconversion of experimentally infected primates. Cynomolgus macaques ('cynos') infected with Soviet or Burmese patient faeces (positive for 32–34 nm VLPs) were shown to acquire antibody to 32–34 nm VLPs in the Tashkent number 1435 faeces suspension. One tamarin infected with the Burma isolate was also shown by IEM to have antibody against the larger 32–34 nm VLPs. Paritally purified 32–34 nm VLPs derived from the faeces of a patient with hepatitis E in Telixtac, Mexico, were also shown to react with acute-phase antibody in sera from humans and primates infected with non-A, non-B hepatitis (NANBH) (Bradley et al 1988). Sera from patients in the Soviet Union, Pakistan, Nepal, Burma, Borneo, Somalia and Mexico were all capable of aggregating 32–34 nm VLPs in the Telixtac number 14 stool; antibody coating on these particles was very heavy and was rated 4+ (scale: 0–4+). Seroconversion of experimentally infected primates was also clearly documented. It is equally important to note that selected cynos from the first, second and third passage of a Burma ET-NANBH isolate were shown to acquire virus-specific antibody, thus reinforcing the notion that hepatitis E can be successfully passaged in this species of non-human primate and that animals infected with one isolate readily acquire antibody against another geographically distinct isolate.

In short, it is clear that one virus or class of serologically related viruses is responsible for disease worldwide, including Soviet Asia, Asia, South-East Asia, North Africa and North America. Limited cross-challenge studies conducted in cynos suggest further that animals convalescent from a bout of hepatitis E induced by an Asian (Burma/Miyanmar) isolate are protected from reinfection by a second (Mexican) isolate (D Bradley, unpublished data). This finding is in agreement with the serological (IEM) data showing that geographically distinct virus isolates react with antisera from a variety of outbreaks. Figure 25.1 shows antibody-aggregated 32–34 nm VLPs typical of those found in stools of ET-NANBH patients in Borneo, Burma, Mexico, Pakistan, Somalia and the former Soviet Union.

IDENTIFICATION OF HEV-Ag IN HEPATOCYTES

An antigen associated with hepatitis E (HEVAg) has been identified in the cytoplasm of hepatocytes of experimentally infected cynomolgus macaques (Krawczynski & Bradley 1989). HEVAg was found in hepatocytes of infected cynos, chimpanzees and aotus monkeys inoculated with faeces preparations derived from the Burma, Pakistan and Mexico outbreaks. The specificity of this antigen for hepatitis E was determined by blocking experiments with the use of acute- and convalescent-phase serum samples and by absorption experiments (normal liver and immunoglobulins). Positive results in the fluorescent (FA) antibody-blocking assay were found to be concordant with immune aggregation of 32–34 nm

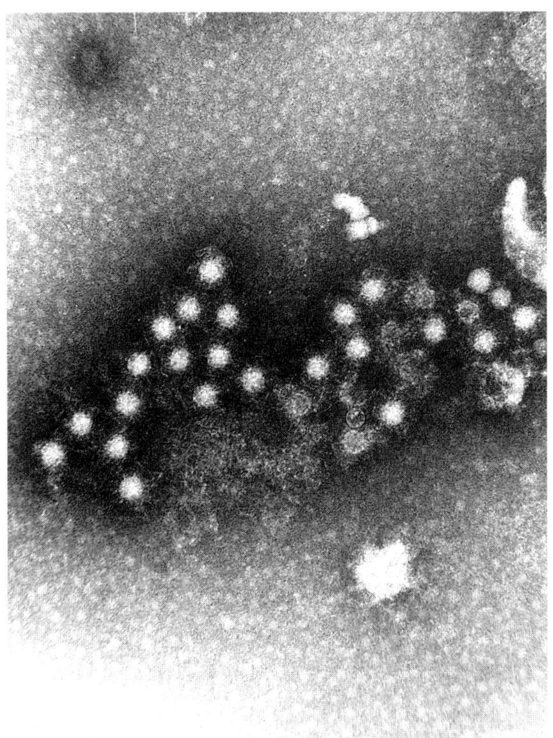

Fig. 25.1 Electron micrograph of typical 32-nm virus particles recovered from faeces from a patient with ET-NANBH in Telixtac, Mexico, during a 1986 outbreak. Particles are morphologically indistinguishable from those recovered from patients in Borneo, Burma, India, Somalia and Tashkent.

HEV particles and suggested the existence of common antigenic determinants of HEVAg observed in hepatocytes. It is concluded also that HEVAg detected in liver cells by FA reflects the presence of HEV particles or their subcomponents.

'FIRST-GENERATION' SEROLOGICAL ASSAYS AND IMMUNE RESPONSE

Attempts to develop a conventional radioimmunoassay (RIA) or enzyme-linked immunoassay (EIA) for HEV-associated antigen using acute-phase IgM or convalescent-phase IgG respectively have not been successful. Also, analysis of faeces and sucrose gradient fractions rich in virus particles has not revealed any specific, positive result. The reproducibility of these results may have been complicated by the lability of the virus, although even faeces and sucrose gradient fractions rich in particles failed to give a positive signal in tests. In fact, RIA analysis of separate gradient fractions containing equal numbers of HAV and HEV particles (by IEM) showed that HAV could be easily detected using a conventional antibody 'sandwich' assay, while no HEV-associated antigen could be found by this method. These results indicated that, while antibody in some sera may be adequate for IEM or immunofluorescent antibody (FA) analysis, these same antibodies lack the avidity to function in conventional RIA and EIA assays. This presumption was supported further by the finding that an IgG fraction of a convalescent serum obtained from a patient with hepatitis E in Mexico could be labelled with fluoroscein isothiocyanate and used to detect HEV-associated antigen in liver tissue of infected cynos (see above) (Krawczynski & Bradley 1989). In 1989, a fluorescent antibody (FA)-blocking assay was developed by Krawczynski and co-workers as a prototype test for the identification and titration of anti-HEV in serum samples. The prevalence of anti-HEV in groups of patients from well-defined and geographically isolated outbreaks of hepatitis E in Asia, Africa and North America varied from 77% to 100% (Krawczynski et al 1991). Although a relatively small number of serum samples was evaluated by FA for anti-HEV, an immunological relationship between sera obtained from geographically isolated outbreaks of hepatitis E was established. This finding is in complete agreement with previous IEM studies. The serological relatedness of geographically distinct outbreaks of hepatitis E has also been demonstrated by the seroconversion of primates that had been infected individually with three different isolates of HEV (Burma, Pakistan and Mexico). Seroconversion to anti-HEV was observed in cynos in each of five passages of hepatitis E in tamarins and in two passages of hepatitis E in chimpanzees (K Krawczynski, unpublished data).

Approximately 71% of sporadic cases of non-transfusion-transmitted acute NANBH in Nepal, i.e. a geographical region where HEV infection is endemic, were positive for anti-HEV. In contrast, sporadic cases of acute, non-transfusion-transmitted NANBH in the USA, Japan and Italy were found to be serologically unrelated to HEV infection. Most 'sporadic' cases of acute non-A, non-B hepatitis found in the USA have been observed in individuals who had visited endemic areas, including northern Mexico. The results of recent serological tests, Western blotting for anti-HEV antibody and reverse transcription–polymerase chain reaction (RT–PCR) for HEV RNA in serum (see below) further indicate that some cases of fulminant hepatic failure (FHF) in England and the USA appear to be associated with HEV infection. It is important to note that most of these FHF patients had *not* travelled to regions known to be endemic for HEV.

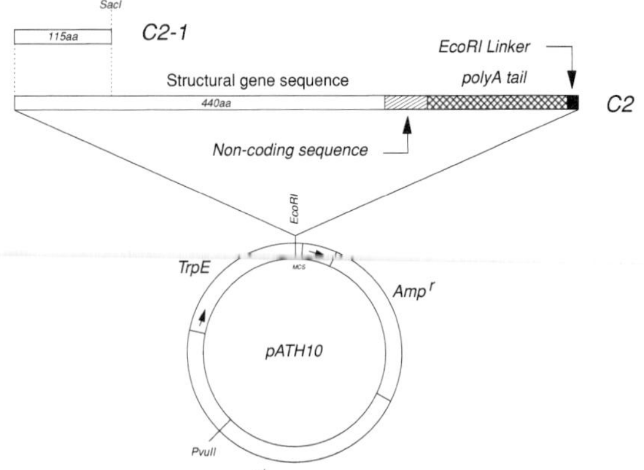

Fig. 25.2 Construction of the *trpe*–C2 fusion protein used for Western blot analysis of human and primate sera; the *trpE* portion of the fusion protein is a 37 000-dalton enzyme contained within the bacterial tryptophan operon. The fusion protein is expressed in bacteria as an insoluble product that can be readily recovered in a relatively pure state by low-speed centrifugation of the bacterial lysate.

'SECOND-GENERATION' SEROLOGICAL ASSAYS AND CROSS-REACTIVITY

HEV isolates from geographically distinct regions of the world have been shown by IEM to possess at least one major cross-reactive epitope (Bradley et al 1991). Acute- and convalescent-phase sera from well-documented cases of hepatitis E occurring in China, Somalia, Burma, the Soviet Union, Mexico, Borneo, India, Pakistan and Greece also have been shown to 'block' antibody binding in a fluorescent antibody (FA) test that utilizes a fluorescein isothiocyanate (FITC)-labelled IgG probe (Mexico) and liver sections from a HEV Burma-infected cyno (Krawczynski et al 1991). These findings imply that a sero-diagnostic assay for HEV-specific antibody can be developed if recombinant expressed proteins containing the immunodominant (or broadly cross-reactive) epitope of HEV are utilized. In fact, a sensitive and specific Western blot (WB) assay for both IgM and IgG anti-HEV has been developed at the Centers for Disease Control (CDC) (Purdy et al 1992). This assay makes use of a *trpE*–HEV fusion protein (expressed in *Escherichia coli* as an insoluble protein, *trpE*-C2) that contains the carboxy-terminal two-thirds of open reading frame 2 (ORF2), or the region that encodes a portion of the putative structural protein (see Fig. 25.2). This assay has been shown to be capable of detecting anti-HEV in acute- and convalescent-phase case sera collected from outbreaks worldwide. In contrast to the earlier IEM and FA assays for virus-specific antibody, the Western blot procedure has been shown to be capable of detecting IgG anti-HEV for up to 2 years after the acute phase of illness (Purdy et al 1992). Alternative configurations of the Western blot procedure that incorporate β-galactosidase fusion proteins (representing portions of HEV ORF2 or ORF3) as antigens have shown that the Burma and Mexico HEV isolates contain both type-common and type-specific epitopes (Reyes et al 1991, Yarbough et al 1991). HEV isolates can be broadly divided into two sero-types, one represented by the Mexico archetype and the other represented by the Burma isolate. The latter 'serotype' appears to be the most common, since all isolates cloned and sequenced, with the exception of the Mexico isolate, demonstrate a high degree of homology at both the nucleotide and amino acid level (see Ch. 23). Although it would appear that at least two different serotypes of HEV exist, cross-challenge studies conducted in cynos have shown that animals infected with the Burma isolate are immune to reinfection by the Mexico isolate (D Bradley, unpublished findings).

RT–PCR FOR HEV RNA IN FAECES AND SERUM

HEV can be detected in many acute-phase case

faeces specimens and sera by a newly developed reverse transcription–polymerase chain reaction (RT–PCR) method that incorporates the use of a silicon dioxide (glass) matrix to efficiently absorb RNA extracted from patient materials (McCaustland et al 1991). Following the reverse transcription of the viral RNA, PCR primers specific for a portion of the HEV RDRP (RNA-dependant RNA polymerase) can be used to amplify target cDNA (usually 230–275 bp in length). The PCR product (separated on an agarose gel) is visualized by either ethidium bromide staining of the DNA or hybridization of a labelled probe to the DNA followed by fluorography. Some acute-phase sera may not be positive for HEV RNA because maximum viraemia often precedes both the peak of ALT activity and clinical symptoms of disease (CDC, unpublished data).

REFERENCES

Bradley D W, Andjaparidze A, Cook E H et al 1988 Aetiological agent of enterically transmitted non-A, non-B hepatitis. Journal of General Virology 69: 731–738

Bradley D W, Krawczynski K, Beach M J, Purdy M A et al 1991 Non-A, non-B hepatitis: towards the discovery of hepatitis C and E viruses. Seminars in Liver Disease 11: 128–146

Kane M A, Bradley D W, Shrestha S M et al 1984 Epidemic non-A, non-B hepatitis in Nepal: recovery of a possible etiologic agent and transmission studies in marmosets. Journal of the American Medical Association 252: 3140–3145

Krawczynski K, Bradley D W 1989 Enterically transmitted non-A, non-B hepatitis: identification of virus-associated antigen in experimentally infected cynomolgus macaques. Journal of Infectious Diseases 159: 1042–1049

Krawczynski K, Bradley D, Ajdukiewicz A et al 1991 Virus-associated antigen and antibody of epidemic non-A, non-B hepatitis: Serology of outbreaks and sporadic cases. In: Shikata T, Purcell R H, Uchida T (eds) Viral hepatitis C, D and E. Elsevier Scientific Publishers, Amsterdam, pp 229–236

McCaustland K A, Shengli B, Purdy M A, Bradley D W 1991 Application of two RNA extraction methods prior to amplification of hepatitis E virus nucleic acid by the polymerase chain reaction. Journal of Virological Methods 35: 331–342

Purdy M A, McCaustland K A, Krawczynski K et al 1992 Expression of a hepatitis E virus (HEV)–*trpE* fusion protein containing epitopes recognized by antibodies in sera from human cases and experimentally infected primates. Archives of Virology (in press)

Reyes G R, Huang C-C, Yarbough P O et al 1991 Hepatitis E virus (HEV): epitope mapping and detection of stain variation. In: Shikata T, Purcell R H, Uchida T (eds) Viral hepatitis C, D and E. Elsevier Science Publishers, Amsterdam, pp 237–245

Yarbough P O, Tam A W, Fry K E et al 1991 Hepatitis E virus: identification of type-common epitopes. Journal of Virology 65: 5790–5797

SECTION 6

Diagnosis of viral hepatitis

26. Diagnostic approach

Paul Martin   Lawrence S. Friedman   Jules L. Dienstag

Viral hepatitis enters into the differential diagnosis of both acute and chronic liver disease. Infection caused by all five currently identified hepatitis viruses (A – E) can present as acute viral hepatitis, whereas only hepatitis B (HBV), C (HCV) and D (HDV, delta) viruses are important causes of chronic liver disease. The recent identification of HCV and hepatitis E virus (HEV), the two viruses previously grouped under the descriptive term 'non-A, non-B hepatitis', as well as the application of molecular biological techniques, including polymerase chain reaction (PCR) amplification (see Ch. 27), have enhanced the sensitivity and sophistication of diagnostic testing in viral hepatitis. Specific serological identification of each of the five types of viral hepatitis must be guided by both an appreciation of the clinical circumstances and a recognition of the limitations of currently available diagnostic tests.

HEPATITIS A

Hepatitis A virus (HAV), which causes acute but not chronic hepatitis, is spread almost exclusively by the faecal–oral route. Although direct detection of HAV antigen and HAV RNA is available as a research technique (Lemon 1985), as detailed below, in clinical practice a diagnosis of acute hepatitis A is achieved by serological detection of specific viral antibodies. Moreover, by the time a patient presents with symptoms of acute hepatitis, virus levels in faeces and blood are markedly diminished or undetectable.

Antibody to HAV of the IgM class (IgM anti-HAV) is usually detectable in serum at the time of onset of symptoms and is a reliable marker of acute or recent HAV infection (Fig. 26.1). Typically, IgM anti-HAV persists for about 3–6 months after acute illness, very rarely up to 18 months (Locarnini 1977). False-negative IgM anti-HAV results are uncommon, but occasionally the duration of IgM anti-HAV positivity is as short as several days (Tassopoulos et al 1987). False-positive IgM anti-HAV results have been described and are attributable to confounding binding in the immunoassay, such as may occur in the presence in serum of rheumatoid factor or hyperglobulinaemia (Hoofnagle & Di Bisceglie 1991). In a small proportion of cases, hepatitis A recurs several weeks to several months after apparent recovery. Such relapses are associated with recurrent faecal excretion of HAV (Sjögren et al 1987) and, theoretically, infectivity. In patients with relapsing hepatitis A, IgM anti-HAV may reappear in serum after its initial disappearance; however, in most cases, relapses occur during the period of IgM anti-HAV positivity associated with the initial expression of hepatitis (Tanno et al 1988). The primary immune response to HAV is of the IgM class; however, antibody to HAV of the IgG class (IgG anti-HAV) also appears in serum following HAV infection, but its concentration rises more gradually than does that of IgM anti-HAV. After HAV infection, IgG anti-HAV persists indefinitely and confers permanent protection against reinfection. Both radioimmunoassays (RIAs) and enzyme-linked immunoassays (EIAs) are available for detecting total and IgM anti-HAV antibodies (Decker et al 1989); recently microparticle-based, automated fluorescence immunoassays have been introduced as well. The presence of IgG anti-HAV is signified by the

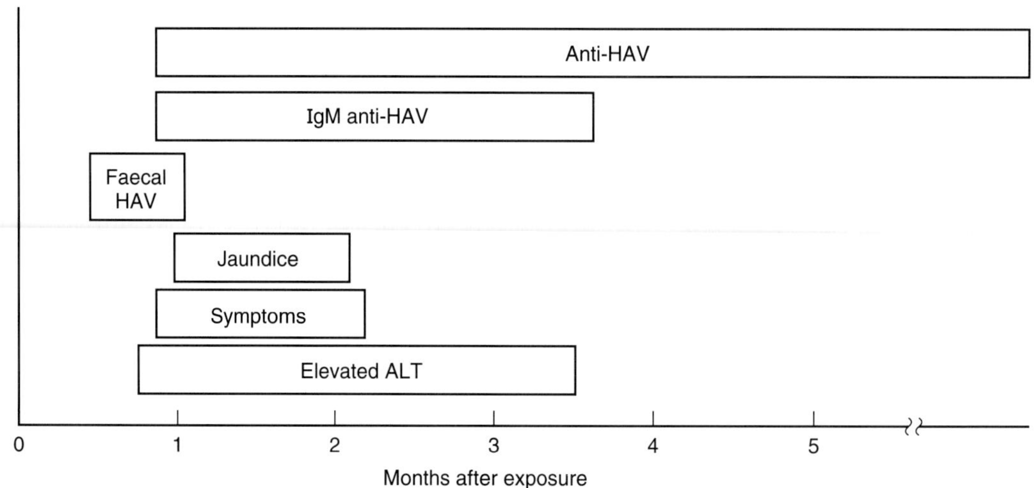

Fig. 26.1 Typical course of acute hepatitis A.

detection of total anti-HAV in the absence of IgM anti-HAV, whereas acute or recent hepatitis A is characterized by the presence of both total and IgM anti-HAV.

A number of experimental methods are also available to detect HAV infection (Lemon 1985). Hepatitis A virus antigen can be detected in faeces by RIA during the incubation period and early symptomatic phase of the illness. Similarly, HAV antigen can be detected by immunofluorescence techniques in liver tissue during acute illness; however, because liver biopsy is generally not indicated for uncomplicated acute hepatitis A, liver tissue is rarely available. In addition, HAV RNA can be detected in faeces, serum, and liver by molecular hybridization (Sjögren et al 1987), and PCR promises to increase the sensitivity of detecting HAV RNA; however, the likelihood that these sophisticated techniques will be applied to routine clinical testing is low.

Generally, the diagnosis of acute hepatitis A is not difficult or challenging, except in the rare patient with rheumatoid factor activity and false-positive IgM anti-HAV activity. Patients who have received prophylactic normal human immunoglobulin (passive immunization) may have low levels of detectable serum IgG anti-HAV for several weeks, although protective activity tends to last for several months, outlasting detectable anti-HAV. Active immunization with hepatitis A vaccines induces an initial IgM anti-HAV response as well as a later, secondary IgG anti-HAV response. Once these HAV vaccines are introduced into practice, the differential diagnosis of a positive IgG anti-HAV result will include previous vaccination in addition to recovery from past infection.

HEPATITIS B

The complexity of the organization and replicative cycle of HBV (Miller et al 1989), a DNA virus, is reflected by the complexity of its antigenic expression and associated antibody responses. Hepatitis B virus causes a sizeable proportion of all cases of both acute and chronic viral hepatitis. Currently, routine serological diagnosis relies on the detection of three pairs of antigens and antibodies: hepatitis B surface antigen (HBsAg) and its corresponding antibody (anti-HBs), hepatitis B e antigen (HBeAg) and its corresponding antibody (anti-HBe), and antibody to hepatitis B core antigen (anti-HBc) (hepatitis B core antigen (HBcAg), against which anti-HBc is directed, does not circulate freely in the serum). Recently, an assay to detect HBV DNA by molecular hybridization has also been introduced as a commercially available kit (see Ch. 27). Experimental application of PCR can demonstrate HBV DNA in the absence of other conventional markers of viral replication, such as HBeAg or HBV DNA detected by regular (slot or dot-blot) molecular hybridization (Kaneko et al 1990). Additional viral markers that circulate in serum during HBV infection can be detected by experimental techniques; these include HBV DNA polymerase and pre-S1 and pre-S2 antigens and their antibodies (anti-pre-S1 and anti-pre-S2).

Hepatitis B surface antigen, the product of the S gene of HBV, circulates at very high serum concentrations (up to 10^{13} particles per ml) during HBV infection (Froesner et al 1982). This virus protein comprises the outer coat or envelope of the virion and, in addition, is produced in excess as non-virion 22-nm spheres and tubules, which outnumber intact virions by several orders of magnitude. Intact-virion-associated HBsAg differs from smaller, non-virion-associated spherical forms in containing more pre-S gene product. Circulating HBsAg can be detected readily in serum by commercial RIA or EIA 1 to 10 weeks after infection with HBV and 2–8 weeks before the onset of clinical hepatitis (Fig. 26.2). In less than 5% of cases of acute hepatitis B, HBsAg may be undetectable at the time of presentation, because levels of HBsAg either never reached or had already declined below the detection threshold of the assay. Typically, false-positive HBsAg results are borderline or only weakly positive.

Although anti-HBs appears early during acute infection, marked antigen excess prevents routine detection of anti-HBs until HBsAg disappears. Typically, with the resolution of acute hepatitis B, HBsAg becomes undetectable as anti-HBs becomes detectable (Krugman et al 1979). Because of the sensitivity of current assays, the previously described 'window period' between the disappearance of HBsAg and the appearance of anti-HBs in serum is rarely, if ever, observed nowadays. Antibody to HBsAg is a neutralizing antibody, which, when present, is associated with lifelong immunity and is the antibody produced in response to hepatitis B vaccination with current vaccines composed entirely of HBsAg (Scolnick et al 1984); at present, anti-HBs levels of at least 10 MIU/ml are regarded as protective. Failure of acute HBV infection to resolve and the development of chronic HBV infection are

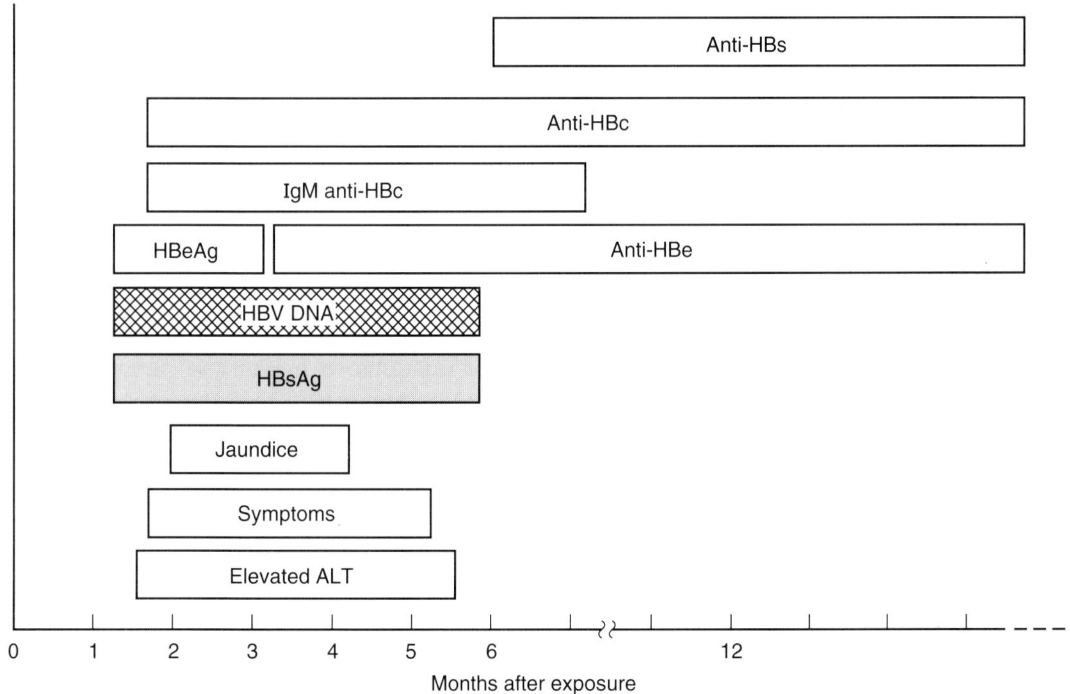

Fig. 26.2 Typical course of acute hepatitis B.

suggested by persistence of circulating HBsAg and absence of detectable anti-HBs.

Hepatitis B core antigen is a particulate non-secreted nucleocapsid protein which, rather than circulating in serum, remains cell associated and virion associated. Although free HBcAg is not detected in serum during HBV infection, the corresponding antibody, anti-HBc, is an important marker of HBV infection, whether current or remote (Krugman et al 1979). Antibody to HBcAg, which circulates in patients with ongoing HBV infection, has not been felt to be a neutralizing antibody; however, chimpanzees immunized with HBcAg have been protected against HBV challenge, and the T-cell immune response to HBcAg has been shown to provide help in promoting the humoral immune response to HBsAg. Antibody to the nucleocapsid protein (anti-HBc) appears early in the course of infection (just after HBsAg) and persists indefinitely. As was true for immunoglobulin classes of anti-HAV, the class of anti-HBc can be used to distinguish recent from remote HBV infection. Antibody to HBcAg of the IgM class (IgM anti-HBc), which appears in high titre early during acute infection and is readily detectable by commercial RIA or EIA (Chau et al 1983), is useful in establishing a diagnosis of acute or recent HBV infection. The presence of IgM anti-HBc is a helpful diagnostic adjunct when the time of onset of HBV infection is not known (for example in the blood donor found to harbour HBsAg) or in the unusual cases in which HBsAg levels fall beneath the detection threshold or in which the disappearance of HBsAg has not been followed by the prompt appearance of anti-HBs, the so-called 'window period'. Typically, in acute resolving cases of hepatitis B, IgM anti-HBc declines to levels undetectable by commercial assays approximately 6 (with a range of 3–12) months after the onset of infection. As the primary IgM response to HBcAg declines, anti-HBc of the IgG class (IgG anti-HBc) becomes the predominant class of anti-HBc; it appears shortly after the beginning of acute infection, at which time it is overshadowed by IgM anti-HBc, rises slowly in titre, and persists indefinitely, through recovery or into chronic infection. Thus, IgG anti-HBc in patients with HBsAg is a marker of HBV infection with an onset in the remote past (longer than 6 months ago). The presence of IgG anti-HBc is a particularly reliable marker of previous HBV infection and may persist even when anti-HBs titres decline to undetectable levels many years following recovery from HBV infection.

Hepatitis B e antgen (HBeAg), like HBcAg, is a product of the nucleocapsid (core) gene of HBV but, unlike HBcAg, is a soluble, non-particulate protein that is secreted in serum (Ou et al 1986); for HBeAg to be expressed, the pre-core region of the C gene must be intact and translated. Detectable by commercial RIA or EIA, HBeAg is a convenient marker of high virus replicative activity, which, in turn, is associated with a high level of infectivity and liver injury. Invariably, HBeAg is detectable early in the course of acute hepatitis B, coincident with or immediately following the appearance of HBsAg, and generally disappears within several weeks in acute, resolving cases. When HBeAg persists beyond the first 3–4 months, however, protracted HBV infection is predictable. In patients with chronic hepatitis B, HBeAg tends to persist for many months or even years, constituting the active replicative phase of chronic HBV infection; when HBeAg disappears, as it does at a rate of 10–15% per year in patients with chronic hepatitis B, virus replication falls dramatically to undetectable or nearly undetectable levels (Hoofnagle et al 1981). For routine diagnostic purposes, testing for HBeAg is not necessary in most cases of acute hepatitis B. Testing for HBeAg is of value, instead, primarily in patients with chronic hepatitis B, in whom HBeAg is an important marker of viral replication that correlates qualitatively with more quantitative markers of active replication, such as serum HBV DNA detected by molecular hydridization. However, the absence of HBeAg does not preclude active viral replication (see below).

Antibody to HBeAg becomes detectable when HBeAg antigen is lost (Krugman et al 1979), and the appearance of anti-HBe in acute hepatitis B implies a high likelihood that HBV infection will resolve spontaneously (Hoofnagle et al 1981). In some cases, anti-HBe may not be detectable after the loss of HBeAg.

Other serological markers of HBV infection are undergoing evaluation. These include pre-S1 and pre-S2 antigens, coded for by regions upstream of the component of the S gene that codes for HBsAg, and their corresponding antibodies. The pre-S proteins on the viral envelope are involved in viral attachment to hepatocytes (Neurath et al 1985, 1986, Pontisso et al 1989), code for envelope proteins that are more heavily represented in complete virions than in small, non-virion HBsAg particles and can enhance immunological responsiveness to S-only (HBsAg) proteins. In acute hepatitis B, the appearance of both pre-S antibodies precedes the appearance of anti-HBs and correlates (although not reliably so) with resolving infection (Budkowska et al 1990). In contrast, persistence of the pre-S antigens and the absence of detectable pre-S antibodies has been suggested as a marker predictive that chronic hepatitis B will ensue. Similarly, the subsequent appearance of pre-S antibodies during the course of chronic hepatitis B has been found to predict the eventual cessation of viral replication and, in some cases, the ultimate loss of HBsAg (Budkowska et al 1990, 1992). Perhaps in the future, testing for pre-S antibodies will be a useful adjunct in predicting the likelihood that HBV infection will ultimately resolve. At present, however, these markers remain a research tool only, the predictive value of which has not been adequately confirmed. Assays for hepatitis B X antigen and antibody (HBxAg and anti-HBx) are also available as research tools, but the clinical import and utility of these markers remain uncertain.

A commercially available molecular hybridization assay is now available for the routine detection of HBV DNA in serum. The presence of HBV DNA detected in this manner signifies ongoing replication of HBV in hepatocytes (Kuhns 1990). The available dot-blot or liquid hybridization HBV DNA assays can detect DNA concentrations of 10^6 genome equivalents per ml. These assays provide a quantitative determination of the level of HBV replication and supplement qualitative HBeAg testing. Consequently, these assays are particularly helpful in patients who have lost detectable HBeAg, despite the fact that viral replication is felt to be continuing, as suggested, for example by the persistence of elevated serum aminotransferase levels and ongoing hepatic inflammatory activity. Naturally, quantitative assays for HBV DNA can be used to identify patients likely to respond to interferon therapy (HBV DNA levels $\leq$200 pg/ml) and to monitor HBV replication during antiviral therapy.

More recently, the ultrasensitive technique of polymerase chain reaction (PCR) has been applied to the study of HBV replication (Kaneko et al 1990). This technique allows the amplification of minute quantities of viral nucleic acid and can detect HBV DNA in quantities as low as 10–50 genomes/ml. Whereas detection of HBV DNA by molecular hybridization implies active viral replication and a high probability of active liver disease, detection of HBV DNA by PCR alone signifies ongoing HBV infection with little active replication (Hoofnagle et al 1981). The technique suffers from oversensitivity, resulting in false-positive results if contamination of serum samples is not avoided scrupulously.

Another experimental method used in the past to detect HBV replication is the measurement of serum HBV DNA polymerase activity; however, this assay has been superseded for the most part by the more quantitative molecular hybridization assays for HBV DNA (Kuhns 1990).

With the use of conventional serological markers plus molecular assays for HBV DNA, we can distinguish between two phases of chronic HBV infection (Hoofnagle et al 1987) (Fig. 26.3). The early 'replicative' phase is characterized by the presence of circulating HBeAg and high levels of serum HBV DNA and infectious virions. Clinically, patients are often symptomatic, have elevated serum aminotransferase levels, demonstrate histological evidence of liver injury and are highly infectious for their contacts. Eventually, patients may enter the 'non-replicative' phase, characterized by loss of HBeAg, appearance of anti-HBe and a marked decrease in serum levels of HBV DNA, which may remain detectable only by PCR. An improvement in symptoms as well as biochemical and histological indicators of necroinflammatory activity and a marked reduction in infectivity follow. Often the change from the replicative to the non-replicative phase

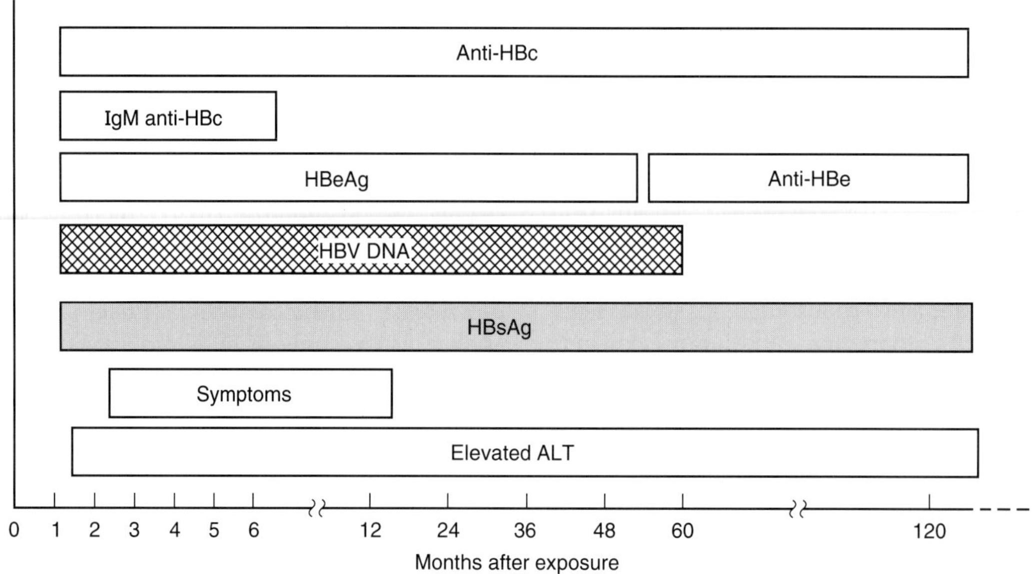

Fig. 26.3 Typical course of acute hepatitis B progressing to chronic hepatitis B (with ultimate conversion from replicative to non-replicative phase).

is accompanied by a clinical exacerbation of chronic hepatitis, with a transient marked elevation in serum aminotransferase levels and perhaps an exacerbation of symptoms. Very rarely, primarily in patients with slightly compensated chronic liver disease, this clinical exacerbation can resemble fulminant hepatitis and lead to hepatic failure. Once the infection has entered a non-replicative phase, liver injury is unlikely; however, subsequent spontaneous or immunosuppression-induced reactivation of HBV replication is still possible. Such reactivations of replicative HBV may result in a recurrence of active liver disease and are reflected serologically by the reappearance of HBeAg and high levels of HBV DNA in serum (Davis & Hoofnagle 1987). Unfortunately, because the reappearance of IgM anti-HBc during such reactivations is variable, occurring in some cases but not others, the absence of IgM anti-HBc cannot be relied upon to distinguish reactivation of chronic hepatitis B from acute hepatitis B (Davis & Hoofnagle 1985). During the course of chronic HBV infection, transition to the non-replicative phase is associated with integration of HBV DNA into the host genome of infected hepatocytes, a process that sets the stage (i.e. is necessary but not necessarily sufficient in and of itself) for the later development of primary hepatocellular carcinoma (Popper et al 1987).

An important exception to the typical serological profile described above is a variant of HBV that results in severe liver disease and active virus replication in the absence of HBeAg in serum. This 'e-minus' variant form of HBV results from a single nucleotide mutation in the pre-core region of the viral genome, which in effect inserts a 'stop codon', a termination signal, that prevents the synthesis of HBeAg (Carman et al 1989) (see Ch. 7). Patients infected with this HBe-minus (or pre-core) variant have high levels of HBV DNA in serum despite the absence of HBeAg and presence of anti-HBe in serum. The clinical course in patients with such HBV mutants has been described as being characterized by particularly severe chronic hepatitis B with the rapid progression to cirrhosis and with limited responsiveness to antiviral therapy. This variant form of HBV, most prevalent in Mediterranean and Far Eastern countries, may arise during the course of infection by 'wild-type' HBV, presumably the result of a 'non-lethal' (to the virus) nucleotide mutation in the setting of evolutionary immunological pressure. In addition, sporadic cases and outbreaks of fulminant acute hepatitis B in Israel and Japan have been attributed to the HBe-minus mutant (Carman et al 1991, Kosaka et al 1991, Liang et al 1991, Omata et al 1991). Although initial reports identified these pre-core mutants in patients with severe hepatitis B, more recent analyses indicate that these pre-core mutants, as well as a variety of other mutations throughout the HBV genome, are quite common even in 'garden variety' and mild cases of hepatitis B. Therefore, the ultimate impact of HBV mutations on the natural history and pathogenicity of HBV remains to be better defined.

Another specific HBV mutant that may complicate routine serodiagnosis and that may have implications for immunoprophylactic strategies has been described. An HBV mutant has been described in which the '*a*' determinant of HBsAg undergoes a conformational change as a result of a single amino acid substitution in a critical epitope. This leads to the loss of neutralizing activity by anti-HBs. This particular mutant has been described in a small number of HBV vaccine recipients (Carman et al 1990) and in a patient with HBV infection undergoing liver transplantation and receiving monoclonal anti-HBs (Fung et al 1991). Detection of such mutant forms of HBV requires sequencing of the HBV genome after amplification by PCR, which is laborious; therefore, extensive analysis of the HBV genome in successfully vaccinated persons has not been carried out.

Routine diagnosis of HBV infection generally depends on the detection of HBsAg in serum; however, the presence of HBsAg does not distinguish between acute and chronic HBV infection. The additional presence of IgM anti-HBc generally signifies acute infection, whereas the presence of IgG anti-HBc without IgM anti-HBc signifies chronic HBV infection. As can be inferred from earlier comments, a patient with acute hepatitis cannot be assumed to have acute hepatitis B merely because of the presence in serum of HBsAg. The possibility must also be considered that such a patient has chronic hepatitis B with a superimposed acute hepatic insult. The differential diagnosis includes the following: (1) transient exacerbation of chronic hepatitis B associated with conversion from the replicative to the non-replicative phase; (2) acute reactivation of previously quiescent anti-HBe-positive chronic hepatitis B with the reappearance in serum of HBeAg and HBV DNA (and sometimes IgM anti-HBc); (3) acute superinfection with another hepatitis virus (HAV, HCV, HDV) or another virus that may cause hepatitis as part of a systemic illness, such as Epstein–Barr virus or cytomegalovirus; (4) the new onset of hepatocellular carcinoma; and (5) acute drug-induced hepatitis, alcoholic liver injury, shock liver, passive hepatic congestion secondary to right heart failure, Budd–Chiari syndrome, or some other acute hepatitis-like illness.

Immunoperoxidase staining of liver tissue can be used to detect HBsAg, HBcAg, and even HBeAg in hepatocytes during HBV infection (Mathiesen et al 1979). Immunoperoxidase staining, however, adds little to the routine diagnosis of HBV infection; generally, information about HBV infection and replication can be derived from noninvasive serologic assays.

HEPATITIS C

Hepatitis C is characterized by a 50% rate of chronicity following acute infection, a propensity for progression to cirrhosis and an associated risk after protracted infection of primary hepatocellular carcinoma. Although HCV transmission has been characterized most thoroughly following blood transfusion, non-percutaneous spread of HCV is thought to account for some sporadic cases of hepatitis C. Perinatal and sexual transmission of HCV are uncommon, however, and covert spread remains unexplained in many cases (Everhart et al 1990, Resnick et al 1990).

The recent identification of HCV (Choo et al 1989, Kuo et al 1989), an RNA virus responsible for most, if not all, cases of post-transfusion and sporadic (non-epidemic) non-A, non-B hepatitis, was followed by the rapid development of serological tests. The first-generation RIAs and then EIAs introduced were designed to detect antibody directed against C100-3, a recombinant polypeptide derived from a non-structural region of the viral genome. Typically, anti-HCV can be detected by first-generation EIA no earlier than several weeks, usually several months, after the onset of acute hepatitis and may not become detectable at all in 30–40% of patients with acute, self-limiting cases of hepatitis C (Alter et al 1989). Even in patients with chronic transfusion-related non-A, non-B hepatitis shown by other techniques (see below) to be caused by HCV, anti-HCV may be undetectable by first-generation EIA in approximately 20% of cases. Therefore, because of the relative insensitivity of the assay, and because of the delay in appearance of antibody detectable with the assay, the absence of anti-HCV by first-generation EIA does not preclude a diagnosis of either acute or chronic HCV infection. In addition, the EIA tests currently available for routine clinical diagnosis provide no information about the duration of infection. In acute resolving hepatitis C, anti-HCV detectable by EIA tends to disappear shortly after acute illness, but in chronic hepatitis C anti-HCV persists indefinitely (Hoofnagle & Di Bisceglie 1991) (Fig. 26.4). Currently, therefore, clinicians are on reasonable grounds to conclude that all patients with anti-HCV are currently infected with HCV. Distinguishing between acute and chronic hepatitis C must rely on clinical judgment, rather than on the basis of serological testing alone.

A number of more sensitive, second-generation EIA-based tests for HCV are also under evaluation (Alter 1992). An EIA incorporating C200, a polypeptide that is a composite of C100-3 and the adjacent non-structural protein C33c, in addition to C22-3, a nucleocapsid core protein, has recently become available. Typically, antibodies directed against the C22-3 and C33c antigens are detected 30–90 days before antibody to C100-3 during the course of acute hepatitis C (Alter 1992). Moreover, the sensitivity of the second-generation EIA is 10–20% greater than that of the first-generation assay (McHutchison et al 1992). The increased sensitivity of the second-generation anti-HCV EIA is expected to implicate HCV in a substantial proportion of patients with acute and chronic non-A, non-B hepatitis whose sera were non-reactive in the first-generation tests for anti-HCV.

In addition to its relative lack of sensitivity, the first-generation EIA for anti-HCV suffers from limitations in its specificity. For example, false-positive results have been described in patients with autoimmune chronic active hepatitis (McFarlane et al 1990). The finding of an apparently biological false-positive anti-HCV result under these circumstances has been shown to correlate with the hypergammaglobulinaemia characteristic of autoimmune chronic active hepatitis. In such cases, anti-HCV may become undetectable following therapy with corticosteroids, presumably the result of a decrease in gamma globulin levels (Czaja et al 1991, Everhart et al 1990, McFarlane et al 1990). In addition to hypergammaglobulinaemia, other

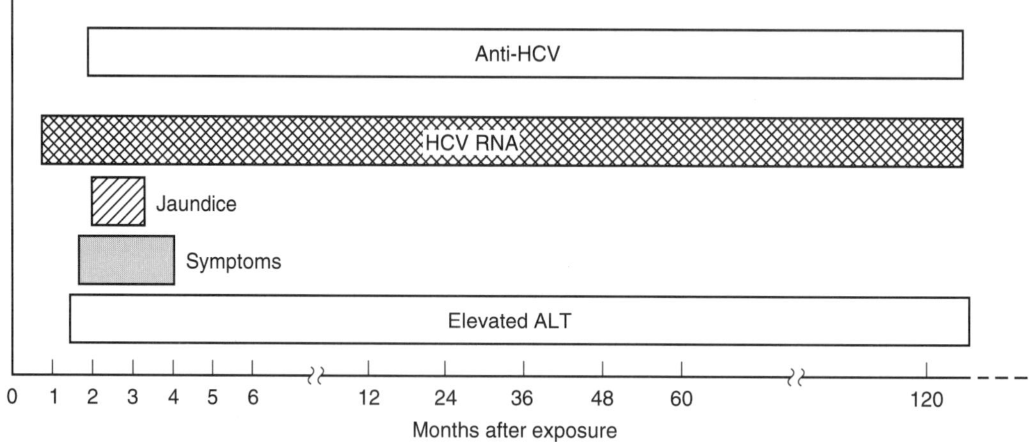

Fig. 26.4 Typical course of acute hepatitis C progressing to chronic hepatitis C.

factors such as prolonged storage of serum specimens may interfere with accurate anti-HCV testing. Simply because the test is characterized by incomplete specificity, persons with a low prior probability of true infection (e.g. normal volunteer blood donors) are likely to have false-positive tests, as has been shown in approximately 50% of this group. In general, detection of anti-HCV by EIA is likely to be truly positive when the level of antibody (based on optical density reading) is high, when the alanine aminotransferase (ALT) is substantially elevated, and when the person tested is in a high-risk group for infection and has chronic liver disease (high prior probability of true positivity); most false-positive results are characterized by low or borderline EIA optical density readings and tend to occur in patients with normal ALT levels, in those who are not part of high-risk groups for infection and, as stated above, in patients with autoimmune disorders.

Confidence in the specificity of EIA testing for anti-HCV can be improved by supplementary testing with a recombinant immunoblot assay (RIBA) recently introduced into clinical use. The first version of this assay consisted of a nitrocellulose strip with separate bands containing the polypeptides C100-3 (recombinant yeast derived) and 5-1-1 (recombinant bacteria derived), which are the products of overlapping non-structural segments of the HCV genome, as well as superoxide dismutase, a fusion protein with which C100-3 is expressed in its yeast vector and which may account for some false-positive EIA reactivity (Ebeling et al 1990). A larger panel of HCV antigens, incorporating both first- and second-generation EIA proteins (C100-3, 5-1-1, C33c from the non-structural region, C22-3 from the HCV core-associated region, as well as superoxide dismutase), has been introduced in a second-generation 'RIBA-II' test. The major use of RIBA testing has been to confirm (technically speaking to 'supplement') EIA reactivity. Typically, anti-HCV EIA results with a high optical density reading are RIBA reactive also, whereas low or equivocal results tend to be RIBA non-reactive. Supplementary RIBA testing is useful in 'confirming' EIA reactivity in low-risk populations, such as asymptomatic blood donors with normal serum aminotransferase levels, of whom half to three-quarters may have false-positive EIA anti-HCV reactivity (Hsu et al 1991). In persons at high risk of having HCV infection, RIBA-II testing, similar to second-generation EIA testing, improves the sensitivity of detecting HCV infection. For example, of 100 patients with a clinical diagnosis of non-A, non-B hepatitis reported by Marcellin et al (1991), 76 were anti-HCV EIA positive, but an additional 20 were RIBA-II positive. The impact of second-generation assays for anti-HCV on the specificity of anti-HCV testing remains to be documented.

Use of polymerase chain reaction (PCR) amplification has enhanced the sensitivity of testing for HCV infection, has provided information about virus replication, and has yielded important insights into the natural history of HCV infection (Farci et al 1991) (see Ch. 27). In patients with acute hepatitis C, HCV RNA can be detected in serum earlier than any other virological or biochemical event – before the onset of symptoms, elevated serum aminotransferase activity and the appearance of anti-C100-3 in serum. In addition, almost all patients with chronic HCV infection also have HCV RNA in serum, usually continuously but occasionally intermittently (Farci et al 1991). Because the level of HCV RNA is low, standard molecular hybridization by Northern blot analysis is usually inadequate to detect viraemia, and PCR is required. This technique may be particularly useful in certain populations such as organ transplant recipients, in whom, because of the effect of immunosuppression, HCV infection in the absence of detectable anti-HCV is not uncommon (Poterucha et al 1991). The use of PCR, however, is confined to a limited number of research laboratories, and rigid precautions must be taken, and appropriate controls used, to avoid non-specificity related to contamination of the reaction by minute quantities of HCV RNA from other laboratory sources. Another research technique that enhances the sensitivity of testing for HCV infection is immunohistochemical staining of liver tissue for HCV antigens. As is the case for serum HCV RNA testing, HCV antigens can be detected by immunofluorescence microscopy in hepatocytes prior to the appearance of anti-HCV in serum and is demonstrable in both acute and chronic hepatitis C (Krawczynski et al 1989).

Because of the limitations of anti-HCV testing discussed above, and because PCR and similar techniques are not available for routine diagnostic testing, the diagnosis of HCV infection at present requires a synthesis of virological and clinical data. In a patient with acute hepatitis, a diagnosis of acute hepatitis C can be made with a commercial EIA by the demonstration of anti-HCV seroconversion. However, the absence of first- and even second-generation anti-HCV EIA positivity does not exclude acute hepatitis C, especially in the appropriate clinical setting (e.g. after transfusion). Similarly, because of limitations in the specificity of anti-HCV testing, and because of the inability of currently available EIAs for anti-HCV to distinguish current from remote infection, all the clinical features of a case should be considered before attributing liver dysfunction to HCV infection. For example, in apparent cases of chronic hepatitis C with anti-HCV EIA seropositivity, other confounding factors such as rheumatoid factor activity or hypergammaglobulinaemia secondary to autoimmune chronic active hepatitis should be excluded. Supplementary testing with the RIBA-II assay, or its equivalent, is desirable in such cases to exclude false-positive anti-HCV EIA reactivity. A history of parenteral exposure to HCV before the onset of liver dysfunction, such as an antecedent blood transfusion or intravenous drug abuse, is also helpful diagnostically. As noted above, a substantial minority of patients with typical clinical features of HCV infection are negative for anti-HCV by EIA; in these patients, a diagnosis of HCV infection can only be presumed, and these persons should be re-evaluated periodically. Widespread availability of second-generation EIAs and supplementary blot assays for anti-HCV will enhance the sensitivity and specificity of routine HCV diagnosis (Alter 1992).

HEPATITIS D (DELTA)

Hepatitis D virus (HDV), or the delta agent, is an RNA virus that requires the helper function of HBV to complete its replicative cycle; therefore, HDV infection is not encountered in the absence of HBV infection. Infection caused by HDV can occur either simultaneously with acute HBV infection (co-infection) or, more commonly, superimposed on chronic HBV infection (superinfection) (Di Bisceglie & Negro 1989). The importance of HDV infection, especially superinfection, is that it may result in more severe liver disease than HBV alone. Whereas patients co-infected with HDV and HBV often have acute resolving hepatitis no more severe than, and indistinguishable from, that caused by HBV alone (with occasional exceptions) (Govindarajan et al 1984), those with HDV superinfection are more likely to have severe hepatitis with rapid progression to cirrhosis, and even to have fulminant hepatitis, than are persons with chronic hepatitis B alone (Rizzetto et al 1983).

The diagnosis of HDV infection in clinical practice rests on the detection of antibody to HDV antigen (anti-HDV) by commercial EIA or RIA. Total anti-HDV, however, generally in low titre (<1:100), is undetectable in over 90% of cases of acute HDV infection (Aragona et al 1987). The time to first appearance of anti-HDV is variable, and repeated testing may be necessary to confirm the diagnosis. Moreover, anti-HDV tends to persist for only a short time beyond the resolution of acute hepatitis D and may disappear subsequently, leaving no marker of previous infection (Fig. 26.5). In patients with chronic hepatitis B who become superinfected with HDV, anti-HDV appears early, reaches high titres, and persists indefinitely; serodiagnosis of HDV infection in this setting is quite reliable (Fig. 26.6). Assays are available in Europe to detect IgM anti-HDV, which may be detectable in high titre during acute HDV infection. The presence of IgM anti-HDV, however, does not distinguish acute from chronic HDV infection; IgM anti-HDV also persists in chronic infection, and high titres are often found in patients with severe liver inflammation (Hoofnagle & Di Bisceglie 1991).

Of limited availability, EIA and RIA methods have been developed for the detection of HDV antigen (HDAg) in serum. With these immunoassays, HDAg can be detected in many patients with early acute infection but is detected rarely in patients with chronic HDV infection (Hoofnagle

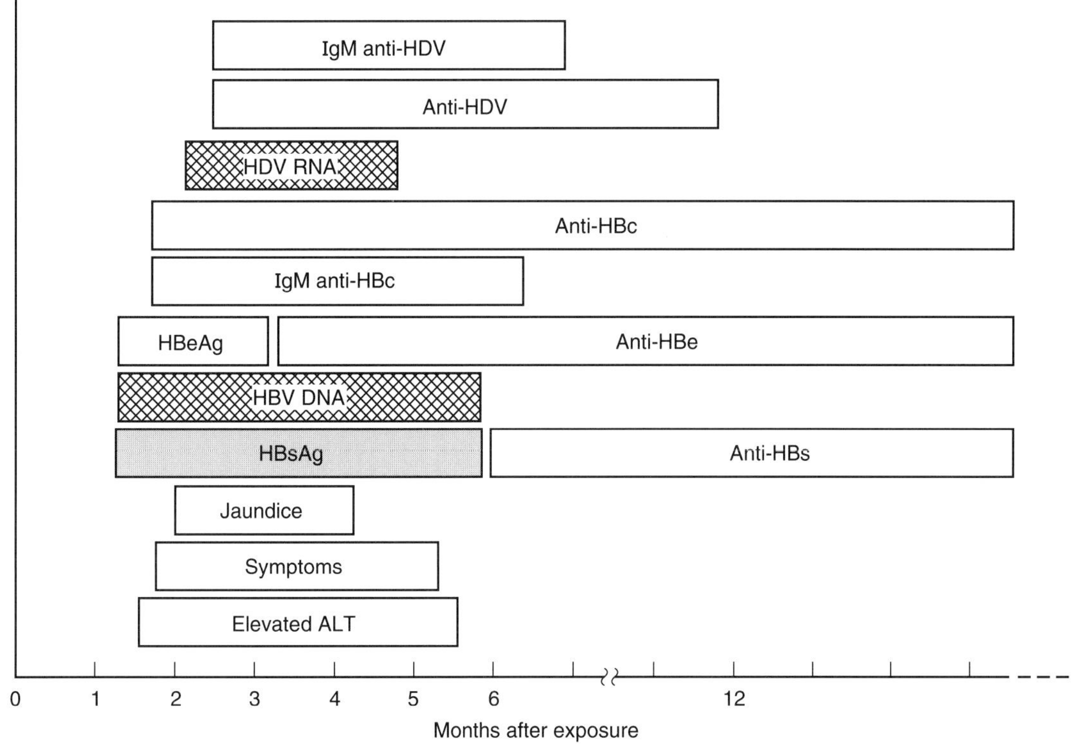

Fig. 26.5 Typical course of acute HDV co-infection.

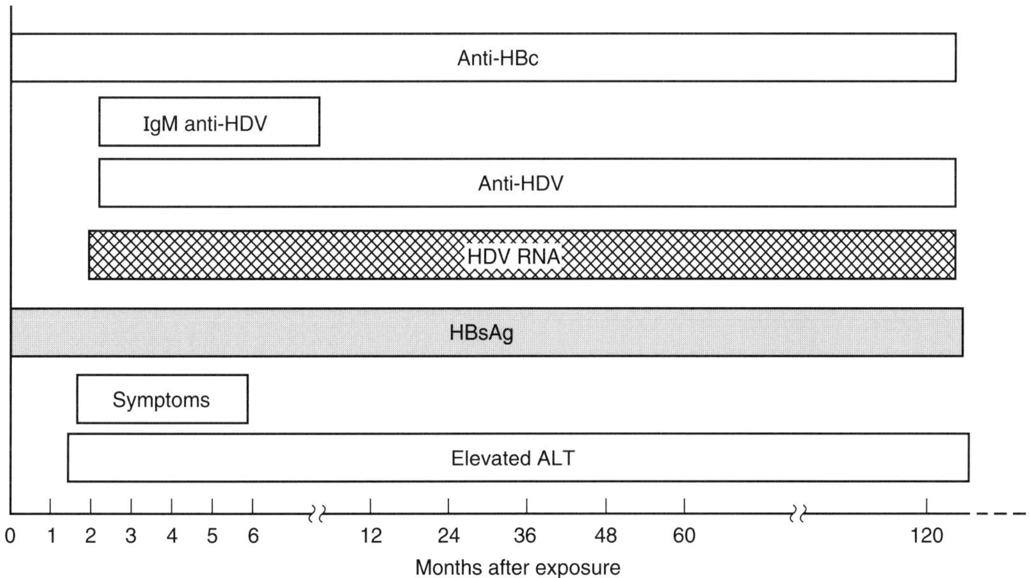

Fig. 26.6 Typical course of chronic HDV superinfection.

& Di Bisceglie 1991). In contrast, HDAg can be detected by Western blot in over 70% of cases of chronic HDV infection (Buti et al 1989). Technically difficult, cumbersome and not readily adaptable for routine diagnostic purposes, however, Western blotting for HDAg remains a research tool confined to a small number of specialized laboratories.

Other research tools have been applied to the evaluation of HDV infection. Hepatitis D RNA (HDV RNA) can be detected in serum by molecular hybridization transiently during acute HDV infection and persistently in chronic HDV infection (Smedile et al 1986). Although testing for HDV RNA remains a limited availability research tool currently, in the future testing of serum HDV RNA levels will be used to monitor responsiveness to antiviral therapy in patients with chronic hepatitis D (Farci et al 1990). Research techniques for detection of intrahepatic HDV include demonstration of HDV RNA by in situ hybridization (Negro et al 1989) and of HDAg by immunofluorescence or immunoperoxidase staining in frozen sections or formalin-fixed sections respectively (Hoofnagle & Di Bisceglie 1991). Because reagents and techniques for these immunohistochemical techniques have not been standardized, they are not done routinely in clinical diagnostic pathology laboratories; however, if appropriate reagents and positive-control tissue are available, these techniques can be adapted for routine diagnostic purposes and can be relied upon for the definitive diagnosis of HDV infection.

Routine diagnosis of acute simultaneous HBV HDV co-infection is based on the detection of anti-HDV in serum in association with IgM anti-HBc. Because HDV suppresses HBV replication, loss of HBsAg from serum may be accelerated in HDV co-infection, and, occasionally, IgM anti-HBc may be the only marker of acute HBV infection in this setting (Hoofnagle & Di Bisceglie 1991). A diagnosis of HDV superinfection in a patient with chronic hepatitis B is supported serologically by the presence of anti-HDV in a patient who harbours HBsAg and IgG anti-HBc. Persistence of high-titre anti-HDV for more than 6 months also supports a diagnosis of chronic HDV infection.

HEPATITIS E

Hepatitis E virus (HEV) is an RNA virus, with features most closely resembling those of caliciviruses, which causes acute, but not chronic, hepatitis. Similar in some ways to HAV (Hoofnagle & Di Bisceglie 1991), HEV is spread by the faecal–oral route and is an important cause of sporadic, endemic and epidemic hepatitis in certain Third World countries (Gust & Purcell 1990, Kane et al 1984). Hepatitis E virus is not indigenous to the USA, but 'imported' cases have been reported in travellers returning from endemic areas, including Pakistan and Mexico. For unknown reasons, acute hepatitis E has a particularly high mortality rate in pregnant women during the third trimester of pregnancy (up to 20%). Routine serological testing for HEV is not available at present; however, immune electron microscopy and immunofluorescence are currently employed as research tools to detect HEV antigen or antibody. Now that the entire HEV genome has been cloned (Balayan et al 1983, Reyes et al 1990), molecular approaches to the diagnosis of HEV infection are possible; again, these techniques are unlikely to become routinely available for diagnostic purposes, but such advances will engender practical immunoassays, and these are in the process of development.

During acute hepatitis E, HEV antigen can be identified in faeces, bile, and liver by immune electron microscopy during the incubation and symptomatic phases of infection (Balayan et al 1983). Antibody to HEV antigen (anti-HEV) can also be detected in liver by immune electron microscopy (Gust & Purcell 1990) or in serum by 'blocking immunofluorescence' (inhibition by anti-HEV in a patient's serum of the binding by a standard, known amount of anti-HEV binding to HEV antigen in primate livers) (Krawczynski et al 1988) during the acute phase of illness. None of these techniques is readily applicable for routine diagnostic use.

Currently the diagnosis of HEV infection is made on the basis of an appropriate travel history and exclusion of other specific causes of acute viral hepatitis. Specific diagnostic techniques are available as research tools only.

DIAGNOSTIC APPLICATIONS OF SEROLOGICAL TESTS

All five major hepatitis viruses can cause acute hepatitis, but only three of these – HBV, HDV and HCV – also cause chronic hepatitis. Therefore, serological diagnosis of viral hepatitis should be tailored to the particular clinical circumstances. As noted above, diagnostic testing for HEV is available on a research basis only. Infection with HDV does not occur in the absence of HBV infection, and testing for HDV should generally not be part of a first-line panel.

In suspected cases of acute viral hepatitis, appropriate initial tests should be directed towards detection of acute hepatitis A, B, or C (Fig. 26.7) with an initial diagnostic panel consisting of IgM anti-HAV, HBsAg, IgM anti-HBc, and anti-HCV. The diagnosis of acute hepatitis A is established by detection of IgM anti-HAV. For the diagnosis of acute hepatitis B, HBsAg as well as IgM anti-HBc should be detectable. The presence of IgM anti-HBc suggests that, if HBsAg is present, HBV infection is acute or that, if HBsAg is absent, the patient has acute resolving hepatitis B or acute hepatitis B with a level of HBsAg beneath the detection threshold of the immunoassay. If there are additional epidemiological or clinical features to suggest HDV infection, such as an unusually severe episode of acute hepatitis or a known risk factor such as intravenous drug abuse, testing for anti-HDV should be done. Finally, testing for anti-HCV should be done, especially in a patient with post-transfusion hepatitis or a history of intravenous drug use. Because of the low sensitivity of anti-HCV testing, particularly early in acute hepatitis C, repeated testing for anti-HCV is appropriate if no other cause for acute hepatitis has been identified. If this initial battery of serological tests is negative, the diagnosis of acute viral hepatitis should be reconsidered. Other possible causes of acute liver dysfunction, such as drug hepatotoxicity, biliary tract disease, cardiac failure or

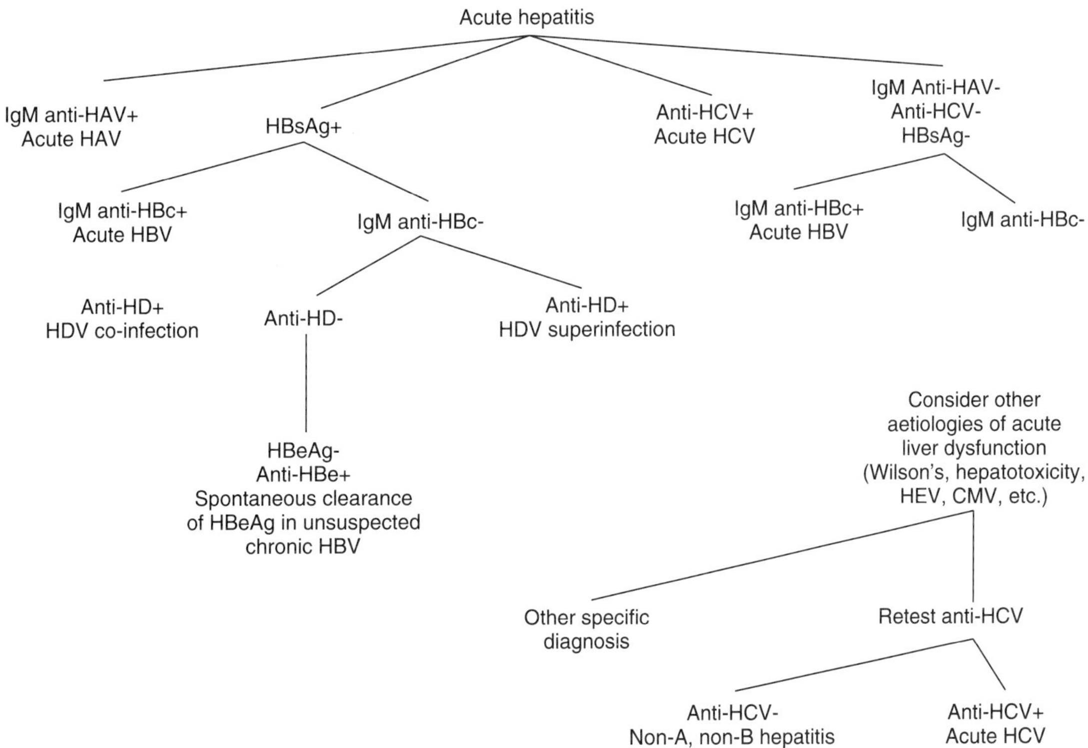

Fig. 26.7 Diagnostic approach to the patient with acute viral hepatitis.

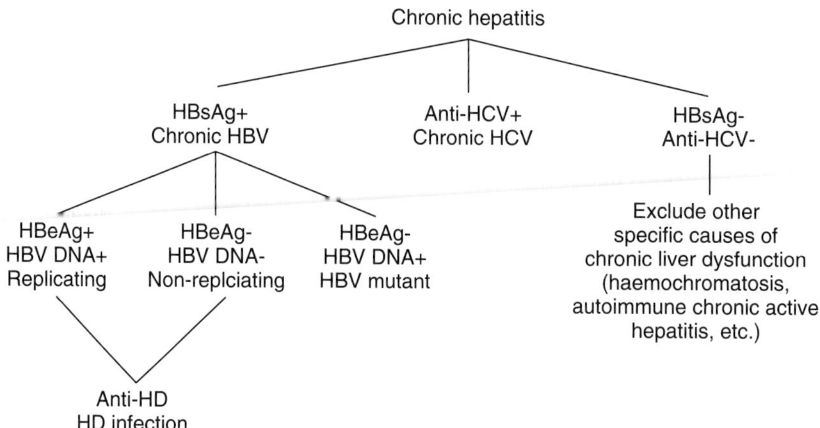

Fig. 26.8 Diagnostic approach to the patient with chronic viral hepatitis.

involvement of the liver in a multisystem disease, such as infectious mononucleosis or metastatic malignancy, should be considered.

In chronic liver disease, neither HAV nor HEV is included in the differential diagnosis. Testing for HBV and HCV infection should be accomplished initially by immunoassays for HBsAg and anti-HCV respectively (Fig. 26.8). If HBsAg is present, detection of IgG anti-HBc in the absence of IgM anti-HBc excludes acute hepatitis B and confirms chronic hepatitis B. Additional information about HBV infection may be obtained by testing for HBeAg, to document the presence of active viral replication, as well as anti-HDV, to establish the presence of associated HDV infection, particularly if the clinical features of liver disease are severe or risk factors such as intravenous drug abuse exist. In a patient with a high risk of percutaneous exposure to HCV, the detection of anti-HCV by EIA usually confirms a diagnosis of chronic HCV infection; however, if doubt exists about the interpretation of the anti-HCV result (either falsely negative or falsely positive), supplementary testing with RIBA-II should be performed. Although liver biopsy generally is not indicated purely for diagnosis in chronic viral hepatitis, demonstration of viral antigens in liver tissue provides additional confirmation of a specific viral infection; however, apart from immunofluorescence to detect intrahepatic HBV antigens, these techniques are not widely available.

Common serological patterns and their interpretations are illustrated in Table 26.1.

Unusual serological patterns

There are a number of limitations to serological diagnostic testing for viral hepatitis. As discussed above, these limitations include a lack of sensitivity and to a lesser extent specificity for currently available anti-HCV assays and a lack of sensitivity for anti-HDV testing in acute hepatitis D. However, the serological patterns that tend to cause the most diagnostic confusion are related to HBV.

Occasionally, anti-HBc, in the absence of HBsAg and anti-HBs, is the sole marker in the serum of people tested for HBV markers. Some of these cases may result from false-positive anti-HBc reactivity. In other cases, however, the isolated anti-HBc result represents a true-positive finding. For example, rarely in acute HBV infection, anti-HBc, typically IgM anti-HBc, may be the only marker of acute HBV infection, when levels of circulating HBsAg do not reach a detectable threshold, or of recent HBV infection after the disappearance of HBsAg and before the appearance of anti-HBs (Lemon et al 1981). Follow-up testing should confirm this interpretation. Even more rarely, anti-HBs fails to appear and becomes detectable or appears long after resolution of acute hepatitis B (McMahon et al 1981). Additionally, anti-HBs levels may become undetectable many years after resolution of HBV infection, and an isolated anti-HBc (of the IgG class) persists as the only marker of past HBV infection (Seeff et al 1987). Recent studies

Table 26.1 Common serological patterns and their interpretation

Virus	Pattern	Interpretation
Hepatitis A	IgM anti-HAV	Acute infection
	IgG anti-HAV	Remote infection
Hepatitis B	HBsAg with IgM anti-HBc	Acute infection
	HBsAg and anti-HBs –, IgM anti-HBc +	Acute infection
	HBsAg with IgG anti-HBc	Chronic infection
	HBsAg, IgG anti-HBc, HBV DNA +, HBeAg–	Chronic 'e-minus' infection
	HBsAg, IgG anti-HBc, HBV DNA +, HBeAg+	Replicative chronic infection
	HBsAg, IgG antiHBc+, HBV DNA, HBeAg–	Non-replicative chronic infection
	HBsAg –, IgG anti-HBc and anti-HBs +	Resolved infection
Hepatitis D	Anti-HDV and HBsAg+	HDV infection
	IgM anti-HBc +	co-infection
	IgM anti-HBc –	superinfection
Hepatitis C	Anti-HCV	HCV infection

Anti-HAV, antihepatitis A virus antibody; HBsAg, hepatitis B surface antigen; HBV DNA, hepatitis B virus DNA; HBeAg, hepatitis B e antigen; anti-HBc, antihepatitis B core antibody; anti-HDV, antihepatitis D (delta) antibody; anti-HCV, antihepatitis C virus antibody.

using PCR to detect HBV DNA have suggested that some cases of an isolated anti-HBc may in fact represent persistent low-level HBV replication, but because patients with this virological pattern do not have clinical or biochemical liver disease the significance of HBV DNA detectable by PCR in such cases is uncertain (Luo et al 1991). Passive acquisition of anti-HBc from donor blood units is now unlikely in the USA, for anti-HBc-positive units are discarded (Koff 1991). Transmission of anti-HBc from mothers to infants has been reported, and the antibody can persist for several months in the infant (Stevens et al 1987).

Successful immunization against HBV with currently available vaccines results in the appearance in serum of anti-HBs without anti-HBc. Isolated anti-HBs can also be acquired passively from hepatitis B normal human immunoglobulin or other blood products (Devine et al 1989). Some chronic carriers of HBV have both HBsAg and anti-HBs in serum. The antibody is directed against HBsAg epitopes not present on the circulating HBsAg and is thus not protective (Sheih et al 1987).

ACKNOWLEDGEMENT

The authors are grateful to Ms Kerry Porter for her assistance in the preparation in this manuscript.

REFERENCES

Alter H J 1992 New kit on the block: evaluation of second-generation assay for detection of antibody to the hepatitis C virus. Hepatology 15: 350–353

Alter H J, Purcell R H, Shih J W et al 1989 Detection of antibody to hepatitis C virus in prospectively followed transfusion recipients with acute and chronic non-A, non-B hepatitis. New England Journal of Medicine 321: 1494–1500

Aragona M, Macano S, Caredda F et al 1987 Serological response to the hepatitis delta virus in hepatitis C. Lancet i: 478–480

Balayan M S, Andzhaparidze A G, Savinskaya S S et al 1983 Evidence for a virus in non-A, non-B hepatitis transmitted via the fecal oral route. Intervirology 20: 23–31

Budhkowska A, Dubreuil P, Maillard P et al 1990 A biphoric pattern of anti-pre-S responses in acute hepatitis B virus infection. Hepatology 12: 1271–1277

Budkowska A, Dubreuil P, Poynard T et al 1992 Anti-pre-S responses and viral clearance in chronic hepatitis B virus infection. Hepatology 15: 26–31

Buti M, Esteban R, Jardi R et al 1989 Chronic delta hepatitis: detection of hepatitis delta virus in serum by immunoblot and correlation with other markers of delta viral replication. Hepatology 10: 907–910

Carman W F, Jacyna M R, Hadziyannis S et al 1989 Mutation preventing formation of hepatitis B e antigen in patients with chronic hepatitis B infection. Lancet 335: 588–591

Carman W F, Zanetti A R, Karayiannis P et al 1990 Vaccine-induced escape mutant of hepatitis B virus. Lancet 336: 325–329

Carman W F, Hadziyannis S, Karayiannis P et al 1991 Association of the precore variant of HBV with acute and fulminant hepatitis B infection. In: Hollinger F B, Lemon S M, Margolis H S (eds) Viral Hepatitis and Liver Disease, Williams and Wilkins, Baltimore, p 216–219

Chau K H, Hargie M P, Decker R H et al 1983 Serodiagnosis of recent hepatitis B infection by IgM class anti-HBc. Hepatology 3: 142–149

Choo Q-L, Kuo G, Weiner A J et al 1989 Isolation of a cDNA clone derived from a blood-borne non-A, non-B viral hepatitis genome. Science 244: 359–362

Czaja A J, Taswell H F, Rakela J, Schumek C M 1991 Frequency and significance of antibody to hepatitis C virus in severe corticosteroid-treated autoimmune chronic active hepatitis. Mayo Clinic Proceedings 66: 572–582

Davis G L, Hoffnagle J H 1985 Reactivation of chronic type B hepatitis presenting as acute viral hepatitis. Annals of Internal Medicine 102: 762–765

David G L, Hoofnagle J H 1987 Reactivation of chronic hepatitis B virus infection. Gastroenterology 92: 2028–2031

Decker R H, Kosakowski S M, Vanderbilt A S et al 1981 Diagnosis of acute hepatitis A by HAVAB-M, a direct radioimmunoassay for IgM anti-HAV. American Journal of Clinical Pathology 76: 140–148

Devine P, Taswell H F, Moore S B et al 1989 Passively acquired antibody of hepatitis B surface antigen: pitfall is evaluating immunity to hepatitis B viral infection. Archives of Pathology and Laboratory Medicine 113: 529–531

Di Bisceglie A M, Negro F 1989 Diagnosis of hepatitis delta virus infection. Hepatology 10: 1014–1016

Ebeling F, Naukkarinen R, Leikola J 1990 Recombinant immunoblot assay for hepatitis C virus antibody as predictor of infectivity. Lancet 335: 982–983

Everhart J E, Di Bisceglie A M, Murray L M et al 1990 Risk for non-A, non-B (type C) hepatitis through sexual or household contact with chronic carriers. Annals of Internal Medicine 112: 544–545

Farci P, Mandos A, Lai M E et al 1990 Treatment of chronic delta hepatitis with high and low doses of interferon alpha-2a. A randomized controlled trial (abstract). Hepatology 12: 869

Farci P, Alter H, Wong D et al 1991 A long-term study of hepatitis C virus replication in non-A, non-B hepatitis. New England Journal of Medicine 325: 98–104

Froesner G G, Schomerus H, Wiedmann K H et al 1982 Diagnostic significance of quantitative determination of hepatitis B surface antigen in acute and chronic hepatitis B infection. European Journal of Clinical Microbiology 1: 52–58

Fung J, Ostberg L, Shapiro R et al 1991 Human monoclonal antibody against hepatitis B surface antigen in preventing hepatitis B following transplantation. In: Hollinger FB, Lemon SM, Margolis HS (eds) Viral hepatitis and liver disease. Williams & Wilkins, Baltimore, p 651

Govindarajan S, Chin K P, Redeker A G et al 1984 Fulminant B viral hepatitis: role of delta agent. Gastroenterology 86: 1417–1420

Gust I D, Purcell R H 1990 Report of a workshop: waterborne non-A, non-B hepatitis. Science 248: 1335–1339

Hoofnagle J H & Di Bisceglie A M 1991 Serologic diagnosis of acute and chronic viral hepatitis. Seminars in liver disease 11(2): 73–83

Hoofnagle J H, Dusheiko G M, Seeff L B et al 1981 Seroconversion from hepatitis B e antigen to antibody in chronic type hepatitis. Annals of Internal Medicine 94: 744–748

Hoofnagle J H, Shafritz D A, Popper H 1987 Chronic type B hepatitis and the 'healthy' HBsAg carrier state. Hepatology 7: 758–763

Hsu H H, Gonzalez M, Foung S K H, Feinstone S M, Greenberg H B 1991 Antibodies to hepatitis C virus in low-risk blood donors: implications for counseling positive donors. Gastroenterology 101: 1724–1727

Kane M A, Bradley D W, Shrestha S M et al 1984 Epidemic non-A, non-B hepatitis in Nepal. Recovery of a possible etiologic agent and transmission studies in marmosets. Journal of the American Medical Association 252: 3140–3145

Kaneko S, Miller R H, Di Bisceglie A M et al 1990 Detection of hepatitis B virus DNA in serum by polymerase chain reaction. Gastroenterology 99: 799–804

Koff RS 1991 Difficult serologic diagnosis in viral hepatitis. In: Hollinger F B, Lemon S M, Margolis H S (eds) Viral hepatitis and liver disease. Williams & Wilkins, Baltimore, pp 790–791

Kosaka Y, Takase K, Kojima M et al 1991. Fulminant hepatitis B: induction by hepatitis B virus mutants defective in the precore region and incapable of enacting HBeAg. Gastroenterology 324: 1087–1094

Krawczynski K, Bradley D W, Kane M A 1988 Virus associated antigen of epidemic non-A, non-B hepatitis and specific antibodies in outbreaks and in sporadic cases of NANB hepatitis. Hepatology 8: 1223

Krawczynski K, Kuo G, Di Bisceglie A et al 1989 Blood-borne non-A, non-B hepatitis (PT-NANB): immunohistochemical identification of disease and hepatitis C virus-associated antigen(s) (abstract). Hepatology 10: 580

Krugman S, Overby L R, Mushahwar I K et al 1979 Viral hepatitis, type B. Studies on the natural history and prevention reexamined. New England Journal of Medicine 300: 101–105

Kuhns M C 1990 Monitoring hepatitis B virus replication. Journal of Hepatology 11 (suppl. 1): 590–594

Kuo G, Choo Q-L, Alter H J et al 1989 An assay for circulating antibodies to a major etiologic virus of human non-A, non-B hepatitis. Science 244: 362–364

Lemon S 1985 Type A viral hepatitis. New developments in an old disease. New England Journal of Medicine 313: 1059–1967

Lemon S M, Gates W L, Simms T E, Barcroff W H 1981 IgM antibody to hepatitis core antigen as a diagnostic parameter of acute infection with hepatitis B virus. Journal of Infectious Diseases 143: 803–804

Liang T J, Haseqaura K, Rimon N et al 1991 A hepatitis B virus mutant associated with an epidemic of fulminant hepatitis. New England Journal of Medicine 324: 1705–1709

Locarnini S, A Ferris A A, Lehmann N F et al 1977 The antibody response following hepatitis A infection. Intervirology 8: 309–318

Luo K X, Zhou R, He C et al 1991 Hepatitis B virus DNA in sera of viral carriers positive exclusively for antibodies to the hepatitis B core antigen. Journal of Medical Virology 35: 55–59

McFarlane I G, Smith H M, Johnson P J et al 1990 Hepatitis C virus antibodies in chronic active hepatitis: pathogenetic factor or false-positive result? Lancet 335: 754–757

McHutchison J G, Person J L, Govindarajan S et al 1992

Improved detection of hepatitis C virus antibodies in high-risk populations. Hepatology 15: 19–25
McMahon B, Bender T R, Berquist K R et al 1981 Delayed development of antibody to hepatitis B surface antigen after symptomatic infection with hepatitis B virus. Journal of Clinical Microbiology 14: 130–134
Marcellin P, Martino-Perynoy M, Boyer N et al 1991 Second generation (RIBA) test in diagnosis of chronic hepatitis C. Lancet 337: 551–552
Mathiesen L R, Fauerholt L, Moller A M et al 1979 Immunofluorescence studies for hepatitis A virus and hepatitis B surface and core antigen in liver biopsies from patients with acute viral hepatitis. Gastroenterology 77: 623–628
Miller R H, Keneko S, Chung C T et al 1989 Compact organization of the hepatitis B virus genome. Hepatology 9: 322–327
Negro F, Bonino F, Di Bisceglie A et al 1989 Intrahepatic markers of hepatitis delta virus infection: a study by *in situ* hybridization. Hepatology 10: 916–920
Neurath A R, Kent S B H, Strick N et al 1985 Hepatitis B virus contains pre-S gene-encoded domains. Nature 315: 154–156
Neurath A R, Kent S B H, Parker K et al 1986 Antibodies to a synthetic peptide from the pre-S 120–145 region of the hepatitis B virus neutralizing. Vaccine 4: 35–37
Omata M, Ehata T, Yokosuka O et al 1991 Mutation in the precore region of hepatitis B virus DNA in patients with fulminant and severe hepatitis. New England Journal of Medicine 324: 1699–1704
Ou J, Laub O, Rutter W 1986 Hepatitis B virus gene function: the precore region targets the core antigen to cellular membranes and causes the secretion of the e antigen. Proceedings of the National Academy of Sciences of the USA 83: 1578–1582
Pontisso P, Ruvioletto M G, Yerlich W H et al 1989 Identification of an attached site for human liver plasma membranes on hepatitis B virus particles. Virology 137: 523–530
Popper H, Shafritz D A, Hoofnagle J H 1987 Relation of the hepatitis B virus carrier state to hepatocellular carcinoma. Hepatology 7: 764–772
Poterucha J, Rakela J, Taswell H et al 1991 Diagnosis of chronic hepatitis C after liver transplantation using polymerase chain reaction. Gastroenterology 100: 786 (abstract)
Resnick H W, Wong V C W, Ip H M H et al 1990 Mother-to-infant transmission and hepatitis C virus. Lancet 335: 1216–1217
Reyes G R, Prudy M A, Kim J P et al 1990 Isolation of a cDNA from the virus responsible for enterically treated non-A, non-B hepatitis. Science 248: 1335–1340
Rizzetto M, Verme G, Recchia S et al 1983 Chronic HBsAg hepatitis with intrahepatic expression of delta antigen: an active and progressive disease unresponsive to immunosuppressive therapy. Annals of Internal Medicine 98: 437–441
Scolnick E M, McLean A A, West D J et al 1984 Clinical evaluation in healthy adults of a hepatitis B vaccine made by recombinant DNA. Journal of the American Medical Association 251: 2812–2815
Seeff L B, Bebe G W, Hoofnagle J H et al 1987 A serologic follow up of the 1942 epidemic of post-vaccination hepatitis in the United States Army. New England Journal of Medicine 316: 965–970
Sheih M T, Taswell H F, Czaja A J et al 1987 Frequency and significance of concurrent hepatitis B surface antigen and antibody in acute and chronic hepatitis B. Gastroenterology 93: 675–680
Sjögren M H, Tanno H, Fay O et al 1987 Hepatitis A virus in stool during clinical relapse. Annals of Internal Medicine 106: 221–226
Smedile A, Rizzetto M, Denistan K et al 1986 Type D hepatitis: the clinical significance of hepatitis D virus DNA in serum as detected by a hybridization based assay. Hepatology 6: 1297–1302
Stevens C E, Taylor P E, Tong MJ et al 1987 Prevention of perinatal hepatitis B infection with hepatitis B immune globulins and hepatitis B vaccine. In: Zuckerman A J (ed) Viral hepatitis and liver disease. Alan R. Liss, New York, pp 982–987
Tanno H, Fay O H, Rojman J A, Palazzi J 1988 Biphasic form of hepatitis A virus infection: a frequent variant in Argentina. Liver 8: 53–57
Tassopoulos N C, Roumeliotou-Karayannis A, Sakka M et al 1987 An epidemic of hepatitis A in an institution for young children. American Journal of Epidemiology 125: 302–307

27. Application of molecular biology to diagnosis

Christian Brechot

The diagnosis of viral hepatitis has been markedly improved by a combination of four factors:

1. the development of sensitive serological tests for viral antigens;
2. the identification of new causative agents (hepatitis viruses D, C and E);
3. the cloning of the viral genomes, opening the way to diagnostic procedures based on molecular biology;
4. the improvement and simplification of molecular hybridization techniques and the development of the polymerase chain reaction (PCR).

This review will focus on the advantages and limitations of these approaches for the diagnosis of infection by hepatitis viruses B and C.

THE TECHNIQUES

Purification of viral nucleic acids

DNA or RNA can be extracted from serum, plasma, mononuclear blood cells and tissue by means of routine techniques (phenol–chloroform extraction for DNA, guanidinum thiocyanate for RNA). New, faster procedures are also available (Boom et al 1991). It should, however, always be kept in mind that poorly purified nucleic acids will not be suitable for further analysis. A balance must therefore be struck between the rapidity of the extraction and the efficiency of the detection procedures (see, for example, our protocols described in Bréchot et al 1981a, b, Scotto et al 1983a, Zignego et al 1990, Dény et al 1991, Gerken et al 1991b, Féray et al 1992,Thiers et al 1992b). DNA and RNA can also be extracted from paraffin-embedded liver sections (Lo et al 1989, Lampertico et al 1990, M L Chen et al 1991, Shindo et al 1991) as long as they have been fixed with paraformaldehyde; other fixatives may nonetheless be suitable, but picric acid solution alters nucleic acids and should be avoided.

Detection of viral genomes (Table 27.1)

The viral genome can be detected by hybridization on either a solid support or in a liquid medium (Bréchot 1987, Krosgaard 1988, Gerken et al 1992).

Detection on solid supports can be performed using a filtration assay through a nylon membrane (referred to as spot or dot assays) or with the Southern blot test. The slot blot is simply a variation of the dot blot in which the DNA solution is loaded into a linear well (Bonino et al 1981, Berninger et al 1982, Lieberman et al 1982, Lin et al 1989, Weller et al 1982, Hadziyannis et al 1983, Scotto et al 1983a, Feinman et al 1984, Shimizu et al 1984, Dusheiko et al 1985, Gmelin et al 1985, Harrison et al 1985, Imazeki et al 1985, Morace et al 1985, Chaussade et al 1986, Diegutis et al 1986, Bréchot 1987, Krogsgaard 1988, Thiers et al 1988a, Zarski et al 1989). The dot test is simple, meaning that general departments can have access to the detection of HBV DNA and it is suited to the analysis of large numbers of samples.

With prior migration on an agarose gel, Southern assay separates the viral molecules according to their molecular weight. As a result, it can be used to determine the state of the viral DNA in liver cells. This is not a difficult procedure but it requires excellent technical conditions to

Table 27.1 Comparison of different procedures for detecting HBV DNA

	Samples to be analysed	Amount of sample*	Sensitivity	Risk of cross-contamination	Duration of the assay	Specific advantages
(a) *Without amplification of nucleic acids*						
1. Dot or spot test	Serum or plasma	50–100 μl	10^4–10^5-HBV particles	Limited	3–5 days+	• Reliability • Possibility of semiquantification
2. Liquid hybridization (microtitre plates columns)	Serum or plasma	50–100 μl	10^4–10^5 HBV particles	Limited	1–2 days	Easier quantification
3. Southern blot	Liver peripheral blood mono-nuclear cells (PBMCs)	10–30 μg of DNA 5×10^6–10^7 PBMCs	1–10 pg of HBV DNA	Limited ‡	1 week	Can determine the state of the viral DNA
(b) *With prior amplification of nucleic acids: PCR*						
1. Dot Liquid hybridization	As in (a)	10–100 μl of serum or plasma	1–10 particles/ml 1 ng of HBV DNA	Major ζ	2–4 days+	• Sensitivity • Semiquantification
2. Southern Blot	As in (a)	1–5μg of DNA or RNA	One copy of HBV DNA per 10^5 cells	Major ζ	2–4 days+	As above plus detection of viral genome rearrangements

* Average from the literature.
+ 1–3 days' exposure with radioactive probes; redued by using non-radioactive probes to 1 day.
‡ But risk of false-positive results in liver samples contaminated by liver bacterial plasmids.
ζ Higher in nested than in single-step PCR.

be really informative, i.e. to detect 1 pg of HBV DNA and to clearly identify weak, HBV specific, bands. Its interpretation may be hampered by contamination of the cellular DNA with plasmid DNA from bacteria contained in the liver; these DNA will hybridize to the vector plasmid DNA (including the HBV DNA probe), which will remain present in the HBV DNA solution despite all purification steps and thus will also be labelled, together with the HBV insert. As a control the same filter is rehybridized with a probe made only of the plasmid DNA without the insert.

The Southern blot assay can also be used to analyse amplified products after PCR and, by evaluating the size of the amplified DNA, to search for rearrangements in the viral genome (Fig. 27.1).

Probes

Radioactive probes have been extensively used following the development of nick translation and random priming labelling procedures, with good reliability and sensitivity. These qualities are now also obtained with non-radioactive probes although, in our experience, their use is still limited in the classical Southern blot assay by lower sensitivity. In contrast, such probes will be advantageous in the analysis of amplified DNA or RNA (Negro & Chiaberge 1985, Larzul et al

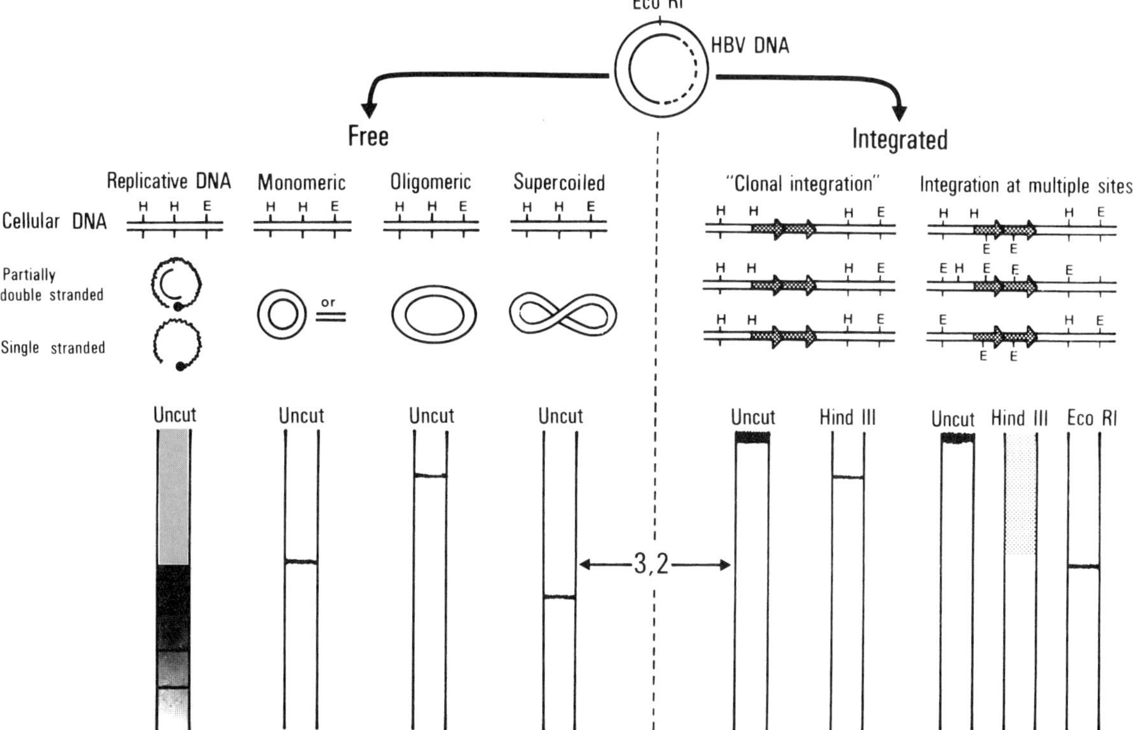

Fig. 27.1 Schematic representation of the results obtained from HBV DNA detection with Southern blot. Digestion of liver cellular DNA by various restriction enzymes, with or without a restriction site in the HBV DNA, allows the different forms of the viral DNA in the liver cells to be distinguished.
Free HBV DNA. The presence of replicative HBV DNA is generally associated with secretion of complete, infectious, Dane particles; in contrast monomeric and oligomeric HBV DNA do not reflect a productive viral infection. The supercoiled HBV DNA is involved in the persistence of the viral infection. *Integrated HBV DNA.* The Southern blot pattern on uncut or undigested liver DNA can show clonal proliferation of the infected cells, a finding generally restricted to tumour samples of patients with HCC or to some cirrhotic tissues. Integration without detection of cellular clones is generally observed in HBV chronic carriers without HCC as well as in a few cases of acute hepatitis.

1987, 1989, Casacubetta et al 1988, Quibriac et al 1989, Santantonio et al 1990, Valentine-Thon et al 1990, 1991, Guo & Bowden 1991, Mantero et al 1991, Nakagami et al 1991, Gerken et al 1992).

Quantification

The quantification of the results obtained with these procedures is still problematic. The following approaches have been used:

- semiquantification based on visual estimation after autoradiography *or* densitometric analysis.
- counting of the hybridized filters.
- liquid hybridization (Fagan et al 1985, Thiers et al 1986, Kuhns et al 1988, 1989, Zarski et al 1989, Keller et al 1990, Banerjee & Khandekar 1991), an interesting alternative approach: single- or double-stranded DNA can be separated after hybridization on a column. Alternatively, liquid hybridization can be carried out on microplates for fast and simple resolution.

One of the most difficult points is still however the choice of controls for quantification:

- cultured cell lines containing a known amount of HBV DNA can be used to test the sensitivity of classical Sourthern blot or PCR.

- in dot assays, purified DNA, without the associated proteins, will behave differently from that in intact particles.
- recombinant phage particles may be an interesting alternative by mimicking HBV particles.
- serum from infected patients or chimpanzees can also be used, but their titration will only provide a rough estimation. Furthermore, it should be kept in mind that the serum of infected individuals contains a mixture of defective and complete viral particles, leading to an overestimation of the number of infectious particles.

Polymerase chain reaction (Fig. 27.2)

The polymerase chain reaction (PCR) gives selective amplification of short DNA or RNA sequences. These sequences can subsequently be identified and cloned by conventional hybridization and recombinant DNA procedures. The technique has several advantages: (1) only small quantities of material (serum or tissue) are required, as 1–5 μg of DNA or RNA is sufficient; (2) amplification is generally extremely efficient (10^6–10^9); (3) the procedure is quick, taking only 1–3 days; (4) the amplified nucleic acid can readily be cloned and/or sequenced for fast and precise characterization.

A PCR test involves a series of amplification cycles (normally between 20 and 40). Each cycle consists of three phases. The first is denaturation of the nucleic acid, the second is hybridization of short oligonucleotides (20–30 bases; referred to as primers) to the target DNA and the third is the extension of the primers using the *Taq* polymerase (a thermoresistant DNA polymerase), which synthesizes complementary DNA molecules. It has been recently shown that the initiation of PCR at a high temperature (referred to as 'hot-start PCR') enhances the specificity and sensitivity of the test by minimizing non-specific hybridization of the primers. If the substrate is RNA there is an additional step: a strand of cDNA complementary to the target RNA molecule is synthesized from the antisense primer; this is followed by the normal PCR procedure after the addition of the second primer. Alternatively, the cDNA can be synthesized by means of random priming, with subsequent addition of the two specific primers.

Optimal design of the primers is critical for the success of the PCR technique. The sequence of a primer is chosen according to the following rules:

- the length of the primer should be between 20 and 30 bases.
- comparison of all available sequences allows primers to be designed so that they are complementary to genomic regions conserved between different viral isolates. This should minimize the possibility of false-negative results caused by genetic variations.
- the two primers should not include sequences complementary to each other, as this would result in the primers annealing. Were this to occur, these dimers, rather than the target DNA or RNA, would be amplified during the PCR resulting in so-called 'primer dimers', and this would significantly reduce the efficiency of the assay.

Analysis of amplification products

Amplified DNA sequences can be visualized by ethidium bromide staining after electrophoresis on agarose gels. However, transfer to a filter and hybridization with a specific probe (Sourthern blot) is necessary to check the specificity of the procedure. Southern blotting gives an indication as to the length of the product and thus allows separation of the specific amplified products from primers and non-specifically amplified sequences.

It is important to realize that, when analysing tissue cellular DNA, PCR will not allow the state of the viral DNA in the infected cells to be determined. However, the use of a combination of different primers can provide some indirect information on this; new procedures, based on PCR, have been also proposed to clone cellular sequences adjacent to the HBV DNA integration sites, and are currently being evaluated.

Finally, PCR can also be performed on liver tissue to identify viral DNA and RNA. The technique is suitable for paraffin-embedded and frozen samples, despite a significant loss of sensitivity in the former, around 10-fold (Lo et al

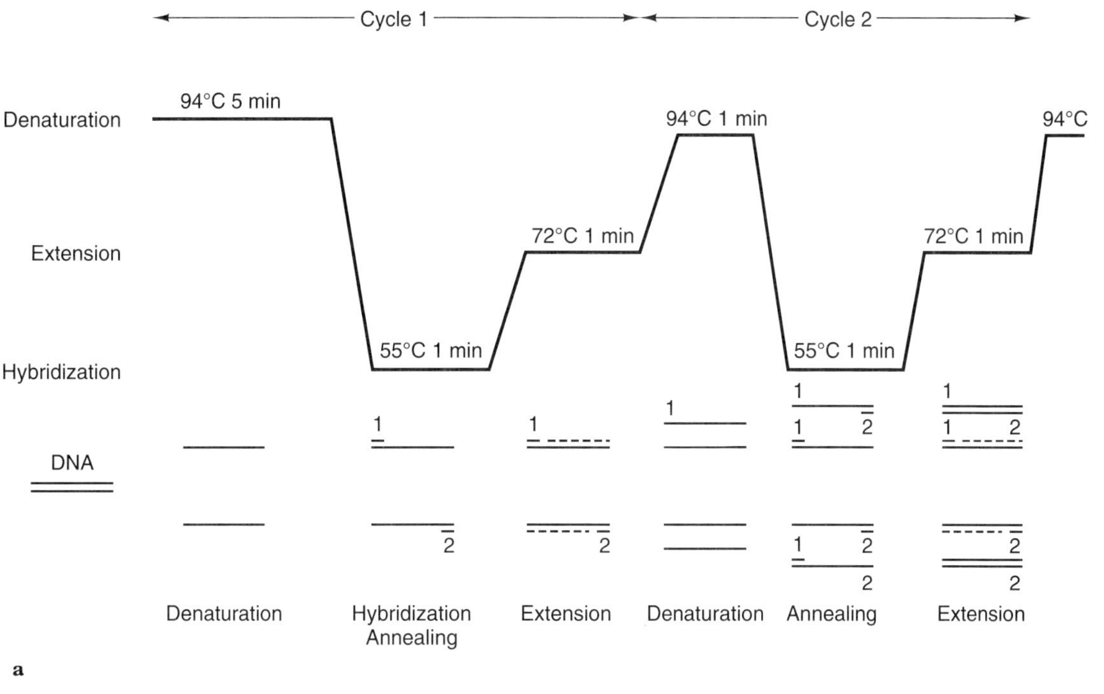

a

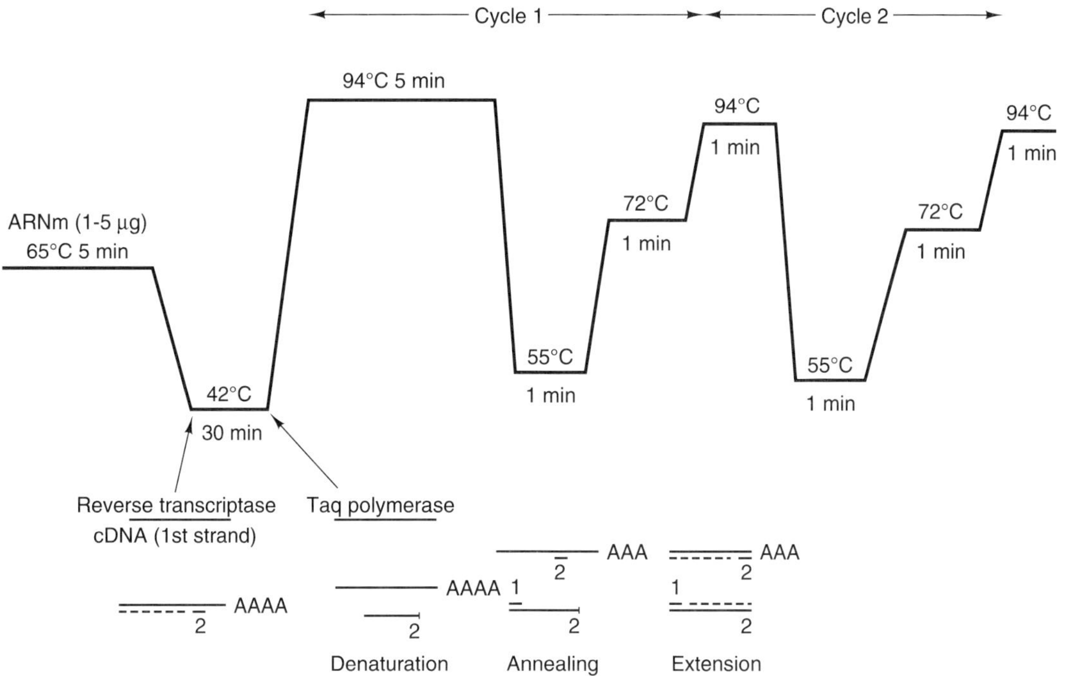

b

Fig. 27.2 Schematic representation of the polymerase chain reaction (PCR). (a) Amplification of HBV DNA. (b) Amplification of HBV RNA.

1989, Lampertico et al 1990, Chen et al 1991).

The risk of false-positive results, due to contaminants generated from aerosols, must be kept in mind at all times. False-negative results, due to inhibitors of amplification, should always also be taken into account. These issues can be addressed with appropriate controls:

- PCR performed in parallel with primers specific for cellular DNA (HLA) or RNA sequences.
- inclusion of several negative controls at each step of the procedure (including nucleic acid extraction).
- drastic physical separation of the different amplication phases.

The results should also be interpreted taking into account the possibility that the viral genome is present in defective as well as complete viral particles (this is true for all molecular biology techniques).

The quantification of the amplification is still an unresolved issue despite several approaches. Serial dilutions have been generally used with comparison to internal standards; this procedure does provide semiquantitative information, but its interpretation is markedly hampered by a lack of reproducibility. Co-amplification of HCV RNA, together with an internal control including the same sequences to be annealed with the primers, is attractive but raises the issue of artefacts due to these co-amplifications. In fact, one of the major difficulties is linked to the variable efficiency of the RNA extraction procedures, a major point to be evaluated.

In situ hybridization

This combination of liver histology and molecular biology provides both detection of the viral genome and localization of the infected cells. It is now also possible to use either radioactive or non-radioactive probes. In addition, cDNA, RNA and oligonucleotide probes *are* suitable. It is, however, important to note that in situ hybridization is highly dependent on both the amount and the complexity of the viral genome. It is therefore necessary to define precisely the experimental conditions for each viral infection (as an example, the conditions used to detect HCV RNA in our laboratory are shown in Lamas et al 1992).

Thus, in situ hybridization cannot yet be viewed as a true diagnostic test, but it can provide important information on the cell types infected and, thus, on the pathogenesis of virus-induced liver diseases (Fournier et al 1982, Negro & Chiaberge 1985, Rijntjes et al 1985, Hadchouel et al 1988, Tay et al 1990, Lau et al 1991). A further problem with this approach is the preservation of liver cell morphology during the hybridization steps. Finally, it has been recently reported that PCR can be applied to in situ detection. This could have major implications but has only been demonstrated on isolated cell preparations (Bagasra et al 1992).

HEPATITIS B VIRAL (HBV) DNA DETECTION

HBV DNA detection, without prior amplification, in spot (or dot) tests

The classical spot test is still a reference method for direct, sensitive detection of viral DNA in serum of plasma. This is based on the results of a large number of studies:

1. the viral DNA, detected in the serum, is present in viral particles.
2 spot tests detect around 10^5 particles per ml (radioactive and non-radioactive probes now provide similar sensitivity).
3. tests based on liquid hybridization are now available and provide a semiquantitative estimation of viral DNA. As stated on p. 416 there is still no reliable method for direct and precise quantification. However, semi-quantitative estimation is sufficient for the follow-up of patients on antiviral therapy (a major application of this method) (Kuhns et al 1988, 1989).
4. the detection of HBV DNA has permitted a direct appraisal of the course of infection and has significant advantages over the detection of HBe-Ag and the corresponding antibody (anti-HBe).

Table 27.2 HBV DNA in HBsAg- and anti-HBe-positive chronic HBV carriers: detection by spot test without PCR

Geographical origin	Liver disease	HBV DNA in serum	References
North Europe	Asymptomatic carriers	1/18	Krogsgaard et al 1986
		3/65	Thiers et al 1986
		0/42	Gerken et al 1991b
		2/34	Chemin et al 1991
	Chronic liver disease	1/18	Karayannis et al 1985
		6/24	Thiers et al 1986
		0/10	Gerken et al 1991b
		0/12	Loriot et al 1992
		14/46	Baker et al 1991
South Europe	Asymptomatic carriers	0/63	Negro & Chiaberge 1985
		0/81	Bonino et al 1991
	Chronic liver disease	28/34	Negro et al & Chiaberge 1985
		28/37	Bonino et al 1986
		16/32	Lieberman et al 1982
		5/24	Karayannis et al 1985
		14/18	Hadziyannis et al 1983
Asia	Asymptomatic carriers	4/22	Wu et al 1986
		4/24	Chen et al 1986
		17/95	Matsuyama et al 1985
	Chronic liver disease	9/47	Wu et al 1986
		14/22	Chen et al 1986
		7/12	Karayannis et al 1985
		2/9	Kaneko et al 1989b
		3/13	Yokosuka et al 1985
Africa and Middle East	Asymptomatic carriers	4/111	Tur-Kuspa et al 1984
		26/116	Dusheiko et al 1985
		0/59	Dazza et al 1991
	Chronic liver disease	3/13	Karayannis et al 1985
		6/45	Karayannis et al 1985
		7/12	Karayannis et al 1985

Hepatitis B surface antigen-positive patients (Tables 27.2, 27.3)

Studies based on Southern blot and spot test assays, as well as those using immunohistochemistry and in situ hybridization, have delineated the kinetics of HBV multiplication and the state of viral DNA during the course of infection (reviewed in Bréchot 1987, Gerken et al 1992) (Figs 27.1, 27.3). Southern blot can identify productive HBV infection on the basis of the presence of free, cytoplasmic, HBV DNA replication intermediates together with serum HBV DNA contained in the infectious Dane particles (Bréchot et al 1981a, Weller et al 1982, Scotto et al 1983b, 1985, Fowler et al 1984, Yokosuka et al 1985, Pontisso et al 1986, Lok et al 1991). It can also detect the integration of the viral DNA into the host genome, the restriction DNA patterns being consistent or not with clonal expansion of infected cells (Yokosuka et al 1985, Lin et al 1989). Supercoiled HBV DNA, which is involved in the persistence of viral DNA in cells, can also be detected if proteinase K is omitted from the lysis buffer. Other molecules can be visualized too; they include free monomeric HBV DNA that is detected in the liver when viral replication is coming to an end (Bréchot et al 1981a, Lok et al 1985, Pontisso et al 1986, Bréchot 1987), and free oligomeric viral DNA (of unknown significance) that has been found in some subjects with acute hepatitis (Lugassy et al 1987).

Table 27.3 Serum HBV DNA in HBsAg and antiHBe-positive subjects: detection with or without amplification

	HBV DNA		References
	Dot blot	PCR	
Chronic hepatitis	2/9	9/9*	Kaneko et al 1989b
	0/33		
	0/12	8/12*	Loriot et al 1992
	2/11	11/11	Chemin et al 1991
	0/10	8/10	Gerken et al 1991b
	ND	23/32	Coursaget et al 1991
	3/13	12/13	Yokosuka et al 1991
	14/46	36/46	Baker et al 1991
	21/134	137/174	
Asymptomatic carriers	2/34	25/34	Chemin et al 1991
	0/42	22/42	Gerken et al 1991b
	ND	1/31	Ljunggren et al 1991
	2/76	46/107	
Resolved acute hepatitis (> 12 months)		0/6	Kaneko et al 1989b
		0/10	Gerken et al 1991b
		0/12*	Loriot et al 1992
		0/28	

*6/12 and 3/12 positive results, 6 and 12 months after acute HBV infection.

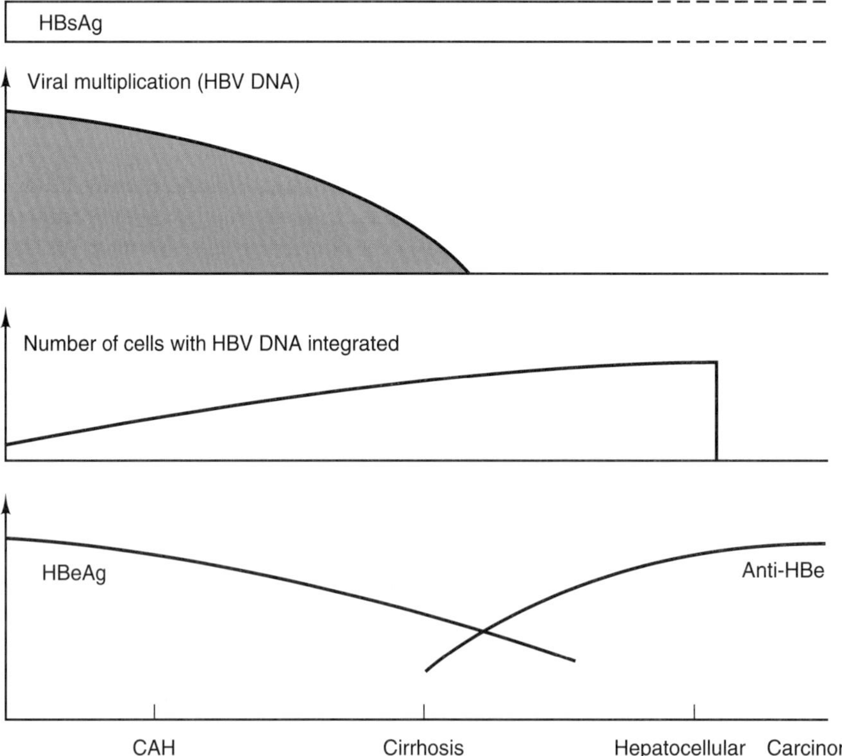

Fig. 27.3 Schematic representation of the course of HBV infection. The results of the HBeAg and HBV DNA tests are indicated, together with the putative evolution in the liver of the state of the viral DNA.

Integrated HBV DNA sequences are found in tumours tissues from most patients with hepatocellular carcinoma (HCC); integration precedes tumour development and has been identified in patients with chronic hepatitis. We have even found integrated HBV DNA in some patients with severe acute hepatitis. However, HBV integration is not involved in viral replication and often only affects a small percentage of infected cells. It is tempting to speculate that integration might be related to liver cell regeneration (cellular DNA replication) and expansion of some infected cells could be due to the site of integration in the genomic DNA and/or to viral gene expression. DNA patterns observed in some patients with cirrhosis tend to support such clonal proliferation. Finally, the existence of preferential integration sites in cellular DNA is still hypothetical.

Both free and integrated HBV DNA can be identified in a given liver sample, although abundant free viral DNA will hamper detection of integrated forms. In situ hybridization has provided a further approach to this issue, with the identification of hepatocytes containing cytoplasmic HBA DNA replication molecules (integrated viral DNA is generally undetectable with these techniques).

The detection of HBV DNA in various cell types has led to the suggestion that the virus might have a much wider cellular tropism than first thought. HBV DNA has been detected in human bone marrow, peripheral mononuclear cells, pancreas, skin, sperm and kidney (Romet Lemonne et al 1983, Dejean et al 1984, Pontisso et al 1985, Lauré et al 1987, Hadchouel et al 1988, Zignego et al 1988, Choi 1990, Féray et al 1990, Lobbiani et al 1990, Pasquinelli et al 1990, Baginski et al 1991, Repp et al 1991, Poterucha et al 1992). The state of the viral DNA in these cells has not been determined, although free monomeric HBV DNA is most frequently identified. It is also noteworthy that there is little information on the cell types involved or the pathological implications of these results. In particular, the clinical relevance of the detection of HBV DNA in extrahepatic cells is unknown.

HBeAg-positives subjects. Most individuals who are serum HBeAg positive have active viral DNA replication, as shown by the presence of HBV DNA in the serum and replicative DNA intermediate molecules in the liver (H J Alter et al 1976, Bréchot et al 1981b, Kaw et al 1982, Alberti et al 1983, Scotto et al 1983b, Tur-Kaspa et al 1984, Karayiannis et al 1985, Matsuyama et al 1985, Moestrup et al 1985, Chu et al 1985a, Carloni et al 1986, D J Chen et al 1986, Gowans 1986, Grenfield et al 1986, Lee et al 1986, Feinman et al 1988, Govindarajan et al 1988, Krosgaard 1988, Kuhns et al 1988, Michikata et al 1988, Peng et al 1988, Zarski et al 1989, Pol et al 1990, Scott et al 1990, Pontisso et al 1992). However, a significant proportion of these subjects have no detectable serum HBV DNA. The frequency of this finding is mostly related to the duration and severity of the liver disease (Chu et al 1985a, b, Karayiannis et al 1985, Chaussade et al 1986, Wu et al 1986, 1987). It has been estimated that around 10% of HBeAg-positive subjects with chronic active hepatitis are negative for HBV DNA; in contrast, up to 30% of patients with cirrhosis have been found to be HBV DNA negative, mostly around the Mediterranean Basin and in Africa (possibly as a result of early contamination in these areas). This dissociation between the results of the HBeAg and HBV DNA tests is generally transient, and is followed by the disappearance of HBeAg and the appearance of anti-HBe. However, in a few cases, patients may be persistently HBV DNA negative despite HBeAg positivity and the absence of treatment; it is unclear whether this reflects a low level of HBV DNA replication or, possibly, synthesis of HBeAg from integrated HBV DNA, without encapsidation. In Asia, most infected subjects still have ongoing viral replication when cirrhosis and hepatocellular carcinoma occur. The reasons for these geographical differences are unclear; in particular, there is no evidence for a link with viral mutations.

A dissociation between the HBe and HBV DNA test results is also frequently observed in the acute stage of infection; HBV DNA is detectable in approximately 30–70% of patients with acute benign hepatitis (Krogsgaard et al 1985, Lok et al 1985, Lugassy et al 1987, Pontisso et al 1986, Wood et al 1988) but only 10% of cases of fulminant hepatitis (Bréchot et al 1984, De Cock et al 1986, Govindarajan et al 1986) at admission to hospital. The persistence of serum HBV DNA is predictive of the development of a chronic carrier state (Fig. 27.4).

Anti-HBe-positive individuals. One of the most informative findings obtained with HBV DNA tests has been the identification of subjects with ongoing, often intense, viral DNA replication despite anti-HBe positivity (Lok et al 1984, Chu et al 1985a, Karayiannis et al 1985, Pontisso et al 1985, Bonino et al 1986, Chaussade et al 1986, Grenfield et al 1986, Lee at al 1986, Wu et al 1986, 1987, Fattovich et al 1988, Govindarajan et al 1988, Krosgaard 1988, Norder et al 1989, Scott et al 1990, Naoumov et al 1992). This phenomenon also varies according to the geographic origin of the patients, but is present in all areas.

In Northern Europe, 10–20% of anti-HBe-positive patients with chronic hepatitis have serum HBV DNA; in contrast, only 1–5% of chronic carriers with normal laboratory liver tests are positive for HBV DNA. These latter subjects might already have chronic active hepatitis (CAH) despite normal liver test results or be at a risk of developing CAH during follow-up. In the Mediterranean Basin and Asia the prevalence of this finding is much higher (up to 40 or 50% of cases).

It is now established that anti-HBe-and HBV DNA-positive individuals can transmit the virus (including mother-to-child transmission). In addition, they are at risk of severe liver diseases and are being considered for treatment programmes.

Follow-up of HBsAg-positive chronic carriers. Combined tests for HBe-Ag, anti HBe and HBV DNA (spot tests and Southern blot assay) have allowed two major events during the course of HBV infection to be characterized.

1. Termination of viral multiplication. This can occur spontaneously or during antiviral treatment and is generally associated with HBe–anti-HBe seroconversion. As mentioned earlier, this is part of the natural history of the infection and may be a late or early event. In

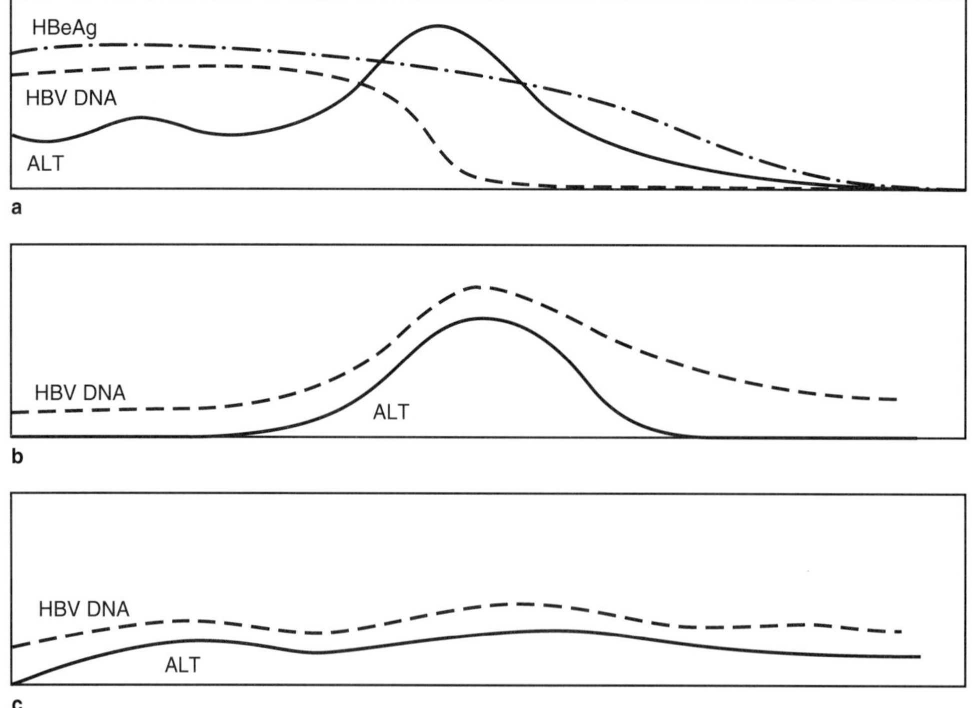

Fig. 27.4 Dissociation between HBeAg and HBV DNA during HBV chronic infection. (a) Delayed HBeAg anti-HBe seroconversion; (b) reactivation of HBV multiplication in anti-HBe+ patients; (c) persistent HBV multiplication in anti-HBe+ patients.

some patients a marked elevation of aminotransferase precedes the arrest of HBV DNA replication; in this case, there is often a period in which HBV DNA is no longer detected, despite the persistence of HBeAg; HBeAg disappears later and anti-HBe then emerges.

2. Reactivation of viral multiplication (Hess et al 1988, Liaw et al 1988, Krosgaard et al 1990). This can occur at various times after the disappearance of HBV DNA, and clearly identified risk factors are rare. The reactivation of viral DNA replication can be associated with the reappearance of HBeAg but can also occur despite the persistence of anti-HBe.

Tests for HBV DNA are thus mandatory for the interpretation of increased transaminases in chronic carriers, as they can help to distinguish between the arrest of viral multiplication and the reactivation of HBV DNA replication and to analyse modifications of HBV viraemia in the context of co-infections with hepatitis D (Bas et al 1988, Wu et al 1988), hepatitis C (HCV) or human type 1 immunodeficiency virus (HIV-1) (Housset et al 1992). Testing for HBV DNA is also of special interest in the follow-up of patients undergoing liver transplantation (Féray et al 1990, Repp et al 1991); a positive test for HBV DNA prior to liver transplantation indicates a major risk of reinfection of the graft despite immunotherapy, while patients without detectable replication may benefit from anti-HBs immunoglobulins. In addition, because of the immunosuppressive therapy, the serological profile of these patients is difficult to interpret.

Hepatitis B surface antigen-negative patients

HBV DNA sequences can be identified in the serum, liver and peripheral blood mononuclear cells (PBMCs) of patients with acute and chronic hepatitis, as well as those with primary liver cancer (PLC), who lack the standard HBV serological markers (Bréchot et al 1981a, 1985, Scotto et al 1983b, Tassopoulos et al 1986, Bréchot 1987, Pol et al 1987, Thiers et al 1988a, 1988b, ME Lai et al 1989, Mariyama et al 1989, M–Y Lai 1990, Rumi et al 1990, Tanaka et al 1990, Fagan et al 1991, Luo et al 1991, Marcellin et al 1991, Nalpas et al 1992a). It is likely that several factors are involved in these unusual patterns. The number of viral particles identified in serum and cells containing HBV DNA is low (around 10^4–10^5/ml, 0.01% of total liver cells), while genetic variations in viral DNA and modifications in the host immune response may also be important.

The first studies were performed using Southern blot and spot test procedures. In the liver, the results were consistent with the presence of both free and integrated viral DNA (also reviewed in Bréchot 1987). However, in patients with PLC only a small percentage of tumour cells contained viral DNA and no clear evidence for clonal proliferation of the infected liver cells was obtained. It is important to note that none of these experiments gave evidence of an increase in the hybridization signal after lowering the stringency of hybridization conditions. The size of the hybridizing DNA bands was that of regular HBV DNA (3.2 kb). The results thus suggested the presence of HBV or HBV with minor genetic variations in the tissue and serum samples.

However, different results have been obtained by several authors, who failed to detect HBV DNA in HBsAg-negative individuals. This led to discussions on the differences between the patients and the existence of false-negative or -positive results due, respectively, to the small amount of viral DNA and liver contamination by plasmids.

Using PCR, we and several other groups have confirmed the presence of HBV DNA sequences in serum and liver samples from HBsAg-negative individuals and determined the nucleotide sequences of some isolates. In view of the small amount of viral DNA in these subjects, the identification of HBsAg-negative, HBV DNA-positive subjects is now best done by means of PCR. The clinical implications of these results are discussed on p. 423.

Detection of HBV DNA by means of PCR

Single-step PCR is sufficient to detect HBV DNA (Mack & Sninsky 1988, Bréchot 1990) or

RNA and there is no need for nested PCR. In addition, the high degree of homology between the nucleotide sequences from different HBV subtypes markedly simplifies primer design. It is clear, however, that the efficiency can be very different and that appropriate controls must be used.

As mentioned above, PCR should not be viewed as a routine diagnostic test for HBV infection, but there is a need for more sensitive tests to identify HBV DNA sequences:

1. HBsAg-positive blood donors or mothers have been shown to transmit HBV, despite being serum anti-HBe positive and HBV DNA negative (Shiraki et al 1980, De Virgiliis et al 1985, Krosgaard et al 1986, Lee et al 1986).
2. Some patients with HBsAg-positive and anti-HBe positive CAH have active liver disease despite serum HBV DNA negativity and the absence of HDV or HCV co-infection, auto-immune liver disease or liver disease of other aetiologies.
3. It is important to obtain precise follow-up data for patients on antiviral therapy, to evaluate partial or complete responses and the risk of reactivation.
4. PCR is necessary for subsequent sequencing of amplified products (either directly or after cloning) (Bréchot 1990). PCR has provided a 'window' on the genetic variability of HBV (Orito et al 1989), the precise typing of HBV DNA, the potential implications of mutations in the pre-C, C and pre-S/S sequences in the persistence of HBV infection, the severity of liver disease and the response to treatment (Okamoto et al 1987, 1990b, Carman et al 1989, Brunetto et al 1990, Kremsdorf et al 1990, Liang et al 1990, 1991b, Yatsumoto et al 1990, Ehata et al 1991, Gerken 1991a, Kosaka et al 1991, Lin et al 1991, Ljunggren et al 1991, Omato et al 1991, Tran et al 1991, Wakita et al 1991, Yokosuka et al 1991, Brown et al 1992, Naoumov et al 1992).
5. The reliable detection of HBV DNA sequences in HBsAg-negative patients is markedly facilitated by PCR.

Hepatitis B surface antigen-positive subjects (Fig. 27.5, Table 27.3)

Several studies have shown that PCR can be used for HBV DNA detection in serum, plasma, liver and PBMCs (Larzul et al 1988, 1989, 1990, Mack & Sninsky 1988, Kaneko et al 1989a, b, Sumazaki et al 1989, Ulrich et al 1989, Féray et al 1990, 1993, Kaneko & Miller 1990, Keller et al 1990, Quint et al 1990, Shih et al 1990, Baginski et al 1991, Baker et al 1991, Barlet et al 1991, Carman et al 1991, Chemin et al 1991, Cheyrou et al 1991, Gerken et al 1991b, Loriot et al 1992). The detection limit is 10–100 molecules per ml. Comparative analysis of sera by PCR and inoculation into chimpanzees showed that PCR could be used to detect HBV DNA in the last infectious dilution. It must be noted, however, that the HBV DNA sequences identified by PCR may not always be included in viral particles but rather correspond to minute amounts of leucocyte DNA contaminating the most carefully prepared serum or plasma samples. A potential approach to this problem is the amplification, from the same sample, of a cellular locus such as an HLA gene; a positive PCR result obtained for HBV and not for the HLA primers would demonstrate viraemia. An alternative solution is to capture viral particles prior to the amplification, by using anti-HBs antibodies.

Table 26.2 shows a compilation of the results obtained so far. Figure 27.5 shows a representative result obtained in our laboratory; around 50% of HBsAg-positive and anti-HBe-positive asymptomatic carriers who were HBV DNA negative in a regular spot test had HBV DNA identified by PCR. In contrast, HBV DNA was detected in almost all HBsAg-positive subjects with CAH and none of those with resolved acute hepatitis or negative controls.

This observation has two main implications:

1. PCR is highly sensitive, detecting as few as 10 HBV particles per ml.
2. PCR is not positive for all HBV carriers and the results may thus have prognostic implications.

It is, however, clear that quantitative tests will be necessary to evaluate the real value of the test in

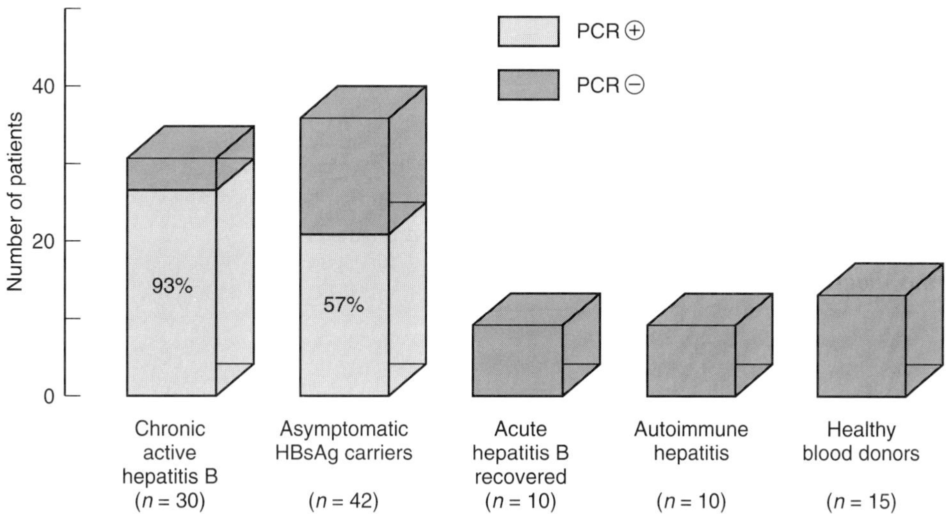

Fig. 27.5 PCR assay for the detection of HBV DNA: representative results obtained in HBV carriers (from: Gerken et al 1991b).

chronic HBV infection. In particular, it would not be wise to initiate antiviral therapy in all patients who are HBV DNA positive by PCR but negative by spot test assays. Some of our recent results indicate that at least a semiquantitative estimation of HBV DNA can be obtained, which is a promising result for more precise follow-up of antiviral therapy and prediction of future relapse of viral multiplication.

Given its sensitivity, PCR can be extremely useful in determining the efficacy of antiviral treatment; PCR has indeed given negative results for the serum of some patients a long time after interferon therapy (Korenman et al 1991). Not surprisingly, HBV DNA was still detectable in the liver of such patients despite clearance of serum HBsAg (Marcellin et al 1990). It will also be important to evaluate the time required for the HBV DNA assay to become negative after resolution of acute hepatitis or termination of HBV multiplication.

HBV DNA and RNA have both been detected by PCR in PBMCs, confirming results obtained without amplification. The technique is interesting for the appraisal of HBV infection after liver grafting, indicating in some cases a 'window', during which the liver graft is not yet reinfected although HBV DNA is present in PBMCs; this is often followed by reinfection of the liver, probably from PBMC (Fezay et al 1990).

Finally, although PCR is not necessary for routine diagnosis of HBV mother-to-child transmission, it can be used for direct evaluation, and to identify the HBV strains contaminating the newborn (Mitsuda et al 1989, Lin et al 1990).

Hepatitis B surface antigen-negative patients (Table 27.4)

The possibility of amplifying the viral DNA and RNA prior to detection has enabled previous reports of HBV DNA in HBsAg-negative subjects to be confirmed (Thiers et al 1988b, 1992, Kaneko et al 1989b, Kremsdorf et al 1990, Paterlini et al 1990, Coursaget et al 1991, Dazza et al 1991, Liang et al 1991a, Wang et al 1991, Féray et al 1993, Loriot et al 1992, Pontisso et al 1992, Wright et al 1992). In addition, transmission experiments to chimpanzees demonstrated that the viral DNA sequences were contained in infectious transmissible particles, with the serological profiles in the infected animals providing clues as to the nature of these HBV genomes. Two patterns were identified; in some animals serum HBsAg became clearly detectable with regular assays during acute hepatitis, thus demonstrating that a small amount of circulating HBV DNA was present in the patient whose serum was used for injection. This resembled the situation in infections by the so-called 'HBV-2'

Table 27.4 HBV DNA in serum HBsAg-negative patients: detection by PCR

	HBV DNA (PCR)	Geographical	References
Chronic hepatitis	3/11*	Japan	Kaneko et al 1989b
	2/13	France	Loriot et al 1992
	4/9	Sénégal	Coursaget et al 1991
	2/36	France	Porchon et al 1992
	3/26	France	Barlet et al 1991
	0/11	Japan	Yokosuka et al 1991
	4/8	Japan	Kaneko et al 1989b
	21/67$^+$	Israël	Liang et al 1991a
	39/217		
Primary liver (hepatocarcinoma: HCC)	2/3 HCC	Italy	Pontisso et al (in press)
	0/6 Hepatoblastomas		
	18/31 HCC ǂ	Sénégal	Coursaget et al 1991
	10/19 HCC	France/Italy	Paterlini et al 1990
	6/8 HCC	South Africa	
	36/61		
Asymptomatic carriers	9^ζ/206	Taïwan	Wang et al 1991
	7/42	Sénégal	Coursaget et al 1991
	8/107	Taïwan	Shih et al 1990
Acute	1/19	France	Thiers et al (in press)
post-transfusional	1/19	Taïwan	Wang et al 1991
fulminant	6/12 (liver)	France, USA	Wright et al 1992

*Patients HBsAg+ with subsequent negativation of serum HBsAg during follow-up.
+11.21 without any HBV serological marker.
ǂ6/13 without any HBV serological marker.
ζ2/9 without any HBV serological marker.

(Coursaget et al 1987), in which the unusual serological pattern (anti-HBc negativity) mostly reflects abnormal host immune response. In contrast, other animals with acute hepatitis did not develop the usual HBV serological markers, and some were infected despite the presence of anti-HBs before inoculation; this raised the issue of mutations in the viral genome modifying HBV epitopes.

PCR has recently provided access to the nucleotide sequence of these variants. We have determined the complete sequence of two HBV DNAs isolated from infected chimpanzees. Extensive homology was found, with only a few point mutations (less than 1%) relative to the regular HBV subtype *ayw*. Some of these mutations had previously been identified in other HBV subtypes. The majority were located on the third base of the codon and did not lead to amino acid changes. None was located in the enhancer element of HBV or in the viral gene promoters. They did not induce a stop codon in the gene coding for polymerase activity. It is important to note that the chimpanzees were negative for HBV by PCR assay before injection of the HBV DNA-positive sera and were therefore free of latent HBV infection.

The low rate of mutation observed in these isolates is thus striking. However, previous results have shown that a single point mutation in the S antigenic region can induce either a change from one HBV subtype to another of the loss of expression of a subtype determinant. It is also important to note that the amino acid substitutions observed in this study were located in antigenic regions of the pre-S and S regions and might have been involved in the negative serological results. Amino acid substitutions were observed in the pre-C/C coding sequence, and these mutations might have led to modifications in the antigenicity of the viral particles. These findings are also reminiscent of the identification of single amino acid variations in the S protein of 'escape mutants' recently reported in vaccination programmes.

We were recently able to extend these results by transfection of the viral envelope gene into mouse fibroblast L cells. Pre-S2/S/encoding sequences, under the control of an SV40 regulatory element, from two HBsAg isolates were analysed. Transfection of these constructs into mouse L cells led to the detection in the supernatant of HBsAg and pre-S2 epitopes in a regular assay (Kremsdorf et al, in press). These observations indicate that the negativity of the serum for HBsAg cannot be solely explained by genetic variations that would modify the structure of HBsAg. Further experiments will be required to test whether modification of the surface antigen could account for the apparent non-protection by anti-HBs in some chimpanzees during the inoculation experiments. It should also be noted that, in addition to genetic variations, quantitative modifications in the expression of the different viral genes might be involved in the serological response of the host. In this regard, we have always observed, in both HBsAg-negative humans and chimpanzees, a low level of HBV multiplication. Recently, there have been other reports of nucleotide sequences of HBV DNA from HBsAg-negative subjects. For one of these isolates, transfection experiments indicated a low level of replication, probably as a result of point mutations in the polymerase gene.

Additional explanations should also be considered, bearing in mind the importance of the immune response to the virus. Circulation of HBsAg in immune complexes has been demonstrated in the serum of HBsAg-negative individuals. Further, a minor or absent immune response to HBsAg has been documented after vaccination, and this may also be the case for HBsAg. Taken together, these different observations suggest that it is a combination of various viral and/or host factors that result in unexpected serological profiles.

Finally, the detection of HBV DNA in HBsAg-negative alcoholics points to a further possibility. Alcohol has been shown to modify the exportation of several proteins by the liver and it is tempting to speculate that this might be also the case for HBsAg secretion. Recent experiments performed on HBsAg-producing transgenic mice indeed indicated that alcohol might reduce the secretion of HBsAg into the serum (Nalpas et al 1992a).

Clinical implications of HBV in HBsA-negative individuals: interplay with hepatitis C virus (HCV) infection

Acute and chronic hepatitis. HBV DNA sequences have been identified in serum and liver of patients with acute and chronic hepatitis (mostly sporadic but also post-transfusional), and primary liver cancer. Although this does not demonstrate a role for the virus in these liver diseases, it indicates that a productive infection (i.e. with ongoing viral multiplication) persist in these individuals. It is, in particular, likely that HBV can still be involved in some cases of PTH (Baginski et al 1992, Thiers et al 1992), and this is consistent with the detection of HBV DNA in HBsAg-negative blood donors in various geographical areas. By contrast, we were unable to detect viral DNA in the serum of patients with resolved acute hepatitis B. Thus, persistence of viral DNA is not always observed after HBV infection, further suggesting that it might be relevant to hepatitis and liver carcinogenesis.

On the other hand, it is now clear that infection by hepatitis C virus (HCV) is a major aetiological factor in non-A, non-B acute and chronic hepatitis. In a recent study (Porchon et al 1992), 73% of our patients with post-transfusional and sporadic chronic hepatitis were found to be anti-HCV positive in RIBA-2 tests, most also being HCV RNA positive. Individuals co-infected by HCV and HBV, as shown by both serological and PCR tests, have now been identified in this group of non-A, non-B hepatitis, as well as in some HBsAg-positive carriers. It has been suggested that HCV infection might lower the rate of HBV multiplication, and possibly also lead to negative serum HBsAg test results in some cases. In contrast, the effect of HBV on HCV expression is not known.

HBsAg-negative primary liver cancer. We have recently confirmed by means of PCR that HBV DNA can be detected in the tumour tissue of HBsAg-negative subjects (including completely seronegative individuals) (Paterlini et al 1990). Careful comparative analysis of the results obtained in serum, and non-tumorous and tumorous liver samples from the same patients, yielded defective forms of HBV DNA in the tumour, while apparently intact viral genomes were identified in the serum and non-tumorous tissues (Paterlini et al 1992). This indicated that, although present in only a small percentage of tumour cells, the viral DNA is integrated into a clonally expanded population of liver cells. The results were not merely due to contamination by circulating serum virions or non-tumorous cells, and thus support the hypothesis that HBV induces at least one of the steps in liver carcinogenesis. Further studies will aim to test whether molecular mechanisms similar to those discussed in HBsAg-positive HCC may occur and whether HBV and HCV have synergistic effects.

In summary: The routine use of PCR for the detection of HBV DNA is still limited to the following settings:

1. detection of HBV replication in HBsAg+, anti-HBe+ patients with active liver disease, despite a negative spot test for HBV DNA.
2. appraisal of HBsAg-negative liver diseases.
3. follow-up of HBV infection in liver transplantation programmes.

Other potential applications are:

- follow-up of antiviral treatment (pending quantitative assays).
- detection of HBV DNA in blood donors (pending automatization).

DETECTION OF HEPATITIS C VIRUS (HCV) RNA

Hepatitis C virus is the major aetiological agent of sporadic and post-transfusional non-A, non-B hepatitis (C E Alter et al 1989, Choo et al 1989, Aach et al 1991, Houghton et al 1991, Kremsdorf et al 1991, Kuroki et al 1991). It is an RNA virus related to the flaviviruses and pestiviruses (Miller & Purcell 1990, Houghton et al 1991). The viral genome is approximately 10 kb long and encodes a large polyprotein that is secondarily processed into structural and non-structural proteins (Harada et al 1991, Houghton et al 1991). The diagnosis of HCV infection is based on the detection of antibodies to some of the structural and non-structural proteins (Miyamura et al 1990, Houghton et al 1991, Kuroki et al 1991, Van der Poel et al 1991). Several assays made by various companies are now available; they are based on either expressed viral proteins or synthetic peptides. Despite significant improvements, serological assays still have serious limitations:

- seroconversion to HCV is generally delayed after the acute infection.
- HCV infection can occur in chronically infected patients, despite persistent seronegativity.
- some serological results are difficult to interpret (e.g. the 'indeterminate' RIBA).
- there is no serological test for HCV antigens or HCV multiplication.
- mother-to-child HCV transmission is difficult to demonstrate because of the persistence of maternal anti-HCV.

PCR for HCV RNA detection

A large number of studies have shown the value of PCR for the detection of HCV RNA, since it overcomes the problems raised by the use of conventional methodology for detecting very low-level HCV viraemia (10^4–10^5 viral particles per ml). PCR can be performed on RNA purified from serum, plasma, liver tissue or PBMCs. However, some technical considerations must be borne in mind:

- storage of the RNA: rapidly frozen, unthawed samples will yield more reliable results. It has been shown that heparin may inhibit PCR, and plasma should be collected with EDTA (Hsu et al 1991).
- material: 100–200 μl is generally used.
- design of primers: this is of major importance in view of the genetic variability of HCV. Four HCV types have been described but, given the conservation of the 5' non-coding region, primers synthesized from this sequence are undoubtedly the most efficient (Christiano et al 1990, Kato et al 1990, Cha et al 1991, Choo et al 1991, Houghton et al 1991, Ogata et al 1991, Bukh et al 1992, P J Chen et al

1992, Féray et al 1992, Hibbs et al 1992, Okamoto et al 1992, 1990a). The core sequence has also been used in some studies. In addition, HCV variants have been described in which even the 5' non-coding sequence diverges; it may therefore be useful to retest some negative samples by using a combination of primers, including the NS3, NS4 and NS5 regions of the HCV genome (Christiano et al 1990).

- Nested PCR has been proposed (Garson et al 1990a, Féray et al 1992) for a further enhancement of the sensitivity of the assay; it consists of two steps with four primers that markedly increase the specificity and, thus, the sensitivity of the assay. There is, however, a major risk of contamination with this procedure, linked to the aerosols generated by opening the test tube. We use two protocols with the same overall sensitivity (Fig. 27.6):
  — nested PCR in a single tube,
  — single-step PCR with three primers (one for cDNA synthesis and two for amplication).

PCR can also be used to detect (depending on the primers used to initiate cDNA synthesis) both positive ('genomic') and negative viral RNA strands (Fong et al 1991); the significance of the negative strand is not yet clear but, by analogy with flaviviridae replication, it probably represents replicative intermediates. It has recently been suggested that, in the absence of complete inactivation of reverse transcriptase after cDNA synthesis, false-positive results might be obtained when detecting negative HCV RNA (Tahekara et

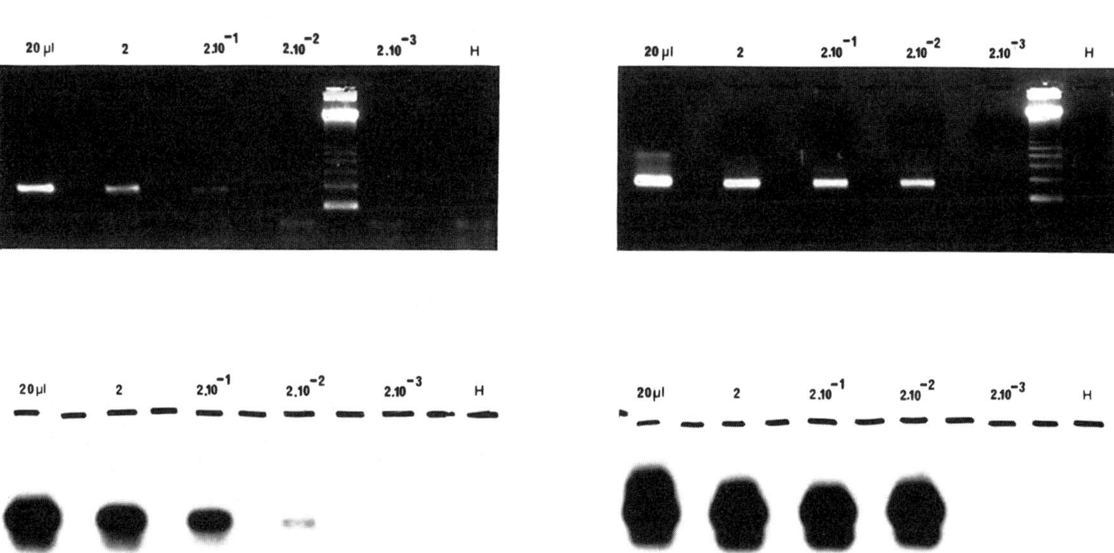

Fig. 27.6 Detection of the HCV RNA through PCR. Two different procedures, used in our laboratory with the same overall sensitivity, are shown. The single-step PCR, using three different primers, avoids the use of the nested PCR; it is however necessary to have the same sensitivity as nested PCR to hybridize the amplified products. Nested PCR allows a direct visualization of the amplified products but induces a high risk of contamination; thus we use a 'one-tube' nested PCR (see Féray et al 1992a).

al 1992). This is an important issue since these negative RNA molecules have been detected in serum and PBMCs, as well as in liver samples. Negative RNA in the serum might correspond to replicative intermediates encapsidated and secreted prior to completion of HCV RNA replication (a finding already reported for HBV but not previously explored for the flaviviruses and pestiviruses). We have recently been able to confirm the presence of these negative HCV RNA molecules in serum and mononuclear cells (Paterlini et al 1990, Zignego et al 1992).

HCV RNA detection in serum and plasma (Tables 27.5, 27.6)

Anti-HCV-positive patients

Acute infection (Shimizu et al 1990, Zanaro et al 1990, Farci et al 1991, Beach et al 1992). HCV viraemia can be detected as soon as a few days after contamination. HCV RNA becomes undetectable after resolution of acute hepatitis, while it persists if chronic infection develops.

Chronic infection. (Gerritzen & Scholt 1990, Garson et al 1990b, Kato et al 1990b, Weiner et al 1990, Allain et al 1991a, b, Inchauspe et al 1991, Lucey & Traber 1991, Tedder et al 1991, Féray et al 1992, Hagiwara et al 1992, Porchan et al 1992, Takehara et al 1992). Most anti-HCV-positive patients with chronic hepatitis have detectable HCV RNA in the serum or plasma. A few subjects score negative but the viral RNA can be identified in the liver; it is not clear if this reflects intermittent viraemia in these patients. A positive test for anti-HCV is also generally associated with HCV viraemia in other clinical situations; chronic alcoholics have been shown to have an increased prevalence of anti-HCV positivity (around 15% in our experience) (Nalpas et al 1991, Nishiguchi et al 1991). We have recently shown that HCV RNA is detected in the serum of the vast majority of these subjects, the viral infection possibly worsening the liver disease (Nalpas et al 1992b). This is also the case in most of anti-HCV-positive patients under haemodialysis (Pol et al 1992).

Detection of HCV viraemia can also be very useful in patients with CAH associated with markers of autoimmunity. Adults with anti-LKM1 autoantibodies have a high prevalence of anti-HCV. HCV RNA has been identified in the serum of most of these patients, a finding that confirmed serological test results and raised the issue of IFN treatment of these subjects (Magrin et al 1991). Other autoimmune diseases are associated with HCV infection, e.g. thyroiditis, cryoglobulinaemia and Sjögren's syndrome (Haddad et al 1992). HCV viraemia status will again be of major importance for the choice of therapeutic approaches.

On the other hand, PCR does not yet provide much information on the efficacy of IFN treatment. Serum HCV RNA parallels transaminase levels after therapy, being undetectable in case of remission and reappearing when relapse

Table 27.5 Serum and liver HCV RNA detected by PCR

Number of patients	Anti-HCV		References
	+	–	
Serum			
40	13+/16	7+/14	Kato et al 1990b
40	31+/36	4+/4	Cristiano et al 1990
156	121+/129	15+/27	Hagiwara et al 1992
30	19+/20	5+/10	Brillantini et al 1991
36	22+/27	5+/9	Porchon et al 1992
22 (HCC)	11+/22	0/11	Paterlini et al (in press)
Liver			
16	7+/10	2+/6	Weiner et al 1990
19	12+/19	ND	Shiëh et al 1991

Table 27.6 PCR for HCV RNA detection in patients with chronic hepatitis

	Anti-HCV +ve		Anti-HCV –ve	
	HCV RNA +ve	HCV RNA –ve	HCV RNA +ve	HCV RNA –ve
	299		75	
Serum	275 (92%)	24 (8%)	30 (48%)	39(52%)
Liver	24	12	2	8
	36		10	

Sources: Brillantini et al (1991), Cristiano et al (1990), Hagiwara et al (1992), Kato et al (1990), Paterlini et al (1993), Porchon et al (1992), Romeo et al (unpublished results), Weiner et al (1990), Shieh et al (1991).

occurs (Brillantini et al 1991). As a result, it gives no further clues as to the prediction of relapses. Assays providing a fast and at least semi-quantitative estimation of viraemia are clearly necessary before PCR can be used for monitoring in therapeutic protocols.

Anti-HCV-positive blood donors. Several studies have shown that most are potentially infectious (Garson et al 1990a, Ulrich et al 1991, Widell et al 1991). However, the status of blood donors who consistently have normal levels of transminases is not yet clear. We have recently shown that they actually constitute a heterogeneous group with regard to HCV viraemia: only some (4/27 in our study) have detectable serum HCV RNA. In view of the reports of chronic hepatitis in anti-HCV-positive blood donors with normal transaminase levels, PCR might be of value in identifying those who warrant more extensive investigation and, possibly, treatment.

Anti-HCV-negative patients

Acute, benign and fulminant hepatitis. As mentioned earlier, there is a delay in seroconversion to HCV; HCV RNA is the only marker of infection during the lag period.

There is no solid evidence that HCV infection alone is a cause of fulminant hepatitis (Féray et al 1992b). We recently studied subjects with HBsAg-positive and -negative fulminant hepatitis. Anti-HCV and HCV RNA were not detected in the serum or liver of the HBsAg-negative patients, and none originated from areas at risk for hepatitis E virus (HEV) infection. These results are similar to those reported in the USA (Wright et al 1991a, b) and UK but differ from a report in Japan (Yanagi et al 1991), where a significant proportion of patients with fulminant hepatitis had both HCV RNA and anti-HCV in the serum; it is not clear, however, if these Japanese subjects, in an area with a high rate of HCV infection, were really acutely infected or rather chronic carriers of HCV with a superimposed hepatitis of another origin. Altogether, these findings raise the unsolved issue of 'non-A, non-B, non-C, non-D, non-E' viruses.

In contrast to the negative results obtained among HBsAg-negative patients, we and others have shown that a large number of patients with HBs-Ag-positive fulminant hepatitis have detectable HCV RNA in the serum and/or liver. This suggests that HBV and HCV co-infections or superinfections may be involved in the pathogenesis of fulminant hepatitis.

Chronic hepatitis. HCA RNA has been found in the serum or liver of anti-HCV-negative subjects in all studies performed so far. This, in fact, has even been the case of blood donors with normal transaminase levels (Villa et al 1991, Sagitani et al 1992) and confirms that anti-HCV negative blood donors can transmit HCV infection. As also discussed for HBV, it is not known whether this seronegativity is related to genetic variability, low viral gene expression, the host immune response or a combination of these factors. In contrast, immunosuppressive therapy is clearly involved after liver transplantation and PCR is mandatory for the appraisal of HCV infection (given the high frequency of reinfection of the liver graft) (Féray et al 1992, Poterucha et al 1992).

Mother-to-child HCV transmission

PCR is of great value for the direct identification of infection in neonates. Maternal anti-HCV antibodies persist for an average of 12 months. Viral RNA has been detected in infants' sera by several investigators (Mitsuda et al 1989, Degos et al 1991, Inoue et al 1991, Kuroki et al 1991, Thaler et al 1991, Novati et al 1992), demonstrating the existence of this mode of transmission; the frequency of transmission seems to be related to the level of HCV viraemia in the mother. HCV RNA is rarely detected in neonates of anti-HCV-positive mothers without chronic hepatitis (F Roudot Thoraval, personal communication), in contrast to the high rate in mothers with chronic liver disease and/or HCV and HIV co-infection. We have also found a transient pattern of HCV viraemia in some infants, the implications of which remain to be determined (Novati et al 1992); this might in part explain discrepancies in the results of different studies.

PCR for the rapid identification of an HCV strain; implications of HCV genetic variability

Comparison of nucleotide sequences from the published HCV genomes in Japan, the USA and Europe shows the existence of distinct subtypes of HCV. The 5' non-coding and, to a lesser extent, the core and NS3–NS4 regions of the viral genome are well conserved (Houghton et al 1991, Nishigushi et al 1991, Ogata et al 1991, Martell et al 1992, Okamoto et al 1992, Weiner et al 1992) among different isolates. In contrast, the open reading frames encoding E1 and E2/NS1 – likely envelope proteins – are much less conserved. In the 5' part of the E2/NS1 sequence is a 'hypervariable' domain (HVR). It is possible to take advantage of this HVR to identify an HCV strain and its mutations during follow-up. This is achieved by amplification of the HVR using primers located on both sides on the E2/NS1 sequence, followed by nucleotide sequence analysis of the HVR. The main applications will be as follows.

Demonstration of reinfection of liver grafts by the original HCV strain

We have recently validated PCR as the most reliable test to identify HCV infection after liver transplantation. It has also been possible to demonstrate the recurrence of HCV infection on the liver graft by the original HCV strain (Féray et al 1992).

Analysis of mother-to-child and sexual HCV transmission

PCR can be used to demonstrate the identity of viral strains in different individuals.

Follow-up analysis of HCV RNA during IFN treatment

The cloning of the amplified products can show, in the serum of a given patient, a mix of different HCV RNA molecules derived from the same original strain (Martell et al 1992). A comparison of these molecules during the course of the infection may lead to the identification of particles that are selected (spontaneously or during treatment). This approach may be valuable for the identification in vivo of epitopes involved in the immune response to the virus (Weiner et al 1992).

PCR for the detection of HCV RNA in tissues and PBMCs

Liver samples

RNA extracted normally from frozen liver samples is suitable for PCR (Weiner et al 1990, Shibata et al 1991, Shieh et al 1991, Paterlini et al 1992). This approach can be useful in patients with chronic hepatitis and no detectable serum HCV RNA. The detection of the viral RNA in liver is also interesting for studies of the association between chronic HCV infection and primary liver cancer. The HCV genome does not integrate into cellular DNA. We have recently investigated French patients with HCC and found both ongoing HCV viraemia and the persistence of viral RNA in tumorous and non-tumorous tissues

(Paterlini et al 1992). This is in accordance with results from Japan (Yoneyama et al 1990, Chou et al 1991). Taken together, our investigations underline the association of HCC in HBsAG-negative patients in France with both HCV and HBV infections. It is not known whether the viral genome exerts a direct effect in liver cell transformation, but it has recently been shown that HCV RNA, like HBV DNA, can be detected in paraffin-embedded liver sections, enlarging the scope of tumours accessible to analysis.

A general problem in tumour studies with PCR is the risk of contamination by minute amounts of serum or non-tumour cells. To avoid this problem it is possible to take advantage of HCV genetic variability and, by amplifying the E2/NS1 hypervariable domain, to analyse comparatively the HCV RNA molecules present in the tumour and non-tumour samples. Using this approach, we were recently able to demonstrate significant sequence variations, showing the presence of the viral RNA in the tumour, which are probably due to a different rate of replication in tumour and non-tumour cells.

Peripheral mononuclear blood cells (PBMCs)

HCV RNA has been detected in the PBMCs of patients with chronic hepatitis. In most cases, HCV RNA was also detectable in the serum, raising the possibility of viral particles adsorbed to PBMCs. This problem has been addressed in our laboratory by using two complementary approaches (Zignego et al 1992):

- short-term cultures of PBMCs stimulated with mitogens (phytohaemagglutinin, PMA) showed an increase in the number of positive HCV RNA strands and detection of negative HCV RNA molecules.
- in situ hybridization has recently allowed us to confirm this observation (J Moldvay et al, unpublished results).

It is important to note, however, that other investigators, while detecting HCV RNA in PBMCs, failed to identify negative HCV RNA in these cells, in contrast to liver samples. It therefore remains to be established whether or not HCV replicates in uncultured PBMCs and which mononuclear cell populations are infected.

Infection of mononuclear blood cells by HCV may be involved in the immunopathology of liver cell necrosis, as well as in the persistence of the viral infection; it may also be of particular importance in infection of liver grafts and be involved in the emergence of HCV variants, as previously discussed for lymphocytic choriomeningitis virus (LCMV) and HIV. Finally, in view of these results, the role of HCV in aplastic anaemias has been raised; recent evidence indicates a minor role for HCV in this disease (Hibbs et al 1992, Pol et al 1990).

In situ hybridization for HCV RNA detection

It is possible to detect the viral RNA in liver sections, but the number of infected cells is controversial. It has been reported to be high in acutely infected chimpanzees. This is not our experience with samples from chronically infected patients, where only a few hepatocytes (diffusely distributed in the lobules) scored clearly as HCV RNA positive, a finding consistent with other reports. Furthermore, we also identified infected mononuclear blood cells in these liver section. Again, the level of HCV viraemia in the individual might account for the prevalence of positive results; indeed, we have only obtained unambiguous results so far in patients who are co-infected by HIV and HCV. Differences in the results might also reflect technical problems inherent to this method, including the use of RNA or oligonucleotide HCV probes. This issue will be of importance, as will viral antigen detection, for the appraisal of HCV immunopathology.

SUMMARY

Molecular biology has significantly improved our understanding of viral infections of the liver. HBV DNA and HCV RNA should be now viewed as reliable markers with real clinical applications. Marked improvements in non-radioactive probes and the development of convenient test formats will allow laboratories with limited expertise in the field to take advantage of these procedures. It is, however, important to consider them as complementary to serological assays (Tables 27.7, 27.8).

The place of PCR in these diagnostic tests is not yet settled, but there is no doubt that PCR is of major importance for the diagnosis of HCV infection. However, its widespread use remains presently severely restricted by several technical considerations, and the standardization programmes that have been now initiated are essential to validate investigations from different laboratories. Finally, the interpretation of a positive HCV RNA test may be difficult since the detection of the HCV RNA molecule per se does not always indicate infectivity. This will be important to consider when discussing, for example, the implications of detecting HCV RNA in saliva (Hsu et al 1991, Takamatsu et al 1990) or other biological fluids (Hsu et al 1991). Quantitative interpretation of PCR results is indeed a difficult task. But should be facilitated by ongoing progress with non-radioactive probes. Finally, the results of HCV RNA testing will have to be compared with those of new serological tests, particularly if assays for HCV antigens become available.

Despite all these reservations, PCR will benefit in the near future from significant improvements, such as automated handling of amplified products, amplification in microplates, simplified nucleic acid extraction procedures, to name but a few.

Table 27.7 Polymerase chain reaction (PCR) in viral hepatitis

Sensitive estimation of viral multiplication (too sensitive?), HBV, HCV, HDV

- Evaluation of infectivity?
- Follow-up of antiviral therapy

→

- PCR not always positive?
- Quantification?

Detection of HBV DNA and HCV RNA in seronegative patients
- Delayed seroconversion in acute HCV infection
- Seronegative chronic carriers (HBV and HCV)

Direct evaluation of mother to child HIV transmission

Analysis of genetic variability and its implications (HBV, HCV)

Table 27.8 PCR: limitations of the assay

1. Technical
   - False-positive (contamination) and false-negative (quality of DNA and RNA)
     — PCR with HLA (DNA) or cyclin (RNA) primers
     — Amount of serum or plasma used; conservation
   - Design of primers (prediction of efficacy on sequence analysis?)
   - Single-step (three primers) or nested PCR (one-tube assay)?
   - Quantification?
2. Interpretation
   - Intact or defective genomes?
     — 'Capture' with anti-HBs (HCV?) before PCR?
     — Comparison with infectious doses
   - Contamination of PBMCs or tissue samples by serum particles?
     — In situ hybridization
     — PCR profile with different primers
     — Sequence comparison

ACKNOWLEDGMENTS

I would like to thank Patricia Paterlini, Dina Kremsdorf and Valérie Thiers for critical reading of this chapter and David Young and Marianne Wagner for editing the manuscript.

REFERENCES

Aach R D, Stevens C E, Hollinger B et al 1991 Hepatitis C virus infection in post-transfusion hepatitis. An analysis with first and second generation assays. New England Journal of Medicine 1325–1329

Alberti A, Tremolada F, Fattovich G, Bartolotti F, Realdi G 1983 Virus replication and liver disease in chronic hepatitis B virus infection. Digestive Disease and Science 28: 962–966

Allain J P, Coghlan P J, Kenrick K G et al 1991a Prediction of hepatitis C virus infectivity in seropositive Australian blood donors by supplemental immunoassays and detection of viral RNA. Blood 78: 2462–2468

Allain J P, Dailey S H, Laurian Y, Vallari D S, Rafowicz A, Desai S M, Devare S G 1991b Evidence for persistent hepatitis C virus (HCV) infection in hemophiliacs. Journal of Clinical Investigation 88: 1672–1679

Alter C E, Stevens G E, Tegtmeier et al 1989 An assay for circulating antibodies to a major etiologic virus of human non-A, non-B hepatitis. Science 244: 362–364

Alter H J, Seeff, L B, Kaplan, P M et al 1976 Type B hepatitis: the infectivity of blood positive for e antigen DNA polymerase after accidental needlestick exposure. New England Journal of Medicine 295: 904–915

Bagasra O, Hauptman S P, Lischner H W, Sachs M,

Pomeranz, R J 1992 Detection of human immunodeficiency virus type I provirus in mononuclear cells by in situ polymerase chain reaction. New England Journal of Medicine 326: 1385–1391
Baginski I, Chemin I, Bouffard P, Hantz and Trepo C 1991 Detection of polyadenylated RNA in hepatitis B virus infected peripheral blood mononuclear cells by polymerase chain reaction. Journal of Infectious Diseases 163: 996–1000
Baginski I, Chemin I, Hantz O et al 1992 Transmission of serologically silent hepatitis B virus along with hepatitis C virus in two cases of posttransfusion hepatitis. Transfusion: 32: 215–220
Baker B L, Di Bisceglie M, Kaneko S, Miller R, Feinstone S M, Waggoner J G, Hoofnagle J H 1991 Determination of hepatitis B virus DNA in serum using the polymerase chain reaction: clinical significance and correlation with serological and biochemical markers. Hepatology 13: 632–636
Banerjee K, Khandekar P 1991 A bacteriophage M13 based sandwich hybrization assay for the detection of hepatitis B virus in human blood. Journal of Biochemistry and Biophysics 28: 93–95
Bas C, Bartolome J, La Banda F, Porres J C, Quiroga J A, Mora I, Carreno V 1988 Assessment of hepatitis B virus DNA levels in chronic HBsAg carriers with or without hepatitis delta virus superinfection. Journal of Hepatology 6: 208–213
Barlet V, Zarski J P, Thelu M A, Seigneurin J M 1991 Advantage of PCR for detecting low amounts of HBV DNA in patients' sera. Research in Virology 142: 373–379
Beach M J, Meeks E L Mimms L T et al 1992 Temporal relationships of hepatitis C virus RNA and antibody responses following experimental infection of chimpanzees. Journal of Medical Virology 36: 226–237
Berninger M, Hammer M, Hoyer B, Gerin J L 1982 An assay for the detection of the DNA genome of hepatitis B virus in serum. Journal of Medical Virology 9: 57–68
Bréchot C 1987 Hepatitis B virus (HBV) and hepatocellular carcinoma. HBV DNA status and its implications. Journal of Hepatology 4: 269–279
Bréchot C 1990 Polymerase chain reaction. A new tool for the study of viral infections in hepatology. Journal of Hepatology 11: 124–129
Bréchot C, Hadchouel M, Scotto J et al 1981a State of hepatitis B virus DNA in hepatocytes of patients with hepatitis B surface antigen-positive and negative liver diseases. Proceedings of the National Academy of Sciences of the USA 78: 3906
Bréchot C, Scotto J, Charnay P et al 1981b Detection of hepatitis B virus DNA in liver and serum: a direct appraisal of the chronic carrier state. Lancet 765–767
Bréchot C, Bernuau J, Thiers V et al 1984 Multiplication of hepatitis B virus in fulminant hepatitis B. British Medical Journal 288: 270–271
Bréchot C, Degos F, Lugassy C et al 1985 Hepatitis B virus DNA in patients with chronic liver disease and negative tests for hepatitis B surface antigen. New England Journal of Medicine 312: 270–276
Bonino F, Hoyer B, Nelson J, Engle R, Verme G, Gerin J 1981 Hepatitis B virus DNA in the sera of HBsAg carriers: a marker of active hepatitis B virus replication in the liver. Hepatology 1: 386–391
Bonino F, Rosina F, Rizzeto M et al 1986 Chronic hepatitis in HBsAg carriers with serum HBV-DNA and anti-HBe. Gastroenterology 90: 1268–1273
Boom R, Sol C J, Heijtink R, Wertheim-van Dillen P M, van der Noorda, J 1991 Rapid purification of hepatitis B virus DNA from serum. Journal of Clinical Microbiology 29: 1804–1811
Brillantini S, Garson J A, Tuke P W et al 1991 Effect of a-interferon therapy on hepatitis C viraemia in community-acquired chronic non-A, non-B hepatitis: a quantitative polymerase chain reaction study. Journal of Medical Virology 34: 136–141
Brown J L, William F, Carman F, Thomas H C 1992 The clinical significance of molecular variation within the hepatitis B virus genome. Hepatology 15: 144–148
Brunetto M R, Stemler M, Bonino F et al 1990 A new hepatitis B virus strain in patients with severe anti-HBe positive chronic hepatitis B. Journal of Hepatology 10: 258–261
Bukh J, Purcell H, Miller R 1992 Importance of primer selection for the detection of hepatitis C virus RNA with the polymerase chain reaction assay. Proceedings of the National Academy of Sciences of the USA 89: 187–191
Carloni G, Delfini C, Colloca D, Alfani E, Taliani G De Bac 1986 Incidence of hepatitis B virus DNA and DNA-polymerase in sera of Italian asymptomatic carriers with the serological markers of HBV. Archives of Virology 87: 97–105
Carman W F, Hadziyannis S, McGarvey M J, Jacyna M R, Karayiannis P, Makris A, Thomas H C 1989 Mutation preventing formation of hepatitis B e antigen in patients with chronic hepatitis B infection. Lancet i: 588–590
Carman W F, Zanetti A R, Karayiannis P et al 1990 Vaccine-induced mutant of hepatitis B virus. Lancet 336: 325–329
Carman W F, Dourakis S, Karayiannis P, Crossey M, Drobner R, Thomas H C 1991 Incidence of hepatitis B viraemia, detected using the polymerase chain reaction, after successful therapy of hepatitis B virus carriers with interferon alpha. Journal of Medical Virology 34: 114–118
Casacubetta J M, Jardi R, Buti M, Puigdomenech P, Segundo B S 1988 Comparison of different non-isotopic methods for hepatitis B virus detection in human serum. Nucleic Acids Research 16: 11834
Cha T A, Kolberg J, Irvine B et al 1991 Use of a signature nucleotidesequence of hepatitis C virus for detection of viral RNA in human serum and plasma. Journal of Clinical Microbiology 2528–2534
Chaussade S, Thiers V, Bréchot C, Boboc B, Berthelot P, Degos F 1986 L'antigenè HBe et l'ADN VHB chez les malades atteints d'hépatite chronique active. Gastroenterology and Clinical Biology 10: 744–747
Chemin I, Baginski I, Petit M A et al 1991 Correlation between HBV DNA detection by polymerase chain reaction and Pre S1 antigenemia in symptomatic and asymptomatic hepatitis B virus infections. Journal of Medical Virology 33: 51–57
Chen D S, Lai M Y, Lee S C, Yang P M, Sheu J C, Sung J L 1986 Serum HBsAg, HBeAg, anti HBe, and hepatitis B viral DNA in asymptomatic carriers in Taïwan. Journal of Medical Virology 19: 87–94
Chen M L, Shieh Y S, Shim K S, Gerber M A 1991 Comparative studies on the detection of hepatitis B virus DNA in frozen and paraffin sections by the polymerase chain reaction. Modern Pathology 4: 555–558
Chen P J, Lin M H, Tai K F, Liu P C, Chen D S 1992 The

Taiwanese hepatitis C virus genome: sequence determination and mapping the 5' termini of viral genomic and antigenomic RNA. Virology 188: 102–113

Cheyrou A, Guyomartch C, Jasserand P, Blouin P 1991 Improved detection of HBV DNA by PCR after microwave treatment of serum. Nucleic Acids Research 19: 4006

Choi Y J 1990 Persistent hepatitis B virus infection of mononuclear blood cells without concomitant liver infection. The liver transplantation model. Transplantation 49: 1155–1158

Choo Q L, Kuo G, Weiner A J, Overby L R, Bradley D W, Houghton M 1989 Isolation of a cDNA clone derived from a blood-borne non-A, non-B viral hepatitis genome. Science 244: 359–361

Choo Q L, Richman K H, Han J H et al 1991 Genetic organization and diversity of the hepatitis C virus. Proceedings of the National Academy of Sciences of the USA 88: 2451–2455

Chou W H, Yoneyama T, Takeuchi K, Harada H, Saito I, Miyamura T 1991 Discrimination of hepatitis C virus in liver tissues from different patients with hepatocellular carcinomas by direct nucleotide sequencing of amplified cDNA of the viral genome. Journal of Clinical Microbiology 29: 2860–2864

Chu C M, Karayiannis P, Fowler M J F, Monjardino J, Liaw Y F, Thomas H C 1985a Natural history of chronic hepatitis B virus infection in Taïwan: studies of hepatitis B virus DNA in serum. Hepatology 5: 431–434

Chu C H M, Liaw Y F, Sheen I S, Chen T J 1985b Correlation of age with the status of hepatitis B virus replication and histological changes in chronic type B hepatitis. Liver 5: 177–122

Coursaget P, Bourdil C, Adamowicz P et al 1987 HBsAg positive reactivity in man not due to hepatitis B virus. Lancet 12: 1354–1357

Coursaget P, Le Cann P, Leboulleux D, Diop M T, Bao O, Coll A M 1991 Detection of hepatitis B virus DNA by polymerase chain reaction in HBsAg negative Senegalese patients suffering from cirrhosis or primary liver cancer. FEMS Letters, 35–38

Cristiano K, Bisceglie A M, Hoofnagle J H, Feinstone S M 1990 Hepatitis C viral RNA in serum of patients with chronic non-A, non-B hepatitis: detection by the polymerase chain reaction using multiple primer sets. Hepatology 14: 51–55

Dazza M C, Meneses L V, Girard P M, Paterlini P, Villaroel C, Bréchot C 1991 Polymerase chain reaction for detection of hepatitis B virus DNA in HBsAg seronegative patients with hepatocellular carcinoma from Mozambique. Annals of Tropical Medicine and Parasitology. 85: 277–279

De Cock K M, Govindarajan S, Valinluck B, Redeker A G 1986 Hepatitis B virus DNA in fulminant hepatitis B. Annals of Internal Medicine 105: 546–547

Degos F, Thiers V, Erlinger S, Maisonneuve P, Noël L, Bréchot C, Benhamou J P 1991 Neonatal transmission of HCV from mother with chronic hepatitis. Lancet 338: 758

Dejean A, Lugassy C, Zafrani S, Tiollais P, Bréchot C 1984 Detection of hepatitis B virus DNA in pancreas, kidney and skin of two human carriers of the virus. Journal of General Virology 651–655

Dény P, Zignego A L, Rascalou N, Ponzetto A, Tiollais P, Bréchot C 1991 Nucleotide sequence analysis of three different hepatitis delta viruses isolated from a woodchuck and humans. Journal of General Virology 72: 735–739

Diegutis P S, Keirnan E, Burnett L, Nightingale B N, Cossart Y E 1986 False-positive results with hepatitis B virus DNA dot-hybridization in hepatitis B surface antigen negative specimens. Journal of Clinical Microbiology 23: 797–799

De Virgiliis S, Frau S, Sanne G et al 1985 Perinatal hepatitis B virus detection by hepatitis B virus-DNA analysis. Archives of Disease in Childhood 60: 56–58

Dittmann S, Roggendorf M, Dürkop J, Wiese M, Lorbeer B, Deinhardt F 1991 Long-term persistence of hepatitis C virus antibodies in a single source outbreak. Journal of Hepatology 13: 323–327

Dusheiko G M, Bowyer S M, Sjogren M H, Ritchie M J, Santos A P, Kew M C 1985. Replication of hepatitis B virus in adult carriers in an endemic area. Journal of Infectious Diseases 152: 566–571

Ehata T, Omata M, Yokosuka O, Hosoda K, Ohto M 1991 Variations in codons 84 101 in the core nucleotide sequence correlate with hepatocellular injury in chronic hepatitis B virus infection. Journal of Clinical Investigation 89: 332–338

Fagan E A, Guarner P, Perera S D K et al 1985 Quantitation of hepatitis B virus DNA (HBV-DNA) in serum using the spot hybridization technique and scintillation counting. Journal of Virological Methods 12: 251–262

Fagan E A, Davidson F D, Trowbridge R, Carman W F, Smith H M, Tedder R, Willimas R 1991 Detection of hepatitis B virus DNA sequences in liver in HBsAg seronegative patients with liver disease with and without anti-HBe antibodies. Quarterly Journal of Medicine 78: 123–134

Farci P, Alter H J, Wong D, Miller R H, Shih J W, Jett B, Purcell R H 1991 A long term study of hepatitis C virus replication in non-A, non-B hepatitis. New England Journal of Medicine 325: 98–104

Fattovich G, Brollo L, Alberto A, Pontisso P, Giustina G, Realdi G 1988 Long term follow-up of anti HBe positive chronic active hepatitis B. Hepatology 8: 1651–1654

Féray C, Zignego A L, Samuel D, Bismuth A, Reynes A, Bismuth H, Bréchot C 1990 Persistent hepatitis B virus liver infection: the liver transplantation model. Transplantation 49: 1155–1158

Féray C, Samuel D, Thiers V et al 1992 Reinfection of liver graft by hepatitis C virus (HCV) after liver transplantation. Journal of Clinical Investigation 89: 1361–1365

Féray C, Gigou M, Samuel D et al 1993 Hepatitis C virus RNA and hepatitis B virus DNA in serum and liver of patients with fulminant hepatitis. Gastroenterology 104: 549–555

Feinman S V, Berris B, Guha A et al 1984 DNA: DNA hybridization method for the diagnosis of hepatitis B infection. Journal of Virological Methods 8: 199–206

Feinman S V, Berris B, Fay O, Sooknanan R, Tanno H E, Tung W W, Lieberman H M 1988 Serum HBV-DNA (hepatitis B virus DNA) in acute and chronic hepatitis B infection. Clinical and Investigative Medicine 11: 286–91

Fong T L, Shindo M, Feinstone S M, Hoofnagle J H, and Di Bisceglie A M 1991 Detection of replicative intermediates of hepatitis C viral RNA in liver and serum of patients with chronic hepatitis C. Journal of Clinical Investigation 88: 1058–1060

Fournier J G, Kessous A, Richer G, Bréchot C and Simard R 1982 Detection of hepatitis B viral RNAs in human liver tissues by in situ hybridization. Biology of the Cell 43: 225–228

Fowler M J F, Monjardino J, Weller I V D, Lok A S F,

Thomas H C 1984 Analysis of the molecular state of HBV DNA in the liver and serum of patients with chronic hepatitis or primary liver cell carcinoma and the effect of therapy with adenine arabinoside. Gut 25: 611–618

Garson J A, Tuke P W, Makris M, Briggs M, Machin S J, Preston F E, Tedder R S 1990a Demonstration of viraemia patterns in haemophiliacs treated with hepatitis C virus contaminated factor VIII concentrates. Lancet 336: 1022–1025

Garson J A, Tedder R S, Briggs M et al 1990b Detection of hepatitis C viral sequences in blood donations by 'nested' polymerase chain reaction and prediction of infectivity. Lancet 335: 1419–1422

Gerritzen A, Scholt B 1990 A nonradiactive riboprobe assay for the detection of hepatitis B virus DNA in human sera. Journal of Virological Methods 30: 311–318

Gerken G, Gerlich W H, Bréchot C, Thomas H C, Bonino F de Moura C, Meyer Zum Buschenfelde K H 1992 Biological standards for hepatitis B virus assays Journal of Hepatology 15: 251–255

Gerken G, Kremsdorf D, Capel F et al 1991a Hepatitis B defective virus with rearrangements in the PreS gene during chronic HBV infection. Virology 183: 555–565

Gerken G, Paterlini P, Manns M et al 1991b Assay of hepatitis B virus DNA by polymerase chain reaction and its relationship to Pre S and S encoded viral surface antigens. Hepatology 13: 158–1166

Gmelin K, Theilman L, Will H, Czygan P, Doerr H W, Kommerel B 1985 Determination of HBV DNA by a simplified method of spot hybridization. Hepatogastroenterology 32: 117–120

Govindarajan S, DeCock K M, Valinluck B, Ashcavi M 1986 Serum hepatitis B virus DNA in acute hepatitis B. American Journal of Clinical Pathology 86: 352–354

Govindarajan S, Fong T L, Valinluck B, Edwards V, Redeker A G 1988 Markers of viral replication in patients with chronic hepatitis B virus infection. American Journal of Clinical Pathology 89: 233–237

Gowans E J 1986 Relationship between HBeAg and HBV DNA in patients with acute and persistent hepatitis B infection. Medical Journal of Australia 145: 439–441

Grenfield C, Osidinia V, Karayiannis P et al 1986 Perinatal transmission of hepatitis B virus in Kenya: its relation to the presence of serum HBV-DNA and anti-HBe in the mother. Journal of Medical Virology 19: 135–142

Guo K J, Bowden D S 1991 Digoxigenin-labeled probes for the detection of hepatitis B virus DNA in serum. Journal of Clinical Microbiology 29: 506–509

Hadchouel M, Pasquinelli C, Fournier J G, Hugon R N, Scotto J, Bernard O, Bréchot C 1988 Detection of mononuclear cells expressing hepatitis B virus in peripheral blood from HBsAg positive and negative patients by in situ hybridization. Journal of Medical Virology 24: 27–32

Haddad J, Deny P, Munz-Gotheil C et al 1992 Lymphocytic sialadenitis of Sjögren's syndrome associated with chronic hepatitis C virus liver disease. Lancet 339: 321–323

Hadziyannis S J, Lieberman H M, Karvountzis G G, Shafritz D A 1983 Analysis of liver disease, nuclear HBcAg, viral replication, and hepatitis B virus DNA in liver serum of HBeAg vs. anti-HBe positive carriers of hepatitis B virus DNA in serum. Hepatology 3: 656–662

Hagiwara H, Hayashi N, Mita E et al 1992 Detection of hepatitis C virus RNA in chronic non-A, non-B liver disease. Gastroenterology 102: 692–694

Harada S, Watanabe Y, Takeuchi K et al 1991 Expression of processed core protein of hepatitis C virus in mammalian cells. Journal of Virology 65: 3015–3021

Harrison T J, Bal V, Wheeler E G, Meacock T J, Harrison J F Zuckerman A J 1985 Hepatitis B virus DNA and e antigen in serum from blood donors in the United Kingdom positive for hepatitis B surface antigen. British Medical Journal 290: 6469

Hess G, Gerken G, Weber C, Manns M, Meyer Zum Buschenfelde K H 1988 Reactivation of chronic type B hepatitis: the effect of expression of serum HBV-DNA and pre-S encoded proteins. Journal of Medical Virology 25: 197–204

Hibbs J R, Fricklofen N, Rosenfeld S J et al 1992 Aplastic anemia and viral hepatitis non-A, non-B, non-C. Journal of the American Medical Association 267: 2051–4

Houghton M, Weiner A, Han J, Kuo G, Choo Q L 1991 Molecular biology of the hepatitis C viruses: implications for diagnosis, development and control of viral disease. Hepatology 2: 381–388

Housset C, Pol C, Carnot F 1992 Interactions between human immunodeficiency virus-1, hepatitis delta virus and hepatitis B virus in 260 chronic carriers of hepatitis B virus. Hepatology 15: 578–583

Hsu H H, Wright T L, Luba D et al 1991 Failure to detect hepatitis C virus genome in human secretions with the polymerase chain reaction. Hepatology 14: 763–767

Imazeki F, Omata M, Yokosura O, Matsuyama Y, Ito Y, Okuda K 1985 Analysis of DNA polymerase reaction products for detecting hepatitis B virus in serum: comparison with spot hybridization technique. Hepatology 5: 783–788

Inchauspe G, Abe K, Zebedee S et al 1991 Use of conserved sequences from hepatitis C virus for the detection of viral RNA in infected sera by polymerase chain reaction. Hepatology 14: 595–600

Inoue Y, Miyamura T, Unayama T, Takahashi K, Saito I 1991 Maternal transfer of HCV. Nature 353: 609

Kaneko S, Miller R H 1990 Characterization of primers for optimal amplification of hepatitis B virus DNA in the polymerase chain reaction assay. Journal of Virological Methods 29: 225–229

Kaneko S, Feinstone S M, and Miller R H 1989a Rapid and sensitive method for the detection of serum hepatitis B virus DNA using the polymerase chain reaction technique Journal of Clinical Microbiology 27: 1930–1933

Kaneko S, Miller R H, Feinstone S M, Unoura M, Kobayashi K, Hattori N, Purcell R H 1989b Detection of serum hepatitis B virus DNA in patients with chronic hepatitis using the polymerase chain reaction assay. Proceedings of the National Academy of Sciences of the USA 86: 312–316

Karayiannis P, Fowler M J F, Lok A S F, Greenfield C, Monjardino J, Thomas H C 1985 Detection of serum HBV DNA by molecular hybridization. Correlation with HBeAg/antiHBe status, racial origin, liver histology and hepatocellular carcinoma. Journal of Hepatology 1: 99–106

Kato N, Hijikata M, Oostsuyama Y, Nakagawa M, Ohkoshi S, Sugimura T, Shimothono K 1990a Molecular cloning of the human hepatitis C virus genome from Japanese patients with non-A, non-B hepatitis. Proceedings of the National Academy of Sciences of the USA 87: 9524–9528

Kato N, Yokosuka O, Omata M, Hosoda K, Ohto M 1990b Detection of hepatitis C virus ribonucleic acid in the serum by amplification with polymerase chain reaction. Journal of Clinical Investigation 86: 1764–1767

Kaw W, Rall L B, Smuckler E A, Schmid R, Rutter W J 1982 Hepatitis B viral DNA in liver and serum of asymptomatic carriers. Proceedings of the National Academy of Sciences of the USA 79: 7522–7526

Keller G H, Huang D P, Shih J W, Manak M M 1990 Detection of hepatitis B virus DNA in serum by polymerase chain reaction amplification and microtiter sandwich hybridization. Journal of Clinical Microbiology 28: 1411–1416

Korenman J, Baker B, Waggoner J, Everhart J E, Di Bisceglie A M, Hoofnagle J H 1991 Long term remission of choronic hepatitis B after alpha-interferon therapy. Annals of Internal Medicine 114: 629–634

Kosaka Y, Takase K, Kojima M et al 1991 Fulminant hepatitis B: induction by hepatitis B virus mutants defective in the precore region and incapable of encoding e antigen. Gastroenterology 100: 1087–1094

Kremsdorf D, Thiers V, Garreau F et al 1990 Nucleotide sequence analysis of three hepatitis B virus genomes isolated from serologically negative patients. In: Hollinger F B, Lemon S M, Margolis H S (eds) Viral hepatitis and liver disease. Williams & Wilkins, Baltimore, pp 222–226

Kremsdorf D, Porchon C, Kim J P, Reyes G R, Bréchot C 1991 Partial nucleotide sequence analysis of a french hepatitis C virus: implications for HCV genetic variability in the E2/NS1 protein. Journal of General Virology 72: 2557–2561

Kremsdorf D, Garreau F, Duclos H, Thiers V, Schellekens H, Petit M A, Bréchot C Complete nucleotide sequence in viral envelope protein expression of a hepatitis B virus DNA derived from a hepatitis B surface antigen-seronegative patient. Journal of Hepatology (in press)

Krosgaard K 1988 Hepatitis B virus DNA in serum applied molecular biology in the evaluation of hepatitis B infection. Liver 8: 1–27

Krosgaard K, Aldershvile J, Kryger P, Andersson P, Nielsen J O, Hansson B G The Copenhagen Hepatitis Acuta Programme 1985 Hepatitis B virus DNA, HBeAg and delta infection during the course from acute to chronic hepatitis B virus infection. Hepatology 5: 778–782

Krosgaard K, Wantzin P, Aldershville J, Kryger P, Andersson P, Nielsen J O 1986 Hepatitis B virus DNA in hepatitis B surface antigen-positive blood donors: relation to the hepatitis B e system and outcome in recipients. Journal of Infectious Diseases 153: 298–303

Krosgaard K, Aldershville J, Kryger P 1990 Reactivation of viral replication in anti-HBe positive chronic HBsAg carriers. Liver 10: 54–58

Kuhns M C, McNamara A L, Cabal C M, Decker R H, Thiers V, Bréchot C, Tiollais P 1988. A new assay for the quantitative detection of hepatitis B viral DNA in human serum. In: Hollinger F B, Lemon S H, Margolis H S (eds) Viral hepatitis and liver disease. Alan R Liss, New York, pp 258–262

Kuhns M C, McNamara A L, Perrillo R P, Cabal C M, Campbel C R 1989 Quantitation of hepatitis B viral DNA by solution hybridization: comparison with DNA polymerase and hepatitis B e antigen during antiviral therapy. Journal of Medical Virology 27(4): 274–281

Kuroki T, Nishiguchi S, Fukuda K et al 1991 Mother-to-child transmission of hepatitis C virus. Journal of Infectious Diseases 164: 427–428

Lai M E, Farci P, Figus A, Balestrieri A, Arnone M, Vyas G N 1989 Hepatitis B Virus DNA in the serum of Sardinian blood donors negative for the hepatitis B surface antigen. Blood 73: 17–19

Lai M Y, Chen P–J, Yang P–M, Sheu J–C, Sung J–L, Chen D–S 1990 Identification and characterization of intrahepatic hepatitis B virus DNA in HBsAg-seronegative patients with chronic liver disease and hepatocellular carcinoma in Taïwan. Hepatology 12: 575–581

Lamas L, Baccarini P, Housset C, Kremsdorf D, Bréchot C 1992 Detection of hepatitis C virus (HCV) RNA sequences in liver tissue by in situ hybridization. Journal of Hepatology (in press)

Lampertico P, Malter J S, Colombo M and Gerber M A 1990 Detection of hepatitis B virus DNA in formalin-fixed, paraffin-embedded liver tissue by the polymerase chain reaction. American Journal of Pathology 253–258

Larzul D, Thiers V, Courouce A M, Bréchot C, Guesdon J L 1987 Non-radioactive hepatitis B virus DNA probe for detection of HBV-DNA in serum. Journal of Hepatology 1987, 5: 199–204

Larzul D, Guigue F, Sninsky J J, Mack D H, Bréchot C, Guesdon J L 1988 Detection of hepatitis B virus sequences in serum by using in vitro enzymatic amplification. Journal of Virological Methods 20: 227–237

Larzul D, Chevrier D, Guesdon J L 1989 A non radioactive diagnostic test for the detection of HBV DNA sequences in serum at the single molecule level. Molecular Cellular Probes 3 (1): 45–47

Larzul D, Chevrier D, Thiers V, Guesdon J L 1990 An automatic modified polymerase chain reaction procedure for hepatitis B virus detection. Journal of Virological Methods 27: 49–60

Lau J Y, Naoumova N V, Alexander G J, Williams R 1991 Rapid detection of hepatitis B virus DNA in liver tissue by in situ hybridisation and its combination with immunohistochemistry for simultaneous detection of HBV antigens. Journal of Clinical Pathology 44: 905–908

Lauré F, Chatenoud L, Pasquinelli C et al 1987 Frequent lymphocytes infection by hepatitis B virus in haemophiliacs. British Journal of Haematology 65: 181–185

Lee S D, Lo K J, Wu J C et al 1986 Prevention of maternal-infant hepatitis B virus transmission by immunization: the role of serum hepatitis B virus DNA. Hepatology 6: 369–373

Liang J T, Isselbacher K J, Wu J C et al 1989 Rapid identification of low level hepatitis B-related viral genome in serum. Journal of Clinical Investigation 84: 1367–1377

Liang T J, Blum H E, Wands J R 1990 Characterization and biological properties of a hepatitis B virus isolated from a patient without hepatitis B virus serologic markers. Hepatology 12: 204–212

Liang T J, Baruch Y, Ben-Porath E et al 1991a Hepatitis B virus infection in patients with idiopathic liver disease. Hepatology 1991, 13: 1044–1051

Liang T J, Hasegawa K, Rimon N, Wands J R, Ben-Porath E 1991b A hepatitis B virus mutant associated with an epidemic of fulminant hepatitis. New England Journal of Medicine 324: 1705–1709

Liaw Y F, Pao C C, Chu C M 1988 Changes of serum HBV-DNA in relation to serum transaminase level during acute exacerbation in patients with chronic type B hepatitis. Liver 8: 231–235

Lieberman H M, LaBrecque D R, Kew M C, Hadziyannis S J, Shafritz D A 1982 Detection of hepatitis B virus DNA directly in human serum by a simplified molecular hybridization test: comparison to HBeAg/anti-HBe status in HBsAg carriers. Hepatology 3: 285–291

Lin H J, Chung H T, Lai C L, Leong S, Tam O S 1989 Detection of supercoiled hepatitis B virus DNA and related forms by means of molecular hybridization to an oligonucleotide probe. Journal of Medical Virology 29 (4): 284–288

Lin H J, Lai C L, Lau J Y, Chung H T, Lauder I J, Fong M W 1990 Evidence for intrafamilial transmission of hepatitis B virus from sequence analysis of mutant HBV DNAs in two Chinese families. Lancet 336: 208–212

Lin H J, Lai C L, Lauder I J, Wu P C, Lau T K and Fong M W 1991 Application of hepatitis B virus (HBV) DNA sequence polymorphisms to the study of HBV transmission. Journal of Infectious Diseases 164: 284–288

Ljunggren K, Kidd A H 1991 Enzymatic amplification and sequence analysis of precore/core DNA in HBsAg positive patients. Journal of Medical Virology 34: 179–183

Lucey M, Traber P G 1991 Detection of hepatitis C viral RNA by the polymerase chain reaction. Hepatology 13: 193–195

Lo Y M D, Mehgal W Z, Fleming K A 1989 In vitro amplification of hepatitis B virus sequences from liver tumor DNA and from paraffin wax embedded tissues using the polymerase chain reaction. Journal of Clinical Pathology 42: 840–846

Lobbiani A, Lallatta F, Lugo F, Colucci G 1990 Hepatitis B virus transcripts and surface antigen in human peripheral blood lymphocytes. Journal of Medical Virology 31: 190–194

Lok A S F, Hadziyannis S J, Weller I V D et al 1984 Contribution of low level HBV replication to continuing inflammatory activity in patients with anti-HBe positive chronic hepatitis B virus infection. Gut 25: 1283–1287

Lok A S F, Karayiannis P, Jowett T P et al 1985 Studies of HBV replication during acute hepatitis followed by recovery and acute hepatitis progressing to chronic disease. Journal of Hepatology 1: 671–679

Lok A S, Ma O C, Lau J Y 1991 Interferon alfa therapy in patients with chronic hepatitis B virus infection. Effects on hepatitis B virus DNA in the liver. Gastroenterology 100: 756–761

Loriot M A, Marcellin P, Bismuth E 1992 Demonstration of hepatitis B virus DNA by polymerase chain reaction in the serum and the liver after spontaneous or therapeutically induced HBeAg to anti HBe or HBsAg to anti-HBs seroconversion in patients with chronic hepatitis B. Hepatology 15: 32–36

Lugassy C, Bernuau J, Thiers V et al 1987 Sequences of hepatitis B virus DNA in the serum and liver of patients with acute benign and fulminant hepatitis. Journal of Infectious Diseases 155: 64–71

Luo K X, Zhou R, He C, Liang Z S, Jiang S 1991 Hepatitis B virus DNA in sera of virus carriers positive exclusively for antibodies to the hepatitis B core antigen. Journal of Medical Virology 35: 55–59

Mack D H, Sninsky J J 1988 A sensitive method for the identification of uncharacterized viruses related to known virus groups: hepadnavirus model system. Proceedings of the National Academy of Sciences of the USA 85: 6977–6981

Magrin S, Craxi A, Fabiano C et al 1991 Hepatitis C virus replication in 'autoimmune' chronic hepatitis. Journal of Hepatology 13: 364–367

Mantero G, Zonaro A, Albertini A, Bertolo P, Primi D 1991 DNA enzyme immunoassay: general method for detecting products of polymerase chain reaction. Clinical Chemistry 37: 422–429

Marcellin P, Martinot-Peignoux M, Loriot M A, Giostra E, Boyer N, Thiers V, Benhamou J P 1990 Persistence of hepatitis B virus DNA demonstrated by Polymerase chain reaction in serum and liver after loss of HBsAg induced by antiviral therapy. Annals of Internal Medicine 112: 3

Marcellin P, Calmus Y, Takahashi H et al 1991 Latent hepatitis B virus (HBV) infection in systemic necrotizing vasculitis. Clinical and Experimental Rheumatology 9: 23–28

Martell M, Esteban J I, Quer J 1992 Hepatitis C virus (HCV) circulates as a population of different but closely related genomes: quasispecies nature of HCV genome distribution. Journal of Virology 66: 3225–3229

Matsuyama Y, Omata M, Yokosuka O, Imazeki F, Ito Y, Okuda K 1985 Discordance of hepatitis B e antigen/antibody and hepatitis B virus deoxuribonucleic acid in serum. Gastroenterology 89: 1104–1108

Michikata K, Horiike N, Nadano S, Onji M, Ohta Y 1988 Change of hepatitis B virus DNA distribution associated with the progression of chronic hepatitis. Liver 8: 247–253

Miller R H, Purcell R H 1990 Hepatitis C virus shares amino acid sequence similitary with pestiviruses and flaviviruses as well as members of two plant virus of human supergroups. Proceedings of the National Academy of Sciences of the USA 87: 2057–2061

Mitsuda T, Yokota S, Mori et al 1989 Demonstration of mother-to-infant transmission of hepatitis B virus by means of polymerase chain reaction. Lancet 335: 302

Miyamura T, Saito I, Katayama T et al 1990 Detection of antibody against antigen expressed by molecularly cloned hepatitis C virus cDNA: application to diagnosis and lood screening for post-transfusion hepatitis. Proceedings of the National Academy of Sciences of the USA 87: 983–987

Moestrup T, Hansson B G, Widell A, Blomberg J, Nordenfelt E 1985 Hepatitis B virus DNA in the serum of patients followed-up longitudinally with acute and chronic hepatitis B. Journal of Medical Virology 17: 337–344

Morace G, Von Der Helm K, Jilg W, Deinhardt F 1985 Detection of hepatitis B virus DNA by a rapid filtration-hybridization assay. Journal of Virological Methods 12: 235–242

Moriyama K, Ishibashi H, Kashiwagi S, Asayama R 1989 Presence of HBV DNA and HBeAg in serum of an anti-HBs-Positive individual. Gastroenterology 97: 1068–1069

Nakagami S, Matsunaga H, Oka N, Yamane A 1991 Preparation of enzyme-conjugated DNA probe and application to the universal probe system. Annals of Biochemistry 198: 759

Nalpas B, Driss F, Pol S, Hamelin B, Housset C, Bréchot C, Berthelot P 1991 Association between HCV and HBV infection in hepatocellular carcinoma and alcoholic liver disease. Journal of Hepatology 12: 70–74

Nalpas B, Pourcel C, Feldman G et al 1992a Chronic alcohol intoxication decreases the serum level of hepatitis B surface antigen transgenic mice. Journal of Hepatology 15: 118–124

Nalpas B, Thiers V, Pol S, Driss F, Thepot V, Berthelot P, Bréchot C 1992b Hepatitis C viremia and anti-HCV antibodies in alcoholics. Journal of Hepatology 14: 381–384

Naoumov N V, Schneider R, Grötzinger T, Jung M C, Miska S, Pape G R, Will H 1992 Precore mutant hepatitis B virus infection and liver disease. Gastroenterology 102: 538–543

Negro F, Chiaberge E 1985 Detection of HBV DNA by in situ hybridization using a biotin-labeled probe. Journal of Medical Virology 15: 373–382

Nishigushi S, Kuroki T, Yabusako T et al 1991 Detection of hepatitis C virus antibodies and hepatitis C virus RNA in patients with alcoholic liver disease. Hepatology 14: 985–989

Nishigushi S, Kuroki T, Yabusako T et al 1991 Detection of hepatitis C virus antibodies and hepatitis C virus isolated from a human carrier: comparison with reported isolates for conserved and divergent regions. Journal of General Virology 72: 2697–2704

Norder H, Brattstrom C, Magnius L 1989 High frequency of hepatitis B virus DNA in anti HBe positive sera on longitudinal follow-up of patients with renal transplants and chronic hepatitis B. Journal of Medical Virology 27 (4): 322–328

Novati R, Thiers V, D'Arminio Monforte A et al 1992 Mother to child transmission of hepatitis C virus detected by nested polymerase chain reaction. Journal of Infectious Diseases 1992; 165: 720–723

Ogata N, Alter H J, Miller R H, Purcell R H 1991 Nucleotide sequence and mutation rate of the H strain of hepatitis C virus. Proceedings of the National Academy of Sciences of the USA 88: 3392–3396

Okamoto H, Tsuda F, Mayumi M 1987 Defective mutants of hepatitis B virus in the circulation of symptom-free carriers. Japanese Journal of Experimental Medicine 57: 217–221

Okamoto H, Yotsumoto S, Akahane Y et al 1990b Hepatitis B viruses with precore region defects prevail in persistently infected hosts along with seroconversion to the antibody against e antigen. Journal of Virology 64: 1298–1303

Okamoto H, Okada S, Sugiyama Y et al 1990a The 5' terminal sequence of the hepatitis C virus genome. Japanese Journal of Experimental Medicine 60: 167–177

Okamoto H, Kurai K, Okada S I 1992 Full length sequence of a hepatitis C virus genome having poor homology to reported isolates: comparative study of four distinct genotypes. Virology 188: 331–341

Omata M, Ehata T, Yokosuka O, Hosoda K, Ohto M 1991 Mutations in the precore region of hepatitis B virus DNA in patients with fulminant and severe hepatitis. New England Journal of Medicine 324: 1699–1704

Orito E, Mizokami M, Ina Y, Moriyama E N, Kameshima N, Yamamoto M, Gojobori T 1989 Host-independent evolution and a genetic classification of the hepadnavirus family based on nucleotide sequences. Proceedings of the National Academy of Sciences of the USA 86: 7059–7062

Pasquinelli C, Melegari M, Villa E 1990 Hepatitis B virus infection of peripheral blood mononuclear cells in common in acute and chronic hepatitis. Journal of Medical Virology 31: 135–140

Paterlini P, Gerken G, Nakajima E et al 1990 Polymerase chain reaction to detect hepatitis B virus DNA and RNA sequences in primary liver cancers from patients negative for hepatitis B surface antigen. New England Journal of Medicine 323: 80–85

Paterlini P, Franco D, Driss F, Nalpas B, Pisi E, Berthelot P, Bréchot C 1993 Persistence of hepatitis B and hepatitis C viral genomes in primary liver cancers from HBsAg-negative patients: a study of low endemic area. Hepatology 17: 20–29

Peng H W, Su T S, Han S H, Ho C K, Ho C H, Ching K N, Chiang B N 1988 Assessment of HBV persistent infection in an adult population in Taïwan. Journal of Medical Virology 24: 405–412

Pol S, Thiers V, Nalpas B et al 1987 Monoclonal anti-HBs antibodies: radioimmunoassay and serum HBV-DNA hybridization as diagnostic tools of HBV infection: relative prevalence among HBsAg-negative alcoholics, patients with chronic hepatitis or hepatocellular carcinomas and blood donors. European Journal of Clinical Investigation 17: 515–521

Pol S, Driss F, Devergie A, Bréchot C, Berthelot P, Gluckman E 1990 Is hepatitis C virus involved in hepatitis-associated aplastic anemia? Annals of Internal Medicine 113: 435–437

Pol S, Legendre C, Saltiel C et al 1992 Hepatitis C virus kidney recipients. Epidemiology and impact on renal transplantation. Journal of Hepatology 15: 202–206

Pontisso P, Chemello L, Fattovitch G, Alberti A, Realdi G, Bréchot C 1985 Relationship between HBcAg in serum and liver and HBV replication in patients with HBsAg positive chronic liver disease. Journal of Medical Virology 17: 145–152

Pontisso P, Bortolotti F, Schiavon E, Chemello L, Alberti A, Realdi G 1986 Serum hepatitis B virus DNA in acute hepatitis type B. Digestion 34: 46–50

Pontisso P, Morsica G, Ruvoletto M G et al 1992 Latent hepatitis B virus infection in childhood hepatocellular carcinoma, analysis by polymerase chain reaction. Cancer 69: 2731–2735

Porchon C, Kremsdorf D, Pol S et al 1992 Serum hepatitis C virus RNA and hepatitis B virus DNA in non-A, non-B post transfusional and sporadic chronic hepatitis. Journal Hepatology 16: 184–189

Poterucha J J, Rakela J, Lumeng L et al 1992 Diagnosis of chronic hepatitis C after liver transplantation by the detection of viral sequences with polymerase chain reaction. Hepatology 15: 42–45

Quibriac M, Petijean J, Thiers V, Tiollais P, Bréchot C, Freymuth F 1989 Comparison of a non-radioactive hybridization assay for detection of hepatitis B virus DNA with the radioactive method. Molecular and Cellular Probes 3: 209–212

Quint W G V, De Bruijn I, Kruining H, Heijtink R A 1990 HBV–DNA detection by gene amplification in acute hepatitis B. Hepatology 12: 653–656

Repp R, Mance A, Bertram U, Nieman H, Gerlich W H, Lampert F 1991 Persistent hepatitis B virus replication in mononuclear blood cells as a source of reinfection of liver transplants. Transplantation 52: 5

Rijntjes P J M, Van Ditzhuijsen J M, Van Loon A M, Van Haelst U J G M, Bronkhorst F B, Yap S H 1985 Hepatitis B virus DNA detected in formalin-fixed liver specimens and its relation to serologic markers and histopathologic features in chronic liver disease. American Journal of Pathology 120: 411–418

Romet Lemonne J L, MacLane M F, Elfassi E, Haseltine W A, Azocar J, Essex M 1983 Hepatitis B virus infection in cultured human lymphoblastoid cells. Science 221: 667–669

Rumi M G, Colombo M, Romeo R et al 1990 Serum hepatitis B virus DNA detects cryptic hepatitis B virus infections in multitransfused hemophiliac patients. Blood 75: 1654–1658

Sagitani M, Inchauspé G, Shindo M, Prince A M 1992

Sensitivity of serological assays to identify blood donors with hepatitis C viraema. Lancet 339: 1018

Santantonio T, Pontisso P, Milella M, Chemello L, Luchena N, Pastore G 1990 Detection of hepatitis B virus DNA in serum by spot hybridization technique: sensitivity and specificity of radiolabeled and biotin-labeled probes. Virology 177: 367–371

Scott J S, Pace R A, Sheridan J W, Cooksley W G 1990 Discordance of hepatitis B e antigen and hepatitis B viral deoxyribonucleic acid. Hepatology 13: 627–631

Scotto J, Hadchouel M, Hery C, Yvart J, Tiollais P, Bréchot C 1983a Detection of hepatitis B virus DNA in serum by a simple spot hybridization technique: comparison with results for other viral markers. Hepatology 3: 279–284

Scotto J, Hadchouel M, Hery C et al 1983b Hepatitis B virus DNA in children's liver diseases: detection by blot hybridisation in liver and serum. Gut 24: 618–624

Scotto J, Hadchouel M, Wain-Hobson S, Sonigo P, Courroucé A M, Tiollais P, Bréchot C 1985 Hepatitis B virus DNA in Dane particles: evidence for the presence of replicative intermediates. The Journal of Infectious Diseases 151: 610–617

Shibata M, Morishima T, Kudo T et al 1991 Detection of hepatitis C virus sequences in liver tissue by the polymerase chain reaction. Laboratory Investigation 65: 408–411

Shieh Y S, Shim K S, Lampertico P et al 1991 Detection of hepatitis C virus sequences in liver tissues by the polymerase chain reaction. Laboratory Investigation 65: 408–411

Shih L N, Sheu J C, Wang J T 1990 Detection of hepatitis B viral DNA by polymerase chain reaction in patients with hepatitis B surface antigen. Journal of Medical Virology 30: 159–162

Shimizu Y, Ida S, Matsukura T, Yuasa T 1984 Determination of hepatitis B virus DNA in serum by molecular hybridization. Microbiology and Immunology 28: 117–123

Shimizu Y K, Weiner A J, Rosenblatt J et al 1990 Early events in hepatitis C virus infection of chimpanzees. Proceedings of the National Academy of Sciences of the USA 87: 6441–6444

Shindo M, Okuno T, Arai K et al 1991 Detection of hepatitis B virus DNA in paraffin embedded liver tissues in chronic hepatitis B or non-A, non-B hepatitis using the polymerase chain reaction. Hepatology 13: 167–171

Shiraki K, Yoshihara N, Sakurai M, Eto T, Kawana T 1980 Acute hepatitis B in infants born to carrier mothers with the antibody to hepatitis B e antigen. Journal of Pediatrics 97: 768–770

Sumazaki R, Motz M, Wolf H, Heinig J, Jilg W, Deinhardt F 1989 Detection of hepatitis B virus in serum using amplification of viral DNA by means of the polymerase chain reaction. Journal of Medical Virology 27(4) 304–308

Tahekara T, Hayashi N, Mita E et al 1992 Detection of minus strand of hepatitis C virus RNA by reverse transcription and polymerase chain reaction. Implication for hepatitis C virus replication in infected tissue. Hepatology 15: 387–390

Takamatsu K, Koyanagi Y, Okita K et al 1990 Hepatitis C virus RNA in saliva (letter). Lancet 336: 1515

Tanaka Y, Esumi M, Shikata T 1990 Persistence of hepatitis B virus DNA after serological clearance of hepatitis B virus. Liver 10: 6–10

Tassopoulos N C, Papaevangelou G J, Roumeliotou-Karayannis A, Ticehurst J R, Feinstone S M, Purcell R H 1986 Search of hepatitis B virus DNA in sera from patients with acute type B or non-A, non-B hepatitis. Journal of Hepatology 2: 410–418

Tay N, Chan S H, Ren E C 1990 Detection of integrated hepatitis B virus DNA in hepatocellular carcinoma cell lines by non radioactive in situ hybridization. Journal of Medical Virology 30: 266–271

Tedder R S, Briggs M, Ring C et al 1991 Hepatitis C antibody profile and viraemia prevalence in adults with severe haemophilia. British Journal of Haematology 79: 512–515

Thaler M M, Park C K, Landers D V 1991 Vertical transmission of hepatitis C virus. Lancet 338: 17–18

Thiers V, Bouchardeau F, Courouce A M, Tiollais P, Bréchot C 1986 L'ADN du virus de l'hépatite B comme marqueur de multiplication virale comparison avec l'antigéne HBe et l'anticorps anti-HBe. Nouvelle Press Médicale 15: 1219–1222

Thiers V, Fujita Y, Takahashi H et al 1988a In: Hollinger F B, Lemon S M, Margolis H S (eds) Hepatitis B virus DNA sequences in the serum of HBsAg-negative patients with chronic liver. Viral hepatitis and liver disease. Alan R Liss, New York, pp 553–557

Thiers V, Nakajima E, Kremsdorf, D et al 1988b Transmission of hepatitis B from hepatitis B seronegative subjects. Lancet 1273–1276

Thiers V, Lunel-Fabiani F, Valla D et al 1992 Post transfusional anti-HCV negative non-A, non-B hepatitis: serological and polymerase chain reaction analysis for hepatitis C and hepatitis B viruses. Journal of Hepatology (in press)

Tran A, Kremsdorf D, Capel F, Housset C, Dauguet C, Petit M A, Bréchot C 1991 Emergence of and takeover by hepatitis B virus (HBV) with rearrangements in the Pre-S/S and pre-C/C genes during chronic HBV infection. Journal of Virology 65: 3566–3574

Tur-Kaspa R, Keshet E, Eliakakim M, Shouval D 1984 Detection and characterization of hepatitis B virus DNA in serum of HBe antigen-negative HBsAg carriers. Journal of Medical Virology 14: 17–26

Ulrich P P, Bhat R A, Seto B, Mack D, Sninsky J, Vyas G N 1989 Enzymatic amplification of hepatitis B virus DNA in serum compared with infectivity testing chimpanzees. Journal of Infectious Diseases 160: 37–43

Ulrich P P, Romeo J M, Lane P K, Kelly I, Daniel L J, Vyas G N 1991 Detection, semiquantification, and genetic variation in hepatitis C virus sequences amplified from the plasma of blood donors with elevated alanine aminotransferase. Journal of Clinical Investigation 86: 1609–1614

Valentine-Thon E, Steinman J, Arnold W 1990 Evaluation of the commercially available HepProbe kit for detection of hepatitis B virus DNA in serum. Journal of Clinical Microbiology 28: 39–42

Valentine-Thon E, Steinman J, Arnold W 1991 Detection of hepatitis B virus DNA in serum with nucleic acid probes labelled with^{32} P, biotin, alkaline phosphatase or sulphone. Molecular and Cellular Probes 5: 299–305

Van Der Poel C L, Cuypers H T M, Reesink H W et al 1991 Confirmation of hepatitis C virus infection by new four-antigen recombinant immunoblot assay. Lancet 337: 317–319

Villa E, Feretti I, De Palma M et al 1991 HCV RNA in

serum of asymptomatic blood donors involved in post-transfusion hepatitis (PTH). Journal of Hepatology 13: 256–259

Wakita T, Kakumu S, Shibata M et al 1991 Detection of pre-C and core region mutants of hepatitis B virus in chronic hepatitis B virus carriers. Journal of Clinical Investigation 88: 1793–1801

Wang J T, Wang T H, Sheu J C et al 1991 Detection of hepatitis B virus DNA by polymerase chain reaction in plasma of volunteer blood donors negative for hepatitis B surface antigen. Journal of Infectious Diseases 163: 397–399

Weller I V D, Fowler M J F, Monjardino J, Thomas H C 1982 The detection of HBV DNA in serum by molecular hybridisation: a more sensitive method for the detection of complete HBV particles. Journal of Medical Virology 9: 273–280

Weiner A J, Kuo G, Bradley D W et al 1990. Detection of hepatitis C viral sequences in non-A, non-B hepatitis. Lancet 335: 1–3

Weiner A J, Geysen H M, Christopherson C et al 1992 Evidence for immune selection of hepatitis C virus (HCV) putative envelope glycoprotein variants: potential role in chronic HCV infections. Proceedings of the National Academy of Sciences of the USA 89: 3468–3472

Widell A , Mansson A S, Sunstrom G et al 1991 Hepatitis C virus RNA in blood donor sera detected by the polymerase chain reaction: comparison with supplementary hepatitis C antibody assays. Journal of Medical Virology 35: 253–258

Wood J R, Taswell H F, Czaja A J, Rabe D 1988 Pattern duration of HBV DNA seropositivity in acute hepatitis B. Digestive Disease and Science 33: 477–480

Wright T L, Hsu H, Donegan E et al 1991 Hepatitis C virus not found in fulminant non-A, non-B hepatitis. Annals of Internal Medicine 115: 111–112

Wright T L, Mamish D, Combs C et al 1992 Hepatitis B virus and appearent fulminant non-A, non-B hepatitis. Lancet 339: 952–955

Wu J C, Lee S D, Wang L Y et al 1986 Analysis of the DNA of hepatitis B virus in the sera of Chinese patients infected with hepatitis B. Journal of Infectious Diseases 153: 974–977

Wu J C, Lee S D, Wang J Y et al 1987 Correlation between hepatic hepatitis B core antigen serum hepatitis B virus-DNA levels in patients with chronic hepatitis B virus infections in Taïwan. Archives of Pathology and Laboratory Medicine 111: 181–184

Wu J C, Lee S D, Tsay Y T, Chan C Y, Huang Y S, Lo K J, Ting L P 1988 Symptomatic anti-HBe positive chronic hepatitis B in Taïwan with special reference to persistent HBV replication and HDV superinfection. Journal of Medical Virology 25: 141–148

Yanagi M, Kaneko S, Unoura M et al 1991 Hepatitis C virus fulminant hepatic failure. New England Journal of Medicine 324: 1895

Yokosuka O, Omata M, Hosoda K et al 1991 Detection and direct sequencing of hepatitis B virus genome by DNA amplification method. Gastroenterology 100: 175–181

Yokosuka O, Omata M, Imazeki F, Okuda K and Summers J 1985 Changes of hepatitis B virus DNA in liver and serum caused by recombinant leukocyte interferon treatment: analysis of intrahepatic replicative hepatitis B virus DNA. Hepatology 5: 728–734

Yoneyama T, Takeuchi K, Watanabe Y et al 1990 Detection of hepatitis C virus cDNA sequence by the polymerase chain reaction in hepatocellular carcinoma tissues. Japanese Journal of Medical Science and Biology 43: 89–94

Yotsumoto S, Okamoto H, Tsuda F, Miyakawa Y, Mayumi M 1990 Subtyping hepatitis B virus DNA in free or integrated forms by amplification of the S-gene sequences by the polymerase chain reaction and single-track sequencing for adenine. Journal of Virological Methods 28: 107–116

Zarski J P, Kuhns M, Berck L, Degos F, Schalm S W, Tiollais P, Bréchot C 1989 Comparison of a quantitative standardized HBV–DNA assay and a classical spot hybridization test in chronic active hepatitis B patients undergoing antiviral therapy. Research in Virology 140: 283–291

Zignego A L, Samuel D, Gugenheim J 1988 Hepatitis B virus replication and mononuclear blood cell infection after liver transplantation. In: Hollinger F B, Lemon S M, Margolis H S (eds) Viral hepatitis and liver disease. Alan Liss, New York, pp 808–809

Zignego A L, Dény P, Feray C, Ponzetto A, Gentilini P, Tiollais P, Bréchot C 1990 Amplification of hepatitis delta virus RNA sequences by Polymerase chain reaction: a tool for viral detection and cloning. Molecular and Cellular Probes 4: 43–51

Zignego A L, Macchia D, Monti M, Thiers V, Mazzeti M, Foschi M, Maggi E, Romagnani S, Gentilini P, Bréchot C 1992 Infection of peripheral mononuclear blood cells by hepatitis C virus. Journal of Hepatology 15: 382–386

Zonaro A, Puoti M, Fiordalisi G, Mantero G, Castelnuovo F, Primi D, Cariani E 1990 Detection of serum hepatitis C virus RNA in acute non-A, non-B hepatitis. Journal of Infectious Diseases 163: 923–924

UPDATE

- *Importance of HCV RNA detection in the serum of anti-HCV positive blood donors*: Several papers indicate that, indeed, blood donors with normal levels of transaminase but detectable HCV viraemia, may frequently show histological features of chronic hepatitis if a liver biopsy is performed. Thus, PCR should be useful for the evaluation of blood donors.

  Romeo R, Thiers V, Driss F, Berthelot P, Nalpas B, Bréchot C Hepatitis C virus (HCV) RNA in serum blood donors with or without elevated transaminase levels. Transfusion (in press)

Alberti A, Morsica G, Chemello L, Cavalletto D, Noventa F, Pontisso P, Ruol A 1992 Hepatitis C viraemia and liver disease in symptom-free individuals with anti-HCV. Lancet 340: 697–698

Sagitani M, Inchauspé G, Shindo M, Prince A M 1992 Sensitivity of serological assays to identify blood donors with hepatitis C viraemia. Lancet 339: 1018–1019

- *Detection of HCV RNA in paraffin-embedded liver biopsy*: a recent report suggests that HCV RNA might be detected not only on frozen liver biopsies, but also on paraffin-embedded samples. This would allow a much wider access to retrospective studies.

Bresters D, Cuypers H T M, Reesink H W, Chaumuleau R A F M, Schipper M E I, Boeser-Nunnink B D M, Lelie P N, Jansen P L M 1992 Detection of hepatitis C viral RNA sequences in fresh and paraffin-embedded liver biopsy specimens of non-A, non-B hepatitis patients. Journal of Hepatology 1–5

- *Genotyping of HCV by PCR*: the genetic variability of HCV has now been well characterized. Some recent reports suggest an association between infection by some of the HCV genotypes and the severity of the liver disease as well as the response or non-response to treatment by interferon alpha. Some procedures have been proposed which would allow a rapid genotyping using PCR with specific primers, without the need for sequence analysis. This evaluation will be of major importance for the investigation of the role of HCV genotypes in the course of HCV chronic infection.

Okamoto H, Sugiyama Y, Okada S et al 1992 Typing hepatitis C virus polymerase chain reaction with type-specific primers:application to clinical surveys and tracing infectious sources. Journal of General Virology 73: 673–679

Takada N, Takase S, Enomoto N, Takada A, Date T 1992 Clinical backgrounds of the patients having different types of hepatitis C virus genomes. Journal of Hepatology 14: 35–40

Yoshioka K, Kakumu S, Wakita T et al 1992 Detection of hepatitis C virus by Polymerase Chain Reaction and response to interferon-alpha therapy: relationship to genotypes of hepatitis C virus. Hepatology 16: 293–299

- *Quantification of HCV RNA in the serum*: a number of reports are now using either serial dilutions or, more precisely, internal standards for determination of HCV RNA quantification. The use of internal standards shows promising results, although the number of samples evaluable with this approach is still limited.

Kaneko S, Murakami S, Unoura M, Kobayashi K 1992 Quantification of hepatitis C virus RNA by competitive Polymerase Chain Reaction. Journal of Medical Virology 37: 278–282

SECTION 7

Clinical aspects

28. Treatment of fulminant viral hepatitis

Phillip M. Harrison Johnson Y.N. Lau Roger Williams

Acute liver failure is the broad term used to describe the development of encephalopathy within 6 months of the onset of symptoms related to liver disease. It can be further subdivided to reflect variations in clinical features and prognosis. Fulminant hepatic failure describes the subgroup of patients with the most rapid progression of symptoms, and it is variously defined as the onset of encephalopathy within 4 weeks (Mathieson et al 1980) or 8 weeks (Trey & Davidson 1970) of the onset of symptoms, or alternatively within 2 weeks of the onset of jaundice (Bernuau et al 1986a). Patients whose encephalopathy occurs some 8 weeks to 6 months after the onset of symptoms are described as having late-onset hepatic failure (Gimson et al 1986). All of the definitions require the presence of encephalopathy, although it has been argued that a coagulopathy alone should be taken as adequate evidence of severe hepatic dysfunction (Bernuau et al 1986). In this chapter the term fulminant hepatic failure will be confined to those patients fulfilling the criteria of Trey & Davidson (1970), namely the onset of encephalopathy within 8 weeks of the onset of symptoms of liver disease in a patient with a previously normal liver. The term acute liver failure will be used when the broader definition is required.

AETIOLOGY

Any virus that causes an acute hepatitis can also cause fulminant hepatic failure, although the relative proportion of cases due to the different viruses varies geographically (Table 28.1). Viruses are the commonest cause of acute liver failure worldwide, although in the UK they account for only 31% of cases because of the very high incidence of paracetamol overdose (Fig. 28.1). Fulminant hepatitis A is more common in countries where there is overcrowding and poor standards of sanitation, as shown by the recent major outbreak in China. Although the risk of developing fulminant hepatitis A is low in the UK, it appears to rise with increasing age. The predisposing factors for the development of fulminant hepatitis B appear to differ between countries. The incidence of post-transfusion fulminant hepatitis B has decreased drastically since the exclusion of blood donors seropositive for hepatitis B surface antigen (Gimson et al 1983). Females appear to be more commonly affected than heterosexual males, but whether homosexual males are more at risk of developing fulminant hepatitis B is uncertain (Bernuau et al 1986). Clustering of cases of fulminant hepatitis B occurs in groups of intravenous drug abusers and their sexual contacts.

Table 28.1 The relative frequencies of the three main viral causes of fulminant hepatic failure in the reported series of patients worldwide

	HAV (%)	HBV (%)	NANB (%)
UK	20	44	36
France	6	60	34
Denmark	20	32	48
Greece	2	74	24
USA	2	60	38
Japan	2	74	24

Sequence analysis of viral DNA, amplified from the plasma of patients with hepatitis B using the polymerase chain reaction (PCR), has revealed the existence of a variant of the hepatitis B virus

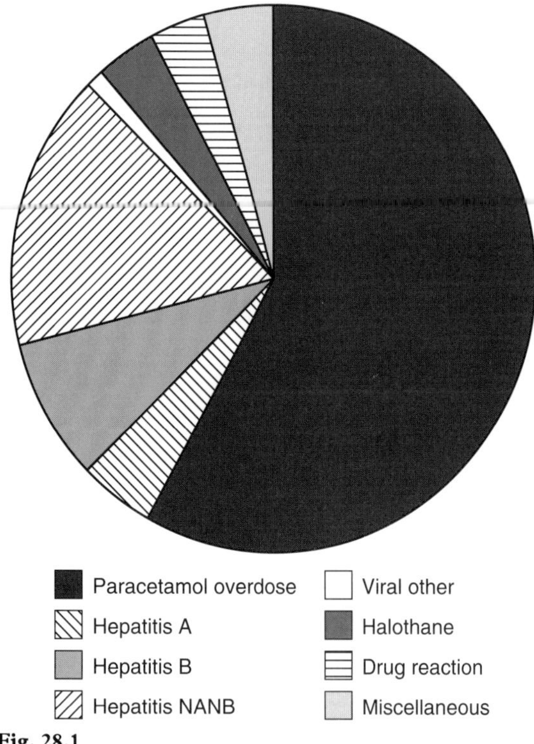

Fig. 28.1

with a mutation in the pre-core region of the viral genome. Hepatocytes infected with this virus cannot produce HBeAg as a point mutation from guanine to adenine at nucleotide 83 in the pre-core region converts the codon for tryptophan (TGG) to a stop codon (TAG), although the HBeAg-negative virus particles produced are still infectious. Fulminant hepatic failure has developed in patients contracting hepatitis B virus from individuals negative for the HBe antigen (HBeAg), although the absence of HBeAg from plasma in some patients with hepatitis B-induced fulminant hepatic failure had been attributed to the rapid clearance of the virus. Carman et al (1991) have now demonstrated that the majority of patients with fulminant hepatitis B negative for HBeAg are infected with the mutant virus, whereas patients who are HBeAg positive are infected with the wild-type virus. Fulminant hepatic failure caused by the pre-core mutant virus appears to be due to transmission of this mutant virus rather than a rapid mutation of an infecting wild-type virus (Kojima et al 1991, Liang et al 1991, Omata et al 1991, Terazawa et al 1991). The mutant virus may be more likely to cause a hepatitis with a fulminant course than the wild-type virus (Kosaka et al 1991, Omata et al 1991), although the outcome from fulminant hepatic failure is not necessarily worse (Carman et al 1991). It will be important to determine whether the mutant virus causes liver injury by the same mechanism as the wild-type virus or is directly cytopathic. Both hepatitis B and hepatitis D virus co-infection and superinfection of hepatitis D virus in chronic hepatitis B virus carriers have been documented to be associated with acute liver failure.

Serological tests for hepatitis C virus have demonstrated that it is the main cause of chronic non-A, non-B viral hepatitis, but its role in causing fulminant hepatic failure has only recently been investigated. Japanese workers reported that, out of a series of 21 patients with fulminant hepatic failure, six (29%) had antibodies to hepatitis C virus and seven (33%) had detectable hepatitis C viral RNA in serum (Yanagi et al 1991). However, although four out of seven patients with presumed non-A, non-B hepatitis were either anti-hepatitis C virus or hepatitis C viral RNA positive, one out of three patients with hepatitis A and four out of eight cases of hepatitis B were also positive. The significance of the detection of multiple viral agents was unknown, but may it may have been important to the development of acute liver failure. In contrast, in the USA (Wright et al 1991) and in the UK (Sallie et al 1991) evidence of hepatitis C virus infection has not been found in patients with fulminant hepatitis.

Hepatitis E viral genome has been detected in the serum of patients with fulminant non-A, non-B hepatitis (Sallie et al 1991). It is well established that pregnant women are at increased risk of developing fulminant hepatitis due to an enteric non-A, non-B hepatitis virus and this is probably hepatitis E virus. Less than 50 cases of acute hepatitis due to herpes simplex have been reported, but the severity of the disease is striking, with more than 90% mortality (Bernuau et al 1986). Both type 1 and 2 herpesviruses have been implicated, with type 2 found most commonly in women in their third trimester. Recently, herpesvirus type 6 has also been reported to cause fulminant hepatitis.

CLINICAL FEATURES AND MANAGEMENT OF FULMINANT HEPATIC FAILURE

The treatment of patients with fulminant hepatic failure is centred upon intensive support of all failing organs in order to provide the optimal environment to promote liver regeneration and, in those awaiting liver transplantation, to maintain the patient until a graft is available. The natural history of fulminant hepatic failure is characterized by the development of encephalopathy and coagulopathy. The time course for the onset of these features is variable. Cardiovascular, pulmonary and renal complications are common and their development denotes the onset of a multiple-organ failure syndrome. Complications can be analysed according to the system effected, although in reality there is an interdependence between such systems.

Encephalopathy

Hepatic encephalopathy is a complex neuropsychiatric disorder fundamental to the diagnosis of acute liver failure (Trey & Davidson 1970) and is graded clinically on a scale from 0 to 4 (Table 28.2). The severity may fluctuate in the early stages of the illness, especially in those patients with late-onset hepatic failure. Many patients do not progress beyond grade 2 encephalopathy, and in these individuals the prognosis is very good. The rate of onset and deterioration of encephalopathy is variable and the time interval between the appearance of jaundice and encephalopathy has prognostic significance.

Hepatic encephalopathy is thought to be caused by the accumulation of toxins that impair neuronal function and damage the blood–brain barrier. Increased gamma-aminobutyric acid (GABA) neurotransmission has been implicated in the pathogenesis of hepatic encephalopathy (Jones et al 1987), although GABAergic agonists do not appear to be increased and GABA receptor numbers and affinity are normal. Recent studies in animals with encephalopathy due to acute liver failure suggest that GABAergic neurotransmission may be increased by the presence of elevated concentrations of benzodiazepine agonists such as diazepam and *N*-desmethyldiazepam (Olasmaa et al 1990, Basile 1991). Endogenous benzodiazepine receptor ligands have now been found in cerebrospinal fluid from patients with hepatic encephalopathy (Olasmaa et al 1990) and in frontal cortex of some patients dying from paracetamol-induced fulminant hepatic failure (Basile et al 1991). In an open study of the effects of intravenous infusion of flumazenil, a benzodiazepine receptor antagonist, 5 out of 11 episodes of encephalopathy in 10 patients with fulminant hepatic failure improved. The favourable clinical response was also accompanied by an improvement of somatosensory evoked potentials (Ferenci & Grimm 1990). However, in the patients who did not respond to flumazenil or had normal concentrations of benzodiazepine receptor ligands, other mechanisms must have been involved in the evolution of the encephalopathy.

Table 28.2 Clinical features of the grades of hepatic encephalopathy

Grade	Clinical features
0	Not encephalopathic
I	Mild or episodic drowsiness, impaired intellect and concentration but rousable and coherent
II	Increased drowsiness with confusion and disorientation but rousable and conversant
III	Very drowsy, disorientated, responds to simple verbal commands but often agitated and aggressive
IV	Unresponsive to verbal commands but may move on painful stimulus

A number of other substances have been proposed as putative toxins, including ammonia, medium-chain fatty acids and mercaptans, which have all been shown to induce coma in animal models. They can act synergistically to precipitate coma in normal animals (Zieve et al 1984, Fick et al 1989), although the relative contribution of each of these toxins is still as yet unknown. Whatever the mechanism of encephalopathy, the gut flora is thought to play a role in its pathogenesis and measures such as a reduction in dietary protein and the administration of lactulose are used in the early stages, especially in late-onset hepatic failure. However, there is little evidence that these measures are effective in acute liver failure.

Coagulopathy

The liver is the site of synthesis of the majority of the factors involved in the coagulation process. It is, therefore, not surprising that bleeding is a major complication of fulminant hepatic failure as levels of most of the clotting factors fall rapidly at its onset (Lechner et al 1977). Platelets are intimately involved in coagulation and are responsible for formation of the initial haemostatic plug. They adhere to damaged vascular endothelium by the interaction of platelet glycoproteins with part of the factor VIII complex, the von Willebrand factor. This interaction induces a conformational change in the platelet and stimulates both the production of thromboxane A_2 from arachidonic acid and the release of granule contents. A high local concentration of these platelet products recruits further platelets, which then aggregate at the site of injury, activating and binding the coagulation factors. Although platelet numbers are usually only moderately reduced early on in fulminant hepatic failure when encephalopathy first appears, their function is grossly abnormal. The aggregation response is poor and is probably an acquired defect within the platelet. In contrast, platelet adhesion is enhanced, as evidenced by increased levels of platelet-specific proteins released from granules, e.g. β-thromboglobulin (Langley et al 1982), and this may be the consequence of the increased levels of von Willebrand factor that are found in fulminant hepatic failure (Langley et al 1985). The liver clears the activated coagulation factors and old platelets from the circulation through the reticuloendothelial system. Its function is greatly reduced in fulminant hepatic failure (Imawari et al 1985), allowing the activated products of the clotting process to remain in circulation. This leads to further consumption of clotting factors and can progress to microthrombus formation (Gazzard et al 1975a) and sludging in the microcirculation (Fujiwara et al 1988a).

Severe bleeding occurs in about 30% of patients with fulminant hepatic failure, and the most common site of haemorrhage is from mucosal erosions in the upper gastrointestinal tract. The incidence of bleeds from this site has been shown to be reduced by decreasing the acid output from the stomach with H_2 receptor blockade (Macdougall & Williams 1978) and may be reduced by instilling sucralfate into the stomach to protect the mucosa against acid and pepsin attack. Blood is used to replace that lost through haemorrhage. As fresh blood is rarely practicably available, stored blood is given with clotting factors in the form of fresh-frozen plasma. Cryoprecipitate is added if the fibrinogen levels are low. Vitamin K supplements, although routinely given, have little or no effect on the rate of synthesis of coagulation factors, in acute hepatic necrosis. The correction of the prothrombin time with fresh-frozen plasma is essential if the patient is bleeding but is of no benefit in reducing morbidity nor mortality if undertaken prophylactically (Gazzard et al 1975), it also deprives the clinician of the use of a valuable prognostic indicator. The prophylactic administration of factor IX concentrate led to severe complications; patients who were given it developed a marked intravascular coagulation and a few died of major bleeds (Gazzard et al 1984). Usually a platelet count of $>20 \times 10^9/l$ is sufficient to prevent or stop bleeding, but in acute liver failure, because of the factors already discussed, bleeding occurs at higher counts. It was shown that patients who suffered a major bleed had mean platelet counts of $53 \times 10^9/l$ whereas non-bleeders had counts around $91 \times 10^9/l$ (Gazzard et al 1975). It would seem reasonable therefore to maintain the platelet count $>50 \times 10^9/l$ by platelet transfusion. The levels of the coagulation inhibitors antithrombin III and protein C (Langley & Williams 1988) are low in fulminant hepatic failure, and their supplementation has been suggested in order to halt the consumption of coagulation factors. Both inhibitors have been shown to reverse the lethal effects of shock in animal models, and an uncontrolled study has suggested that maintaining normal plasma antithrombin III levels prolongs survival time in acute liver failure (Fujiwara et al 1988) and can prevent the development of the microcirculatory failure.

Cardiovascular system

A severe circulatory disturbance is characteristic of fulminant hepatic failure, although the haemodynamic and metabolic changes are similar to those seen in septic shock. There is a low systemic vascular resistance and mean arterial pressure is maintained by a compensatory increase in cardiac output (Rueff & Benhamou 1973). Hypotension occurs in 60% of patients and is caused by a further fall in systemic vascular resistance or drop in cardiac output. Patients require a high cardiac output to maintain mean arterial pressure and a fall is usually due to a reduction in left ventricular filling pressure. A relative hypovolaemia is common at presentation and volume is replaced by a combination of whole blood and 4.5% albumin solution, in order to maintain the haemoglobin at between 12 and 14 g/dl. Left and right heart filling pressures are monitored by a pulmonary artery flotation catheter in order to monitor and optimize the volume expansion. Cardiac arrythmias are rare and are usually attributable to a precipitating event such as the insertion of a central venous catheter or the development of hypoxia, hypo- or hyperkalaemia.

The pathogenesis of the low systemic vascular resistance is unclear and unlikely to be attributable to a single agent. Serum octopamine is elevated and it was thought that this false neurotransmitter might compete with endogenous catecolamines, leading to vasodilatation (Chase et al 1977). However, levels correlate directly with mean arterial pressure and are actually higher in those patients with a normal systemic vascular resistance (Trewby et al 1977). Local administration of cytokines such as tumour necrosis factor (TNF) has been shown to dilate small arterioles in an animal model in vivo (Vicaut et al 1991), and when injected into healthy animals TNF induces systemic haemodynamic changes similar to those observed in fulminant hepatic failure (Tracey et al 1986, Remick et al 1987). Production of TNF and interleukin 1 (IL-1) is high in fulminant hepatic failure (Muto et al 1988), and high levels of interleukin 6 (IL-6) have been reported in the sera in acute liver failure (Shiratori et al 1991).

In animals, administration of plasma bacterial lipopolysaccaride (endotoxin), TNF or IL-1 causes vasodilatation and hypotension by increasing production of endothelium-derived relaxing factor (EDRF) (Thiemermann & Vane 1990, Klabunde & Ritger 1991, Nava et al 1991). Nitric oxide, synthesized from L-arginine (Palmer et al 1988), accounts for the biological properties of EDRF (Palmer et al 1987). L-Citrulline is the co-product of the formation of nitric oxide from L-arginine (Moncada et al 1991), and raised plasma levels of citrulline have been found in fulminant hepatic failure (Chase et al 1978). Nitric oxide has a very short half-life in vivo as it is quickly converted to nitrite and nitrate. Plasma levels of these stable end products are thought to reflect nitric oxide synthesis (Ochoa et al 1991), and nitrite levels are high in fulminant hepatic failure (Table 28.3). The effects of nitric oxide are mediated by the activation of the cytoplasmic soluble guanylate cyclase, through the formation of a nitrosyl–haem complex at the activator site of the enzyme, with the consequent elevation of intracellular levels of cyclic 3',5'-guanosine monophosphate (cGMP) (Arnold et al 1977). The appearance of cGMP in the plasma, following its egression from cells, is used as a marker of the biological activity of nitric oxide. The stimulation of particulate guanylate cyclase by atrial natriuretic peptide (ANP) also raises plasma cGMP, and in normal subjects plasma cGMP is thought to reflect the egression of cGMP from cells following the stimulation of particulate guanylate cyclase by ANP (Jespersen et al 1990, Sagnella et al 1990, Vorderwinkler et al 1991) rather than the activity of soluble guanylate cyclase. However, a dissociation between high cGMP production and normal ANP levels has been reported in patients with severe chronic liver disease (Miyase et al 1990) and fulminant hepatic failure (Harrison et al 1992). It is possible, therefore, that the vasodilatation in fulminant hepatic failure is due to the induction of EDRF synthesis by cytokines, although this requires further investigation. The role of arachadonic acid metabolites ie prostaglandins and leukotrienes is also undefined.

Although the liver might be a major source of

Table 28.3 Plasma levels of cyclic 3',5'-guanosine monophosphate (cGMP), nitrite and atrial natriuretic peptide (ANP) in 21 patients with fulminant hepatic failure (13 had taken a paracetamol overdose, five had presumed non-A, non-B viral hepatitis and three hepatitis caused by hypersensitivity to prescribed medication) and 14 normal controls, before and after infusion of *N*-acetylcysteine

		Fulminant hepatic failure (*n*=21)	Controls (*n*=14)
cGMP (nmol/l)	Baseline	7 (1.2–120)*	1.9 (1.2–5.5)
	N-acetylcysteine	11 (1.1–115)†	—
Nitrite (μmol/l)	Baseline	18.3 (8.9–35.9)**	0.1 (0.02–0.46)
	N-acetylcysteine	15.1 (5.4–23.7)	—
ANP (pmol/l)	Baseline	14.0 (9.3–36.0)*	6.8 (3.7–14.3)
	N-acetylcysteine	15.0 (9.5–37.5)	—

Values given are median with range: *P<0.01 and **P<0.001 compared with control values;

cytokines, Devergne et al (1991), using in situ hybridization to detect RNA, found that both interleukin 1 and interleukin 6 were not expressed in liver from patients with fulminant hepatitis B viral infection, which suggests that the liver does not produce cytokines in fulminant viral hepatitis. Further studies to investigate the site of production of cytokines are required.

Even in patients with an apparently adequate mean arterial pressure and arterial oxygenation, tissue hypoxia (Bihari et al 1985a, 1986) and lactic acidosis (Bihari et al 1986b) are common and are associated with a poor outcome. Tissue hypoxia occurs because tissue oxygen uptake becomes dependent on the delivery of oxygen to the tissues, so that even though oxygen delivery is usually raised it is often inadequate for tissue requirements (Bihari et al 1987). The pathogenesis of the impaired tissue oxygen extraction is poorly understood, but it may be the consequence of abnormal blood flow in the microcirculation (Bihari et al 1985a). An impairment of hepatic microcirculation may compound liver injury in fulminant hepatic failure (Horney & Galambos 1977). Indeed, liver congestion in the presence of endotoxaemia may lead to acute hepatic necrosis without any other stimulus (Shibayama 1987). Tissue hypoxia contributes to the development of multiorgan failure in critically ill patients (Shoemaker et al 1988a, 1989) and it is associated with a poor prognosis as outcome is inversely related to the number and duration of dysfunction of failing organs (O'Grady et al 1988).

Covert tissue hypoxia is customarily detected by measuring oxygen transport variables before and after an increase in cardiac output. This is usually accomplished by the administration of either intravenous fluid (Haupt et al 1985), inotropic agents such as dobutamine (Vincent et al 1990) or microcirculatory vasodilators like prostacyclin (Bihari et al 1987). In patients demonstrated to have 'supply-dependent oxygen consumption' early in the course of their illness, it has been suggested that maintaining adequate oxygen transport variables is crucial to prevent the development of tissue hypoxia and to improve survival (Shoemaker et al 1988a, 1989). Recently a prospective controlled trial (Shoemaker et al 1988b) and a historically controlled study (Edwards et al 1989) have both shown that the optimization of oxygen transport variables, utilizing judicious volume loading and inotropic support, can significantly increase the survival of patients with sepsis and multiorgan failure.

Work with murine models has shown that *N*-acetylcysteine protects hepatocytes from oxygen free radical damage induced by interferon (Ghezzi et al 1985) and endotoxin (Ghezzi et al 1986). In addition, *N*-acetylcysteine, at concentrations obtainable in vivo, impairs the chemotaxis and generation of oxygen radicals by neutrophils (Lucht et al 1987, Kharazmi et al 1988), which potentially could prevent secondary organ damage by activated neutrophils. In a porcine model of endotoxin-induced multiorgan failure, *N*-acetylcysteine significantly attenuated all monitored haematological and pathophysiological changes (Modig & Sandin 1988). The authors concluded that inhibition of leucocyte and platelet aggregation and improvement of haemodynamic parameters by *N*-acetylcysteine contributed to a beneficial effect on outcome in this model. Another group examined the role of intravenous *N*-acetylcysteine in a sheep model of adult respiratory distress syndrome. They also found that the response to endotoxin was markedly blunted in sheep treated with *N*-acetylcysteine (Bernard et al 1984). It markedly attenuated the endotoxin-induced alterations in lung mechanics and diminished the rise in lung lymph flow.

Encouraged by the results of their animal studies, this group investigated patients with adult respiratory distress syndrome and multiorgan failure and found that they had depressed plasma and red cell glutathione concentrations. In a randomized, double-blind, controlled clinical study, these levels were substantially increased by intravenous *N*-acetylcysteine and there was a measurable clinical response to treatment with regard to an improvement in lung compliance and resolution of pulmonary oedema, as measured by gas exchange and on radiological findings (Bernard 1990). It was not clear whether these effects were directly attributable to the *N*-acetylcysteine or were the result of to repletion of glutathione. Both act as a scavengers of oxygen free radicals (Aruoma et al 1989), which have been implicated in the diffuse lung injury leading to the adult respiratory distress syndrome (Brigham 1990).

N-acetylcysteine has been shown to improve survival when administered in a controlled trial of patients with established fulminant hepatic failure following paracetamol overdose (Keays et al 1991), and a further study suggested that the improved survival might have been caused by *N*-acetylcysteine enhancing tissue oxygen transport variables (Harrison et al 1991). The effect of *N*-acetylcysteine on systemic haemodynamics and oxygen transport in viral fulminant hepatic failure is now known to be similar to that seen in patients with paracetamol-induced disease. A study in 15 patients with viral fulminant hepatic failure, due to non-A, non-B viral hepatitis in 13 and hepatitis A in the other two, is presented below.

Acute viral hepatitis was diagnosed by testing for the presence of specific IgM antibody against the common causes of virus hepatitis: hepatitis A virus, hepatitis B virus (core antigen), delta virus and Epstein–Barr virus. Non-A, non-B viral hepatitis was diagnosed by exclusion of all other causes. In all cases a pulmonary artery flotation catheter (7 French, Edward Laboratories, Irvine, CA, USA) and a radial arterial line had been inserted as part of the routine cardiovascular monitoring of patients with fulminant hepatic failure. When necessary, the pulmonary capillary wedge pressure had been increased ≥ 8 mmHg by infusion of 4.5% human albumin solution prior to the study; no further colloid was administered during the study period. Cardiovascular pressures were measured with reference to the mid-axillary line. Cardiac outputs were performed in triplicate and the mean value taken (thermodilution method, 10 ml of 5% dextrose as injectate at room temperature; COM-1 computer, Edward Laboratories). All patients had been haemodynamically stable up to the point of study and no other vasoactive drugs were administered concurrently.

At the start of the study, haemodynamic measurements were made, followed immediately by withdrawal of mixed venous and radial arterial blood samples. Each sample was analysed immediately for oxygen and carbon dioxide tensions (ABL 2000; Radiometer, Copenhagen, Denmark), along with haemoglobin content and oxygen saturation (Instrumentation laboratory oximeter 282, Lexington, MA, USA). After baseline data had been obtained, *N*-acetylcysteine (Parvolex; Duncan Flockhart, Greenford, UK) was infused in accordance with the standard intravenous regimen following paracetamol overdose: 150 mg/kg in 250 ml over 15 mins, then 50 mg/kg in 500 ml over 4 h (Prescott et al 1979). All measurements were repeated after 30 min of this regimen. The haemodynamic data obtained before and after infusion of *N*-acetylcysteine are given in Table 28.4. Infusion of *N*-acetylcysteine for

Table 28.4 The effects of intravenous *N*-acetylcysteine on systemic haemodynamics in 15 patients with acute liver failure (13 due to non-A, non-B viral hepatitis and two due to hepatitis A). Values are median (range)

	Baseline	*N*-acetylcysteine
Mean arterial pressure (mmHg)	80 (48–113)	89 (40–118)
Heart rate (beats/min)	96 (53–170)	98 (57–170)*
Cardiac index (l/min^{-1} m^{-2})	4.8 (2.4–14.0)	5.4 (2.9–15.0)***
Stroke volume index (ml/m^2)	50 (28–150)	55 (31–153)**
Left ventricular stroke work index (g $beat^{-1}$ m^2)	48 (19–139)	55 (17–160)**
Systemic vascular resistance index (dyn s cm^{-5} m^{-2})	1318 (434–2611)	1090 (453–2507)**
Pulmonary vascular resistance index (dyn s cm^{-5} m^{-2})	130 (6–361)	138 (11–529)
Right atrial pressure (mmHg)	10 (2–18)	10 (0–19)
Pulmonary capillary wedge pressure (mmHg)	13 (8–22)	13 (6–23)

*$P<0.05$, **$P<0.01$, ***$P<0.001$

30 min produced a significant fall in systemic vascular resistance ($P<0.01$), although pulmonary vascular resistance was unchanged. Cardiac index rose ($P<0.001$), associated with an increase in stroke volume index ($P<0.01$) and a small increase in heart rate ($P<0.05$). There was an increase in left ventricular stroke work index ($P<0.01$). However, there were no changes in mean arterial, right atrial or pulmonary capillary wedge pressures and no significant changes in calculated alveolar–arterial oxygen tension gradient [median 175 (range 17–413) mmHg before versus 184 (2–391) mmHg during infusion] or pulmonary shunt [median 20 (range 14–39)% before versus 20 (11–38)% during infusion]. There was an improvement in oxygen delivery ($P<0.0001$), a striking increase in oxygen consumption in all patients ($P<0.0001$) and a rise in the oxygen extraction ratio ($P<0.0001$) (Table 28.5).

Further prospective studies are underway to determine whether the effects of *N*-acetylcysteine on tissue oxygen uptake do reduce the incidence of organ failure. If this is the case then *N*-acetylcysteine should reduce mortality in viral fulminant hepatic failure. A controlled trial will then be required to examine the effect of *N*-acetylcysteine on survival in patients with viral or drug-induced acute liver. Assuming the same level of improvement in survival as seen in the patients with paracetamol-induced fulminant hepatic failure, the trial will need to enrol around 160 patients to avoid a type II error. Any single centre cannot complete such a trial in a sensible period of time because of the large numbers involved and a multicentre study will, therefore, be required.

The development of hypotension due to a further fall in systemic vascular resistance is associated with a poor prognosis. The administration of dobutamine is ineffective at increasing mean arterial pressure and, therefore, the vasopressor agents adrenaline and noradrenaline are frequently administered, commencing at a dose of 0.1 $\mu g\, kg^{-1}\, min^{-1}$, in an attempt to maintain perfusion of vital organs. However, in a recently reported study, although infusion of noradrenaline in patients with severe septic shock refractory to other therapies reversed the hypotension, the effects on tissue oxygen transport were highly variable and in many cases detrimental (Meadows et al 1988). In fulminant hepatic failure, vasopressor agents can also further compromise tissue oxygenation. Infusion of either adrenaline or noradrenaline was shown to increase mean arterial pressure, however oxygen extraction fell, resulting in a fall in oxygen uptake. Vasopressors

Table 28.5 Oxygen transport variables before and during infusion of *N*-acetylcysteine in 15 patients with acute liver failure (13 due to non-A, non-B viral hepatitis and two due to hepatitis A). Values are median (range)

	Baseline	*N*-acetylcysteine
Oxygen delivery ($ml\ min^{-1}m^{-2}$)	580 (331–1547)	680 (353–1624)***
Oxygen consumption ($ml\ min^{-1}m^{-2}$)	102 (66–294)	134 (96–316)***
Oxygen extraction ratio (%)	19 (8–31)	22 (9–31)***

***$P<0.0001$ compared with baseline values

are not, therefore, always of benefit to the patient (Wendon et al 1992). Monitoring blood pressure alone is now known to be inadequate to predict those patients who will develop tissue hypoxia, and the measurement of oxygen delivery to and oxygen consumption by the tissues should form part of the routine assessment. The success of any intervention should be assessed by its effect not only on cardiac output and blood pressure but also on oxygen transport indices.

Cerebral oedema

Patients who progress to grade IV encephalopathy with fulminant hepatic failure have an 80% chance of developing intracranial hypertension (Ede et al 1986), and this is still a major cause of death (O'Grady et al 1989). In contrast, only 9% of patients with late-onset hepatic failure develop cerebral oedema (Gimson et al 1986). The increase in intracranial pressure could result from the expansion of either the cerebrospinal fluid (CSF), blood volume or brain tissue. Changes in volume of CSF have not been measured in fulminant hepatic failure, but imaging studies have shown that the ventricles are collapsed and, therefore, it is unlikely that an increase in volume of the CSF is the initiating event (Munoz et al 1991). Increased cerebral blood flow was proposed as a pathogenic mechanism (Ede et al 1988), however it has now been shown that cerebral blood flow is decreased in all stages of encephalopathy and is independent of the aetiology of the fulminant hepatic failure (Almdal et al 1989, Sari et al 1990). Available evidence suggests that cerebral oedema initiates the raised intracranial pressure, and this is supported by work in animal models (Dixit & Chang 1990, Traber et al 1986, 1989).

The pathogenesis of cerebral oedema remains unclear, but two mechanisms have been elucidated – vasogenic and cytotoxic. In vasogenic cerebral oedema, a damaged blood–brain barrier leads to increased permeability with extravasation of a protein-rich oedema fluid into the extracellular space. Increased blood–brain barrier permeability does occur in animal models of fulminant hepatic failure (Horowitz et al 1983, Zaki et al 1984), but the endothelium appears intact (Traber et al 1987) and cytoplasmic vesicles appear to be responsible for the increased transport of substances (Kato et al 1989). The presence of increased numbers of endothelial cell vacuoles has been confirmed in a recently reported study of the ultrastructure of brain capillaries in patients dying from fulminant hepatic failure (Kato et al 1992). However, although this study suggested that vasogenic mechanisms play a role in cerebral oedema formation, the electron micrographs also showed marked intravascular swelling of perivascular astroglial foot processes pointing to cytotoxic causes being the most important. Cytotoxic cerebral oedema is due to intracellular swelling. It can be induced by ammonia or by inhibition of the Na^+, K^+-ATPase pump and serum from patients with fulminant hepatic failure was found to significantly decrease ouabain-sensitive Na^+,K^+-ATPase activity (Seda et al 1984). The two mechanisms of cerebral oedema formation are not mutually exclusive, and there is evidence that both play a role in causing the cerebral oedema of fulminant hepatic failure (Traber et al 1989).

The raised intracranial pressure due to cerebral

oedema is manifested clinically as systemic hypertension, decerebrate posturing, abnormal pupillary reflexes and ultimately impairment of brain stem function. However, these features are only apparent once raised intracranial pressure is established and cerebral oedema can occur in the absence of clinical symptoms. Papilloedema is rarely observed. The appearance of clinical signs is usually paroxysmal and they are often precipitated by tactile stimuli. Early detection of patients with cerebral oedema is required, as this will allow prompt administration of proven therapeutic modalities to prevent a fatal rise in intracranial pressure. Munoz et al (1991) assessed the efficacy of computed tomography scans of the brain to determine the presence of cerebral oedema in 15 patients with acute liver failure, comparing the findings to the direct measurement of intracranial pressure obtained from an epidural pressure monitor. Only 33% of patients with an elevated intracranial pressure were found to have evidence of cerebral oedema on the scans. It was concluded that CT scans are a poor indicator of raised intracranial pressure in patients with acute liver failure. Currently the insertion of an intracranial pressure monitoring device is the only method available to establish the diagnosis and monitor the response to therapy, although the impact of intracranial pressure monitoring on survival is as yet unknown. An extra- or subdural pressure sensor can be inserted, under local anaesthetic, through a frontal burr hole made over the non-dominant cerebral hemisphere. The procedure can be performed without correcting the coagulopathy, however at the Institute of Liver Studies we infuse platelets before making the burr hole in patients whose platelet count is $<50 \times 10^9$/l. Direct measurement of intracranial pressure allows cerebral perfusion pressure to be calculated (mean arterial pressure - intracranial pressure) and management is directed to maintaining the latter at greater than 50 mmHg. Susceptible patients are nursed at less than 20° head up (Davenport et al 1990) and tactile stimuli kept to a minimum. Immediate treatment of a fall in cerebral perfusion pressure before the development of pupillary abnormalities is expedient. In the absence of intracranial pressure monitoring, a rapid rise in the systolic blood pressure to above 150 mmHg is taken as indicative of intracranial hypertension (Ede et al 1986).

Mannitol (0.3–0.4 g/kg), by rapid bolus infusion, is the first line of treatment if raised intracranial pressure is compromising cerebral perfusion pressure (Canalese et al 1982a) and can be repeated, if necessary, unless the plasma osmolarity rises above 310 mosmol/l. In patients with incipient or established renal failure, or in those who do not have a diuresis to mannitol, ultrafiltration is commenced to remove about three times the given volume of the mannitol bolus over the subsequent 30 min. Thiopentone may be useful in the management of cerebral oedema that is resistant to mannitol therapy (Forbes et al 1989). Prolonged hyperventilation is not beneficial in controlling cerebral oedema (Ede et al 1986), and the role of acute hyperventilation to reduce cerebral blood flow in order to control sudden surges of intracranial hypertension is now under review, as it reduces cerebral oxygen consumption and increases cerebral lactate production, suggesting that it causes cerebral ischaemia (Wendon et al 1993). The prophylactic administration of steroids was found to be ineffective in reducing cerebral oedema (Canalese et al 1982). Vasopressor agents are administered when required in order to maintain an adequate mean arterial pressure and maintain the cerebral perfusion pressure at greater than 50 mmHg.

Although the clinical signs of raised intracranial pressure due to cerebral oedema in fulminant hepatic failure have been attributed to coning, coning is found in only 25% of these patients at autopsy (Ware et al 1971). Therefore, there is increasing interest in the role of cerebral hypoxia in the evolution of the pupillary abnormalities in fulminant hepatic failure, as it is known that cerebral oxygen consumption is markedly reduced (Sari et al 1990). If this is confirmed, the cerebral hypoxia must be reversible, at least in some patients, as those who recover from fulminant hepatic failure complicated by cerebral oedema have a low incidence of permanent neurological sequelae (O'Brien et al 1987).

In a controlled trial of intravenous *N*-acetylcysteine in patients with established fulminant hepatic failure following paracetamol overdose, there was a lower incidence of clinical signs of raised intracranial pressure in the treated group (Keays et al 1991). In order to determine whether this might be related to improvements in cerebral oxygen transport, cerebral blood flow and oxygen consumption were measured in 12 patients with fulminant hepatic failure in grade IV coma using the intravenous xenon-133 technique. Cerebral blood flow following infusion of *N*-acetylcysteine rose from 31.5 to 40 ml $min^{-1}100g^{-1}$ ($P<0.01$), associated with a rise in cerebral oxygen consumption from 0.89 to 1.21 ml $min^{-1}100g^{-1}$ ($P<0.01$) (Wendon et al 1992b). The response to *N*-acetylcysteine was independent of the aetiology of the liver failure (Table 28.6). The mechanism by which *N*-acetylcysteine improves tissue oxygenation is unknown, but there is some evidence to suggest that *N*-acetylcysteine may have improved tissue blood flow by enhancing the local effects of endothelium-derived relaxing factor (Harrison et al 1992), producing a rise in plasma cGMP (Table 28.3).

Respiratory complications

When patients progress to grade IV encephalopathy intubation is usually required to protect the airway. In addition, the risk of aspiration of gastric contents is not inconsiderable in patients with grade II–III encephalopathy, who frequently vomit, and airway protection with an endotracheal tube is advised before transportation of such patients to a specialist centre. Poor gas exchange leading to arterial hypoxaemia can develop as a result of a combination of lobar pneumonia, intrapulmonary haemorrhage, the adult respiratory distress syndrome, atelectasis and intrapulmonary shunting. The hypoxaemia is managed utilizing volume-controlled mechanical ventilation while the patient receives a continuous intravenous infusion of muscle relaxant, usually atracurium at 50 mg/h. Adjuvant positive end-expiratory pressure is frequently used in an attempt to improve arterial oxygenation. However, it can accentuate the haemodynamic instability and, although theoretically beneficial, it has never conclusively been shown to be of benefit.

Table 28.6 Cerebral blood flow and cerebral metabolism in patients with fulminant hepatic failure and grade IV encephalopathy (seven following paracetamol overdose and five patients with acute non-A, non-B viral hepatitis), before and after infusion of *N*-acetylcysteine:

	Paracetamol overdose (*n*=7)	Acute non-A, non-B viral hepatitis (*n*=5)
Cerebral blood flow (ml 100 g^{-1} min^{-1})		
Baseline	33 (24–60)	30 (27–54)
N-acetylcysteine		
Oxygen consumption (ml 100 g^{-1} min^{-1})		
Baseline	0.85 (0.33 – 2.03)	0.93 (0.66–1.59)
N-acetylcysteine		
Oxygen extraction ratio (%)		
Baseline	17.9 (4.2–40.5)	24.3 (7.6–48.8)
N-acetylcysteine		
Metabolic rate for lactate (µmol 100 g^{-1} min^{-1})		
Baseline	0 (-12–15.6)	-2.0 (-37.8–8.1)
N-acetylcysteine		
Metabolic rate for glucose (µmol 100 g^{-1} min^{-1})		
Baseline	22 (3–30)	15 (2–27)
N-acetylcysteine		

Values given are median with range.
There were no statistical differences between the two aetiological groups.

Bronchoscopy and lavage may be required to remove mucous plugs causing hypoventilation of a lung or segment, or to establish the cause of infection. Chest physiotherapy is used, however this may need to be withheld temporarily if the patient develops raised intracranial pressure.

Renal failure and metabolic disorders

Renal failure requiring dialysis (anuria or oliguria with a urine output <300 ml/24 h and a serum creatinine >300 µmol/l) occurs in about 30% of patients in grade IV encephalopathy resulting from fulminant viral hepatitis (O'Grady et al 1988). It is caused by a combination of functional renal failure and acute tubular necrosis; the latter is caused by poor renal perfusion. Renal blood flow is reduced because of the formation of local vasoconstrictors and low perfusion pressure secondary to the loss of circulating volume, which occurs early in the course of fulminant hepatic failure. Impaired urea synthesis in acute liver failure results in a marked disparity between the serum urea and creatinine levels and the former is a very unreliable guide to renal function.

The use of a low-dose dopamine infusion (2.5 $\mu g\,kg^{-1}\,h^{-1}$) may prevent a further deterioration in renal function and is routinely given, although it has never been shown to be effective in a prospective, controlled study. The use of high-dose loop diuretics is not advised as this does not improve or prevent a deterioration in renal function and can exacerbate the hepatorenal failure. Nephrotoxic drugs, such as mannitol and aminoglycosides, may have to be given, but their use should be monitored with considerable care. Renal replacement therapy is instituted if acidosis, fluid overload, hyperkalaemia or a creatinine of greater than 400 µmol/l occurs. Intermittent machine haemodialysis is often problematical in these patients and can cause a deterioration in cerebral oedema (Davenport et al 1989a). Continuous arteriovenous haemodiafiltration may have considerable advantages (Davenport et al 1989b) and it is considered the treatment of choice in patients requiring renal replacement therapy who are haemodynamically unstable or at risk of developing cerebral oedema. Anticoagulation is necessary despite the coagulopathy and it is normally achieved with heparin, but prostacyclin may be used to reduce platelet activation.

Hypoglycaemia is a consequence of increased circulating insulin, impaired gluconeogenesis and inability to mobilize glycogen stores. Blood glucose levels are monitored hourly and 50 ml of 50% glucose is administered intravenously if the blood level falls below 3.5 mmol/l. In patients with frequent hypoglycaemia, a continuous infusion of 10 or 20% glucose is more appropriate. Hypophosphataemia is common in patients with acute liver failure who are continuing to pass urine and it is treated by appropriate intravenous replacement.

The development of a metabolic acidosis that does not respond to intravenous volume loading develops in around 10% of patients with viral acute liver failure and is associated with a very poor prognosis as it reflects profound tissue hypoxia. As already discussed management of this problem centres upon improving tissue oxygen delivery. The administration of intravenous sodium bicarbonate is not beneficial, and haemodialysis or continuous arteriovenous haemodiafiltration can remove hydrogen ions but does not treat the underlying problem and rarely corrects the arterial pH. Plasma lactate levels are frequently raised in fulminant hepatic failure and are due to a combination of anaerobic metabolism by hypoxic tissues and reduced lactate clearance by the failing liver (Bihari et al 1985b). Although they are frequently used as a guide to the development of tissue hypoxia, it is important to remember that tissue hypoxia can occur before the change to anaerobic respiration (Robin 1980) and lactic acid production (Cohen & Woods 1976).

Sepsis

Bacterial infection is found in more than 80% of patients (Rolando et al 1990). The prevalent organisms are *staphylococci*, *streptococci* and *coliform* bacteria (Rolando et al 1990). Fungi are frequently isolated, predominantly *Candida* species (Rolando et al 1990), but *Aspergilla* has also been reported as a common pathogen (Watanabe et al 1987). The high incidence of infection is related to impaired cell-mediated and humoral immunity. Neutrophil adherence and phagocytosis (Altin et al 1983) and Kupffer cell function are compromised (Imawari et al 1985). The latter may limit the clearance of endotoxin and allow the passage of bacteria translocated from the gut into the systemic circulation. The importance of Kupffer cell function to outcome from fulminant hepatic failure is emphasized by a study that demonstrated that in a group of patients with a similar degree of hepatocyte dysfunction survival was related to the degree of Kupffer cell dysfunction, as measured by microaggregated albumin clearance (Canalese et al 1982). The deficiency of fibronectin production exacerbates the defect in host immunity by reducing opsonization (Imawari et al 1985, Almasio et al 1986, Anand et al 1989). Antibiotics are commenced in patients where there is a clinical suspicion of bacterial infection and the choice of antimicrobial directed by the results of daily cultures which should be taken from all sites. No response after 48 h suggests a fungal aetiology and appropriate therapy should be added. A 14-day course of amphotericin B with 5-flucytosine is usually adequate treatment. The benefit of prophylactic administration of broad-spectrum antibiotics with or without selective gastrointestinal tract decontamination is as yet unproven.

LIVER TRANSPLANTATION AND ASSESSMENT OF PROGNOSIS

Survival from acute liver failure is improving as a result of constant refinements to the intensive medical care outlined above (Fig. 28.2). However, it is recognized that some patients will not survive with medical therapy alone, and these cases require orthotopic liver transplantation (Bismuth et al 1987, Peleman et al 1987, Vickers et al 1987, O'Grady et al 1988, Emond et al 1989). Recent reports are encouraging with a 1-year survival of around 70% (O'Grady et al 1988). This topic is covered in more detail elsewhere in this volume.

The availability of orthotopic liver transplantation as a management option in acute liver failure has necessitated the development of methods of accurately assessing the prognosis in individual patients early in the clinical course. The aetiology of the liver failure has a major influence on outcome. Those patients with either hepatitis A or B viruses have survival rates of between 40 and 68% with intensive medical care alone, whereas those with non-A, non-B hepatitis have a survival rate of only 20% without liver transplantation (Fig. 28.2).

However, aetiology alone is insufficient to predict accurately the outcome in an individual, and other prognostic indicators are required. Many variables have been used to assess outcome in fulminant hepatic failure (Christensen et al 1984) and coagulation studies are established as prognostic indicators (Tygstrup & Ranek 1986). In an early study from the Institute of Liver Studies, the factor VII level was shown to provide a good indication of prognosis (Dymock et al 1975), and later serial factor VII levels were shown to improve the predictive power of this test (Gazzard et al 1976). Benhamou's group in Paris, using a multivariate analysis, found that a reduced factor V level was the most sensitive prognostic indicator in patients with fulminant hepatitis B infection (Bernuau et al 1986). However, the assay of individual clotting factors is not a routine investigation in most laboratories, whereas the prothrombin time is reproducible and is nearly always available. Data have shown that a prothrombin time >50 s (control 15 s) is associated with a poor outcome in viral-induced fulminant hepatic failure, as are a bilirubin >300 μmol/l, age under 10 years and over 40 years, and an interval of >7 days between the onset of jaundice and the development of encephalopathy (O'Grady et al 1989).

UNSUCCESSFUL THERAPEUTIC INTERVENTIONS

The results of randomized, controlled trials of corticosteroid therapy in fulminant hepatic failure show that this treatment is of no benefit, and it may even increase mortality (Rakela et al 1991). Some patients with late-onset hepatic failure are steroid responsive, but these patients are hard to identify and the use of steroids greatly increases the chance of sepsis. Continuous infusions of

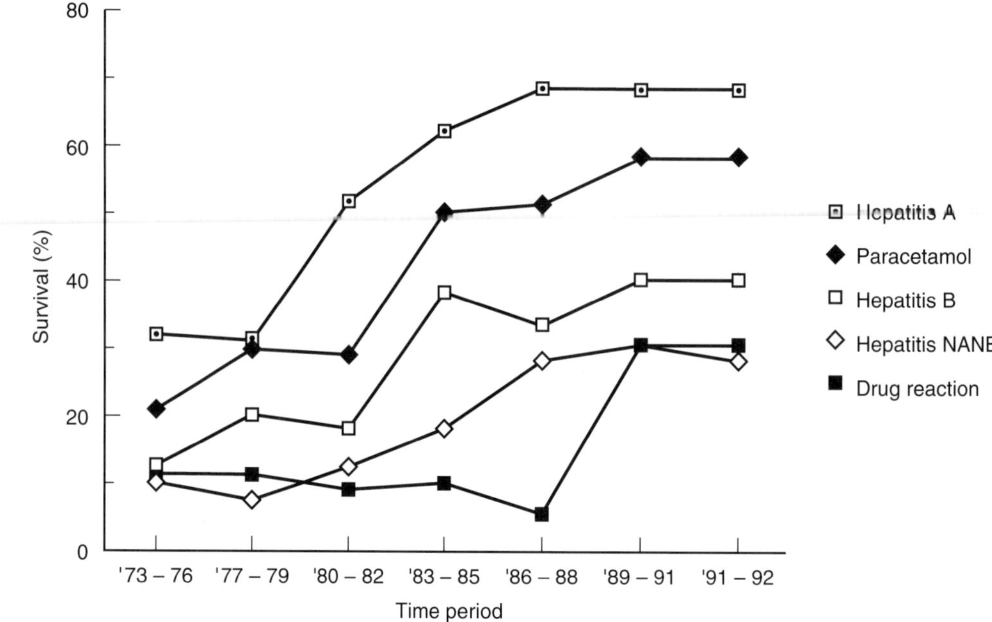

Fig. 28.2

insulin and glucagon, in order to promote liver regeneration, have been tried, and in uncontrolled studies this therapy appeared to increase survival. However, Woolf & Redeker (1991) completed a randomized, controlled trial of insulin and glucagon infusion in 38 patients and showed that mortality was not significantly different in control and treatment groups (67% and 82% respectively). These results confirm those of another recent controlled trial from the Institute of Liver Studies (Harrison et al 1990) and demonstrate that the combination of insulin and glucagon is not useful in the treatment of acute liver failure.

Charcoal is an effective adsorbent for a wide range of potentially toxic substances including mercaptans, aromatic amino acids and inhibitors of the Na^+, K^+ ATPase. Significant reductions in the circulating levels of these substances have been demonstrated in patients treated by charcoal haemoperfusion, and early results in patients treated in grade III rather than grade IV encephalopathy pointed to an improved survival, although in a subsequent controlled trial no improvement in survival was found comparing 10 h of charcoal haemoperfusion daily to conventional intensive care (O'Grady et al 1988). However, the relatively small numbers of patients in each of the different aetiological groups in this study does mean that the possibility of a type II error was quite high.

NEW THERAPEUTIC AGENTS

Mortality in fulminant hepatic failure, as in other causes of multiorgan failure, is directly related to the number of failing organs (O'Grady et al 1988); with support recovery of organ function is possible and the liver's remarkable capacity for regeneration means that patients who recover do so completely. New therapies are required that would, when administered in fulminant hepatic failure due to any cause, be effective in reducing hepatic necrosis, promote recovery of liver function and prevent or attenuate the multiorgan failure. A number of potential therapeutic agents are discussed below.

There are only a few studies on the use of antiviral drugs, and these are limited to uncontrolled trials using small numbers of patients. In most cases of fulminant hepatitis B and D, active viral replication appears to be low compared with uncompensated acute hepatitis B viral infection and may have ceased before admission. In some patients the extent of liver damage may be so great that liver regeneration is impossible even if further replication were inhibited by antiviral therapy.

In patients with fulminant viral hepatitis, peripheral blood mononuclear cells were demonstrated to be unable to produce interferons and circulating interferon was markedly low (Levin & Hahn 1985). Therefore, interferon has been administered to patients with fulminant hepatic failure in the hope that it might confer a benefit. In an uncontrolled study of 32 patients (due in 17 to hepatitis A virus, in 7 to hepatitis B virus, in 6 to non-A, non-B virus and in one each to herpes and cytomegalovirus) treated with human alpha interferon at an i.m. dose of 3×10^6 U/day (70 000 U kg^{-1} day^{-1} for infants) for mean 88 ± 3 days, 16 patients (50%) recovered, including 9 of 22 (41%) who were in grades III–IV coma when treatment was started. In patients who recovered, improvement was often noted on about the fifth day of interferon treatment (Levin et al 1989). However, in a multicentre study of 16 patients with fulminant viral hepatitis, fibroblast interferon was shown to offer no significant benefit (Milazzo et al 1985), and in another study of 10 patients with fulminant viral hepatitis (hepatitis A, 1; hepatitis B, 2; hepatitis B and hepatitis D co-infection, 7) treated with recombinant alpha interferon, only one patient survived (Sanchez-Tapias et al 1987). Therefore, the role of interferon in fulminant viral hepatitis remains unproven and no controlled studies have been reported to date. Antagonism of endogenous opioids by naloxone has been shown to improve the haemodynamic disturbance, attenuate lactic acidosis and increase survival during endotoxin shock (Law & Ferguson 1988). In an anecdotal report, naloxone improved the circulatory disturbance in fulminant hepatic failure (De et al 1983) but no further data on its efficacy are available.

In animal models of toxic and viral acute liver failure, prostaglandins of the E series have been shown to offer cytoprotection to the liver (Alp & Hickman 1987) and brain (Dixit & Chang 1987). Also, prostacyclin has been shown to attenuate liver damage in rats treated with galactosamine (Noda et al 1986). In clinical studies, the treatment of fulminant viral hepatitis with prostaglandins of the E series has been reported to be of some benefit in comparison with historical controls (Sinclair & Levy 1991). However, two studies from Benhamou's group in Paris have not confirmed these findings in fulminant hepatic failure due to either hepatitis B virus, or non-A, non-B hepatitis. The results of controlled studies are needed before routine therapy with prostaglandin E becomes established.

Oxpentifylline is a dimethylxanthine derivative that has been shown to counter the lethal effects of endotoxin in an animal model of septic shock (Schönharting & Schade 1989). It inhibited the production of TNF in mononuclear cells both in vitro (Waage et al 1990) and in vivo in man (Zabel et al 1989), following endotoxin challenge, an effect that was probably mediated by decreasing TNF mRNA. The effect was selective as IL-6 production was unaffected. In view of the possible role of TNF in mediating some of the pathophysiological changes in fulminant hepatic failure, oxpentifylline is potentially beneficial. However, to date there have been no studies of the effects of oxpentifylline in acute liver failure.

The development of monoclonal antibodies to endotoxin and TNF and IL-1 receptor antagonists offers another possible therapeutic approach. A randomized, double-blind, placebo-controlled trial of an antiendotoxin monoclonal antibody (HA-1A) in patients with Gram-negative sepsis, showed that HA-1A was of some benefit (Ziegler et al 1991). However, HA-1A has recently been withdrawn due to a concern over its safety in some sub-groups of patients. Also, an IL-1 receptor antagonist has proved effective in a rabbit model of septic shock (Ohlsson et al 1990). However, again there have been no studies examining the effects of these agents in acute liver failure.

Recently, research has focused on methods of transplantation of hepatocytes and hepatocytes immobilized in cell reactors, the so-called bioartificial liver. Transplantation of hepatocytes into the spleen or lung has proved successful in animal models, but these techniques are unlikely to be adopted for the treatment of patients with fulminant hepatic failure. Workers have attached hepatocytes to microcarriers as a support and injected them into the intraperitoneal cavity, however transplanted hepatocytes underwent complete necrosis in 3 days, indicating the need for other methods of metabolic support. Microencapsulation of hepatocytes within semipermeable membranes prior to transplantation may be a better method for maintaining cell viability and reducing the need for immunosuppression. Free hepatocytes isolated from rats and microencapsulated with collagen within an alginate copolymer membrane were transplanted into the peritoneal cavity of Gunn rats, which are congenitally deficient in bilirubin conjugation, and serum bilirubin was reduced for up to 1 month. No inflammatory reaction was observed and the hepatocytes remained intact in the microcapsules (Dixit et al 1990). This approach could be more practical for application in liver failure.

Demetriou has developed an extracorporeal circuit with hepatocytes in a hollow fibre membrane. Direct perfusion of blood or preferably plasma over microcarrier-attached hepatocytes in an extracorporeal device may be a better approach than retaining hepatocytes by membranes, though the biocompatibility of the microcarrier needs to be considered. Hemoperfusion over hepatocytes immobilized on Biosilon microcarriers significantly improved the survival rate of rats with liver failure induced by galactosamine compared with haemoperfusion with microcarriers alone (Shnyra et al 1991). It remains to be seen which method will prove best for clinical use, but there is little doubt that in the future the bioartificial liver will play an important role in the treatment of fulminant hepatic failure, both as a bridge to transplantation and as a support until the patient's own liver regenerates.

SUMMARY

Acute liver failure is no longer invariably fatal and survival rates continue to improve. Medical management relies on meticulous intensive care with attention to the specific systems as outlined above. At the time of initial presentation, and subsequently, the patient must be assessed with regard to their likely prognosis and, hence, their requirement for orthotopic liver transplantation. This has been facilitated by the development of prognostic indicators that can identify those patients in need of urgent liver grafting early in the course of the illness. Patients with acute live failure should be transferred early to liver centres experienced in the management of such patients and with facilities for transplantation. Patients should not be transferred and assessed for transplantation once intensive care has failed, as these patients are frequently too sick to undergo the grafting procedure. The improved outcome of all aetiological groups with fulminant hepatic failure treated at the Institute of Liver Studies since 1973 (Fig. 28.2) not only demonstrates the value of a coordinated management approach but also the long-term reward of continued research and development.

REFERENCES

Almasio P L, Hughes R D, Williams R 1986 Characterization of the molecular forms of fibronectin in fulminant hepatic failure. Hepatology 6: 1340–1345

Almdal T, Schroeder, Ranek L 1989 Cerebral blood flow and liver function in patients with encephalopathy due to acute and chronic liver diseases. Scandinavian Journal of Gastroenterology 24: 299–303

Alp M H, Hickman R 1987 The effect of prostaglandins, branched-chain amino acids and other drugs on the outcome of experimental acute porcine hepatic failure. Journal of Hepatology 4: 99–107

Altin M, Rajkovic I A, Hughes R.D, Williams R 1983 Neutrophil adherence in chronic liver disease and fulminant hepatic failure. Gut 24: 746–750

Anand A C, Irshad M, Acharya S K, Gandhi B M, Joshi Y K, Tandon B N 1989 Fibronectin in acute and subacute hepatic failure. Journal of Clinical Gastroenterology 11: 314–319

Arnold W P, Mittal C K, Katsuki S, Murad F 1977 Nitric oxide activates guanylate cyclase and increases guanosine 3',5'- cyclic monophosphate levels in various tissue preparations. Proceedings of the National Academy of Sciences of the USA 74: 3203–3207

Aruoma O, Halliwell B, Hoey B, Butler J 1989 The antioxidant action of N-acetylcysteine: its reaction with hydrogen peroxide, hydroxyl radical, superoxide, and hypochlorous acid. Free Radical Biology and Medicine 6: 593–597

Basile A S 1991 The contribution of endogenous benzodiazepine receptor ligands to the pathogenesis of hepatic encephalopathy. Synapse 7: 141–150

Basile A S, Hughes R D, Harrison P M et al 1991 Elevated brain concentrations of 1,4-benzodiazepines in fulminant hepatic failure. New England Journal of Medicine 325: 473–478

Bernard G R 1990 Potential of N-acetylcysteine as treatment for the adult respiratory distress syndrome European Respiratory Journal (suppl.)

Bernard G R, Lucht W D, Niedermeyer M E, Snapper J R, Ogletree M L, Brigham K L 1984 Effect of N-acetylcystein on the pulmonary response to endotoxin in the awake sheep and upon in vitro granulocyte function. Journal of Clinical Investigation 73: 1772–1784

Bernuau J, Goudeau A, Poynard T et al 1986 Multivariate analysis in fulminant hepatitis B. Hepatology 6: 648–651

Bernuau J, Rueff B, Benhamou J P 1986 Fulminant and subfulminant liver failure: definitions and causes. Seminars in Liver Disease 6: 97–106

Bihari D, Gimson A E, Waterson M, Williams R 1985a Tissue hypoxia during fulminant hepatic failure. Critical Care Medicine 13: 1034–1039

Bihari D, Gimson A E, Lindridge J, Williams R 1985b Lactic acidosis in fulminant hepatic failure. Some aspects of pathogenesis and prognosis. Journal of Hepatology 1: 405–416

Bihari D J, Gimson A E, Williams R 1986 Cardiovascular, pulmonary and renal complications of fulminant hepatic failure. Seminars in liver Disease 6: 119–128

Bihari D, Smithies M, Gimson A,Tinker J 1987 The effects of vasodilation with prostacyclin on oxygen delivery and uptake in critically ill patients. New England Journal of Medicine 317: 397–403

Bismuth H, Samuel D, Gugenheim J et al 1987 Emergency liver transplantation for fulminant hepatitis. Annals of Internal Medicine 107: 337–341

Brigham K L 1990 Oxidant stress and adult respiratory distress syndrome. European Respiratory Journal (suppl) 11: 482S–484S

Canalese J, Gimson A E S, Davis C et al 1982 Controlled trial of dexamethasone and mannitol for the cerebral oedema of fulminant hepatic failure. Gut 23: 625–629

Canalese J, Gove C D, Gimson A E S, Wilkinson S P, Wardle E N, Williams R 1982. Reticuloendothelial system and hepatocyte function in fulminant hepatic failure. Gut 23: 265–269

Carman W F, Fagan E A, Hadziyannis S et al 1991 Association of a precore genomic variant of hepatitis B virus with fulminant hepatitis. Hepatology 14: 219–222

Chase R, Trewby P, Davis M, Williams R 1977 Serum octopamine, coma and charcoal haemoperfusion in fulminant hepatic failure. European Journal of Clinical Medicine 7: 351–354

Chase R, Davies A M, Trewby M A, Silk D B A, Williams R 1978 Plasma amino acid profiles in patients with fulminant hepatic failure treated by repeated polyacrylonitrile membrane hemodialysis. Gastroenterology 75: 1033–1040

Christensen E, Bremmelgaard A, Bahnsen M et al 1984 Prediction of fatality in fulminant hepatic failure. Scandinavian Journal of Gastroenterology 19: 90–96

Cohen R D, Woods H F 1976 Clinical and biochemical aspects of lactic acidosis. Blackwell Scientific Publications, Oxford

Devenport A, Will E J, Davison A M 1990 Effect of posture on intracranial pressure and cerebral perfusion pressure in patients with fulminant hepatic and renal failure after acetaminophen self-poisoning. Critical Care Medicine 18: 286–289

Davenport A, Will E J, Davison A M et al 1989a Changes in intracranial pressure during machine and continuous haemofiltration. International Journal of Artificial Organs 12: 439–444

Davenport A, Will E J, Davison A M et al 1989b Changes in intracranial pressure during haemofiltration in oliguric patients with grade IV hepatic encephalopathy. Nephron 53: 142–146

De G G, Schalm S W, Dirksen R, Valk K C, Boks A L 1983 Effect of naloxone on shock in a patient with fulminant hepatic failure. Netherlands Journal of Medicine 26: 77–79

Devergne O, Peuchmaur M, Humbert M et al 1991 In vivo expression of IL-1 beta and IL-6 genes during viral infections in human. European Cytokine Network 2: 183–194

Dixit V, Chang T M 1987 Effects of prostaglandin E2 on brain edema and liver histopathology in a galactosamine-induced fulminant hepatic failure rat model. Biomaterials, Artificial Cells and Artificial Organs 15: 559–573

Dixit V, Darvasi R, Arthur M, Brezina M, Lewin K, Gitnick G 1990 Restoration of liver function in Gunn rats without immunosuppression using transplanted microencapsulated hepatocytes. Hepatology 12: 1342–1349

Dymock I W, Tucker J S, Woolf I L et al 1975 Coagulation studies as a prognostic index in acute liver failure. British Journal of Haematology 29: 385–395

Ede R J, Gimson A E, Bihari D, Williams R 1986 Controlled hyperventilation in the prevention of cerebral oedema in fulminant hepatic failure. Journal of Hepatology 2: 43–51

Ede R, Gove C, Williams R 1988 Increased cerebral blood flow in fulminant hepatic failure due to paracetamol overdose. In: Soeters P, Wilson J, Meijer A, Hahn E (eds) Advances in ammonia metabolism and hepatic encephalopathy. Elsevier, Amsterdam, pp 301–305

Edwards J D, Brown G C, Nightingale P, Slater R M, Faragher E B 1989 Use of survivors' cardiorespiratory values as therapeutic goals in septic shock. Critical Care Medicine 17: 1098–1103

Emond J C, Aran P P, Whitington P F et al 1989 Liver transplantation in the management of fulminant hepatic failure. Gastroenterology 96: 1583–1588

Ferenci P, Grimm G 1990 Benzodiazepine antagonist in the treatment of human hepatic encephalopathy. Advances in Experimental Medicine and Biology 272: 255–265

Fick T E, Schalm S W, de V M 1989 Continuous intravenous ammonia infusion as a model for the study of hepatic encephalopathy in rabbits. Journal of Surgical Research 46: 221–225

Forbes A, Alexander G J, O'Grady J G et al 1989 Thiopental infusion in the treatment of intracranial hypertension complicating fulminant hepatic failure. Hepatology 10: 306–310

Fujiwara K, Ogata I, Ohta Y et al 1988 Intravascular coagulation in acute liver failure in rats and its treatment with antithrombin III. Gut 29: 1103–1108

Fujiwara K, Okita K, Akamatsu K et al 1988 Antithrombin III concentrate in the treatment of fulminant hepatic failure. Gastroenterologica Japonica 23: 423–427

Gazzard B G, Henderson J M, Williams R 1975 Early

changes in coagulation following a paracetamol overdose and a controlled trial of fresh frozen plasma therapy. Gut 16: 617–620
Gazzard B G, Rake M O, Flute P T, Williams R 1975 Bleeding in relation to the coagulation defect of fulminant hepatic failure. Artificial liver support. Pitman Medical Publishing, London
Gazzard B G, Henderson J M, Williams R 1976 Factor VII levels as a guide to prognosis in fulminant hepatic failure. Gut 17: 489–491
Gazzard B G, Lewis M L, Ash G, Williams R 1984 Coagulation factor concentrate in the treatment of the haemorrhagic diathesis of fulminant hepatic failure. Gut 15: 993–998
Ghezzi P, Bianchi M, Gianera L, Landolfo S, Salmona M 1985 Role of reactive oxygen intermediates in the interferon-mediated depression of hepatic drug metabolism and protective effect of N-acetylcysteine in mice. Cancer Research 45: 3444–3447
Ghezzi P, Saccardo B, Bianchi M 1986 Role of reactive oxygen intermediates in the hepatotoxicity of endotoxin. Immunopharmacology 12: 241–244
Gimson A E S, White Y S, Eddleston A L W F, Williams R 1983 Clinical and prognostic differences in fulminant hepatitis type A, B, and non-A, non-B. Gut 24: 1194–1198
Gimson A E S, O'Grady J, Ede R J et al 1986 Late-onset hepatic failure: clinical, serological and histological features. Hepatology 6: 288–294
Harrison P M, Hughes R D, Forbes A, Portmann B, Alexander G J M, Williams R 1990 Failure of insulin and glucagon to stimulate liver regeneration in fulminant hepatic failure. Journal of Hepatology 10: 332–336
Harrison P M, Wendon J A, Gimson A E, Alexander G J, Williams R 1991 Improvement by acetylcysteine of hemodynamics and oxygen transport in fulminant hepatic failure. New England Journal of Medicine 324: 1852–1857
Harrison P M, Wendon J A, Williams R 1992 Increase in plasma cyclic 3',5'-guanosine monophosphate but not atrial natriuretic factor in response to N-acetylcysteine infusion in fulminant hepatic failure (abstract). Journal of Vascular Research 29: 129
Haupt M T, Gilbert E M, Carlson R W 1985 Fluid loading increases oxygen consumption in septic patients with lactic acidosis. American Review of Respiratory Disease. 131: 912–916
Horney J, Galambos J 1977 The liver during and after fulminant hepatitis. Gastroenterology. 73: 639–645
Horowitz M E, Schafer D F, Molnaret P et al 1983 Increased blood–brain transfer in a rabbit model of acute liver failure. Gastroenterology 84: 1003–1011
Imawari M, Hughes R D, Gove C D, Williams R 1985 Fibronectin and Kupffer cell function in fulminant hepatic failure. Digestive Disease and Science 30: 1028–1033
Jespersen B, Jensen L, Sorensen S S, Pedersen E B 1990 Atrial natriuretic factor, cyclic 3',5'-guanosine monophosphate and prostaglandin E2 in liver cirrhosis: relation to blood volume and changes in blood volume after furosemide. European Journal of Clinical Investigation 20: 632–641
Jones D B, Mullen K D, Roessle M, Maynard T, Jones E A 1987 Hepatic encephalopathy. Application of visual evoked responses to test hypotheses of its pathogenesis in rats. Journal of Hepatology 4: 118–126
Kato M, Sugihara J, Nakamura T, Muto Y 1989 Electron microscopic study of the blood–brain barrier in rats with brain edema and encephalopathy due to acute hepatic failure. Gastroenterologica Japonica 24: 135–142
Kato M, Hughes R D, Keays R, Williams R 1992 Electron microscopic study of brain capillaries in cerebral edema from fulminant hepatic failure. Hepatology 15: 1060–1066
Keays R, Harrison P M, Wendon J A et al 1991 Intravenous acetylcysteine in paracetamol induced fulminant hepatic failure: a prospective controlled trial. British Medical Journal 303: 1026–1029
Kharazmi A, Nielsen H, Schiotz P 1988 N-acetylcysteine inhibits human neutrophil and monocyte chemotaxis and oxidative metabolism. International Journal of Immunopharmacology 10: 39–46
Klabunde R E, Ritger R C 1991 NG-monomethyl-l-arginine (NMA) restores arterial blood pressure but reduces cardiac output in a canine model of endotoxic shock. Biochemical and Biophysical Research Communications 178: 1135–1140
Kojima M, Shimizu M, Tsuchimochi T et al 1991 Posttransfusion fulminant hepatitis B associated with precore-defective HBV mutants. Vox Sanguinis 60: 34–39
Kosaka Y, Takase K, Kojima M et al 1991 Fulminant hepatitis B: induction by hepatitis B virus mutants defective in the precore region and incapable of encoding e antigen. Gastroenterology 100: 1087–1094
Langley P G, Williams R 1988 The effect of fulminant hepatic failure on protein C antigen and activity. Thrombosis and Haemostasis 59: 316–318
Langley P G, Hughes R D 1982 Platelet adhesiveness to glass beads in liver disease. Acta Haematologica 67: 124–127
Langley P G, Hughes R D, Williams R 1985 Increased factor VIII complex in fulminant hepatic failure. Thrombosis and Haemostasis 54: 693–696
Law W R, J L Ferguson 1988 Naloxone alters organ perfusion during endotoxin shock in conscious rats. American Journal of Physiology 54: H1023–1029
Lechner K, Niessner H, Thaler 1977 Coagulation abnormalities in liver disease. Seminars in Thrombosis and Haemostasis 4: 40–56
Levin S, Hahn T 1985 Interferon deficiency syndrome. Clinical and Experimental Immunology 60: 267–273
Levin S, Leibowitz E, Torten J, Hahn T 1989 Interferon treatment in acute progressive and fulminant hepatitis. Israeli Journal of Medicine and Science 25: 364–372
Liang T J, Hasegawa K, Rimon N, Wands J R, Ben P E 1991 A hepatitis B virus mutant associated with an epidemic of fulminant hepatitis. New England Journal of Medicine 324: 1705–1709
Lucht W, English D, Bernard G, Serafin W, Brigham K 1987 Prevention of release of granulocyte aggregants into sheep lung lymph following endotoxemia by N-acetylcysteine. American Journal of Medicine and Science 294: 161–167
Macdougall B R D, Williams R 1978 H2 receptor antagonist in the prevention of acute upper gastrointestinal haemorhage in fulminanthepatic failure. Gastroenterology 74: 464–465
Mathieson L R, Shivoj P, Nielsen J P, Purcell R H, Wong D, Ranek L 1980 Hepatitis type A, B and non-A, non-B in fulminant hepatitis. Gut 21: 72–77
Meadows D, Edwards J D, Wilkins R G et al 1988 Reversal of intractable septic shock with norepinephrine therapy. Critical Care Medicine 16: 663

Milazzo F, Galli M, Fassio P G et al 1985 Attempted treatment of fulminant viral hepatitis with human fibroblast interferon. Infection 13: 130–133

Miyase S, Fujiyama S, Chikazawa H, Sato T. 1990 Atrial natriuretic peptide in liver cirrhosis with mild ascites. Gastroenterologica Japonica 25: 356–362

Modig J, Sandin R 1988 Haematological, physiological and survival data in a porcine model of adult respiratory distress syndrome induced by endotoxaemia. Effects of treatment with N-acetylcysteine. Acta Chirugica Scandinavica 154: 169–177

Moncada S, Palmer R M J, Higgs E A 1991 Nitric Oxide: physiology, pathophysiology and pharmacology. Pharmacological Reviews 43: 109–142

Munoz S J, Robinson M, Northrup B et al 1991 Elevated intracranial pressure and computed tomography of the brain in fulminant hepatocellular failure. Hepatology 13: 209–212

Muto Y, Nouri A K, Meager A, Alexander G J, Eddleston A L, Williams R 1988 Enhanced tumour necrosis factor and interleukin-1 in fulminant hepatic failure. Lancet ii: 72–74

Nava E, Palmer R M, Moncada S 1991 Inhibition of nitric oxide synthesis in septic shock: how much is beneficial. Lancet 338: 1555–1557

Noda Y, Hughes R D, Williams R 1986 Effect of prostacyclin (PG12) and a prostaglandin analogue BW245C on galactosamine-induced hepatic necrosis. Journal of Hepatology. 2: 53–64

O'Brien C J, Wise R J, O'Grady J G, Williams R 1987 Neurological sequelae in patients recovered from fulminant hepatic failure. Gut 28: 93–95

Ochoa J B, Udekwu A O, Billiar T R et al 1991 Nitrogen oxide levels in patients after trauma and during sepsis. Annals of Surgery 214: 621–626

O'Grady J, Alexander G J M, Thick M, Potter D, Calne R Y, Williams R 1988. Outcome of orthotopic liver transplantation in the aetiological and clinical variants of acute liver failure. Quarterly Journal of Medicine 69: 817–824

O'Grady J G, Gimson A E, O'Brien C J, Pucknell A, Hughes R D, Williams R 1988 Controlled trials of charcoal hemoperfusion and prognostic factors in fulminant hepatic failure. Gastroenterology 94: 1186–1192

O'Grady J, Alexander G J M, Hayllar K M, Williams R 1989 Early indicators of prognosis in fulminant hepatic failure. Gastroenterology 97: 439–445

Ohlsson K, Björk P, Bergenfeldt M, Hageman R, Thompson R C 1990 Interleukin-1 receptor antagonist reduces mortality from endotoxin shock. Nature 348: 550–552

Olasmaa M, Rothstein J D, Guidotti A et al 1990 Endogenous benzodiazepine receptor ligands in human and animal hepatic encephalopathy. Journal of Neurochemistry. 55: 2015–2023

Omata M, Ehata T, Yokosuka O, Hosoda K, Ohto M 1991 Mutations in the precore region of hepatitis B virus DNA in patients with fulminant and severe hepatitis. New England Journal of Medicine 324: 1699–1704

Palmer R M, Ferrige A G, Mocanda S 1987 Nitric oxide release accounts for the biological activity of endothelium-derived relaxing factor. Nature 327: 524–526

Palmer R M, Ashton D S, Moncada S 1988 Vascular endothelial cells synthesize nitric oxide from L-arginine. Nature 333: 664–666

Peleman R R, Gavaler J S, Van Thiel D H et al 1987 Orthotopic liver transplantation for acute and subacute hepatic failure in adults. Journal of Hepatology 7: 484–489

Prescott L F, Illingworth R N, Critchley J A J H, Stewart M J, Adam R D, Proudfoot A T 1979 Intravenous N-acetylcysteine: the treatment of choice for paracetamol poisoning. British Medical Journal 2: 1097–1100

Rakela J, Mosley J W, Edwards V M, Govindarajan S, Alpert E 1991 A double-blinded, randomized trial of hydrocortisone in acute hepatic failure. The Acute Hepatic Failure Study Group. Digestive Disease and Science 36: 1223–1228

Remick D G, Kunkel R G, Larrick J W, Kunkel S L 1987 Acute in vivo effects of human recombinant tumor necrosis factor. Laboratory Investigation 56: 583–590

Robin E D 1980 Of men and mitochondria: coping with hypoxic dysoxia. American Review of Respiratory Disease 122: 517–531

Rolando N, Harvey F, Brahm J et al 1990 Prospective study of bacterial infection in acute liver failure: an analysis of fifty patients. Hepatology 11: 49–53

Rueff B, Benhamou J P 1973 Acute hepatic necrosis and fulminant hepatic failure. Gut 14: 805–815

Sagnella G A Singer D R, Markandu N D et al 1990 Atrial natriuretic peptide – cyclic GMP coupling and urinary sodium excretion during acute volume expansion in man. Canadian Journal of Physiology and Pharmacology 68: 535–588

Sallie R, Tibbs C J, Silva A E, Sheron N, Eddleston A L W F, Williams R 1991 Detection of hepatitis E but not C in sera of patients with fulminant NANB hepatitis (abstract). Hepatology 14: 68A

Sanchez-Tapias L M, Mas A, Costas J et al 1987 Recombinant alpha 2c-interferon therapy in fulminant viral hepatitis. Journal of Hepatology 5: 205–210

Sari A, Yamashita S, Ohosita S et al 1990 Cerebrovascular reactivity to CO_2 in patients with hepatic or septic encephalopathy. Resuscitation 19: 125–134

Schönharting M M, Schade U F 1989 The effect of pentoxifylline in septic shock – new pharmacologic aspects of an established drug. Journal of Medicine 20: 97–105

Seda H W, Hughes R D, Gove C D, Williams R 1984 Inhibition of rat brain Na^+, K^+-ATPase activity by serum from patients with fulminant hepatic failure. Hepatology 4: 74–79

Shibayama Y 1987 The role of hepatic venous congestion and endotoxaemia in the production of fulminant hepatic failure secondary to congestive heart failure. Journal of Pathology 151: 133–138

Shiratori Y, Moriwaki H, Kawashima Y et al 1991 Elevated interleukin-6 levels in sera of patients with fulminant hepatitis. Gastroenterologica Japonica 26: 233

Shnyra A, Bocharov A, Bochkova N, Spirov V 1991 Bioartificial liver using hepatocytes on biosilon microcarriers: treatment of chemically-induced acute hepatic failure in rats. Artificial Organs 15: 189–197

Shoemaker W C, Appel P L, Kram H B 1988a Tissue oxygen debt as a determinant of lethal and nonlethal postoperative organ failure. Critical Care Medicine 16: 1117–1120

Shoemaker W, Appel P, Kram H, Waxman K, Lee T S 1988b Prospective trial of supranormal values as therapeutic goals in high-risk surgical patients. Cher 94: 1176–1186

Shoemaker W C, Appel P L, Kram H B 1989 Tissue oxygen debt as a determinant of postoperative organ failure. Progress in Clinical Biology Research 308: 133–136

Sinclair S B, G A Levy 1991 Treatment of fulminant viral hepatic failure with prostaglanin E- A preliminary report. Digestive Disease and Science 36: 791–800

Terazawa S, Kojima M, Yamanaka T et al 1991 Hepatitis B virus mutants with precore-region defects in two babies with fulminant hepatitis and their mothers positive for antibody to hepatitis B e antigen. Pediatric Research 29: 5–9

Thiemermann C, Vane J 1990 Inhibition of nitric oxide synthesis reduces the hypotension induced by bacterial lipopolysaccharides in the rat in vivo. European Journal of Pharmacology 182: 591–595

Traber P G, Ganger D R, Blei A T 1986 Brain edema in rabbits with galactosamine-induced fulminant hepatitis. Regional differences and effects on intracranial pressure. Gastroenterology 91: 1347–1356

Traber P G, Dal C M, Ganger D R, Blei A T 1987 Electron microscopic evaluation of brain edema in rabbits with galactosamine-induced fulminant hepatic failure: ultrastructure and integrity of the blood–brain barrier. Hepatology 7: 1272–1277

Traber P, DalCanto M, Ganger D, Blei A T 1989 Effect of body temperature on brain edema and encephalopathy in the rat after hepatic devascularization. Gastroenterology 96: 885–891

Tracey K J, Beutler B, Lowry S F et al 1986 Shock and tissue injury induced by recombinant human cachectin. Science 234: 470–474

Trewby P, Chase R, Davis M, Williams R 1977 The role of the false neurotransmitter octopamine in the hypotension of fulminant hepatic failure. Clinical Science 52: 305–310

Trey C, Davidson C S 1970 The management of fulminant hepatic failure. In Popper H, Shaffner F (eds) Progress in liver disease, Vol. 3. Grune & Stratton, New York, pp 282–298

Tygstrup N, Ranek L 1986 Assessment of prognosis in fulminant hepatic failure. Seminars in Liver Disease 6: 129–137

Vicaut E, Hou X, Payen D, Bousseau A, Tedgui A 1991 Acute effects of tumor necrosis factor on the microcirculation in rat cremaster muscle. Journal of Clinical Investigation. 87: 1537–1540

Vickers C, Neuberger J, Buckels J, McMaster P, Elias E 1987 Liver transplantation for fulminant hepatic failure. Gut 28: A1345

Vincent J, Roman A, De Backer D, Kahn R J 1990 Oxygen uptake/supply dependency: effects of short-term dobutamine infusion. American Review of Respiratory Disease 142: 2–7

Vorderwinkler K P, Artner D E, Jakob G et al 1991 Release of cyclic guanosine monophosphate evaluated as a diagnostic tool in cardiac diseases. Clinical Chemistry 37: 186–190

Waage A, Sørensen M, Stødal B 1990 Differential effect of oxpentifylline on tumour necrosis factor and interleukin-6 production. Lancet 335: 543

Ware A J, D'Agostino A N, Combes B 1971 Cerebral oedema: a major complication of massive hepatic necrosis. Gastroenterology 61: 877–884

Watanabe A, Fujiwara M, Nagashima H 1987 Aspergillosis in acute hepatic failure. Journal of Medicine 18: 17–22

Wendon J A, Harrison P M, Keays R, Gimson A E S, Alexander G J M, Williams R 1992 The effects of vasopressor agents and epoprostenol on systemic hemodynamics and oxygen transport in fulminant hepatic failure. Hepatology 15: 1067–1071

Wendon J A, Harrison P M, Keays R, Williams R 1993 Cerebral blood flow and metabolism in fulminant hepatic failure. Hepatology (in press)

Woolf G M, Redeker A G 1991 Treatment of fulminant hepatic failure with insulin and glucagon. A randomized, controlled trial. Digestive Disease and Science. 36: 92–96

Wright T L, Hsu H, Donegan E et al 1991 Hepatitis-C virus not found in fulminant non-A, non-B hepatitis. Annals of Internal Medicine 115: 113–115

Yanagi M, Kaneko S, Unoura M et al 1991 Hepatitis C virus in fulminant hepatic failure (letter). New England Journal of Medicine. 324: 1895–1896

Zabel P, Wolter D T, Schönharting M, Schade U F 1989 Oxpentifylline in endotoxaemia. Lancet 334: 1474–1477

Zaki A E, Ede R J, Davis M, Williams R 1984 Experimental studies of blood brain barrier permeability in acute hepatic failure. Hepatology 4: 359–363

Ziegler E, Fisher C, Sprung C, Staube R et al 1991 Treatment of gram negative bacteriaemia and septic shock with HA-1A human monoclonal antibody against endotoxin. New England Journal of Medicine. 324: 429–436

Zieve L Doizaki W M, Lyftogt C 1984 Brain methanethiol and ammonia concentrations in experimental hepatic coma and coma induced by injections of various combinations of these substances. Journal of Laboratory and Clinical Medicine 104: 655–664

UPDATE

- Although non-A, non-B (NANB) viral hepatitis has been implicated as an aetiology of fulminant hepatitis, HCV has not been shown to result in acute hepatic failure and hepatitis E virus HEV has predominantly been associated with fulminant hepatitis among pregnant women. 17 patients with sporadic fulminant or subfulminant hepatitis of presumed NANB viral aetiology were studied. The diagnosis of acute NANB viral hepatitis was made based on clinical information, serological tests, biochemical profiles, and pathological features. All 17 patients were negative for anti-HEV IgM antibodies and HEV RNA in either serum and/or liver. HCV RNAs were detected in 2 patients although anti-HCV antibodies were negative in all of them. It was shown that HCV is infrequently associated with and HEV is not an identifiable cause of presumed NANB fulminant or subfulminant hepatitis in this patient population. Although further studies will be required for identification of the causative agent, it is possible that another agent is responsible for the occurrence of sporadic NANB fulminant or subfulminant hepatitis (Liang et al 1993).
- REFERENCE:

Liang T J, Jeffers L, Reddy R K et al 1993 Fulminant or subfulminant non-A, non-B viral hepatitis: the role of hepatitis C and E viruses. Gastroenterology 104, 2: 556–562

29. Transfusion-associated hepatitis

Harvey J. Alter Leonard B. Seeff

Transfusion-associated hepatitis (TAH) is the most common serious consequence of blood transfusion therapy. Although transfusion-associated acquired immunodeficiency disease (AIDS) (TA-AIDS) has captured the world's attention in recent years because of its devastating clinical syndrome and universal fatality, the number of cases of TA-AIDS is miniscule as compared with TAH. Once a screening test for the human immunodeficiency virus (HIV-1) was developed and implemented in 1985, the risk of TA-AIDS fell to approximately 1 case per 100 000 transfusion recipients (0.001%), while the simultaneous rate for TAH was 4–8 cases per 100 recipients (4–8%). Nonetheless, TA-AIDS focused attention on the serious and sometimes mortal risks of blood transfusion in ways that hepatitis had never done. The fear engendered by AIDS resulted in changes in the blood donor constituency that not only reduced the risk of AIDS but also had a dramatic impact on the more prevalent TAH because of overlap in the high-risk populations capable of transmitting both diseases. Measures introduced since 1985 have markedly reduced the incidence of TAH, although the observed decline has been documented in only a limited number of prospective studies. (Feinman et al 1988, Mattsson et al 1989, Esteban et al 1991, Donahue et al 1992).

In this chapter, we will chronicle the history of TAH and describe the fall in TAH prevalence from rates that exceeded 30% in the 1960s to rates that may be below 1% in the 1990s. Among the landmark events in this chronology (Alter 1987) are the identification of the inordinate risk from donors who receive payment for their blood; the discovery of the hepatitis B virus (HBV) and the introduction of HBsAg screening in 1971; the development of radioimmunoassays for HBsAg and their introduction in 1975; the recognition of an additional human hepatitis agent(s), non-A, non-B (NANB); the recognition that surrogate markers (alanine aminotransferase, anti-HBc) could reveal donors at risk of transmitting NANB hepatitis; and, most recently, the cloning of the hepatitis C virus (HCV) followed by the introduction of a specific assay to detect HCV carriers (anti-HCV).

The transfusion setting has been the paradigm for our understanding of hepatitis viruses B and C and may be the basis for identification of hepatitis non-A, non-B, non-C. Blood transfusion provides a unique opportunity to define precisely the date and source of exposure and hence provides an ideal setting in which to study viral epidemiology and serology and to define the sequential events that follow hepatitis virus exposure. In this chapter we will examine this unique experiment in nature to elucidate the causes of TAH and the measures that have so effectively led to the near eradication of this untoward transfusion event.

TRANSFUSION-ASSOCIATED HEPATITIS PRIOR TO THE RECOGNITION OF SPECIFIC HEPATITIS AGENTS

Viral hepatitis is believed to be almost as old as recorded history. Ancient writings indicate that the disease was probably known during the Biblical period and that Hippocrates seemed to be aware of the entity (Zuckerman 1972). In the Middle Ages and more recent centuries, references were made to outbreaks of 'epidemic jaundice', occurring particularly during times of war. The circumstances surrounding these epidemics, namely the unhygienic and crowded living conditions of wartime, suggest that what was being described was probably infection with either the oral-faecally transmitted hepatitis A virus (HAV) or perhaps even the hepatitis E virus (HEV). The origin and evolution of the parenterally transmitted hepatitis B virus (HBV) and hepatitis C virus (HCV) is unknown, but conceivably these agents, too, have existed for centuries, perhaps propagated by ritual scarification or by insect vectors. It is highly likely that the frequency of both HBV and HCV infections, the latter in particular, has increased in this century as medical technology has advanced, especially with the advent of the hypodermic needle and the science of blood transfusions.

The first generally accepted reference to parenterally transmitted hepatitis is that of an outbreak of 'jaundice' in 1885 that affected approximately 15% of a group of 1289 Bremen shipyard workers (Lurman 1885). Lurman, a thoughtful and perceptive German public health official who studied the outbreak, attributed it to the earlier receipt by these workers of smallpox vaccine containing glycerinated lymph of human origin. This mini epidemic was regarded initially as an isolated and unique event. However, percutaneously transmitted hepatitis was identified again in the early part of the present century among patients attending diabetic, venereal disease and arthritis clinics, where the needles used to administer medication or to draw blood were non-discardable and ineffectively sterilized (Flaum 1926, Hartfall 1937, Biggar 1943, MacCallum 1945). The jaundice noted among these clinic patients was at first ascribed to the toxic effects of the drugs used for treatment, such as salvarsan, arsenic and bismuth. Later, however, consideration began to be given to hepatitis as the aetiology. This view was reinforced by reports soon thereafter of jaundice following other instances of percutaneous injections – in children who had received measles convalescent serum and among British troops who had been given mumps convalescent serum (Propert 1938, Beeson et al 1944). Introduction at about this time of the terms, 'homologous serum', 'post-inoculation', and 'syringe' jaundice now constituted clear acknowledgement of the entity.

A dramatic epidemic in 1942 of icteric hepatitis involving 50 000 US servicemen represented the final proof of the existence of parenterally transmissible hepatitis (Sawyer et al 1943). The epidemic followed shortly after the receipt of specific lots of yellow fever vaccine that had been 'stabilized' with pooled human sera, mimicking a smaller outbreak that had occurred among yellow fever vaccinees in Brazil a short time earlier (Findlay & MacCallum 1937, Fox et al 1942). Subsequent interviews with blood donors to the pool revealed that some had had a recent bout of 'catarrhal jaundice' and that at least one was ill at the time of donation (Walker 1945). The outbreak was proven to be of HBV origin through a serological analysis conducted 40 years later among selected individuals who had been involved in the original vaccine programme (Seeff et al 1987). Also established in that long-term follow-up study was that approximately 300 000 additional vaccinees had developed undetected anicteric hepatitis B. This dramatic event thus constitutes the largest ever recognized epidemic of percutaneously transmitted hepatitis.

One year after this outbreak, Beeson (1943) and Morgan & Williamson (1943) reported for the first time the development of hepatitis following the transfusion of whole blood. 'Post-transfusion hepatitis' was now an established fact and of great concern because World War II was being waged and whole blood and plasma were increasingly in demand. For this reason and because of the inability to culture a hepatitis virus or to identify a susceptible animal model, human inoculation experiments were considered justifiable and studies of this nature were begun both in the UK (MacCallum & Bauer 1944) and in the USA (Havens et al 1944, Neefe et al 1946).

These experiments, using nasopharyngeal washings, faecal suspensions, urine and serum samples, appeared to confirm the prevailing view that there were two, and only two, viruses capable of inducing hepatitis. The one form, transmitted both orally and parenterally, produced disease after an incubation period of 2–4 weeks, and seemed to be relatively mild and transient. The other could be transmitted by the percutaneous route only, inducing disease with a longer incubation period of 1–6 months. This form of the disease appeared to be more severe and to persist for a longer period than that induced by the first agent. The two illnesses, previously referred to by a variety of names, were now relabelled 'infectious' and 'serum' hepatitis, terms that were subsequently changed to 'hepatitis A' and 'hepatitis B' respectively. In 1977, the latter nomenclature was adopted by the World Health Organization Committee on Viral Hepatitis (World Health Organization 1977). Prior to the identification of HBV and the ability to test for this agent, the terms 'serum hepatitis, 'hepatitis B' and 'post-transfusion hepatitis' were used interchangeably, implying that hepatitis following transfusion was invariably related to HBV infection.

Early studies of prevalence of transfusion-associated hepatitis

Although the first efforts to determine the frequency of transfusion-associated hepatitis were begun shortly after the end of World War II, particular attention was directed to the problem in the later part of the 1950s and the early 1960s. Studies at this time were handicapped, however, by the fact that a diagnosis of hepatitis depended on the identification of jaundice or on the development of certain non-specific symptoms, such as fatigue, malaise or anorexia. Because of the vague nature of such symptoms, accuracy of diagnosis was obviously limited. Furthermore, as is now apparent, acute hepatitis commonly develops without symptoms; asymptomatic and anicteric hepatitis exceeds overt hepatitis by a factor of 2–7 (Hampers et al 1964, Walsh et al 1970, Seeff et al 1975a). Accordingly, the data accrued were useful largely for the trends that they described, for comparative purposes, and for efforts to define risk factors rather than for establishing true and accurate incidence figures. Among five representative studies undertaken between 1946 and 1962, when only a clinical diagnosis was possible, the hepatitis attack rate, based on the review of medical records, was reported to range from 0.1–0.6%, expressed at that time as cases of hepatitis per 100 units transfused (Jennings et al 1957, Hoxworth et al 1959, Kunin 1959, Allen & Sayman 1962, Grady & Chalmers 1964).

The recognition of serum enzymes in the mid-1950s, particularly the aminotransferases, as sensitive measures of acute hepatocellular necrosis, constituted a dramatic and ground-breaking diagnostic milestone (Wroblewski & LaDue 1955, Wroblewski et al 1956). For the first time, it was possible to define the full spectrum of acute hepatic disease. Accordingly, during the decade of the 1960s, several relatively small-scale studies were undertaken to determine attack rates of TAH through serum enzyme testing of recipients (Shimizu & Kitamoto 1963, Hampers et al 1964, Creutzfeldt et al 1966, Walsh et al 1970, National Transfusion Hepatitis Study 1972). Comparison of these figures with the data reported from the previous decade is not strictly appropriate because the hepatitis prevalence was now being expressed as cases of hepatitis per 100 *patients* transfused rather than per 100 *units* transfused. Regardless, the attack rate, ranging in five representative studies from 14.0–65.0%, was markedly higher than had previously been reported, clearly a consequence of the improved diagnostic capability (Table 29.1). The utility of serial enzyme testing was particularly well illustrated by the data of the large National Transfusion Hepatitis Study that was begun in the late 1960s and completed in the early 1970s. For most of that study, the diagnosis was established by questionnaire surveys of the transfused subjects; however, among the last 10% of study subjects,

Table 29.1 Early studies of transfusion-associated hepatitis diagnosed by serum enzyme measurements

Reference	No. of patients	Attack Rate/100 transfused persons (%)
Shimizu et al 1963	175	64.8
Hampers et al 1964	56	17.8
Creutzfeldt et al 1966	309	14.0
Walsh et al 1970	110	38.1*
National Transfusion Hepatitis Study 1972+	5142	2.9≠ 10.9δ

*51% in 82 recipients of commercial blood; 0% in 28 recipients of only volunteer donor blood.
+National Transfusion Hepatitis Study
≠Questionnaire only
δSerial SGPT

the diagnosis was based on results of serial serum glutamic pyruvate transaminase (SGPT) measurements. The frequency of hepatitis, 2.9% in the questionnaire phase of the study, was found to be 10.9% among the group subjected to serial enzyme screening. The stage was now set for the initiation of large-scale, prospective, enzyme-monitored surveys.

TRANSFUSION-ASSOCIATED HEPATITIS FOLLOWING IDENTIFICATION OF THE HEPATITIS B VIRUS

As thoughts were germinating regarding new prospective studies, another event was unfolding that would revolutionize our understanding of viral hepatitis and forever change the direction of research of the disease. Blumberg et al (1965), while searching for diagnostic genetic markers, had unexpectedly identified a lipoprotein precipitate using an agarose gel immunodiffusion (ID) system. The significance of this precipitin line, termed the 'Australia antigen' because serum from an Australian aborigine had been its source, was at first unclear. Within a relatively short time, however, it was linked first to viral hepatitis in general (Blumberg et al 1967) and then to hepatitis B specifically (Giles et al 1969). When it became apparent that what was being detected was, in fact, the outer shell of the hepatitis B virus, the term 'Australia antigen' was abandoned and, after some terminological modification, replaced with the designation hepatitis B surface antigen (HBsAg).

The natural next step after initial identification of this antigen was to apply the gel ID system to the investigation of TAH. Gocke and colleagues (Gocke & Kavey 1969, Gocke et al 1969, 1970, Gocke 1972) began a series of studies of both donors and recipients, demonstrating a clear association between the presence of HBsAg in donor blood and the development of hepatitis B or the antigen or its antibody in the recipient. Their studies led them to conclude that hepatitis B had probably never accounted for more than 20–25% of all cases of icteric TAH (Gocke et al 1970, Gocke 1972), a view expressed also by other investigators (Holland et al 1973).

UNITED STATES PROSPECTIVE STUDIES

Against this background, a series of prospective, enzyme-monitored studies were undertaken in the USA, beginning in the late 1960s and lasting through much of the 1970s, with two primary goals in mind. The first was to establish true incidence figures for TAH and to define risk factors for the disease (Alter et al 1975, 1978a, Aach et al 1978); the second was to evaluate the efficacy of immune globulin preparations in the prevention or attenuation of the disease (Knodell et al 1976, Seeff et al 1977, 1978a). Not recognized at the time of their initiation was that these studies would also become the vehicles for identification of non-A, non-B (NANB) hepatitis, since they overlapped the discovery of both HBV (Blumberg et al 1965) and HAV (Feinstone et al 1973). The serological tests utilized for HBV were in the process of evolution as the studies were proceeding, progressing from the initial insensitive gel ID test, through counterelectrophoresis (CEP), culminating finally with passive haemagglutination and several generations of radioimmunoassay (RIA). By 1972, federal law required that all donor blood be screened for HBsAg (Federal Register 37), and in late 1975 the use of a third-generation assay became mandatory.

Among the five studies conducted in the USA during the decade of the 1970s, three focused on the issue of immunoprophylaxis (Knodell et al 1976, Seeff et al 1977, 1978a). Two of them were Veterans Administration (VA) Cooperative Studies and the third was undertaken at the Walter Reed Army Hospital in Washington DC. Because they were large trials, they generated information that related not only to the value of prophylaxis (see later) but also to hepatitis attack rates and risk factors. The other two studies were designed with the specific aim of defining the annual incidences of TAH. One of them, at the Department of Transfusion Medicine of the National Institutes of Health (NIH), has been ongoing from 1963 to the present (Alter et al 1978a). The other, a multicentre study, referred to as the Transfusion Transmitted Viruses Study (TTVS), was unique in that it involved the determination of both the TAH rate and of the 'background' hepatitis rate by evaluating transfusion recipients as well as non-transfused hospital controls (Aach et al 1978). All five studies employed similar, although not identical, selection criteria, methods of patient evaluation and diagnostic criteria for hepatitis.

Together, these five studies evaluated well over 4000 consecutive blood recipients, many of whom had undergone coronary artery bypass surgery. As shown in Figure 29.1, the rates of hepatitis were found to range from a low of 9.1% in the TTVS study to a high of 18.3% in the study at the Walter Reed Army Hospital. Screening of donors and recipients for HBsAg was performed by CEP during the first VA cooperative study and during part of the NIH and Walter Reed Army Hospital studies; RIA was utilized in the other studies. Based on these assays, HBV was determined to be responsible for only 3–22% of the total cases of hepatitis that developed. The differences among these studies in the proportionate contribution of HBV to the overall hepatitis frequencies appeared to be attributable to the variable sensitivities of the HBV donor screening assays employed. In the first VA trial, in which HBsAg-positive blood donors were excluded on the basis of CEP screening, HBV was found to be responsible for 22% of hepatitis cases among the recipients (Seeff et al 1977). In the second VA trial that utilized RIA for donor screening from the outset, only 3% of the hepatitis cases could be ascribed to HBV infection (Seeff et al 1978a). Similar results were found in the NIH study; the total frequency of HBV-related TAH was noted to decline from 4.8% at the time of ID screening to 3.7% when CEP was employed, and finally to 0.6% shortly after the introduction of the third-generation RIA (Alter et al 1972).

The origin of the non-B cases of hepatitis at first remained obscure, since it seemed doubtful on epidemiological grounds that hepatitis A could account for the majority of patients with TAH. Indeed, Prince et al (1974), concluded after studying the clinical characteristics of 36 non-B TAH cases that HAV was highly unlikely to be the responsible agent. Proof of this view came later that year with the identification of the specific virus of hepatitis A by Feinstone et al (1973). Serological analysis of stored sera from the above-described studies for the presence of

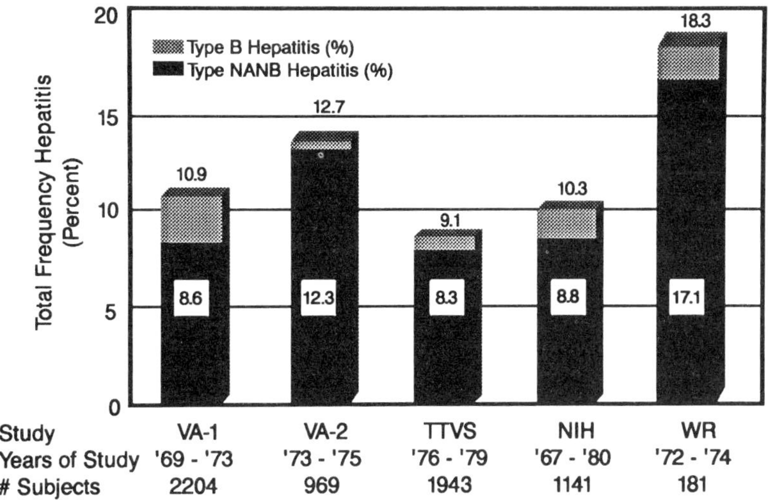

Fig. 29.1 Frequencies of transfusion-associated hepatitis in five prospective, serum-monitored studies in the USA, 1967–80. The number above the bars represents the total hepatitis frequency (%); the number in the lower, solid portion of the bar represents the frequency of type non-A, non-B hepatitis (%); the upper cross-hatched portion of the bar represents the frequency of type B hepatitis. VA, Veterans Administration Cooperative Study; TTVS, Transfusion Transmitted Viruses Study, NIH, National Institutes of Health Blood Bank Study; WR, Walter Reed Army Hospital Study.

HAV revealed, to widespread surprise, that *none* of the cases of transfusion-associated hepatitis could be attributed to this virus (Feinstone et al 1975). Thus, by 1975, the entity of transfusion-associated NANB hepatitis had been recognized. An early concern that the illness may not have been caused by a virus at all was dispelled within a short time through experiments confirming transmission to inoculated chimpanzees (Tabor et al 1978, Alter et al 1978b, Bradley et al 1979).

European prospective studies

Smaller studies were in progress in Europe during the 1970s at about the same time as those being performed in the USA. Six representative examples are shown in Table 29.2. As noted, the frequencies ranged from zero in Germany and Switzerland (Sugg et al 1976, Frey-Wettstein 1977) where RIA screening was being utilized, to 15.7% in Greece, where screening was performed by passive haemagglutination (Hadziyannis 1978). Of interest is that NANB hepatitis accounted for none of the cases in Germany and the Netherlands (Brandt et al 1963, Sugg et al 1976), but for approximately 80% of those in the English and Greek studies (Working Party of Post-Transfusion Hepatitis 1974, Hadzyannis 1978). The impact of the increasing sensitivity of the HBsAg assays was noted in these European studies, too. In one study from Germany, prior to screening of blood donors, the incidence of TAH was 13.9% (Creutzfeldt et al 1966). This figure declined to 4.1% after CEP screening was introduced and to zero after RIA became available (Sugg et al 1976).

RISK FACTORS IDENTIFIED IN PROSPECTIVE STUDIES

Efforts to seek factors that might increase the likelihood of hepatitis transmission were begun soon after the recognition of this transfusion-associated disease. Attention focused initially on donor blood characteristics. Factors that were shown to correlate with hepatitis transmission included the type of blood product transfused, the source of the blood and the numbers of units administered.

Blood products identified as carrying a high risk for hepatitis transmission included fibrinogen and pooled plasma (both now withdrawn from use because of this threat), as well as factor IX complex, factor VIII complex (antihaemophilic factor) and multiple donor platelet concentrates. Products of average risk were found to be whole blood; fresh-frozen plasma; single-donor platelet concentrates; single-donor granulocyte concentrates; and single-unit cryoprecipitate. An initial suggestion that washed or frozen red blood cells decreased the risk of hepatitis transmission (Tullis et al 1970) could not be corroborated in subsequent studies (HJ Alter et al 1978c, Haugen 1979).

Blood products that have appeared to be safe are those that are either heat treated for 10 h at 60°C, such as albumin, or prepared by cold ethanol Cohn fractionation, such as immune or hyperimmune globulins. There have been rare reports, however, of transmission of hepatitis by immune globulin prepared outside the USA (Petrilli et al 1979, Tabor & Gerety 1979, John et al 1979). More recently, clotting factor concentrates have been rendered safe by a variety of

Table 29.2 European prospective studies of transfusion-associated hepatitis during the 1960s and 1970s

Reference (country)	HBsAg screening	Incidence of hepatitis	Non-A, non-B hepatitis (%)
Creutzfeldt et al 1966 (Germany)	None	13.9	—
	CEP	4.1	—
Sugg et al 1976 (Germany)	RIA	0	—
Brandt et al 1963 (Netherlands)	None	3.1	—
Frey-Wettstein 1977 (Switzerland)	RIA	0	—
Working Party 1974 (England)	PHA	5.6	80
Hadziyannis 1978 (Greece)	PHA	15.7	80

CEP, Counterelectrophoresis; RIA, radioimmunoassay; PHA passive haemagglutination.

virus inactivation procedures including pasteurization, dry heating, treatment with solvent detergent and photochemical decontamination (H J Alter 1987).

Prior to the advent of hepatitis serological assays, by far the most important hepatitis risk factor identified was the origin of the donor blood. As early as the 1960s, investigators had noted that paid (commercial) blood was much more likely to be associated with subsequent hepatitis in the recipient than was blood that had been voluntarily donated (Kunin 1959, Allen & Sayman 1962). Even stronger support for this observation emerged from numerous studies conducted during the 1970s, including the prospective studies described above (Walsh et al 1970, HJ Alter et al 1972, Goldfield et al 1975, Seeff et al 1977, 1978a, Aach et al 1978). In every study in which this risk was investigated, the frequency of hepatitis was found to be far greater in recipients of commercial donor blood than in recipients of volunteer donor blood (Table 29.3). Especially noteworthy were the results of the early phase of the NIH Blood Bank study (HJ Alter et al 1972), in which it was shown that combined exclusion of all commercial and HBsAg-positive donors resulted in a fall in hepatitis frequency from 33% to 10%; it was estimated, however, that three-quarters of the observed decline was due to exclusion of paid blood rather than HBsAg testing. Equally compelling were the data from the extensive first VA cooperative study (Seeff et al 1977). In this trial, the frequency of hepatitis was noted to increase sequentially with the number of commercial units received from 6.9% among those who had received 1 unit to 40.6% among recipients of 11 or more units. This study also demonstrated clearly the value of interdiction of commercial donor blood (Seeff et al 1975a, b). At one of the participating hospitals in Illinois, where over 90% of blood used at the inception of the study was of commercial origin, the hepatitis rate was 20.8%. As the study proceeded, a Blood Labelling Act was promulgated in the State of Illinois. In consequence, the proportion of commercial units administered fell to 4.1% of the total, paralleled by a decline in the hepatitis frequency to 6.2%. At these same time, in three other states (New Jersey, Florida and Pennsylvania) in which the proportion of commercial donor blood used remained consistently high, the hepatitis frequency also persisted at the same high level. Based on this accumulated evidence, as well as on studies showing that commercial donors were more likely than volunteer donors to harbour HBsAg (Cherubin & Prince 1971) and HBeAg (Tabor et al 1980), it was declared mandatory in 1978 in the USA to label the origin of all donor blood, namely whether derived from a paid or from a volunteer donor (Federal Register 43 (1978)).

Another risk factor, suggested first by Allen & Sayman (1962) as well as by other investigators soon thereafter (Shimizu & Kitamoto 1963, Hampers et al 1964), was that the hepatitis rate correlated with the number of units transfused. This view received limited support from other studies (National Transfusion Hepatitis Study 1972, Aach et al 1978, Seeff et al 1977, Japanese Red Cross 1991). In the National Transfusion Hepatitis Study, there was a tendency for the hepatitis rate to increase modestly as the number

Table 29.3 Comparison in frequency of transfusion-associated hepatitis between recipients of volunteer and recipients of commercial (paid) donor blood

	Volunteer donors		Commercial donors	
	No. of recipients	Per cent with NANB hepatitis	No. of recipients	Per cent with NANB hepatitis
Walsh et al 1970	28	0	82	51.0
Prince 1975	83	7.2	13	53.8
Goldfield et al 1975	364	7.7	288	28.7
Aach et al 1978	389	6.5	26	34.4
Seeff et al 1978a	439	6.9	267	17.2

of units of blood administered reached 8 or more, but these results were not corrected for HBV serology or donor source. As pointed out, the latter may be especially important. In the VA cooperative study, the hepatitis frequency was noted to increase in proportion to the numbers of units administered, but this relationship was observed almost exclusively among recipients of paid donor blood (Seeff et al 1977). Among recipients of volunteer donor blood, the frequency remained unchanged at approximately 2.5% until 11 or more units had been given, at which point the frequency trebled. Most recently, the Japanese Red Cross (1991) have reported a prevalence of 4.9% among those who had received 1–10 units of blood and of 16.3% among those given 11–20 units. A similar, although lesser, increase was noted in this survey even after donor screening for antibody to hepatitis C (anti-HCV) had been implemented.

HBV markers as a risk factor:

HBsAg

Following the identification of HBsAg, numerous paired donor–recipient studies were performed demonstrating that this antigen is a highly specific marker of HBV infectivity (Gocke & Kavey 1969, Okochi et al 1970, Cherubin 1971, Szmuness et al 1973, 1975). With improvement of the sensitivity of the serological assays, as described above, and the requirement by federal regulation in 1975 that all blood donors be screened for this antigen by third-generation assays, the frequency of HBV-related TAH has declined to 0.3% or less, but has not reached zero.

Several theoretical explanations have been advanced for the continued existence of HBV-related transfusion-induced hepatitis despite routine screening for HBsAg (Hoofnagle 1990). First is the possibility that technical errors may confound routine testing; this explanation is regarded as highly unlikely because of the rigours of quality assurance. Second is the possibility that the disease might not have derived from the transfusion episode, also believed to be unlikely, based in part on the results of the TTV study that demonstrated a rate of HBV-related hepatitis of 1.7% in transfusion recipients but of only 0.14% in the non-transfused, hospital controls (Aach et al 1978). Third is the consideration that the disease might have derived from an infectious donor who was incubating hepatitis B but had not yet become HBsAg positive. This explanation, too, is believed unlikely because of the infrequency of HBV infection in US volunteer donors and the fact that donor follow-up evaluation uncommonly reveals acute hepatitis B. Fourth is the possibility that a donor may be HBsAg-negative yet a low-level HBV carrier. Support for this consideration comes from chimpanzee studies, which demonstrate that inoculation with known HBsAg-positive serum diluted to the point of RIA negativity is still capable of transmitting the disease (Barker et al 1970, 1975) and that HBV DNA may occasionally be identified in HBsAg-negative serum by the technique of polymerase chain reaction (PCR) (Kaneko et al 1989), a finding that requires validation.

Anti-HBc

Currently, the more acceptable marker of potential low-level HBV infectivity is anti-HBc, a sensitive indicator of HBV replication (Hoofnagle et al 1974). Theoretically, this antibody is present alone in the 'window' period of acute resolving hepatitis B, between the loss of HBsAg and the first appearance of anti-HBs. Efforts have been directed, therefore, toward determining whether receipt of donor blood positive solely for anti-HBc might be associated with recipient hepatitis (Hoofnagle et al 1978, Lander et al 1978, Katchaki et al 1979, Rakela et al 1980, Dike 1981, Hopkins et al 1982, Larsen et al 1990). This association has been deduced for at least 24 cases, although others have failed to show the same relationship (Tabor et al 1981, Koziol et al 1986, Sugg et al 1976). An interesting report in this regard has come from the Mayo Clinic transplantation group (Motschman et al 1989). They found that two cases of hepatitis B had developed in patients who had undergone a liver transplantation despite the fact that blood transfusions that they had received has been screened for both HBsAg and anti-HBc, and that the liver donors had been tested for HBsAg. Retrospective testing of stored blood samples revealed the presence of anti-HBc alone in the two liver donors whose recipients had developed hepatitis. Currently, all blood donors in the USA are being screened for anti-HBc as a 'surrogate' test to reduce NANB hepatitis; it remains to be seen whether this measure will also eradicate transfusion-related HBV infection. The efficacy of anti-HBc testing has already been demonstrated in Japan, where the post-testing incidence of transfusion-associated hepatitis B has fallen to levels that now approximate zero (Nishioka 1991).

Anti-HBs

Another early supposition was that anti-HBs might define potentially infectious donor blood by revealing HBV carriers in whom HBsAg is masked by HBsAg–anti-HBs immune complexes (Koretz et al 1976). Other studies, however, do not support this theoretical consideration (Reinicke et al 1973, Seeff et al 1977, Koziol et al 1986).

TRANSFUSION-ASSOCIATED HEPATITIS IN THE 1980s

The decade of the 1980s represented an arid period in the USA for prospective studies of TAH. However, numerous studies were performed during this time in other countries, establishing that TAH has a global distribution, albeit with a varying frequency, ranging from 0.3% to almost 19%. Table 29.4 demonstrates that hepatitis following transfusion was reported from several European countries (Katchaki et al 1981, Grillner et al 1982, Tremolada et al 1983, Collins et al 1983, Hernandez et al 1983, Aymard et al 1986, Colombo et al 1987, Sirchia et al 1991, Barrera et al 1991, Contreras et al 1991), from the Middle East (Tur-Kaspa et al 1983), Australia (Cossart et al 1982) Canada (Feinman et al 1988), Taiwan (Wang et al 1991) and Japan (Tateda et al 1979, Japanese Red Cross 1991). The lowest rates were detected in England (Collins et al 1983, Contreras et al 1982), the Netherlands (Katchaki et al 1981) and Australia (Cossart et al 1982),

Table 29.4 Frequency of transfusion-associated hepatitis during the 1980s

Reference	Country	No. of patients	Hepatitis frequency (%)	Total cases caused by hepatitis B (%)
Tateda 1979	Japan	676	11.6	7
Katchaki et al 1981	Netherlands	380	3.4	0
Cossart et al 1982	Australia	842	2.0	18
Grillner et al 1982	Sweden	74	18.9	0
Tremolada et al 1983	Italy	297	18.5	4
Collins et al 1983	England	248	2.4	0
Tur-Kaspa et al 1983	Israel	50	8.0	0
Hernandez et al 1983	Spain	230	16.9	26
Aymard et al 1986	France	64	6.3	0
Colombo et al 1987	Italy	676	14.0	3
Widell 1987	Sweden	173 (83)*	5.2	0
		739 (84–85)	2.4	0
Feinman et al 1988	Canada	576	9.2	0
Sirchia et al 1990	Italy	780	6.7	0
		155 (86)	10.9	0
		228 (87)	6.6	0
		234 (88)	5.6	0
		163 (89)	4.3	0
Barrera et al 1991	Spain	250	16.0	0
Red Cross et al 1991	Japan	1581 (<89)	7.7	0.25
		908 (>89)	2.1	0
Contreras et al 1991	England	387	0.3	0
Wang et al 1991	Taiwan	296	12.5	2.7

* Numbers in parentheses represent the year of the study.

and the higher rates in Sweden (Grillner et al 1982), Italy (Tremolada et al 1983, Colombo et al 1987, Sirchia et al 1991), Spain (Hernandez et al 1983, Barrera et al 1991), Taiwan (Wang et al 1991) and Japan (Tateda et al 1979). In the vast majority of these studies, none of the cases could be defined as the consequence of HBV infection. Even in Taiwan, where HBV is endemic, almost all the cases were of non-B hepatitis origin (Wang et al 1991). In only two of the studies did hepatitis B contribute appreciably to the total hepatitis frequency; in a study from Australia (Cossart et al 1982), 18% of the total cases were hepatitis B, and in a study from Spain (Hernandez et al 1983) 26% of the total cases were diagnosed as hepatitis B. These discrepancies are probably attributable to the fact that the studies with higher hepatitis B frequencies used early-generation HBV serological assays to screen blood donors.

Noteworthy is that the one study with geographic proximity to the USA (Toronto, Canada, Feinman et al 1988) described a frequency for total hepatitis and hepatitis B that closely approximated the figures established in the US prospective studies conducted in the 1970s. Presumably, the almost 10% hepatitis rate detected in this Canadian study, performed between the years 1983 and 1985, is a good representation of the TAH frequency in the USA during that period, given the similarity of the population traits of the two countries.

FAILED EFFORTS AT SEROLOGICAL AND VIROLOGICAL DETECTION: THE DECADE OF FRUSTRATION 1975–85

The awkward designation non-A, non-B hepatitis was applied because at the time of discovery it was uncertain whether the illness was of viral origin or related to some other post-surgical event. Further, if caused by a virus, it was unknown how many agents might be involved. In the latter instance, it was felt that viral assays would rapidly evolve and that a specific viral designation could then replace the exclusionary designation, non-A, non-B. This logic proved to be overly optimistic as more than a decade elapsed before the first specific non-A, non-B agent (hepatitis C virus) was identified. The intervening years produced a series of false hopes as one putative NANB test after another was reported and subsequently disproved (Alter 1983, Dienstag 1983). None of the more than 50 published reports could be substantiated in independent laboratories, and none of the assays was able to distinguish sera proven to transmit NANB hepatitis from non infectious control sera using coded panels distributed by the NIH. The failure of these tests generally reflected the detection of host proteins, some of which may have been induced by the virus, but none of which was sufficiently reproducible to serve as a reliable indirect index of viral presence. It is of interest in this regard that the NANB agent did seem capable of inducing non-immune host responses including the production of cytoplasmic tubular structures (Shimizu et al 1979) and a host antigen (Shimizu et al 1985) in experimentally infected chimpanzees, the production of an aberrant IgM in humans (Shiraishi et al 1985) and, most recently, the induction of antibody to a host protein designated GOR (Mishiro et al 1990).

During this decade of diagnostic uncertainty, theories abounded as to the nature of the agent causing NANB hepatitis. One of the most prominent views was that the NANB hepatitis agent was a cryptic form of the HBV based on reactions of NANB hepatitis sera with monoclonal antibodies directed against HBV (Shafritz et al 1982), and upon the finding of HBV DNA in the hepatocytes of patients with NANB hepatitis (Brechot et al 1981). Another view was that the NANB agent was a retrovirus based on the finding of reverse transcriptase in the serum of patients with NANB hepatitis (Seto et al 1984). The hepatitis B virus theory, however, was not supported by other epidemiological or serological studies including the demonstrated lack of cross-immunity between HBV and NANB in both human and chimpanzee studies, the lack of homology between HBV DNA and the nucleic acid derived from sera known to transmit NANB hepatitis and, most conclusively, by the cloning of HCV, which showed it to be in a viral class totally distinct from HBV and other hepadnaviruses. The retroviral theory also was dispelled when other laboratories could not confirm the presence of reverse transcriptase activity in

NANB hepatitis sera and when the reporting laboratory could not reliably distinguish NANB hepatitis sera from controls in coded panels. As with HBV, the retroviral theory was conclusively disproved when HCV was cloned and shown to be in the family of flaviviridae rather than the retroviruses.

The difficulty in developing a specific NANB hepatitis assay lay not in the effort expended, but in the nature of the virus and the immune response that it elicited. Unlike HBV, the NANB agent is present in very low titre. This was demonstrated in chimpanzee transmission studies in which HBV-containing sera were shown to have infectivity titres frequently in excess of 10^8 chimpanzee dosed infectious (CID_{50}/ml), whereas NANB inocula generally had titres less than 10^3 CID_{50}/ml (Feinstone et al 1981). Only one human serum and one chimpanzee serum have been shown to have an infectivity titre as high as 10^6 CID_{50}/ml. This low titre of infectious virus would obviate detection of viral antigen in human sera unless the antigen were produced in enormous excess of that required to coat virions. The fortuitous overproduction of surface antigen that occurs in HBV infection allowed detection of viral antigen with a technique as insensitive as agar gel diffusion. We were not to be that fortunate again.

Attention therefore shifted to the detection of antiviral antibody, but this raised the dilemma of how to identify an antibody in the absence of a known viral antigen or an observed virus particle. In addition, clinical studies of TAH had shown that at least 50% of patients developed chronic hepatitis (H J Alter 1989), suggesting that the frequency of persistent NANB hepatitis infection was even higher than 50% and that persistent infection might reflect the absence of an appropriate antibody response. In the absence of a known antigen or antibody, an observed particle or a tissue culture system, blind serological screening was pursued, using sera of known infectivity as a source of antigen and sera from patients with chronic infection or presumed recovery from infection as a source of antibody. In one such experiment at the NIH (Shiraishi et al 1985), the most highly pedigreed infectious sera were pelleted to concentrate contained virus, the best pedigreed convalescent sera were fractionated into IgG and IgM components, and the reactants were tested by radioimmunoassay, then the most sensitive serological technique available. This study epitomized the frustration of the preceding decade; no viral-specific assay evolved, but an anomalous IgM resulted in reactivity that mimicked true antibody. It seemed at the time (1984) that no further serological approaches were likely to be successful and the search for a NANB agent lay relatively dormant until the advent of molecular biology (see below).

Despite the absence of a serological assay and the inability to grow the virus in culture or observe the virus by electron microscopy, a great deal was learned about the NANB agent through chimpanzee transmission studies. After the initial transmission of NANB hepatitis to the chimpanzee using a wide variety of inocula (Alter et al 1978b, Tabor et al 1978, Bradley et al 1979, Hollinger et al 1978), it was possible to use this animal model as the end-point of experiments; pedigreed sera were used to determine the size of the particle by filtration, determine the existence of a viral envelope by its sensitivity to lipid solvents and to assess viral inactivation by a variety of physical techniques. These studies demonstrated that the NANB agent was lipid enveloped (Feinstone et al 1983, Bradley et al 1983) and relatively small in diameter, probably in the range of 30–40 nm (He et al 1987, Yuasa et al 1991). Chimpanzee studies also showed that the virus could be inactivated by lipid solvents (Prince et al 1986), now one of the major means of ensuring the safety of factor VIII concentrates, and that it could be inactivated by heat (Hollinger et al 1984), providing the rationale for the long established safety of heat-treated albumin. Later studies also revealed that normal human immune globulin fractions were rendered free of NANB infectivity by virtue of the Cohn fractionation process (Biswas et al 1991).

Hence, even without a viral assay, it was possible to characterize the NANB agent as a small, lipid-enveloped virus. These physical characteristics narrowed the potential number of viral families to which the virus could belong and suggested that it was either in the family of togaviruses (now flaviviridae) or that it represented a new class of viral agents. Cloning of the agent, as described below, revealed that the major NANB hepatitis agent is indeed in the family of flaviviraidae, representing a new genus within that family.

Despite cloning and relatively complete genomic characterization, the hepatitis C virus has still not been visualized or grown in culture. There are, however, early reports of a short-term liver culture supporting the growth of HCV (Jacob et al 1991). This finding has not been independently confirmed and the particle observed in tissue culture is pleomorphic and on the average larger (39–60 mm) than that predicted for HCV in prior filtration studies (He et al 1987, Yuasa et al 1991).

RATIONALE AND EFFICACY OF SURROGATE ASSAYS FOR THE DETECTION OF NANB CARRIERS

In the mid-1980s, when TAH prevalence was 4–8% and when it appeared that a test for NANB hepatitis agents might never be developed, the concept of using surrogate tests for the detection of NANB virus carriers became a controversial issue in blood transfusion medicine. The concept evolved from a retrospective analysis of two prospective studies conducted in the 1970s. In 1981, the Transfusion Transmitted Virus Study (TTVS) group first reported a significant association between elevated serum alanine transaminase (ALT) in the donor and the development of hepatitis in the recipient (Aach et al 1981). From their data, it was predicted that the exclusion of donors with elevated ALT might prevent 30% of NANB hepatitis cases at the loss of approximately 3% of the donor supply. A simultaneous prospective study at the NIH (H J Alter et al 1981) found an almost identical outcome, predicting that donor exclusion based on ALT might prevent 29% of TAH at the loss of approximately 1.5% of the donor population. Because these data represented reassessments of previously conducted studies rather than randomized prospective studies, the derived estimates represented predicted efficacy rather than established efficacy. A randomized, controlled trial was planned, but never initiated and, to the present time, the efficacy of ALT testing for the prevention of NANB hepatitis has been implied, but never proved.

In 1985 and 1986, these same studies were reanalysed and paradoxically showed a significant association between the presence of hepatitis B core antibody (anti-HBc) in the donor and the subsequent development of NANB hepatitis in the recipient. In the TTVS (Stevens et al 1984), recipients of at least 1 unit of anti-HBc positive blood had a 19% frequency of NANB hepatitis compared to 7% among recipients of only anti-HBc-negative blood ($P<0.001$). In the NIH study (Koziol et al 1986), recipients of anti-HBc-positive blood had an 11.9% prevalence of TAH compared with 4.2% among recipients of only anti-HBc negative blood ($P<0.001$). Hence, in both studies, recipients of anti-HBc positive blood had an approximate threefold increased risk of contracting TAH. These US studies were supported by a third study conducted in Germany (Sugg et al 1988), which measured the impact of adding anti-HBc testing to the screening of a donor population already tested for ALT. This study demonstrated that recipients of anti-HBc positive blood had a fivefold greater risk of developing TAH than recipients of anti-HBc-negative blood. The investigators predicted that the introduction of routine anti-HBc testing would reduce the TAH prevalence by 40% over that already achieved by ALT testing. In composite, these three studies comprised over 2000 patients, and each demonstrated that both elevated ALT and the presence of anti-HBc in the donor correlated strongly with the development of hepatitis in the recipient. The combined data were sufficiently compelling to convince the major blood organizations of these countries and many others throughout the world that these tests should be routinely implemented for purposes of blood screening. In the USA, ALT testing was implemented in 1986 and anti-HBc testing in 1987.

It appeared that both surrogate tests were detecting a cohort of high-risk NANB hepatitis virus carriers, one test because it defined biochemical evidence of liver disease and the other because it established prior exposure to hepatitis viruses; it was presumed that subjects exposed to HBV might also be more likely to be exposed to the NANB virus. Although these assumptions are still felt to be correct, studies revealed a surprisingly uncommon concordance of these markers in the donor population; donors with elevated ALT rarely had anti-HBc and, conversely, donors with anti-HBc most frequently had normal ALT values. This disparity is not totally explained, but may be accounted for in part by the fact that both tests generate false-positive results that, in the case of ALT, are due to non-viral causes of hepatocellular injury and, in the case of anti-HBc, to inadequacies of the test procedure itself. Because the surrogate assays did not correlate well in any given donor, and because each assay appeared independently to be efficacious, there was no way to select one surrogate assay in preference to the other; hence both were adopted. Anti-HBc testing has the additional potential advantage of detecting some HBV carriers whose HBsAg titres are below the level of detectability and of serving as a surrogate marker for HIV-1 carriers, since the prevalence of anti-HBc is very high among each of the groups known to be at highest risk for developing AIDS.

The impact of ALT testing has never been directly assessed in a prospective, randomized, controlled trial. The impact of anti-HBc testing has been assessed in only one prospective, controlled study. In that study (Esteban et al 1991), conducted in Spain, anti-HBc testing of donors did not decrease the TAH incidence. However, the frequency of anti-HBc in this donor population was very high (15%), implying a high level of HBV endemicity. In a population where HBV is endemic, transmission may more commonly be through heterosexual, intrafamilial and maternon-fetal contact rather than by homosexual activity or intravenous drug use. In such a population, the spread of HBV might not parallel the spread of NANB/HCV and hence anti-HBc might not serve efficiently as a surrogate marker.

The TTVS and NIH studies predicted that the combined use of ALT and anti-HBc testing would prevent 40–50% of TAH. There is now some indirect corroboration of this prediction. In the clinical trial of the first licensed anti-HCV assay it was shown that among 350 donors with a true positive anti-HCV result as confirmed by an immunoblot assay, 43% had a surrogate marker, whereas only 3.9% of 3247 donors with a false-positive anti-HCV assay had either an elevated ALT or a positive test for anti-HBc. These data imply that the surrogate assays would have excluded 43% of infectious donors identified by specific anti-HCV testing and are in agreement with the predictions generated in the TTVS and NIH studies. Further, Nelson et al (1992) assessed anti-HCV seroconversion in almost 1000 patients prior to surrogate marker testing and a similar number after surrogate marker and showed a 60% decrease in seroconversion rate after these tests were introduced. Although other changes were occurring in the donor population simultaneously with the introduction of the surrogate tests, it seems from both these analyses that surrogate marker testing did accomplish its goal of recognizing a significant number of hepatitis C virus carriers and hence of preventing as much as 50% of TAH. Now that specific, sensitive markers for HCV are in routine use, there is room for debate as to whether surrogate marker testing should be retained considering the 2–4% loss of donors that these assays engender. This is a complicated issue that will not be readily resolved, but is currently being addressed.

DISCOVERY OF THE HEPATITIS C VIRUS

The strategy and methodology that eventuated in the cloning of HCV will be described in detail in a separate chapter. However, they are so essential to this discussion of TAH and the specific viral assays used to screen donors that they will be briefly summarized herein.

The cloning of HCV was a collaborative effort between the Centers for Disease Control (CDC) and the Chiron Corporation, relying upon infectivity studies that the CDC had conducted for over a decade. A chimpanzee was identified that had an unusually high titre (10^6 CID_{50}/ml) of an agent that reproducibly transmitted NANB hepatitis. Plasmapheresis units were obtained at the time of recurrent ALT elevations in this animal and litres of this plasma were pelleted to concentrate any contained virus. Nucleic acid was then extracted from the pellet. Because it was not known if the virus was DNA or RNA, a denaturation step was included before the synthesis of complementary DNA (cDNA) so that either DNA or RNA could serve as a template; conversion of RNA into cDNA involved reverse transcription with random primers. The resultant cDNA was inserted into a cloning vector, -gt11, and expressed in *Escherichia coli*. Clones were lysed so that expressed proteins could adhere to overlying filter paper and the filters were in turn layered with serum from a patient with NANB hepatitis and then with radiolabelled antiglobulin. A single clone, designated 5-1-1, was reactive by autoradiography. A larger clone, C100-3, was then assembled from overlapping clones and expressed in yeast as a fusion protein using superoxide dismutase sequences to facilitate expression. The C100-3 antigen was then utilized to coat microtitre plates and became the basis for the first licensed assay to detect the complementary antibody in HCV carriers.

In addition to the overall brilliance of the cloning strategy there were three critical elements to this experiment. First was the availability of large volumes of starting plasma with an unusually high titre of infectious virions. There was no similar human supply of this plasma, and it was only these meticulously conducted chimpanzee studies that permitted identification of a substrate suitable for cloning. Second was the use of an expression vector that not only amplified the viral genome but expressed the proteins coded by that genome. The third element was the assumption that people infected with the agent of NANB hepatitis would have circulating antibody even though such antibody had never been detected through the intensive investigations outlined above. The essence of the experiment was thus blind immunoscreening of expressed proteins from the amplified genome of a previously unrecognized virus. This contrasts with standard cloning procedures, which require that the viral genome be identified prior to amplification by cloning. Indeed, the fundamental value of this experiment goes beyond the discovery of HCV in that it provides a method for the identification of other elusive viruses that have escaped serological detection, in vitro propagation and microscopic visualization.

By using overlapping clones and 'walking the genome', Houghton and associates at Chiron rapidly determined the nucleotide sequence of the entire HCV genome and compared the sequence with that of previously identified viruses (Choo et al 1989). HCV was found to represent a single-stranded, positive-sense RNA virus of approximately 9500 nucleotides coding for 3000 amino acids. HCV is genomically distinct from any known virus, but shares minor homology with and is structurally related to members of the flaviviridae family, which includes the yellow fever virus, the dengue fever virus and several animal viruses in the genus pestivirus.

The genomic structure of the virus is shown in Figure 29.2 and is relevant to interpretation of anti-HCV screening assays. The genome contains a 5' non-coding (untranslated) region, followed by the core (nucleocapsid) and envelope structural regions and then by five non-structural domains. The original 5-1-1 antigen contains amino acid sequences derived from non-structural region 4 (NS4) and the expanded antigen, C100-3, contains both NS4 and NS3 sequences. C100 was the sole viral antigen in the first generation of anti-HCV assays. Second-generation assays include two new antigens, C33c, a non-structural protein from the NS3 region, and C22-3, a structural protein from the core (nucleocapsid) region. As indicated below, the addition of these new antigens considerably increases the sensitivity of the assay, as evidenced by earlier appearance of antibody after transfusion exposure and by increased ability to detect HCV infection in both donors and recipients.

DETECTION OF HEPATITIS C VIRUS INFECTION

First-generation antibody assays

Although HCV RNA can be measured in serum following amplification in the polymerase chain reaction (PCR), the presence of HCV is generally indirectly assessed by the detection of anti-HCV antibody. In the prototype assay (Kuo et al 1989), anti-HCV was detected by radioimmunoassay, but the assays that have been licensed and are in wide clinical application are enzyme immunoassays (EIAs). As indicated above, there have thus far been two generations of anti-HCV EIAs

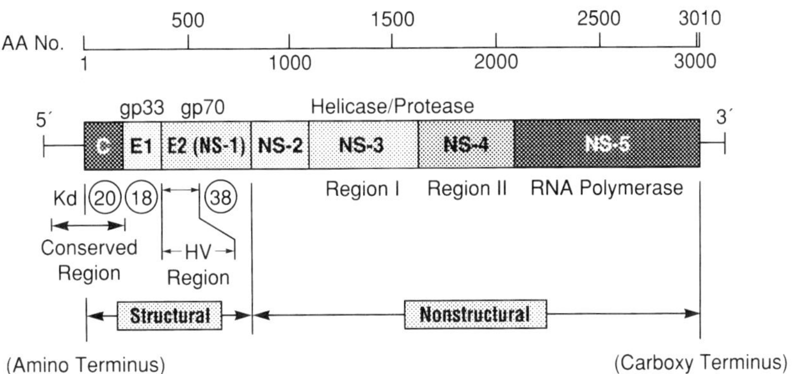

Fig. 29.2 Putative structure of the HCV genome. The genome consists of approximately 10 000 nucleotide bases coding for 3000 amino acids. Structural genes are located at the 5' end of the genome and include the core or nucleocapsid (C) and the envelope (E1, E2) regions. Five non-structural regions (NS1 to NS5) extend to the 3' end of the genome. Highly conserved sequences are found in the 5' untranslated region and in the core. A hypervariable region is found in the E2 (NS1) domain. First-generation anti-HCV assays utilize a protein (C100–3) in the NS3 region. Second-generation assays will fuse an additional non-structural protein, C33c, to C100–3 to form a new composite antigen designated C200. In addition, second-generation assays will detect antibody to a nucleocapsid antigen, C22–3. (Figure courtesy of Michael Houghton PhD, Chiron Corporation, Emeryville, CA, USA.)

distinguished by the number of recombinant antigens adherent to the solid phase. EIA-1 contained the C100-3 antigen and EIA-2 adds C33C and C22. Most of the information available to date was generated by EIA-1, and the information relevant to blood transfusion is summarized below.

First, the prevalence of anti-HCV was found to be remarkably constant throughout the world, ranging from 0.3% in Canada and northern Europe to 0.6% in the USA and central Europe, and to 1.2–1.5% in southern Europe and Japan. This is in contrast to the prevalence of the primary marker for active hepatitis B infection (HBsAg), which varies markedly by geographic area, ranging from 0.1% in the USA to as high as 20% in some regions of Asia and Africa. There is currently no epidemiological explanation for the global distribution of HCV at such a constant and relatively low level of endemicity. This pattern of HCV prevalence defies established routes of viral transmission and suggests that neither socioeconomic status, age, climate, insect vectors, social mores nor sexual practices significantly influences the spread of HCV.

Second, the prevalence of anti-HCV was found to be very high in patients transfused with blood or blood products with rates of 60–80% in those with chronic transfusion-associated NANB hepatitis (H J Alter et al 1989, Esteban et al 1990), 50% in patients with acute, resolving NANB hepatitis and 60–90% in haemophiliacs receiving commercial clotting factor concentrates (Brettler et al 1990, Allain et al 1991, Blanchette et al 1991). In contrast, haemophiliacs receiving only virus-inactivated blood products or single-donor cryoprecipitate were generally anti-HCV negative (Blanchette et al 1991). The prevalence of anti-HCV was also high in patients who sustained intravenous exposure through illicit drug use (60–90%) or renal dialysis (15–20%) (Genesca et al 1991, Gitnick 1991, Hayashi et al 1991); the HCV prevalence among dialysis patients is consistent with their history of blood transfusion rather than suggestive of inadvertent HCV spread within the dialysis setting.

Third, HCV prevalence was similar in patients with NANB hepatitis associated with blood transfusion and in those with NANB hepatitis unrelated to parenteral exposure (sporadic hepatitis), suggesting that both epidemiological forms of NANB hepatitis are due to the same agent (M J Alter et al 1990, McHutchinson et al 1991). This had been previously implied by the fact that transfusion-associated and sporadic NANB hepatitis had similar clinical patterns, particularly their frequent progression to chronic hepatitis. Since approximately 50% of clinically apparent cases of sporadic hepatitis C have no identified parenteral source of exposure (M J Alter, 1991), it has been inferred that HCV must be spread by non-parenteral routes. Such routes have not been well defined, although it has been suggested that HCV may be spread through sexual contact (M J Alter et al 1989, 1990). In the setting of whole-blood transfusion, there has been no evidence that patients with transfusion-associated hepatitis C transmit this infection to their sexual partners; in two studies (Esteban et al 1989, Everhart et al 1990) involving 61 patients with TAH, no sexual contact was anti-HCV positive and none had a history of hepatitis. In the haemophilia setting, transmission of HCV to sexual partners appears to relate to the HIV status of the index case; in a study of 200 anti-HCV-positive haemophiliacs (Eyster et al 1991), none of 30 heterosexual partners was anti-HCV positive when the haemophiliac was infected with HCV but not HIV, whereas 7 of 170 (4%) partners were anti-HCV positive when the index case was co-infected with HCV and HIV. It has been postulated that the average titre of HCV in infected individuals is so low as to render sexual transmission very inefficient; co-infection with HIV and its associated immunodeficiency may enhance the replication of HCV and facilitate its spread by sexual and perhaps other non-parenteral routes.

Lastly, first-generation anti-HCV assays served not only to define the proportion of NANB hepatitis cases that are HCV related, but also to clarify the sequential events in HCV infection. As indicated above, the proportion of patients with transfusion-associated NANB hepatitis who are anti-HCV reactive ranged from 50–80%, the range dependent primarily upon the duration of infection and the certainty of diagnosis. In the prospective studies conducted at the NIH, 79% of 97 patients who developed NANB hepatitis after open heart surgery were anti-HCV positive. The proportion rose to 88% in those who progressed to chronic hepatitis and fell to 50% in patients who sustained an acute episode that rapidly resolved. Distinct differences in the clinical spectrum of disease were noted between anti-HCV-positive and anti-HCV-negative patients. Anti-HCV-positive patients were twice as likely to have severe disease, as judged by the peak serum aminotransferase or bilirubin level, and twice as likely to progress to chronic liver disease. There are several possible explanations for these differences. The most intriguing is that there are two distinct NANB hepatitis agents: HCV, which causes more severe disease that is likely to become chronic, and a 'non-C' agent that, conversely, causes milder disease that is likely to resolve. Alternatively, it is possible that some proportion of anti-HCV-negative cases with low-level ALT elevations are incorrectly classified as NANB hepatitis. Such misclassification is inherent in diagnoses that are derived by serological exclusion and become increasingly likely when the observed abnormalities are mild and transient. Although some degree of misdiagnosis is inevitable considering the myriad of medications and clinical events that beset post-operative patients, it is unlikely to account completely for the large number of NANB cases that prove to be anti-HCV negative. A third possibility is that some of these anti-HCV negative cases are indeed HCV related, but fail to be detected because of the relative insensitivity of first-generation assays. As indicated below, the increased sensitivity of second-generation EIAs will confirm that an additional 10–20% of patients that test anti-HCV negative by first-generation EIA are indeed HCV related. Still additional cases will be shown to be HCV related when liver tissue is examined for HCV antigens by immunofluorescence and for HCV RNA by PCR or in situ hybridization. Thus, the proportion of transfusion-associated NANB hepatitis cases that are due to HCV infection will continue to increase as diagnostic capabilities improve. Nonetheless, preliminary testing with these more sensitive techniques suggests that a small proportion of bonafide NANB hepatitis cases are probably due to an agent other than HCV. It is anticipated that these 'non-A, non-B, non-C' cases will constitute less than 15% of the total burden of TAH.

Confirmatory Testing

Enzyme immunoassays are prone to false-positive reactions when testing low-risk populations, such as routine blood donors. This was very evident in the case of HIV assays, for which the Western blot demonstrated that almost 90% of EIA-reactive samples represented false-positive results. A Western blot has not been developed for HCV because the virus has not been propagated in culture and a whole viral lysate cannot be prepared. However, a recombinant immunoblot assay (RIBA) has been developed. In this method, a series of recombinant HCV proteins are attached to a nitrocellulose strip, which is then reacted with patient serum. The recombinant proteins placed on the strip include the original 5-1-1 antigen, C100-3, C33c and the core protein, C22. In addition, the strip has two levels of gamma-globulin that control for anti-human antibody reactions and provide the basis for quantitating the strength of anti-HCV reactivity. An additional control is a superoxide dismutase (SOD) band, utilized because SOD is fused to the recombinant proteins to enhance cloning efficiency. A variation of RIBA is the matrix assay, which utilizes similar recombinant proteins fixed to a solid support, but uses chemiluminescence as the end-point, allowing for semiquantitation of the reactions. In addition, one can confirm specificity by simple neutralization. These assays have been called supplemental rather than confirmatory tests because they utilize the same antigens as employed in the screening assay and hence do not provide independent confirmation of specificity. Nonetheless, because of their format as multiple discrete bands or dot blots, they have proved very useful in discriminating true from false-positive EIA reactions and they correlate well with determinations of HCV RNA by PCR; in the RIBA and EIA-2 clinical trials, more than 90% of RIBA-positive samples were also PCR positive, approximately 20% of RIBA-indeterminate samples were PCR positive and RIBA-negative samples were uniformly PCR negative. When there is corroborating evidence of HCV infection, such as clinical NANB hepatitis, implication in hepatitis transmission or a positive surrogate marker, then the RIBA assay generally confirms the initial EIA reactivity (Kleinman et al 1992). In contrast, when such corroborating evidence is absent, as in most random blood donors, then the supplemental assays fail to confirm the initial EIA reaction 50–75% of the time. In this instance, where most EIA reactivity in blood donor samples represents false positivity, it is important that supplemental testing be performed before donors are notified of their anti-HCV result. The message to the donor is very different for these two circumstances, a specific reaction calling for further medical evaluation and a false-positive reaction requiring no medical attention.

Comparison of first- and second-generation assays

Although the introduction of first-generation anti-HCV assays represented a dramatic advance in our ability to detect HCV carriers and to proportionately decrease the incidence of TAH, this assay was less than optimal in that the duration from exposure to antibody seroconversion was very long (average 22 weeks), and in that only 75% of HCV cases had an antibody-positive donor identified in retrospective analysis (H J Alter et al 1989). The second-generation EIA has substantially improved the assay in both these deficient parameters. Clinical trials of the second-generation assay reveal that antibody to C22-3 and/or C33c appears earlier than antibody to C100-3 in 75% of transfusion-related and community-acquired hepatitis C cases. Generally, anti-HCV is detected 30–90 days earlier by the second-generation assays and, in rare instances, as much as 40 weeks earlier.

In the NIH series (H J Alter et al 1991, 1992), in which only 63% of TAH cases were EIA-1 positive by post-transfusion week 20, 100% were positive by week 20 using EIA-2; 50% of cases were anti-HCV positive by post-transfusion week 10 in EIA-2 compared with only 12% by EIA-1. Thus, the period from virus exposure to antibody detection has been considerably narrowed, diminishing the probability that an infectious donor could present during the seronegative window. The narrowed interval to antibody seroconversion is also very important in the clinical diagnosis of hepatitis cases. With the second-generation assay, approximately 40% of hepatitis C patients have antibody detectable at the time of the first observed ALT elevation compared with only 6% by EIA-1; 78% have antibody within 5 weeks of the onset of hepatitis, making this a powerful acute-phase diagnostic tool.

In cases of acute transfusion-associated or sporadic NANB hepatitis, second-generation assays detect anti-HCV in approximately 20% more patients than first-generation assays. Enhanced detection is less evident in chronic cases, in which the incidence is already high, but even here approximately 10% more cases are found to be HCV-related using EIA-2. In the NIH series (H J Alter et al 1991, 1992), 89% of 18 chronic cases demonstrated anti-HCV seroconversion by EIA-2 compared with 78% by EIA-1. Overall, 71% of 24 TAH cases were anti-HCV positive by EIA-2; interestingly, in this study, EIA-2 detected anti-HCV seroconversion in only one of six (17%) acute, resolving cases of NANB hepatitis. As mentioned above, this raises the possibility of a non-A, non-B, non-C infectious agent; however, there are alternative explanations, including non-viral causes of ALT elevation and insufficient sensitivity, even of the second-generation assay. In the large, prospective TTV study (Aach et al 1991), among 111 recipients with NANB hepatitis, EIA-1 detected anti-HCV in 46% compared with a 60% detection rate by EIA-2. When the hepatitis frequency was corrected for the occurrence of NANB hepatitis in non-transfused controls, then only 74 of the TTVS cases were attributable to transfusion and, of these, 64 (91%) demonstrated anti-HCV seroconversion by EIA-2.

From the perspective of donor detection, among 14 068 donors in the USA EIA-2 clinical trial (Kleinman et al 1992), 11 (0.08%) true-positive (RIBA reactive) donor samples were detected by both first- and second-generation assays, whereas 16 additional true positives were detected only by the second-generation assay, for an overall detection rate of 0.19%. In the TTVS study (Aach et al 1991), of 59 recipients with type C TAH, 48 (81%) had received an anti-HCV positive unit of blood as tested by EIA-1 and 55 (93%) had received a positive unit as assessed by EIA-2.

In summary, the introduction of second-generation anti-HCV assays will increase the frequency of anti-HCV detection in groups at high risk for hepatitis transmission, will detect anti-HCV in a considerably higher proportion of acute and chronic NANB cases whether transfusion associated or sporadic, will detect antibody seroconversion earlier, thus decreasing the seronegative window of infectivity and enhancing the diagnostic value of the assay in acute hepatitis.

Impact of anti-HCV testing

The previous section outlined the increased sensitivity of the second-generation anti-HCV assay. This section will deal with the established and anticipated impact of these assays on the prevention of transfusion-related hepatitis C infection. To determine efficacy, it is important to establish the infectivity of RIBA-confirmed anti-HCV positive blood units. In three prospective studies of TAH, 78% (H J Alter et al 1991), 90% (Esteban et al 1990) and 92% (Aach et al 1991) of recipients of RIBA-confirmed, anti-HCV-positive blood developed hepatitis in temporal relation to their transfusion. The failure of some patients to develop hepatitis after receipt of anti-HCV positive blood may reflect pre-existing protective immunity by virtue of previous exposure or indicate that the donor is no longer infectious despite the presence of specific antibody. The latter instance has been documented in that anti-HCV may persist in the serum for years after viral RNA, and presumed infectivity, has cleared (H J Alter et al 1991). Overall, it is probable that at least 90% of confirmed anti-HCV-positive donors are infectious. For purposes of discussing test efficacy, we will assume that interdiction of an anti-HCV 'true'-positive donor is equivalent to the prevention of a hepatitis case.

In a serological reanalysis of previously conducted prospective studies using EIA-2, an anti-HCV-positive donor was identified in 84% of hepatitis cases in the NIH study and in 93% of hepatitis cases in the TTV study. Hence at least 85% of hepatitis C cases could have been prevented had this test been available at the time of these prospective studies. The only contemporaneous, prospective study of TAH to directly assess test efficacy was performed in Barcelona, Spain (Esteban et al 1991). An ongoing prospective study in Barcelona was terminated when anti-HCV testing first became available and a new prospective study was instituted in which all blood units were screened for anti-HCV by EIA-1 and discarded if positive. While test efficacy was not measured in a randomized, controlled procedure, the only known difference between these two immediately consecutive studies was the introduction of anti-HCV donor screening. In the first study, prior to HCV testing, the hepatitis incidence was 9.6% among multiply transfused recipients. Following the introduction of anti-HCV screening, the hepatitis incidence fell to 1.8%. This represents an 80% reduction in overall hepatitis incidence.

An additional approach to estimating efficacy was taken in a prospective seroconversion study conducted in the USA (Nelson et al 1992). In this study, anti-HCV seroconversion rather than biochemical evidence of hepatitis was assessed by measurement of anti-HCV in a pretransfusion and 6-month post-transfusion sample. The study had enhanced statistical power because of the large number of donor exposures (25 832 units administered to 2415 patients) analysed and because analysis could be related to sequential changes in donor screening. Prior to the introduction of surrogate assays as an indirect measure of NANB hepatitis carriers, 3.83% of blood recipients seroconverted for anti-HCV antibody. This rate fell to 1.53% after the introduction of surrogate assays ($P<0.01$) and to 0.57% after the addition of anti-HCV testing ($P=0.08$). The authors estimated that the residual risk of TAH is 1 in 3 333 units transfused (0.03%).

Still another method to assess efficacy is to measure the additional hepatitis reduction effected by the introduction of the second-generation EIA. In the EIA-2 clinical trial (Kleinman et al 1992), PCR was used to determine the minimum number of RIBA-positive, EIA-positive donations that were infectious. EIA-1 detected 0.8 infectious donors per 1000 tested, whereas EIA-2 detected 2.2 infectious donors per 1000 tested. When corrected for surrogate marker status, EIA-2 detected one infectious donor per 1000 who would otherwise have been found eligible to donate by all donor screening measures, including EIA-1. When projected to a national level, based on 18 million transfused products in the USA per year, the introduction of EIA-2 testing will prevent approximately 18 000 TAH cases per year or 50 cases per day. Thus, by any parameter measured, donor screening for anti-HCV is highly efficacious. It is estimated that the post-screening hepatitis incidence will fall to under 2% and perhaps to as low as 0.5%. The risk per unit of fully screened blood may be between 1 in 3000 (0.03%) to 1 in 1000 (0.1%).

CHRONIC SEQUELAE OF TRANSFUSION-ASSOCIATED HEPATITIS

Chronic hepatitis B

Acute hepatitis B commonly culminates in chronic hepatitis, particularly in the Far East, where HBV is predominantly a perinatally transmitted virus (Beasley et al 1981a, Stevens et al 1982). Infected newborns in these countries become HBV carriers in 90% or more of instances. In the USA and other western countries, where HBV is more commonly an adult-acquired illness, it is believed that chronic hepatitis evolves in 5–10% of acute cases. Data on the outcome of transfusion-associated hepatitis B are not available because of the sparcity of cases from any one centre or study group. Indeed, with one exception, there is no information on the frequency of progression from acute to chronic hepatitis B in adults infected through percutaneous exposure.

The exception is the dramatic epidemic of yellow fever vaccine-associated hepatitis B that involved over 300 000 US servicemen in 1942. This outbreak, the largest ever recorded point-source epidemic of hepatitis B, was established more than 40 years later to be the result of HBV infection (Seeff et al 1987). A careful follow-up study over this 40-year period has revealed no remarkable differences in all-cause mortality between the servicemen who developed icteric or anicteric hepatitis and carefully matched non-infected control subjects, although a slight excess mortality from primary hepatocellular carcinoma was found among the anicteric cases (J E Norman, G W Beebe, J H Hoofnagle, L B Seeff, in press). This unexpectedly low hepatitis B-related mortality derives from the evidence that the carrier rate in the outbreak was determined to be only 0.3% rather than the anticipated 5–10% (Seeff et al 1987). The reason suggested for the remarkably low carrier rate was that the outbreak resulted from a single exposure and that it involved young, healthy, immunocompetent men. However, it seems unlikely that this relatively benign outcome can be anticipated for patients who develop transfusion-related hepatitis B, since transfusions are commonly multiple and obviously are administered to subjects with compromised health status. Fortunately, any concern regarding this issue is offset by the fact that transfusion-related hepatitis B is virtually a problem of the past.

Chronic hepatitis C

The overriding concern in transfusion-associated hepatitis NANB/C is the development of persistent viraemia and the frequent progression to chronic liver disease. Indeed, acute transfusion-associated hepatitis NANB/C is symptomatic in only 25% of cases, is generally mild even in symptomatic cases and is very rarely fulminant. Were it not for the chronic sequelae, morbidity and mortality would be minimal. However, some chronic manifestation occurs in at least 50% of both transfusion-associated and sporadic cases, making NANB/C hepatitis one of the most common forms of chronic liver disease in the world.

The chronic sequelae of NANB hepatitis have been repeatedly documented and extensively reviewed (H J Alter 1989). It has been the uniform observation that at least 50% of prospectively followed patients with transfusion-associated NANB hepatitis develop biochemical and histological evidence of chronic hepatitis (Mattsson et al 1989, Di Bisceglie et al 1991). In a composite of eight studies (Dienstag 1983), involving 339 patients prospectively followed after transfusion, 47% had biochemical evidence of chronic liver disease and 102 were biopsied. Biopsy revealed chronic active hepatitis (CAH) in 41% and cirrhosis in 20%. It is noteworthy that the CAH was often mild and the cirrhosis often associated with minimal inflammation. Nonetheless, it is apparent from these and other studies (Realdi et al 1982) that approximately 20% of patients with chronic TAH have histological evidence of cirrhosis. This was observed also in a comprehensive study (Aledort et al 1985) of 155 biopsies from patients with haemophilia, of whom 15% had cirrhosis and 7% had severe CAH that probably would progress to cirrhosis. Also apparent from prospective studies is that repetitive biopsies have documented progression from lesser forms of chronic hepatitis to increasingly severe CAH and cirrhosis. In an NIH series (Di Bisceglie et al 1991), of 20 patients with repeat liver biopsies over the course of 8–20 months, the histological diagnosis remained unchanged in nine (45%), worsened in four (20%), three of whom developed cirrhosis, and improved in seven (35%). A total of eight patients in the original cohort of 39 developed cirrhosis (20%), and two of these patients died of liver failure, while two others have decompensated cirrhosis. Four other patients with cirrhosis have no clinical evidence of liver disease. In an Italian study (Realdi et al 1983), five patients with CAH on initial biopsy demonstrated cirrhosis on repeat biopsy. Additional studies in Japan (Omata et al 1981) and Sweden (Iwarson et al 1979) have documented histological progression from acute hepatitis to cirrhosis, substantiating that the cirrhosis evolved from the acute post-transfusion hepatitis rather than from a pre-existing condition.

Despite this documentation of frequent cirrhosis and occasional mortality, the general course of chronic TAH is very indolent and symptom free. In a retrospective–prospective analysis of patients presenting with chronic liver disease, investigators in Japan found that the average interval between blood transfusion and the clinical presentation of chronic hepatitis was 13.6 years, that the interval to clinical cirrhosis was 17.8 years and that the interval to transfusion-associated hepatocellular carcinoma (HCC) was 23.4 years (Kiyosawa et al 1982). This slow evolution to clinical disease may account, in part, for the recent finding in a large collaborative study that among 1552 patients followed an average of 17 years, there was no increased mortality among the 568 that had developed TAH as compared with the 984 control subjects who had received blood transfusion, but had not developed hepatitis (Seeff 1991). Hence, while the progression of TAH to cirrhosis is unequivocal, the clinical significance of the cirrhosis has been questioned (Koretz et al 1980, Seeff 1991). The divergence between the frequent objective histological evidence of cirrhosis and the relatively rare clinical evidence of cirrhosis has been a paradox perhaps best explained by the relatively advanced age of most transfusion recipients and by the very slowly progressive nature of the hepatic lesion. While there is no doubt that some patients with chronic TAH do poorly and succumb to their transfusion-induced cirrhosis, the vast majority of such patients have such indolent chronic liver disease that they die of other causes before the cirrhosis becomes clinically manifest. Age at hepatitis onset may be an important factor in this equation, not only in determining the expected lifespan in which a slowly progressive lesion could become clinically evident and the probability that other fatal medical events will occur before cirrhosis, but also in determining susceptibility to progressive liver disease. Sanchez-Tapias et al (1990) in a study of 306 patients with chronic NANB hepatitis found that age and initial histological grade were the only variables influencing progression to cirrhosis. After a mean follow-up of 8 years, cirrhosis developed in only 19% of those younger than 50 at disease onset compared with 39% in those older than 50. Similarly, Mattson et al (1989) found that, among 92 patients with NANB hepatitis, 64% of those older than 30 had chronic hepatitis compared with 33% of those younger than 30; follow-up biopsies after a mean of 5 years showed progression to cirrhosis in 27% of TAH cases whose mean age was 54 compared with none of the sporadic cases whose mean age was less than 40.

Thus, many transfusion recipients who are infected with HCV do not live sufficiently long to manifest the more serious chronic consequences of their transfusion-associated hepatitis. Nonetheless, TAH can lead to clinical cirrhosis, end-stage liver disease and probably hepatocellular carcinoma (see below); a subset of approximately 5% of TAH patients manifest these untoward and sometimes fatal sequelae (Dienstag 1983, H J Alter 1989).

Transfusion-associated hepatocellular carcinoma

The exceedingly strong association between HBV infection and the subsequent development of HCC (Beasley et al 1981b) generated speculation that the agent of NANB hepatitis might be similarly implicated. This was supported by several case reports (Gilliam et al 1984, Kiyosawa et al 1984) documenting the histological progression from chronic TAH to cirrhosis to HCC. Subsequently, Kiyosawa et al (1990) reported the progression from acute post-transfusion hepatitis to HCC in 21 individuals; the sequential development of chronic hepatitis, cirrhosis and then HCC was documented by biopsy in most cases. Okuda et al (1984) studied 113 patients with HCC unrelated to alcohol; 20% had no hepatitis B markers and an additional 49% had hepatitis B markers that implied recovery from infection. It thus appeared that at least 20% of HCC cases and perhaps as many as 70% might be related to NANB hepatitis. This inference is now substantiated by HCV serology, which demonstrates an inordinately high rate of anti-HCV positivity among HCC patients in Japan (Nishioka et al 1991); in Japanese patients with HCC, in the absence of a history of alcoholism or of HBsAg, the crude prevalence of anti-HCV is 70% compared with a background prevalence of 1.5%. Similarly high prevalences of anti-HCV have been found in HCC patients in eastern Europe (Columbo et al 1989, Bruix et al 1989). This dramatic seroprevalence in HCC cases is perhaps the greatest surprise from the application of HCV serology. The prevalence of anti-HCV in HCC cases in the USA and Africa has not been as high (30–50%) (Kew et al 1990), suggesting that there may be genetic or environmental co-factors that influence the role that HCV plays in the development of HCC.

A true association between HCV and HCC has not yet been established by appropriate epidemiological studies, but HCV RNA sequences have been detected in both cancerous and non-cancerous tissue in most seropositive cases examined (Chou et al 1991). It is probable that HCV will prove to be an important aetiological agent in the development of HCC. It is unknown whether this is the result of a direct oncogenic effect of the virus or the result of malignant transformation of cells undergoing excessive mitotic activity during the rapid regeneration that accompanies evolving cirrhosis. The latter hypothesis would link the mechanisms of malignant degeneration in alcohol- and viral-induced liver diseases and would place cirrhosis as the common denominator of this event, although rare cases appear to occur in the absence of established cirrhosis.

PREVENTION STRATEGIES INDEPENDENT OF SEROLOGY

Risk-behaviour intervention

Despite all the advances in hepatitis virus serology since 1965, the measures that have had the greatest impact on hepatitis prevention have been those directed toward proper donor selection through volunteerism and appropriate medical history. As indicated earlier in this chapter, the transition from paid donors to volunteer donors resulted in a dramatic decline in hepatitis incidence and has probably been the most significant effector of a safe blood supply instituted thus far. While payment per se does not render a donor dangerous, the inducement of remuneration draws segments of the population that have hepatitis risks at least 10-fold higher than that of the general population.

The next major non-serological influence on blood safety was the introduction of questions relating to high-risk sexual and addictive behaviour. Such questions had previously seemed too sensitive to ask donors, but in the wake of the AIDS endemic these personal questions became essential and acceptable — and also effective. Between 1985 and 1990, prior to anti-HCV screening, TAH prevalence in the USA fell from 8% to approximately 3%. While anti-HIV and surrogate marker screening was important in this process, the main determinant of the fall in hepatitis incidence was the self-exclusion of individuals having experienced even a single male homosexual encounter, those ever having used intravenous drugs and those having sexual contact with a prostitute or any person known to be in a high-risk group for AIDS transmission. As indicated earlier, any measures that reduce AIDS transmission also serve to reduce hepatitis transmission because the same individuals harbour multiple viruses. It has been estimated that self-exclusion based on explicit instructions to donors, direct donor questioning regarding high-risk behaviour and the promulgation of autologous donor programmes and intraoperative blood salvage have reduced the risk of transfusion-transmitted hepatitis by 40–60%.

Despite these advances in donor selection, it is apparent that many donors still do not provide accurate information regarding high-risk behaviour or do not consider themselves at sufficient risk to warrant deferral. In an ongoing study of donors excluded because they tested anti-HCV positive, approximately 85% had a known parenteral exposure, more than half of which involved the sharing of needles in illicit drug use (Conry-Cantilena et al 1992). The majority of these individuals are not current drug addicts, but had experimented with intravenous drugs at some time in their life. Because of the duration between this activity and the time of donation, they did not consider the activity relevant to the safety of their blood. There is considerable need to educate donors that such activities place them and their blood recipients at lifetime risk and there is need to redesign donor questionnaires and interview processes so that all risk behaviours, whether current or remote, result in donor exclusion.

Autologous blood programmes

The threat of AIDS was sufficiently alarming that, for the first time, blood recipients and practitioners were willing to engage in programmes that avoided the use of homologous blood. Medical practitioners became more judicious in their ordering of blood products and patients were willing, where medically feasible, to predonate their own blood prior to elective surgery. Blood collection facilities established autologous blood programmes and, in some regions, up to 15% of blood needs are met solely by autologous products. In addition, intraoperative salvage of surgical blood loss has become almost universally accepted in many surgical procedures and has greatly reduced the need for homologous blood and thus the risk for hepatitis and AIDS transmission. There is still room for expansion of autologous blood programmes and for advances in salvage techniques; however, there are practical limits to this approach because often blood use cannot be predetermined and because salvage cannot generally be performed in surgical procedures that might allow for the recovery of malignant cells or bacterial organisms. Despite these limitations, autologous blood programmes have been a major advance in blood safety.

Viral inactivation

The technological limits of viral assay sensitivity and the extreme sensitivity of the biological model, namely the blood recipient, suggest that serological assays will always fall short of ensuring absolute blood safety. The optimal means of protecting the blood supply would be to apply a comprehensive inactivation process that would destroy all blood-transmitted viruses. This idealized process or 'magic bullet' has actually evolved for the inactivation of some plasma products such as factor VIII, but pitfalls remain for other products because the inactivation procedure may simultaneously destroy the functional properties of non-viral proteins and/or the integrity of the cellular elements of blood.

Multiple methods have been employed to inactivate or physically remove viruses from plasma. Those of more universal applicability and immediate relevance are: (1) heat inactivation; (2) inactivation with beta-propiolactone (BPL) and ultraviolet light; (3) membrane-active lipid solvents and detergents; and (4) photochemical inactivation. It has long been accepted that pasteurization (heating solutions to 60°C for 10 h) could render albumin safe for transfusion. While rigorous controlled trials have not been performed to establish safety, the long record of clinical safety leaves little doubt that fractionation followed by pasteurization renders albumin virtually free of human hepatitis and retroviral agents. However, pasteurization inactivates many labile plasma proteins and destroys the functional integrity of all cellular elements. It is thus necessary to stabilize the labile proteins during the heating process or to heat the products after lyophilization (dry heat). Dry heating of clotting factor concentrates has had a chequered history appearing safe in chimpanzee studies (Hollinger et al 1984), but sometimes unsafe in humans even when noninfectious in the chimpanzee (Colombo et al 1985). However, more recently formulated products, in which dry heating has been conducted at higher temperatures and for longer intervals (80°C for 72 h), appear to completely inactivate HCV; no cases of hepatitis and no anti-HCV seroconversions have been observed after the infusion of these dry-heated products (Study Group of UK Haemophilia Centre 1988, Preston et al 1990, Skidmore et al 1990). In addition, products pasteurized in the presence of glycine and sucrose to stabilize factor VIII (Schimpf et al 1987), second-generation factor VIII concentrates purified with an additional step of anionic-exchange chromatography and pasteurization (Manucci et al 1990) and products purified by combined heating and immunoaffinity chromatography using monoclonal antibodies to factor VIII (Michael & Garret 1990) have not been implicated in hepatitis transmission or anti-HCV seroconversion.

Lipid solvents and detergents that destroy the envelope of lipid-encapsidated viruses, such as HBV, HCV and HIV, have had considerable success in inactivating these agents. The largest accumulated experience has been in the use of tri-(*n*-butyl)-phosphate (TNBP) in combination with the detergent sodium cholate. Studies in chimpanzees showed that this method inactivates both HBV and HCV suspended in factor VIII concentrates (Prince et al 1986). Subsequent use in humans has revealed no instances of hepatitis virus infection (Horowitz et al 1988), and this method is now commonly used in the preparation of clotting factor concentrates.

Methods that employ photochemical inactivation of nucleic acid rather than denaturation of proteins (heating) or destruction of membranes (solvent/detergent) have particular appeal because they theoretically should not affect the integrity of red cells or platelets. Two such methods have been utilized; these include beta-propiolactone (BPL) in combination with ultraviolet light (Prince et al 1985) and psoralen in combination with long-range UV light (Alter et al 1988). Both methods inactivate a broad range of viruses, including single- and double-stranded RNA and DNA viruses. Both BPL and psoralen in combination with the appropriate light source have been shown to inactivate 10^4–10^5 chimpanzee infectious doses 50 (CID_{50}) of HCV and HBV in a variety of media including factor VIII concentrates and preparations of prothrombin complex (Prince et al 1985, H J Alter et al 1988). BPL is currently in use in Europe and has an established record of clinical safety, but has not been licensed in the USA. Psoralen/UV is not licensed for blood products, but has been approved for the treatment of psoriasis and epidermal T-cell lymphoma. Its safety will have to be further established before it can be licensed for use in blood products, and practical methods for the delivery of effective long-range UV light to blood cells will have to be developed before this method can realize its potential of rendering the cellular elements of blood virus-free and functionally sound.

The complete safety of some clotting factor concentrates has already been achieved; patients with severe haemophilia A, who previously were almost uniformly infected with HBV, HCV and HIV as a result of clotting factor replacement therapy, face a future in which virtually no newly diagnosed patients should be infected with these agents. The potential to inactivate cellular blood products is an exciting prospect that would leap the final hurdle to complete eradication of viruses from transfused products. This prospect, fantasy only a decade ago, now seems a realistic and achievable goal.

Passive imunoprophylaxis for transfusion-associated hepatitis

Prior to the 1970s, 11 field trials had been conducted to evaluate the efficacy of immune globulin for the prevention of transfusion-related hepatitis (Seeff 1990). A beneficial effect was reported in 6 of the 11 studies. Most of these studies, however, were performed in a manner inconsistent with current rigorous principles that require a randomized, double-blind, controlled trial. The most compelling of these studies, one that did adhere to accepted practice and involved large numbers, unfortunately assessed most of the subjects through a questionnaire survey rather than through serial enzyme testing (National Transfusion Hepatitis Study 1972). The investigators of this study concluded that normal human immune globulin (NHIG) was without benefit. In view of the conflicting results, four additional well-controlled trials were conducted in the early 1970s to determine the efficacy of IG for the prevention of transfusion-associated hepatitis (Kuhns et al 1975, Seeff et al 1977, 1978a, Knodell et al 1976). While there were many similarities in these studies, they did not utilize a common protocol.

As shown in Table 29.5, two of the trials compared the relative efficacies of placebo and NHIG (Kuhns et al, 1975, Seeff et al 1977), one involved comparison of NHIG and HBIG (Seeff et al 1978a), and one utilized a three-arm approach – placebo, NHIG and HBIG (Knodell et al 1976). None of them showed beneficial effect for NHIG in the prevention of transfusion-associated hepatitis B. The efficacy of HBIG in preventing hepatitis B could not be determined because this form of the disease had been virtually eliminated through donor screening by the time of initiation of the HBIG trials.

Relevant to these data are the results of immunoprophylaxis studies involving lesser forms of percutaneous exposure, namely accidental needlestick injury. Conflicting results have emerged from two major controlled trials. In one study, Grady, et al (1978) found that among 435 persons exposed to HBV by 'needlestick', 9.8% of those who received two 3-ml injections of HBIG (anti-HBs titre 1 : 500 000) developed hepatitis B, compared with 12.3% of those who received NHIG (anti-HBs titre 1 : 50), a non-significant difference. In contrast, in a similar VA cooperative study (Seeff et al 1978b) that administered two 5-ml doses of NHIG, hepatitis B developed in 1.4% of HBIG (anti-HBs) titre 1 : 100 000) recipients and in 5.9% of NHIG (no

Table 29.5 Efficacies of normal human immune globulin (NHIG) and hepatitis B immune globulin (HBIG) in prevention of transfusion-associated hepatitis (TAH), type B

Reference	No. of patients	HBsAg screening	Incidence of TAH-B		
			Placebo	NMIG	HBIG
Kuhns et al 1975	195	No	7.8	7.5	—
Knodell et al 1976	279	No	1.1	1.1	0.0
Seeff et al 1977	2204	No	2.6	2.1	—
Seeff et al 1978a	969	Yes	—	0.4	0.4

anti-HBs) recipients; this difference was significant. Subsequent analysis suggested that HBIG had merely modified the presentation of the disease, acting through passive–active immunization to decrease only the overt, icteric form of hepatitis B (Hoofnagle et al 1979). Supported by data of an uncontrolled trial from Britain (Combined Medical Research Council and Public Health Laboratory Service Report 1980), and by the data from a study involving sexual exposure to hepatitis B (Redeker et al 1975), HBIG was licensed for use in the USA for type B hepatitis post-exposure prophylaxis.

An unexpected dividend was that the entity of non-A, non-B hepatitis was recognized during the course of these studies, permitting evaluation of the effects of immunoprophylaxis for this form of viral disease (Table 29.6). No beneficial effect of NHIG was found in the study of Kuhns et al (1975), a significant reduction only in icteric hepatitis was noted among NHIG recipients in the VA Cooperative Study (Seeff et al 1977), and a significant reduction in both acute and chronic non-A, non-B hepatitis was reported by Knodell et al (1976). In the VA Cooperative Study, the most prominent risk factor was the use of paid donor blood. After correcting for this factor, the benefit of NHIG was no longer discernible.

These uncertain results have led to equivocation with regard to recommending routine passive immunoprophylaxis for TAH, now known to be predominantly related to HCV. Recently, a randomized study from Spain has provided additional information in support of the routine use of NHIG (Sanchez-Qiijano et al 1988). As in the study of Knodell et al (1976), two injections of NHIG were administered, the first one predating receipt of the transfusion. The investigators reported that NHIG reduced the frequency of non-A, non-B hepatitis by 72.7% and that NHIG appeared to diminish progression to chronic liver disease. Similar results have emerged from a randomized study from Scandinavia involving cardiac surgery patients with cardiopulmonary bypass (al-Khaja et al 1991). Here, too, NHIG was given prior to (at the time of premedication) and following (at the third postoperative day) transfusion in a small dose of 2 ml

Table 29.6 Efficacy of normal human immune globulin (NHIG) in the prevention of transfusion-associated non-A, non-B hepatitis (TAH-NANB)

Reference	No of patients	Prevalence of NANB hepatitis (%)			
		Anicteric		Icteric	
		Placebo	NHIG	Placebo	NHIG
Kuhns et al 1975	195	8.8	11.8	7.8	6.4
Seeff et al 1977	2204	7.7	6.9	1.8	0.8*
Knodell et al 1976	279	5.3	4.9	7.4	1.1*

*$P < 0.05$.

i.m. on each occasion. The prevalence of hepatitis in the controls (not double-blinded) was 10% and in NHIG recipients less than 2%.

Fortunately, the incidence of transfusion-associated non-A, non-B hepatitis is in the process of rapid decline as donors are subjected to increasingly rigorous historical and serological screening. Were this not the case, further consideration might be given to the routine administration of NHIG both prior to and following each transfusion episode.

SUMMARY

Reductions in TAH incidence have depended on both the introduction of specific and non-specific assays to detect the virus carrier state and on increasing restrictions on donor eligibility based on high-risk behaviour practices. The psycho-social measures have been more effective than the serological measures, particularly the exclusion of paid donors beginning in the 1970s and the intensive efforts to promote self-exclusion of donors at high risk for AIDS transmission in the 1980s. Fortunately, the overlap between groups at risk for AIDS and groups at risk for viral hepatitis is so marked that a single exclusionary process diminishes both occurrences.

There have been no recent large prospective studies in the USA that have precisely defined the current incidence of TAH. The proportion of recipients developing hepatitis must thus be inferred from prior incidence determinations and from the projected impact of a variety of screening measures including the exclusion of donors with high-risk behaviour and the recent introduction of anti-HCV testing. Data from prospective studies at NIH suggested that the incidence of TAH had diminished to the range of 6.5–8% in the years just prior to the introduction of anti-HIV and other AIDS-related measures. The impact of these AIDS-related measures was not directly assessed in the USA, but in Canada TAH prevalence fell from 9% prior to 1965 to 2% after 1965 (Feinman et al 1988). This dramatic decline in TAH incidence was not related to any specific or non-specific hepatitis screening measure, but solely to the increased restrictions on blood donation engendered by concern for transfusion-transmitted AIDS. In the USA, the introduction of ALT and anti-HBc as surrogate assays for the detection of NANB hepatitis carriers, combined with AIDS-related interventions, resulted in a fall in TAH prevalence to approximately 3%, as measured in an ongoing NIH prospective study (unpublished). In an ongoing study of anti-HCV seroconversion rates, Nelson et al (1992) demonstrated a fall in seroconversion incidence from 3.8% to 0.6% after the sequential introduction of surrogate assays and anti-HCV screening.

It is felt that anti-HCV donor screening will decrease TAH prevalence throughout the world by 50–70%, as already evidenced in Barcelona, where TAH incidence fell from 9.6% to 1.9% immediately after the introduction of anti-HCV screening (Esteban et al 1991). Similarly, TAH incidence in the ongoing NIH study has fallen to under 1.5% after introduction of anti-HCV testing.

Thus, wherever measured, TAH rates appear to be under 2% and perhaps as low as 0.5% per transfusion episode, a dramatic decline from rates in excess of 10% in the early 1980s, 20% in the 1970s and 30% in the 1960s. Coupled with the complete inactivation of viruses in factor VIII concentrates and other blood components and the potential that even cellular blood products may be amenable to viral inactivation procedures, the goal of zero hepatitis risk in the blood supply appears to be an obtainable end, rather than an obtuse vision.

REFERENCES

Aach R D, Lander J J, Sherman L A et al 1978 Transfusion-transmitted viruses: interim analysis of hepatitis among transfused and nontransfused patients. In: Vyas G N, Cohen S N, Ahmid R (eds) Viral hepatitis. Franklin Institute Press, Philadelphia, pp 383–396

Aach R D, Szmuness E, Mosley J W et al 1981 Serum alanine aminotransferase of donors in relation to the risk of non-A, non-B hepatitis in recipients; the transfusion-transmitted viruses study. New England Journal of Medicine 304: 989–994

Aach R D, Stevens C E, Hollinger F B et al 1991 Hepatitis C virus infection in post-transfusion hepatitis. New England Journal of Medicine 325: 1325–1329

al-Khaja N, Roberts D G, Belboul A et al 1991 Gamma globulin prophylaxis to reduce post-transfusion non-A, non-B hepatitis after cardiac surgery with cardiopulmonary by-pass. Scandinavian Journal of Thoracic and Cardiovascular Surgery 25: 7–12

Aledor T L M, Levine P H, Hilgartner M, et al 1985 A study of liver biopsies and liver disease among hemophiliacs. Blood 66: 367–372

Allain J P, Dailey S H, Laurian Y et al 1991 Evidence for persistent hepatitis C virus (HCV) infection in hemophiliacs. Journal of Clinical Investigation 88: 1672–1679

Allen J C, Sayman W A 1962 Serum hepatitis from transfusion of blood: epidemiologic study. Journal of the American Medical Association 180: 1079–1085

Alter H J 1983 Characteristics of NANB viruses. In Overby L R, Deinhardt F (eds) Viral hepatitis: Second International Max von Pettenhoffer Symposium Marcel Dekker, New York, pp 53–56

Alter H J 1987 You'll wonder where the yellow went: a 15-year retrospective of posttransfusion hepatitis. In: Moore S B (ed) Transfusion-transmitted viral diseases. American Association of Blood Banks, Arlington pp 53–86

Alter H J 1989 Chronic consequences of non-A, non-B hepatitis. In: Seeff L B, Lewis J H (ed) Current prospective in hepatology. Plenum Publishing Corporation, New York, pp 83–97

Alter H J 1992 New kit on the block: evaluation of second generation assays for detection of antibody to the hepatitis C virus. Hepatology 15: 130–136

Alter H J, Holland P V, Purcell R H, Lander J J, Feinstone S M, Morrow A G, Schmidt P J 1972 Transfusion hepatitis after exclusion of commercial and hepatitis-B antigen-positive donors. Annals of Internal Medicine 77: 691–699

Alter H J, Purcell R H, Holland P V, Feinstone S M, Morrow A G, Moritsugu Y 1975 Clinical and serological analysis of transfusion-associated hepatitis. Lancet ii: 838–841

Alter H J, Purcell R H, Feinstone S M, Holland PV, Morrow A G 1978a Non-A/non-B hepatitis: a review and interim report of an ongoing prospective study. In: Vyas G N, Cohen S N, Schmid R (eds) Viral hepatitis. Franklin Institute Press, Philadelphia, pp 359–381

Alter H J, Purcell R H, Holland P V, Popper H 1978b Transmissible agent in 'non-A, non-B' hepatitis. Lancet i: 459–463

Alter H J, Tabor E, Merryman H T et al 1978c Transmission of hepatitis B virus infection by transfusion of frozen-deglycerolized red blood cells. New England Journal of Medicine 298: 637–642

Alter H J, Purcell R H, Holland P V, Alling D W, Koziol D E 1981 The relationship of donor transaminase (ALT) to recipient hepatitis: impact on blood transfusion services. Journal of the American Medical Association 246: 630–634

Alter H J, Purcell R H, Feinstone S M, Tegtmeier G E 1982 Non-A, non-B hepatitis: its relationship to cytomegalovirus, to chronic hepatitis and to direct and indirect test methods. In: Szmuness W, Alter H J, Maynard J E (eds) Viral hepatitis: 1981 International Symposium. Franklin Institute Press, Philadelphia, pp 279–294

Alter H J, Creagan R P, Morel P A et al 1988 Photochemical decontamination of blood components containing hepatitis B and non-A, non-B virus. Lancet ii: 1446–1450

Alter H J, Purcell R H, Shih J W et al 1989 Detection of antibody to hepatitis C virus in prospectively followed transfusion recipients with acute and chronic non-A, non-B hepatitis. New England Journal of Medicine 321: 1494–1500

Alter H J, Jett B W, Polito A J et al 1991 Analysis of the role of hepatitis C virus in transfusion-associated hepatitis. In: Hollinger F B, Lemon S M, Margolis H (eds) Viral hepatitis and liver disease. Williams & Wilkins, Baltimore, pp 396–402

Alter M J 1991 Epidemiology of community-acquired hepatitis C. In: Hollinger F B, Lemon S M, Margolis H (eds). Viral hepatitis and liver disease. Williams & Wilkins, Baltimore, pp 410–413

Alter M J, Coleman P J, Alexander J et al 1989 Importance of heterosexual activity in the transmission of hepatitis B and non-A, non-B hepatitis. Journal of the American Medical Association 262: 1201–1205

Alter M J, Hadler S C, Judson F N, Hu P Y et al 1990 Risk factors for acute non-A, non-B hepatitis in the United States and association with hepatitis C infection. Journal of the American Medical Association 264: 2231–2235

Aymard J P, Janot C, Gayet C, Guillemin C, Canton P, Gaucher P, Streiff F 1986 Post-transfusion non-A, non-B hepatitis after cardiac surgery: prospective analysis of donor blood anti-HBc activity as a predictor of the occurrence of non-A, non-B hepatitis in recipients. Vox Sanguinis 51: 236–238

Barker L F, Shulman R, Murray R, Hirschman R J, Ratner D, Diefenbach W C, Geller H M 1970 Transmission of serum hepatitis. Journal of the American Medical Association 211: 1509–1512

Barker L F, Maynard J E, Purcell R H 1975 Viral hepatitis, type B, in chimpanzees: titration of subtypes. Journal 132: 451–458

Barrera J M, Bruguera M, Ercilla G, et al 1991 Incidence of non-A, non-B hepatitis after screening blood donors for antibodies to hepatitis C virus and surrogate markers. Annals of Internal Medicine 115: 595–600

Beasley R P, Hwang L-Y, Lin C-C et al 1981a Hepatitis B immune globulin (HBIG) efficacy in the interruption of perinatal transmission of hepatitis B virus carrier state. Lancet 2: 388–393.

Beasley R P, Hwang LY, Lin CC et al 1981b Hepatocellular carcinoma and hepatitis B virus: a prospective study of 22,707 men in Taiwan. Lancet ii: 1006–1008

Beeson P B 1943 Jaundice occurring one to four months after transfusion of blood or plasma: report of seven cases. Journal of the American Medical Association 121: 1332–1334

Beeson P B, Chesney G, McFarlane A M 1944 Hepatitis following injection of mumps convelescent serum. I. Use of plasma in mumps epidemic. Lancet ii: 814–815

Biggar J W 1943 Jaundice in syphilitics under treatment: possible transmission of virus. Lancet i: 457–458

Biswas R, Mitchell F, Wilson L, Tankersley D, Finalayson J, Nedjars 1991 Hepatitis C and therapeutic immunolobulin product safety: a chimpanzee study. Abstracts of the Third International Symposium on HCV (Strasbourg, France) 115

Blanchette V S, Vortsman E, Shore A et al 1991 Hepatitis C infection in children with hemophilia A and B. Blood 78: 285–289

Blumberg B S, Alter H J, Visnich S 1965 A new antigen in leukemia serum. Journal of the American Medical Association 66: 924–931

Blumberg B S, Gerstley B J S, Hungerford D A, London W T, Sutnick Al 1967 A serum antigen (Australia Antigen) in Down's Syndrome, leukemia and hepatitis. Annals of Internal Medicine 66: 924–931

Bradley D W, Cook E H, Maynard J E, et al 1979 Experimental infection of chimpanzees with antihemophilic (factor VIII) materials. recovery of virus like particles associated with non-A, non-B hepatitis. Journal of Medical Virology 3: 253–269

Bradley D W, Maynard J E, Popper H, et al 1983 Post-transfusion non-A, non-B hepatitis: physico-chemical properties of two distinct agents. Journal of Infectious Disease 148: 254–265

Brandt K H, Meulendijk P N, Poulie N J, Schalm L, Schultz M J, Zanan H C 1963 De warde van de transaminasem-bepalingin donorbloed Geneesk. 107: 2313–1232

Brechot C, Hadchouel M, Scotto J et el 1981 State of hepatitis B virus DNA in hepatocytes of patients with hepatitis B surface antigen-positive and -negative liver disease. Proceedings of the National Academy of Sciences of the USA 78: 3906–3910

Brettler D B, Alter H J, Dienstag J L, Forsberg A D, Levine P H 1990 Prevalence of hepatitis C virus antibody in a cohort of hemophilia patients. Blood 76: 254–256

Bruix J, Calvet X, Costa J et al 1984 Prevalence of antibodies to hepatitis C virus in Spanish patients with hepatocellular carcinoma and hepatic cirrhosis. Lancet 2: 1004–1006

Cherubin C E 1971 Risk of post-transfusion hepatitis in recipients of blood containing S H antigen in Harlem Hospital. Lancet 1: 627–300

Cherubin C E, Prince A M 1971 Serum hepatitis specific antigen (SH) in commercial and volunteer sources of blood. Transfusion 11: 25–27

Choo Q-L, Kuo G, Weiner A J, Overby L R, Bradley D W, Houghton M 1989 Isolation of a cDNA clone derived from a blood-borne non-A, non-B hepatitis genome. Science 244: 359–362

Chou W H, Yoneyama T, Takeuchi K, Harada H, Saito I, Miyamura T 1991 Discrimination of hepatitis C virus in liver tissues from different patients with hepatocellular carcinomas by direct nucleotide sequencing of amplified cDNA of the viral genome. Journal of Clinical Microbiology 29: 2860–2864

Collins J D, Bassendine M F, Codd A H, Colins A, Ferner R E, James O F 1983 Prospective study of post-transfusion hepatitis after cardiac surgery in a British Centre. British Medical Journal 287: 1422–1424

Colombo M, Oldani S, Donato M F et al 1987 A multicenter, prospective study of posttransfusion hepatitis in Milan. Hepatology 7: 709–712

Colombo M, Mannuci P M, Carnelli V, Saridge G F, Gazengci C, Schimpf K 1985 Non-A, non-B hepatitis by heat-treated factor VIII concentrates. Lancet ii: 1–6

Colombo M, Oldani S, Donato M F et al 1987 A multicenter, prospective study of posttransfusion hepatitis in Milan. Hepatology 7: 709–712

Combined Medical Research Council and Public Health Laboratory Service Report 1980 The incidence of hepatitis B infection after accidental exposure and anti-HBs immunoglobulin prophylaxis. Lancet i: 6

Conry-Cantilena, Viladomiu L, Melpolder J et al 1992 Hepatitis C virus infection in a U.S. urban blood donor population. Abstracts of the American Association of Blood Banks. Transfusion (in press)

Contreras M, Barbara J A, Anderson C C et al 1991 Low incidence of non-A, non-B post-transfusion hepatitis in London confirmed by hepatitis C virus serology. Lancet 337: 753–757

Cossart Y E, Kirsch S, Ismay S L 1982 Post-transfusion hepatitis in Australia: report of the Australian Red Cross Study. Lancet i: 208–213

Creutzfeldt W, Severidt H-I, Schmitt H et al 1966 Incidence and course of icteric and anicteric transfusion hepatitis. German Medical Monthly 11: 469–476

Di Bisceglie A M, Goodman Z D, Ishak K G, Hoofnagle J H, Melpolder J J, Alter H J 1991 Long-term clinical and histopathological follow-up of chronic postransfusion hepatitis. Hepatology 14: 969–974

Dienstag J L 1983 Non-A, non-B hepatitis. I. Recognition, epidemiology, and clinical features. Gastroenterology 85: 439–462

Dike A E 1981 Post-transfusion hepatitis B transmitted by HbsAg-negative blood containing anti-HBc. Medical and Laboratory Sciences 38: 415–417

Donahue J G, Munoz A, Ness P M 1992 The declining risk of post-transfusion hepatitis C virus infection. New England Journal of Medicine 327: 369–373

Esteban J I, Esteban R, Viladomiu L et al 1989 Hepatitis C virus antibodies among risk groups in Spain. Lancet ii: 294–297

Esteban J I, Gonzalez A, Hernandez J M et al 1990 Evaluation of antibodies to hepatitis C virus in a study of transfusion-associated hepatitis. New England Journal of Medicine 323: 1107–1112

Esteban J I, Gonzalez A, Hernandez J M et al 1991 Open prospective efficacy trial of anti-HCV screening of blood donors to prevent posttransfusion hepatitis. In: Hollinger F B, Lemon S M, Margolis H S (eds) Viral hepatitis and liver disease. Williams & Wilkins, Baltimore, pp 431–433

Everhart J E, Di Bisceglie A M, Murray L M et al 1990 Risk for non-A, non-B, (type C) hepatitis through sexual or household contact with chronic carriers. Annals of Internal Medicine 112: 544–555

Eyster M E, Alter H J, Aledort L M, Quan S, Hatzakis A, Goedert J J 1991 Heterosexual co-transmission of hepatitis C virus (HCV) and human immunodeficiency virus (HIV). Annals of Internal Medicine 115: 764–768

Federal Register 37: 106, Title 42, Part 73.775, p 10937

Federal Register 1978 43: 9: 2142

Feinman S V, Berris B, Bojarski S 1988 Posttransfusion hepatitis in Toronto, Canada. Gastroenterology 95: 464–469

Feinstone S M, Kapikian A Z, Purcell R H 1973 Hepatitis A detection by immune electron microscopy of a virus-like antigen associated with acute illness. Science 182: 1026–1028

Feinstone S M, Kapikian A Z, Purcell R H, Alter H J, Holland P V 1975 Transfusion-associated hepatitis not due to viral hepatitis type A or B. New England Journal of Medicine 292: 767–770

Feinstone S M, Alter H J, Dienes H P et al 1981 Non-A, non-B hepatitis in chimpanzees and marmosets. Journal of Infectious Diseases 144: 588–598

Feinstone J M, Mihalik K B, Kamimura J, Alter H J, London W T, Purcell R H 1983 Inactivation of hepatitis B virus and non-A, non-B virus by chloroform. Infection and Immunity 4: 816–821

Findley G M, MacCallum F O 1937 Note on acute hepatitis and yellow fever immunization. Transactions of the Society of Tropical Medicine and Hygiene 31: 297–308

Flaum A Malmross H, Persson E 1926 Eine nosocomiale Ikterus Epidemic. Acta Medica Scandinavica 16 (suppl.): 544–553

Fox J P, Manso C, Penna H A, Madereira P 1942 Observations on the occurrence of icterus in Brazil following vaccinations against yellow fever. American Journal of Hygiene 36: 63–116

Frey-Wettstein 1977 How frequent is post-transfusion hepatitis after the introduction of 3rd generation donor screening for hepatitis B? What is the probable nature? Vox Sanguinis 32: 352–353

Genesca J, Esteban J I, Alter H J 1991 Blood-borne non-A, non-B hepatitis: hepatitis C. Seminars in Liver Disease 11: 147–164

Giles J P, McCollum R W, Berndtson L W Jr 1969 Viral hepatitis: relation of Australia/SH antigen to the Willowbrook MS-2 strain. New England Journal of Medicine 281: 119–122

Gilliam J H, Geissinger K R, Richter J E 1984 Primary Hepatocellular carcinoma after chronic non-A, non-B post-transfusion hepatitis. Annals of Internal Medicine 101: 794–795

Gitnick G 1991 Current hepatitis risks to dialysis patients. Proceedings of the Third International Symposium on HCV, Strasbourg, France. p 42

Gocke D J 1972 Journal of the American Medical Association 1972 A prospective study or posttransfusion hepatitis: the role of the Australia antigen. Journal of the American Medical Association 219: 1165–1170

Gocke D J, Kavey N B 1969 Hepatitis antigen: correlation with disease and infectivity of blood. Lancet i: 1055–1069

Gocke D J, Greenberg H B, Kavey N B 1969 Hepatitis antigen: detection of infectious blood donors. Lancet 2: 248–249

Gocke D J, Greenberg H B, Kavey N B 1970 Correlation of Australia antigen with posttransfusion hepatitis. Journal of the American Medical Association 212: 877–879

Goldfield M, Black H C, Bill J, Srihongse S, Pizzuti W 1975 The consequences of administering blood pretested for HBsAg by third generation techniques: a progress report. American Journal of Medical Science 270: 335–342

Grady G F, Chalmers T C 1964 Risk of post-transfusion viral hepatitis. New England Journal of Medicine 271: 337–342

Grady G F, Lee V A, Prince A M et al 1978 Hepatitis B immune globulin for accidental exposures among medical personnel: final report of a multicenter controlled trial. Journal of Infectious Disease 138: 625–638

Grillner L, Bergdahl S, Jyrala A 1982 Non-A, non-B after open-heart surgery in Sweden. Scandanavian Journal of Infectious Diseases 14: 171–175

Hadziyannis P 1978 Post-transfusion hepatitis: thesis, Athens

Hampers C I, Prager D, Senior J R 1964 Post-transfusion anicteric hepatitis. New England Journal of Medicine 271: 747–754

Hartfall S J, Garland H G, Goldie W 1937 Gold Treatment of arthritis: a review of 900 cases. Lancet ii: 784–788

Haugen R K 1979 Hepatitis after transfusion of frozen red cross and red cells and washed red cells. New England Journal of Medicine 301: 393–395

Havens W P, Ward D, Drill V A et al 1944 Experimental production of viral hepatitis by feeding icterogenic materials. Proceedings of the Society for Experimental Biology and Medicine 57: 206–208

Hayashi J, Nakashima K, Kajiyama W et al 1991 Prevalence of antibody to hepatitis C virus in hemodialysis patients. American Journal of Epidemiology 134: 651–657

He L F, Alling D, Popkin T, Shapiro M, Alter H J, Purcell R H 1987 Non-A, non-B hepatitis virus: determination of size by filtration. Journal of Infectious Diseases 156: 636–640

Hernandez J M, Pigueras J, Carrera A, Triginer J 1983 Posttransfusion hepatitis in Spain: a prospective study. Vox Sanguinis 44: 231–237

Holland P V, Alter H J, Purcell R H, Walsh J J, Morrow A G, Schmidt P J 1973 The infectivity of blood containing the Australia antigen. In: Prier J E, Friedman H (eds) Australia antigen. University Press, Baltimore, pp 191–203

Hollinger F B, Gitnick G L, Aach R D et al 1978 Non-A, non-B hepatitis transmission in chimpanzees: a project of the Transfusion-Transmitted Viruses Study Group. Intervirology 10: 60–68

Hollinger F B, Dolana G, Thomas W, Gyorkey F 1984 Reduction in risk of hepatitis transmission by heat-treatment of a human factor VIII concentrate Journal of Infectious Diseases 150: 250–262

Hoofnagle J H 1990 Postransfusion hepatitis B. Transfusion 30: 384–386

Hoofnagle J H, Gerety R J, Ni L Y 1974 Antibody to hepatitis B core antigen: a sensitive indicator of hepatitis B virus replication. New England Journal of Medicine 290: 1336–1340

Hoofnagle J H, Seeff L B, Bales Z B, Zimmerman H J 1978 Type B hepatitis after transfusion with blood containing antibody to hepatitis B core antigen. New England Journal of Medicine 298: 1379–1383

Hoofnagle J H, Seeff L B, Bales Z B 1979 Passive–active immunity from hepatitis B immune globulin: re-analysis of a Veterans Administration cooperative study of needle-stick hepatitis. Annals of Internal Medicine 91: 813

Hopkins R, Kane E, Robertson A E, Haase G 1982 Hepatitis B virus transmitted by HBsAg-negative blood containing anti-HBc. Medical and Laboratory Science 39: 61–62

Horowitz M S, Rooks C, Horowitz B, Hilgartner M W 1988 Virus safety of solvent/detergent-treated anti-hemophiliac factor concentrate. Lancet ii: 186–188

Hoxworth P I, Haesler W E Jr, Smith H Jr 1959 The risk of hepatitis from whole blood and stored plasma. Surgery in Gynecology and Obstetrics 109: 30–42

Iwarson S, Lindberg J, Lundin P 1979 Progression of hepatitis non-A, non-B to chronic active hepatitis: a histologic follow-up of two cases. Journal of Clinical Pathology 32: 351–355

Jacob J R, Sureau C, Burk K H, Eichberg J W, Dreesman G R, Landford R E 1991 In vitro replication of non-A, non-B hepatitis virus In: Hollinger F B, Lemon S M, Margolis H S (eds) Viral hepatitis and liver disease. Williams & Wilkins, Baltimore, pp 387–392

Japanese Red Cross 1991 Non-A, non-B hepatitis research group. Effect of screening for hepatitis C virus antibody and hepatitis B virus core antibody on incidence of post-transfusion hepatitis. Lancet 338: 1040–1041

Jennings E R, Hindman W M, Zak B et al 1957 The thymol turbidity test in screening of blood donors. American Journal of Clinical Pathology 27: 489–502

John T J, Nina G T, Rajagapolalan M S et al 1979 Epidemic

hepatitis B caused by commercial human immunoglobulin. Lancet i: 1074

Kaneko S, Miller R H, Feinstone S M 1989 Detection of serum hepatitis B DNA in patients with chronic hepatitis utilizing the polymerase chain reaction assay. Proceedings of the National Academy of Sciences of the USA 86: 312–316

Katchaki J N, Siem T H, Brouwer R, van Loon A M, van der Logt 1979 Hepatitis B core antibody in volunteer blood donors: comparison of radioimmunoassay and indirect immunofluorescence. Journal of Medical Virology 3: 275–280

Katchaki J N, Siem Th, Brouwen R 1981 Post-transfusion non-A, non-B hepatitis in the Netherlands. British Medical Journal 282: 197–198

Kew M C, Houghton M, Choo Q L, Kuo G 1990 Hepatitis C virus antibodies in southern African blacks with hepatocellular carcinoma. Lancet 335: 873–874

Kiyosawa K, Akahane Y, Nogata A et al 1982 Significance of blood transfusion in non-A, non-B chronic liver disease in Japan Vox Sanguinis 43: 45–52

Kiyosawa K, Akahane Y, Nagata A, Furate S 1984 Hepatocellular carcinoma after non-A, non-B post-transfusion hepatitis. American Journal of Gastroenterology 79: 777–781

Kiyosawa K, Sodeyama T, Tanaka E et al 1990 Interrelationship of blood transfusion, non-A, non-B hepatitis and hepatocellular carcinoma. Analysis by detection of antibody to hepatitis C virus. Hepatology 12: 671–675

Kleinman S, Alter H J, Busch M et al 1992 Increased detection of HCV infected blood donors using a multiple antigen HCV enzyme immunoassay. Transfusion 32: 805–813

Knodell R G, Conrad M E, Ginsberg A L, Bell C J, Flannery E P 1976 Efficacy of prophylactic gamma-globulin in preventing non-A, non-B post-transfusion hepatitis. Lancet i: 557–561

Koretz R L, Overby L R, Gitnick G L 1976 Post-transfusion hepatitis: the role of hepatitis B antibody. Gastroenterology 70: 556–561

Koretz R H, Stone O, Gitnick G 1980 The long-term course of non-A, non-B post-transfusion hepatitis. Gastroenterology 79: 893–898

Koziol D E, Holland P V, Alling D W et al 1986 Antibody to hepatitis B core antigen as a paradoxical marker for non-A, non-B hepatitis agents in blood. Annals of Internal Medicine 184: 488–495

Kuhns W J, Prince A M, Brotman B, Hazzi C, Grady G F 1975 A clinical and laboratory evaluation of immune serum globulin from donors with a history of hepatitis: attempted prevention of post-transfusion hepatitis. American Journal of Medicine and Science 272: 255–261

Kunin C M 1959 Serum Hepatitis from whole blood: incidence and relation to source of blood. American Journal of Medicine and Science 237: 293–303

Kuo G, Choo Q-L, Alter H J et al 1989 An assay for circulating antibodies to a major etiologic virus of human non-A, non-B hepatitis. Science 244: 362–364

Lander J T, Gitnick G L, Gelb L H, Aach R D 1978 Anticore antibody screening of transfused blood. Vox Sanguinis 34: 77–80

Larsen J, Hetland G, Skaug K 1990 Posttransfusion hepatitis B transmitted by blood from a hepatitis B surface antigen-negative hepatitis B virus carrier. Transfusion 30: 431–432

Lurman A 1885 Eine Icterusepidemia. Berliner Klinische Wochenschrift 2–2: 20–23

MacCallum F O,Bauer D J 1944 Homologous serum jaundice transmission experiments with human volunteers. Lancet 1: 622–627

MacCallum F O 1945 Transmission of arsenotherapy jaundice by blood: failure with faeces and nasopharyngeal washings. Lancet i: 1342

McHutchinson J G, Kuo G, Houghton M, Choo Q, Redeker A G 1991 Hepatitis C virus antibodies in acute icteric and chronic non-A, non-B hepatitis. Gastroenterology 101: 1117–1119

Manucci P M, Schimpf K, Brettler B et al 1990 Low risk for hepatitis C in hemophiliacs given a high-purity, pasteurized factor VIII concentrate. Annals of Internal Medicine 113: 27–32

Mattsson L, Weiland O, Glaumann H 1989 Chronic non-A, non-B hepatitis developed after transfusion, illicit self injections or sporadically. Outcome during long-term follow-up. Liver 9: 120–127

Michael B R, Garret E B 1990 Safety of monoclonal antibody purified factor VIII. Lancet 336: 188

Mishiro S, Hoshi Y, Takeda K et al 1990 Non-A, non-B specific antibodies directed at host-derived epitope: implication for an autoimmune process. Lancet 336: 1400–1403

Morgan H W, Williamson D A 1943 Jaundice following administration of human blood products. British Medical Journal 1: 750–753

Motschman T L, Taswell H F, Brecher M E 1989 Intraoperative blood loss and patient and graft survival in orthotopic liver transplantation: their relationship to clinical and laboratory data. Mayo Clinic Proceedings 64: 346–355

National Transfusion Hepatitis Study 1972 Risk of posttransfusion hepatitis in the United States: a prospective cooperative study. Journal of the American Medical Association 220: 692–701

Neefe J R, Gellis S S, Stokes J Jr 1946 Homologous serum hepatitis and infectious (serum) hepatitis. Studies in volunteers bearing on immunologic and other characteristics of the etiologic agent. American Journal of Medicine 1: 3–22

Nelson K E, Donahue J C, Munoz A et al 1992 The risk of transfusion transmission of hepatitis C virus (HCV) and effectiveness of donor screening. Abstracts of the 5th National Forum on AIDS, Hepatitis, and other Blood-Borne Diseases; Altanta, GA. p 70

Nishioka K, Watanabe J, Furuta S, et al 1991 A high prevalence of antibody to the hepatitis C virus in patients with hepatocellular carcinoma in Japan. Cancer 67: 429–433

Norman J E, Beebe G W, Hoofnagle J H, Seeff L B 1992 Mortality follow-up of the 1942 epidemic of hepatitis B in the United States Army. Annals of Internal Medicine (in press)

Okochi K S, Murakami S, Ninomiya K et al 1970 Australia antigen, transfusion and hepatitis. Vox Sanguinis 18: 289–300

Okuda H, Obata H, Motoike Y et al 1984 Clinicopathological features of hepatocellular carcinoma: comparison of seropositive and seronegative patients. Hepatogastroenterology 31: 64–68

Omata M, Iwama S. Sumida M et al 1981 Clinico-pathological study of acute non-A, non-B post-transfusion hepatitis: Histological features of liver biopsies in acute phase. Liver 1: 201–208

Petilli F L, Crovari P, DeFlora S 1977 Hepatitis B in subjects treated with a drug containing immunoglobulins. Journal of Infectious Diseases 135: 252–258

Preston F E, Makris M, Triger D R, Underwood J C E 1990 Prevention of hepatitis C virus infection in haemophiliacs. Lancet 336: 62–63

Prince A M, Grady G F, Hazzi C, Brotman B, Kuhns W J, Levine R W, Millian S J 1974 Long-incubation post-transfusion hepatitis without serologic evidence of exposure to hepatitis-B virus. Lancet ii: 241–246

Prince A M, Horowitz B, Brotman B, Huima T, Richardson L, van der Ende M C 1984 Sterilization of Hepatitis and HTLV-III viruses by exposure to tri (n-Butyl) phosphate and sodium cholate. Lancet i: 706–709

Prince A M, Stephan W, Dichtelmuller H, et al 1985 Inactivation of the Hutchinson strain of non-A, non-B hepatitis virus by combined use of beta-propriolactone and ultra-violet irradiation. Journal of Medical Virology 16: 119–125

Prince A M, Horowitz B, Brotman B 1986 Sterilization of hepatitis and HTLV-III viruses by exposure to tri (n-butyl) phosphate and sodium cholate. Lancet i: 706–709

Propert S A 1938 Hepatitis after prophylactic serum. British Medical Journal ii: 677–678

Rakela J, Mosley J W, Aach R D, Gitnick G L, Hollinger B, Stevens C, Szumuness W 1980 Viral hepatitis after transfusion with blood containing antibody to hepatitis B core antigen. Gastroenterology 78: 1318

Redeker A G, Mosley J W, Goche D J 1975 Hepatitis immune globulin as a prophylactic measure for spouses exposed to acute type B hepatitis. New England Journal of Medicine 293: 1055

Reinicke V, Poulsen H, Banke O, Dybkjaer E 1973 The significance of Australia-antibody in blood donors: study of liver histology in donors and post-transfusion hepatitis in recipients. Acta Pathologica et Microliologica Scandinavica 81: 753–756

Realdi G, Alberti A, Rugge M et al 1982 Long term follow-up of acute and chronic non-A, non-B post-transfusion hepatitis: evidence of progression to liver cirrhosis Gut 23: 270–275

Realdi G, Tremolada F. Bortolotti F et al 1983 The natural history of post-transfusion and sporadic non-A, non-B hepatitis in Italy. in: Verme G, Bonino G, Rizzetto M (eds) Viral hepatitis and delta infection. Alan R. Liss, New York, pp 55–66

Sanchez-Quijano A, Pineda J A, Lissen E et al 1988 Prevention of post-transfusion non-A, non-B hepatitis by non-specific immunoglobulin in heart surgery patients. Lancet 1: 1245–1249

Sanchez-Tapias J M, Barrera J, Costa J et al 1990 Hepatitis C virus infection in patients with nonalcoholic chronic liver disease. Annals of Internal Medicine 112: 921–924

Sawyer W A, Meyer K F, Eaton M D, Bauer J H, Putnam P, Schwentker F F 1943 Jaundice in Army personnel in the western region of the United States and in relation to vaccination against yellow fever. American Journal of Hygiene 39: 337–430

Schimpf K, Manucci P M, Kreutz W, et al 1987 Absence of hepatitis after treatment with a pasteurized factor VIII concentrate in patients with hemophilia and no previous transfusion. New England Journal of Medicine 316: 918–922

Seeff L B 1990 Diagnosis, therapy, and prognosis of viral hepatitis. In: Zakim D, Boyer TD (eds). Hepatology: Textbook of liver disease. Philadelphia, W B Saunders, pp 958–1025

Seeff L B 1991 Mortality of non-A, non-B transfusion-associated hepatitis in the U.S. 18 years after infection. Hepatology 14: 90A

Seeff L B, Wright E C, Zimmerman H J, McCollum R W 1975a Members of the V A Hepatitis Cooperative Studies Group. Veterans Administration cooperative study of post-transfusion hepatitis, 1969–1974: incidence and characteristics of hepatitis and responsible risk factors. 270: 355–362

Seeff L B, Zimmerman H J, Greenlee H B 1975b Rates of post-transfusion hepatitis (letter). New England Journal of Medicine 532–533

Seeff L B, Zimmerman H J, Wright E C et al 1977 A randomized, double-blind, controlled trial of the efficacy of immune serum globulin for the prevention of post-transfusion hepatitis. A Veterans Administration cooperative study. Gastroenterology 72: 111–121

Seeff L B, Wright E C, Zimmerman H J et al 1978a Post-transfusion hepatitis, 1973–1975: a Veterans Administration cooperative study. In: Vyas G N, Cohen S N, Schmid R (eds) Viral hepatitis. Franklin Institute Press, Philadelphia, 219–242

Seeff L B, Wright E C, Zimmerman H J et al 1978b Type B hepatitis after needle-stick exposure: prevention with hepatitis B immune globulin. Annals of Internal Medicine 88: 285–293

Seeff L B, Beebe G B, Hoofnagle J H et al 1987 A serologic follow-up of the 1942 epidemic of post-vaccination hepatitis in the United States Army. New England Journal of Medicine 316: 965–970

Seto B, Coleman W G, Iwarson S et al 1984 Detection of reverse transcriptase activity in association with non-A, non-B hepatitis agent(s) Lancet ii: 941–942

Shafritz D A, Lieberman H M, Isselbacher K J, Wands J R 1982 Monoclonal radioimmunoassays for hepatitis B surface antigen: demonstration of hepatitis B virus DNA or related sequences in serum and viral epitopes in immune complexes. Proceedings of the National Academy of Sciences of the USA 79: 5675–5679

Shimizu Y, Kitamoto O 1963 The incidence of viral hepatitis after blood transfusions. Gastroenterology 4: 740–744

Shimizu Y K, Feinstone S M, Purcell R H, Alter H J, London W T 1979 Non-A, non-B hepatitis: ultrastructural evidence for two agents in experimentally infected chimpanzees. Science 205: 197–200

Shimizu Y K, Omura M, Abe K et al 1985 Production of antibody associated with non-A, non-B hepatitis in a chimpanzee lymphoblastoid cell line established by a vitro transformation with Epstein–Barr virus. Proceedings of the National Academy of Sciences of the USA 82: 2138–2142

Shiraishi H, Alter H J, Feinstone S M, Purcell R H 1985 Rheumatoid factor-like reactants in sera proven to transmit Non-A, Non-B hepatitis: a potential source of false positive reactions in Non-A, Non-B assays. Hepatology 5: 181–187

Sirchia G, Giovanetti A M, Paravicini A, Bellobuono A, Mozzi F, Pizzi M N, Almini D 1991 Prospective evaluation of posttransfusion hepatitis. Transfusion 31: 299–302

Skidmore S J, Pasi K J, Mawson S J et al 1990 Serological evidence that dry heating of clotting factor concentrates prevents transmission of non-A, non-B hepatitis. Journal of Medical Virology 30: 50–52

Stevens C E, Beasley R P, Lin C-C et al 1982 Perinatal hepatitis B virus infection: use of hepatitis B immune globulin. In: Szmuness W, Alter H J, Maynard J E (eds) Viral hepatitis – 1981 international symposium, Philadelphia, Franklin Institute Press, pp 527–535

Stevens C E, Aach R D, Hollinger F B, et al 1984 Hepatitis B virus antibody in blood donors and the occurrence of non-A, non-B hepatitis in transfusion recipients: an analysis of the transfusion-transmitted viruses study. Annals of Internal Medicine 104: 488–495

Study Group of the UK Haemophilia Centre 1988 Effect of dry heating of coagulation factor concentrates at 80°C for 72 hours on transmission of non-A, non-B hepatitis. Lancet ii: 814–816

Sugg U, Frosner G G, Schneider W, Stunkat R 1976 Hepatitisshaufgheit nach Transfusion von HBsAg negativem und anti-HBs positivem Blut: Klinische Wochenschrift 53: 1133–1136

Sugg U, Erhardt S, Morgenroth T, Flehmig B 1983 Is the use of the term post-transfusion hepatitis type B in its conventional sense still justified? Vox Sanguinis 44: 305–311

Sugg U, Schenzle D, Hess G 1988 Antibodies to hepatitis B core antigen in blood donors screened for alanine aminotransferase level and hepatitis non-A, non-B in recipients. Transfusion 1988; 28: 386–388

Szmuness W, Prince A M, Brotman B, Hirsch A L 1973 Hepatitis B Antigen and antibody in blood donors: an epidemiologic study. Journal of Infectious Diseases 127: 17–25

Szmuness W, Hirsch R L, Prince A M 1975 Hepatitis B surface antigen in blood donors: further observations. Journal of Infectious Disease 131: 111–118

Tabor E, Gerety R J 1979 Transmission of hepatitis B by immune serum globulin. Lancet ii: 1293

Tabor E, Gerety R J, Drucker J A et al 1978 Transmission of non-A, non-B hepatitis from man to chimpanzee. Lancet i: 463–466

Tabor E, Goldfield M, Black H C 1980 Hepatitis Be antigen in volunteer and paid blood donors. Transfusion 20: 192–198

Tabor E, Hoofnagle J H, Barker L F, Pineda-Tamondong G, Nath N, Smallwood L A, Gerety R J 1981 Antibody to hepatitis B core antigen in blood donors with a history of hepatitis. Transfusion 21: 366–371

Tateda A, Kikuchi K, Numazaki Y, Shirachi R, Ishida N 1979 Non-B hepatitis in Japanese recipients of blood transfusions: laboratory screening of donor blood for hepatitis B surface antigen. Journal of Infectious Disease 139: 511–518

Tremolada F, Ciapetti F, Noventa F, Valfre C, Ongaro G, Realdi G 1983 Prospective study of posttransfusion hepatitis in cardiac surgery patients receiving only blood or also blood products. Vox Sanguinis 44: 25–30

Tullis J L, Hinman J, Sproul M T, Nickerson R J 1970 Incidence of post-transfusion hepatitis in previously frozen blood. Journal of the American Medical Association 214: 719–723

Tur Kaspa R, Shimon D V, Shalit M et al 1983 Posttransfusion non-A, non-B hepatitis after cardiac surgery: a prospective study. Vox Sanguinis 45: 312–315

Wang T H, Wang J T, Lin J T, Sheu J C, Sung J L, Chen D S 1991 A prospective study of post transfusion hepatitis in Taiwan. Journal of Hepatology 13: 38–43

Walker D M 1945 Some epidemiological aspects of infectious hepatitis in the US Army. American Journal of Tropical Medicine and Hygiene 25: 75–82

Walsh J H, Purcell R H, Monour A G, Chanock A G, Schmidt P J 1970, Post-transfusion hepatitis after open-heart operation: incidence after administration of blood from commercial and volunteer donor populations. Journal of the American Medical Association 211: 261–265

Working Party on Post-Transfusion Hepatitis in a London Hospital 1974 Results of a two year prospective study. J Hyg 73: 173–176

World Health Organization 1977 Advances in Viral Hepatitis. Report of the WHO Expert Committee on Viral Hepatitis. WHO Technical Report Series No. 602. Geneva

Wroblewski F, LaDue J S 1955 Serum glutamic oxalacetic transminase activity as an index of liver cell injury: a preliminary report. Annals of Internal Medicine 43: 345–360

Wroblewski F, Jervis G, LaDue S 1956 The diagnostic, prognostic, and edimiologic significance of alterations in serum glutamic pyruvic (SGP-T) transminase in hepatitis. Annals of Internal Medicine 45: 782–800

Yuasa T, Ishikawa G, Manabe S, Sekiguchi S, Takeuchi K, Miyamura T 1991 The particle size of hepatitis C virus estimated by filtration through microporous regenerated cellulose fiber. Journal of General Virology 72: 2021–2024

Zuckerman A J 1972 Hepatitis-associated antigen and viruses, Elsevier, New York

UPDATE

- REFERENCES

Bresters D, Zaauer H L, Cuypers H T M et al 1993 Recombinant immunoblot assay reaction patterns and hepatitis C virus RNA in blood donors and non-A, non-B hepatitis patients. Transfusion 33, 8: 634–638

Chemello L, Cavalletto D, Pontisso P et al 1993 Patterns of antibodies to hepatitis C virus in patients with chronic non-A, non-B hepatitis and their relationship to viral replication and liver disease. Hepatology 17: 179–182

Dodd R Y 1993 The risk of transfusion-transmitted infection. New England Journal of Medicine 327: 419–420

Gill P 1993 Transfusion-associated hepatitis C: reducing the risk. Transfusion Medicine Review 7,2: 104–111

Hagiwara H, Hayashi N, Mita E et al 1993 Quantitation of hepatitis C virus RNA in serum of asymptomatic blood donors and patients with type C chronic liver disease. Hepatology 17: 545–550

Koretz R L, Brezina M, Polito A J et al 1993 Non-A, non-B posttransfusion hepatitis: comparing C and non-C hepatitis. Hepatology 17: 361–365

Romeo J M, Ulrich P P, Busch M P, Vyas G N 1993 Analysis of hepatitis C virus RNA prevalence and surrogate markers of infection among seropositive voluntary blood donors. Hepatology 17: 188–195

Romeo R, Thiers V, Driss F, Berthelot P, Nalpas B, Bréchot C 1993 Hepatitis C virus RNA in serum of blood donors with or without elevated transaminase level. Transfusion 33: 629–632

Serfaty L, Giral P, Elghouzzi M H, Jullien A M, Poupon R 1993 Risk factors for hepatitis C virus antibody ELISA-positive blood donors according to RIBA-2 status: a case-control survey. Hepatology 17: 183–187

Troisi C L, Hollinger F B, Hoots E K et al 1993 A multicenter study of viral hepatitis in a United States hemophilic population. Blood 81: 412–418

30. Hepatitis and haemophilia

Christine Lee Geoffrey Dusheiko

There are two types of haemophilia, A and B, which are identical in their clinical manifestations and mode of inheritance. In haemophilia A, the more common variety, bleeding is caused by a deficiency of factor VIII in the blood. In haemophilia B, factor IX is deficient. The clinical severity of haemophilia correlates with the level of circulating factor VIII/IX. Patients with severe disease (< 2 u/dl) suffer from repeated, spontaneous and painful bleeding into muscles and joints which, if untreated, rapidly leads to crippling. Uncontrolled bleeding in other sites, such as the brain, causes premature death.

Although the first report of blood transfusion being used to treat haemophilia was as early as 1840 (Lane 1840), effective therapy for the disease has only become widely available in the last 20 years. As recently as 1937, Birch described 113 patients with haemophilia, of whom 82 died before the age of 15 years, often as a result of trivial injury (Birch 1937). Fresh-frozen plasma improved management of the condition and was the main treatment during the 1950s and 60s (Biggs 1967). However it was the introduction of clotting factor concentrates from the late 1960s that revolutionized the treatment of haemophilia, realizing the prospect of a near normal life for many patients.

The description of a method for the production of a high-potency concentrate of anti-haemophilic globulin in a closed-bag system (cryoprecipitate) (Pool & Shannon 1965) made home treatment a possibility. This concentrate now accounts for less than 5% of factor VIII usage in the UK. Although it has the advantages of simplicity of manufacture and low donor exposure for patients, the latter advantage may be lost in patients with severe haemophilia, who usually need very frequent transfusions. In most western countries, lyophilized clotting factor concentrates are now preferred for the routine treatment of haemophilia. These products are usually manufactured on an industrial scale, from plasma pools to which many thousands of donors have contributed. Their convenience and efficacy has led to a rapid escalation of use (Fig. 30.1). Most countries remain dependent upon imported commercial preparations, largely derived from paid donors in the USA, because demand outstrips the capacity of voluntary blood services. Although not the case now, there is no doubt that in the past commercially obtained concentrates were associated with higher risks of viral transmission than products derived from voluntary donors (Hollinger et al 1981).

Patients with haemophilia have been considered to be at high risk of developing viral hepatitis because of the use of high-risk pooled human blood products.

Transfusion-associated jaundice was first described in the 1940s (Beeson 1943, Spurling et al 1946) and became increasingly recognized as a complication of haemophilia treatment following the introduction of plasma product therapy in subsequent years (McMillan et al 1961). By the 1970s overall estimates of the rate of symptomatic acute hepatitis with jaundice in haemophiliacs ranged from 2 to 6% of treated patients per year, being particularly recognized in those patients who had previously received little or no treatment with blood products (Kasper & Kipnis 1972, Biggs 1974).

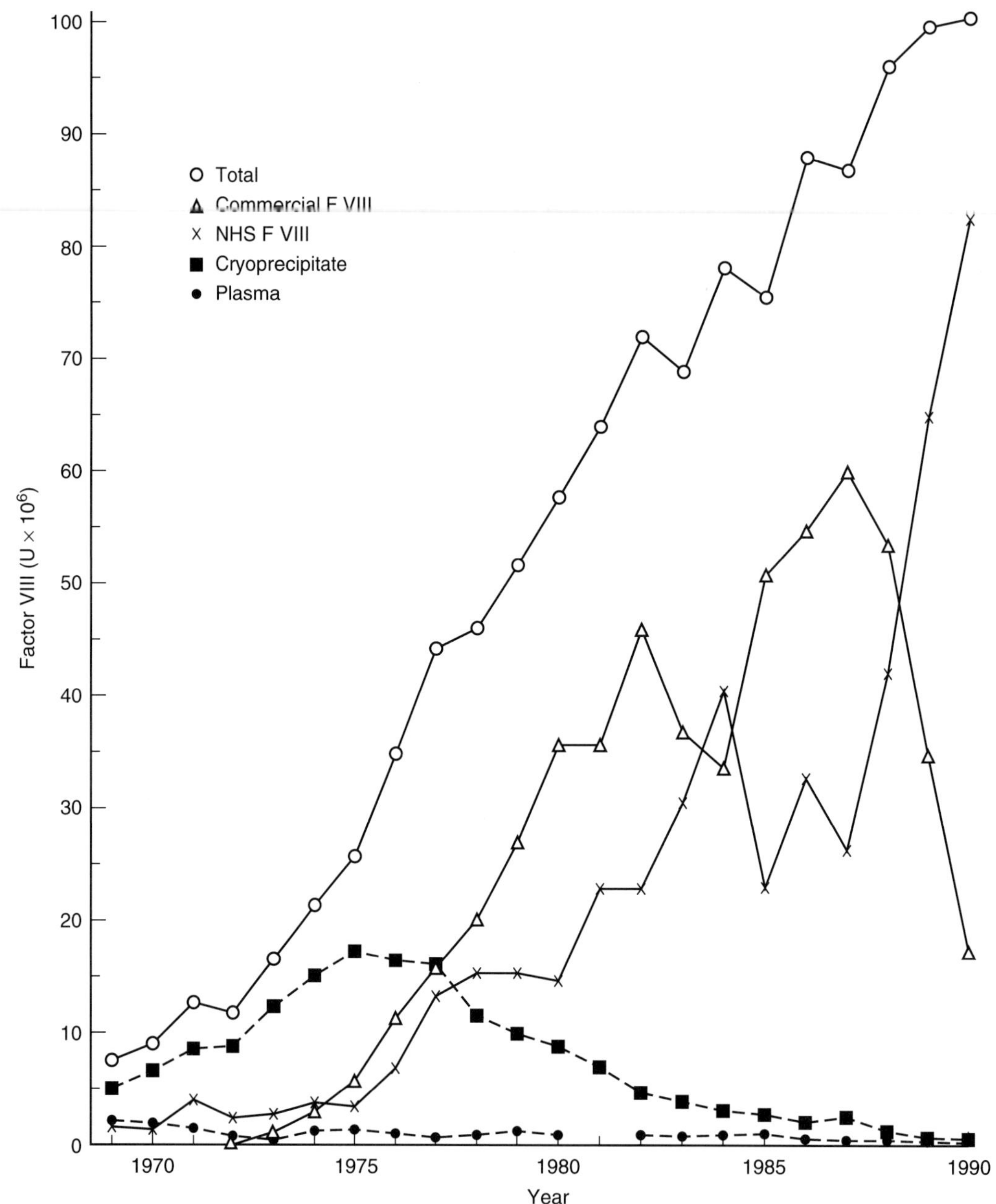

Fig. 30.1 UK haemophilia treatment.

CHRONIC LIVER DISEASE

A high proportion of patients with haemophilia have prolonged or intermittent mild to moderate increase in serum transaminases. Many studies carried out from the mid-1970s showed that 50–90% multitransfused haemophiliacs had abnormal serum aminotransferases (Mannucci et al 1975, Hasiba et al 1977, Hilgartner & Giardina 1977, Levine et al 1977). These abnormalities were frequently persistent and therefore by definition represented the development of chronic liver disease. In most patients the major cause of chronic liver disease was thought to be non-A, non-B (NANB) hepatitis and was not accounted for by alcohol, drugs or biliary tract disease.

There has been accumulating evidence from liver biopsy studies that significant histopathological liver disease is found in many haemophiliacs. An international collaborative panel of distinguished histopathologists examined samples obtained either by biopsy or at post-mortem from 155 patients worldwide (Aledort et al 1985). 15% of samples were judged to show cirrhosis, and a further 7% chronic active hepatitis (CAH). Thus 22% of patients had progressive liver disease. The majority of patients had histological evidence of chronic hepatitis, usually borderline between chronic persistent hepatitis and chronic–active hepatitis. It was apparent that even patients without major abnormalities of liver function tests could have serious histopathological liver disease. A number of smaller studies have also indicated that a proportion of haemophiliacs have morphological abnormalities (Mannucci et al 1978, Preston et al 1978, Spero et al 1978, Bamber et al 1981).

The natural history of chronic viral hepatitis varies; the concept of chronic persistent and chronic active hepatitis and their progression to cirrhosis has been challenged. Relatively benign liver disease, termed chronic persistent hepatitis (CPH), may progress to serious disease if viral replication continues. In one reported case a single infusion of concentrate was followed by acute NANB hepatitis and then histologically proven cirrhosis 4 years later (Preston et al 1982). Sequential biopsies in haemophiliacs have shown progression of CPH to CAH and cirrhosis in four of six patients within 4–6 years (Hay et al 1985).

Liver biopsy in haemophiliacs carries increased risks of bleeding, and sequential biopsies to assess progression in this group are precluded. In the international collaborative study cited above (Aledort et al 1985) 12.5% of cases were complicated by bleeding, necessitating prolonged hospitalization and/or increased concentrate usage, and there was a fatality rate of 1% compared with 0.01% in non-haemophiliacs. Infusion of factor VIII to raise factor VIII levels or plugged or transjugular biopsies may allow the procedure, but the risk of biopsy always has to be weighed against the information it can provide, and the cost. Efforts have therefore been made to find non-invasive methods of assessment of chronic liver disease. Clinical evidence, such as hepatomegaly, or biochemical parameters are unreliable indicators of the severity of hepatitis in most patients. Using CT scanning with or without contrast 28/47 patients (60%) with abnormal liver function tests were found to have splenomegaly and 7/28 (25%) to have oesophageal varices (Miller et al 1988). Serum procollagen III peptide levels may be helpful in the assessment of hepatic fibrogenesis.

HEPATITIS A

Hepatitis A virus (HAV) is only rarely transmitted by transfusion (Hollinger et al 1983, Sheretz et al 1984) and has formerly not been a problem for recipients of blood product therapy. However, outbreaks of hepatitis A have recently been reported from Italy (Mannucci 1992), Germany (Gerritzen et al 1992), the Republic of Ireland (Temperley 1993) and Belgium (Peerlinck 1983). In the Italian epidemic, a total of 50 cases were all associated with a high-purity factor VIII concentrate sterilized by solvent detergent (Octa VI). This product was also associated with 13 HAV infections in 46 susceptible haemophilic patients at the Bonn Haemophilia Centre, 15 patients in the Republic of Ireland and 6 cases in Belgium. Two of four of the German factor VIII preparations were found to be positive by nested polymerase chain reaction (PCR), and one of these PCR-positive batches was administered to four haemophiliacs who had acute HAV infection (Normann et al 1992). It is thought that these outbreaks of hepatitis A are due to the particular factor VIII because of the wide geographical distribution spread over time and the fact that no case of jaundice has been reported among those treated with commercial concentrates prepared by other virucidal methods (pasteurization, steam heating). Since HAV is non-enveloped, it would not be inactivated by solvent/detergent. It may be significant that HAV has not been transmitted by similarly sterilized factor IX concentrates. Clearly susceptible patients with haemophilia should be vaccinated with hepatitis A vaccine.

HEPATITIS B AND DELTA INFECTION

The discovery in the mid-1960s of the 'Australia antigen', against which multitransfused haemophiliacs developed precipitating antibodies, led to the identification of the several specific serological markers that are now available for characterization of HBV infection and the recognition that HBV was a cause of transfusion-transmitted hepatitis. The majority of intensively treated older haemophiliacs have serological evidence of previous HBV infection – over 90% in a series reported from our centre (Lee et al 1985a) – and most of these infecions were probably subclinical followed by a state of acquired immunity. A small minority of infected patients have in the past become chronic carriers of HBsAg with or without anti-HBe. In our practice the prevalence of HBsAg carriers amongst severely affected patients is 5%, and half of these patients carry HBeAg. The advances made in blood donor screening and concentrate sterilization have largely stopped HBV transmission to haemophiliacs. However, such patients are at higher risk of receiving unsterilized blood products, and therefore hepatitis B vaccination is practised.

Hepatitis D virus (HDV, delta agent) requires the presence of HBV for its propagation. Superinfection with HDV can occur in chronic HBV infection, and co-infection in acute hepatitis B. It has been shown that among individuals who receive multiple transfusions of blood and blood products, haemophiliacs have the highest risk of acquiring infection with HDV (Rizzetto et al 1982, Jacobson et al 1985). Rosina et al (1985) reported an anti-HD prevalence of 34% among 79 HBsAg-positive haemophiliacs who had received commercial clotting factor concentrates in Western Europe and the USA. However, in this study, there was no evidence of HDV infection among 24 HBsAg-positive haemophilic patients from Brazil, Germany (former GDR) and Australia who had received factor concentrated prepared locally (Rosina et al 1985).

A similar low prevalence of HDV infection among Australian haemophiliacs (only 1 in 192 HBsAg carriers) has also been reported (Dimitrikakis & Gust 1988). However, we have described a patient who seroconverted for anti-HDV after receiving only a single infusion of National Health Service (NHS) factor IX concentrate (Lee et al 1985b). Thus the agent was clearly present in the UK volunteer donor population in the early 1980s.

Lemon et al (1991) instituted a prospective multicentre clinical study at seven North American institutions in order to obtain a better understanding of the prevalence of HDV infections among haemophiliacs. Of 61 HBsAg-positive haemophiliacs studied, 21 were positive for anti-HD. Using a 1-kb cloned HDV RNA probe (Wang et al 1986), 2 of 33 (6%) anti-HD-negative HBsAg carriers also had HDV RNA detected. Thus it is likely that a small proportion of HBsAg carrier haemophiliacs are chronically infected with HDV despite the absence of anti-HD. This may reflect poor B-lymphocyte function owing to concomitant HIV infection. (H C Lane et al 1983). The presence of HDV infection in this cohort of HBsAg-positive haemophiliacs correlated with a past history of acute hepatitis and with evidence of chronic liver disease. Thus one-half of the HDV-positive patients had a history of acute hepatitis compared with only 12% of those who did not have anti-HD antibody or HDV RNA in their serum.

Haemophilic patients infected with HDV may have rapidly progressive liver disease. Three of 22 HDV-infected patients (of whom 20 were anti-HD positive and two HDV RNA positive) died of liver disease (Table 30.1).

Although haemophilic patients who have received clotting factor concentrates in the past have been at significant risk of infection with HDV, it is unlikely that sterilized clotting factor concentrates continue to transmit HDV (Lee 1992).

HEPATITIS C

Before the introduction of heat treatment of clotting factor concentrates in the mid-1980s, virtually 100% patients who received a first exposure to clotting factor concentrate developed

Table 30.1 Mortality and HDV status among HBsAg-positive haemophiliacs (n = 60)

	HDV RNA or anti-HD (+)	Anti-HD (–)
n	22	38
Mean follow-up (months)	26.7	26.3
Death	4 (18%)	3 (8%)
Hepatitis, fulminant	1 (5%)	—
Hepatitis, chronic	2 (9%)	—
AIDS-related	—	2 (5%)
Cancer (non-HCC)	—	1 (3%)
Heart disease	1 (5%)	—

From Lemon et al (1991).

non-A, non-B hepatitis (Fletcher et al 1983, Kernoff et al 1985). This was formerly diagnosed by exclusion of hepatitis A, hepatitis B, cytomegalovirus and Epstein–Barr virus. Typically, acute NANB hepatitis was clinically mild and usually anicteric, but appeared to progress to chronicity in at least 50% of cases. Many cases of acute and chronic NANB were apparently asymptomatic. Therefore reported frequencies based on clinical criteria alone led to gross underestimates of the prevalence, and it is of interest that as early as 1943 Beeson commented that 'the real frequency of this complication of transfusion (hepatitis) will be known only when there has been an concerted effort by physicians to recognise such cases.' Until the isolation of the major blood-borne NANB agent designated hepatitis C virus (HCV) (Kuo et al 1989) and the development of serological tests for HCV, no reliable tests fo NANB were available, and realistic estimates of incidence and chronicity rates could only be derived from prospective studies in which serum transaminases were monitored at frequent intervals. The similarities between the clinical expression and histological features of NANB and the liver disease found in haemophilia have led to the widely held view that NANB infection not confirmed to be hepatitis C, is largely responsible for the hepatic problems of haemophiliacs (Aledort 1985).

Although generally the reported mortality from liver disease in haemophiliacs has not been high, chronic hepatitis is not necessarily benign in this group. Differences in the spectrum of disease reported in these patients may reflect differences in patient selection and patient age, which may be important in determining severity.

Estimates of the seroprevalence of anti-C100-3 among patients who have regularly received clotting factor concentrates vary considerably in different geographical regions, although most estimates fall within the 55–85% range (Esteban et al 1989, Ludlam et al 1989, Noel et al 1989, Roggendorf et al 1989, Makris et al 1990) (Fig. 30.2). It is apparent that the first-generation anti-C100 test has underestimated the extent of HCV infection in haemophiliacs. Kudesia et al (1992) have found using second-generation assays 38% of first generation anti-HCV-negative samples to be positive. Tedder et al (1991) tested sera from 21 patients who had received large amounts of unheated factor VIII concentrate. These workers tested for anti-C100-3 and antibodies to recombinant structural (core) and non-structural (replicase) HCV proteins expressed in baculoviruses. Antibodies to core epitopes of HCV were detected in 100% of the sera, but only 62% and 19% were positive for anti-C100 and replicase antibodies. Furthermore, hepatitis C viraemia was demonstrated in 90% of the patients by polymerase chain reaction amplification of the 5' untranslated region of the HCV genome. It was concluded that the prevalence of hepatitis C infection in haemophiliacs may have been underestimated previously and that indeed almost all HCV-infected patients have evidence of ongoing viral replication (Watson et al 1992).

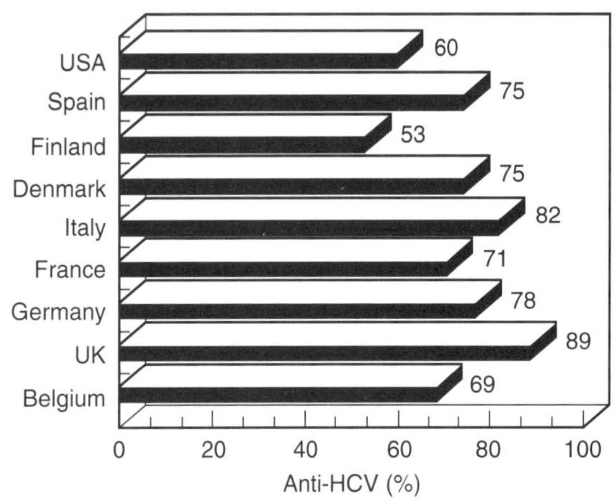

Fig. 30.2 Anti-HCV in haemophilia patients worldwide.

We have also found that detection of anti-C100 antibody alone underestimates the incidence of HCV infection in anti-HIV positive haemophiliacs, who, as a result of receiving clotting factor concentrates, must have been infected with non-A, non-B hepatitis (Fletcher et al 1983, Kernoff et al 1985). In a patient with severe haemophilia previously reported (patient 1 in Lim et al 1991) (Fig. 30.3), there was a fall in anti-C100 coincident with progression of HIV disease. We tested sera from 125 haemophiliacs who had seroconverted between 1979 and 1985 (Lee et al 1989). Although 18% of the HIV infected haemophiliacs were anti-C100-3 negative, this was not related to the progression of HIV disease. However, there was a 96% prevalence of HCV infection when anti-C22 and anti-C33 were assayed, and it would seem likely that virtually all recipients of unheated clotting factor concentrate will have been infected with HCV (Sabin et al 1993). HCV viraemia is significantly more frequent in HIV-positive haemophiliacs (Allain 1991).

It has been possible to establish the time to anti-C100 seroconversion in a longitudinal study of haemophiliacs, in which 28 patients with congenital coagulation disorders who had developed NANBH following first exposure to unsterilized clotting factor concentrate were studied (Kernoff et al 1985). The median time interval to aspartate aminotransferase (AST) elevation was 4 weeks (range 1–7) and to anti-HCV seroconversion was 11 weeks (range 7.5–14.5) (Lim et al 1991). This interval is much shorter than in prospectively followed transfusion recipients, in whom the mean time to anti-C100-3 seroconversion was 21.9 weeks (range 10–29) (Alter et al 1989). The shorter period may reflect a higher inoculum of transmitted virus in pooled concentrates compared with single blood donor units.

It is not clear at present whether all HCV-infected haemophilic patients remain viraemic. Using nested PCR, three temporal patterns of viraemia have been observed in sequential serum samples from previously untreated haemophiliacs in whom hepatitis C developed after treatment

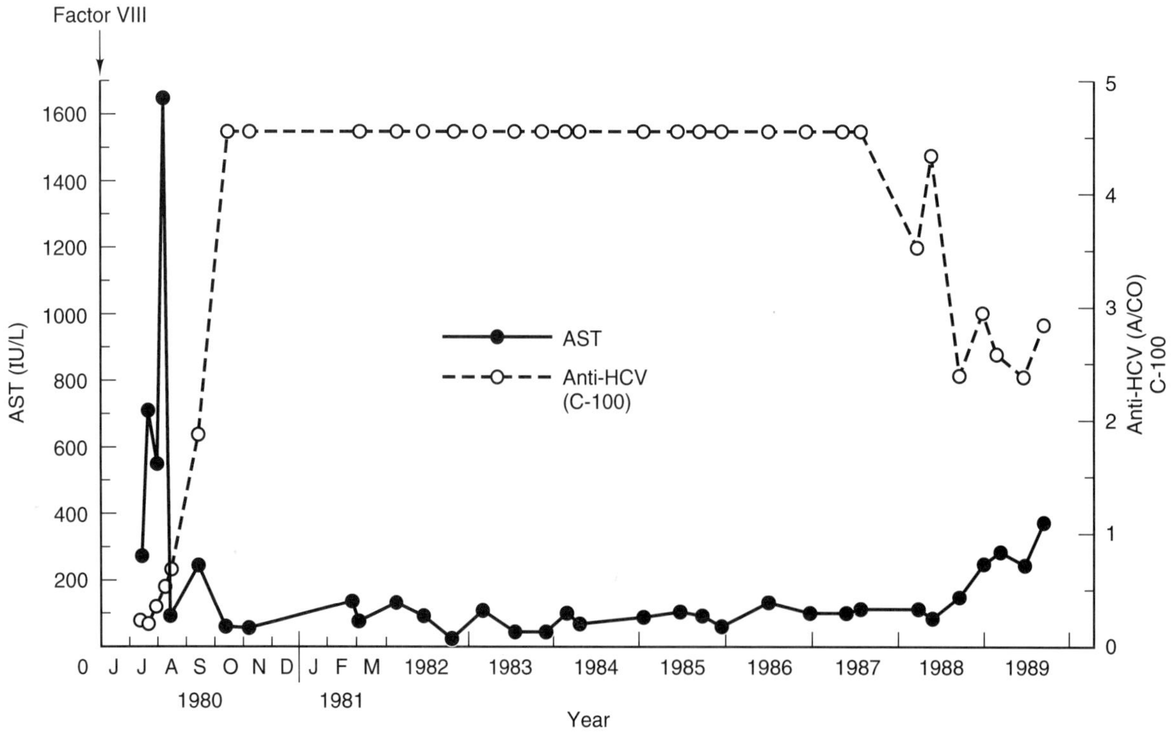

Fig. 30.3 HIV and HCV in haemophilia.

with factor VIII concentrate: transient viraemia in acute resolving hepatitis C; viraemia lasting for several years in chronic hepatitis C; and intermittent viraemia in chronic hepatitis C (Garson et al 1990).

Although the majority of haemophiliacs have persistently detectable anti-HCV for at least 8 years (Lim et al 1991), the antibody may disappear after a variable interval. These findings are similar to post-transfusion hepatitis C (Alter et al 1989). It may be that, although almost all HCV-infected patients have evidence of ongoing viral replication (Tedder et al 1991), a minority of patients with haemophilia may lose anti-HCV and are not viraemic.

Sequence analysis of HCV genomes have shown interesting differences. Phylogenetic analysis of HCV was performed in blood products, haemophiliacs and drug users in Scotland by Simmonds et al (1991). HCV sequences were divided into three distinct groups: intravenous drug users (il-5), locally infected haemophiliacs (hl-3) and haemophiliacs who received commercial factor VIII concentrates (fl–5) (Fig. 30.4). The finding of related sequences in intravenous drug users was thought to be related to transmission by needle sharing. However, it was surprising that there was a close identity between HCV sequences obtained from five batches of factor VIII from different manufacturers because the paid donations of plasma had been collected from a wide geographical area. It was thought that a group h1–3 identified in three of five haemophiliacs from Edinburgh represented an HCV variant common in Scotland 25 years ago. Typing in Japanese haemophiliacs using a universal sense primer and a mixture of four type-specific primers (antisense) has shown a mixture of types in those receiving imported concentrate (Okamato 1992).

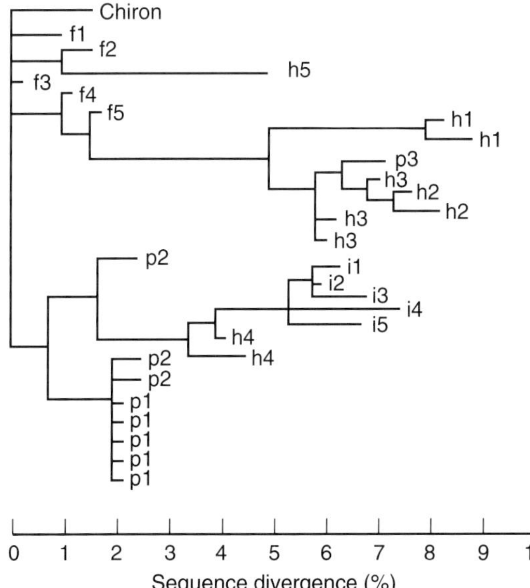

Fig. 30.4 Sequence diversity of HCV. Chiron, published sequence: f1–5, five commercial factor VIII batches; h1–5, five haemophiliacs; i1–5, five intravenous drug abusers from Edinburgh; p1–3, three Scottish plasma pools. (From Simmonds et al 1991.)

It has been demonstrated that essential mixed cryoglobulinaemia is associated with HCV (Pascual et al 1990, Casato et al 1991). We have reported a patient who developed cryoglobulinaemia in association with vasculitis, arthritis and nephritis following a first exposure to factor VIII concentrate. This coincided with an acute NANBH which has since been serologically proven to be hepatitis C (Lee et al 1985c).

The transmission rate of HCV has been studied in the female sexual partners of antibody-positive haemophilic males (Brettler et al 1992). Amongst 106 sexual partners from Europe, America and Australia there was an overall prevalence of 2.7%. This suggests that the efficiency of heterosexual transmission of HCV is poor.

MULTIPLE VIRAL INFECTIONS

Multiple viral infections can occur in haemophiliacs. As a result, complex viral interactions develop and it is sometimes difficult to disentangle the modulating influences of different hepatotropic viruses.

Figure 30.5 shows acute HCV and HBV infections in a patient who received a first exposure to NHS factor IX concentrate (Lee et al 1985b, Lim et al 1991) In this patient the level of anti-C100 declined at the onset of HBV infection and there was a delay in the appearance of serological markers to HBV. This is the phenomenon of viral interference previously observed in experimental animals by Brotman et al (1983). Watson et al (1992) have shown negative or indeterminate

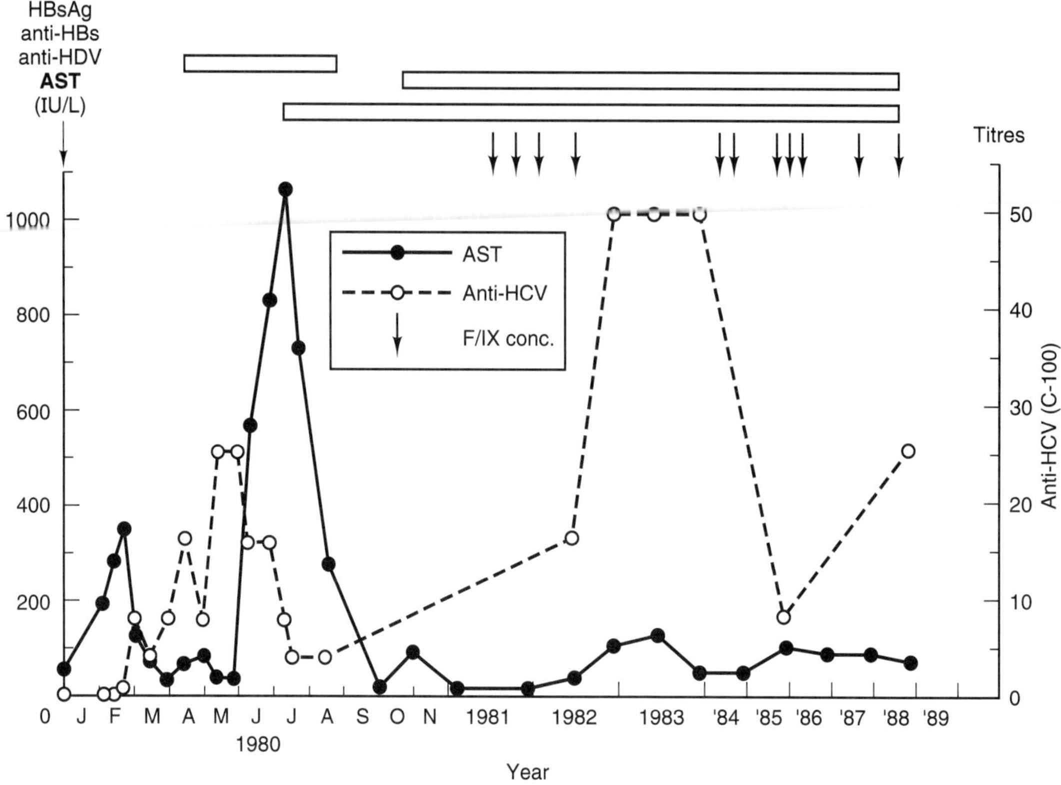

Fig. 30.5 Viral interference.

HCV serology in two HBsAg-positive carriers with haemophilia. This correlated with a finding of a decreased prevalence of anti-HCV in HBsAg-positive patients with hepatocellular carcinoma and cirrhosis (Tanaka et al 1991). These studies suggest that concurrent infection with HCV and HBV interferes with viral replication.

A further example of viral interaction is shown in Figure 30.6 (Lee et al 1985b). This patient was first exposed to factor VIII concentrate in 1976 when he developed acute 'non-B' hepatitis. He continued to receive factor VIII and in 1977–78 had a presumed subclinical attack of HBV infection that resulted in him becoming an HBsAg/HBeAg-positive carrier. In early 1980 he seroconverted from HBeAg to antiHBe, and this was accompanied by a severe exacerbation of the hepatitis that was attributed to clearance of virus from infected hepatocytes. Retrospective testing showed that anti-HDV became detectable shortly after this episode, and it seems more likely that the exacerbation was due to HDV superinfection. This conclusion was supported by the finding of HDAg in the liver biopsy. It may also be relevant that the patient seroconverted to anti-HIV at the onset of the exacerbation of hepatitis. It is possible that he acquired HDV and HIV from the same batch of concentrate and that a coincident HIV infection may have contributed to the severity of the exacerbation.

Hatzakis et al (1987) have shown a prevalence of 1.2% of concurrent HBsAg, anti-HD and anti-HIV in a population of 247 studied Greek haemophiliacs. They point out that the prognosis for such patients is unknown. It has been suggested that HIV accelerates the progression of chronic HCV disease (Martin et al 1989). In our own cohort of HIV-infected haemophiliacs there have been four deaths from hepatocellular failure

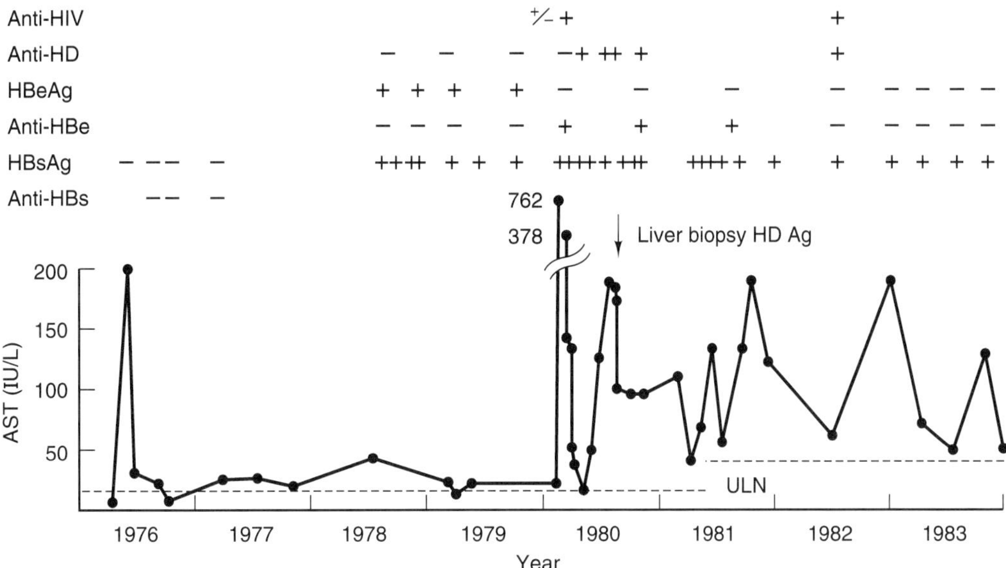

Fig. 30.6 The relationship between HBV and delta agent in a patient with haemophilia A. ULN, upper limit of normal. (From Lee et al 1985x.)

in a cohort of 111 patients (Sabin et al 1993), whereas in more than 100 HCV-infected patients there have been no deaths from liver failure.

HEPATOCELLULAR CARCINOMA

Approximately 50–90% of multitransfused haemophilic patients show abnormalities of serum transaminases and therefore evidence of chronic liver disease, and 30% of them show histological signs of cirrhosis (Lee & Kernoff 1990, Triger & Preston 1990), the major causes of cirrhosis being the hepatitis C virus and, to a lesser extent, hepatitis B. Post-mortem reports and prospective cohort studies in non-haemophilic patients with chronic liver disease have provided clear evidence that patients with cirrhosis are at risk of developing hepatocellular carcinoma (HCC) (Kew & Popper 1984, Johnson & Williams 1987).

Colombo et al (1991) carried out a questionnaire-based survey among large haemophilia centres worldwide in order to obtain more information on the incidence of HCC in haemophilia. In April 1990, 89 centres (46 in the USA and 43 in Europe) were first contacted to ascertain whether or not they had seen a case of HCC. Centres that gave positive answers were then asked to fill out a more detailed questionnaire. 10 cases of HCC were reported from eight centres, including 11 801 male patients worldwide. This represented a crude rate of HCC of 3.2/100 000 patients per year. The crude rate of HCC among the haemophiliacs is at least 30 times higher than the corresponding age-adjusted background incidence of this tumour in the USA, Germany and Italy (the countries of origin of the patients (Munoz & Bosch 1987). The epidemiological, clinical and serological characteristics and outcome of the 10 patients with hepatocellular carcinoma are shown in Table 30.2. The frequency of transfusion-transmitted hepatitis in haemophilia was relatively low until the 1970s when commercial clotting factor concentrates were used on a large scale (Lee & Kernoff 1990). Thus it is unlikely that HCC in haemophilia has hitherto been overlooked since the average incubation period for transfusion-associated HCC is thought to be 20–30 years (Kiyosawa et al 1990). A clinically important observation in this worldwide survey was that all patients with HCC also had cirrhosis (Table 30.2). It is probable that hepatitis viruses and alcohol were the causes of the cirrhosis since 8 of 10 patients had HBsAg or anti-HCV, and 4 of 10 had a history of alcohol

Table 30.2 Epidemiological and clinical characteristics and outcome of 10 patients with hepatocellular carcinoma

Case	Centre	Patient age (years)	Serum markers				Liver cirrhosis	Alcohol abuse	Presenting symptoms	Tumour characteristics	Therapy	Present status
			HBsAg	Anti-HCV	Anti-HIV	AFP (ng/ml)						
1	Worcester, MA, USA	74	Pos	NA	Pos	NA	Yes	Yes	None†	Diffuse	None	Dead‡
2	Padua, Italy	46	Pos	NA	Neg	1060	Yes	NA	Abdominal pain	Multifocal	None	Dead
3	Padua, Italy	51	Pos	NA	Neg	171	Yes	NA	Ascites	Multifocal	None	Dead
4	Miami, FL, USA	56	Neg	Pos	Pos	1399	Yes	No	Abdominal pain	Unifocal	Cisplatin	Dead
5	Milan, Italy	55	Neg	Pos	Pos	NA	Yes	No	Jaundice	Unifocal	None	Dead
6	Venice, Italy	39	Neg	Neg	Neg	25	Yes	Yes	Jaundice	Multifocal	None	Dead‡
7	Frankfurt, Germany	49	Pos	Pos	Neg	1200	Yes	Yes	None	Multifocal	OLT	Alive
8	Frankfurt, Germany	52	Neg	Pos	Pos	807	Yes	No	None	Unifocal	Resection	Alive
9	Providence, RI, USA	49	NA	NA	NA	NA	NA	Yes	None	Lung metastases	None	Dead
10	Chapel Hill, NC, USA	42	Pos	NA	NA	NA	Yes	No	None†	Multifocal	None	Dead

NA, information not available; OTP, orthotopic liver transplantation.

*These patients also had anti-IID.
†In these patients HCC was incidentally diagnosed at autopsy.
‡These patients died of causes other than HCC, which was incidentally discovered at autopsy.

From Colombo et al (1991).

abuse. It is significant that 2 of the 10 patients in whom asymptomatic HCC was detected by ultrasound scan were alive and tumour-free several months after hepatic resection or orthotopic liver transplantation. Unfortunately, diagnosis of cirrhosis in haemophilic patients is difficult because percutaneous liver biopsy – the hepatologist's gold standard – cannot be routinely performed because of haemorrhagic risks associated with this procedure. The serum alphafetoprotein level is not an infallible diagnostic marker of early HCC, but in order to detect small HCC it is suggested that haemophilic patients who had persistently elevated transaminases should be screened annually by means of ultrasound scanning.

TREATMENT OF CHRONIC LIVER DISEASE

The beneficial effect of alpha interferon (IFN-α) on aminotransferases and liver histology was first shown to be effective in post-transfusion NANBH by Hoofnagle et al (1986). This has now been confirmed by several large randomized trials (Davis et al 1989, Di Bisceglie et al 1989). None of these studies included patients with haemophilia.

Makris et al (1991) have now shown that low-dose recombinant IFNα is effective in normalizing transaminases and improving the histological appearances in at least 50% of haemophiliacs with chronic hepatitis C. In this study 10 patients received 3 MU subcutaneously thrice weekly for a year and eight were untreated. Biopsies were performed at entry on all 20 patients and on 17 at conclusion of the study. Biopsy appearances in the treated group of patients were significantly improved compared with controls. It is interesting that improvement in liver histology was also noted in three HIV antibody-positive patients in this study since the progression of HCV chronic liver disease may be accelerated in the presence of HIV (Martin et al 1989).

There are however potential hazards of performing liver biopsy in haemophilic patients as well as the cost of clotting factor concentrate to cover the procedure. Thus, even though histological examination of the liver is the ideal method of assessing response to treatment with interferon, it is unlikely to be performed routinely in haemophilic patients. Further trials are required to establish the ideal dose, frequency of administration and length of treatment with interferon.

It has been pointed out that interferon is a useful therapy in the multitransfused haemophilic patient in that it can be self-administered intravenously (Lee et al 1989a). Furthermore in such patients, it may stop the replication of more than one virus and control some of the associated phenomena of HIV infection.

Ribavarin, a guanosine analogue, is the first drug to offer a potentially effective oral treatment for chronic hepatitis C (Reichard et al 1991). Multicentre trials that include haemophiliacs to further evaluate this drug have begun. It is likely that further trials will be designed to evaluate combination therapy with IFN-α in the hope of providing cure for some individuals with chronic hepatitis C virus infection.

LIVER TRANSPLANTATION

Liver transplantation in haemophilic patients with end-stage liver disease has been shown not only to reverse the hepatic failure, but also to correct the coagulation defect of patients with haemophilia A (Bontempo et al 1987). It has been demonstrated by immunohistological techniques that FVIII:C is primarily located in hepatic sinusoidal cells (Kwast et al 1986) and it is likely that the hepatocyte is the site of synthesis because it contains messenger RNA (Wion et al 1985). Amongst the four patients reported by Bontempo et al (1987) the synthesis of factor VIII occurred as early as 6 h after the re-establishment of circulation through the new liver.

There have more recently been reports of orthoptic liver transplantation to treat haemophilia A (Gibas et al 1988), haemophilia B (Merion et al 1988) and combined haemophilia A and B (Delorme et al 1990). In all these cases both the coagulation defect and the transfusion-related liver disease have been reversed by transplantation.

However, the application of liver transplantation to the haemophilic population is complicated by the high prevalence of HIV infection in multitransfused haemophiliacs. Five of 10 non-haemophilic recipients of a liver transplant who were or became anti-HIV positive died of infection shortly after transplantation – an early mortality rate far higher than that in anti-HIV negative patients (Rubin et al 1987).

It has been suggested by some (Gibas et al 1988) that as the success of liver transplantation continues to improve early liver transplantation might be advocated even in the absence of liver failure. For the present, liver transplantation must be carefully considered for the multitransfused haemophilic patient with liver failure or cirrhosis who is also infected with HIV.

PREVENTION OF HEPATITIS

Virucidal sterilization

A variety of methods of sterilizing clotting factor concentrates, including long dry heat, pasteurization and solvent/detergent, have been shown to be virucidal (Lee 1992). More recently both factor VIII and factor IX concentrates have been produced by monoclonal antibody purification and there has been no transmission of hepatitis C in virgin patient studies (unpublished data). Following the cloning and expression of the factor VIII gene in 1984, a recombinant factor VIII has been produced by recombinant DNA technology and has undergone clinical trial (Schwartz et al 1990). There has been no hepatitis transmission by this product.

Hepatitis B vaccination

Despite the advances that have been made in blood donor screening and concentrate sterilization, haemophiliacs continue to be at above average risk of acquiring HBV infection. This is not only because of the residual risk of concentrates, but also because other therapeutic products, such as cryoprecipitate and the cellular components of blood, cannot be effectively sterilized. Vaccination against HBV is therefore regarded as mandatory in patients without serological evidence of immunity.

Currently licensed HBV vaccines are either derived from formalin-inactivated plasma obtained from HBsAg carriers or produced in yeast by recombinant DNA technologies. Hepatitis B vaccine is conventionally given intramuscularly. However, because this route may cause serious bleeding in haemophiliacs, subcutaneous administration has generally been preferred and is well tolerated (Desmyter et al 1983, Miller et al 1989, Mannucci et al 1989). A study using yeast recombinant vaccine in haemophiliacs has shown that this is satisfactorily immunogenic (Mannucci et al 1988a) with seroconversion rates similar to those for plasma-derived vaccines.

Although it was initially thought that a protective level of anti-HBs (>10 IU/l) would usually be retained for at least 5 years, evidence from haemophiliacs and other groups indicates that it may be lost much earlier. Those infected with HIV respond to vaccine with lower initial anti-HBs titres and/or lose anti-HBs more quickly (Zanetti et al 1986, Drake et al 1987, Miller et al 1989). The duration of antibody response is dependent on initial peak anti-HBs titres. However in a series of 67 anti-HIV negative haemophiliacs, even though there was a progressive decline in titres, anti-HBs was still detectable at year 4 (Mannucci et al 1989). If the decline of anti-HBs over time was extrapolated to 10 mIU/ml, it appeared from these data that patients with maximal antibody titres of less than 5000 mIU/ml should not need revaccination for 5–6 years. For patients with higher maximal titres (more than 5000 mIU/ml) revaccination should not be needed for as long as 10–12 years (Mannucci et al 1989).

It is important to note that anti-HIV seropositive patients known to have been previously anti-HBc positive remain at risk of acquiring HBV infection by transfusion. Williams et al (1988) reported acute hepatitis B in 11 of 27 haemophilic boys who received a common batch of factor VIII. Two previously immune children who were also HIV positive became infected with HBV.

Patients with severe haemophilia and other lifelong bleeding disorders should therefore be vaccinated immediately after diagnosis because, in spite of sterilization, concentrates can still be infectious (Mannucci et al 1988b). In newly diagnosed infants, immunization should be started immediately after birth (Moyes et al 1987). It is our policy to check anti-HBs levels in all vaccinated patients at yearly intervals with a view to maintaining levels above 10 IU/l. In poor responders, and in some patients with low levels of naturally acquired anti-HBs, a booster injection or a repeated course with 40 µg of vaccine is given (Lee & Kernoff 1990).

REFERENCES

Aledort L M, Levine P H, Hilgartner M et al 1985 A study of liver biopsies and liver disease among haemophiliacs. Blood 66: 367–372

Allain J P, Dailey S H, Laurian Y, Vallari D S, Rafowicz A, Desai S M, Devare S G 1991 Evidence for persistent hepatitis C virus (HCV) infection in haemophiliacs. Journal of Clinical Investigation 88: 1672–1679

Alter H J, Purcell R H, Shih J W, Melpolder J C, Houghton M, Choo Q L, Kuo G 1989 Detection of antibody to hepatitis C virus in prospectively followed transfusion recipients with acute and chronic non-A non-B hepatitis. New England Journal of Medicine 321: 1494–1500

Bamber M, Murray A, Arborgh B A M, Scheuer P J, Kernoff P B A, Thomas H C V, Sherlock S 1981 Short incubation non-A, non-B hepatitis transmitted by factor VIII concentrates in patients with congenital coagulation disorders. Gut 22: 854–859

Beeson P B 1943 Jaundice occurring one to four months after transfusion of blood or plasma. Journal of the American Medical Association 121: 1332–1334

Biggs R 1967 Thirty years of haemophilia treatment in Oxford. British Journal of Haematology 13: 452–463

Biggs R 1974 Jaundice and antibodies directed against factors VIII and IX in patients treated for haemophilia or Christmas disease in the United Kingdom. British Journal of Haematology 26: 313–329

Birch C L 1937 Hemophilia, Clinical and Genetic Aspects. Urbana, University of Illinois

Bontempo F A, Lewis J H, Gorenc T J, Spero J A, Ragni M V, Scott J P, Starzl T E 1987 Liver transplantation in hemophilia A. Blood 69: 1721–1724

Brettler D B, Mannucci P M, Gringeri A et al 1992 The low risk of hepatitis C virus transmission among sexual partners of hepatitis C-infected haemophilic males: an international, multicenter study. Blood 80: 540–543

Brotman B, Prince A M, Huima T, Richardson L, van den Ende M C, Pfeifer U 1983 Interference between non-A and non-B and hepatitis B virus infection in chimpanzees. Journal of Medical Virology 11: 191–205

Casato M, Taliani G, Pucillo L P, Gothredo F, Lagana B, Bonomo L 1991 Cryoglobulinaemia and hepatitis C virus. Lancet 337: 1047–1048

Colombo M, Mannucci P M, Brettler D B et al 1991 Hepatocellular carcinoma in haemophilia. American Journal of Hematology 37: 243–246

Davis G L, Balart L A, Schiff E R et al 1989 Treatment of chronic hepatitis C with recombinant Interferon alpha: a multicenter randomized, controlled trial. New England Journal of Medicine 321: 1501

Delorme M A, Adams P C, Grant D, Ghent C N, Walker I R, Wall W J 1990 Orthotopic liver transplantation in a patient with combined hemophilia A and B. American Journal of Hematology 33: 136–138

Desmyter J, Colaert J, Verstraete M, Vermylen J 1983 Hepatitis B vaccination of haemophiliacs. Scandinavian Journal of Infectious Diseases 38 (suppl.): 42–45

Di Bisceglie A M, Martin P, Kassianides C et al 1989 Recombinant interferon alpha therapy for chronic hepatitis C. A randomized, double-blind, placebo-controlled trial. New England Journal of Medicine 321: 1506–1510

Dimitrikakis M, Gust I 1988 Prevalence of delta infection in Australia and the Western Pacific Region. In: Zuckerman A J (ed.) Viral hepatitis and liver disease. Alan R Liss, New York, pp 433–435

Drake J H, Parmley R T, Britton H A 1987 Loss of hepatitis B antibody in human immunodeficiency virus-positive haemophilia patients. Pediatric Infectious Diseases 6: 1051–1054

Esteban J I, Esteban R, Viladomiu L, Lopez-Talavera J C, Gonzales A, Hernandez J M 1990 Hepatitis C virus antibodies among risk groups in Spain. Lancet ii: 294–297

Fletcher M L, Trowell J M, Craske J, Pavier K, Rizza C R 1983 Non-A non-B hepatitis after transfusion of factor VIII in infrequently treated patients. British Medical Journal 287: 1754–1757

Garson J A, Tuke P W, Makris M, Briggs M, Machin S J, Preston F E, Tedder R S 1990 Demonstration of viraemia patterns in haemophiliacs treated with hepatitis-C-virus contaminated factor VIII concentrates. Lancet 336: 1022–1025

Gerritzen A, Schneweis K E, Brachmann H H, Oldenburg J, Hanflana P, Gerlich W H, Caspari G 1992 Acute hepatitis A in haemophiliacs. Lancet 340: 1231–1232

Gibas A, Dienstag J L, Schafer A I et al 1988 Cure of hemophilia A by orthotopic liver transplantation. Gastroenterology 95: 192–194

Hasiba U W, Spero J A, Lewis J H 1977 Chronic liver dysfunction in multitransfused haemophiliacs. Transfusion 17: 490–494

Hatzakis A, Hadziyannis S, Maclure M, Louizoun C, Yannitsiotis A, Mandalaki T 1987 Concurrent hepatitis B, delta and human immunodeficiency virus infection in hemophiliacs. Thrombosis and Haemostasis 58: 791

Hay C R M, Preston F E, Triger D R, Underwood J C E 1985 Progressive liver disease in haemophilia: an understated problem? Lancet i: 1495–1498

Hilgartner M W, Giardina P 1977 Liver dysfunction in patients with hemophilia A, B and von Willebrand's disease. Transfusion 17: 495–499

Hollinger F B, Alter H J, Holland P V, Aach R D 1981 Non-A, non-B posttransfusion hepatitis in the United States. In:

Gerety R J (ed.) Non-A, non-B hepatitis. Academic Press, New York, pp 49–70

Hollinger F B, Kahn N C, Oefinger P E, Yawn D H, Schmulen A C, Dressman G R, Melnick J L 1983 Post-transfusion hepatitis type A. Journal of the American Medical Association. 250: 2313–2317

Hoofnagle J H, Mullen K D, Jones D B et al 1986 Treatment of chronic non-A non-B hepatitis with recombinant human alpha Interferon: a preliminary report. New England Journal of Medicine 315: 1575–1578

Jacobson I M, Dienstag J L, Werner B G, Brettler D B, Levine P H, Mushahwar I K 1985 Epidemiology and clinical impact of hepatitis D virus (delta) infection. Hepatology 5: 188–191

Johnson P J, Williams R 1987 Cirrhosis and the aetiology of hepatocellular carcinoma. Journal of Hepatology 4: 140–147

Kasper C K, Kipnis S A 1972 Hepatitis and clotting-factor concentrates. Journal of the American Medical Association 221: 510

Kernoff P B A, Lee C A, Karayiannis P, Thomas H C 1985 High risk of non-A non-B hepatitis after a first exposure to volunteer or commercial clotting factor concentrates: effects of prophylactic immune serum globulin. British Journal of Haematology 60: 469–479

Kew M C, Popper H 1984 Relationship between hepatocellular carcinoma and cirrhosis. Seminars in Liver Disease 4: 136–146

Kiyosawa K, Sodeyama T, Tanaka et al 1990 Interrelationship of blood transfusion, non-A non-B hepatitis and hepatocellular carcinoma: analysis by detection of antibody to hepatitis C virus. Hepatology 12: 671–675

Kudesia G, Chapman S, Makris M, Preston F E 1992 Need for second-generation anti-HCV testing in haemophilia. Lancet 339: 501–502

Kuo G, Choo Q L, Alter H J et al 1989 An assay for circulating antibodies to a major etiologic virus of human non-A non-B hepatitis. Science 244: 362–364

Kwast T H, Stel H V, Cristen E, Bertina R M, Veerman E C I 1986 Localization of factor VIII-procoagulent antigen: an immunohistological survey of the human body using monoclonal antibodies. Blood 67: 222–227

Lane H C, Masur H, Edgar L C, Whalen G, Rook A H, Fauci A S 1983 Abnormalities of B-cell activation and immunoregulation in patients with the acquired immunodeficiency syndrome. New England Journal of Medicine 309: 453–458

Lane S 1840 Haemorrhagic diathesis. Successful transfusion of blood. Lancet i: 185–188

Lee C A 1992 Coagulation factor replacement therapy. In: Hoffbrand A V, Brenner M K (eds) Recent advances in haematology. Churchill Livingstone, Edinburgh pp 73–88

Lee C A, Bofill M, Janossy G, Thomas H C, Rizza C R, Kernoff P B 1985a Relationships between blood product exposure and immunological abnormalities in English haemophiliacs. British Journal of Haematology 60: 161–172

Lee C A, Kernoff P B A 1990 Viral hepatitis and haemophilia. British Medical Bulletin 46: 408–422

Lee C A, Kernoff P B A, Peters D K 1985c Cryoglobulinaemia in haemophilia. British Medical Journal 290: 1947–1948

Lee C A, Kernoff P B A, Karayiannis P, Thomas H C 1989a Interferon therapy for chronic non-A non-B and chronic delta liver disease in haemophilia. British Journal of Haematology 72: 235–238

Lee C A, Phillips A, Elford J, Miller E J, Bofill M, Griffiths P D, Kernoff P B A 1989b The natural history of human immunodeficiency virus infection in a haemophilic cohort. British Journal of Haematology 73: 228–234

Lee C, Chrispeels J, Telfer P, Dusheiko G 1992 Hepatitis C antibody profile in adults with haemophilia and their sexual partners. British Journal of Haematology 81: 133–134

Lee C A, Kernoff P B A, Karayiannis P, Farci P, Thomas H C 1985b Interactions between hepatotropic viruses in patients with haemophilia. Journal of Hepatology 1: 379–384

Lemon S M, Becherer P R, Wang J G et al 1991 Hepatitis delta infection among multiple-transfused hemophiliacs. In: Gerin J L (ed.) The hepatitis delta virus. Wiley-Liss, New York, pp 351–360

Levine P H, McVerry B A, Attock B, Dormandy K M 1977 Health of the intensively treated hemophiliac with special reference to abnormal liver chemistries and splenomegaly. Blood 50: 1–9

Lim S G, Lee C A, Charman H, Tilsed G, Griffiths P D, Kernoff P B 1991 Hepatitis C antibody assay in a longitudinal study of haemophiliacs. British Journal of Haematology 78: 398–402

Ludlam C A, Chapman D, Cohen B, Litton P A 1989 Antibodies to hepatitis C virus in haemophilia. Lancet ii: 560–561

McMillan C W, Diamond L K, Surgenor D M 1961 Treatment of classic haemophilia: the use of fibrinogen rich in factor VIII for haemorrhage and for surgery. New England Journal of Medicine 265: 223–230, 277–283

Makris M, Preston F E, Triger D R, Underwood J C E, Choo Q L, Kuo G, Houghton M 1990 Hepatitis C antibody and chronic liver disease in haemophilia. Lancet 335: 1117–1119

Makris M, Preston F E, Triger D R, Underwood J C E, Westlake L, Adelman M I 1991 A randomized controlled trial of recombinant Interferon-*a* in chronic hepatitis C in hemophiliacs. Blood 78: 1672–1677

Mannucci P M 1992 Outbreak of hepatitis A among Italian patients with haemophilia. Lancet 339: 819

Mannucci P M, Capitanio A, Del Ninno E, Colombo M, Pareti F, Ruggeri Z M 1975 Asymptomatic liver disease in haemophiliacs. Journal of Clinical Pathology 28: 620–624

Mannucci P M, Ronchi G, Rota L, Colombo M 1978 Liver biopsy in hemophilia. Annals of Internal Medicine 88: 429–430

Mannucci PM, Gringeri A, Morfini M et al 1988a Immunogenicity of a recombinant hepatitis B vaccine in hemophiliacs. American Journal of Hematology 29: 211–214

Mannucci P M, Zanetti A R, Colombo M and the Study Group of the Fondazione dell'Emofilia 1988b Prospective study of hepatitis after factor VIII concentrate exposed to hot vapour. British Journal of Haematology 68: 427–430

Mannucci P M, Zanetti A R, Gringeri A et al 1989 Long-term immunogenicity of a plasma-derived hepatitis B vaccine in HIV seropositive and HIV seronegative haemophiliacs. Archives of Internal Medicine 149: 1333–1337

Martin P, Di Bisceglie A M, Kassianides C, Lisker-Melman M, Hoofnagle J H 1989 Rapidly progressive non-A non-B hepatitis in patients with human immunodeficiency virus infection. Gastroenterology 97: 1559–1561

Merion R M, Delius R E, Campbell D A, Turcotte J G 1988 Orthoptic liver transplantation totally corrects factor IX deficiency in hemophilia B. Surgery 104: 929–931

Miller E J, Lee C A, Karayiannis P, Hamilton-Dutoit S J, Dick R, Thomas H C, Kernoff P B A 1988 Non-invasive investigation of liver disease in haemophiliac patients. Journal of Clinical Pathology 41: 1039–1043

Miller E J, Lee C A, Karayiannis P, Holmes S, Thomas H C, Kernoff P B A 1989 Immune response of patients with congenital coagulation disorders to hepatitis B vaccine. Suboptimal response and human immunodeficiency virus infection. Journal of Medical Virology 28: 96–100

Moyes C D, Milne A, Dimitrakakis M, Goldwater P N, Pearce N 1987 Very low-dose hepatitis B vaccine in newborn infants: an economic option for control in endemic areas. Lancet i: 29–31

Munoz N, Bosch X 1987 Epidemiology of hepatocellular carcinoma. In: Okuda K, Ishak K (eds) Neoplasms of the liver Springer Verlag Tokyo, pp 3–19

Noel L, Guerois C, Maisonneuve P, Verroust F, Laurian Y 1989 Antibodies to hepatitis C virus in haemophilia. Lancet ii: 560

Normann A, Graff J, Gerritzen A, Brackmann H-H, Flehmig B 1992 Detection of hepatitis A virus RNA in commercially available factor VIII preparation. Lancet 340: 1232–1233

Okamoto H, Sugiyama Y, Okada S et al 1992 Typing hepatitis C virus by polymerase chain reaction with type-specific primers: application to clinical surveys and tracing infectious sources. Journal of General Virology 73: 673–679

Pascual M, Perrin L, Giostra E, Schifferli J A 1990 Hepatitis C virus in patients with cryoglobulinaemia type II. Journal of Infectious Diseases 162: 569–570

Pool J G, Shannon A E 1965 Production of high-potency concentrates of antihemophilic globulin in a closed-bag system. New England Journal of Medicine 273: 1443–1447

Preston F E, Triger D R, Underwood J C E, Bardhan G, Mitchell V E, Stewart R M, Blackburn E K 1978 Percutaneous liver biopsy and chronic liver disease in haemophiliacs. Lancet ii: 592–594

Preston F E, Triger D R, Underwood J C E 1982 Blood product concentrates and chronic liver disease. Lancet i: 565

Reichard O, Andersson J, Schvarcz R, Weiland O 1991 Ribavirin treatment for chronic hepatitis C. Lancet 337: 1058–1061

Rizzetto M, Morello C, Mannucci P M 1982 Delta infection and liver disease in haemophilic carriers of hepatitis B surface antigen. Journal of Infectious Diseases 145: 18–22

Roggendorf M, Deinhardt F, Rasshofer R et al 1989 Antibodies to hepatitis C virus. Lancet ii: 324–325

Rosina F, Saracco G, Rizzetto M 1985 Risk of post-transfusion infection with the hepatitis delta virus: a multicenter study. New England Journal of Medicine 312: 1488–1491

Rubin R H, Jenkins R L, Shaw B W et al 1987 The acquired immunodeficiency syndrome and transplantation. Transplantation 44: 1–4

Sabin C, Phillips A, Elford J, Griffiths P, Janossy G 1993 The progression of HIV disease in a haemophilic cohort followed for 12 years. British Journal of Haematology 83: 330–333

Schwartz R S, Abildgaard C F, Aledort L M et al 1990 Human recombinant DNA-derived antihaemophilic factor (factor VIII) in the treatment of haemophilia A. New England Journal of Medicine 323: 1800–1805

Sherertz R J, Russell B A, Reuman P D (1984) Transmission of hepatitis A by transfusion of blood products. Archives of Internal Medicine 144: 1579–1580

Simmonds P, Zhang L Q, Watson H G et al 1990 Hepatitis C quantification and sequencing in blood products, haemophiliacs, and drug users. Lancet 336: 1469–1472

Spero J A, Lewis J H, Van Thiel D H, Hasiba U, Rabin B S 1978 Asymptomatic structural liver disease in haemophilia. New England Journal of Medicine 298: 1373–1378

Spurling N, Shone J, Vaughan J 1946 The incidence, incubation period and symptomatology of homologous serum jaundice. British Medical Journal 2: 409–412

Tanaka K, Hirohata T, Koga S et al 1991 Hepatitis C and hepatitis B in the aetiology of hepatocellular carcinoma in the Japanese population. Cancer Research 51: 2842–2847

Tedder R S, Briggs M, Ring C et al 1991 Hepatitis C antibody profile and viraemia prevalence in adults with severe haemophilia. British Journal of Haematology 79: 512–515

Temperley I J, Cotter K P, Walsh T J, Power J, Hillary I B 1992 Clotting factors and hepatitis A. Lancet 340: 1466

Triger D R, Preston F E 1990 Chronic liver disease in haemophiliacs. British Journal of Haematology 74: 241–245

Wang K S, Choo Q L, Weiner A J et al 1986 Structure, sequence and expression of the hepatitis delta (δ) viral genome. Nature 323: 508–514

Watson H G, Ludlam C A, Rebus S, Zhang L Q, Peutherer J F, Simmonds P 1992 Use of several second generation serological assays to determine the true prevalence of hepatitis C virus infection in haemophiliacs treated with non-virus inactivated factor VIII and IX concentrates. British Journal of Haematology 80: 514–518

Williams M D, Boxall E H, Hill F G H 1988 Change in immune response to hepatitis B in boys with haemophilia. Journal of Medical Virology 25: 317–327

Wion K L, Kelly D, Summerfield J A, Tuddenham E G, Lawn R M 1985 Distribution of factor VIII m-RNA and antigen in human liver and other tissues. Nature 317: 726–729

Zanetti A R, Mannucci P M, Tanzi E et al 1986 Hepatitis B vaccination of 113 haemophiliacs: lower antibody response in anti-HAV/HTLV-III positive patients. American Journal of Hematology 23: 339–345

UPDATE

- REFERENCES

Temperly I J, Cotter K P, Walsh T J, Power J, Hillary I B 1992 Clotting factors and hepatitis A. Lancet 340: 1466

Peerlinck K, Vermylen J 1993 Acute hepatitis A in patients with haemophilia A. Lancet 341: 179

Eyster M E, Diamondstone L S, Lien J-M et al 1993 Natural history of hepatitis C virus infection in multitransfused haemophiliacs: Effect of coinfection with human immunodeficiency virus. Journal of Acquired Immune Deficiency Syndromes 6: 602–610

31. Occupational aspects of hepatitis

A. Cockcroft

The hepatitis viruses are an important cause of occupational infectious disease. The occupational hazard is increased by the frequently long carrier phase when infected individuals are relatively well but nevertheless able to transmit infection. Viral hepatitis is recognized as an occupational risk in certain occupations and, on the other hand, individuals with hepatitis infection may pose a risk of transmission to others in the course of their work. Discussion of viral hepatitis in relation to occupation includes consideration of the evidence for occupational transmission risk in different circumstances, the modes of transmission of hepatitis in the occupational setting, theoretical and practical aspects of prevention of occupational transmission and management of individuals with hepatitis in relation to their work. There is a large body of published material about hepatitis B and occupation, and rather less evidence about other forms of viral hepatitis and occupation. This chapter will therefore first consider the occupational aspects of hepatitis B infection and then more briefly discuss the available information for the other types of viral hepatitis.

Hepatitis B and occupation

It is well recognized that hepatitis B can be transmitted via infected blood and other body fluids, either during acute infection or from individuals who have become virus carriers. This is known to happen by sexual contact, by sharing needles for intravenous drug use, by transfusion of infected blood and by accidental exposures to infected blood or other body fluids. It is the transmission by blood exposure incidents that is particularly relevant to occupational risk.

RISK OF OCCUPATIONAL TRANSMISSION OF HEPATITIS B TO WORKERS

Evidence of risk in different occupational groups

A number of surveys, mainly reflecting occupational exposures before the widespread availability of hepatitis B immunization, have shown an increased prevalence of hepatitis B infection markers in workers exposed to blood and body fluids, especially health care workers. West (1984) reviewed evidence from a number of seroprevalence studies in the USA and concluded that the overall risk to people employed in health-related fields was four times that of the general adult population; physicians and dentists were at 5–10 times the risk of the general population, and groups with over 10 times the risk included surgeons, clinical workers in dialysis units and mental handicap units and laboratory workers having frequent contact with blood samples.

More recent studies have confirmed these findings. The prevalence of hepatitis B markers among a group of emergency physicians was found to be about five times greater than in the general population in the USA (Iserson & Criss 1985). The risk is not restricted to health care workers in urban areas: staff with frequent blood contact in community hospitals in the USA have also been shown to have an excess of hepatitis B infection markers (McLean et al 1987). A study of workers in five hospitals found an overall prevalence of hepatitis B infection markers of 14%, related to race, sex, age, frequent blood contact and frequency of needlestick injuries (Hadler et al 1985). The excess risk of hepatitis B infection among

USA oral surgeons was confirmed in a seroprevalence study of 434 individuals; 26% had evidence of previous infection, including two who were positive for hepatitis B surface antigen (HBsAg) (Reingold et al 1988). A group of occupational health nurses, many of whom had little contact with blood and needles, was nevertheless found to have a small excess of hepatitis B infection markers compared with the general USA population (Strickler & Bradshaw 1987). A recent study from Stockholm of health care workers enrolling for hepatitis B immunization found a prevalence of hepatitis B markers of 4%, not greater than in the general population but related to age, duration of health care work and history of blood exposure incidents (Struve et al 1992).

In the USA, the Centers for Disease Control (1989) have estimated that 12,000 health care workers whose jobs entail exposure to blood become infected with hepatitis B each year, that 500–600 of them require hospital admission as a result of the infection, and that 700–1200 of those infected become hepatitis B carriers. They also estimate that about 250 of the infected workers will die from fulminant hepatitis, cirrhosis or liver cancer. Not all of these infections among health care workers will have been acquired occupationally. In the UK, examination of laboratory reports of acute hepatitis B infections has revealed an excess rate among health care workers compared with the general population. In 1975–79 the average annual rate for men in the whole population was 4 per 100 000 while health care workers had rates of up to 36 per 100 000 (Polakoff & Tillett 1982). In 1980–84 the average annual rate in men in the general population was 6 per 100 000 and again up to 37 per 100 000 among health care workers (Polakoff 1986a).

Even in countries where hepatitis B infection is endemic, there is evidence of additional occupational risk among health care workers. Among 234 dentists in the Philippines, the prevalence of hepatitis B infection markers was found to be 58%, similar to the prevalence in the general population but increasing with the number of years in dental practice (Lim et al 1986). In Japan, a seroprevalence study found that over a third of hospital workers had evidence of previous hepatitis B infection, about the same prevalence as a group of healthy controls, but that nurses and surgeons had significantly higher seroprevalences than other staff or the controls (Kashiwagi et al 1985). A study in Cairo revealed a higher prevalence of hepatitis B infection markers among non-professional staff (60%) than among doctors and nurses, presumably as a result of non-occupational infection in early life, but still found a relationship between infection markers and blood exposures and years of practice among the physicians (Goldsmith et al 1989). Among hospital employees in Israel, those born in countries with high endemicity of hepatitis B infection had a higher prevalence of hepatitis B infection markers but there was also evidence of increased risk of infection among occupational groups with more frequent exposure to blood and sharp instruments (Donchin & Shouval 1992).

Occupations allied to health care may also carry a risk of hepatitis B infection. A serosurvey of 133 embalmers (Turner et al 1989) found that they had hepatitis B infection markers at about twice the rate of a blood donor comparison group and commonly gave a history of needlestick injuries at work. A Canadian study reported that 13% of staff (and more than 20% of specialized teachers) in a day school for mentally handicapped children had markers of hepatitis B infection (Remis et al 1987). Emergency medical workers, such as emergency ambulance staff and paramedics, have been reported to have an increased risk of hepatitis B infection (Kunches et al 1983, Valenzuela et al 1985, Pepe et al 1986). Other studies of groups of emergency workers and public-safety workers have not found an excess of hepatitis B infection markers. Morgan-Capner & Wallice (1990) found no excess of hepatitis B markers among Lancashire ambulance personnel compared with blood donors; their subjects undertook both routine and emergency work. Other studies of police officers (Peterkin & Crawford 1986, Morgan-Capner & Hudson 1988, Welch et al 1988), prison officers (Radvan et al 1986) and firemen (Crosse et al 1989) have not documented an increased risk of hepatitis B infection.

Occupational hepatitis B infection has also been reported in professions unrelated to health care or the emergency services. Outbreaks of hepatitis B have been reported in butchers' shops (Gerlich

& Thomssen 1982, Mijch et al 1987), apparently spread from infected employees to colleagues as a result of frequent cuts sustained at work. A review of collected statistics on hepatitis B infection in Scotland revealed an excess among hairdressers and suggested that dermatitis and small cuts from scissors and other sharp instruments may be the route of entry of the virus in this occupational setting (Watt 1987). Several studies have reported an excess of hepatitis B infection among naval personnel and merchant seamen; this can be partly explained by work in a health care setting for some personnel but appears to be related mainly to paraoccupational factors such as drug abuse, casual sexual contact in foreign ports and tattooing (Dembert et al 1987, Hyams et al 1989, Siebke et al 1989).

Modes of occupational transmission of hepatitis B

The most important means of transmission of hepatitis B in the occupational setting is by inoculation of infected blood, either by stab injuries with blood-contaminated needles (so-called needlestick injuries) or by cuts with scalpels or other sharp instruments contaminated with blood (sharps injuries). Evidence of the risk of transmission of hepatitis B after accidental inoculation of infected blood comes from several studies (Table 31.1). Direct comparison of the rates of transmission reported from the different studies is difficult because some included all cases in which there was evidence of hepatitis B transmission, including asymptomatic seroconversions, while others included only clinical cases of hepatitis. Also, the data come from studies whose main purpose was to examine the efficacy of post-exposure prophylaxis with hepatitis B immune globulin (HBIG), using those treated with normal human immunoglobulin (NHIG) as a comparison group and not including a totally untreated control group. All the reported studies found that the transmission rate was significantly greater if the source patient was HBeAg positive: the transmission risk from HBeAg-positive source patients was between 19% and 31%, while for HBeAg-negative source patients it was 1–6% (Table 31.1). HJ Alter et al (1976) compared cases of hepatitis B transmission after needlestick injury from HBsAg-positive source patients with cases where transmission did not occur: in 14 cases of transmission, all the source patients were positive for HBeAg; while in 17 cases without transmission, 12 of the source patients were negative for HBeAg. There is some evidence from the study of Masuko et al (1985) of the risk of transmission when no treatment is given; three staff who had needlesticks

Table 31.1 Rate of transmission of hepatitis B after needlestick injuries from HBsAg-positive source patients

Reference	Percentage of recipients developing hepatitis B		
	HBeAg-positive source patients (*n*)	HBeAg-negative source patients (*n*)	All source patients (*n*)
Seeff et al 1978*	22 [51]	1 [146]	6 (203)
Grady et al 1978 †	31 [42]	6 [99]	14 (141)
Werner & Grady 1982 ‡	19 [234]	2 [156]	12 (390)
Hansen et al 1981 §	—	—	3 (101)
Masuko et al 1985 ¶	20 [56]	0 [43]	11 (99)

* The recipients of HBeAg-positive needlesticks shown are those who were given NHIG. All hepatitis B cases among these were clinically apparent. Some of the recipients of HBeAg-negative needlesticks had received HBIG.

† The recipients of needlesticks shown were those who had received normal titre globulin (NHIG). Subclinical cases of hepatitis B are included.

‡ The recipients of needlesticks had received globulin of varying anti-HBs content. Subclinical cases of hepatitis B are included.

§ HBeAg status was not determined. Only clinical cases of hepatitis B were recorded and all recipients had been treated with HBIG.

¶ Cases of subclinical hepatitis B are included. All the needlestick recipients shown were given HBIG; of three others with HBeAg-positive needlesticks, two developed hepatitis B.

from HBeAg-positive source patients did not receive HBIG for technical reasons and two of them (67%) developed hepatitis B. There is no study of a larger group without any post-exposure prophylaxis to confirm this figure.

Data to allow an estimate of the risk of hepatitis B transmission following other exposures to infected blood are not available. It is likely that the risk of transmission is less than after inoculation injuries. In a study of oral surgeons, those who wore gloves less than 10% of the time were no more likely than those who wore gloves more than 90% of the time to have markers of hepatitis B infection; this emphasizes the major importance of frequent puncture wounds and lacerations, rather than contact of possibly non-intact skin with blood-stained saliva, as the means of virus transmission to operators (Reingold et al 1988). This contrasts with an earlier study of hepatitis B in haemodialysis units, which reported that wearing gloves protected staff from infection (Pattison et al 1973). There seems to be little direct evidence of transmission of hepatitis B by means of contact of infected blood with open wounds, non-intact skin or mucous membranes. This may be because workers did not notice or report such minor incidents of blood exposure until recent years, when fear of contracting human immunodeficiency virus (HIV) in these circumstances has led to more attention being paid to the risks of blood contact. With the availability of HBIG and hepatitis B immunization during this period of increased awareness of minor blood exposures, demonstration of hepatitis B transmission in these circumstances is now fortunately unlikely. There are documented case studies of HIV seroconversion among health care workers following non-parenteral exposure to infected blood, including contamination of non-intact skin and of the eyes and mouth (Centres for Disease Control 1987a, Gioannini et al 1988). By analogy, they provide evidence that hepatitis B can be transmitted in the same way.

Reports from the era before the availability of hepatitis B immunization provide indirect evidence of hepatitis B transmission by non-inoculation blood contact. Over a 40-month period, Hansen et al (1981) recorded cases of clinical hepatitis B infection among employees in a medical centre: there were 23 cases among employees who had not reported exposures to blood or body fluids; one case in a laboratory technician who reported accidents in which serum touched open cuts on her hands when she was working with an automated chemistry analyser (she may well have handled samples that were infected with hepatitis B); and only three cases among staff who had reported inoculation injuries with blood positive for hepatitis B surface antigen. The authors suggest that unreported, and perhaps unnoticed, blood exposures could be responsible for transmission of hepatitis B in the medical setting. Pattison et al (1974) report five cases of clinical hepatitis (at least four of which were hepatitis B) over a 6-month period among staff in a hospital laboratory. Further investigations revealed that 36% of staff in the blood bank and specimen control areas had serological markers of hepatitis B infection, compared with only 10% in other laboratory areas. They found that the staff with clinical hepatitis were significantly more likely to have sustained minor cuts with computer test request cards than staff without hepatitis B markers and concluded that blood contaminations of minor cuts could explain the risk of hepatitis B among laboratory staff.

Bryan et al (1973) reported 12 cases of hepatitis B among clinical staff in a children's hospital; 10 had been contacts of a child with hepatitis B and a bleeding disorder. None of the 10 staff recalled needlestick injuries associated with the child, but they had frequent hand contact with his blood and did not routinely wear gloves; none of the ENT staff who dealt with the child's frequent nose bleeds developed hepatitis B, but it was noted that they wore gloves for this work.

Other body fluids also pose a potential risk for transmission of hepatitis B, including amniotic fluid, pericardial fluid, peritoneal fluid, synovial fluid, cerebrospinal fluid, semen and vaginal secretions (Centers for Disease Control 1988, Department of Health 1990). There are no documented cases of transmission of hepatitis B following inoculation injuries or other exposures to non-blood-stained faeces, nasal secretions, sputum, sweat, tears, urine and vomitus (Centers for Disease Control 1988, Department of Health 1990). Saliva is also not believed to pose a risk unless it is blood stained, as is commonly the case in the dental setting. Hepatitis B transmission has been reported following human bites

(MacQuarrie et al 1974, Hamilton et al 1976, Cancio-Bello et al 1982), presumably related to some inoculation of the biter's blood-stained saliva. This is the sort of exposure that may be experienced by workers with mentally disturbed or subnormal patients or by policemen and prison officers.

Transmission of hepatitis B by inhalation of droplets or aerosols of infected blood has not been reported. However, exposure to environments contaminated with blood in clinical laboratories may be contributing to the documented excess risk of hepatitis B infection among laboratory workers (Anderson & Woodfield 1982, Follett & Sleigh 1980); a study from the USA National Institutes of Health involving 800 environmental samples from 10 laboratories found hepatitis B surface antigen in 31 samples from 11 work stations (Evans et al 1990). Similarly, 7 of 163 environmental samples in a haemodialysis unit were found to be positive for HBsAg, including samples from a table, a nurse's glove and a refrigerator door handle (Dankert et al 1976).

Magnitude of risk of occupational transmission of hepatitis B

The risk of transmission of hepatitis B to workers, taking the health care setting as the best-documented example, depends on several variables: the prevalence of hepatitis B carrier state among the patient population; the frequency of needlestick injuries or other blood exposures among health care workers; the risk of transmission following an exposure to infected blood; and the level of immunity to hepatitis B within the population of health care workers. The risk of transmission following an exposure to infected blood or other body fluids has been considered in the previous section, and the level of immunity to hepatitis B is considered in the section on hepatitis B immunization of workers at risk of occupational hepatitis B infection.

Prevalence of hepatitis B carriers among patient populations

The prevalence of the carrier state in the patient population will vary considerably in different areas. It will be higher in areas with high endemicity of hepatitis B infection. The Department of Health (1990) have estimated that the prevalence of hepatitis B carriers (people who are HBsAg positive for more than 6 months) in the general UK adult population is about 1 in 500, with 5–10% of these being HBeAg positive. In the USA, there are estimated to be about 300 000 hepatitis B infections per year, with 6–10% becoming carriers (Centers for Disease Control 1989). The situation in the UK is changing, with a rise in the number of laboratory reports of acute hepatitis B infections between 1980 and 1984 and a steady reduction between 1985 and 1988, giving an average annual incidence of infection in adults of 4 per 100 000 for men and 2 per 100 000 for women in the period 1985–89 (Polakoff 1989). Figures for the overall population are likely to be an underestimate of the prevalence of hepatitis B carriers in a patient population, since groups at high risk for hepatitis B infection, such as intravenous drug users and patients with bleeding disorders or who have required blood transfusion, are over-represented among hospital outpatients and inpatients.

In the UK, the prevalence of hepatitis B infection is also reported to be higher among patients in hospitals for the mentally handicapped: 8% of patients were reported to be HBsAg positive in one hospital (Kingham et al 1978), between 1 and 12% in a survey of seven hospitals (Clarke et al 1984), and 2% in a hospital in Wales (McGregor et al 1988). However, another study of 220 patients in a hospital for the mentally handicapped in the north of England found only one man who had antibodies to hepatitis B core antigen and no other patients with hepatitis B markers (Thomson et al 1989).

Frequency of blood exposures among health care workers

Blood exposure incidents, including needlestick and other sharps injuries and blood contamination of broken skin or mucous membranes, are common in the health care setting. The risk of transmission of HIV (Henderson et al 1990) by such incidents has led to an increased number of studies of their incidence and causation in recent years. Not surprisingly, operating theatres are high-risk areas for blood exposures. Lowenfels et al (1989) reported a median rate of puncture injuries among surgeons in New York, contacted by letter or telephone, of 4.2 per 1000 operating room hours, with 25% of the surgeons having injury rates of nine or more per 1000 operating room hours. Hussain et al (1988) asked 18 surgeons in Saudi Arabia to record all accidental injuries during surgery and reported that sharps injuries occurred in 5.6% of operations. An observational study of 1307 surgical procedures at San Francisco General Hospital revealed accidental blood exposures in 6.4% of procedures and parenteral exposure to blood in 1.7%. The risk of blood exposure was highest for procedures lasting more than 3 h, when blood loss exceeded 300 ml and for major vascular and gynaecological procedures (Gerberding et al 1990). The authors believe that the lower rate of injuries in San Francisco may reflect greater attention to safe practices because of the high rate of HIV infection among the patients. However, in a more recent prospective observational study in four hospitals in the USA, sharps injuries were noted in 6.9% of procedures (Tokars et al 1991) and injuries were recorded by operating theatre staff in Glasgow at a rate of 1.6% per surgeon per operation, calculated to give 4.6% per operation overall (Camilleri et al 1991a). These authors considered that this rate of injuries could explain the excess of hepatitis B infections in surgeons compared with physicians.

Blood exposures other than sharps injuries are common in surgical practice. These include glove tears and perforations (Brough et al 1988, Camilleri et al 1991b, Wright et al 1991) and eye splashes with blood and other body fluids (Brearley & Buist 1989, Porteous 1990, Hinton et al 1991). It has recently been reported that even minor suturing procedures undertaken in the accident and emergency department are associated with one or more glove perforations in 11% of cases (Richmond et al 1992).

The risk of blood exposures is not confined to surgery. Sharps injuries and other blood and body fluid exposures have been found to be frequent among embalmers (Beck-Sague et al 1991). Collins & Kennedy (1987) have reviewed a number of studies of sharps injuries among groups of health care workers and compared the results in terms of needlestick injuries per 100 employee–years for different occupational groups. Widely varying figures come from the different studies reviewed (Table 31.2). Nurses appear to suffer the highest number of injuries, even allowing for the number of nurses employed. Other groups at risk include domestic and portering staff, who get injured from needles and other sharp instruments improperly disposed of, and laboratory staff. Relatively few injuries in the reported studies were to doctors.

Surveys of routinely reported incidents must be interpreted with caution because of the general belief that there is considerable under-reporting, particularly among doctors. Some authors have attempted to quantify this under-reporting. Astbury & Baxter (1990), using questionnaire responses to estimate the incidence of sharps injuries and bites and scratches over the preceding year, found that only 5% of injuries had been reported by staff to the hospital occupational health service. The low (45%) response rate to their questionnaire may have biased their results. McGeer et al (1990) reported a less than 5% reporting rate for sharps injuries among medical students, interns and residents in Toronto but they asked respondents to recall incidents occurring over several previous years, which may have led to inaccuracies. A recent questionnaire study of 158 operating department staff at the Royal Free Hospital in London (Williams et al 1993) recorded 26 sharps injuries and 240 other blood exposure incidents during the preceding

Table 31.2 Incidence of needlestick injuries per 100 employee years. Data from eight surveys

Survey no.	Nurses (all grades)	Laboratory staff	Domestics and Porters
1	1.65	–	1.04
2	13.0	10.8	16.9
3	9.26	10.47	12.7
4	0.86	0.62	1.71
5	61.1	12.5	34.4
6	23.0	18.0	12.0
7	9.95	6.65	10.89
8	2.96	–	5.4

From Collins & Kennedy (1987).

month; only 15% of the sharps injuries and none of the other blood exposures were reported to occupational health (or to anywhere else).

RISK OF TRANSMISSION OF HEPATITIS B FROM INFECTED WORKERS

The main area of concern when considering the risk of transmission of hepatitis B from an infected worker is the health care setting because of the potential for blood of the worker to come into contact with a patient's circulation or open tissues, for example during surgery. Infected workers may occasionally pose a risk in other settings; outbreaks of hepatitis B infection among butchers have been attributed to transmission from an infected worker (Gerlich & Thomssen 1982, Mijch et al 1987). It is clearly important for workers in any occupation where cuts and other injuries leading to bleeding are common to be trained in proper methods of treating wounds and cleaning up any blood spillages. Patients seem to have become more concerned about their risk of contracting hepatitis B from health care workers recently, probably following on from anxieties about contracting HIV from health care workers. This reflects public fears of HIV infection rather than actual risk, since HIV is very much less transmissible (Henderson et al 1990) than HBV (see Table 36.1).

Evidence of hepatitis B transmission from infected workers

Indirect evidence of transmission to patients comes from reports of cases of hepatitis B infection. In the years 1985–88, 3% of the cases of acute hepatitis B notified to the Public Health Laboratory Communicable Diseases Surveillance Centre had a history of recent surgical or dental treatment (Polakoff 1989). There is also a considerable body of direct evidence of hepatitis B transmission to patients. A recent review considered 12 outbreaks of hepatitis B infection transmitted from infected surgical staff in the UK between 1975 and 1990, with a total of 91 infections among patients (Heptonstall 1991). The review stresses that recognized and reported outbreaks are an underestimate of the total number of cases of hepatitis B infection acquired by patients through surgical procedures. Many infections may be subclinical and the long incubation period may make tracing to a common source difficult. Heptonstall (1991) reviews transmission rates in five outbreaks where this information was available; the results are summarised in Table 31.3. The proportion of patients found to have acquired acute icteric hepatitis B was between 1 and 2%. For the three outbreaks in which evidence of recent anicteric infection was also sought, the overall transmission rates were between 4 and 9%.

The USA Centers for Disease Control (1991) identified 20 published reports of hepatitis B infection clusters from infected health care workers worldwide since the early 1970s, involving over 300 infected patients. Eight of the reported clusters involved infected gynaecological (5) or cardiothoracic (3) surgeons; the remaining 12 clusters involved dentists or oral surgeons (9), a general practitioner, an inhalation therapist, and a cardiopulmonary bypass pump technician.

Table 31.3 Transmission rates for outbreaks of hepatitis B infection associated with infected surgical staff

Specialty	Exposed patients selected for follow-up	Number (%) of patients followed up	Number (%) of acute icteric infections	Number (%) of acute anicteric infections	Overall transmission rate (%)
Gynaecology	646	589 (91)	8 (1.4)	ND	–
Gynaecology	–	1020	9 (0.9)	ND	–
Gynaecology	268	247 (92)	5 (2.0)	17 (6.8)	9
Cardiothoracic Surgery	361	279 (77)	5 (1.8)	12 (4.3)	6
Cardiothoracic Surgery	128	123 (95)	2 (1.6)	3 (2.4)	4

ND, not determined.
From Heptonstall (1991).

It is possible to identify particular circumstances that increase the risk of transmission of hepatitis B from an infected health care worker to patients. Certain surgical specialities are over-represented among the reported outbreaks; obstetrics and gynaecology and cardiothoracic surgery seem to be particularly likely to be associated with transmission to patients (Heptonstall 1991, Centers for Disease Control 1991). Transmission of infection is more likely during major surgery, particularly when manipulation of needles or other sharp instruments in the body cavity without clear vision or in a restricted space is necessary. In one outbreak, the transmission rate from an infected surgeon performing major obstetric or gynaecological surgery was 20% and less than 1% from the same surgeon performing medium or low-risk procedures (Welch et al 1989). The Centers for Disease Control (1991) describe 'exposure-prone' surgical and dental procedures, in which there is a risk of percutaneous injury to the health care worker and in which, if such injury does occur, the worker's blood is likely to contact the patient's tissues or mucous membranes.

The risk of transmission from health care workers to patients appears to be restricted to those workers who are HBeAg positive. Heptonstall (1991) reports that in 11 of 12 outbreaks of transmission to patients the source health care worker was HBeAg positive; the HBeAg status was not determined in the remaining case. Similarly, in the USA report of 20 infection clusters among patients, HBeAg was positive in the source health care worker in every case that it was determined (17 out of 20) (Centers for Disease Control 1991). Some of the source health care workers had a history of recent acute hepatitis B; others were chronic carriers.

Magnitude of risk of hepatitis B transmission from infected workers

What is the risk to a patient undergoing a surgical or dental procedure of contracting hepatitis B from a member of the operating team during the procedure? The risk depends upon the prevalence of infective hepatitis B carriers among populations of health care workers undertaking invasive procedures and the frequency of incidents where their blood comes into contact with the patient's circulation or open tissues. Some of the studies of prevalence of hepatitis B markers among health care workers discussed above have included prevalence of HBsAg. In the review by West (1984), seroprevalences of HBsAg of about 1–2% were reported among groups of dentists, and rather less among groups of doctors and nurses. The current prevalence of HBsAg among health care workers in the USA and UK is unknown. Indirect evidence suggests that it is low. At the Royal Free Hospital in London, several thousand staff have been immunized against hepatitis B in the last 5 years, and only a handful have been found to be HBsAg positive among non-responders to immunization. Most of these were workers originating in areas of high hepatitis B endemicity; one was a doctor involved in invasive procedures with a history of hepatitis abroad. None was HBeAg positive.

The frequency of needlestick and other sharps injuries to health care workers, especially during surgical procedures, has been discussed above. When considering transmission risk to the patient, what is relevant is the frequency of incidents in which exposure of the patient to the operator's blood is also likely. A recent observational study in the USA (Tokars et al 1991) found a high rate of injuries to surgical staff during operative procedures and noted that in one-third of the incidents the needle or other sharp object recontacted the patient's tissues. It seems likely that oral surgeons and dentists also have a high rate of sharps injuries (Reingold et al 1988) and that their work in the confined space in and around the mouth will lead to the sharp object recontacting the patient's tissues quite frequently, but no observational studies have been reported to confirm this.

On the basis of the observations of Tokars et al (1991), and using estimates of the probability of transmission from an infected surgeon in such an incident, Bell et al (1991) calculated that the probability of a surgeon who is HBeAg positive transmitting to at least one patient over a 7-year period is 57–100%. Using estimates of the prevalence of HBeAg-positive surgeons and dentists in the USA, they further calculated that between 1980 and 1990 478–4773 patients may have acquired hepatitis B infection from infected surgeons and dentists in the USA. It should be stressed that these calculations are based on multiplying several estimated figures and could therefore be quite inaccurate. On the basis of laboratory reports of acute hepatitis B between 1980 and 1983, Polakoff (1986b) estimated that the risk of a patient developing acute hepatitis B as part of a cluster caused by staff during surgical procedures was one in a million operations and that the transmission of hepatitis B from health care workers to patients was rare in the UK.

PREVENTION OF OCCUPATIONAL TRANSMISSION OF HEPATITIS B

Given the availability of an effective vaccine against hepatitis B, it should be possible to eliminate occupational transmission of hepatitis B almost entirely. In general, anything that reduces the risk of transmission *to* workers will also reduce the risk of transmission *from* workers, by decreasing the number of infected workers and making transmission from any that are infected less likely. The aspects to consider in the prevention of occupational transmission of hepatitis B, and indeed other blood-borne infections such as hepatitis C, include: safe practices to reduce hazardous exposures, immunization programmes for workers at risk, management of blood exposure incidents and management of workers known to be infected.

Safe practices for prevention of occupational transmission of hepatitis B

There are two general approaches to safe practice with regard to prevention of transmission of blood-borne infections: the 'traditional' infection control approach and the more recent universal precautions approach. In the traditional approach, patients or specimens known or suspected to be infected are identified and special precautions are taken in their care or processing. This approach was advocated for reducing the risk of transmission of hepatitis B in the era before immunization became available (Hansen et al 1981) and continues to be recommended by some authorities in relation to both hepatitis B and HIV infection in laboratories (Advisory Committee on Dangerous Pathogens 1990, Health Services Advisory Committee 1991a) and in operating theatres (Royal College of Surgeons of England 1990). Other official guidance in both the USA and the UK favours the universal precautions approach (Centers for Disease Control 1985, 1987b, 1988, Department of Health 1990). Professional bodies representing surgical specialties are moving towards recommending universal precautions, although still suggesting additional precautions for 'high-risk' patients (Royal College of Obstetricians and Gynaecologists 1990, British Orthopaedic Association 1991). The concept of universal precautions arose mainly as a result of the HIV epidemic and is based on the concept that patients with blood-borne infections cannot be reliably identified on the basis of their histories so that the blood of all patients should be treated as potentially infectious; the level of precautions to be taken should depend upon a risk assessment of the procedures being undertaken rather than of the patient's infection status.

The arguments for the two approaches in relation to HIV infection have been rehearsed recently (Shanson & Cockcroft 1991). Those in favour of the traditional approach argue that health care workers have a right to 'know what they are dealing with' so that they can protect themselves appropriately. It is also argued that financial constraints mean that a high level of protection can only be afforded in some cases and therefore those cases where it is necessary should be identified. A universal high standard of protection is not considered justified except in areas with very high seroprevalences of hepatitis B or HIV. But there are serious problems with the traditional approach. Firstly, identification of patients infected with HIV or hepatitis B on the basis of history is not reliable (Gordin et al 1990, Parry et al 1991) so that compulsory testing of patients would be required, which would be expensive and divert money away from safer equipment and protective clothing. In areas of low seroprevalence of HIV and hepatitis B a screening programme would not be efficient, and in areas of high prevalence treating all patients as infected is sensible. Awaiting test results is not feasible in emergency situations, the very situations where exposure to blood is likely.

Perhaps the most important criticism of relying on identification of 'high-risk' patients for hepatitis B and HIV infection to determine the level of precautions to be taken is that knowledge of patients' 'high-risk' status does not seem to reduce the risk of blood exposures during surgical procedures. Gerberding et al (1990) found no difference in the rate of blood exposures overall, or in sharps injuries specifically, between known or suspected 'high-risk' patients and others. In another study (Panililio et al 1991) there was a lower rate of blood exposures during surgery in identified 'high-risk' patients, but the numbers were very small and the difference could well have occurred by chance. In the operating department at San Francisco General Hospital (Gerberding et al 1990), universal precautions were already being practised to a large extent, so that it is clear that this approach is also not sufficient to prevent needlestick injuries and other blood exposures during surgery. There is, however, evidence that practising universal precautions reduces the frequency of non-parenteral blood exposures among trained health care workers (Fahey et al 1991).

Despite the simplicity and logic of universal precautions, several authors have reported that health care workers do not practise them even when it is official policy to do so (Baraff & Talan 1989, Kelen et al 1990). Reasons given for not using barrier precautions at all times included lack of time, a feeling that the protective clothing interferes with skilful performance of tasks and complaints that the materials are uncomfortable. Embalmers studied in the USA did not practise universal precautions, but many declined to embalm bodies when there was a known diagnosis of AIDS (Beck-Sague et al 1991). Differential treatment of 'high-risk' cases is still officially recommended in UK mortuaries and post-mortem rooms (Health Services Advisory Committee 1991b). It seems that many health care workers choose to base their practice upon what they know or suspect of a patient's infection status rather than upon the procedure being performed. In a recent study, a majority of clinical medical students and consultants at a London hospital reported changing their clinical practice – mainly by wearing gloves and by taking care with needles – if they knew a patient was infected with a blood-borne virus (Elford & Cockcroft 1991). Perhaps not surprisingly, in the same survey a substantial proportion of both students and consultants were in favour of compulsory testing (in this case for HIV) of patients, presumably because they felt that this would help them to decide what precautions to take with which patients.

A major criticism of universal precautions is that they are expensive and that such an approach could not possibly be afforded in developing countries that may have a high prevalence of hepatitis B and HIV infection. This is a misconception, perhaps because the term 'universal' is misleading, suggesting the same level of precautions for every procedure. The basis of the universal precautions approach should be a risk assessment of procedures, with the level of precautions set accordingly. This can allow scarce resources to be used most effectively, with protective equipment reserved for those procedures for which it is really needed. The UK health service is increasingly cost conscious, so it is hard to justify practices such as washing down the walls of an operating theatre after a lymph node biopsy, simply because the patient was infected with hepatitis B or HIV.

It is clear that preventing inoculation injuries is of prime importance in reducing the risk of occupational transmission of hepatitis B and other blood-borne viruses. This requires a detailed understanding of how and why such injuries occur and the development of new techniques and equipment to reduce the risk. Studies in operating theatres have shown that suturing often leads to glove perforation and needlestick injuries (Brough et al 1988, Hussain et al 1988, Chan & Lewis 1989, Wright et al 1991) and have recommended using instruments to handle needles during suturing, alternative wound closure techniques, such as stapling, and the use of blunt needles for suturing adipose tissue. Other authors have recommended safer surgical techniques including methods of passing instruments between nurse and operator and avoidance of the use of sharp instruments (Raahave & Bremmelgaard 1991, Sim 1991). Camilleri et al (1991b) have suggested that the risk of injuries to junior surgeons could be reduced by compulsory training on surgical rigs. There is evidence that double gloving reduces the rate of perforation of the inner glove (Matta et al 1988), and some authors recommend this as a routine precaution (Gerberding et al 1990).

Protection of operating theatre staff from eye splashes by the use of spectacles or visors (Brearley & Buist 1989, Hinton et al 1991) and from skin contamination by means of impermeable gowns (Smith & Nichols 1991) is recommended. Although there is no evidence of transmission of hepatitis B or HIV by blood aerosols, some surgeons are turning to the use of ventilated hoods during procedures that generate blood aerosols (British Orthopaedic Association 1991).

Effective systems for collecting and disposing of used sharp instruments throughout the health care setting are important in reducing the risk of sharps injuries to all groups of staff (British Medical Association 1990). All staff at risk should be considered: staff in Central Sterile Supplies Departments have a high rate of injuries from returned sharp instruments, and systems to avoid handling these instruments should be devised; and laundry staff risk injury from sharp instruments sent down with used linen and white coats. There is currently considerable interest in developing safer needle and syringe combinations to reduce needle handling (Humphries 1990) and automatically protect the needle after use (Kingston & Brookes 1988). Although reported incidents may be a biased sample of those occurring in a hospital, careful monitoring of reported incidents can be a useful indicator of dangerous procedures as well as ensuring proper management of individual incidents (Oakley et al 1992). During the period reviewed by Oakley et al (1992), it was noted that needlestick injuries to nurses frequently occurred during the procedure of obtaining finger pulp blood samples, whether using a simple stylet or a spring-loaded device; a new disposable device that retracts the used stylet into the hub after use was introduced as a result, and this has been successful in preventing further injuries to staff. It may also protect patients from the risk of hepatitis B transmission that has been reported in association with improper use of the spring-loaded device (Polish et al 1992).

Hepatitis B immunization programmes

A safe, effective vaccine against hepatitis B has been licensed in the UK for a decade, and immunization was recommended for health care workers, ambulance and emergency workers and certain police officers at an early stage (Zuckerman 1984). The Department of Health Joint Committee on Vaccination and Immunisation (1990) recommends hepatitis B immunization for groups of health care workers at risk of exposure to blood likely to be infected with hepatitis B. There have been campaigns by professional bodies to encourage all nurses and doctors to be immunized against hepatitis B (Royal College of Nursing 1987, Hunter 1991). Viral hepatitis is a Prescribed Industrial Disease among workers exposed to blood and body fluids (Benefits Agency 1991); a health care worker with clinical contact who develops hepatitis B can claim Industrial Injuries Benefit and may well be able to sue his or her employer successfully if hepatitis B immunization had not been offered.

Very high rates of seroconversion (95% and above) following hepatitis B immunization given intramuscularly have been reported among health care workers (Fagan et al 1987, Cockcroft et al 1990, Waldron 1990). The poor antibody response after intradermal immunization make this route of administration inappropriate for occupational immunization programmes (Tant et al 1991); there is no saving with intradermal programmes because of the additional antibody tests and booster doses of vaccine that are required (Tant et al 1991). It has been reported from the USA (Mauskopf et al 1991) and from Belgium (Lahaye et al 1987) that the financial benefits of an occupational hepatitis B immunization programme outweigh the costs, even if the prevented pain and suffering of cases are not taken into account.

There is evidence in the UK of a marked fall in the number of cases of acute hepatitis B among health care workers between 1985 and 1988, much of which can be attributed to immunization programmes (Polakoff 1989). Employers have a responsibility to protect workers against occupational hazards; in the UK hepatitis B as a biological hazard is covered by the Control of

Substances Hazardous to Health (COSHH) Regulations (Statutory Instruments 1988) which specify assessment of work processes to assess risk to health and provision of necessary training and protection against recognized risks. In this case, provision of immunization would be one of the protective measures. Despite this, provision of immunization for health care workers and students is not universal in developed countries. A survey of hospitals in the USA found that 75% had hepatitis B immunization programmes for staff, with programmes being more common in large urban hospitals (Alexander et al 1990). In the UK, some hospitals provide a full hepatitis B immunization programme but some recommend staff and students to request immunization from their general practitioners, some provide immunization only for staff in certain areas considered to be at particularly high risk, and some provide immunization but do not subsequently check for an antibody response. A survey of hospital occupational health departments in 1988 revealed that many of their programmes of hepatitis B immunization for staff were limited by the cost of the vaccine and the resources of the departments (Baddick & Aw 1989). The majority of medical (Department of Health, personal communication, 1991) and dental (Scully & Matthews 1990) students are now offered immunization early in their training.

Defining groups of workers at different levels of risk of occupational hepatitis B, as is required with limited immunization programmes, is very difficult because staff tend to move between areas and because some groups without direct patient contact may nevertheless have a high rate of needlestick injuries, such as portering and domestic staff. Ideally, an immunization programme should include all staff with direct or indirect contact with patients or their blood (Cockcroft et al 1990). Most people would agree that emergency ambulance workers should be offered immunization, but there has been debate about whether police officers, prison officers and firemen are at sufficiently increased risk of hepatitis B infection in their work to warrant their being offered hepatitis B immunization. The Centres for Disease Control (1989) recommend that if the duties of such workers bring them into contact with blood and body fluids they should be included in hepatitis B immunization programmes.

Even when immunization programmes are available, not all health care workers participate. A number of recent studies have found incomplete hepatitis B immunization among groups of health care workers (Table 31.4). Reported reasons for the low uptake rates include apathy, lack of knowledge about vaccine efficacy, fears about vaccine safety, and lack of knowledge about hepatitis B transmission. Among surgeons there was also a fear that being a non-responder may lead to career problems. In the study by Spence & Dash (1990), immunization was not provided to the workers on site, and this may explain their low immunization rate. Similarly, the very low rate in the study by Astbury & Baxter (1990) may be because immunization was not provided by the hospital; staff had to obtain it from their general practitioners. It has been suggested that the only way to increase immunization uptake among health care workers is to make immunization or proof of immunity mandatory (Harris et al 1991). Another study found that workers' beliefs about vaccine safety and efficacy were the most important predictors of vaccine acceptance and concluded that educating workers about these issues would be the best way to increase programme participation rates (Bodenheimer et al 1986).

It may be that immunization rates among staff reporting blood exposure incidents are not representative of those among the whole population of workers at risk. Newman & Hambling (1992) suggest that workers who know themselves to be successfully immunized may be less likely to report incidents so that the immunization rate among reporters is an underestimate. Gompertz (1990) found that medical students who had been advised to be immunized against hepatitis B recalled fewer needlestick injuries than those who had not been so advised; he suggests that this could indicate that education results in safer practice. In the Royal Free study of operating theatre staff (Williams et al 1993) those who knew themselves to be immune to hepatitis B following immunization were significantly *more* likely to report sharps injuries than others, perhaps reflecting that they are individuals who are aware

Table 31.4 Hepatitis B immunization rates among groups of health care workers

Reference	Occupational group	Number studied	Percent immunized	Percent antibody checked*
Berridge et al 1990	Vascular surgeons	206	64%	45%
J R Williams & Flowerdew 1990	General surgeons	76	87%	47%
Porteous 1990	Orthopaedic surgeons	800	69%	–
Williams et al 1993	Operating theatre staff	158	78%	81%
Astbury & Baxter 1990	Hospital staff	803	25%	–
Spence & Dash 1990	Nurses in 'high-risk' areas	169	42%	–
Wood 1989	GP principals	416	35%	–
	GP Trainees	32	69%	–
Van-Damme et al 1990	Belgian GPs	149	44%	–
	Belgian Dentists	126	71%	–
Choudhury & Cleator 1992	Clinical medical students	172	95%	83%
Ellinghouse C 1992†	Preclinical medical students	99	97%	89%
Newman & Hambling 1992	Hospital staff in blood exposures	2975	49%	Checked at time of incident
Oakley et al 1992	Hospital staff in blood exposures	438	71%	Checked at time of incident

* Percentage of those immunized who had anti-HBs response measured.
† Unpublished data from Royal Free Occupational Health Service.

of infection risks at work. Indeed, there is no published evidence to support the idea that fewer blood exposure incidents are reported since hepatitis B immunization of health care workers has become widespread in recent years. Probably concern about hepatitis B risk has been replaced by greater concern about HIV risk; there is evidence that doctors and medical students consider themselves at greater risk of HIV infection in their work than in their personal lives, with a significant minority believing themselves to be at 'great' risk at work (Elford & Cockcroft 1991).

There is debate about whether testing for hepatitis B markers is necessary before immunization of health care workers. Dienstag & Ryan (1982) suggested that the presence of anti-HBs without anti-HBc in some health care workers may indicate natural immunization rather than infection, owing to low-level, continuous exposure to hepatitis B. However, others have found that the presence of anti-HBs alone, especially at low levels, may not indicate immunity (Werner et al 1985) and prescreening should include anti-HBc. Prescreening is only cost-effective in populations with a high risk of infection markers (Perrillo 1985); this will not include health care workers unless they come from areas of high hepatitis B endemicity. In South Africa, for example, it was calculated that it was cost-effective to prescreen Black nursing and laboratory personnel but not their White counterparts (Schoub et al 1991).

Despite the high response rate to immunization, testing for antibody response is appropriate among workers occupationally exposed to hepatitis B. The presence of anti-HBc can be sought in all with a low or absent anti-HBs response; those with anti-HBc without anti-HBs can then be counselled and tested for HBsAg, and those without anti-HBc can be offered further doses of vaccine. Identification of hepatitis B carriers among health care workers undertaking invasive procedures is important for occupational as well as clinical reasons (see below). Persistent non-responders need to be made aware that they are not protected against hepatitis B and to understand the importance of safe practice and immediate reporting of blood exposure incidents so that post-exposure prophylaxis can be given if necessary. It may be possible for non-responders to avoid certain duties; for example, porters who do not respond should not collect sharps boxes. Non-responders undertaking invasive procedures should perhaps be tested for HBsAg at intervals to ensure that they have not become carriers.

For people with a continuing occupational risk of hepatitis B infection, maintaining adequate levels of protection after immunization is important. Authors disagree about the time course of decay of antibody levels in individuals after successful immunization and about how to determine the timing of booster doses of vaccine (Jilg et al 1984, Gesemann & Scheiermann 1989, Gilks et al 1989, Nommensen et al 1989). It has been suggested that it is only necessary to test antibody levels if a blood exposure is reported (Morris 1989), but this seems unreliable given the evidence of gross under-reporting of exposure incidents (Collins & Kennedy 1987). The antibody level required for protection against infection with hepatitis B is not known; there is evidence of protection even after antibody levels have fallen below 10 mIU/ml (Hadler et al 1986). However, estimates have been revised upwards for those occupationally exposed, and currently many believe that a titre of 100 mIU/ml should be the target among health care workers (A J Zuckerman, personal communication, 1991). The procedure followed at the Royal Free Hospital in London is to test for antibody response 1 month after the third injection of vaccine and thereafter at 2-yearly intervals, giving booster doses of vaccine if the antibody level is below 100 mIU/ml.

Management of blood exposure incidents

Proper management of blood exposure incidents can reduce the risk of hepatitis B transmission, even if the worker involved has not been previously immunized against hepatitis B. Management should include establishing the worker's hepatitis B immune status, testing known source patients for HBsAg (and HBeAg) and administering HBIG and hepatitis B vaccine if necessary. For non-immunized workers, the use of HBIG is recommended, together with the first dose of vaccine. HBIG alone is clearly not completely effective; in the study by Masuko et al (1985), 20% of staff who had sustained needlesticks from HBeAg-positive source patients developed hepatitis B, despite receiving HBIG within 48 h. There are no reported studies of the effects of adding vaccine to the post-needlestick-exposure prophylaxis regimen, but there is evidence that small amounts of HBsAg in the NHIG used by Grady et al (1978) led to active immunization against hepatitis B in the recipients and therefore improved the protection given by this preparation (Hoofnagle et al 1979).

As the protection conferred by post-exposure prophylaxis in non-immune individuals is likely to be incomplete, it is important that they should be followed up, especially if the source patient is HBeAg positive. The use of HBIG seems to delay seroconversion by two to three times, so that it may be over 8 months before there is evidence of infection (Masuko et al 1985). Post-exposure active immunization following all incidents (even when the source patient is known not to be infected with hepatitis B) is important for future protection, since individuals reporting incidents are clearly at risk.

Management of blood exposure incidents should be undertaken by a specified department, ideally the Occupational Health Department if there is one available, and the arrangements for reporting incidents should be widely publicized among all employees. The management of incidents should be regularly reviewed so that problems can be identified and dealt with. Oakley et al (1992) reviewed more than 400 reported incidents over 2½ years and noted that only about half the known source patients were tested for HBsAg as a result of the incident, although a request for testing was explicit policy. Failure to test was mainly for logistic reasons and the rate of testing increased during the period. In a few cases, the source patient was not tested for HBsAg even though the injured worker was not immune to hepatitis B; identifying this problem has led to a modification of policy. Monitoring time trends is also important; the Royal Free study has revealed that the proportion of workers reporting incidents who are immune to hepatitis B has risen significantly over a 3-year period (Fig 31.1).

Management of health care workers with hepatitis B infection

In the light of the evidence, discussed above, that hepatitis B has been transmitted from infected

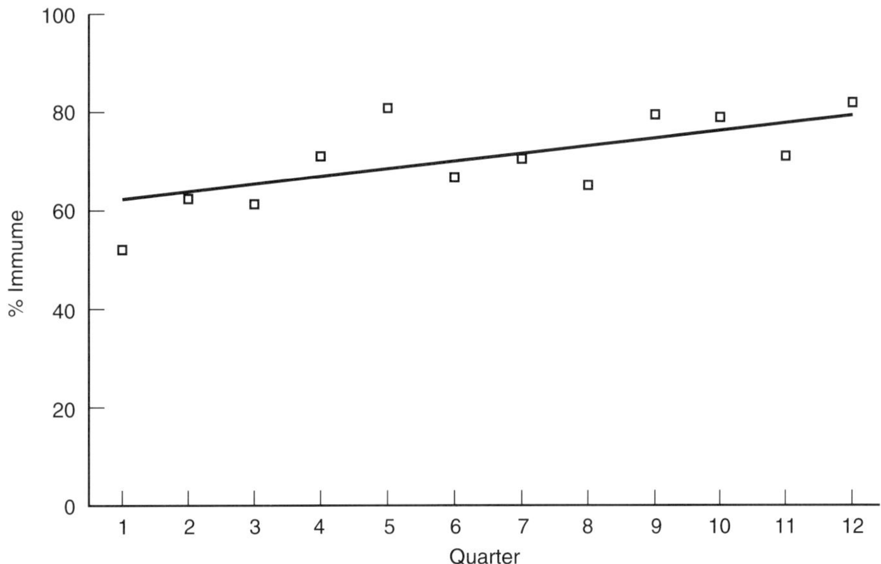

Fig. 31.1 Proportion of staff reporting blood exposure incidents who were immune to hepatitis B 1989–91, Royal Free Hospital. Some of the data contributing to this figure have been published previously (Oakley et al 1992).

health care workers to patients during invasive procedures, it seems reasonable to protect patients against this small risk by ensuring that health care workers who are HBeAg positive do not undertake procedures in which transmission is likely. This will only be effective if all individuals who are HBeAg positive are identified; relying on chance discovery of HBeAg status is not enough. Hepatitis B immunization, with testing of antibody reponse, allows non-responders to be identified and tested for carrier status. There have been calls to make hepatitis B immunization and evidence of response, or at least of lack of HBeAg, a condition of employment for workers undertaking invasive procedures (O'Dowd & O'Dowd 1990). Certainly the current UK guidelines, which only recommend restrictions on practice when transmission from a health care worker has been demonstrated (Department of Health 1981), seem no longer tenable (Cockcroft 1991).

New guidelines from the USA (Centers for Disease Control 1991) recommend that health care workers who perform certain 'exposure-prone' invasive procedures should either have evidence of immunity following hepatitis B immunization or should know their HBeAg status; if HBeAg positive, they should not generally be allowed to continue these invasive procedures. In the UK, new guidance is imminent and is expected to recommend that health care workers who are HBeAg positive should not participate in invasive procedures and that immunization should be a condition of employment in invasive specialities. It will be relatively easy to implement these guidelines for new employees, even more so in the future as hepatitis B immunization and antibody testing become universal among students. The few medical and dental students who have acquired hepatitis B before starting their training can be given career guidance at an early stage to steer them away from invasive specialities. But there will be some cases of hardship, such as a senior surgical registrar who is required to be tested when applying for a consultant post and finds himself to be HBeAg positive.

The guidelines do not specify how to solve the problem of staff already in post. They should not be forced to be tested for hepatitis B infection but should be encouraged to have immunization and antibody testing and can be advised that it is very unlikely that they will find themselves to be hepatitis B carriers after not responding to vaccine. The few surgeons and dentists who do discover themselves to be HBeAg positive need informed and confidential advice. A reasonable approach is to consider with surgeons the type of operations that they perform and advise avoidance of those procedures in which transmission has been shown to be likely. Which procedures come into this category needs to be agreed between surgeons and other professionals such as virologists, infection control specialists and occupational physicians. Advice may be available from expert panels in both the UK and the USA in difficult cases. Restrictions of practice may only be needed temporarily, as some individuals will become HBeAg negative either with time or as a result of treatment.

Modification of practice has been reported to prevent further transmission in some cases (Carl et al 1982) but is not always successful (Lettau et al 1986). It may be necessary therefore to redeploy surgical workers into work such as teaching or research, with protected income. The question of compensation may arise; hepatitis B is a Prescribed Industrial Disease among health care workers and the affected surgeon may wish to sue if it seems likely that the infection was acquired occupationally and that the employer had not offered reasonable protection, including immunization. Health care employers need to develop policies for management of employees with hepatitis B infection, covering medical, ethical and practical issues (S Williams & Cockcroft 1992); in the UK employers can afford to treat infected employees generously since they will be rare and it is important to retain their skills within the organisation. The existence of clear, accepted policies within an organization for the management of employees with hepatitis B infection can help to avoid some of the confusion and conflicting advice that is common at present (Kennedy 1991).

OCCUPATION AND OTHER FORMS OF VIRAL HEPATITIS

Hepatitis C

Occupational transmission of hepatitis C

Modes of occupational transmission of hepatitis C appear to be similar to those of hepatitis B. However, there is much less evidence on which to base estimates of occupational risk. Several studies have reported on the prevalence of hepatitis C antibodies or the frequency of non-A, non-B hepatitis among occupational groups exposed to blood. M J Alter et al (1990) reported that 2% of patients with non-A, non-B hepatitis in their sentinel counties surveillance in the USA had occupational exposure to blood. Abb (1991) found hepatitis C antibodies in 8 of 738 health care workers (1%), compared with much higher seroprevalences among certain patient groups. Mortimer et al (1989) found that none of 100 hospital staff reporting inoculation injuries was anti-HCV positive. H Hofmann & Kunz (1990) reported a 2% prevalence of antibodies to hepatitis C among 294 health care workers from different departments but concluded that the risk of occupational infection was generally low, although apparently higher among staff with direct patient contact. In another study, although only 0.58% of 1033 hospital employees had antibodies to hepatitis C, this prevalence was significantly greater than the 0.24% of 2113 blood donor controls (Jochen 1992).

Klein et al (1991) found antibodies to hepatitis C among 2% of 456 dentists in New York compared with 0.1% of 723 controls; among a small group of oral surgeons the prevalence was 9%. Dentists who had antibodies to hepatitis C reported having treated more intravenous drug users in the previous month than did seronegative dentists. Among those dentists who had not been immunized against hepatitis B, 25% had anti-HBsAg, and 6% of these had antibodies to hepatitis C, compared with only 2% among those who were anti-HBsAg negative. This suggests a common mode of transmission for the two viruses, though with a lower risk for hepatitis C. A study of 94 dental surgeons in South Wales (Herbert et al 1992) found none to have antibodies to hepatitis C, despite up to 45 years in practice, sometimes without wearing gloves.

There are case reports of transmission of hepatitis C after needlestick injuries (Schlipkoter et al 1990, Vaglia et al 1990, Cariani et al 1991, Seeff 1991). Mayo-Smith (1987) reports a case in which apparently both non-A, non-B hepatitis and hepatitis B were transmitted to a medical student by a single needlestick. Transmission of hepatitis C by a human bite has also been reported

(Dusheiko et al 1990). A recent prospective study has attempted to estimate the risk of seroconversion after a needlestick injury from a source patient with anti-HCV antibodies (Kiyosawa et al 1991). 200 injuries to 196 health care workers were studied; in 110 the source patient had anti-HCV antibodies. Four health care workers developed hepatitis after an anti-HCV-positive needlestick (4%; 95% CI 19%); in three of these anti-HCV seroconversion occurred. The incubation period was around 40 days. There were no seroconversions without biochemical or clinical evidence of hepatitis. Clearly, the risk of hepatitis C infection following accidental inoculation of infected blood is much less than the risk of hepatitis B infection after inoculation of HBeAg-positive blood, probably because of the relatively low titre of the virus in human blood.

Presumably transmission of hepatitis C from an infected health care worker to a patient during an invasive procedure is possible, by analogy with hepatitis B, but there are no reports of such transmission having occurred. The apparently lower infectivity of hepatitis C than hepatitis B from inoculation injuries suggests that any risk to patients from infected workers is likely to be very small.

Prevention of occupational transmission of hepatitis C

As a form of viral hepatitis, hepatitis C is a Prescribed Industrial Disease among workers exposed to blood (Benefits Agency 1991). The most important means of prevention is avoidance of needlestick injuries and other blood exposures. The incidence of blood exposures among health care workers and approaches to safe practice are discussed above in relation to hepatitis B. The development of a test for hepatitis C antibodies has strengthened the case for the universal precautions approach; it is now clear that many patients not treated as posing a risk from blood inoculation, because they did not have HBsAg or antibodies to HIV, were infected with hepatitis C, which could be transmitted to carers. Patients with haemophilia, intravenous drug users and patients on renal dialysis units seem especially likely to be infected with hepatitis C, but safe practice assumes that any patient could be infected. In a retrospective study of sera from 528 source patients in needlestick injuries, Cummins & Tedder (1992) found antibodies to hepatitis C in 14 samples (2.7%); in this series, hepatitis C infection was more common than either hepatitis B or HIV infection.

The value of post-exposure prophylaxis for hepatitis C infection is uncertain. It has been suggested that gamma-globulin should be given, and there is evidence from a Spanish group (Sanchez-Quijano et al 1988) that NHIG reduced the risk of post-transfusion non-A, non-B hepatitis in heart surgery patients. In this study, the treated group received NHIG before as well as 1 week after the blood transfusion. However, there is no published evidence of efficacy of either NHIG or HBIG given after inoculation incidents with anti-HCV positive blood, in some areas the titre of anti-HCV in NHIG and HBIG is very low (J Heptonstall, personal communication, 1991), and the antibody detected by current tests is not neutralizing. Antiviral agents used to treat hepatitis C infection may have a role in prophylaxis, but there is no evidence to support their use at present.

Hepatitis D

Hepatitis D infection is rarely of occupational relevance, except in particular circumstances. Staff who work with animals experimentally infected with hepatitis D should be screened for hepatitis B infection before starting the work and immunized against hepatitis B. This is in order to protect them, indirectly, from hepatitis D infection which they can only contract if they already have hepatitis B infection, contracted by any means. Staff working with patients who might have hepatitis D infection should in any case be immunized against hepatitis B.

Hepatitis A

Occupational transmission of hepatitis A

Workers occupationally exposed to faecal material are reported to have an increased risk of hepatitis A infection. A study of 93 sewage workers in Germany found them to have a seroprevalence of anti-HAV antibodies 3–4 times that of the general population of the same age; 36% in those less than 30 years old and 85% in those aged 50 years and above (Chriske et al 1990). Similarly, among Copenhagen municipal employees, significantly more sewer workers than gardeners or clerks had antibodies to hepatitis A (Skinhoj et al 1981). Edgar & Campbell (1985) report a sewage worker who contracted hepatitis A after falling into a sewage tank; six nurses looking after him also became jaundiced.

Occupations that require frequent travel to areas where hygiene conditions are poor may be expected to lead to an excess rate of hepatitis A infection. A study among Norwegian merchant seamen found that the prevalence of hepatitis A antibodies increased with years in foreign trade (Siebke et al 1989). A study in the Canadian armed forces, however, could not find a relationship between anti-HAV seroprevalence and posting at home or abroad (Embil et al 1989). Contaminated food and water were found to be important causes of hepatitis A among US Navy and Marine personnel (Dembert et al 1987).

Outbreaks of hepatitis A infection have been reported among both patients and staff in certain health care settings. An outbreak in an institution for the mentally retarded affected 47 patients and 13 staff members; there was a high anti-HAV seroprevalence among the staff and the outbreak was thought to be caused by infected staff from another institution (Helmsing et al 1980). Outbreaks of hepatitis A in child care centres have been described, with transmission related to contact with non-toilet-trained children (Benenson et al 1980, Vernon et al 1982). In a study of an outbreak of hepatitis A in a neonatal intensive care unit, Rosenblum et al (1991) found that risk factors for infection among the nurses included care of a primary infant patient, drinking beverages in the unit, and not wearing gloves when taping an intravenous line. Infants who were cared for by nurses who cared for primary infant patients during the same shift were at greater risk of infection. In another study of an outbreak of hepatitis A on a paediatric intensive care unit (Drusin et al 1987), the source patient was thought to be a child who became incontinent of faeces prior to his death; it was also noted that staff who shared food, drink and cigarettes with patients or their families were at increased risk of infection.

Kitchen workers may be at risk of contracting hepatitis A through handling raw food, as suggested by a German study that found a high anti-HAV seroprevalence among hospital kitchen workers (F Hofmann et al 1990). Infected food handlers can be a source of outbreaks of hepatitis A infection, especially if they do not follow proper food hygiene procedures (Lowry et al 1989).

Prevention of occupational transmission of hepatitis A

Until recently, the only means of preventing occupational transmission of hepatitis A were strict adherence to hygiene measures and the use of gamma-globulin when work required foreign travel. The short-lived protection from gamma-globulin made it inconvenient for frequent travellers or for those with a continuing occupational risk. Now that an effective vaccine against hepatitis A is available (Tilzey et al 1992), it should be considered for groups of workers at risk of acquiring or transmitting infection. These will include: sewage workers and others dealing with human faecal material, such as plumbers in hospitals; military personnel and others whose work requires them to travel to areas of high endemicity (including medical students on electives); food handlers; and health care workers, especially those working with children or the mentally handicapped. It is not yet clear how long the antibodies induced by immunization will last before booster doses are required in workers with continuing exposure. The use of vaccine against hepatitis A should not mean that training of workers in hygiene measures to prevent faecal–oral spread of infection is relaxed, as such measures are essential to prevent transmission of other faecal organisms.

Hepatitis E

There is little information about occupational associations with hepatitis E infection. It may pose a risk for individuals whose work takes them to areas of endemicity and poor hygiene, as for hepatitis A. An outbreak of acute hepatitis E virus infection has been described among military personnel in Ethiopia (Tsega et al 1991).

REFERENCES

Abb J 1991 Prevalence of hepatitis C virus antibodies in hospital personnel. International Journal of Medical Microbiology 274: 543–547

Advisory Committee on Dangerous Pathogens 1990 HIV – the causative agent of AIDS and related conditions: second revision of guidelines. HMSO, London

Alexander P G, Johnson R, Williams W W, Hadler S C, White J W, Coleman P J 1990 Hepatitis B vaccination programmes for health care personnel in U.S. hospitals. Public Health Report 105: 610–616

Alter H J, Seeff L B, Kaplan P M et al 1976 Type B hepatitis: the infectivity of blood positive for e antigen and DNA polymerase after accidental needlestick exposure. New England Journal of Medicine 295: 909–913

Alter M J, Hadler S C, Judson F N et al 1990 Risk factors for acute non-A, non-B hepatitis in the United States and association with hepatitis C virus infection. Journal of the American Medical Association 264: 2231–2235

Anderson R A, Woodfield D G 1982 Hepatitis B virus infections in laboratory staff. New Zealand Medical Journal 95: 69–71

Astbury C, Baxter P J 1990 Infection risks in hospital staff from blood: hazardous injury rateas and acceptance of hepatitis B immunization. Journal of the Society of Occupational Medicine 40: 92–93

Baddick M R, Aw T-C 1989 Immunisation against hepatitis B among NHS staff in West Midlands Regional Health Authority. British Medical Journal 299:607

Baraff L J, Talan D A 1989 Compliance with universal precautions in a university hospital emergency department. Annals of Emergency Medicine 18: 654–657

Beck-Sague C M, Jarvis W R, Fruehling J A, Ott C E, Higgins M T, Bates F L 1991 Universal precautions and mortuary practitioners: influence on practices and risk of occupationally acquired infection. Journal of Occupational Medicine 33: 874–878

Bell D M, Martone W J, Cuiver D H et al 1991 Risk of endemic HIV and hepatitis B virus (HBV) transmission to patients during invasive procedures . Proceedings of the Seventh International Conference on AIDS, Florence, 16–21 June 1991, p 37

Benefits Agency 1991 If you have an industrial disease: industrial injuries disablement benefit (NI 2, August 1989, revised October 1991). HMSO, London

Benenson M W, Takafuji E T, Bancroft W H, Lemon S M, Callahan M C, Leach D A 1980 A military community outbreak of hepatitis type A related to transmission in a child care facility. American Journal of Epidemiology 112: 471–481

Berridge D C, Galea M H, Evans D F, Pugh S, Hopkinson B R, Makin G S 1990 Hepatitis B immunisation in vascular surgeons. British Journal of Surgery 77: 585–586

Bodenheimer H C, Fulton J P, Kramer P D 1986 Acceptance of hepatitis B vaccine among hospital workers. American Journal of Public Health 76: 252–255

Brearley S, Buist L J 1989 Blood splashes: an underestimated hazard to surgeons. British Medical Journal 299: 1315

British Medical Association 1990 A code of practice for the safe use and disposal of sharps. British Medical Association, London

British Orthopaedic Association 1991 Guidelines for the prevention of cross-infection between patients and staff in orthopaedic operating theatres with special reference to HIV and the blood-borne hepatitis viruses. British Orthopaedic Association, London

Brough S J, Hunt T M, Barrie W W 1988 Surgical glove perforations. British Journal of Surgery 75: 317

Bryan J A, Carr H E, Gregg M B 1973 An outbreak of nonparenterally transmitted hepatitis B. Journal of the American Medical Association 223: 279–283

Camilleri A E, Murray S, Imrie C W 1991a Needlestick injuries in surgeons: what is the incidence? Journal of the Royal College of Surgeons of Edinburgh 36: 317–318

Camilleri A E, Murray S, Squair J L, Imrie C W 1991b Epidemiology of sharps accidents in general surgery. Journal of the Royal College of Surgeons of Edinburgh 36: 314–316

Cancio-Bello T P, de Medina M, Shorey J, Valledor M D, Schiff E R 1982 An institutional outbreak of hepatitis B related to a human biting carrier. Journal of Infectious Diseases 146: 652–656

Cariani E, Zonaro A, Primi D et al 1991 Detection of HCV RNA and antibodies to HCV after needlestick injury. Lancet 337: 850

Carl M, Blakey D L, Francis D P, Maynard J E 1982 Interruption of hepatitis B transmission by modification of a gynaecologist's surgical technique. Lancet i: 731–733

Centers for Disease Control 1985 Recommendations for protection against viral hepatitis. Morbidity and Mortality Weekly Report 34: 313–324, 329–335

Centers for Disease Control 1987a Human immunodeficiency virus infections in health care workers exposed to blood of infected patients. Morbidity and Mortality Weekly Report 36: 285–289

Centers for Disease Control 1987b Recommendations for prevention of HIV transmission in health-care settings. Morbidity and Mortality Weekly Report 36 (suppl. 2S): 1–18

Centers for Disease Control 1988 Update: universal precautions for prevention of transmission of human immunodeficiency virus, hepatitis B virus and other blood borne pathogens in health care settings. Morbidity and Mortality Weekly Report 37: 377–388

Centers for Disease Control 1989 Guidelines for prevention of transmission of human immunodeficiency virus and hepatitis B virus to health-care and public-safety workers. Morbidity and Mortality Weekly Report 38 (S–6): 1–37

Centers for Disease Control 1991 Recommendations for preventing transmission of human immunodeficiency virus and hepatitis B virus to patients during exposure-prone procedures. Morbidity and Mortality Weekly Report 40: 2–3

Chan P, Lewis A A M 1989 Influence of suture technique on surgical glove perforation. British Journal of Surgery 76: 1208–1209

Choudhury R P, Cleator, S J 1992 An examination of needlestick injury rates, hepatitis B vaccination uptake and instruction on 'sharps' technique among medical students. Journal of Hospital Infection 22: 143–148

Chriske H W, Abdo R, Richrath R, Braumann S 1990 Risk of hepatitis A infection among sewage workers. Arbeitsmedizin, Sozialmedizin, Praventivmedizin 25: 285–287

Clarke S E R, Caul E O, Jancar J, Gordon-Russell J B 1984 Hepatitis B in seven hospitals for the mentally handicapped. Journal of Infection 8: 34–43

Cockcroft A 1991 Surgeons who test positive for the e antigen of hepatitis B should be transferred to low-risk duties. Reviews in Medical Virology 1: 195–200

Cockcroft A, Soper P, Insall C et al 1990 Antibody response following hepatitis B immunization in a group of health care workers. British Journal of Industrial Medicine 47: 199–202

Collins C H, Kennedy D A 1987 Microbiological hazards of occupational needlestick and 'sharps' injuries. Journal of Applied Microbiology 62: 385–402

Crosse B A, Teale C, Lees E M 1989 Hepatitis B markers in West Yorkshire firemen. Epidemiology and Infection 103: 383–385

Cummins A J, Tedder R S 1992 Inadequate information on needlestick accidents. Lancet 339: 1178–1179

Dankert J, Uitentuis J, Houwen B et al 1976 Hepatitis B surface antigen in environmental samples from haemodialysis units. Journal of Infectious Diseases 134: 123–127

Dembert M L, A-Shaffer R, Baugh N L, Berg S W, Zajdowicz T 1987 Epidemiology of viral hepatitis among US navy and marine personnel, 1984–85. American Journal of Public Health 77: 1446–1447

Department of Health 1981 Chief Medical Officer's Letter (CMO (81) 11). Department of Health, London

Department of Health 1990 Guidance for clinical health care workers: protection against infection with HIV and hepatitis viruses. HMSO, London

Department of Health, Joint Committee on Vaccination and Immunisation 1990 Immunisation against infectious disease. HMSO, London

Dienstag J L, Ryan D M 1982 Occupational exposure to hepatitis B virus in hospital personnel: infection or immunization? American Journal of Epidemiology 115: 26–39

Donchin M, Shouval D 1992 Occupational and non-occupational hepatitis B virus infection among hospital employees in Jerusalem: a basis for immunisation strategy. British Journal of Industrial Medicine 49: 620–625

Drusin L M, Sohmer M, Groshen S L, Spiritos M D, Senterfit L B, Christenson W N 1987 Nosocomial hepatitis A infection in a paediatric intensive care unit. Archives of Disease in Childhood 62: 690–695

Dusheiko G M, Smith M, Scheuer P J 1990 Hepatitis C virus transmitted by human bite. Lancet 336: 503–504

Edgar W M, Campbell A D 1985 Nosocomial infection with hepatitis A. Journal of Infection 10: 43–47

Elford J, Cockcroft A 1991 Compulsory HIV antibody testing, universal precautions and the perceived risk of HIV: a survey among medical students and consultant staff at a London teaching hospital. AIDS Care 3: 151–158

Embil J A, Manley K, White L A 1989 Hepatitis A: a serological study in the Canadian armed forces. Military Medicine 154: 461–465

Evans M R, Henderson D K, Bennett J E 1990 Potential for laboratory exposures to biohazardous agents found in blood. American Journal of Public Health 80: 423–427

Fagan E A, Tolley P, Smith H M et al 1987 Hepatitis B vaccine: immunogenicity and follow-up including two year booster doses in high risk health care personnel in a London teaching hospital. Journal of Medical Virology 21: 49–56

Fahey B J, Koziol D E, Banks S M, Henderson D K 1991 Frequency of nonparenteral occupational exposures to blood and body fluids before and after universal precautions training. The American Journal of Medicine 90: 145–153

Follett E A, Sleigh J D 1980 Hepatitis B as a hazard to laboratory staff: a reappraisal. Journal of Clinical Pathology 33: 1017–1020

Gerberding J L, Littell C, Tarkington A, Brown A, Schecter W P 1990 Risk of exposure of surgical personnel to patients' blood during surgery at San Francisco General Hospital. New England Journal of Medicine 322: 1788–1793

Gerlich W H, Thomssen R 1982 Outbreak of hepatitis B at a butcher's shop. Deutsche Medizin Wochenschrift 107: 1627–1630

Gesemann M, Scheiermann N 1989 Timing of booster doses of hepatitis B vaccine. Lancet ii: 1274

Gilks W R, Hall A J, Day N E 1989 Timing of booster doses of hepatitis B vaccine. Lancet ii: 1273–1274

Gioannini P, Sinicco A, Cariti G, Lucchini A, Paggi G, Giachino O 1988 HIV infection acquired by a nurse. European Journal of Epidemiology 4: 119–120

Goldsmith R S, Zakaria S, Zakaria M S et al 1989 Occupational exposure to hepatitis B virus in hospital personnel in Cairo, Egypt. Acta Trop 46: 283–290

Gompertz S 1990 Needle-stick injuries in medical students. Journal of the Society of Occupational Medicine 40: 19–20

Gordin F M, Gibert C, Harold H P, Willoughby A 1990 Prevalence of human immunodeficiency virus and hepatitis B virus in unselected hospital admissions: implications for mandatory testing and universal precautions. Journal of Infectious Diseases 161: 14–17

Grady G F, Lee V A, Prince A M et al 1978 Hepatitis B immune globulin for accidental exposures among medical personnel: final report of a multicenter controlled trial. Journal of Infectious Diseases 138: 625–638

Hadler S C, Doto I L, Maynard J E et al 1985 Occupational risk of hepatitis B infection in hospital workers. Infection Control 6: 24–31

Hadler S C, Francis D P, Maynard J E et al 1986 Long-term immunogenicity and efficacy of hepatitis B vaccine in homosexual men. New England Journal of Medicine 315: 209–214

Hamilton J D, Larke B, Qizilbash A 1976 Transmission of hepatitis B by a human bite: an occupational hazard. Canadian Medical Association Journal 115: 439–440

Hansen J P, Falconer J A, Hamilton J D, Herpok F J 1981 Hepatitis B in a medical center. Journal of Occupational Medicine 23: 338–342

Harris A A, Daly-Gawenda D, Hudson E K 1991 Vaccine choice and programme participation rates when two hepatitis B vaccines are offered. Journal of Occupational Medicine 33: 804–807

Health Services Advisory Committee 1991a Safety in health service laboratories: safe working and the prevention of infection in clinical laboratories. HMSO, London

Health Services Advisory Committee 1991b Safety in health service laboratories: safe working and the prevention of infection in the mortuary and post-mortem room. HMSO, London

Helmsing P J, Duermeyer W, Van Hattem G C A M, Wielaard F 1980 Outbreak of hepatitis A in an institution for the mentally retarded. Journal of Medical Virology 5: 143–150

Henderson D K, Fahey B J, Willy M W 1990 Risk for

occupational transmission of human immunodeficiency virus type 1 (HIV-1) associated with clinical exposures: a prospective evaluation. Annals of Internal Medicine 113: 740–746
Heptonstall J 1991 Outbreaks of hepatitis B virus infection associated with infected surgical staff. Communicable Disease Report 1: R81–R85
Herbert A-M, Walker D M, Davies K J, Bagg J 1992 Occupationally acquired hepatitis C virus infection. Lancet 339: 305
Hinton A E, Herdman R C, Timms M S 1991 Incidence and prevention of conjunctival contamination with blood during hazardous surgical procedures. Annals of the Royal College of Surgeons of England 73: 239–242
Hofmann F, Koster D, Schrenk C, Wehrle G, Berthold H 1990 Hepatitis A: an occupational risk for health service employees? Arbeitsmedizin, Sozialmedizin, Praventivmedizin 25: 76–79
Hofmann H, Kunz C 1990 Low risk of health care workers for infection with hepatitis C virus. Infection 18: 286–288
Hoofnagle J H, Seeff L B, Bales Z B, Wright E C, Zimmerman H J 1979 Passive–active immunity from hepatitis B immune globulin. Annals of Internal Medicine 91: 813–818
Humphries P J 1990 Safe blood collection. Laboratory Practice 39: 91–92
Hunter S 1991 Hepatitis jabs are injection of common sense. Hospital Doctor 3 October: 21
Hussain S A, Latif A B A, Choudhary A A A A 1988 Risk to surgeons: a survey of accidental injuries during operations. British Journal of Surgery 75: 314–316
Hyams K C, Palinkas L A, Burr R G 1989 Viral hepatitis in the US navy, 1975–1984. American Journal of Epidemiology 130: 319–326
Iserson K V, Criss E A 1985 Hepatitis B prevalence in emergency physicians. Annals of Emergency Medicine 14: 119–122
Jilg W, Schmidt M, Deinhardt F, Zachoval R 1984 Hepatitis B vaccination: how long does protection last? Lancet ii: 458
Jochen A B B 1992 Occupationally acquired hepatitis C infection. Lancet 339: 304
Kashiwagi S, Hayashi J, Ikematsu H et al 1985 Prevalence of immunologic markers of hepatitis A and B infection in hospital personnel in Miyazaki Prefecture, Japan. American Journal of Epidemiology 122: 960–969
Kelen G D, DiGiovanni T A, Celentano D D et al 1990 Adherence to universal (barrier) precautions during interventions on critically ill and injured emergency department patients. Journal of Acquired Immune Deficiency Syndromes 3: 987–994
Kennedy S 1991 An elementary mistake? British Medical Journal 302: 1614
Kingham J G C, McGuire M, Paine D H D, Wright R 1978 Hepatitis B in a hospital for the mentally subnormal in southern England. British Medical Journal ii: 594–596
Kingston P J, Brookes B L 1988 An NHS hospital and district based field trial of the 'sterimatic safety needle': a device designed to prevent needlestick injuries (STD/88/17). Department of Health, London
Kiyosawa K, Sodeyama T, Tanaka E et al 1991 Hepatitis C in hospital employees with needlestick injuries. Annals of Internal Medicine 115: 367–369
Klein R S, Freeman K, Taylor P E, Stevens C E 1991 Occupational risk for hepatitis C virus infection among New York City dentists. Lancet 338: 1539–1542
Kunches L M, Craven D E, Werner B G, Jacobs L M 1983 Hepatitis B exposure in emergency medical personnel: prevalence of serologic markers and need for immunization. American Journal of Medicine 75: 269–272
Lahaye D, Strauss P, Baleux C, Van Ganse W 1987 Cost–benefit analysis of hepatitis-B vaccination. Lancet ii: 441–443
Lettau L A, Smith J D, Williams D et al 1986 Transmission of hepatitis B with resultant restriction of surgical practice. Journal of the American Medical Association 255: 934–937
Lim D J, Lingao A, Macasaet A 1986 Sero-epidemiological study on hepatitis A and B virus infection among dentists in the Philippines. International Dental Journal 36: 215–218
Lowenfels A B, Wormser G P, Jain R 1989 Frequency of puncture injuries in surgeons and estimated risk of HIV infection. Archives of Surgery 124: 1284–1286
Lowry P W, Levine R, Stroup D F, Gunn R A, Wilder M H, Konigsberg C 1989 Hepatitis A outbreak on a floating restaurant in Florida, 1986. American Journal of Epidemiology 129: 155–164
McGeer A, Sinor A E, Low D E 1990 Epidemiology of needlestick injuries in house officers. Journal of Infectious Diseases 162: 961–964
McGregor M A, Cowie V A, Wassef E, Veasey D, Munro J 1988 Hepatitis B in a hospital for the mentally subnormal in South Wales. Journal of Mental Deficiency Research 32: 75–77
McLean A A, Monahan G R, Finkelstein D M 1987 Public health briefs: Prevalence of hepatitis B serologic markers in community hospital personnel. American Journal of Public Health 77: 998–999
MacQuarrie M B, Forghani B, Wolochow D A 1974 Hepatitis B transmitted by a human bite. Journal of the American Medical Association 230: 723–724
Masuko K, Mitsui T, Iwano K et al 1985 Factors influencing postexposure immunoprophylaxis of hepatitis B virus infection with hepatitis B immune globulin. Gastroenterology 88: 151–155
Matta H, Thompson A M, Rainey J B 1988 Does wearing two pairs of gloves protect theatre staff from skin contamination? British Medical Journal 297: 597–598
Mauskopf J A, Bradley C J, French M T 1991 Benefit–cost analysis of hepatitis B vaccine programs for occupationally exposed workers. Journal of Occupational Medicine 33: 691–698
Mayo-Smith M F 1987 Type non-A, non-B and type B hepatitis transmitted by a single needlestick. American Journal of Infection Control 15: 266–267
Mijch A M, Barnes R, Crowe S M, Dimitrakakis M, Lucas C R 1987 An outbreak of hepatitis B and D in butchers. Scandinavian Journal of Infectious Diseases 19: 179–184
Morgan-Capner P, Hudson P 1988 Hepatitis B markers in Lancashire police officers. Epidemiology of Infection 100: 145–151
Morgan-Capner P, Wallice P D B 1990 Hepatitis B markers in ambulance personnel in Lancashire. Journal of the Society of Occupational Medicine 40: 21–22
Morris D J 1989 Timing of booster doses of hepatitis B vaccine. Lancet ii: 1274–1275
Mortimer P P, Cohen B J, Litton P A et al 1989 Hepatitis C virus antibody. Lancet ii: 798

Newman C P S, Hambling M H 1992 Hazardous incidents and immunity to hepatitis B. Communicable Disease Report 2: R30–R31

Nommensen F E, Go S T, MacLaren D M 1989 Half-life of HBs antibody after hepatitis B vaccination: an aid to timing of booster vaccination. Lancet ii: 847–849

Oakley K, Gooch C, Cockcroft A 1992 Review of management of incidents involving exposure to blood in a London teaching hospital 1989–91. British Medical Journal 304: 949–951

O'Dowd T C, O'Dowd S M M 1990 Precautions taken by orthopaedic surgeons to avoid infection with HIV and hepatitis B virus. British Medical Journal 301: 440–441

Panililio A L, Foy D R, Edwards J R et al 1991 Blood contacts during surgical procedures. Journal of the American Medical Association 265: 1533–1537

Parry C M, Harries A D, Beeching N J, Rothburn M M 1991 Phlebotomy in inoculation risk patients: a questionnaire survey of knowledge and practices of hospital doctors in Liverpool. Journal of Hospital Infection 18: 313–318

Pattison C P, Maynard J E, Berquist K R et al 1973 Serological and epidemiological studies of hepatitis B in haemodialysis units. Lancet 2: 172–174

Pattison C P, Boyer K M, Maynard J E, Kelly P C 1974 Epidemic hepatitis in a clinical laboratory: possible association with computer card handling. Journal of the American Medical Association 230: 854–857

Pepe P E, Hollinger F B, Troisi C L, Heiberg D 1986 Viral hepatitis risk in urban emergency medical services personnel. Annals of Emergency Medicine 15: 454–457

Perrillo R P 1985 Screening of health care workers before hepatitis B vaccination: more questions than answers. Annals of Internal Medicine 103: 793–795

Peterkin M, Crawford R J 1986 Hepatitis B vaccine for police forces? Lancet ii: 1458–1459

Polakoff S 1986a Acute viral hepatitis B: laboratory reports 1980–4. British Medical Journal 293: 37–38

Polakoff S 1986b Acute hepatitis B in patients in Britain related to previous operations and dental treatment. British Medical Journal 293: 33–36

Polakoff S 1989 Acute viral hepatitis B: laboratory reports 1985–8. Communicable Diseases Report 29: 3–6

Polakoff S, Tillett H E 1982 Acute viral hepatitis B: laboratory reports 1975–9. British Medical Journal 284: 1881–1882

Polish L B, Shapiro C N, Bauer F et al 1992 Nosocomial transmission of hepatitis B virus associated with the use of a spring-loaded finger-stick device. New England Journal of Medicine 326: 721–725

Porteous M J LeF 1990 Operating practices of and precautions taken by orthopaedic surgeons to avoid infection with HIV and hepatitis B virus during surgery. British Medical Journal 301: 167–169

Raahave D, Bremmelgaard A 1991 New operative technique to reduce surgeons' risk of HIV infection. Journal of Hospital Infection 18: 177–183

Radvan G H, Hewson E G, Berenger S, Brookman D J 1986 The Newcastle hepatitis B outbreak: observations on cause, management, and prevention. Medical Journal of Australia 144: 461–464

Reingold A L, Kane M A, Hightower A W 1988 Failure of gloves and other protective devices to prevent transmission of hepatitis B virus to oral surgeons. Journal of the American Medical Association 259: 2558–2560

Remis R S, Rossignol M A, Kane M A 1987 Hepatitis B infection in a day school for mentally retarded students: transmission from students to staff. American Journal of Public Health 77: 1183–1186

Richmond P W, McCabe M, Davies J P, Thomas D M 1992 Perforation of gloves in an accident and emergency department. British Medical Journal 304: 879–880

Rosenblum L S, Villarino M E, Nainan O V et al 1991 Hepatitis A infection in a neonatal intensive care unit: risk factors for transmission and evidence of prolonged viral excretion among preterm infants. Journal of Infectious Diseases 164: 476–482

Royal College of Nursing 1987 Introduction to hepatitis B and nursing guidelines for infection control. Report of the RCN Safety Representatives Conference Coordinating Committee. RCN, London

Royal College of Obstetricians and Gynaecologists 1990 HIV infection in maternity care and gynaecology. Royal College of Obstetricians and Gynaecologists, London

Royal College of Surgeons of England 1990 A statement by the college on AIDS and HIV infection. Royal College of Surgeons of England, London

Sanchez-Quijano A, Pineda J A, Lissen E et al 1988 Prevention of post-transfusion non-A, non-B hepatitis by non-specific immunoglobulin in heart surgery patients. Lancet i: 1245–1249

Schlipkoter U, Roggendorf M, Cholmakow K, Weise A, Deinhardt F 1990 Transmission of hepatitis C virus (HCV) from a haemodialysis patient to a medical staff member. Scandinavian Journal of Infectious Diseases 22: 757–758

Schoub B D, Johnson S, McAnerney J, Blackburn N K, Padayachee G N 1991 Exposure to hepatitis B virus among South African health care workers: implications for pre-immunisation screening. South African Medical Journal 79: 27–29

Scully C, Matthews R 1990 Uptake of hepatitis B immunisation among United Kingdom dental students. Health Trends 22: 92

Seeff L B 1991 Hepatitis C from a needlestick injury. Annals of Internal Medicine 115: 411

Seeff L B, Wright E C, Zimmerman H J et al 1978 Type B hepatitis after needle-stick exposure: prevention with hepatitis immune globulin. Final report of the Veterans Administration: Cooperative Study. Annals of Internal Medicine 88: 285–293

Shanson D C, Cockcroft A 1991 Forum: Testing patients for HIV antibodies is useful for infection control purposes. Reviews in Medical Virology 1: 5–9

Siebke J C, Wessel N, Kvandal P, Lie T 1989 The prevalence of hepatitis A and B in Norwegian merchant seamen: a serological study. Infection 17: 77–80

Sim A J W 1991 Towards safer surgery. Journal of Hospital Infection 18: 184–190

Skinhoj P, Hollinger F B et al 1981 Infectious liver diseases in three groups of Copenhagen workers: correlation of hepatitis A infection to sewage exposure. Archives of Environmental Health 36: 139–143

Smith J W, Nichols R L 1991 Barrier efficiency of surgical gowns: are we really protected from our patients' pathogens? Archives of Surgery 126: 756–763

Spence M R, Dash G P 1990 Hepatitis B: perceptions, knowledge and vaccine acceptance among registered nurses

in high-risk occupations in a university hospital. Infection Control in Hospitals and Epidemiology 11: 129–133
Statutory Instruments 1988 The control of substances hazardous to health regulations. HMSO, London
Strickler A C, Bradshaw E D 1987 Prevalence of hepatitis B markers in occupational health nurses. Journal of Occupational Medicine 29: 685–687
Struve J, Aronsson B, Frenning B, Forsgren M, Weiland O 1992 Prevalence of hepatitis B virus markers and exposure to occupational risks likely to be associated with acquisition of hepatitis B virus among health care workers in Stockholm. Journal of Infection 24: 147–156
Tant M, Gerkin R, Englender S J et al 1991 Inadequate immune response among public safety workers receiving intradermal vaccination against hepatitis B – United States, 1990–1991. Morbidity and Mortality Weekly Report 40: 569–572
Thomson R G, Rawlins M D, James O F W, Tyrer S P, Codd A 1989 Low prevalence of hepatitis B in mental handicap hospital. Lancet i: 44–45
Tilzey A J, Palmer S J, Barrow S et al 1992 Clinical trial with inactivated hepatitis A vaccine and recommendations for its use. British Medical Journal 304: 1272–1276
Tokars J, Bell D, Marcus R et al 1991 Percutaneous injuries during surgical procedures. Proceedings of the VII International Conference on AIDS, Vol 2, Florence, Italy, p 83
Tsega E, Krawczynski K, Hansson B-G et al 1991 Outbreak of acute hepatitis E virus infection among military personnel in Northern Ethiopia. Journal of Medical Virology 34: 232–236
Turner S B, Kunches L M, Gordon K F, Travers P H, Mueller N E 1989 Public health briefs: Occupational exposure to human immunodeficiency virus (HIV) and hepatitis B virus among embalmers: a pilot seroprevalence study. American Journal of Public Health 79: 1425–1426
Vaglia A, Nicolin R, Puro V, Ippolito G, Bettini C, de Valla F 1990 Needlestick hepatitis C virus seroconversion in a surgeon. Lancet 336: 1315–1316
Valenzuela T D, Hook E W, Copass M K, Corey L 1985 Occupational exposure to hepatitis B in paramedics. Archives of Internal Medicine 145: 1976–1977
Van-Damme P, de-Cock G, Cramm M, Eylenbosch W 1990 Precautions taken by orthopaedic surgeons to avoid infection with HIV and hepatitis B virus. British Medical Journal 301: 611
Vernon A A, Schable C, Francis D 1982 A large outbreak of hepatitis A in a day-care center. American Journal of Epidemiology 115: 325–331
Waldron H A 1990 Antibody response to hepatitis B vaccination. British Journal of Industrial Medicine 47: 354–355
Watt A D 1987 Hairdressers and hepatitis B: a risk of inapparent parenteral infection. Journal of the Society of Occupational Medicine 37: 124–125
Welch J, Tilzey A J, Bertrand J, Bott E C A, Banatvala J E 1988 Risk to Metropolitan police officers from exposure to hepatitis B. British Medical Journal 297: 835–836
Welch J, Webster M, Tilzey A J, Noah N D, Banatvala J E 1989 Hepatitis B infections after gynaecological surgery. Lancet i: 205–207
Werner B A, Grady G F 1982 Accidental hepatitis B surface antigen positive inoculations. Annals of Internal Medicine 97: 367–369
Werner B A, Dienstag J L, Kuter B J et al 1985 Isolated antibody to hepatitis B surface antigen and response to hepatitis B vaccination. Annals of Internal Medicine 103: 201–205
West D J 1984 The risk of hepatitis B infection among health professionals in the United States: a review. The American Journal of the Medical Sciences 287: 26–33
Williams J R, Flowerdew A D S 1990 Uptake of immunisation against hepatitis B among surgeons in Wessex Regional Health Authority. British Medical Journal 301: 154
Williams S, Gooch C, Cockcroft A 1993 Hepatitis B immunization and exposure to blood among surgical staff. British Journal of Surgery 80: 714–716
Williams S, Cockcroft A 1992 Policies for HIV and hepatitis B infected health care workers. Occupational Health Review 36: 12–14
Wood A 1989 Hepatitis B vaccination and GPs. Practitioner 233: 1067–1068
Wright J G, McGeer A J, Chyatte D, Ransohoff D F 1991 Mechanisms of glove tears and sharp injuries among surgical personnel. Journal of the American Medical Association 266: 1668–1671
Zuckerman A J 1984 Who should be immunised against hepatitis B? British Medical Journal 289: 1243–1244

UPDATE

- New UK guidelines about hepatitis B and health care workers were published in August 1993:

  Department of Health 1993 Protecting health care workers and their patients from hepatitis B. Department of Health, London

32. Neonatal and paediatric infection

G.V. Gregorio G. Mieli-Vergani A.P. Mowat

Viral hepatitis in neonates and children constitutes a wide spectrum of disease from an acute asymptomatic infection to widespread necrosis and inflammation leading to hepatic failure. The clinical symptoms and the course of hepatitis are influenced by the age of the patient and the status of the immune system. Most cases of viral hepatitis are caused by hepatotropic viruses considered in detail elsewhere in this volume. This chapter will concentrate on paediatric aspects of such infections.

Of greatest practical significance is the frequently ineffective immune response to hepatitis B virus (HBV) infection during the first 2 years of life with a propensity to produce an asymptomatic chronic carrier state with all its sequelae in more than 80% of those infected. Liver involvement may also occur as part of a disseminated viral disease (Table 32.1). The susceptibility of the fetus and infant to infection makes viral agents an important cause of hepatitis syndrome of infancy (Table 32.2). In certain geographic areas, the exotic viruses may cause clinically important hepatic disease in children. Developments in our knowledge of hepatic aspects of both forms of infection are reviewed.

HEPATITIS A VIRUS (HAV)

Prevalence

The distribution of the disease is worldwide. It is endemic in early childhood in areas with poor living conditions and low socioeconomic status. Seropositivity to HAV was noted in 70% of children 3–4 years of age in Liberia (Prince et al 1985) and in 76% of children between 9 and 11 years in Venezuela (Amesty-Valbuena et al 1991).

Table 32.1 Hepatic pathology occurring with viral infections in children

Aetiology	Acute liver disease	Fulminant hepatic failure	Chronic liver disease	Cirrhosis	Hepatocellular carcinoma
Hepatitis A virus	+	+	–	–	–
Hepatitis B virus	+	+	+	+	+
Hepatitis C virus	+	+	+	+	–
Hepatitis D virus*	+	+	+	+	–
Hepatitis E virus	+	+	–	–	–
Cytomegalovirus	+	+	+	+	–
Epstein–Barr virus	+	+	+	–	–
Herpes simplex	+	+	–	–	–
Varicella zoster	+	+	–	–	–
Coxsackie	+	+	–	–	–
Adenovirus	+	+	–	–	–
Rubella	+	–	–	–	–

* In association with hepatitis B virus.
+, reported; –, not reported.

Table 32.2 Infections associated with hepatitis syndrome of infancy

Aetiological agent	Antecedent history	Diagnostic investigations	Extrahepatic manifestations	Remarks
Primary hepatotrophic viruses				
Hepatitis A virus (HAV)	Neonatal intensive care (NICU) epidemics	Anti-HAV IgM	None reported	Usually asymptomatic
Hepatitis B virus (HBV)	HBsAg-positive mothers	HBsAg	None reported	Usually asymptomatic; rarely acuteicteric or fulminant hepatitis
Hepatitis C virus (HCV)	Anti-HCV-positive mothers; infants of HIV and i.v. drug abusers	HCV by PCR; demonstration of HCV antigen in the liver		More common if with maternal co-infection with HIV
Hepatitis D virus (HDV)	Anti-HDV-positive mothers	Anti-HDV IgM; HDV antigen in the hepatocytes		Needs co-infection with HBV to manifest the disease
Cytomegalovirus (CMV)	Maternal primary or recurrent CMV infection	CMV-specific IgM; viral isolation in urine or saliva; cytomegalic inclusion bodies in hepatocytes	Microcephaly; intracranial calcifications; choreoretinitis	
Epstein–Barr virus (EBV)	Maternal primary or recurrent EBV infection	Anti-EBV IgM	Low birth weight; congenital anomalies	
Systemic viruses				
Rubella	Maternal infection, especially in the first trimester of pregnancy	Anti-rubella IgM; viral isolation from pharyngeal secretions, urine, CSF	'Blueberry skin lesions'; cataract; heart disease	
Herpes simplex virus (HSV)	Maternal HSV, especially in the genitalia	HSV-specific IgM; viral isolation from vesicular fluid, CSF, liver	Skin vesicles; keratoconjunctivitis; encephalitis	
Varicella zoster virus (VZV)	Maternal varicella less than 5 days before to 7 days after delivery	VZV-specific IgM, viral isolation from vesicular fluid, liver	Skin vesicles; pneumonitis	
Adenovirus	Vaginal delivery; premature rupture of membrane; maternal upper respiratory tract infection	Neutralizing or complement-fixing antibody to adenovirus; viral isolation in the liver	Thrombocytopaemia; coagulopathy; pneumonia	
Coxsackie	Epidemics of enteroviral disease in the community	Viral isolation in faeces, blood, CSF	Myocarditis; meningoencephalitits; pneumonitis; generalized myositis	
Human immuno-deficiency virus (HIV)	HIV-positive mothers	Anti-HIV IgM	Lymphadenopathy; intrauterine growth retardation	

The mean age of infection increases with improvement in sanitation. In Thailand, with its economic growth and improved levels of public sanitation over the last 15 years, the antibody prevalence to hepatitis A among children 10–15 years old has fallen from 50–70% in 1977 to 20–25% in 1992 (Innis et al 1991, Yong 1992). In Hong Kong the prevalence of anti-HAV antibody has declined over the last 10 years from 45% to 17% for children between 11 and 20 years old (Chin et al 1991). In the UK, only 8% of 102 medical students (age 19–31) have serological evidence of past HAV infection (Zuckerman et al 1991).

Transmission of the disease is mainly by faecal contamination of drinking water or food. Epidemics and sporadic cases of HAV in developed countries are usually associated with infected food handlers and contaminated food or water (Gust & Feinstone 1988). Shellfish is frequently implicated (Gust 1988). Outbreaks of hepatitis A have been described in daycare centres (Garcia Puga et al 1989, Hadler & McFarland 1986) and institutions for mentally retarded children (Shimizu et al 1984). Very rarely, parenteral transmission of hepatitis A has been implicated in neonatal intensive care unit (NICU) outbreaks. A single unit of blood transfused caused hepatitis in 11 neonates (Noble et al 1984). In the more recent hepatitis A outbreak in an NICU in Hawaii (Rosenblum et al 1991), the index case was an infant who received a blood transfusion from a donor in the prodromal phase of HAV infection. Both reports have shown a secondary nosocomial faecal–oral transmission to other neonates. A nurse who attended to a patient with HAV infection was implicated in the later study. Prolonged HAV shedding (for up to 4–5 months after infection) among preterms may have contributed.

Transplacental infection with HAV has not been reported. During an epidemic of hepatitis A affecting 431 pregnancies in Shanghai, China, no neonate had detectable anti-HAV IgM (Ye 1990).

Clinical features

Asymptomatic infection has been described in 84% of those infected between 1 and 2 years old (Hadler et al 1980). In a detailed prospective study of 20 000 Thai schoolchildren, aged 2–16 years, eight patients showed clinical or biochemical evidence of liver disease, while 27 had inapparent infections with no elevation of aspartate aminotransferase (AST) detected (Innis et al 1992). The clinical cases of HAV are usually seen in older children, as demonstrated during an epidemic in China where the ratio of clinical to subclinical cases was reported at 1.4:1, with the mean age of clinical and subclinical cases 5.9 (3.4) and 4.5 (2.8) years respectively (Sun et al 1988).

After a prodromal period of 4–10 days, bilirubinuria is usually the first sign of liver disease, followed by jaundice and pale faeces 1–2 days later. The following clinical features were recorded in 281 cases (age 3 months to 12 years): jaundice (99%), tea-coloured urine (85%), anorexia (83%), lethargy (81%), vomiting (72%), abdominal pain (64%), fever (57%), diarrhoea (18%), pale faeces (17%), rash (7%) and arthritis (5%) (Chow et al 1989). Liver function tests returned to normal slowly. 33, 63, 76, 95, 97 and 100% normalized at 1, 3, 6, 9, 12 and 18 months after onset, respectively. Atypically, three children with HAV infection had clinical and ultrasonographic features suggestive of acute cholecystitis (Hermier et al 1985). Enlargement of lymph nodes located in the hepatic hilum, pancreatic area and lesser omentum was demonstrated by abdominal ultrasound in all 58 children who had acute HAV infection (Topper et al 1990). The majority (99.9%) of children with HAV infection recover completely.

Complications

As in adults, the most serious complication of the disease is fulminant hepatic failure, which is heralded by recurrence of initial symptoms, mental confusion, bleeding manifestations and progressively deepening jaundice. In one hospital-based study, fatal fulminant hepatitis A was reported in 3 of 2174 (0.14%) patients. Two were children, aged 5 and 15 years (McNeill et al 1984). The survival of patients with grade III–IV hepatic encephalopathy with specialized intensive care was 67% (O'Grady et al 1988).

In 3–20% of patients with icteric hepatitis, a relapse may occur within 2–12 weeks after initial improvement of their liver function tests (Glikson et al 1992). Such an episode has been described in 23 children who had a second rise in alanine aminotransferase (ALT) levels from 15–90 days after complete resolution of their initial clinical symptoms. In nine patients, there was a third ALT peak 15–40 days after the second rise (Chiriaco et al 1986). During the relapse, only 4 of the 23 children had recurrence of jaundice, and all patients recovered completely after a mean of 81 (33) days. HAV in the stool has been demonstrated during the episode of relapse, implicating HAV as the causative agent of relapsing hepatitis (Sjögren et al 1987).

Fulminant hepatitis requiring liver transplantation has been described during relapse, which suggests an extrahepatic site of viral replication (Fagan et al 1990). Persistent HAV infection was reported in a 4-year-old boy as evidenced by the presence of the HAV antigen in the liver 5 months after infection (van der Anker et al 1988). HAV infection has not been shown to cause a chronic carrier state.

A newly recognized atypical manifestation of HAV infection is the possible triggering of autoimmune chronic active hepatitis (ACAH) (Vento et al 1991). 58 healthy relatives of 13 patients with ACAH were investigated and 14 relatives with no serological evidence of past HAV infection had a defect in the suppressor–inducer T lymphocyte specific for the asialoglycoprotein receptor (ASGPR). During a 4-year follow-up, 3 subclinical cases of acute hepatitis A occurred, but only the 2 with T-cell suppressor inducer defect evolved into icteric autoimmune hepatitis requiring long-term corticosteroid treatment.

Prevention

Active immunization against HAV infection is now possible with the use of formalin-inactivated hepatitis A vaccine derived from the HM175 (Sjögren et al 1991) or CR 325F' virus strains. In 38 000 Thai schoolchildren aged 2–16 years given either HAV or HBV vaccine at 0, 1 and 12 months, HAV vaccine was shown to protect against infection in 97% of recipients (Innis et al 1992). Vaccine protection against both disease and infection occurred 1 month after administration of two doses and persisted for at least a year. The vaccine has been shown to be safe and well tolerated. The most common reaction is soreness at the site of injection.

In a placebo-controlled study in a Jewish community in New York of 1037 healthy children aged 2–16 years, 0.6 ml of a single vaccine, equivalent to 25 units of HAV antigen, completely prevented hepatitis A infection after 21 days. 34 clinical cases occurred in those receiving placebo, with none in the vaccine recipients. Only 1 of 305 recipients had undetectable antibodies 1 month after vaccination (Werzberger et al 1992).

HEPATITIS B VIRUS (HBV)

Prevalence

Hepatitis B infection is a major public health problem with an estimated 300 million HBsAg carriers worldwide. It is primarily a disease of childhood in endemic areas of the world such as Africa and China, where 15–20% of the population are HBsAg carriers (Beasley et al 1982). Infection in the perinatal period or early infancy occurs in 40% of infants in Taiwan, but in only 1–5% in sub-Saharan Africa. The difference is in part explained by the higher prevalence of HBeAg in Chinese (40%) than African (15%) mothers. In Africa, the majority of infections are acquired between 6 months and 6 years of age with other family members implicated as a source of infection (Kiire 1990).

In areas of intermediate endemicity (Italy, Japan, Spain, Greece, Portugal), where 2–10% of the population are HBsAg carriers, infection occurs in both adults and children. In Italy, the HBsAg carrier rate among pregnant women was reported at 5% and the prevalence of hepatitis B markers in children less than 11 years was 1.7%. (Stroffolini et al 1989). In areas of low endemicity (North west Europe, North America, UK, Australia), infection in infancy and childhood is uncommon and <1% of the population has chronic HBV infection (Maynard et al 1988).

Transmission

Infection is either blood-borne or through contaminated body fluids. The mode of transmission is by parenteral (i.e. blood transfusion) or percutaneous exposure (i.e. use of unsterilized instruments, tattooing, acupuncture, ear piercing, etc.). Inapparent spread of infection may also occur through intimate contact with body secretions and skin lesions and sharing of household utensils among family members.

Maternal–infant transmission is an important means by which the virus is sustained in the population. The hepatitis B virus has been shown to be present at birth in 2.5% of infants born to affected mothers, representing in-utero infection (Gussetti et al 1988). One important mode of infection is inoculation of or ingestion by the newborn of infected maternal blood and vaginal secretions around the time of delivery (Lee et al 1978). The risk of infection is 26–40% if the mother is HBsAg positive only but increases to 90% if the mother is HBeAg positive (Beasley et al 1982). In the presence of maternal anti-HBe, the risk of viral transmission to the infant is only 10–20% (Tong et al 1985). Mothers with acute hepatitis B during pregnancy may likewise transmit the virus, in up to 70% if infection occurs during the third trimester of pregnancy and 90% if it occurs within 8 days of delivery (Flower & Tanner 1984). There is no increased risk of abortion or malformation.

Clinical features

More than 80% of infants born to HBeAg– and HBsAg– positive mothers become chronic carriers (Stevens et al 1979). Rarely, infection during the perinatal period may cause an acute icteric or fulminant hepatitis.

Acute hepatitis. For children who develop symptomatic acute hepatitis B infection, by either perinatal or horizontal transmission, clinical features may include jaundice (97%), tea-coloured urine (79%), lethargy (69%), anorexia (55%), fever (52%) and vomiting (45%). The clinical course is more insidious than hepatitis A infection (Chow et al 1989). Extrahepatic manifestations may herald the disease, including arthritis (14%) and skin eruptions (10%), i.e. maculopapular or urticarial rash. The arthritis is symmetrical and polyarticular involving the hands and the knees and may last for about 3 weeks (Schmacher & Ball 1974). The Gianotti–Crosti syndrome has been described with hepatitis B infection and consists of fever, lymphadenopathy, hepatomegaly and a non-pruritic, erythematous papular exanthem of the face and extremities (Kacecioglu Draelos 1986).

The majority (>90%) of children with acute hepatitis B infection recover completely. In 28 hospitalized children age 3 months to 12 years with acute hepatitis B infection followed up for at least 24 months, liver function tests returned to normal in 61% at 6 months and in 86% at 1 year. 96% cleared the HBsAg, and only one patient became a chronic carrier. Anti-HBs seroconversion occurred after 6 months in 77% and in 96% after 1 year (Chow et al 1989). Similarly, in 51 Italian children (mean age 6.3 years) with acute symptomatic hepatitis B infection, chronic evolution was only noted in four (8%) patients after 1 year of follow-up, two of whom were born to an HBsAg-positive mother (Bortolotti et al 1983).

The most dreaded complication of acute hepatitis B infection is fulminant hepatitis, which may occur in <1% but is more frequently observed when there is co-infection or superinfection with the delta agent (Farci et al 1985) (see Hepatitis D section). Fulminant hepatitis secondary to perinatal HBV infection has been shown to occur in infants from 2–6 months of life (Chang et al 1987, Vanclaire et al 1991). Infants born to mothers who are anti-HBe positive are at a particular risk. Six of 17 (35%) Taiwanese children with fulminant hepatitis were born to mothers who were HBsAg positive, five of whom had anti-HBe seroconversion. Mutations in the pre-core region of the HBV DNA have been implicated in fulminant hepatitis B in infancy (Omata et al 1991).

60% of patients with fulminant hepatitis B die unless transplanted (O'Grady et al 1988).

Chronic hepatitis. The probability of developing chronic hepatitis B infection is increased if infection occurs early in life, if it is asymptomatic and if there is a general defect in the immune system (Maggiore et al 1983). More than 80% of infants infected during the first year of life become chronic carriers as compared with a rate of 6–10% if infection occurs after the sixth year of life (Chu et al 1985; Chang et al 1989). In a prospective study of 420 HBsAg carriers in Taiwan in whom infection was detected from <1 month to 17 years of age and observed for 1–12 years, spontaneous loss of HBsAg occurred in only 10 patients (0.6% per year) (Hsu et al 1992). Annual HBsAg clearance rate was significantly higher in those who were anti-HBe positive than those with HBeAg (1.7% *vs.* 0.4%). Carrier children whose mothers were HBsAg negative had a higher incidence of HBsAg clearance (5.6% *vs.* 0.8%). In 78 patients who underwent a liver biospy, 3 of 11 (27%) with chronic active hepatitis *vs.* 1 of 67 (1.5%) with mild histological changes (31 chronic persistent hepatitis, 33 non-specific reactive hepatitis and three with normal histology) became HBsAg negative.

Of infants who acquire HBV infection perinatally, boys have a higher risk of developing histologically aggressive disease with progression to cirrhosis. In a study in Taiwan 91% of children with severe histological changes were males (Hsu et al 1988). Similarly, all 10 Italian children with chronic HBV infection and cirrhosis at presentation were males, seven being less than 4 years of age (Bortolotti et al 1986). A male preponderance (76%) has also been found amongst children with HBV-related hepatocellular carcinoma (Hsu et al 1987).

In a longitudinal study (Lok & Lai 1988) of 51 asymptomatic HBsAg carrier children (median age: 10 years, 34 males) followed up for up to 4 years, 43 had no features of liver disease and eight had hepatomegaly. Serum ALT levels were normal in 80% at presentation and remained within the normal range in 60% during the 4-year study period. The absence of clinical features does not exclude significant pathological change (Bortolotti et al 1986). Chronic HBV infection has been associated with the following histological features at presentation in 292 Italian children: chronic active hepatitis (57%), chronic persistent hepatitis (35%), chronic lobular hepatitis (5%) and cirrhosis (3%). However, none of these 207 children with chronic hepatitis developed features of cirrhosis over a follow-up period of 1–10 years.

HBV infection may have an important role in the development of hepatocellular carcinoma (HCC) in children. In Taiwan, 51 consecutive children with HCC had detectable HBsAg, either in the blood or in the liver tissue (Hsu et al 1987). In Germany, 7 of 11 (64%) cases of HCC in childhood had positive HBsAg serology (Leuschner et al 1988). Integrated HBV DNA sequences have been found in neoplastic liver tissues of children with previous HBV infection (de Potter et al 1987).

Mechanism of liver disease

It is not clear why certain patients progress to chronicity while others clear the HBV after an acute infection. The infected lymphocytes may be unable to mount a normal immune response (Lamelin & Trepo 1990). The presence of HBsAg-specific T-suppressor cells may cause non-responsiveness to HBsAg among chronic carriers (Vento et al 1985). There is also some evidence of a genetic or acquired defect in interferon production (Abb et al 1985). In chronic hepatitis B, defective viral particles are produced in excess. Spontaneous mutation in the genome may explain the variations in the disease expression (Kosaka et al 1991).

Chronic HBV infection is more common in patients with immunodeficiency, Down's syndrome (van-Ditzhuijsen et al 1988), leukaemia (Ratner et al 1986), polyarteritis nodosa and various glomerulopathies (La Manna et al 1985).

Prevention

The administration of hepatitis B immunoglobulin and hepatitis B vaccine has been shown to prevent perinatal transmission of HBV in up to 95% of infants. In Taiwan, the prevalence of HBsAg in children less than 5 years old has decreased from 9.3% (31/332) in 1984 to 2% (9/457) in 1989 as a result of a mass hepatitis B immunization programme (Tsen 1991). Other investigations have shown that hepatitis B vaccine alone given at birth and at 1, 2 and 12 months of life may be effective in preventing perinatal transmission. Only 2 (3.6%) of 55 infants became chronically infected after 13 months of follow-up, one of whom was HBsAg from birth and the other from the first month of life (Poovorawan et al 1989). This scheme of prevention has important economic implications for countries unable to afford hepatitis B immunoglobulin. In Africa, where the majority of infection usually occurs after 5 months of life, integrating HBV vaccination into the routine childhood immunization programme (i.e. DPT series) may be the most cost-effective means of preventing infection in all but 5% of children. In areas of low endemicity the best approach is the screening of all pregnant women for HBsAg and immunization of all newborns of HBsAg-positive mothers, whether HBeAg positive or not, with specific immunoglobulin and HBV vaccine (Immunization Practices Advisory Committee 1988).

The vaccine is ineffective in infants who acquire the infection in-utero and are HBsAg positive at birth. HBV mutant strains may likewise cause HBV infection after immunization (Carman et al 1990).

Treatment

For chronic hepatitis B infection, the goal of treatment is to eradicate the virus and to ameliorate the underlying liver disease. In children as in adults, success in treatment is assessed currently by the rates of clearance of HBeAg and of seroconversion to anti-HBe, rarely to anti-HBs. Agents for which efficacy has been claimed include prednisolone, azathioprine (Giusti et al 1988), laevamisole (Fattovich et al 1982) and interferon (IFN). Only IFN has been assessed in controlled studies (Table 32.3). The different IFN trials are difficult to compare because they have employed different forms of interferon in different doses and for different duration. More important in assessing efficacy may be the difference in rates of viral replication and particularly in disease activity in the patients who were treated. The children reported in studies from Spain, for example, had histologically active disease and high transaminase levels at the beginning of treatment (La Banda et al 1988, Ruiz-Moreno et al 1991, 1992) while the Chinese children (Lai et al 1987, 1991) had inactive liver histology and low transaminase levels. A low rate of spontaneous seroconversion is more likely in the latter.

Recently, better results in Chinese children (age 2–17 years) have been achieved with a combination of prednisolone followed by recombinant alpha interferon (rIFN-α) (Lai et al 1991). In this study, only one patient in the prednisolone–IFN group and one in the control group had elevated transaminase levels prior to treatment, and thus spontaneous seroconversion was unlikely. Preliminary results of a multicentre three-armed study of steroid or placebo treatment for 4 weeks followed by human lymphoblastoid interferon (5 MU/m^2 three times weekly) for 12 weeks, mostly among Caucasian children, has shown anti-HBe seroconversion in 30% of both treatment groups versus 17% of untreated controls (G Mieli-Vergani, personal communication). Based on our present knowledge of the treatment of chronic hepatitis B infection, further studies are needed using different doses and duration of interferon with patients carefully stratified for sex, intensity of viral replication, disease activity and, if possible, duration of infection.

HEPATITIS C VIRUS (HCV)

The epidemiological and clinical features of HCV infection in children reported here are based on studies using the first-generation enzyme-linked immunosorbent assay (ELISA) for detection of antibodies to components of HCV (anti-HCV), except when stated.

Prevalence

A study of 696 children (4–14 years) in Cameroon demonstrated a 14.5% seroprevalence for anti-HCV, which increased steadily with age from 6.6% in those aged 4–6 years to 17.5% for those aged 11–14 years (Ngatchu et al 1992). The prevalence was higher in lower than upper (16% *vs.* 8%) socioeconomic groups and in rural than urban (21% *vs.* 12%) children. A prevalence rate of 0.9% was found among 4496 Saudi Arabian children (1–10 years) (Al-Faleigh et al 1991). A 95% anti-HCV seropositivity was noted among 22 haemophiliacs (age 2.5–11 years) who were regularly transfused with dry heat-treated factor concentrates as compared with no anti-HCV seroconversion in nine children who were given concentrates that were vapour or wet heat treated, effectively inactivating the virus (Blanchette

Table 32.3 Summary of randomized controlled treatment with interferon in children with chronic hepatitis B virus infection

N*	Treatment			Inclusion criteria	Results		Reference
	Drug	Dose	Duration (months)		Loss of HBV DNA (%)	Loss of HBeAg (%)	
Spanish							
8	IFN-α	7.5 MU/m^2	6	HBV DNA (+ve)/ HBeAg (+ve)/ HBsAg (+ve) for 6 months	25	12	La Banda et al 1988
8	IFN-α	10 MU/m^2	6		25	25	
8	(control group)				38	38	
12	IFN-α	5 MU/m^2	6	HBV DNA (+ve)/ increased AST for 1 year; CAH/CPH on liver biopsy	42	42	Ruiz-Moreno et al 1991
12	IFN-α	10 MU/m^2	6		58	50	
12	(control group)				17	17	
12	IFN-α followed by IFN-γ	5 MU/m^2 1 MU/m^2	3 3	HBV DNA (+ve)/ increased AST for 1 year; CAH/CPH on liver biopsy	42	25	Ruiz Moreno et al 1992
11	IFN-γ	1 MU/m^2	6		36	27	
12	(control group)				25	25	
Chinese							
12	alpha-IFN	10 MU/m^2	3	HBsAg/HBeAg/ HBA DNA (+ve)/ for 6 months	17	8.3	Lai et al 1987
12	(control group)				17	8.3	
30	IFN-α	5 MU/m^2	4	HBsAg/HBeAg/ HBV DNA (+ve) for 6 months	6.6	3.3	Lai et al 1991
30	Prednisone followed by IFN-α	0.6 mg/kg 5 MU/m^2	1.5 4		16.6	13.3	
30	(control group)				0	0	

* Number of patients.

et al 1991). In 5 of 27 (18.5%) anti-HCV-positive dialysis patients (age 25.9 ± 1.6 years), the length of time on haemodialysis and hence presumably more units of blood transfused was the most predictive factor for HCV infection (mean of 105 months for those who were anti-HCV positive *vs.* 41 months for the 22 who were anti-HCV negative) (Jonas et al 1992). HCV antibodies were found in 16 of 33 (48%) Italian children with chronic cryptogenic hepatitis (Bortolotti et al 1992). In Taiwan, 14 of 144 (9.7%) children (mean age 3 years, range 1 month to 15 years) with chronic liver disease (Ding-Shinn 1991) and 8 of 22 (36%) with NANB hepatitis were noted to have anti-HCV seroconversion (Shun-Chien et al 1991).

Clinical or laboratory features associated with infection

Asymptomatic HCV infections have been described in four infants born to mothers co-infected with

HCV and the human immunodeficiency virus (HIV), as detected by nested polymerase chain reaction (PCR). Three of the infants were HCV positive at birth but became HCV negative at 2, 7 and 27 months of life. Their transaminase levels were always within the normal range. A fourth infant was HCV negative at birth but became HCV positive with transaminase elevation from the third month of life (Novati et al 1992). Using the second-generation recombinant immunoblot assay, 22 of 43 (51%) infants born to intravenous drug users were documented to be anti-HCV seropositive, 17 infants during the first four postnatal months and five others from 6 to 18 months of life. Four of the 43 (9%) infants who were likewise infected with HIV remained seropositive for anti-HCV after 20–29 months of follow-up, with three having persistent elevation of transaminase. As no apparent source of infection could be identified, it was likely that vertical transmission of HCV occurred (Weintrub et al 1991).

Of 16 anti-HCV-positive Italian children with chronic cryptogenic hepatitis, 11 were asymptomatic at presentation while five had mild nonspecific symptoms (abdominal pain, anorexia and asthenia). Hepatomegaly was noted in six patients, splenomegaly in three. The mean ALT level at presentation was 167 ± 108 IU/l. Nine patients had a liver biopsy that showed chronic lobular/persistent hepatitis (5), chronic active hepatitis (3) and cirrhosis (1). Only 1 of 11 anti-HCV-positive patients normalized ALT on follow-up from 1–14 years (mean 5.3 ± 2.9 years), but no child developed liver failure (Bortolotti et al 1992).

Of 50 leukaemic children in long-term remission observed from 1 to 12 years, 12 (24%) patients were noted to have persistent anti-HCV reactivity using the second-generation recombinant immunoblot assay (RIBA) (Locasciulli et al 1991). In 11 of these 12 (92%) patients, the transaminase remained persistently elevated (mean peak ALT: 780 IU/l) as opposed to transaminase normalization in 10 of 11 patients with transient anti-HCV positivity and in 19 of 27 anti-HCV-negative patients. Accordingly, 14 liver biopsies done in 11 patients who were persistently anti-HCV (+) showed chronic active hepatitis (5) and chronic lobular/persistent hepatitis (9), while in 19 patients who were anti-HCV negative histological diagnosis included chronic active hepatitis (4), chronic lobular/persistent hepatitis (9) and nonspecific reactive hepatitis (6). For this group of patients, therefore, antibodies to HCV appear as markers of ongoing infection and may be useful to predict the severity and course of chronic liver disease.

The presence of HCV antibodies has been described in 80% of patients with liver–kidney microsomal (LKM) antibody type II autoimmune chronic hepatitis (Lenzi et al 1990). However, in a recent report on patients with autoimmune chronic active hepatitis (ACAH) who were anti-LKM positive, antibodies to p450IID6 were present in 13 of 18 (72%) anti-HCV-negative patients but in only 10 of 37 (27%) HCV infected (Ma et al 1993). The difference in the reactivity of LKM-positive patients with or without evidence of HCV infection suggests that they represent two distinct groups, and this has important therapeutic implications. Classical ACAH is treated with immunosuppression, which could exacerbate viral infection, while antiviral agents such as interferon may be used to treat HCV infection but may worsen autoimmune disease. The possible role of HCV infection in autoimmunity remains to be elucidated.

Prevention and treatment

Screening of blood donors for anti-HCV and use of vapour-heated and wet-heated clotting factor concentrates could decrease the risk of HCV transmission. Alpha-lymphoblastoid interferon (3 MU/m^2 three times weekly for 48 weeks) given to seven anti-HCV-positive children caused normalization of transaminase levels in six, which persisted after 1–24 weeks of follow-up (mean 11 weeks) (Iorio et al 1992). Similarly, 6 of 14 (43%) children with thalassaemia major and chronic hepatitis C infection who were treated with recombinant IFN-α (3 MU/m^2 three times weekly for 15 months) normalized ALT from 1 to 15 months from start of treatment with disappearance of HCV RNA from the serum (de Virgilis et al 1992). Longer follow-up will be essential to confirm clinically important benefit.

HEPATITIS D VIRUS (HDV OR DELTA AGENT)

Prevalence

Considerable regional variation in HDV infection has been noted (Bonino et al 1985, Thomas 1985). The role of environmental and genetic factors or HBV strain is unknown. In the Amazon Basin of Brazil, infection rate increases with age from 5% in children less than 10 years of age to 26% in those between 10 and 14 years and >40% in subjects more than 15 years of age (Bensabath et al 1987). Serological evidence of HDV infection was demonstrated in 34 of 270 (12.5%) Italian children who were HBsAg carriers (Farci et al 1985), but in only 4 of 247 (1.6%) Taiwanese children who had acute or chronic HBV infection (Hsu et al 1988). Recent reports have demonstrated that in the Guangzhou area 6 of 44 (13.6%) Chinese children have superinfection with the delta agent, a prevalence rate identical to that in adults (Chen et al 1990).

Clinical features

Asymptomatic infection occurred in an infant whose mother was HBeAg/anti-HDV positive but in none of four infants born to HBsAg-positive mothers with anti-HBe/anti-HDV. The infant remained asymptomatic with normal liver function tests up to 6 months of life (Smedile et al 1981).

In 34 Italian children with serological evidence of HBV-associated delta agent infection (Farci et al 1985), histological features at presentation included chronic active hepatitis (71%), chronic persistent hepatitis (18%) and cirrhosis (12%). 38% showed histological deterioration of liver disease after 2–7 years of follow-up. This is in contrast to 236 delta-negative HBsAg carriers, with improvement in 55% and deterioration in only 7%. In the Amazon Basin, delta virus infection was demonstrated in 74% of patients with fulminant hepatitis (Labrea hepatitis) and in 100% of patients with chronic hepatitis B (Bensabath et al 1987). 32 of the 44 (73%) cases of fulminant hepatitis were in children less than 15 years of age, 31 of whom were males. In the same study, 44 delta virus-negative HBsAg carriers were followed up for 1–5 years; amongst these, four males less than 10 years of age became superinfected with HDV and three developed fulminant hepatitis, fatal in two. Post-mortem studies of patients with fulminant hepatitis showed eosinophilic necrosis and microvesicular steatosis of the liver.

A similar type of fulminant hepatitis with the same epidemiological and histological features as in the Amazon Basin has been described in Columbia (Santa Marta hepatitis) in 81 patients, with the majority (63%) being males and children less than 15 years old (58%). In 69%, the delta antigen was demonstrated in the liver in combination with microvesicular steatosis, granular eosinophilic necrosis, portal lymphocytic inflammation and characteristic morula cells (Buitrago et al 1986).

Prevention and treatment

There is no specific treatment for HDV infection. As the greatest risk of HDV infection occurs in HBV carriers, infection may be prevented by giving only anti-HDV-negative blood or blood products to HBsAg-positive patients. HBV vaccination should prevent and limit the spread of HDV.

PREVALENCE OF HEPATITIS E VIRUS

The disease occurs in the form of water-borne epidemics on the Indian subcontinent, South-East and Central Asia, Africa and North America. In developed countries, sporadic cases are related to HEV infection among people returning from visits to endemic areas. The incubation period is 6 weeks (range 2 – 9 weeks) after primary exposure. It has a low secondary attack rate among exposed household members.

Of 39 Sudanese children with acute hepatitis, 23 (mean age 7.2 ± 3.1 years, range 2–13; 16 males) were found to be IgM anti-HEV positive using a Western blot assay (Hyams et al 1992). Clinically overt disease is observed mostly among young adults between 15 and 40 years of age (2.95%), and the prevalence is only 1.4% in those under 14 years (Bradley 1990). It remains unknown why HEV infection is rarely reported in children despite the fact that it is faecally transmitted.

Clinical features

The clinical features of the disease are similar to those of acute hepatitis A or B. Eight Egyptian children (age 3–8 years, six males) with HEV infection, diagnosed using an ELISA, had the following features at presentation: jaundice (8), fever (8), nausea/vomiting (4) and hepatomegaly (8). The mean bilirubin was 74 µmol/l, ALT 182 IU/l and AST 145 IU/l. Clinical and biochemical features were normal in all children after 12 months of follow-up (Goldsmith et al 1992).

Progression to chronic liver disease has not been observed with HEV infection.

TREATMENT

There is no specific prophylaxis or treatment for HEV infection.

ADENOVIRUS

Adenoviruses are usually respiratory tract pathogens but may cause acute gastroenteritis, haemorrhagic cystitis, meningoencephalitis, hepatitis and myocarditis in the newborn and immunosuppressed patients (Koneru et al 1987; Krilov et al 1990; Salt et al 1990).

Clinical features

Neonatal adenovirus infection produces a sepsis-like picture with hepatomegaly, thrombocytopenia and coagulopathy in the first 10 days of life. In one study, only 2 of 13 reported patients survived (Abzug & Levin 1991). Fatal adenovirus hepatitis has been described in a 7-month-old with severe combined immunodeficiency (Ohbu et al 1987).

Five of 224 (2%) liver transplant recipients (age 10–29 months) had adenovirus hepatitis from 57 to 130 days after transplantation (Cames et al 1992). Initial symptoms included fever (5), enteritis (2), upper respiratory tract infection (2), stomatitis (1) and rash (1). Two patients died of liver failure, while three survived after immunosuppression was discontinued 10–12 days after diagnosis. Another recipient whose donor had intussusception secondary to adenovirus infection also died (Varki et al 1990).

Pathology

There is widespread necrosis of the liver with Feulgen-positive intranuclear target-like inclusions in the hepatocytes. On electron microscopy, paracrystalline arrays of adenovirus virions may be seen.

Treatment

There is no known treatment for adenovirus hepatitis. For allograft recipients, withdrawal or reduction of immunosuppression is essential.

COXSACKIE VIRUS

Coxsackie virus is a human enterovirus causing typically self-limiting gastrointestinal disease. Fatal hepatic necrosis has been reported in a neonate (Kaul et al 1979), in an 11-month-old who presented with a Reye-like syndrome (Hinkle et al 1983) and in a 15-year-old with acute hepatitis (Read et al 1985). In a 14-year-old, it produced a mononucleosis-like syndrome, meningoencephalomyelitis, myocarditis and hepatitis (Begovac et al 1988).

CYTOMEGALOVIRUS

Cytomegalovirus (CMV) is a DNA-containing virus that has the propensity to induce formation of multinucleated giant cells and large intranuclear inclusion bodies (Cowdry type A or Owl's eye) (Fig. 32.1). It is the most common

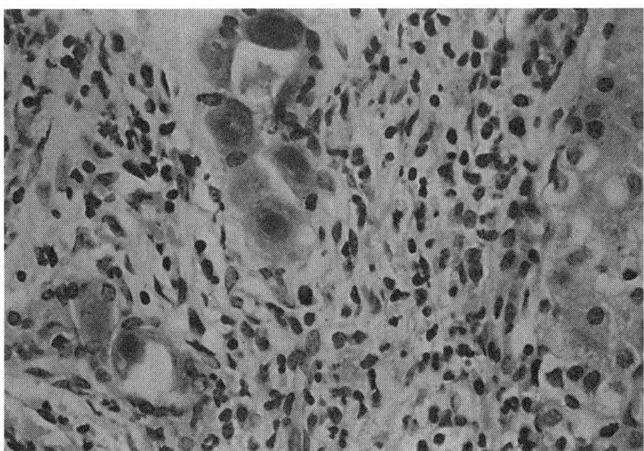

Fig. 32.1 Intranuclear inclusion bodies in CMV infection.

viral agent causing congenital infection in man, occurring in 0.2–2.4% of all live-born infants (Berge et al 1990). In China, seropositivity for CMV increases with age, averaging 52% in those less than 1 year and 60% in those between 4 and 7 years old. A higher rate of CMV antibodies has been observed among urban than rural children, in those who were breast-fed and among day-care centre attendees (Liu et al 1990). Acquisition is later in countries with better socioeconomic conditions.

Primary infection of a pregnant woman could result in symptomatic CMV infection in 5% during the neonatal period (Peckham 1991). Perinatal infection may also occur through infected maternal genital secretions, urine, saliva or breast milk (Wu et al 1989). Following an infection, excretion into the urine and saliva continues for many years and transmission between children may occur through sharing of toys contaminated by infected saliva. Infected blood products or donor organs are likewise important means of CMV transmission.

CMV is not eradicated from the host after a primary infection. It persists in a latent form that can be reactivated many months or years later.

Diagnosis is made by isolation of virus from any site (urine, saliva, bronchoalveolar lavage, blood or liver) or by antibody test demonstrating seroconversion and/or the presence of IgM antibody to CMV (Schultz & Chandler 1991). Immunofluorescence staining using monoclonal antibody to detect the early CMV antigen has been shown to be the most sensitive (84%), while DNA hybridization using the polymerase chain reaction (PCR) is the most specific (100%) method in the diagnosis of CMV hepatitis (Paya et al 1990).

Clinical features

In a review of 106 neonates with symptomatic congenital CMV infection, 70% had petechiae, jaundice and hepatosplenomegaly. The majority has elevated aminotransferase levels (83%) and conjugated hyperbilirubinaemia (81%) that persisted beyond the first month of life (Boppana et al 1992). Recurrent ascites has been associated with intrauterine CMV infection (Levy et al 1989). Perinatal CMV infection has also been shown to progress to cirrhosis (Giacchino et al 1990). Whether in these cases the liver damage had other cause(s) is unknown.

In older children, CMV infection is usually asymptomatic but it may cause symptomatic infection with prolonged fever, exudative pharyngitis, lymphadenopathy and hepatosplenomegaly. In those with jaundice the features are those of viral hepatitis with transaminase up to 20 times normal and jaundice persisting up to 12 weeks. Transient fever with abnormal liver function tests is seen more often in bone marrow transplant patients with CMV infection (Miyajima et al 1990). CMV hepatitis in liver transplant recipients is considered in the presence of spiking fever not explained by other foci of infection and an elevated transaminase level (at least twice normal) with no evidence of rejection on liver biopsy (Salt et al 1990).

Pathology

Various degrees of hepatitis with multinucleated giant cell transformation are seen. Hepatocyte necrosis, cholestasis, extramedullary haematopoiesis and fatty infiltration with minimal inflammatory cells may be demonstrated. Cytomegalic inclusion bodies (CIB) may be detected in the hepatocytes as well as the bile duct epithelium of patients with CMV hepatitis (Kosai et al 1991). Occasionally, portal fibrosis and bile duct proliferation may be seen, similar to findings in extrahepatic biliary atresia (Lurie et al 1987).

Prevention and treatment

Immunocompromised patients should only be given CMV-negative blood or blood products. Efforts are presently directed towards the licensure of an attenuated, live CMV vaccine (Alford et al 1990). Three different prophylactic regimens have been advocated for CMV exposure in liver transplant recipients. Intravenous immune globulin (IgG, 0.5 mg/kg) at weekly intervals for 6 weeks and acyclovir for 3 months after transplantation has been shown to be effective in 16 of 21 (76%) patients (Stratta et al 1991). In another report high-dose acyclovir (800 mg q.d.s. for 3 months) or ganciclovir (5 mg/kg b.d. for 1 week) followed by acyclovir (800 mg q.d.s. for 3 months) was effective in 24 of 39 (62%) and 39 of 57 (69%) transplanted children respectively (Freise et al 1991).

Successful treatment of CMV disease following liver transplantation has been achieved in 60 of 84 (71%) patients after an initial course of ganciclovir (5 mg/kg b.d. for 14 days) (Shaefer et al 1991). Adverse side-effects (neutropenia and thrombocytopenia) occurred in only five (6%) treated patients.

EPSTEIN–BARR VIRUS

Epstein–Barr virus (EBV) is a herpes-type virus causing the sydrome of infectious mononucleosis. The pharynx is the initial site of replication, but the virus disseminates throughout the lymphatic system, where it persists for life and may be periodically reactivated. In developing countries, 90% have been shown to be infected before 4 years of age, while in affluent societies it is a disease of adolescents and adults (Tsai et al 1989). Transmission is by oropharyngeal secretions. The incubation period is 30–40 days.

The diagnosis is made by the finding of atypical lymphocytes in the peripheral blood, a positive heterophile agglutinin test (Paul–Bunnel–Davidsohn absorption method) or by demonstration of IgM antibodies against the specific EBV-induced antigen. Viral isolation may be obtained from throat washings or by identification of EBV DNA genome in tissues using molecular hybridization techniques (Purtillo 1987).

Clinical features

Reactivation of latent, persistent EBV infection during pregnancy has been shown to cause a syndrome of low birth weight, congenital anomalies and neonatal jaundice (Goldberg et al 1981, Fleisher & Bolognese 1983). In children, the infectious mononucleosis syndrome is characterized by persistent or intermittent fever, palatal enanthema, lymphadenopathy and hepatosplenomegaly (Okano et al 1991). An anicteric hepatitis with elevation of transaminase levels occurs in 80%. Jaundice when present may precede, follow or occur simultaneously with the lymph node enlargement. Liver biopsy shows intense portal triad inflammation with mononucleocyte infiltration, Kupffer cell hyperplasia, cholestasis and foci of liver cell necrosis. Progression to hepatic cell necrosis and chronic hepatitis has been reported (Tanaka et al 1986).

Fulminant childhood haemophagocytic syndrome has been described in association with primary EBV infection (Chen et al 1991). Fatal X-linked lymphoproliferative disease (Duncan syndrome) occurs in boys unable to mount a cytolytic T-cell response (Giller & Grose 1989, Su et al 1990). An EBV-associated lymphoproliferative syndrome has been reported in 11 of 253 (4%) children (age 2–15 years, three males) at 3 months to 13 years (mean 17 months) after liver transplantation (Ho et al 1988).

Treatment

There has been no controlled trial on the use of any antiviral agent in the treatment of EBV hepatitis. A combination of intravenous acyclovir and prednisolone has been shown to improve pharyngeal symptoms and fever in 12 of 15 (90%) patients with fulminant mononucleosis (Anderson 1991).

HERPES SIMPLEX VIRUS

Herpes simplex (herpesvirus hominis) (HSV) is a DNA-containing virus that may cause a generalized disease with associated hepatic lesions. Spread of infection may occur by close bodily contact or by trauma or break in the skin. The incubation period is 2–12 days.

Diagnosis is made by demonstration of specific neutralizing antibodies in the sera or intranuclear inclusion bodies and multinucleated giant cells in scrapings or biopsy materials. The virus can be demonstrated immunohistochemically in liver tissue (Tomita et al 1991).

Clinical features

Neonatal HSV infection presents with progressive jaundice, hepatosplenomegaly, raised aminotransferase levels and coagulopathy, most commonly during the second week of life. Skin vesicles are present in 60% of patients (Koskiniemi et al 1989). Fatal herpetic hepatitis has been described in three neonates with no clear risk factor for infection (Benador et al 1990), in a 2-month-old with progressive calcifications of the lungs and the liver (Mannhardt & Schumacher 1991) and in a child with oedematous malnutrition who had pulmonary embolization of necrotic, infected hepatic cell fragment (Brooks et al 1991).

Treatment

Immunosuppressed patients should avoid contact with active herpetic lesions. Acyclovir (10–20 mg/kg per dose every 8 h) is the drug of choice for disseminated HSV infection, and best results are obtained when treatment is started on the first day of illness.

HUMAN IMMUNODEFICIENCY VIRUS

The human immunodeficiency virus (HIV), is a 105- to 120-nm RNA-containing retroviral agent that replicates by reverse transcription. It is the causative organism of acquired immunodeficiency syndrome (AIDS) and impairs the immune system by attacking the helper/inducer (T4) lymphocytes and binding to the CD4 receptor. Transmission may occur by the transplacental or perinatal route or by exposure to infected blood or blood products.

Transient hepatosplenomegaly has been documented in two infants with clinical and laboratory evidence of perinatal HIV infection (Mok et al 1989). An infant born to an HIV seropositive mother with HIV-specific IgM and IgG in the serum presented at 9 months with cholestasis and was found on liver biopsy to have multinucleated giant cell transformation (Witzleben et al 1988).

28 of 30 (93%) children (3 months to 7 years) with AIDS or AIDS-related complex were noted to have the following histopathological findings in the liver: giant cell transformation (23%), cytomegalovirus inclusion (17%), Kaposi sarcoma (13%), lymphoplasmacytic infiltrate (7%) and granulomatous hepatitis secondary to fungal infection (3%). Non-specific liver abnormalities included: steatosis (47%), portal inflammation (24%) and periportal necrosis (10%) (Jonas et al 1989). Chronic active hepatitis with predominantly T8 lymphocytes as determined by tissue immunochemistry were demonstrated in 5 of 12 (42%) children with HIV infection (Kahn et al 1991). The development of primary malignant fibrosarcoma of the liver has been reported in an 8-year-old African girl with HIV infection (Ninane et al 1985).

REOVIRUS

Infection with reovirus type 3 (reo-3) has been suggested as the initial event in the pathogenesis of persistent cholestasis (Glaser et al 1984, Glaser & Morecki 1987, Morecki & Glaser 1989), although this finding was not supported by subsequent studies (Brown et al 1988).

RUBELLA VIRUS

Rubella is a togavirus causing a benign infectious disease in children but associated with an increased incidence of malformations, stillbirths and abortions when infection occurs during the first trimester of pregnancy. Hepatitis and hepatosplenomegaly occur as transient manifestations of congenital rubella, which may be present during the first week of life (Cooper 1985). The liver shows giant cell transformation, cholestasis and focal necrosis. The virus may be isolated in the liver. The persistence of rubella IgG antibody in the sera after 6 months of age and the identification of IgM antibody earlier in life is indicative of congenital rubella infection.

Elevation of transaminase levels was seen in 18 of 241 (7.5%) children with acquired rubella infection. The ALT was shown to increase with the appearance of the rash, peaked on day 3–10 and normalized 8–28 days after onset of rash. Signs of liver involvement were seen in only one patient who had mild hepatomegaly (Sugaya et al 1988). Occasionally, the transaminase elevation may extend for up to 8 weeks or longer (Muraoka et al 1991). In one patient, liver biopsy during the acute phase of infection demonstrated a non-specific reactive hepatitis.

RUBEOLA VIRUS

Rubeola is a 140-nm RNA virus causing febrile exanthem (measles) in children and young adults and transmitted by droplet infection from nasopharyngeal secretions. Neonatal rubeola hepatitis has not been reported. In 52 Israeli children (<14 years) with measles, the AST (31%), ALT (9%) and gamma-glutanyl transferase (GGT) (7%) levels were noted to be abnormal, but no patient developed jaundice and the biochemical parameters normalized after 2–4 weeks (Shalev-Zimels et al 1988). It is not known whether liver involvement is immune mediated or a result of direct viral invasion of the hepatocytes.

VARICELLA ZOSTER

Varicella zoster (herpes varicellidae) is a member of the herpesvirus group, causing a highly contagious disease of childhood, varicella (chicken pox). The infection is spread by direct contact with a patient, who may transmit the disease from 1 day before onset of rash until all the vesicles have become dry. The incubation period is 10–21 days.

Clinical features

Disseminated varicella infection in the neonate usually occurs in the second week of life. The typical lesion is focal necrosis with eosinophilic intranuclear (Cowdry type A) inclusion bodies involving the lungs, liver and other organs. Although hepatitis is present, patients usually die from respiratory failure secondary to interstitial pneumonitis.

In 29 children with normal immunity, varicella zoster infection caused elevation of transaminase levels in a third of patients, but clinical hepatitis was not observed (Myers 1982). In the immunosuppressed, atypical haemorrhagic eruptions may occur (Miliauskas & Webber 1984, Perronne et al 1990). Three recipients of bone marrow transplant were observed to have visceral infection preceding cutaneous lesions believed to be a reactivation rather than a primary varicella zoster infection (Schiller et al 1991). Of 13 paediatric orthoptic liver transplant (OLT) recipients on a maintenance dose of cyclosporine and prednisolone, two died of varicella-related interstitial pneumonitis and hepatic necrosis despite intravenous acyclovir (McGregor et al 1989). Approximately 1 in 30 000 children with chicken pox develops Reye's syndrome (Mowat 1983).

Treatment

Varicella zoster immune globulin (125 units/10 kg) is recommended for newborns whose mother had varicella zoster infection 5 days before to 2 days after delivery and for premature infants with exposure to chicken pox.

For the immunosuppressed, varicella zoster immune globulin (ZIG) should be given within 96 h of exposure to a patient with varicella infection, and acyclovir (500 mg/m^2 t.d.s.) should be started once with apparent infection. Best results are obtained when treatment is started before the third day of illness. If possible, varicella vaccination should be administered prior to transplantation.

FLAVIVIRUS

Dengue virus

Dengue haemorrhagic fever (dengue shock syndrome) is a mosquito-borne infection (*Aedes aegypti*) observed predominantly in the tropical regions of the west Pacific and South-East Asia. The disease is characterized by a sudden onset of fever, myalgia and headache followed 2–3 days later by bleeding diathesis, encephalopathy and cardiovascular collapse. Definitive diagnosis is made by rising titres to dengue antigen.

Hepatitis, manifesting as hepatomegaly and transaminase elevation, is present in 90% of patients as part of multiorgan involvement. AST increases on the third day of illness, reaches peak levels (9x normal) on days 7–8 and normalizes 3 weeks after onset of illness (Wang et al 1990). Pathological lesions in the liver are varying degrees of fatty metamorphosis, focal mid-zonal necrosis, Kupffer cell hyperplasia and the presence of nonnucleated cells with vacuolated acidophilic cytoplasm, resembling Councilman bodies in the sinusoids (Alvarez & Ramirez-Ronda 1985). The dengue viral antigen may be demonstrated in the Kupffer cells.

Two cases of dengue fever in children presenting as fulminant hepatitis, with a fatal outcome in one, have been reported (George et al 1988).

Treatment

Survival is directly related to correction of fluid and electrolyte loss. For prevention, eradication of the mosquito vector is essential.

Yellow fever virus

Yellow fever is a member of the flavivirus (group B arbovirus), a round 35–45 nm particle containing a single-stranded RNA genome (Cunha 1988). It is a disease endemic in West Africa and some parts of South America and is transmitted to man by the mosquito vector, *Aedes aegypti* or *Aedes africanicus*. In the 1986 epidemic in eastern Nigeria, 126 cases of probable yellow fever were identified, one-third of which were in children less than 10 years of age. The highest attack rate (7.9%) occurred in the 20–29 years age group (de Cock et al 1988).

After an incubation period of 3–6 days, the virus is present in the bloodstream of man for 5–10 days. During this time, it may serve as a source of infection for the mosquitoes. The mosquito is then capable of transmitting the virus after an incubation period of 1–2 weeks.

Diagnosis is made by viral isolation or by demonstration of viral antigen in the acute-phase blood samples. Available serological tests for antibody determination include complement fixation, haemagglutination inhibition and ELISA (Monath et al 1984).

Clinical features

The disease varies in severity from subclinical to fatal illness. In the severe form, jaundice, renal and cardiovascular symptoms and bleeding diathesis are present on days 4–5 of illness. The liver is tender, but not enlarged, and splenomegaly is unusual. The mortality rate in hospitalized patients approaches 40–50%. Liver pathology reveals widespread mid-zonal coagulative necrosis with eosinophilic degeneration of hepatocytes (Councilman bodies), microvesicular steatosis and minimal inflammation. For patients who survive, hepatocellular regeneration is rapid and post-necrotic fibrosis does not occur.

Treatment

Treatment of yellow fever is mainly supportive. The disease may be prevented with the administration of a live attenuated vaccine to infants 6 months or older residing in an endemic area. Travellers to endemic areas should be vaccinated at least 10 days before arrival.

ENZOOTIC 'EXOTIC' VIRAL HEPATITIDES

Arenavirus (Lassa fever)

The Lassa fever is a single-stranded RNA-containing virus that is maintained in nature by the African house rat, *Mastomys natalensis*. The rodent excretes the virus in the urine and saliva and man becomes infected by consumption of contaminated food or water. Nosocomial infection may likewise occur by close contact with infected secretions and excretions of patients. Diagnosis is confirmed by viral isolation or by rising antibody titres, which become apparent in the second week of illness.

Epidemics of Lassa fever have been reported in Nigeria, Sierra Leone and Liberia. Lassa fever infection during pregnancy has been reported to cause an 87% fetal and neonatal loss. The risk of maternal death has likewise been shown to be higher if the infection occurred in the third trimester rather than in the first or second trimester of pregnancy (Price et al 1988).

Clinical features

The clinical features are variable and may range from an asymptomatic infection to a fatal disease.

In children, the disease is heralded by a slowly rising temperature, headache, conjunctivitis, pharyngitis, abdominal pain and diarrhoea. Patients either recover or their condition deteriorates with the presence of facial oedema, serous effusion, abdominal swelling (anasarca) and bleeding diathesis.

The liver has been demonstrated as the main target organ in human Lassa virus infection, although jaundice has not been reported. This has been substantiated in animal studies in which higher levels of the virus were detected in the liver than in the serum (Lucia et al 1990). Post-mortem biopsies from 19 patients with fatal Lassa fever infection have demonstrated diffuse hepatocellular necrosis with vigorous macrophage response but with paucity of inflammatory activities. Lassa virus hepatitis has been described to occur in three phases: active hepatocellular injury (<20% necrosis), necrosis and early recovery, and increased mitotic activity and regeneration. All three phases may be present at the time of death (McCormick 1986). Although the morphological changes in the liver may not be sufficient to account for death, it has been proposed that alterations in the metabolic and synthetic capacities of the hepatocytes may occur early in infection in the absence of significant necrosis.

Treatment

Ribavirin (60 mg kg^{-1} day^{-1}), a broad-spectrum antiviral agent, has been shown to be effective for Lassa virus infection (Fernandez et al 1986, Snell 1988).

Infections with bunyavirus and filovirus have not been reported in the paediatric age group and are included in this chapter for completeness. No specific treatment is yet available.

Bunyavirus (Rift valley virus)

The rift valley virus is a round, enveloped, single-stranded RNA particle, 90–100 nm in diameter, which contains a nuclear rod and is transmitted to man by the bite of a Culex mosquito. The disease is endemic in Central and South Africa and is characterized by an acute febrile illness lasting for 3–6 days, associated with headache, myalgia, anorexia, vomiting and lymphadenopathy. Hepatitis is common but jaundice is rare and implies a poor prognosis. Encephalitis and bleeding diathesis may complicate the disease. The liver pathology includes localized or widespread necrosis in the periportal and mid-zonal area with extensive eosinophilic degeneration of the parenchyma.

Nairovirus

The nairovirus is a single-stranded RNA virus that has a similar structure as the rift valley virus but has no nuclear rods. It is a tick-borne disease, causing in man the Crimean Congo haemorrhagic fever (CCHF) (Joubert et al 1985). The disease has been described in Russia, Africa, Pakistan and the Middle East and a nosocomial outbreak has been reported in South Africa (van Eeden et al 1985a, 1985b, 1985c).

Aside from extensive bleeding in the skin, nose, mouth and other parts of the body, patients usually have leucopenia, thrombocytopenia with widespread impairment of liver function but no evidence of hepatic cellular inflammation (van-Eeden et al 1985a, 1985b, 1985c). The liver is usually enlarged but jaundice has not been described. Hepatorenal failure and cardiovascular collapse usually characterize the terminal phase.

Filovirus (Marburg and Ebola viruses)

Marburg and Ebola are enveloped, negative-sense, single-stranded RNA viruses transmitted to man by African green monkeys (*Cercopithicus aethiops*) or by direct contact with blood or skin lesions of infected patients. The disease resembles any febrile haemorrhagic illness, with the liver as the primary target organ. Functional evidence of liver damage is present but jaundice is rare, reported only in 5% of patients with Ebola virus infection. Characteristic findings include hepatic lobular necrosis with eosinophilic cytoplasmic degeneration and lysis of nuclei. There is paucity of inflammatory response and hyperplasia of the Kupffer cells in and around the necrotic area.

REFERENCES

Hepatitis A

Amesty-Valbuena A, Gonzalez-Pirela Y, Rivero M 1989 Seroepidemiologic study of hepatitis A virus among children of Maracaibo, Venezuela. Investigation Clinic 30: 215–228

Chin K P, Lok A S, Wong L S, Lai C L, Wu P C 1991 Current seroepidemiology of hepatitis A in Hong Kong. Journal of Medical Virology 34: 191–193

Chiriaco P, Guadalupi C, Armigliato M, Bortolotti F, Realdi G 1986 Polyphasic course of hepatitis A in children. Journal of Infectious Diseases 153: 378–379

Chow C B, Lau T T Y, Leung N K, Chang W K 1989 Acute viral hepatitis: aetiology and evolution. Archives of Disease in Childhood 64: 211–213

Fagan E A, Yousef G, Brhan J et al 1990 Persistence of hepatitis A virus in fulminant hepatitis and after liver transplantation. Journal of Medical Virology 30: 131–136

Garcia-Puga J M, Toledano Cantero E, Ballesta Rodriguez M 1989 Outbreak of hepatitis A in day nursery: diagnosis and follow-up in a pediatric clinic. Acta Primaria 6: 478–481, 484–485

Glikson M, Galun E, Oren R, Tur-Kapsa R, Shouval D 1992 Relapsing hepatitis A. Review of 14 cases and literature survey. Medicine 71: 14–23

Gust I D 1988 Prevention and control of hepatitis A. In: Zuckerman AJ (ed.) Viral hepatitis and liver disease. Alan R. Liss, New York, pp 77–80

Gust I D, Feinstone SM 1988 Epidemiology of hepatitis A. C R C Press, Boca Raton, pp 163–191

Hadler S C, McFarland L 1986 Hepatitis in day care centers: epidemology and prevention. Review of Infectious Disease 8: 548–557

Hadler S C, Webster H M, Erben J J, Swanson J E, Maynard J E 1980 Hepatitis A in day care centers: a community wide assessment. New England Journal of Medicine 302: 1222–1227

Hermier M, Descos B, Collet J P, Philber M, Pouillaude J P, Pacros J P 1985 Acute cholecystitis disclosing A virus hepatitis. Archives of French Pediatrics 42: 525–529

Innis B L, Snitbhan R, Hoke C H, Munindhorn W, Laorakpongse T 1991 The declining transmission of hepatitis A in Thailand. Journal of Infectious Diseases 163: 989–995

Innis B L, Snitbhan R, Kunasol P et al 1992 Protection against hepatitis A by an inactivated vaccine. Proceedings of the Satellite Symposium of the IX Asian–Pacific Congress of Gastroenterology and the VI Asian–Pacific Congress of Digestive Endoscopy, Bangkok, Thailand, p 16

McNeill M, Hoy J F, Richards M J et al 1984 Aetiology of fatal viral hepatitis in Melbourne: a retrospective study. Medical Journal of Australia 141: 637–640

Noble R C, Kane M A, Reeves S A, Roeckel I 1984 Post-transfusion hepatitis A in a neonatal intensive care unit. Journal of the American Medical Association 252: 2711–2715

O'Grady J G, Gimson A E S, O'Brien C J, Pucknell A, Hughes R, Williams R 1988 Controlled trial of charcoal haemoperfusion and prognostic indicators in fulminant hepatic failure. Gastroenterology 94: 1186–1192

Prince A M, Brotman B, Richardson L, White T, Pollock N, Riddle J 1985 Incidence of hepatitis A virus infection in rural Liberia. Journal of Medical Virology 15: 421–428

Rosenblum L S, Villarino M E, Nainan OV et al 1991 Hepatitis A outbreak in a neonatal intensive care unit: risk factors for transmission and evidence of prolonged viral excretion among preterm infants. Journal of Infectious Diseases 164: 476–482

Shimizu H, Takebayashi T, Goto M, Togashi T 1984 Studies on an outbreak of hepatitis A in an institution for mentally retarded children. Hokkaido Igaku Zasshi 59: 247–253

Sjögren M H, Tanno H, Fay O et al 1987 Hepatitis A virus in stool during clinical relapse. Annals of Internal Medicine 106: 221–226

Sjögren M H, Hoke C H, Binn L N et al 1991 Immunogenicity of an inactivated hepatitis A vaccine. Annals of Internal Medicine 114: 470–471

Sun Y D, Zhang Y C, Ren Y H, Meng Z D 1988 Clinical/subclinical case ratio in hepatitis A. Lancet ii: 1082–1083

Toppet V, Souayah H, Delplace O, Alard S, Moreau J, Levy J, Spehl M 1990 Lymph node enlargement as a sign of acute hepatitis A in children. Pediatric Radiology 20: 249–252

Van den Anker J N, Sukhai R N, Dumas A M 1988 Relapsing hepatitis A in a child, associated with isolation of hepatitis A virus antigen from the liver. European Journal of Paediatrics 147: 333

Vento S, Garofano T, Di Perri G, Dolci L, Concia E, Bassetti G 1991 Identification of hepatitis A virus as a trigger for autoimmune chronic hepatitis type 1 in susceptible individuals. Lancet 337: 1183–1187

Werzberger A, Mensch B, Kuter B et al 1992 A controlled trial of a formalin-inactivated hepatitis A vaccine in healthy children. New England Journal of Medicine 327: 453–457

Ye J Y 1990 Outcome of pregnancy complicated by hepatitis A in the urban districts of Shanghai. Chung-Hua-Fu-Chan-Ko-Tsa-Chih 25: 219–221

Yong P 1992 Epidemiology of hepatitis A. Proceedings of the Satellite Symposium of the IX Asian-Pacific Congress of Gastroenterology and the VI Asian-Pacific Congress of Digestive Endoscopy, Bangkok, Thailand, p 8

Zuckerman J N, Cockcroft A, Griffiths P 1991 Hepatitis A immunization. British Medical Journal 303: 247

Hepatitis B

Abb J, Zachoval R, Eisenburg J, Pape G R, Zachoval U, Deinhardt F 1985 Production of interferon alpha and interferon gamma by peripheral leukocytes from patients with chronic hepatitis B virus infection. Journal of Medical Virology 16: 171–176

Beasley R P, Hwang L Y, Lin C C et al 1982 Incidence of hepatitis B virus infections in preschool children in Taiwan. Journal of Infectious Diseases 142: 198–204

Bortolotti F, Calzia R, Vegnente A et al 1983 Chronic hepatitis in childhood: the spectrum of the disease. Gut 29: 659–664

Bortolotti F, Calzia R, Cadrobbi P et al 1986 Liver cirrhosis associated with chronic hepatitis B virus infection in childhood. Journal of Pediatrics 198: 224–227

Carman W F, Zanetti A R, Karayiannis P et al 1990 Vaccine-induced escape mutant of hepatitis B virus. Lancet 336: 325–329

Chang M H, Lee C Y, Chen D S, Hsu H C, Lai M Y 1987 Fulminant hepatitis in children in Taiwan: the important role of hepatitis B virus. Journal of Pediatrics 111: 34–39

Chang M H, Sung J L, Lee C Y et al 1989 Factors affecting

clearance of hepatitis B e antigen in hepatitis B surface antigen carrier children. Journal of Pediatrics 115: 385–390
Chow C B, Lau T T Y, Leung N K, Chang W K 1989 Acute viral hepatitis: aetiology and evolution. Archives of Disease in Childhood 64: 211–213
Chu C M, Karayiannis P, Fowler M J, Monjardino J, Liaw Y F, Thomas H C 1985 Natural history of chronic hepatitis B virus infection in Taiwan: studies of hepatitis B virus DNA in serum. Hepatology 5: 431–434
de Potter C R, Robberecht E, Laureys G, Cuvelier C A 1987 Hepatitis B related childhood hepatocellular carcinoma. Cancer 60: 414–418
Draelos K Z, Hansen R C, James M A J 1986 Gianotti Crosti syndrome associated with infections other than hepatitis B. Journal of American Medical Association 256: 2386–2388
Farci T, Barbera C, Lavone C et al 1985 Infection with the delta agent in children. Gut 26: 4–7
Fattovich G, Cadrobbi P, Crivellaro C et al 1982 Virological changes in chronic hepatitis type B treated with laevamisole. Digestion 25: 131–135
Giusti G, Piccinino F, Sagnelli E, Ruggiero G, Galanti B, Gallo C 1988 Immunosuppressive therapy of HBsAg positive chronic active hepatitis in childhood. a multicentre retrospective study on 139 patients. Journal of Pediatric Gastroenterology and Nutrition 7: 17–21
Gussetti N, Lagaiolli G, D'Elia R 1988 Absence of maternal antibodies to hepatitis B core antigen and HBV vertical transmission: one case of infection notwithstanding passive-active prophylaxis. Infection 16: 167–170
Hsu H C, Wu M Z, Chang M J, Su I J, Chen D S 1987 Childhood hepatocellular carcinoma develops exclusively in hepatitis B surface antigen carriers in three decades in Taiwan: a report of 51 cases strongly associated with rapid development of liver cirrhosis. Journal of Hepatology 5: 260–267
Hsu H C, Lin Y H, Chang M H, Su I J, Chen D S 1988 Pathology of chronic hepatitis B virus infection in children with special reference to the intrahepatic expression of hepatitis virus antigens. Hepatology 8: 378–382
Hsu H Y, Chang M H, Lee C Y, Chen J S, Hsu H C, Chen D S 1992 Spontaneous loss of HBsAg in children with chronic hepatitis B virus infection. Hepatology 15: 382–386
Immunization Practices Advisory Committee 1988 Prevention of perinatal transmission of hepatitis B virus: prenatal screening of all pregnant women for hepatitis B surface antigen. Mortality and Morbidity Weekly Report 37: 341–346, 351
Kacecioglu Draelos Z et al 1986 Gianotti Crosti syndrome associated with infections other than hepatitis B. Journal of the American Medical Association 256: 2386–2388
Kiire C F 1990 Hepatitis B infection in sub-Saharan Africa. The African Regional Study Group. Vaccine 8: S107–112
Kosaka Y, Takase K, Kojima M et al 1991 Fulminant hepatitis B virus mutants defective in the precore region and incapable of encoding e antigen. Gastroenterology 100: 1087–1094
La Banda F, Ruiz-Moreno M, Carreno V et al 1988 Recombinant α-interferon treatment in children with chronic hepatitis B. Lancet i: 250
Lai C L, Lok A S F, Lin H J et al 1987 Placebo controlled trial of recombinant α-interferon in Chinese HBsAg carrier children. Lancet ii: 877–880
Lai C L, Lin H J, Lau J Y N et al 1991 Effect of recombinant α2 interferon with or without prednisolone in Chinese HBsAg carrier children. Quarterly Journal of Medicine 78: 155–163
La Manna A, Polito C, Del Gado R, Olivieri A N, Di Toro R 1985 Hepatitis B surface antigenaemia and glomerulopathies in children. Acta Paediatrica Scandinavia 74: 122–125
Lamelin J P, Trepo C 1990 The hepatitis B virus and the peripheral blood mononuclear cells: a brief review. Journal of Hepatology 10: 120–124
Lee A K Y, Ip H M H, Wong V C W 1978 Mechanisms of maternal–fetal transmission of hepatitis B virus. Journal of Infectious Diseases 138: 668–671
Leuschner I, Harms D, Schmidt D 1988 The association of hepatocellular carcinoma in childhood with hepatitis B virus infection. Cancer 62: 2363–2369
Lok A S F, Lai C L 1988 A longitudinal follow-up of asymptomatic hepatitis B surface antigen positive Chinese children. Hepatology 8: 1130–1133
Maggiore G, De Giacomo C, Marzani D et al 1983 Chronic viral hepatitis B in infancy. Journal of Pediatrics 103: 749–752
Mynard J E, Kane M A, Alter M H, Hadler SC 1988 Control of hepatitis B by immunization: global perspectives. In: Zuckerman AJ (ed.) Viral hepatitis and liver disease. Alan R. Liss, New York, pp 967–969
O'Grady J G, Gimson A E S, O'Brien C J, Pucknell A, Hughes R D, Williams R 1988 Controlled trials of charcoal haemoperfusion and prognostic factors in fulminant hepatic failure. Gastroenterology 94: 1186–1192
Omata M. Ehata T, Yokosuka O, Hosoda K, Ohto M 1991 Mutations in the precore region of hepatitis B virus DNA in patients with fulminant and severe hepatitis. New England Journal of Medicine 324: 1699–1704
Poovorawan Y, Sanpavat S, Pongpunlert W, Chumdermpadetsuk S, Sentrakul P, Safary A 1989 Protective efficacy of a recombinant DNA hepatitis B vaccine in neonates of HBe antigen positive mothers. Journal of the American Medical Association 261: 3278–3281
Ratner L, Peylan-Ramu N, Wesley R, Poplack D G 1986 Adverse prognostic influence of hepatitis B virus infection in acute lymphoblastic leukemia. Cancer 58: 1096–1100
Ruiz-Moreno M, Rua M J, Molina J et al 1991 Prospective randomized controlled trial of interferon-α in children with chronic hepatitis B. Hepatology 13: 1035–1039
Ruiz-Moreno M, Rua M J, Moraleda G, Guardia L, Moreno A, Carreno V 1992 Treatment with interferon gamma versus interferon alfa and gamma in children with chronic hepatitis B. Pediatrics 90: 254–258
Schmacher H R, Ball E P 1974 Arthritis in acute and chronic hepatitis. American Journal of Medicine 57: 655
Stevens C E, Neurath R E, Beasley R P, Szmuness W 1979 HBeAg and anti-HBe detection by radioimmunoassay: correlation of vertical transmission of hepatitis B virus in Taiwan. Journal of Medical Virology 3: 237–241
Stroffolini T, Franco E, Romano G et al 1989 Hepatitis B virus infection in children in Sardinia, Italy. European Journal of Epidemiology 5: 202–206
Tong M J, Nair P V, Thursby M, Schweitzer I L 1985 Prevention of hepatitis B infection by hepatitis B immunoglobulin in infants born to mothers with acute hepatitis during pregnancy. Gastroenterology 89: 160–164
Tsen Y J, Chang M J, Hsu H Y, Lee C Y, Sung J L, Chen D S 1991 Seroprevalence of hepatitis B virus infection in children in Taipei, 1989: five years after a mass hepatitis B

vaccination program. Journal of Medical Virology 34: 96–99

Vanclaire J, Cornu C H, Sokol E M 1991 Fulminant hepatitis B in an infant born to a hepatitis B e antibody positive, DNA negative carrier. Archives of Disease in Childhood 66: 983–985

Van Ditzhuijsen T J, de Witte van der Shoot E, Van Loon A M, Rijntjes P J, Yap S H 1988 Hepatitis B virus infection in an institution for the mentally retarded. American Journal of Epidemiology 128: 629–638

Vento S, Hegarty J E, Alberti A et al 1985 T-lymphocyte sensitization to HBsAg in hepatitis B virus mediated unresponsiveness to HBsAg in hepatitis B virus related chronic liver disease Hepatology 5: 192–197

Hepatitis C

Al-Faleh F Z, Ayoola E A, Al-Jeffry M et al 1991 Prevalence of antibody to hepatitis C virus among Saudi Arabian children: a community-based study. Hepatology 14: 215–218

Blanchette V S, Vortsman E, Shore A et al 1991 Hepatitis C infection in children with hemophilia A and B. Blood 78: 285–289

Bortolotti F, Vajro P, Cardrobbi P et al 1992 Cryptogenic chronic liver disease and hepatitis C virus infection in children. Journal of Hepatology 15: 73–76

Ding-Shinn C, Kuo G C, Juei-Low S et al 1991 Hepatitis C virus infection in an area hyperendemic for hepatitis B and chronic liver disease: the Taiwan experience. Journal of Infectious Diseases 162: 817–822

de Virgilis S, Clemente M G, Congia M et al 1992 Recombinant interferon alpha treatment in thalassemia major children with chronic hepatitis C and liver iron overload

Iorio R, Guida S, Fariello I, de Rosa E, Porzio S, Vegnente A 1992 Alpha lymphoblastoid interferon (α-Ly-IFN) therapy in 12 children with chronic non-A, non-B hepatitis (CNANBH) (7 anti-HCV+). Proceedings of the Second Joint Meeting of the British and Italian Societies of the Paediatric Gastroenterology and Nutrition. Harwood Academic Publishers, Newmarket, UK, p 65

Hsu S-C, Chang M-H, Chen D-S, Hsu H-C, Lee C-Y 1991 Non-A, non-B hepatitis in children: a clinical, histological and serologic study. Journal of Medical Virology 35: 1–6

Jonas M M, Zilleruelo G E, La Rue S I, Abitbol C, Strauss J, Lu Y 1992 Hepatitis C infection in a pediatric dialysis population. Pediatrics 89: 707–709

Lenzi M, Ballardini G, Fusconi M et al 1990 Type 2 autoimmune hepatitis and hepatitis C virus infection. Lancet 335: 258–259

Locasciulli A, Gornati G, Tagger A et al 1991 Hepatitis C virus infection and chronic liver disease in children with leukemia in long term remission. Blood 78: 1619–1622

Ma Y, Peakman M, Lenzi M et al 1993 Case against subclassification of type II autoimmune chronic active hepatitis. Lancet 341: 60

Ngatchu T, Stroffolini T, Rapicetta M, Chionne P, Lantum D, Chiaramonte M 1992 Seroprevalence of anti-HCV in an urban child population: a pilot survey in a developing area, Cameroon. Journal of Tropical Medicine and Hygiene 95: 57–61

Novati R, Thiers V, Monforte A D et al 1992 Mother-to-child transmission of hepatitis C virus detected by polymerase chain reaction. Journal of Infectious Diseases 165: 720–723

Thaler M M, Park C-K, Landers D V et al 1991 Vertical transmission of hepatitis C virus. Lancet 338: 17–18

Weintrub P S, Veereman-Wauters G, Cowan M J, Thaler M M 1991 Hepatitis C virus infection in infants whose mothers took street drugs intravenously. Journal of Pediatrics 119: 869–874

Hepatitis D

Bensabath G, Hadler S C, Soares M C et al 1987 Hepatitis delta virus infection and Labrea hepatitis. Prevalence and role in fulminant hepatitis in the Amazon Basin. Journal of the American Medical Association 258: 479–483

Bonino F, Caporaso N, Dentico P et al 1985 Familial clustering and spreading of hepatitis delta virus infection. Journal of Hepatology 1: 221–226

Buitrago B, Hadler S C, Popper H et al 1986 Epidemiologic aspects of Santa Marta hepatitis over a 40-year period. Hepatology 6: 1292–1296

Chen G H, Zhang M D, Huang W 1990 Hepatitis delta virus superinfection in Guangzhou area. China Medical Journal 103: 451–454

Farci P, Barbera C, Navone C et al 1985 Infection with the delta agent in children. Gut 26: 4–7

Hsu H Y, Chang M H, Chen D S, Lee C Y 1988 Hepatitis D virus infection in children with acute or chronic hepatitis B virus infection in Taiwan. Journal of Pediatrics 112: 888–892

Smedile A, Dentico P, Zanetti A et al 1981 Infection with HBV associated delta agent in HBsAg carriers. Gastroenterology 81: 992–997

Thomas H C 1985 The delta agent comes of age. Gut 26: 1–3

Hepatitis E

Bradley D W 1990 Enterically-transmitted non-A, non-B hepatitis. British Medical Bulletin 46: 442–461

Goldsmith R, Yarbough P O, Reyes G R et al 1992 Enzyme-linked immunosorbent assay for diagnosis of acute sporadic hepatitis E in Egyptian children. Lancet 339: 328–331

Hyams K C, Purdy M A, Kaur M et al 1992 Acute sporadic hepatitis E in Sudanese children: analysis based on a new Western blot assay. Journal of Infectious Diseases 165: 1001–1005

Adenovirus

Abzug M J, Levin M J 1991 Neonatal adenovirus infection: four patients and review of the literature. Pediatrics 87: 890–896

Cames B, Rahier J, Burtomboy G et al 1992 Acute adenovirus hepatitis in liver transplant recipients. Journal of Pediatrics 120: 33–37

Koneru B, Jaffe R, Esquivel C O et al 1987 Adenovirus infections in pediatric liver transplant recipients. Journal of the American Medical Association 258: 489–492

Krilov L R, Rubin L G, Frogel M et al 1990 Disseminated adenovirus infection with hepatic necrosis in patients with human immunodeficiency virus infection and other immunodeficiency states. Review of Infectious Disease 12: 303–307

Ohbu M, Sasaki K, Okudaira M et al 1987 Adenovirus hepatitis in a patient with severe combined immunodeficiency. Acta Pathologica Japonica 37: 655–664

Salt A, Sutehall G, Sargaison M et al 1990 Viral and toxoplasma gondii infections in children after liver transplantation. Journal of Clinical Pathology 43: 63–67

Varki N M, Bhuta S, Drake T, Porter D D 1990 Adenovirus

hepatitis in two successive liver transplants in a child. Archives of Pathology and Laboratory Medicine 114: 106–109

Coxsackie virus

Begovac J, Puntaric B, Borcic D et al 1988 Mononucleosis-like syndrome associated with a multisystem Coxsackie virus type B3 infection in adolescent. European Journal of Pediatrics 147: 426–427

Hinkle G H, Leonard J C, Krous H F, Alexander J B 1983 Absence of hepatic uptake of Tc-99m sulfur colloid in an infant with Coxsackie B2 viral infection. Clinical Nuclear Medicine 8: 246–248

Kaul A, Cohen M E, Broffman G et al 1979 Reye like syndrome associated with Coxsackie B2 virus infection. Journal of Pediatrics 94: 67–69

Read R B, Ede R J, Morgan-Capner P, Moscoso G, Portmann B, Williams R 1985 Myocarditis and fulminant hepatic failure from Coxsackie virus B infection. Postgraduate Medical Journal 61: 749–752

Cytomegalovirus

Alford C A, Stagno S, Pass R F, Britt W J 1990 Congenital and perinatal CMV infections. Review of Infectious Disease 12: S745–753

Berge P, Stagno S, Federer W et al 1990 Impact of asymptomatic congenital cytomegalovirus infection on size at birth and gestational duration. Pediatric Infectious Disease Journal 9: 170–175

Boppana S B, Pass R F, Britt W, Stagno S, Alford C A 1992 Symptomatic congenital cytomegalovirus infection: neonatal morbidity and mortality. Pediatric Infectious Disease Journal 11: 93–99

Freise C E, Pons V, Lake J et al 1991 Comparison of three regimens for cytomegalovirus prophylaxis in 147 liver transplant recipients. Transplantation Proceedings 23: 1498–1500

Gershon A A 1990 Viral vaccines of the future. Pediatric Clinics of North America 37: 689–707

Giacchino R, Navone C, Ciravegna B, Viscoli C, Ferrea G, Facco F 1990 Liver cirrhosis in childhood. Considerations on 22 cases with different etiology. Pediatrica Medicina Chirurgia 12: 147–152

Griffiths P D, Baboonian C, Rutter D, Peckham C 1991 Congenital and maternal cytomegalovirus infections in a London population. British Journal of Obstetrics and Gynaecology 98: 135–140

Kosai K, Kage M, Kojiro M 1991 Clinicopathological study of liver involvement in cytomegalovirus infection in infant autopsy case. Journal of Gastroenterology and Hepatology 6: 603–608

Levy I, Shoshat M, Levy Y, Alpert G, Nitzhan M 1989 Recurrent ascites in an infant with perinatally acquired cytomegalovirus infection. European Journal of Pediatrics 148: 531–532

Liu Z, Wang E, Taylor W et al 1990 Prevalence survey of cytomegalovirus infection in children in Chengdu. American Journal of Epidemiology 131: 143–150

Lurie M, Elmalach I, Schuger L, Weintraub Z 1987 Liver findings in infantile cytomegalovirus infection: similarity to extrahepatic billary obstruction. Histopathology 11: 1171–1180

Miyajima Y, Fukuda M, Kojima S, Matuyama K 1990 Transient fever with abnormal liver function in patients who underwent bone marrow transplantation – clinical symptoms of cytomegalovirus infection. Rinsho-Kesueki 31: 1670–1673

Paya C V, Holley K E, Wiesner R H et al 1990 Early diagnosis of cytomegalovirus hepatitis in liver transplant recipients: role of immunostaining, DNA hybridization and culture of hepatic tissue. Hepatology 12: 119–126

Peckham C S 1991 Cytomegalovirus infection: congenital and neonatal disease. Scandinavian Journal of Infectious Diseases 80 (suppl.): 82–87

Salt A, Sutehall G, Sargaison M et al 1990 Viral and *Toxoplasma gondii* infections in children after liver transplantation. Journal of Clinical Pathology 43: 63–67

Schultz D A, Chandler S 1991 Cytomegalovirus testing: antibody determinations and viral cultures with recommendations for use. Journal of Clinical Laboratory Analysis 5: 69–73

Shaefer M S, Stratta R J, Markin R S et al 1991 Ganciclovir therapy for cytomegalovirus disease in liver transplant recipients. Transplantation Proceedings 23: 1515–1516

Stratta R J, Shaeffer M S, Cushing K A, Markin R S, Wood R P, Langnas A N 1991 Successful prophylaxis of cytomegalovirus disease after primary CMV exposure in liver transplant recipients. Transplantation 51: 90–97

Wu J, Tang Z Y, Wu Y X, Li W R 1989 Acquired cytomegalovirus infection of breastmilk in infancy. China Medical Journal 102: 124–128

Epstein–Barr virus

Anderson J P 1991 Clinical aspects of Epstein-Barr virus infection. Scandinavian Journal of Infectious Diseases 80 (suppl.): 90–104

Chen R L, Su I J, Lin K H et al 1991 Fulminant childhood hemophagocytic syndrome mimicking histiocytic medullary reticulosis. An atypical form of Epstein–Barr virus infection. American Journal of Clinical Pathology 96: 171–176

Fleisher G, Bolognese R 1983 Persistent Epstein–Barr virus infection and pregnancy. Journal of Infectious Diseases 147: 982–986

Giller R H, Grose C 1989 Epstein–Barr virus: the hematologic and oncologic consequences of virus–host interaction. Critical Review of Oncology and Hematology 9: 149–195

Goldberg G N, Fulginiti V A, Ray G et al 1981 In utero Epstein–Barr virus (infectious mononucleosis) infection. Journal of the American Medical Association 264: 1579–1581

Ho M, Jaffe R, Miller G et al 1988 The frequency of Epstein–Barr infection and associated lymphoproliferative syndrome after transplantation and its manifestation in children. Transplantation 45: 719–727

Okano M, Matsumoto S, Osato T, Sakiyama Y, Thiele G M, Purtilo D T 1991 Severe chronic active Epstein–Barr virus infection syndrome. Clinical Microbiology Review 4: 129–135

Purtilo DT 1987 Epstein–Barr virus: the spectrum of its manifestations in human beings. Southern Medical Journal 80: 943–947

Su I J, Lin D T, Hsieh H C et al 1990 Fatal primary Epstein–Barr virus infection masquerading as histiocytic medullary reticulosis in young children in Taiwan. Hematology Pathology 4: 189–195

Tanaka K, Shimada M, Sasahara A, Yamamoto H, Naruto T, Tomida Y 1986 Chronic hepatitis associated with Epstein–Barr virus infection in an infant. Journal of

Pediatric Gastroenterology and Nutrition 5: 467–471
Tsai W S, Chang M H, Chen J Y, Lee C Y, Liu Y G 1989 Seroepidemiological study of Epstein–Barr infection in children in Taipei. Acta Paediatrica Sinensis 30: 81–86

Herpes simplex virus

Benador N, Mannhardt W, Schranz D et al 1990 Three cases of neonatal herpes simplex virus infection presenting as fulminant hepatitis. European Journal of Pediatrics 149: 555–559
Brooks S E, Taylor E, Golden M H, Golden B E 1991 Electron microscopy of herpes simplex hepatitis with hepatocyte pulmonary embolization in kwashiorkor. Archives of Pathology and Laboratory Medicine 115: 1247–1249
Koskiniemi M, Happonen J M, Jarvenpaa A L, Pettay 0, Vaheri A 1989 Neonatal herpes simplex virus (HSV) infection: a report of 43 patients. Pediatric Infectious Disease 8: 30–35
Mannhardt W, Schumacher R 1991 Progressive calcifications of lung and liver in neonatal herpes simplex virus infection. Pediatric Radiology 21: 236–237
Tomita T, Chiga M, Lenahan M et al 1991 Identification of herpes simplex virus infection by immunoperoxidase and in-situ hybridization methods. Virchows Archives A Pathology, Anatomy, Histopathology 419: 99–105

Human immunodeficiency virus

Jonas M M, Roldan E O, Lyons H J et al 1989 Histopathologic features of the liver in acquired immunodeficiency syndrome. Journal of Pediatric Gastroenterology and Nutrition 9: 73–76
Kahn E, Greco A, Daum F et al 1991 Hepatic pathology in pediatric acquired immunodeficiency syndrome. Human Pathology 22: 1111–1119
Mok J Y Q, Hague R A, Yap P L et al 1989 Vertical transmission of HIV: a prospective study. Archives of Disease in Childhood 64: 1140–1145
Ninane J, Moulin D, Latinne D et al 1985 AIDS in two African children – one with fibrosarcoma of the liver. European Journal of Pediatrics 144: 385–388
Witzleben C L, Marshall G S, Wenner W, Piccoli D A, Barbour S D 1988 HIV as a cause of giant cell hepatitis. Human Pathology 19: 603–605

Reovirus

Brown W R, Sokol R J, Levin M J 1988 Lack of correlation between infection with reovirus 3 and extrahepatic biliary atresia or neonatal hepatitis. Journal of Pediatrics 113: 670–676
Glaser J H, Balistreri W F, Morecki R 1984 Role of reovirus type 3 in persistent infantile cholestasis. Journal of Pediatrics 105: 912–915
Glaser J H, Morecki R 1987 Reovirus type 3 and neonatal cholestasis. Seminars in Liver Disease 7: 100–107
Morecki R, Glaser J 1989 Reovirus 3 and neonatal biliary disease: discussion of divergent results. Hepatology 10: 515–517

Rubella virus

Cooper LZ 1985 The history and medical consequences of rubella. Review of Infectious Diseases 7: S2–10
Muraoka H, Sata M, Hino T et al 1991 A study on hepatic dysfunction associated with rubella infection. Kansenshogaku-Zasshi 65: 597–603
Sugaya N, Nirasawa M, Mitamura K, Murata A 1988 Hepatitis in acquired rubella infection in children. American Journal of Diseases in Children 142: 817–818

Rubeola virus

Shalev-Zimels H, Weizman Z, Lotan C, Gavish D, Ackerman Z, Morag A 1988 Extent of measles hepatitis in various ages. Hepatology 8: 1138–1139

Varicella Zoster

McGregor S R, Zitelli B J, Urbach A H, Malatack J J, Cartner J C 1989 Varicella in pediatric orthotopic liver transplant recipients. Pediatrics 83: 256–261
Miliauskas J R, Webber B L 1984 Disseminated varicella at autopsy in children with cancer. Cancer 53: 1518–1525
Mowat A P 1983 Reye's syndrome – twenty years on. British Medical Journal 286: 1999
Myers M G 1982 Hepatic cellular injury during varicella. Archives of Disease in Childhood 57: 317–319
Paryani S G, Arvin A M 1986 Intrauterine infection with varicella-zoster virus after maternal varicella. New England Journal of Medicine 314: 1542–1546
Perronne C, Lazanas M, Leport C et al 1990 Varicella in patients infected with human immunodeficiency virus. Archives of Dermatology 126: 1086–1088
Schiller G J, Nimer S D, Gajewski J L, Golde D W 1991 Abdominal presentation of varicella-zoster infection in recipients of allogenic bone marrow transplantation. Bone Marrow Transplantation 7: 489–491

Dengue virus

Alvarez M E, Ramirez-Ronda C H 1985 Dengue and hepatic failure. American Journal of Medicine 79: 670–674
George R, Liam C K, Chua C T et al 1988 Unusual clinical manifestations of dengue virus infection. Southeast Asian Journal of Tropical Medicine and Public Health 19: 585–590
Wang L Y, Chang W Y, Lu S N et al 1990 Sequential changes of serum transaminase and abdominal sonography in patients with suspected dengue fever. Kao-Hsiung-I-Hsueh-Ko-Hsueh-Tsa-Chih 6: 483–489

Yellow fever virus

Cunha B A 1988 Systemic infections affecting the liver. Some cause jaundice, some do not. Postgraduate Medicine 84: 148–158
de Cock K M, Monath T P, Nasidi A et al 1988 Epidemic yellow fever in Eastern Nigeria, 1986. Lancet i: 630–632
Monath T P, Nystrom R R 1984 Detection of yellow fever virus in serum by enzyme linked immunoassay. American Journal of Tropical Medicine and Hygiene 33: 151–157

Enzootic 'exotic' viral hepatitides

Fernandez H, Banks G, Smith R 1986 Ribavirin: a clinical overview. European Journal of Epidemiology 2: 1–14
Joubert J R, King J B, Rossouw D J, Cooper R 1985 A nosocomial outbreak of Crimean Congo haemorrhagic fever at Tygerberg hospital. Part III. Clinical pathology and pathogenesis. South African Medical Journal 68: 722–728
Lucia H L, Coppenhaver D H, Harrison R L, Baron S 1990 The effect of an arenavirus infection on liver morphology and function. American Journal of Tropical Medicine and Hygiene 43: 93–98
McCormick J B, Walker D H, King I J et al 1986 Lassa virus

hepatitis: a study of fatal Lassa fever in humans. American Journal of Tropical Medicine and Hygiene 35: 401–407
Price M E, Fisher-Hoch S P, Craven R B, McCormick J B 1988 A prospective study of maternal and foetal outcome in acute Lassa fever infection during pregnancy. British Medical Journal 297: 584–587
Snell N 1988 Ribavirin therapy for Lassa fever. Practitioner 232: 432
van-Eeden P J, Joubert J R, van de Wal B W, King J B, de Kock A, Groenewald J H 1985a A nosocomial outbreak of Crimean Congo haemorrhagic fever at Tygerberg hospital. Part I. Clinical features. South African Medical Journal 68: 711–717
van-Eeden P J, van-Eeden S F, Joubert J R, King J B, van de Wal Michell W L 1985b A nosocomial outbreak of Crimean Congo haemorrhagic fever at Tygerberg hospital. Part II. Management of patients. South African Medical Journal 68: 718–721
van-Eeden P J, Joubert J R, van-Eeden S F, King J B 1985c A nosocomial outbreak of Crimean Congo haemorrhagic fever at Tygerberg hospital. Part IV. Preventive and prophylactic measures. South African Medical Journal 68: 729–732
Woodruff P W, Morrill J C, Burans J P, Hyams K C, Woody J N 1988 A study of viral and rickettsial exposure and causes of fever in Juba, southern Sudan. Transactions of the Royal Society of Tropical Medicine and Hygiene 82: 761–766

UPDATE

- Unexpectedly high anti-HAV prevalence rates were found in a recent community-wide epidemic in a UK city, at 27%, 38% and 22% in 1–4, 5–7 and 8–10-year-olds, respectively. This study also emphasized that the proportion of children developing icteric hepatitis increases with age: only 1 of 43 children less than 5 years became icteric as compared to 1 in 4.7 of those 8–10-years-old. (Stuart et al 1992).
- HEV infection as a trigger for fulminant hepatic failure due to Wilson's disease has been reported in a 6-year-old girl (Sallie et al 1992).
- REFERENCES

Sallie R, Chiyende J, Baldwin D et al 1992 Fulminant hepatic failure due to co-existent Wilson's disease and hepatitis E. Hepatology 16: 516
Stuart J M, Majeed F A, Cartwright K A V et al 1992 Salivary antibody testing in a school outbreak of hepatitis A. Epidemiology Infection 109: 161–166

33. Disinfection and sterilization

Martin S. Favero Walter W. Bond

The purpose of this chapter is to discuss disinfection and sterilization strategies that are used in health care and laboratory settings to prevent the transmission of infectious agents from contaminated medical devices and environmental surfaces to patients and health care workers. Although these strategies are those that are used generally in health care facilities to accomplish disinfection and sterilization for all groups of pathogenic microorganisms, emphasis will be placed on the efficacy of these procedures with the human hepatitis viruses.

The effective use of antiseptics, disinfectants and sterilization procedures in health care settings is important in the prevention of hospital-acquired infections. Historically, the use of physical agents, such as moist heat in the form of steam autoclaves or dry heat sterilizers, has played the predominant role for sterilizing devices, equipment and supplies in hospitals. Gaseous sterilization by ethylene oxide also has become popular for sterilizing items that are heat sensitive. There are a number of newly developed sterilization procedures meant to replace ethylene oxide sterilization, including vapour phase hydrogen peroxide (VPHP), VPHP/gas plasma discharge, peracetic acid and low-temperature steam/formaldehyde. Liquid chemical germicides formulated as sterilants have also been available for many years but primarily are used to disinfect rather than sterilize medical devices (Rutala 1990, Favero & Bond 1991).

The choice of what sterilization or disinfection procedure or which specific chemical germicide should be used for sterilization, disinfection or antisepsis or for environmental sanitization depends on a great many factors. No single chemical germicide or procedure is adequate for all purposes. Factors that should be considered in the selection of a specific sterilization or disinfection procedure include (1) the degree of microbiological inactivation required for the particular device, (2) the nature and physical composition of the device being treated and (3) the cost and ease of using a particular procedure.

REGULATION OF CHEMICAL GERMICIDES

Chemical germicides used as disinfectants or antiseptics in most countries are regulated by the federal or central government and usually by the Public Health Service or Ministry of Health.

In the USA, chemical germicides are regulated by two governmental agencies: the Environmental Protection Agency (EPA) and the Food and Drug Administration (FDA). Chemical germicides formulated as sterilants or disinfectants are initially regulated by EPA, but if a product is marked for use on a specific medical device (e.g. a haemodialysis machine, an endoscope or a high-speed dental handpiece), then the germicide falls under the additional regulatory control of FDA. The EPA requires manufacturers of chemical germicides formulated as sanitizers, disinfectants, hospital disinfectants or sterilant/disinfectants (sporicides) to test these products using specific, standardized assay methods for microbicidal potency, stability and toxicity to humans. For chemical germicides intended for use on medical devices (as opposed to environmental or housekeeping surfaces), the FDA requires that manufacturers submit a premarket application that may include additional specific microbicidal activity data, device/chemical compatibility data and detailed instructions to the user regarding the 'safe and effective use' of the product. FDA also regulates all sterilization devices such as steam or ethylene oxide autoclaves and dry heat ovens.

Chemical germicides that are formulated as antiseptics, preservatives or drugs to be used on or in the human body or as preparations to be used to inhibit or kill microorganisms on the skin are regulated by FDA. This type of chemical germicide is categorized basically by use pattern (e.g. antimicrobial handwashes, patient preoperative skin preparations, skin wound cleansers, skin wound protectants and surgical hand scrubs) and is not regulated or registered in the same fashion that EPA regulates and registers a disinfectant. Currently, data are not available to assess accurately the efficacy of many of the antimicrobial antiseptic formulations on the market; consequently, health care workers must make product selection decisions based on information derived from the manufacturer and published studies in the literature.

The Centers for Disease Control (CDC) do not approve, regulate or test chemical germicides formulated as disinfectants or antiseptics. Rather, the CDC recommends broad strategies for the use of sterilants, disinfectants and antiseptics to prevent transmission of infections in the health care environment (Favero & Bond 1991).

DEFINITIONS

The definitions of sterilization, disinfection, antisepsis and other related terms such as decontamination and sanitization are generally accepted in the scientific community, but some of these terms are misused. It is important not only to understand the definition and implied capabilities of each procedure, but also to understand how to achieve and in some cases monitor each state.

Sterilization and disinfection

The term 'sterilization' is one that students and professionals have memorized and recited seemingly forever. It can be the simplest and the most complex concept depending on how it is viewed and how it is applied. The definition of sterilization can change depending on the user's vantage point. We choose to view this term somewhat like a hologram and will define it in the context of *state* of sterilization, the *procedure* of sterilization, and the *application* of sterilization.

Any item, device or solution is considered to be sterile when it is completely free of all living microorganisms. This *state* of sterility is the objective of the sterilization procedure and, when viewed in this context, the definition is the categorical and absolute definition, i.e. an item is either sterile or it is not.

A sterilization *procedure* is one that kills all microorganisms, including high numbers of bacterial endospores. Sterilization can be accomplished by heat, ethylene oxide gas, radiation (in industry) and by a number of liquid chemical germicides. From an operational standpoint, a sterilization procedure cannot be categorically defined. Rather, the procedure is defined as a process, after which the probability of a microorganisms surviving on an item subjected to the sterilization procedures is less than one in one million (10^{-6}). This is referred to as the 'sterility assurance level', and it is this approach that is used by the medical device industry to sterilize large quantities of medical devices. Some criteria used in the production and labelling of a sterile device are listed in Table 33.1.

The *application* of sterilization principles in industry is much more sophisticated and controlled than sterilization procedures used in hospitals. However, steam autoclaves, ethylene oxide sterilizers and dry heat sterilization ovens used in health care facilities have operational protocols that are verified by the manufacturer to accomplish sterilization, and all the variables that control for the inactivation of microorganisms are

Table 33.1 Criteria used in producing sterile devices

Good manufacturing practices
Validated sterilization process
Sterility testing of a subsample of the batch subjected to the sterilization process
Process controls
Quality control of materials
Post-sterilization testing of devices for function

Table 33.2 Relationship of germicide type and use

Type of germicide	Type of device or surface	Process
Sterilant/disinfectant	Critical (i.v. catheter, spinal needles)	Sterilization (sporicidal chemical, prolonged contact time)
	Semicritical (reusable anaesthesia circuits, endotracheal tubes, laryngoscope)	High-level disinfection (sporicidal chemical, short contact time)
Hospital disinfectant (with label claim for tuberculocidal activity)	Non-critical (blood-contaminated control knobs of anaesthesia machines)	Intermediate-level disinfection
Hospital disinfectant, Sanitizer	Non-critical (exterior of machines, housekeeping, floors)	Low-level disinfection (soap and water)

either automated or built into simple controls in the devices.

The application of the sterilization process takes into account additional considerations. This approach involves the strategy associated with a particular medical device (or medical fluid) and the context of its degree of contact with patients. Spaulding in 1972 (see Favero & Bond 1991) proposed that inanimate surfaces in the medical environment be divided into three general categories based on the theoretical risk of infection if the surfaces are contaminated at time of use. Briefly, medical instruments or devices that are exposed to normally sterile areas of the body require sterilization; instruments or devices that touch mucous membranes may be either sterilized or disinfected; and instruments, medical equipment or environmental surfaces that touch skin or come into contact with the patient only indirectly can be either cleaned and then disinfected with an intermediate-level disinfectant, sanitized with a low-level disinfectant or simply cleaned with soap and water. These instruments or other medical surfaces are termed 'critical', 'semicritical' or 'non-critical' respectively. Selection of the appropriate disinfecting procedure in the last category (non-critical will include consideration of the nature of the surface as well as the type and degree of contamination. (Table 33.2)

In the context of these categorizations, Spaulding (1972) also classified chemical germicides by activity level. The activity levels are listed in Table 33.3 and are as follows.

Table 33.3 Levels of disinfectant action according to type of microorganism*

	Bacteria				Virus	
	Spores	*Mycobacterium* sp.†	Vegetative cells	Fungi‡	Non-lipid and small	Lipid and medium sized
High	+δ ¶	+	+	+	+	+
Intermediate	– ‖	+	+	+	±**	+
Low	–	–	+	±	±	+

* Adapted from Favero & Bond (1991).
† Laboratory potency tests usually employ *M. tuberculosis* var. *bovis*.
‡ Includes asexual spores but not necessarily chlamydospores or sexual spores.
δ Plus sign indicates a killing effect can be expected; a minus sign indicates little or no killing effect.
¶ High-level disinfectants are chemical sterilants (sporicides); inactivation of high numbers of bacterial spores can be expected only when extended exposure times are used, e.g. 6–10 h for sterilization *vs.* 10–30 min for high-level disinfection.
‖ Some intermediate-level disinfectants (e.g. hypochlorites) may show some sporicidal activity, while others (e.g. alcohols, phenolics) have none.
** Some intermediate-level disinfectants (e.g. certain phenolics, isopropyl alcohol) may have limited virucidal activity, even though they readily inactivate *Mycobacterium* spp.

1. *High-level disinfection.* This is a procedure that kills vegetative microorganisms but not necessarily high numbers of bacterial spores. These chemical germicides, by Spaulding's definition, are those that are capable of accomplishing sterilization, that is they kill all microorganisms, including a high number of bacterial spores, when the contact time is relatively long (6–10 h). As high-level disinfectants, they are used for relatively short periods of time (10–30 min). These chemical germicides are very potent sporicides and, in the USA, are those registered with the EPA as sterilant/disinfectants.
2. *Intermediate-level disinfection.* This is a procedure that kills vegetative microorganisms including *Mycobacterium tuberculosis*, all fungi and most viruses. These chemical germicides often correspond to EPA-approved 'hospital disinfectants' that are also 'tuberculocidal'.
3. *Low-level disinfection.* This is a procedure that kills most vegetative bacteria except *M. tuberculosis*, some fungi and some viruses. These chemical germicides are often ones that are approved in the USA by EPA as 'hospital disinfectants' or 'sanitizers'.

General use strategies of sterilization and disinfection using a variety of physical or chemical agents (with specific reference to hepatitis viruses) are shown in Table 33.4.

Spaulding's system for classifying devices and strategies for disinfection and sterilization is quite conservative. There is a direct relationship between the degree of conservatism as expressed by the probability of a microorganism surviving a particular procedure and the microbicidal potency of the physical or chemical germicidal agent. For example, a sterilization procedure accomplished by either steam autoclaving, dry heat or ethylene oxide gas, by design and definition, will result in a one-in-one million probability of a surviving microorganism if the procedure had initially been challenged with 10^6 highly resistant bacterial spores. The risk of infection resulting from the use of an item that was subjected to this type of procedure, assuming that the procedure had been carried out properly, would appear to be zero. Correspondingly, the probability of contamination and the theoretical probability of infection associated with sterilization or high-, intermediate- or low-level disinfection with liquid chemical agents would increase as the overall germicidal potency of the selected germicidal agent or procedure decreased.

A process of liquid chemical sterilization would, at best, be three orders of magnitude less reliable than a conventional heat sterilization procedure. From a practical standpoint, this means that there is a lower level of confidence with such procedures, and if and when mistakes are made there is a higher chance of failure than with a heat sterilization procedure. It also would appear that when procedural errors are made the consequences are magnified when a procedure of lower overall potency is chosen, e.g. chemical disinfection or sterilization *vs.* sterilization by heat. Procedures that contain fewer built-in assurances are procedurally driven and are ones that should be accompanied by very precise protocols, policies and quality assurance monitoring.

Decontamination

Another term quite often used in health care facilities is 'decontamination'. A process of decontamination is one that renders a device, items or materials safe to handle, i.e. safe in the context of being reasonably free from disease transmission risk. In many instances, this process is a sterilization procedure such as steam autoclaving, and this is often the most cost-effective way of decontaminating a device or an item. Conversely, the decontamination process may be ordinary soap and water cleaning of an instrument, a device, or an area. When chemical germicides are used for decontamination, they can range in activity from sterilant/disinfectants, which may be used to decontaminate spills of cultured or concentrated infectious agents in research or clinical laboratories, to low-level disinfectants or sanitizers when general housekeeping of environmental surfaces is the objective.

Antiseptic

The term 'antiseptic' is used to describe a substance that has antimicrobial activity and is for-

Table 33.4 Some physical and chemical methods for inactivating hepatitis viruses*

Class	Class concent or level	Activity
Sterilization		
Heat		
moist heat (steam under pressure)	250°F (121°C), 15 min Prevacuum cycle 270°F (132°C), 5 min	
dry heat	170°C, 1 h 160°C, 2 h 121°C, 16 h or longer	
Gas		
ethylene oxide	450–500 mg/l, 55–60°C	
Liquid†		
glutaraldehyde, aqueous	Variable, usually 1–2%	
hydrogen peroxide, stabilized	6–10%	
formaldehyde, aqueous	8–12%	
Disinfection		
Heat		
moist heat	75–100°C	High
Liquid		
glutaraldehyde, aqueous‡	Variable	High to intermediate
hydrogen peroxide, stabilized	6–10%	High
formaldehyde, aqueousδ	3–8%	High to intermediate
iodophors¶	40–50 mg/l free iodine at use dilution	Intermediate
Chlorine compounds‖	500–5000 mg/l free available chlorine	Intermediate
Phenolic compounds**	0.5–3%	Intermediate
Quaternary ammonium compounds††	0.1–2%	Low

* Comment: Adequate precleaning of surfaces is vital for any disinfecting or sterilizing procedure. Short exposure times may not be adequate to disinfect many objects, especially those that are difficult to clean because of narrow channels or other areas that can harbour organic material. Although alcohols (e.g. isopropanol, ethanol) have been shown to be effective in killing HBV, we do not recommend that they be used generally for this purpose owing to rapid evaporation and consequent difficulty in maintaining proper contact times. Immersion of small items in alcohols could be considered.

† This list of liquid chemical germicides contains generic formulations. Other commercially available formulations based on the listed active ingredients can also be considered for use. Information in the scientific literature or presented at symposia or scientific meetings can also be considered in determining the suitability of certain formulations.

‡ Manufacturer's instructions regarding use should be closely followed.

δ Because of the controversy over the role of formaldehyde as a potential occupational carcinogen, the use of formaldehyde is recommended only in limited circumstances under carefully controlled conditions of ventilation or vapour containment, e.g. disinfection of certain haemodialysis equipment.

¶ Only those iodophors designed as hard-surface disinfectants should be used, and the manufacturer's instructions regarding proper use dilution and product stability should be closely followed. Check product label claims for demonstrated activity against *Mycobacterium* sp. (tuberculocidal activity) as well as a spectrum of lipid and non-lipid viruses.

‖ See text.

** Check product label claims for demonstrated activity against *Mycobacterium* sp. (tuberculocidal activity) as well as a spectrum of lipid and non-lipid viruses.

†† Quaternary ammonium compounds are not tuberculocidal and may not have significant effect against a variety of non-lipid viruses. This class of germicide is used primarily for routine housekeeping throughout health care facilities.

mulated to be used on or in living tissue to remove, inhibit growth of or inactivate microorganisms. Quite often the distinction between an antiseptic and a disinfectant is not made. However, the differences between a disinfectant and an antiseptic are very great and applications are significantly different. A disinfectant is a chemical germicide formulated to be used solely on inanimate surfaces such as medical instruments or environmental surfaces; an antiseptic is formulated to be used solely on or in living tissues. Some chemical agents such as iodophors can be used as active ingredients in chemical germicides that are formulated as both disinfectants and antiseptics. However, the precise formulations are significantly different, use patterns are different and the germicidal efficacy of each formulation differs substantially. Consequently, disinfectants should never be used as antiseptics and vice versa.

FACTORS THAT INFLUENCE GERMICIDAL ACTIVITY

Microorganisms vary widely in their resistance to sterilants and disinfectants. The most resistant microorganisms are bacterial endospores and few, if any, other microorganisms approach the broad resistance of these organisms. A number of factors, some of which are associated with microorganisms themselves and others with the surrounding physical and chemical environment, can significantly influence the antimicrobial efficacy of chemical germicides.

Some factors are more important than others, but all of them should be considered when planning sterilization and disinfection strategies for medical and surgical devices and materials. Briefly, these factors are as follows.

The type of microorganism

Bacterial spores are more resistant than mycobacteria, fungi, vegetative bacteria and viruses; some types of viruses are more resistant to germicides than others. As a general guide, one should define the state or degree of inactivation needed (i.e. sterilization or various levels of disinfection) and then choose the most appropriate procedure.

The number of microorganisms

All other factors being equal, the greater the number of microorganisms present on a device, the longer it takes to inactivate this microbial population. It is for this reason that devices, especially those that are disinfected, should be cleaned prior to being sterilized or disinfected.

The intrinsic resistance of microorganisms

Bacterial spores have already been mentioned, but very few species in the genera *Bacillus* or *Clostridium* are actually responsible for hospital-acquired infections. However, organisms such as *M. tuberculosis* var. *bovis* and non-tuberculous mycobacteria, as well as naturally occurring Gram-negative water bacteria such as *Pseudomonas aeruginosa* and *P. cepacia* can, under some circumstances, be relatively resistant to chemical disinfectants. After bacterial spores, *Mycobacterium* spp. are considered one of the most resistant classes of microorganisms. It is for this reason that chemical germicides that have been approved as 'tuberculocides' are sometimes recommended for purposes of decontamination or disinfection when a higher activity germicide is sought. It is usually not a concern for transmission of *M. tuberculosis* but rather a definition or specification that can be used to describe a germicide with a relatively broad range of germicidal activity. Resistance of certain non-lipid viruses is similar to that of mycobacteria (Prince et al 1991).

Amount of organic soil present on the item to be disinfected or sterilized

Blood, faeces or other organic soil may contribute to failure of a disinfecting or sterilizing procedure in three ways. Organic soil may contain large and diverse microbial populations, may prevent penetration of germicidal agents or may directly inactivate certain germicidal chemicals. This factor, perhaps even more than others, underscores the necessity of precleaning items thoroughly prior to disinfection or sterilization.

Type and concentration of germicide

Generally, with all other factors being constant, the higher the concentration of a germicide, the greater its effectiveness and the shorter the exposure time necessary for disinfection or sterilization. If a chemical agent is reused over a period of time, the product effectiveness may be reduced due to a variety of factors such as dilution or organic contamination.

Time and temperature of exposure

With few exceptions, the longer the exposure time to a given chemical agent, the greater its effectiveness. An increase in temperature will significantly increase germicidal effectiveness, but deterioration or evaporation of the agent along with an increase in corrosiveness may also occur.

Other product- or process-related factors

Presence of organic or inorganic loads, pH and the degree of hydration of biological material may significantly affect the potency of certain chemical germicides. For these as well as other factors given above, care should be taken to examine closely and follow label instructions of proprietary germicides.

Device-related factors

The device or item being disinfected or sterilized must be physically and chemically compatible with the chosen procedure to ensure effectiveness and continued function of the device or item. Also, factors such as ease of access and cleaning as well as the size of the device or item are important considerations. The manufacturer of the item being reprocessed is the best source of pertinent information in this regard.

INACTIVATION OF HEPATITIS VIRUSES

Germicidal activity of physical and chemical agents against the human hepatitis viruses has been difficult to establish because most (HBV, HCV, HDV and HEV) have not yet been grown in tissue culture. With the exception of HAV, comparative virucidal testing, for the most part, has not been performed as it has for other types of viruses that can be conveniently cultured and tested in the laboratory.

Hepatitis A virus

HAV appears to have the same degree of resistance to chemical germicides and reagents as other picornaviruses (Prince et al 1991, Thraenhart 1991). Table 33.5 is adapted, in part, from Thraenhart (1991) and presents activity against HAV by various physical and chemical agents. These data underscore the importance, in practice, of thorough cleaning of surfaces to remove gross organic soil and, at the same time, reduce the level of viral contamination.

Hepatitis B virus

As pointed out in other parts of this book, hepatitis B is a disease of major public health significance. Hepatitis B can be transmitted in health care settings from patient to patient and from patient to staff member, and has been shown to have an environmentally mediated mode of transmission. However, since this virus cannot be grown in tissue culture, data used to verify disinfection and sterilization procedures have been deduced from experiments using human volunteers, blood products that received some degree of treatment and where disease or infection was followed in human recipients, or experiments in which chimpanzees were used to determine HBV inactivation using infectivity as a criterion. In addition, there have been other experimental approaches to demonstrate that certain physical and chemical agents can alter the immunological reactivity of hepatitis B surface antigen (HBsAg) as well as the morphological alteration of various components of the intact virus.

We have used HBsAg as a marker for HBV in order to determine the potential for environmentally mediated modes of transmission as well as inactivation capabilities of various chemical and physical agents (Favero et al 1973, Bond et al 1977). Detection of HBsAg on environmental surfaces does not indicate positively the simultaneous presence of viable HBV but it does serve as an indicator of contamination with potentially infective material. We and others have shown that HBsAg can be quantitated and traced in environmental surfaces as an adjunct to longitudinal or epidemic investigations (Dankert et al 1976, Petersen et al 1976, Bond et al 1977, Lauer et al 1979 Abb et al 1981, Canter et al 1990).

Since there is no evidence to suggest that the resistance level of HBV is equivalent to or even approaches the demonstrated stability of the immunological reactivity of HBsAg, we proposed in 1977 that the immunological reactivity of HBsAg is much more resistant to physical and chemical stresses than is the infectious virion.

Table 33.5 Effects of chemical agents and heat on HAV viability*

Inoculum/exposure conditions	Agent (exposure time)	Result (log reduction)
Tissue culture-derived HAV with 10% faeces added, dry inoculum, 1 min exposure		
	2% glutaraldehyde	>4
	5000 mg/l chlorine	>4
	0.4% quaternary ammonium compound plus 23% hydrochlonic acid	>4
	3000 mg/l available chlorine	<1
	iodophor, 75 mg/l iodine	<1
	Phenolics, with and without alcohol	<1
	Quaternary ammonium compounds, with and without alcohol	<1
	70% ethanol	<1
	3.5% peracetic acid	<1
	6% hydrogen peroxide	<1
Tissue culture-derived HAV, room temperature, liquid inoculum		
	10 mg/l available chlorine (15 min)	3
	3 mg/l iodine (15 min)	3
	300 mg/l peracetic acid (15 min)	<3
	Alcohol (3 min)	2.25
	Alcohol (12 hr)	4.75
HAV + chimpanzee faeces, 18% suspension, 10^6 MID/ml†, marmoset i.v. recovery‡		
	500 mg/l available chlorine (10 min)	<4
	5000 mg/l available chlorine (10 min)	4δ
	75°C wet (10 min)	<5
	75°C wet (30 min)	≥5
	25°C dry, 42% relative humidity (1 month)	<5¶
Tissue culture-derived HAV		
	Room temperature (1 week)	2
	60°C wet, (6–12 h)	<5.25
	85°C wet (1 min)	>5.25

* Modified, in part, from Thraenhart (1991), Tables 26–13, 26–14, 26–16.
† MID, marmoset infective doses.
‡ KA McCaustland, WW Bond & JA Spelbring, unpublished data.
δ 10^4 MID per test, both animals inoculated with treated material were not infected.
¶ from McCaustland et al (1982).

Consequently, those chemical and physical stresses that were shown to destroy the immunological reactivity of HBsAg can be assumed to be effective against HBV. We further proposed that the resistance level of HBV be considered equivalent to that of *Mycobacterium tuberculosis*, i.e. less resistant than bacterial spores but more resistant than most microorganisms. Subsequently, even this assumption was shown to be overly conservative when a number of intermediate- to high-level disinfectants were shown to be effective against HBV.

HBV has been shown to be inactivated by several moderately potent disinfectants, including 0.2% and 0.1% glutaraldehyde, 500 p.p.m. free chlorine from sodium hypochlorite, an iodophor disinfectant and isopropyl or ethyl alcohol. (Bond et al 1983, Kobayashi et al 1984). Table 33.6 gives a summary of some of the inactivation potentials of various physical agents and germicides in tests using titred inocula and chimpanzee infectivity assays.

Since infectivity experiments using chimpanzees are not suitable for the quantitative

Table 33.6 Complete inactivation of HBV inoculum by chemicals and heat *

Inoculum	Treatment	Reference
Human plasma (dry)	10 min, 20°C (all tests)	Bond et al 1983
10^6 CID†	500 mg/l available chlorine sodium hypochlorite	
10^6 CID	70% isopropyl alcohol	
10^6 CID	0.125% glutaraldehyde 0.44% phenol	
10^6 CID	75 mg/l available iodine; iodophor	
10^6 CID	2% glutaraldehyde, pH 8.6	
Human plasma (liquid)		
10^5 CID	5 min, 24°C 1% glutaraldehyde	Kobayashi et al 1984
2.0×10^5 CID	5 min, 24°C 0.1 glutaraldehyde	
3.3×10^5 CID	2 min, 24°C 80% ethyl alcohol	
10^5 CID	2 min, 98C	

* As measured by chimpanzee infectivity tests; titred inocula.
† CID, chimpanzee infective doses.

determination of HBV inactivation, more reliance has been placed on other avenues of experimentation. Thraenhart et al (1978, 1982) developed a test referred to as the 'morphologic alteration and disintegration' test (MADT). This test has been standardized and used in Germany for determining the effect of chemical germicides and physical agents on HBV. The hypothesis of MADT is that the physical destruction of intact HBV virus particles is correlated with the inactivation of infectivity using chimpanzee infectivity tests (Thraenhart et al 1982).

Other Hepatitis Viruses

The effects of physical and chemical agents on other human hepatitis viruses, HCV, HDV and HEV, have not been studied extensively but, as mentioned previously, we are aware of no evidence to suggest that any of these viruses are intrinsically more resistant to physical or chemical agents than most viruses or that the general resistance levels can even approach that of bacterial endospores. Consequently, we continue to propose that the resistance levels of the human hepatitis viruses that have not been studied in great detail be considered near that of *Mycobacterium tuberculosis* var. *bovis* and non-lipid viruses (e.g. poliovirus), but much less than that of bacterial spores.

STERILIZATION, DISINFECTION AND HOUSEKEEPING IN THE LABORATORY

Conventional sterilization procedures such as steam autoclaving or ethylene oxide gas can be relied upon to effectively inactivate all hepatitis viruses. This is also true for liquid chemical disinfectants that are used as sterilants (sporicides). These sterilization procedures are used primarily for medical devices that are reprocessed for use on patients in health care facilities. It is emphasized that chemical germicides capable of being used as sterilants for medical instruments are not appropriate for use on environmental surfaces.

In the context of laboratory settings where liquid chemical germicides may be used to disinfect laboratory worktops or laboratory instruments that have been directly exposed to cultured or concentrated hepatitis viruses or human or animal source specimens containing these agents, it is recommended that chemical disinfectants in their appropriate concentrations and contact times that are capable of producing at least an intermediate level of disinfection activity should be used (see Table 33.4).

For general housekeeping purposes such as cleaning floors, walls and other similar environmental surfaces in the laboratory area, any disinfectant–detergent can be used.

In some high-risk areas, such as laboratories,

haemodialysis units and other health care environments, one is confronted with the problem of decontaminating large and small blood spills, patient care equipment that becomes contaminated with blood and frequently touched instrument surfaces such as control knobs, which may play a role in environmentally mediated transmission of hepatitis B. The strategies for applying the principles of HBV inactivation vary according to the item or surface being considered, its potential role in the risk of hepatitis virus transmission and, to a certain extent, the thermal and chemical lability of the surface or instrument. For example, if a significant spill of blood occurred on the floor or a countertop in a laboratory, the objective of the procedure to inactivate HBV or other blood-borne hepatitis viruses would be one of decontamination or disinfection and not sterilization. Consequently, in such a situation we would recommend that gloves be worn and the blood spill be absorbed with disposable towels. The spill site should be cleaned of all visible blood, and then the area should be wiped down with clean towels soaked in an appropriate intermediate-level disinfectant such as a 1 to 100 dilution of commercially available household bleach (0.05% sodium hypochlorite in final dilution). All soiled towels should be put in a plastic bag or other leakproof container for disposal.

The concentration of disinfectant used depends primarily on the type of surface that is involved. For example, in the case of a direct spill on a porous surface that cannot be physically cleaned before disinfection, 0.5% sodium hypochlorite (5000 mg/l available chlorine) should be used. On the other hand, if the surface is hard and smooth and has been cleaned appropriately, then 0.5% sodium hypochlorite (500 mg/l available chlorine) is sufficient. For commercially available chemical disinfectants, the use concentrations and instructions specified by the manufacturer should be followed.

Other types of environmental surfaces of concern include surfaces that are touched frequently, such as control knobs or panels on laboratory instruments. Ideally, gloves should be worn and manipulated in a manner appropriate not only to avoid skin contact with patient materials but to avoid 'finger painting' of this contamination to a variety of other frequently touched surfaces. Since this ideal is seldom fully realized in a busy laboratory setting, laboratory instrument and equipment surfaces (including fixtures such as light switches and door pulls or push plates) should be routinely cleaned and disinfected. The objective here would be to reduce the level of possible contamination to such an extent that disease transmission is remote. In a practical sense, this could mean that a cloth soaked in either 0.05% sodium hypochlorite or a suitable proprietary disinfectant or disinfectant/detergent could be used. In this context, the element of physical cleaning is as important, if not more important, than the choice of the disinfectant. It is not necessary, cost effective or in many cases even feasible to attempt more powerful germicidal procedures with these types of items or surfaces.

As a rule, routine daily cleaning procedures that are used for general microbiological laboratories can be used for laboratories in which blood specimens are processed. Obviously, special attention should be given to areas or items visibly contaminated with blood or faeces. Furthermore, cleaning personnel must be alerted to the potential hazards associated with blood, serum and faecal contamination. Floors and other housekeeping surfaces contaminated in this manner should be thoroughly cleaned of gross material and then treated with a detergent–disinfectant. Gloves should be worn by cleaning personnel doing these duties. However, in the case of large blood spills as mentioned above, this type of procedure may have to be augmented by specific site decontamination using a more potent chemical agent such as an intermediate-level disinfectant. (see Table 33.4).

SUMMARY

Strategies for disinfection and sterilization used in hospitals and other health care institutions are based on relatively conservative criteria and do not need to be changed because of concern for the presence of hepatitis viruses. These viruses are inactivated by a wide variety of common physical and chemical sterilization and disinfection procedures. The resistance of individual species of hepatitis viruses to heat and chemical germicides varies, but none exceeds the resistance levels of bacterial spores or *M. tuberculosis*.

REFERENCES

Abb J, Deinhardt F, Eisenburg J 1981 The risk of transmission of hepatitis B virus using jet injection inoculation. Journal of Infectious Diseases 144: 179

Bond W W, Petersen N J, Favero M S 1977 Viral hepatitis B: aspects of environmental control. Health Laboratory Science 14: 235–252

Bond W W, Favero M S, Petersen N J, Ebert J W 1983 Inactivation of hepatitis B virus by intermediate-to-high level disinfectant chemicals. Journal of Clinical Microbiology 18: 535–538

Canter J, Mackey K, Good L S et al 1990 An outbreak of hepatitis B associated with jet injections in a weight reduction clinic. Archives of Internal Medicine 150: 1923–1927

Dankert J, Uitentius J, Houwen B, Tegzess A M, van der Hem GR 1976 Hepatitis B surface antigen in environmental samples from hemodialysis units. Journal Infectious Diseases 134: 123–127

Favero M S, Bond W W 1991 Chemical disinfection of medical and surgical materials. In: Block S S (ed.) Disinfection, sterilization and preservation, 4th edn. Lea & Febiger, Philadelphia, pp 617–641

Favero M S, Maynard J E, Petersen N J, Bond W W, Berquist K R, Szmuness W 1973 Hepatitis B antigen on environmental surfaces. Lancet ii: 1455

Kobayashi H, Tsuzuki M, Koshimizu K et al 1984 Susceptibility of hepatitis B virus to disinfectants and heat. Journal of Clinical Microbiology 20: 214–216

Lauer J L, Van Drunen N A, Washburn J W, Balfour H H 1979 Transmission of hepatitis B in clinical laboratory areas. Journal of Infectious Diseases 140: 513–516

McCaustland K A, Bond W W, Bradley D W, Ebert J W, Maynard J E 1982 Survival of hepatitis A virus in feces after drying and storage for one month. Journal of Clinical Microbiology 16: 957–958

Petersen N H, Barrett D H, Bond W W, Berquist K R, Favero M S, Bender T R, Maynard J E 1976 Hepatitis B surface antigen in saliva, impetiginous lesions, and the environment in two remote Alaskan villages. Applied and Environmental Microbiology 32: 572–574

Prince H N, Prince D L, Prince R N 1991 Principles of viral control and transmission. In Block S S (ed.) Disinfection, sterilization and preservation, 4th edn. Lea & Febiger, Philadelphia, pp 411–444

Rutala, W A 1990 Guideline for selection and use of disinfectants. American Journal of Infection Control 18: 99–117

Thraenhart O 1991 Measures for disinfection and control of viral hepatitis. In: Block S S (ed.) Disinfection, sterilization and preservation, 4th edn. Lea & Febiger, Philadelphia, pp 445–471

Thraenhart O, Kuwert E K, Dermietzel R, Scheiermann N, Wendt F 1978 Influence of different disinfection conditions on the structure of hepatitis B virus (Dane particle) as evaluation in the morphological alteration and disintegration test (MADT). Zentralblatt fur Bakteriologie Mikrobiologie und Hygiene (A) 242: 299–314

Thraenhart O, Kuwert E K, Scheiermann N et al 1982 Comparison of the morphological alteration and disintegration test (MADT) and the chimpanzee infectivity test for determination of hepatitis B virucidal activity of chemical disinfectants. Zentralblatt fur Bakteriologie Mikrobiologie und Hygiene (B) 176: 472–484

Index